A guide to... Psychiatric Mental Health Nursing, 7th Edition

Welcome to the challenging, but rewarding world of psychiatric mental health nursing.

Mary C. Townsend guides you step by step, building the knowledge and skills you need to master this often daunting subject. Use the text, the CD-ROM featuring the electronic workbook and test bank, as well as the wealth of learning tools online at DavisPlus to put you on the road to success.

Step 1.
Preview what you'll learn

Chapter Outline, Key Terms, & Core Concepts

Take a look at the **Chapter Outline** and **Key Terms** sections at the beginning of every chapter to see what you will be learning and what **Core Concepts** to focus on.

Objectives

Read the **Objectives** now to see exactly what you'll be learning in each chapter. Then, after you read the chapter, revisit the section and assess your progress. Can you correctly define and explain all of the key points?

Homework Assignment

Take a few moments to review the **Homework Assignment** before you begin the chapter. When you've finished reading the chapter, complete the assignment to reinforce what you've learned.

Step 2.
Prepare for the real world of nursing practice

NEW! Quality and Safety Education for Nurses (QSEN) Activities

Stay up to date—attain the knowledge, skills, and attitudes you need to fulfill the initiative's most current quality and safety competencies.

Case Studies & Care Plans

Enhance your critical-thinking skills with **Case Studies** and **Care Plans** at the end of the disorder chapters to help you prepare for clinical and practice.

Table 25-10 | CARE PLAN FOR THE CLIENT WITH A SUBSTANCE-RELATED DISORDER—cont'd

NURSING DIAGNOSIS: INEFFECTIVE DENIAL
RELATED TO: Weak, underdeveloped ego
EVIDENCED BY: Statements indicating no problem with substance use

OUTCOME CRITERIA	NURSING INTERVENTIONS	RATIONALE
	5. Use confrontation with caring. Do not allow client to fantasize...	5. Confrontation interferes with client's ability to use denial; a caring attitude preserves self-ester... ...and avoids putting the client on th...
	5. Use confrontation with caring. Do not allow client to fantasize ...ut his or her lifestyle (for example: it is my understanding that the last time you drank alcohol, you . . ." or "The lab report shows that you were under the influence of alcohol when you had the accident that injured three people").	
	6. Rationalization and proje... denial that problems exi... client's life because of s... use.	6. ...projec... excus... ...ior on
	7. Encourage participation in group activities.	7. Peer feedback is often... than feedback from a... Peer pressure can be... as can association w... who are experiencir... experienced similar...
	8. Offer immediate positive recognition of client's expressions of insight gained regarding illness and acceptance of responsibility for own behavior.	8. Positive reinforcer... esteem and enco... desirable behavic...

CASE STUDY

SAMPLE CARE PLAN

NURSING HISTORY AND ASSESSMENT

The police bring Dan to the emergency department of the local hospital around 9:00 p.m. His wife, Carol, called 911 when Dan became violent and she began to fear for her safety. Dan was fired from his job as a foreman in a manufacturing plant for refusing to follow his supervisor's directions on a project. When cleaning up after his move, several partially used bottles of liquor were found in his work area.

Carol reports that Dan has been drinking since he came home shortly after noon today. He bloodied her nose and punched her in the stomach when she poured the contents of a bottle from which he was drinking down the kitchen sink. The police responded to her call and brought Dan to the hospital in handcuffs. By the time they arrive at the hospital, Dan has calmed down, and appears drugged and drowsy. His blood alcohol level measures 247 mg/dL. He is admitted to the detoxification unit of the hospital with a diagnosis of Alcohol Intoxication.

Carol tells the admitting nurse that she and Dan have been married for 12 years. He was a social worker before they were married, but his drinking has increased over the years. He has been under a lot of stress at work; hates his job, his boss, and his coworkers; and is depressed a lot of the time. He never had a loving relationship with his parents, who are now deceased. For the past few years, his pattern has been to come home, start drinking immediately, and drink until he passes out for the night. She states that she has tried to get him to go for help with his drinking, but he refuses, and says that he doesn't have a problem.

Carol begins to cry and says to the nurse, "We can't go on like this. I don't know what to do!"

NURSING DIAGNOSES/OUTCOME IDENTIFICATION

From the assessment data, the nurse develops the following nursing diagnoses for Dan:
1. **Risk for injury** related to CNS agitation from alcohol withdrawal.
   a. **Short-Term Goal:** Dan's condition will stabilize within 72 hours.
   b. **Long-Term Goal:** Dan will not experience physical injury.
2. **Ineffective denial** related to low self-esteem, weak ego development, and underlying fears and anxieties.
   a. **Short-Term Goal:** Dan will focus immediate attention on behavioral changes required to achieve sobriety.
   b. **Long-Term Goal:** Dan will accept responsibility for his drinking behaviors, and acknowledge the association between his drinking and personal problems.

PLANNING/IMPLEMENTATION

Risk for Injury

The following nursing interventions may be implemented *in an effort to ensure client safety:*
1. Assess his level of disorientation; frequently orient him to reality and his surroundings.
2. Obtain a drug history.
3. Obtain a urine sample for analysis.
4. Place Dan in a quiet room.
5. Ensure that smoking materials and other potentially harmful objects are stored away.
6. Observe Dan frequently. Take vital signs every 15 to 30 minutes.

NEW! Therapeutic Communication Icon

Look for the **Therapeutic Communication Icon** highlighting talking points and interventions in the care plans to help you feel more comfortable communicating with your patients.

Summary and Key Points

Summary and Key Points

- Cognitive disorders constitute a large and growing public health concern.
- Cognitive disorders include delirium, dementia, and amnestic disorders.
- A delirium is a disturbance of consciousness and a change in cognition that develop rapidly over a short period. Level of consciousness is often affected and psychomotor activity may fluctuate between agitated purposeless movements and a vegetative state resembling catatonic stupor.
- The symptoms of delirium usually begin quite abruptly and often are reversible and brief.
- Delirium may be caused by a general medical condition, substance intoxication or withdrawal, or ingestion of a medication or exposure to a toxin.
- Dementia is a syndrome of acquired, persistent intellectual impairment with compromised function in multiple spheres of mental activity, such as memory, language, visuospatial skills, emotion or personality, and cognition.
- Symptoms of dementia are insidious and develop slowly over time. In most clients, dementia runs a progressive, irreversible course.
- Dementia may be caused by genetics, cardiovascular disease, infections, neurophysiological disorders, and other general medical conditions.
- Amnestic disorders are characterized ___ inability to learn new information ___ ___ normal attention and an inability to recall ___ ___

Summary and Key Points

Too busy to take notes? Refer to the **Summary and Key Points** section at the end of every chapter for a recap of the most important concepts.

Step 3.
Build your confidence

Review Questions & Test Your Critical Thinking Skills

Quiz yourself with multiple-choice, end-of-chapter **Review Questions.**

Then, **Test Your Critical Thinking Skills** with true-to-life scenarios and questions.

TEST YOUR CRITICAL THINKING SKILLS

Kelly, age 23, is ___ gical resident a ___ gling to do well in law school because she wants to make her parents, two prominent local attorneys, proud of her. She had never aspired to do anything but go into law, and that is also what her parents expected her to do.

Kelly's midterm grades were not as high as she had hoped, so she increased the number of hours of study time, staying awake all night several nights a week to study. She started drinking large amounts of coffee to stay awake, but still found herself falling asleep as she tried to study at the library and in her apartment. As final exams approached, she began to panic that she would not be able to continue the pace of studying she felt she needed in order to make the grades she hoped for.

One of Kelly's classmates told her that she needed some "speed" to give her that extra energy to study. Her classmate said, "All the kids do it. Hardly anyone I know gets through law school without it." She gave Kelly the name of a source.

Kelly contacted the source, who supplied her with enough amphetamines to see her through final exams. Kelly was excited, because she had so much energy, did not require sleep, and was able to study the additional hours she thought she needed for the exams. However, when the results were posted, Kelly had failed two courses and would have to repeat them in summer school if she was to continue with her class in the fall. She continued to replenish her supply of amphetamines from her "contact" until he told her he could not get her anymore. She became frantic and stole a prescription blank from her fiancé and forged his name for more pills.

She started taking more and more of the medication in order to achieve the "high" she wanted to feel. Her behavior became erratic. Yesterday, her fiancé received a call from a pharmacy to clarify an order for amphetamines that Kelly had written. He insisted that she admit herself to the chemical dependency unit for detoxification.

On the unit, she appears tired and depressed, moves very slowly, and wants to sleep all the time. She keeps saying to the nurse, "I'm a real failure. I'll never be an attorney like my pare ___ I'm too dumb. I just wish I could die."

Answer the following questions related to Kelly:

1. What is the primary nursing diagnosis for Kelly?
2. Describe important nursing interventions to be impleme ___ with Kelly.
3. In addition to physical safety, what would be the prim ___ short-term goal the nurses would strive to achieve w ___

Review Questions
Self-Examination/Learning Exercise

*Select the answer that is **most** appropriate for each of the following questions:*

1. Mr. White is admitted to the hospital after an extended period of binge alcohol drinking. His wife reports that he has been a heavy drinker for a number of years. Laboratory reports reveal he has a blood alcohol level of 250 mg/dL. He is placed on the chemical dependency unit for detoxification. When would the first signs of alcohol withdrawal symptoms be expected to occur?
   a. Several hours after the last drink.
   b. 2 to 3 days after the last drink.
   c. 4 to 5 days after the last drink.
   d. 6 to 7 days after the last drink.

2. Sympto ___
   a. Euphoria, hyperactivity, and insomnia.
   b. Depression, suicidal ideation, and hypersomnia.
   c. Diaphoresis, nausea and vomiting, and tremors.
   d. Unsteady gait, nystagmus, and profound disorientation.

3. Which of the following medications is the physician most likely to order for a client experiencing alcohol withdrawal syndrome?
   a. Haloperidol (Haldol).
   b. Chlordiazepoxide (Librium).
   c. Methadone (Dolophine).
   d. Phenytoin (Dilantin).

MOVIE CONNECTIONS

Affliction (alcoholism) • Days of Wine and Roses (alcoholism) • I'll Cry Tomorrow (alcoholism) • When a Man Loves a Woman (alcoholism) • Clean and Sober (addiction—cocaine) • 28 Days (alcoholism) • Lady Sings the Blues (addiction—heroin) • I'm Dancing as Fast as I Can (addiction—sedatives) • The Rose (polysubstance addiction)

NEW! Lists of Movies

Take a visual approach—watch the movies listed in every chapter to better understand the conditions and behaviors you may not encounter in clinical.

Multimedia resources make complex concepts crystal clear!

BONUS CD-ROM! (Mac/PC compatible)

Need more practice? Turn to your BONUS CD-ROM for even more tools for success. Rely on these innovative resources to help you retain crucial information…

- **NCLEX-style test bank** with **alternate-item-format questions.**
- **Electronic Workbook in PDF format…**
  - Psychotropic Monographs
  - Client Education Teaching Guides
  - Care Plans
  - Drug Classifications
  - Clinical Tools including…
    - Medication Assessment Tool
    - Cultural Assessment Tool
    - Global Assessment of Functioning (GAF) Scale
    - Mental Status Assessment
    - Glossary

Test Bank

Benzodiazepines

PATIENT MEDICATION INSTRUCTION SHEET

Drug Prescribed

Patient Name
Directions for Use

Examples and Uses of this Medicine:
Benzodiazepines are used to treat moderate to severe anxiety: alprazolam (Xanax), chlordiazepoxide (Librium), clonazepam (Klonopin), clorazepate (Tranxene), diazepam (Valium), lorazepam (Ativan), and oxazepam (Serax). Some are used to treat insomnia (sleeplessness): flurazepam (Dalmane), temazepam (Restoril), estazolam (ProSom), quazepam (Doral), and triazolam (Halcion). Some are used for muscle spasms and to treat seizure disorders.

Before Using this Medicine, Be Sure To Tell Your Doctor if You:
- Are allergic to any medicine
- Are pregnant, plan to be, or are breastfeeding
- Have glaucoma
- Are taking any other medications

Side Effects of this Medicine:
REPORT THE FOLLOWING SIDE EFFECTS TO YOUR DOCTOR IMMEDIATELY:
- Mental confusion or depression
- Hallucinations (seeing, hearing, or feeling things not there)
- Skin rash or itching
- Sore throat and fever
- Unusual excitement, nervousness, irritability, or trouble sleeping

SIDE EFFECTS THAT MAY OCCUR BUT NOT REQUIRE A DOCTOR'S ATTENTION UNLESS THEY PERSIST LONGER THAN A FEW DAYS:
- Blurred vision, or other changes in vision
- Clumsiness, dizziness, lightheadedness, or slurred speech
- Constipation, diarrhea, nausea, vomiting, or stomach pain
- Difficulty in urination
- Drowsiness, headache, or unusual tiredness or weakness

Other Instructions While Taking this Medication:
- Take this medicine only as your doctor has directed. Do not take more of it or do not take it more often than prescribed. If large doses are taken for a prolonged period of time, it may become habit-forming.
- If you are taking this medicine several times a day and you forget a dose, if it is within an hour or so of the missed dose, go ahead and take it. Otherwise, wait and take the next dose at regular time. Do not double up on a dose if you forget one. Just keep taking the prescribed dosage.
- Do not stop taking drug abruptly. Can produce serious withdrawal...

Client Education Teaching Guides

Contents

Client Teaching Guide

Drug Monograph

Psychotropic Drugs: *alprazolam*

alprazolam

(al-**pray**-zoe-lam)

✦Apo-Alpraz, ✦Novo-Alprazol, Niravam, ✦Nu-Alpraz, Xanax, Xanax XR

CLASSIFICATION

Therapeutic: antianxiety agents   **Pharmacologic:** benzodiazepines

Schedule IV

Pregnancy Category D

✦ = Genetic implication.

✦ = Canadian drug name.
Copyright © 2011 by F.A. Davis Company

INDICATIONS
■ Treatment of Generalized Anxiety Disorder (GAD).
■ Panic Disorder.
■ Management of anxiety associated with depression.
■ **Unlabelled Use:**
  ● Management of symptoms of premenstrual syndrome (PMS).
  ● Insomnia, irritable bowel syndrome (IBS) and other somatic symptoms associated with anxiety.
  ● Used as an adjunct with acute mania, acute psychosis.

ACTION
■ Acts at many levels in the CNS to produce anxiolytic effect.
■ May produce CNS depression.
■ Effects may be mediated by GABA, an inhibitory neurotransmitter.
■ Therapeutic Effects:
  ● Relief of anxiety.

PHARMACOKINETICS

Absorption: Well absorbed (90%) from the GI tract; absorption is slower with extended-release tablets.

Distribution: Widely distributed, crosses blood-brain barrier. Probably crosses the placenta and enters breast milk. Accumulation is minimal.

Metabolism and Excretion: Metabolized by the liver (CYP3A4 enzyme system) to an active compound that is subsequently rapidly metabolized.

Half-life: 12–15 hr.

TIME/ACTION PROFILE (sedation)

ROUTE	ONSET	PEAK	DURATION
PO	1–2 hr	1–2 hr	up to 24 hr

Continued on the following page

Psychotropic Drugs | Contents | Help | Print | ◀ 5 ▶

FREE learning and clinical resources online at DavisPlus

From creating your own printable concept maps to examining the intricacies of the brain and quizzing yourself with crossword puzzles and fill-in-the-blank activities—you'll find all of the tools you need to hone your skills with these interactive exercises and clinical resources.

- Interactive Clinical Scenarios
- Interactive Exercises
- Concept Map Care Plans
- Concept Map Generator
- Care Plans
- Psychotropic Drug Monographs
- Neurobiological Illustrations
- Animations
- "Meet the Author"/"Contact the Author" feature

Interactive Clinical Scenarios

Work through the nursing process with client summaries, multiple-choice questions with rationales, drag-and-drop activities, and much more!

---

alprazolam (al-**pray**-zoe-lam)
◆ Apo-Alpraz, ◆ Novo-Alprazol, Niravam, ◆ Nu-Alpraz, Xanax, Xanax XR
Classification
Therapeutic: antianxiety agents
Pharmacologic: benzodiazepines
Schedule IV
Pregnancy Category D

Ⓖ = Genetic implication.
◆ = Canadian drug name.
Copyright © 2011 by F.A. Davis Company

Indications
Treatment of Generalized Anxiety Disorder (GAD). Panic Disorder. Management of anxiety associated with depression. **Unlabeled Use:** Management of symptoms of premenstrual syndrome (PMS). Insomnia, irritable bowel syndrome (IBS) and other somatic symptoms associated with anxiety. Used as an adjunct with acute mania, acute psychosis.

Action
Acts at many levels in the CNS to produce anxiolytic effect. May produce CNS depression. Effects may be mediated by GABA, an inhibitory neurotransmitter. **Therapeutic Effects:** Relief of anxiety.

Pharmacokinetics
Absorption: Well absorbed (90%) from the GI tract; absorption is slower with extended-release tablets.
Distribution: Widely distributed, crosses blood-brain barrier. Probably crosses the placenta and enters breast milk.
Accumulation is minimal.
Metabolism and Excretion: Metabolized by the liver (CYP3A4 enzyme system) to an active compound that is subsequently rapidly metabolized.
Half-life: 12–15 hr.

TIME/ACTION PROFILE (sedation)

ROUTE	ONSET	PEAK	DURATION
PO	1–2 hr	1–2 hr	up to 24 hr

Contraindications/Precautions
Contraindicated in: Hypersensitivity; Cross-sensitivity with other benzodiazepines may exist; Pre-existing CNS depression; Severe uncontrolled pain; Angle-closure glaucoma, obstructive sleep apnea, pulmonary disease; Pregnancy and lactation; Concurrent itraconazole or ketoconazole; **OB/Lactation:** Use in pregnancy or lactation may cause CNS depression, flaccidity, feeding difficulties, and seizures in infant. **Use Cautiously in:** Renal Impairment, Hepatic dysfunction (↓ dose required); Concurrent use with nefazodone, fluvoxamine, cimetidine, fluoxetine, hormonal contraceptives, propoxyphene, diltiazem, isoniazid, erythromycin, clarithromycin, grapefruit juice (↓ dose may be necessary); History of suicide attempt or alcohol/drug dependence; debilitated patients (↓ dose required); **Pedi:** Safety and efficacy not established. Decreased dosage and frequent monitoring required; **Geri:** Elderly patients have increased sensitivity to benzodiazepines. Appears on Beers list and is associated with increased risk of falls (↓ dose required) and excessive CNS effects.

Adverse Reactions/Side Effects (CAPITALS indicate life-threatening; underlines indicate most frequent.)

Psychotropic Drug Monographs

Attach these handy, printable monographs to your care plans or take them into clinical rotations. Patient safety information, classifications, indications, actions, and nursing implications are easy to find on each psychotropic drug monograph from the trusted Davis's Drug Guide for Nurses® database.

SEVENTH EDITION

Psychiatric Mental Health Nursing

Concepts of Care in Evidence-Based Practice

MARY C. TOWNSEND, DSN, PMHCNS-BC
Clinical Specialist/Nurse Consultant
Adult Psychiatric Mental Health Nursing

Former Assistant Professor and Coordinator, Mental Health Nursing Kramer School of Nursing Oklahoma City University Oklahoma City, Oklahoma

F.A. Davis Company • Philadelphia

F. A. Davis Company
1915 Arch Street
Philadelphia, PA 19103
www.fadavis.com

Copyright © 2012 by F. A. Davis Company

Printed in the United States of America

Last digit indicates print number: 10 9 8 7 6 5 4 3 2 1

Publisher, Nursing: Robert G. Martone
Director of Content Development: Darlene D. Pedersen
Senior Project Editor: Padraic J. Maroney
Art and Design Manager: Carolyn O'Brien

As new scientific information becomes available through basic and clinical research, recommended treatments and drug therapies undergo changes. The author(s) and publisher have done everything possible to make this book accurate, up to date, and in accord with accepted standards at the time of publication. The author(s), editors, and publisher are not responsible for errors or omissions or for consequences from application of the book, and make no warranty, expressed or implied, in regard to the contents of the book. Any practice described in this book should be applied by the reader in accordance with professional standards of care used in regard to the unique circumstances that may apply in each situation. The reader is advised always to check product information (package inserts) for changes and new information regarding dose and contraindications before administering any drug. Caution is especially urged when using new or infrequently ordered drugs.

Library of Congress Cataloging-in-Publication Data

Townsend, Mary C., 1941-
    Psychiatric mental health nursing : concepts of care in evidence-based practice / Mary C. Townsend. — 7th ed.
        p. ; cm.
    Includes bibliographical references and index.
    ISBN-13: 978-0-8036-2767-3
    ISBN-10: 0-8036-2767-X
    I. Title.
    [DNLM: 1. Psychiatric Nursing—methods. 2. Evidence-Based Nursing. 3. Mental Disorders—nursing. 4. Psychotherapy—methods. WY 160]
    LC classification not assigned
    616.89'0231—dc23   2011034182

THIS BOOK IS DEDICATED TO:
FRANCIE

God made sisters for sharing laughter
and wiping tears

LOIS ANGELO, MSN, APRN, BC
Assistant Professor
Massachusetts College of Pharmacy and
    Health Sciences
Boston, Massachusetts

CATHY MELFI CURTIS, MSN, RN-BC
Lead Instructor, Psychiatric Nursing
Trident Technical College
Charleston, South Carolina

KARYN I. MORGAN, RN, MSN, CNS
Instructor, Mental Health Nursing
The University of Akron
Akron, Ohio
and
CNS, Intensive Outpatient Psychiatry
Summa Health System
Akron, Ohio

CAROL NORTON TUZO, MSN, RN-BC
Instructor, Psychiatric Nursing
Trident Technical College
Charleston, South Carolina

Theresa Aldelman
Bradley University
Peoria, Illinois

Fredrick Astle
University of South Carolina
Columbia, South Carolina

Carol Backstedt
Baton Rouge Community College
Baton Rouge, Louisiana

Elizabeth Bailey
Clinton Community College
Pittsburgh, New York

Sheryl Banak
Baptist Health Schools Little Rock – School of
    Nursing
Little Rock, Arkansas

Joy A. Barham
Northwestern State University
Shreveport, Louisiana

Barbara Barry
Cape Fear Community College
Wilmington, North Carolina

Carole Bomba
Harper College
Palatine, Illinois

Judy Bourrand
Samford University
Birmingham, Alabama

Susan Bowles
Barton Community College
Great Bend, Kansas

Wayne Boyer
College of the Desert
Palm Desert, California

Joyce Briggs
Ivy Tech Community College
Columbus, Indiana

Toni Bromley
Rogue Community College
Grants Pass, Oregon

Terrall Bryan
North Carolina A&T State University
Greensboro, North Carolina

Ruth Burkhart
New Mexico State University/Dona Ana
    Community College
Las Cruces, New Mexico

Annette Cannon
Platt College
Aurora, Colorado

Deena Collins
Huron School of Nursing
Cleveland, Ohio

Martha Colvin
Georgia College & State University
Milledgeville, Georgia

Mary Jean Croft
St. Joseph School of Nursing
Providence, Rhode Island

Connie Cupples
Union University
Germantown, Tennessee

Karen Curlis
SUNY Adirondack
Queensbury, New York

Nancy Cyr
North Georgia College & State University
Dahlonega, Georgia

Carol Danner
Baptist Health Schools Little Rock – School of
    Nursing
Little Rock, Arkansas

Carolyn DeCicco
Our Lady of Lourdes School of Nursing
Camden, New Jersey

Leona Dempsey
University of Wisconsin Oshkosh
Oshkosh, Wisconsin

Debra J. DeVoe
Our Lady of Lourdes School of Nursing
Camden, New Jersey

Victoria T. Durkee
University of Louisiana at Monroe
Monroe, Louisiana

J. Carol Elliott
St. Anselm College
Fairfield, California

Sandra Farmer
Capital University
Columbus, Ohio

Patricia Freed
Saint Louis University
St. Louis, Missouri

Diane Gardner
University of West Florida
Pensacola, Florida

Maureen Gaynor
Saint Anselm College
Manchester, New Hampshire

Denise Glenore
West Coast University
Riverside, California

Sheilia R. Goodwin
Winston-Salem State University
Winston-Salem, North Carolina

Janine Graf-Kirk
Trinitas School of Nursing
Elizabeth, New Jersey

Susan B. Grubbs
Francis Marion University
Florence, South Carolina

Elizabeth Gulledge
Jacksonville State University
Jacksonville, Alabama

Kim Gurcan
Columbus Practical School of Nursing
Columbus, Ohio

Patricia Jean Hedrick Young
Washington Hospital School of Nursing
Washington, Pennsylvania

Melinda Hermanns
University of Texas at Tyler
Tyler, Texas

Alison Hewig
Victoria College
Victoria, Texas

Cheryl Hilgenberg
Millikin University
Decatur, Illinois

Lori Hill
Gadsden State Community College
Gadsden, Alabama

Ruby Houldson
Illinois Eastern Community College
Olney, Illinois

Eleanor J. Jefferson
Community College of Denver
Platt College
Metropolitan State College
Denver, Colorado

Dana Johnson
Mesa State College/Grand Junction Regional
    Center
Grand Junction, Colorado

Janet Johnson
Fort Berthold Community College
New Town, North Dakota

Nancy Kostin
Madonna University
Livonia, Michigan

Linda Lamberson
University of Southern Maine
Portland, Maine

Irene Lang
Bristol Community College
Fall River, Massachusetts

William S. Pope
Barton College
Wilson, North Carolina

Karen Pounds
Northeastern University
Boston, Massachusetts

Konnie Prince
Victoria College
Victoria, Texas

Susan Reeves
Tennessee Technological University
Cookeville, Tennessee

Debra Riendeau
Saint Joseph's College of Maine
Lewiston, Maine

Sharon Romer
South Texas College
McAllen, Texas

Lisa Romero
Solano Community College
Fairfield, California

Donna S. Sachse
Union University
Germantown, Tennessee

Betty Salas
Otero Junior College
La Junta, Colorado

Sheryl Samuelson
Millikin University
Decatur, Illinois

John D. Schaeffer
San Joaquin Delta College
Stockton, California

Mindy Schaffner
Pacific Lutheran University
Tacoma, Washington

Becky Scott
Mercy College of Northwest Ohio
Toledo, Ohio

Janie Shaw
Clayton State University
Morrow, Georgia

Lori Shaw
Nebraska Methodist College
Omaha, Nebraska

Joyce Shea
Fairfield University
Fairfield, Connecticut

Judith Shindul-Rothschild
Boston College
Chestnut Hill, Massachusetts

Audrey Silveri
University of Massachusetts Graduate School of
　　Nursing
Worcester, Massachusetts

Brenda Smith
North Georgia College & State University
Dahlonega, Georgia

Janet Somlyay
University of Wyoming
Laramie, Wyoming

Charlotte Strahm
Purdue University North Central
Westville, Indiana

Jo Sullivan
Centralia College
Centralia, Washington

Kathleen Sullivan
Boise State University
Boise, Idaho

Judy Traynor
Jefferson Community College
Watertown, New York

Claudia Turner
Temple College
Temple, Texas

Suzanne C. Urban
Mansfield University
Mansfield, Pennsylvania

Dorothy Varchol
Cincinnati State Technical and Community College
Cincinnati, Ohio

Connie M. Wallace
Nebraska Methodist College
Omaha, Nebraska

Sandra Wardell
Orange County Community College
Middletown, New York

Susan Warmuskerken
West Shore Community College
Scotville, Michigan

Roberta Weseman
East Central College
Union, Missouri

Margaret A. Wheatley
Case Western Reserve University, Frances Payne
    Bolton School of Nursing
Cleveland, Ohio

Rodney A. White
Lewis and Clark Community College
Godfrey, Illinois

Jeana Wilcox
Graceland University
Independence, Missouri

Jackie E. Williams
Georgia Perimeter College
Clarkston, Georgia

Rita L. Williams
Langston University School of Nursing & Health
    Professions
Langston, Oklahoma

Vita Wolinsky
Dominican College
Orangeburg, New York

Marguerite Wordell
Kentucky State University
Frankfort, Kentucky

Jan Zlotnick
City College of San Francisco
San Francisco, California

ACKNOWLEDGMENTS

Robert G. Martone, Publisher, Nursing, F. A. Davis Company, for your sense of humor and continuous optimistic outlook about the outcome of this project.

Padraic J. Maroney, Senior Project Editor, Nursing, F.A. Davis Company, for all your help and support in preparing the manuscript for publication.

Berta Steiner, Director of Production, Bermedica Production, Ltd., for your support and competence in the final editing and production of the manuscript.

The nursing educators, students, and clinicians, who provide critical information about the usability of the textbook, and offer suggestions for improvements. Many changes have been made based on your input.

To those individuals who critiqued the manuscript for this edition and shared your ideas, opinions, and suggestions for enhancement. I sincerely appreciate your contributions to the final product.

My daughters, Kerry and Tina, for all the joy you have provided me and all the hope that you instill in me. I'm so thankful that I have you.

My grandchildren, Meghan and Matthew, for showing me what life is truly all about. I am blessed by your very presence.

My furry friends, Chiro, Angel, and Max, for the pure pleasure you bring into my life every day that you live.

My husband, Jim, who gives meaning to my life in so many ways. You are the one whose encouragement keeps me motivated, whose support gives me strength, and whose gentleness gives me comfort.

Mary C. Townsend

CONTENTS

---

*Chapters now contain more comprehensive psychotropic drug information.

The seventh edition of *Psychiatric Mental Health Nursing: Concepts of Care in Evidence-Based Practice* is published at a time of continued change and turmoil in the nursing profession. The United States is in the midst of a nursing shortage that is expected to intensify as baby boomers age and the need for health care grows. Compounding this problem is a shortage of nursing faculty. Qualified applicants to nursing schools are being turned away because of insufficient numbers of faculty. In 2005, the U.S. Department of Labor awarded several million dollars in grants to address the nurse faculty shortage. These new faculty members need assistance in transitioning to the role of nursing educator. It is hoped that this textbook and the accompanying ancillary materials will be of value in facilitating that transition.

Nurses are accountable to their clients to provide the highest quality of care based on knowledge of what is considered best practice. Change occurs so rapidly that what is considered best practice today may not be considered so tomorrow, based on newly acquired scientific data. Included in this seventh edition are a number of research studies that support psychiatric nursing interventions. As nurses, we are bombarded with new information and technological content on a daily basis. Not all of this information yields knowledge that can be used in clinical practice. It is our hope that the information in this new edition will serve to further the movement toward evidence-based practice in psychiatric nursing. There is still a long way to go, and research utilization is the foundation from which to advance the progression. Psychiatric nurses must become involved in nursing research, in disseminating research findings, and in implementing practice changes based on current evidence.

Because most psychiatric nursing students feel uncomfortable and somewhat insecure with the communication aspects of psychiatric nursing, a new emphasis on therapeutic communication is included in the seventh edition. Communication strategies have been expanded within the interventions and care plans. These "communication interventions" are identified by the icon ⬤.

It is our goal to stay on the cutting edge of nursing education. So with this in mind, the topic of *Quality and Safety Education for Nurses (QSEN)* is addressed in this edition. In February 2007, The Robert Wood Johnson Foundation (RWJF) awarded a grant to the University of North Carolina at Chapel Hill School of Nursing to develop a curriculum on quality and safety for nursing schools. The Institute of Medicine (IOM), in its 2003 report, *Health Professions Education: A Bridge to Quality,* challenged faculties of medicine, nursing, and other health professions to ensure that their graduates have achieved a core set of competencies in order to meet the needs of the 21st century health-care system. These competencies include *providing patient-centered care, working in interdisciplinary teams, employing evidence-based practice, applying quality improvement,* and *utilizing informatics.*

Educational associations and accrediting bodies are recommending the inclusion of these competencies in the curricula of nursing schools. Historically, quality care and patient safety have been core concepts of nursing and nursing education. However, it has been suggested that ideas for teaching quality and safety competencies have been sorely lacking. Under the leadership of Principal Investigator Linda R. Cronenwett, the IOM competencies have been adapted for nursing in the hope that they can serve as guidelines to curricular development, and ultimately to "provide a framework for regulatory bodies that set standards for licensure, certification, and accreditation of nursing education programs." The work of Cronenwett and her associates, including competency definitions and an outline of required knowledge, skills, and attitudes associated with each, was published in *Nursing Outlook, 55*(3), and may be found on the website http://www.qsen.org

Definitions of the *quality and safety competencies* as they apply to nursing include the following:

1. **Patient-centered Care.** Recognize the patient or designee as the source of control and full partner in providing compassionate and coordinated care based on respect for patient's preferences, values, and needs.

2. **Teamwork and Collaboration.** Function effectively within nursing and inter-professional teams, fostering open communication, mutual respect, and shared decision-making to achieve quality patient care.

3. **Evidence-based Practice.** Integrate best current evidence with clinical expertise and patient/family preferences and values for delivery of optimal health care.

4. **Quality Improvement.** Use data to monitor the outcomes of care processes and use improvement methods to design and test changes to continuously improve the quality and safety of health care systems.

5. **Safety.** Minimize risk of harm to patients and providers through both system effectiveness and individual performance.

6. **Informatics.** Use information and technology to communicate, manage knowledge, mitigate error, and support decision-making.

Within selected chapters, this textbook includes a number of boxes entitled "QSEN Teaching Strategy." These activities arm the instructor and the student with guidelines for attaining the knowledge, skills, and attitudes necessary for achievement of quality and safety competencies in nursing.

Content and Features New to This Edition

All content has been updated to reflect the current state of the discipline of nursing.

Updated NANDA terminology based on *Nursing Diagnoses: Definitions and Classification 2009–2011* has been used throughout the text.

Homework assignments. At the beginning of each chapter, following the objectives, a new section has been added entitled "Homework Assignment." It is much easier to teach when students come prepared and have read the text before class. However, many students are reluctant readers. One way to encourage students to read before class is to assign homework due *before* class based on the day's topic. Homework questions need to count toward the grade but they don't have to count a lot. Students are motivated by even a small number of points because they know they can complete homework successfully if they try. Grading criteria should be clear, and to minimize grading time, homework could also be assigned "pass-fail." Homework questions are straightforward and, because students will not yet have had a chance to ask questions in class on the topic, are written at

the knowledge and comprehension levels rather than at the application and analysis levels.

Psychopharmacology does not appear as a separate chapter in the seventh edition. Overview content has been moved to Chapter 4, "Concepts of Psychobiology." Content related to specific medications appear in the diagnosis chapter to which the medication applies. This should facilitate understanding of the medication, as well as the study process for the student. An additional chapter entitled "Psychopharmacology," which integrates all of the medication information together, can be found on the F.A. Davis website. All new medications since publication of the previous edition are included.

There is a new emphasis on communication techniques in the seventh edition.

Communication strategies have been expanded within the interventions and care plans. These "communication interventions" are identified by the icon . Many of these interventions appear in "Clinical Pearl" boxes at various sites within the text. These Clinical Pearls also address other specific nursing interventions and information that warrant additional emphasis.

Boxes entitled "QSEN Teaching Strategy" appear within selected chapters. These activities arm the instructor and the student with guidelines for attaining the knowledge, skills, and attitudes necessary for achievement of quality and safety competencies in nursing.

Review questions at the end of each chapter have been updated to reflect the NCLEX format.

New content has been included on **Validity Therapy, Dialectical Behavior Therapy, The Recovery Model,** and **Gender Identity Disorder.**

The chapter on **Mood Disorders** has been divided into two separate chapters: **Mood Disorders—Depression** and **Mood Disorders—Bipolar Disorders.**

The chapter on **Adjustment and Impulse Control Disorders** has been returned to this edition.

New psychiatric assessment scales have been included: **The Abnormal Involuntary Movement Scale (AIMS),** which aids in the early detection of tardive dyskinesia; the **Hamilton Depression Rating Scale;** and the **Hamilton Anxiety Rating Scale.**

Clinical vignettes now introduce all concept map care plans. The concept maps now are specific to the clinical vignettes rather than being standardized, as they were presented in the previous edition.

The diagnostic chapters include a new feature called "**Movie Connections,**" which presents a list of movies that address the subject of the associated chapter. These movies may be used as learning tools to allow students to see on screen the behaviors that they may only read about. The movies provide excellent discussion material.

Features that have been Retained

The major conceptual framework of stress-adaptation has been retained for its ease of comprehensibility and workability in the realm of psychiatric nursing. This framework continues to emphasize the multiple causation of mental illness while accepting the increasing biological implications in the etiology of certain disorders.

Selected research studies with implications for evidence-based practice. (In all relevant clinical chapters.)

The concept of holistic nursing is retained in the 7th edition. An attempt has been made to ensure that the physical aspects .of psychiatric/mental health nursing are not overlooked. In all relevant situations, the mind/body connection is addressed.

Nursing process is retained in the 7th edition as the tool for delivery of care to the individual with a psychiatric disorder or to assist in the primary prevention or exacerbation of mental illness symptoms. The six steps of the nursing process, as described in the American Nurses Association, *Nursing: Scope and Standards of Practice* (2nd edition, 2010), are used to provide guidelines for the nurse. These standards of care are included in the chapters that address *DSM-IV-TR* diagnoses, as well as those on the aging individual, the bereaved individual, and victims of abuse and neglect, and as examples in several of the therapeutic approaches. The six steps include:

Assessment: Background assessment data, including a description of symptomatology, provides an extensive knowledge base from which the nurse may draw when performing an assessment. Several assessment tools are also included.

Diagnosis: Analysis of the data is included, from which nursing diagnoses common to specific psychiatric disorders are derived.

Outcome Identification: Outcomes are derived from the nursing diagnoses and stated as measurable goals.

Planning: Plans of care are presented (either within the text, in care plan format, or both) with selected nursing diagnoses for the *DSM-IV-TR* diagnoses, as well as for the elderly client, the

bereaved individual, victims of abuse and neglect, forensic clients in trauma care and correctional institutions, the elderly homebound client, and the primary caregiver of the client with a severe and persistent mental illness. The planning standard also includes tables that list topics for educating clients and families about mental illness, and sample client teaching guides are presented in Appendix G. Concept map care plans are included for all major psychiatric diagnoses.

Implementation: The interventions that have been identified in the plan of care are included along with rationales for each. Case studies at the end of each *DSM-IV-TR* chapter assist the student in the practical application of theoretical material. Also included as a part of this particular standard is Unit Three of the textbook: *Therapeutic Approaches in Psychiatric Nursing Care.* This section of the textbook addresses psychiatric nursing intervention in depth, and frequently speaks to the differentiation in scope of practice between the basic level psychiatric nurse and the advanced practice level psychiatric nurse.

Evaluation: The evaluation standard includes a set of questions that the nurse may use to assess whether the nursing actions have been successful in achieving the objectives of care.

Internet references for each *DSM-IV-TR* diagnosis, with website listings for information related to the disorder

Tables that list topics for client/family education, (Clinical chapters)

Sample client teaching guides, (Appendix G)

Boxes that include current research studies with implications for evidence-based nursing practice. (Clinical chapters)

Assigning nursing diagnoses to client behaviors. (Diagnostic chapters and Appendix E).

Taxonomy and diagnostic criteria from the *DSM-IV-TR* (2000). Used throughout the text.

All references have been updated throughout the text. Classical references are distinguished from general references.

Boxes with definitions of core concepts appear throughout the text.

An F.A. Davis/Townsend website that contains additional nursing care plans that do not appear in the text, links to psychotropic medications, concept map care plans, and neurobiological content and illustrations.

A Student CD that contains practice test questions, learning activities, concept map care plans, psychotropic drug monographs, and client teaching guides.

Additional Educational Resources

Faculty may also find the following teaching aids that accompany this textbook helpful:

Instructor's Resource Disk (IRD). **This IRD contains:**

- 866 multiple choice questions **(including new format questions reflecting the latest NCLEX blueprint).**

- Lecture outlines **for all chapters**

- Learning activities **for all chapters (including answer key)**

- Answers to the Critical Thinking Exercises **from the textbook**

- PowerPoint Presentation **to accompany all chapters in the textbook**

- Answers to the Homework Assignment Questions **from the textbook**

- 18 case studies for use with student teaching

Additional chapter, "Psychopharmacology," on the F.A. Davis website

Additional chapter, "Client Education," on the F.A. Davis website

Additional chapter, "Psychological Factors Affecting Medical Condition," on the F.A. Davis website

It is hoped that the revisions and additions to this seventh edition continue to satisfy a need within psychiatric/mental health nursing practice. The mission of this textbook has been, and continues to be, to provide both students and clinicians with up-to-date information about psychiatric/mental health nursing. The user-friendly format and easy-to-understand language, for which we have received many positive comments, have been retained in this edition. I hope that this seventh edition continues to promote and advance the commitment to psychiatric/mental health nursing.

Mary C. Townsend

Basic Concepts in Psychiatric/Mental Health Nursing

The Concept of Stress Adaptation

KEY TERMS

"fight or flight" syndrome

general adaptation syndrome

precipitating event

predisposing factors

OBJECTIVES
After reading this chapter, the student will be able to:

1. Define *adaptation* and *maladaptation*.
2. Identify physiological responses to stress.
3. Explain the relationship between stress and "diseases of adaptation."
4. Describe the concept of stress as an environmental event.
5. Explain the concept of stress as a transaction between the individual and the environment.
6. Discuss adaptive coping strategies in the management of stress.

HOMEWORK ASSIGNMENT
Please read the chapter and answer the following questions:

1. How are the body's physiological defenses affected when under sustained stress? Why?
2. In the view of stress as an environmental event, what aspects are missing when considering an individual's response to a stressful situation?
3. In their study, what event did Miller and Rahe find produced the highest level of stress reaction in their subjects?
4. What is the initial step in stress management?

Psychologists and others have struggled for many years to establish an effective definition of the term *stress*. This term is used loosely today and still lacks a definitive explanation. Stress may be viewed as an individual's reaction to any change that requires an adjustment or response, which can be physical, mental, or emotional. Responses directed at stabilizing internal biological processes and preserving self-esteem can be viewed as healthy adaptations to stress.

Roy (1976) defined adaptive response as behavior that maintains the integrity of the individual. Adaptation is viewed as positive and is correlated with a healthy response. When behavior disrupts the integrity of the individual, it is perceived as maladaptive. Maladaptive responses by the individual are considered to be negative or unhealthy.

Various 20th-century researchers contributed to several different concepts of stress. Three of these concepts include stress as a biological response, stress as an environmental event, and stress as a transaction between the individual and the environment. This chapter includes an explanation of each of these concepts.

> ## CORE CONCEPT
>
> ### *Stressor*
>
> A biological, psychological, social, or chemical factor that causes physical or emotional tension and may be a factor in the etiology of certain illnesses.

Stress as a Biological Response

In 1956, Hans Selye published the results of his research concerning the physiological response of a biological system to a change imposed on it. Since his initial publication, he has revised his definition of stress, calling it "the state manifested by a specific syndrome which consists of all the nonspecifically-induced changes within a biologic system" (Selye, 1976). This syndrome of symptoms has come to be known as the "**fight or flight**" **syndrome.** Schematics of these biological responses, both initially and with sustained stress, are presented in Figures 1–1 and 1–2. Selye called this general reaction of the body to stress the **general adaptation syndrome.** He described the reaction in three distinct stages:

1. **Alarm Reaction Stage.** During this stage, the physiological responses of the "fight or flight" syndrome are initiated.

2. **Stage of Resistance.** The individual uses the physiological responses of the first stage as

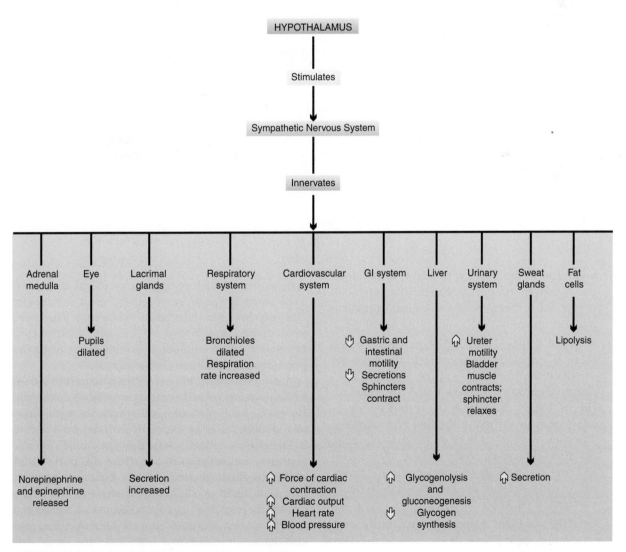

FIGURE 1–1 The "fight or flight" syndrome: the initial stress response.

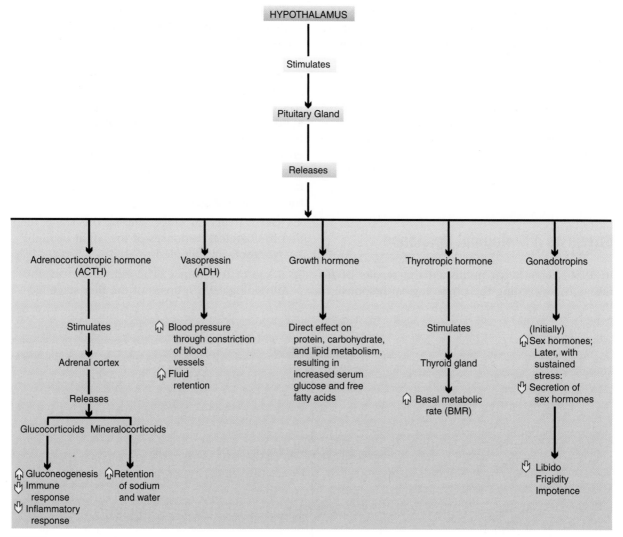

FIGURE 1–2   The "fight or flight" syndrome: the sustained stress response.

a defense in the attempt to adapt to the stressor. If adaptation occurs, the third stage is prevented or delayed. Physiological symptoms may disappear.

3. **Stage of Exhaustion.** This stage occurs when there is a prolonged exposure to the stressor to which the body has become adjusted. The adaptive energy is depleted, and the individual can no longer draw from the resources for adaptation described in the first two stages. Diseases of adaptation (e.g., headaches, mental disorders, coronary artery disease, ulcers, colitis) may occur. Without intervention for reversal, exhaustion, and in some cases even death, ensues (Selye, 1956, 1974).

This "fight or flight" response undoubtedly served our ancestors well. Those *Homo sapiens* who had to face the giant grizzly bear or the saber-toothed tiger as part of their struggle for survival must have used these adaptive resources to their advantage. The response was elicited in emergency situations, used in the preservation of life, and followed by restoration of the compensatory mechanisms to the pre-emergent condition (homeostasis).

Selye performed his extensive research in a controlled setting with laboratory animals as subjects. He elicited the physiological responses with physical stimuli, such as exposure to heat or extreme cold, electric shock, injection of toxic agents, restraint, and surgical injury. Since the publication of his original research, it has become apparent that the "fight or flight" syndrome of symptoms occurs in response to psychological or emotional stimuli, just as it does to physical stimuli. The psychological or emotional stressors are often not resolved as rapidly as some physical stressors, and therefore the body may be depleted of its adaptive energy more readily than it is from physical stressors. The "fight or flight" response may be inappropriate, even dangerous, to the lifestyle of today, in which stress has been described as a psychosocial state that is pervasive, chronic, and relentless. It is this chronic response that maintains the body in the aroused condition for extended periods of time that promotes susceptibility to diseases of adaptation.

CORE CONCEPT

Adaptation

Adaptation is said to occur when an individual's physical or behavioral response to any change in his or her internal or external environment results in preservation of individual integrity or timely return to equilibrium.

Stress as an Environmental Event

A second concept defines stress as the "thing" or "event" that triggers the adaptive physiological and psychological responses in an individual. The event creates change in the life pattern of the individual, requires significant adjustment in lifestyle, and taxes available personal resources. The change can be either positive, such as outstanding personal achievement, or negative, such as being fired from a job. The emphasis here is on *change* from the existing steady state of the individual's life pattern.

Miller and Rahe (1997) have updated the original Social Readjustment Rating Scale devised by Holmes and Rahe in 1967. Just as in the earlier version, numerical values are assigned to various events, or changes, that are common in people's lives. The updated version reflects an increased number of stressors not identified in the original version. In the new study, Miller and Rahe found that women react to life stress events at higher levels than men, and unmarried people gave higher scores than married people for most of the events. Younger subjects rated more events at a higher stress level than older subjects. A high score on the Recent Life Changes Questionnaire (RLCQ) places the individual at greater susceptibility to physical or psychological illness. The questionnaire may be completed considering life stressors within a 6-month or 1-year period. Six-month totals equal to or greater than 300 life change units (LCUs) or 1-year totals equal to or greater than 500 LCU are considered indicative of a high level of recent life stress, thereby increasing the risk of illness for the individual. The RLCQ is presented in Table 1-1.

TABLE 1-1 The Recent Life Changes Questionnaire			
LIFE CHANGE EVENT	**LCU**	**LIFE CHANGE EVENT**	**LCU**
Health		Home and Family	
An injury or illness which:		Major change in living conditions	42
Kept you in bed a week or more, or sent you to the hospital	74	Change in residence:	
		Move within the same town or city	25
Was less serious than above	44	Move to a different town, city, or state	47
Major dental work	26	Change in family get-togethers	25
Major change in eating habits	27	Major change in health or behavior of family member	55
Major change in sleeping habits	26		
Major change in your usual type/amount of recreation	28	Marriage	50
		Pregnancy	67
Work		Miscarriage or abortion	65
Change to a new type of work	51		
		Gain of a new family member:	
Change in your work hours or conditions	35	Birth of a child	66
		Adoption of a child	65
Change in your responsibilities at work:		A relative moving in with you	59
More responsibilities	29		
Fewer responsibilities	21	Spouse beginning or ending work	46
Promotion	31		

Continued

TABLE 1-1 The Recent Life Changes Questionnaire—cont'd

LIFE CHANGE EVENT	LCU	LIFE CHANGE EVENT	LCU
Demotion	42	Child leaving home:	41
Transfer	32	To attend college	
		Due to marriage	41
Troubles at work:		For other reasons	45
With your boss	29	Change in arguments with spouse	50
With coworkers	35		
With persons under your supervision	35	In-law problems	38
Other work troubles	28	Change in the marital status of your parents:	
Major business adjustment	60	Divorce	59
		Remarriage	50
Retirement	52	Separation from spouse:	
Loss of job:		Due to work	53
Laid off from work	68	Due to marital problems	76
Fired from work	79	Divorce	96
Correspondence course to help you in your work	18	Birth of grandchild	43
Personal and Social		Death of spouse	119
Change in personal habits	26	Death of other family member:	
Beginning or ending school or college	38	Child	123
		Brother or sister	102
Change of school or college	35	Parent	100
Change in political beliefs	24	**Financial**	
Change in religious beliefs	29	Major change in finances:	
Change in social activities	27	Increased income	38
		Decreased income	60
Vacation	24	Investment and/or credit difficulties	56
New, close, personal relationship	37	Loss or damage of personal property	43
Engagement to marry	45	Moderate purchase	20
Girlfriend or boyfriend problems	39	Major purchase	37
Sexual difficulties	44	Foreclosure on a mortgage or loan	58
"Falling out" of a close personal relationship	47		
An accident	48		
Minor violation of the law	20		
Being held in jail	75		
Death of a close friend	70		
Major decision regarding your immediate future	51		
Major personal achievement	36		

From Miller, M. A., & Rahe, R. H. (1997). Life changes scaling for the 1990s. Journal of Psychosomatic Research, 43(3), 279–292, with permission.

It is unknown whether stress overload merely predisposes a person to illness or actually precipitates it, but there does appear to be a causal link (Pelletier, 1992). Life changes questionnaires have been criticized because they do not consider the individual's perception of the event. Individuals differ in their reactions to life events, and these variations are related to the degree to which the change is perceived as stressful. These types of instruments also fail to consider the individual's coping strategies and available support systems at the time when the life change occurs. Positive coping mechanisms and strong social or familial support can reduce the intensity of the stressful life change and promote a more adaptive response.

Stress as a Transaction Between the Individual and the Environment

This concept of stress emphasizes the *relationship* between the individual and the environment. Personal characteristics and the nature of the environmental event are considered. This illustration parallels the modern concept of the etiology of disease. No longer is causation viewed solely as an external entity; whether or not illness occurs depends also on the receiving organism's susceptibility. Similarly, to predict psychological stress as a reaction, the properties of the person in relation to the environment must be considered.

Precipitating Event

Lazarus and Folkman (1984) defined *stress* as a relationship between the person and the environment that is appraised by the person as taxing or exceeding his or her resources and endangering his or her well-being. A **precipitating event** is a stimulus arising from the internal or external environment and is perceived by the individual in a specific manner. Determination that a particular person-environment relationship is stressful depends on the individual's cognitive appraisal of the situation. *Cognitive appraisal* is an individual's evaluation of the personal significance of the event or occurrence. The event "precipitates" a response on the part of the individual, and the response is influenced by the individual's perception of the event. The *cognitive response* consists of a primary appraisal and a secondary appraisal.

Individual's Perception of the Event

Primary Appraisal

Lazarus and Folkman (1984) identified three types of primary appraisal: irrelevant, benign-positive, and stressful. An event is judged *irrelevant* when the outcome holds no significance for the individual. A *benign-positive* outcome is one that is perceived as producing pleasure for the individual. *Stress* appraisals include harm/loss, threat, and challenge. *Harm/loss* appraisals refer to damage or loss already experienced by the individual. Appraisals of a *threatening* nature are perceived as anticipated harms or losses. When an event is appraised as *challenging,* the individual focuses on potential for gain or growth, rather than on risks associated with the event. Challenge produces stress even though the emotions associated with it (eagerness and excitement) are viewed as positive, and coping mechanisms must be called upon to face the new encounter. Challenge and threat may occur together when an individual experiences these positive emotions along with fear or anxiety over possible risks associated with the challenging event.

When stress is produced in response to harm/loss, threat, or challenge, a secondary appraisal is made by the individual.

Secondary Appraisal

This secondary appraisal is an assessment of skills, resources, and knowledge that the person possesses to deal with the situation. The individual evaluates by considering the following:

■ Which coping strategies are available to me?

■ Will the option I choose be effective in this situation?

■ Do I have the ability to use that strategy in an effective manner?

The interaction between the primary appraisal of the event that has occurred and the secondary appraisal of available coping strategies determines the quality of the individual's adaptation response to stress.

Predisposing Factors

A variety of elements influence how an individual perceives and responds to a stressful event. These **predisposing factors** strongly influence whether the response is adaptive or maladaptive. Types of predisposing factors include genetic influences, past experiences, and existing conditions.

Genetic influences are those circumstances of an individual's life that are acquired through heredity. Examples include family history of physical and psychological conditions (strengths and weaknesses) and temperament (behavioral characteristics present at birth that evolve with development).

Past experiences are occurrences that result in learned patterns that can influence an individual's adaptation response. They include previous exposure to the stressor or other stressors, learned coping responses, and degree of adaptation to previous stressors.

Existing conditions incorporate vulnerabilities that influence the adequacy of the individual's physical, psychological, and social resources for dealing with adaptive demands. Examples include current health status, motivation, developmental maturity, severity and duration of the stressor, financial and educational resources, age, existing coping strategies, and a support system of caring others.

This transactional model of stress/adaptation will serve as a framework for the process of nursing in this text. A graphic display of the model is presented in Figure 1–3.

CORE CONCEPT

Maladaptation
Maladaptation occurs when an individual's physical or behavioral response to any change in his or her internal or external environment results in disruption of individual integrity or in persistent disequilibrium.

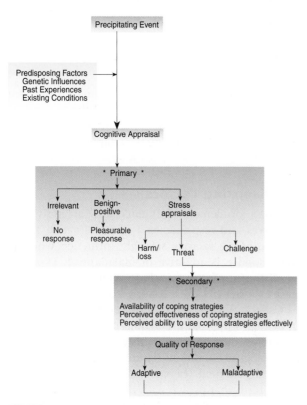

FIGURE 1–3   Transactional model of stress/adaptation.

Stress Management*

The growth of stress management into a multimillion-dollar-a-year business attests to its importance in our society. Stress management involves the use of coping strategies in response to stressful situations. Coping strategies are adaptive when they protect the individual from harm (or additional harm) or strengthen the individual's ability to meet challenging situations. Adaptive responses help restore homeostasis to the body and impede the development of diseases of adaptation.

Coping strategies are considered maladaptive when the conflict being experienced goes unresolved or intensifies. Energy resources become depleted as the body struggles to compensate for the chronic physiological and psychological arousal being experienced. The effect is a significant vulnerability to physical or psychological illness.

Adaptive Coping Strategies

Awareness

The initial step in managing stress is awareness—to become aware of the factors that create stress and the feelings associated with a stressful response. Stress can be controlled only when one recognizes that it is being experienced. As one becomes aware of stressors, he or she can omit, avoid, or accept them.

Relaxation

Individuals experience relaxation in different ways. Some individuals relax by engaging in large motor activities, such as sports, jogging, and physical exercise. Still others use techniques such as breathing exercises and progressive relaxation to relieve stress. (A discussion of relaxation therapy can be found in Chapter 14.)

Meditation

Practiced 20 minutes once or twice daily, meditation has been shown to produce a lasting reduction in blood pressure and other stress-related symptoms (Davis, Eshelman, & McKay, 2008). Meditation involves assuming a comfortable position, closing the eyes, casting off all other thoughts, and concentrating on a single word, sound, or phrase that has positive meaning to the individual. The technique is described in detail in Chapter 14.

---

*Techniques of stress management are discussed at greater length in Unit 3 of this text.

Interpersonal Communication With Caring Other

As previously mentioned, the strength of one's available support systems is an existing condition that significantly influences the adaptiveness of coping with stress. Sometimes just "talking the problem out" with an individual who is empathetic is sufficient to interrupt escalation of the stress response. Writing about one's feelings in a journal or diary can also be therapeutic.

Problem Solving

An extremely adaptive coping strategy is to view the situation objectively (or to seek assistance from another individual to accomplish this if the anxiety level is too high to concentrate). After an objective assessment of the situation, the problem-solving/decision-making model can be instituted as follows:

■ Assess the facts of the situation.

■ Formulate goals for resolution of the stressful situation.

■ Study the alternatives for dealing with the situation.

■ Determine the risks and benefits of each alternative.

■ Select an alternative.

■ Implement the alternative selected.

■ Evaluate the outcome of the alternative implemented.

■ If the first choice is ineffective, select and implement a second option.

Pets

Studies show that those who care for pets, especially dogs and cats, are better able to cope with the stressors of life (Allen, Blascovich, & Mendes, 2002; Barker, Knisely, McCain, & Best, 2005). The physical act of stroking or petting a dog or cat can be therapeutic. It gives the animal an intuitive sense of being cared for and at the same time gives the individual the calming feeling of warmth, affection, and interdependence with a reliable, trusting being. One study showed that, among people who had had heart attacks, pet owners had one-fifth the death rate of those who did not have pets (Friedmann & Thomas, 1995). Another study revealed evidence that individuals experienced a statistically significant drop in blood pressure in response to petting a dog or cat (Whitaker, 2000).

Music

It is true that music can "soothe the savage beast." Creating and listening to music stimulate motivation, enjoyment, and relaxation. Music can reduce depression and bring about measurable changes in mood and general activity.

Summary and Key Points

■ Stress has become a chronic and pervasive condition in the United States today.

■ Adaptive behavior is viewed as behavior that maintains the integrity of the individual, with a timely return to equilibrium. It is viewed as positive and is correlated with a healthy response.

■ When behavior disrupts the integrity of the individual or results in persistent disequilibrium, it is perceived as maladaptive. Maladaptive responses by the individual are considered to be negative or unhealthy.

■ A stressor is defined as a biological, psychological, social, or chemical factor that causes physical or emotional tension and may be a factor in the etiology of certain illnesses.

■ Hans Selye identified the biological changes associated with a stressful situation as the "fight or flight" syndrome.

■ Selye called the general reaction of the body to stress the "general adaptation syndrome," which occurs in three stages: the alarm reaction stage, the stage of resistance, and the stage of exhaustion.

■ When individuals remain in a state of aroused response to stress for an extended period of time, they become susceptible to diseases of adaptation, some examples of which include headaches, mental disorders, coronary artery disease, ulcers, and colitis.

■ Stress may also be viewed as an environmental event. This results when a change from the existing steady state of the individual's life pattern occurs.

■ When an individual experiences a high level of life change events, he or she becomes susceptible to physical or psychological illness.

■ Limitations of this concept of stress include failure to consider the individual's perception of the event, coping strategies, and available support systems at the time when the life change occurs.

■ Stress is more appropriately expressed as a transaction between the individual and the environment that is appraised by the individual as taxing or exceeding his or her resources and endangering his or her well-being.

■ The individual makes a cognitive appraisal of the precipitating event to determine the personal significance of the event or occurrence.

■ Primary cognitive appraisals may be irrelevant, benign-positive, or stressful.

■ Secondary cognitive appraisals include assessment and evaluation by the individual of skills, resources, and knowledge to deal with the stressful situation.

■ Predisposing factors influence how an individual perceives and responds to a stressful event. They include genetic influences, past experiences, and existing conditions.

■ Stress management involves the use of adaptive coping strategies in response to stressful situations in an effort to impede the development of diseases of adaptation.

■ Examples of adaptive coping strategies include developing awareness, relaxation, meditation, interpersonal communication with caring others, problem solving, pets, and music.

 DavisPlus   Additional info available @ davisplus.fadavis.com

Review Questions
Self-Examination/Learning Exercise

Select the answer that is most appropriate for questions 1 through 5. In question 6, identify the category in which each example belongs.

1. Sondra, who lives in Maine, hears on the evening news that 25 people were killed in a tornado in south Texas. Sondra experiences no anxiety upon hearing of this stressful situation. This is most likely because Sondra:
   a. Is selfish and does not care what happens to other people.
   b. Appraises the event as irrelevant to her own situation.
   c. Assesses that she has the skills to cope with the stressful situation.
   d. Uses suppression as her primary defense mechanism.

2. Cindy regularly develops nausea and vomiting when she is faced with a stressful situation. Which of the following is most likely a predisposing factor to this maladaptive response by Cindy?
   a. Cindy inherited her mother's "nervous" stomach.
   b. Cindy is fixed in a lower level of development.
   c. Cindy has never been motivated to achieve success.
   d. When Cindy was a child, her mother pampered her and kept her home from school when she was ill.

3. When an individual's stress response is sustained over a long period, the endocrine system involvement results in which of the following?
   a. Decreased resistance to disease.
   b. Increased libido.
   c. Decreased blood pressure.
   d. Increased inflammatory response.

4. Management of stress is extremely important in today's society because:
   a. Evolution has diminished human capability for "fight or flight."
   b. The stressors of today tend to be ongoing, resulting in a sustained response.
   c. We have stress disorders that did not exist in the days of our ancestors.
   d. One never knows when one will have to face a grizzly bear or saber-toothed tiger in today's society.

Review Questions—cont'd
Self-Examination/Learning Exercise

5. Nancy has just received a promotion on her job. She is very happy and excited about moving up in her company, but she has been experiencing anxiety since receiving the news. Her primary appraisal is that she most likely views the situation as which of the following?
   a. Benign-positive.
   b. Irrelevant.
   c. Challenging.
   d. Threatening.

6. Precipitating stressors, past experiences, existing conditions, and genetic influences are components of the transactional model of stress adaptation, and influence an individual's response to stress. Identify each of these conditions in the following examples.
   a. Precipitating stressor.
   b. Past experience.
   c. Existing conditions.
   d. Genetic influences.

   _____ Mr. T is fixed in a lower level of development.

   _____ Mr. T's father had diabetes mellitus.

   _____ Mr. T has been fired from his last five jobs.

   _____ Mr. T's baby was stillborn last month.

References

Allen, K., Blascovich, J., & Mendes, W. B. (2002). Cardiovascular reactivity and the presence of pets, friends, and spouses: The truth about cats and dogs. *Psychosomatic Medicine, 64,* 727–739.

Barker, S. B., Knisely, J. S., McCain, N. L., & Best, A. M. (2005). Measuring stress and immune response in healthcare professionals following interaction with a therapy dog: A pilot study. *Psychological Reports, 96,* 713–729.

Davis, M. D., Eshelman, E. R., & McKay, M. (2008). *The relaxation and stress reduction workbook* (6th ed.). Oakland, CA: New Harbinger Publications.

Friedmann, E., & Thomas, S. A. (1995). Pet ownership, social support, and one-year survival after acute myocardial infarction in the Cardiac Arrhythmia Suppression Trial. *American Journal of Cardiology, 76,* 1213.

Miller, M. A., & Rahe, R. H. (1997). Life changes scaling for the 1990s. *Journal of Psychosomatic Research, 43,* 279–292.

Pelletier, K. R. (1992). *Mind as healer, mind as slayer: A holistic approach to preventing stress disorders.* New York: Dell.

Whitaker, J. (2000). Pet owners are a healthy breed. *Health & Healing, 10*(10), 1–8.

Classical References

Holmes, T., & Rahe, R. (1967). The Social Readjustment Rating Scale. *Journal of Psychosomatic Research, 11,* 213–218.

Lazarus, R. S., & Folkman, S. (1984). *Stress, appraisal and coping.* New York: Springer.

Roy, C. (1976). *Introduction to nursing: An adaptation model.* Englewood Cliffs, NJ: Prentice Hall.

Selye, H. (1956). *The stress of life.* New York: McGraw-Hill.

Selye, H. (1974). *Stress without distress.* New York: Signet Books.

Selye, H. (1976). *The stress of life* (Rev. ed.). New York: McGraw-Hill.

KEY TERMS

anticipatory grieving	*introjection*	*suppression*
bereavement overload	*isolation*	*undoing*
defense mechanisms	*projection*	humors
compensation	*rationalization*	mental health
denial	*reaction formation*	mental illness
displacement	*regression*	neurosis
identification	*repression*	psychosis
intellectualization	*sublimation*	"ship of fools"

OBJECTIVES
After reading this chapter, the student will be able to:

1. Discuss the history of psychiatric care.
2. Define *mental health* and *mental illness.*
3. Discuss cultural elements that influence attitudes toward mental health and mental illness.
4. Describe psychological adaptation responses to stress.
5. Identify correlation of adaptive/maladaptive behaviors to the mental health/mental illness continuum.

HOMEWORK ASSIGNMENT
Please read the chapter and answer the following quetions:

1. Explain the concepts of *incomprehensibility* and *cultural relativity.*
2. Describe some symptoms of panic anxiety.
3. Jane was involved in an automobile accident in which both her parents were killed. When you ask her about it, she says she has no memory of the accident. What ego defense mechanism is she using?
4. In what stage of the grieving process is the individual with delayed or inhibited grief fixed?

The consideration of mental health and mental illness has its basis in the cultural beliefs of the society in which the behavior takes place. Some cultures are quite liberal in the range of behaviors that are considered acceptable, whereas others have very little tolerance for behaviors that deviate from the cultural norms.

A study of the history of psychiatric care reveals some shocking truths about past treatment of mentally ill individuals. Many were kept in control by means that today could be considered less than humane.

This chapter deals with the evolution of psychiatric care from ancient times to the present. **Mental health** and **mental illness** are defined, and the psychological adaptation to stress is explained in terms of the two major responses: anxiety and grief. A mental health/mental illness continuum and the *Diagnostic and Statistical Manual of Mental Disorders, 4th Edition, Text Revision (DSM-IV-TR)* multiaxial evaluation system are presented.

Historical Overview of Psychiatric Care

Primitive beliefs regarding mental disturbances took several views. Some thought that an individual with mental illness had been dispossessed of his or her soul and that the only way wellness could be achieved was if the soul returned. Others believed that evil spirits or supernatural or magical powers had entered the body. The "cure" for these individuals involved a ritualistic exorcism to purge the body of these unwanted forces. This often consisted of brutal beatings, starvation, or other torturous means. Still others considered that the mentally ill individual may have broken a taboo or sinned against another individual or God, for which ritualistic purification was required or various types of retribution were demanded. The correlation of mental illness to demonology or witchcraft led to some mentally ill individuals being burned at the stake.

The position of these ancient beliefs evolved with increasing knowledge about mental illness and changes in cultural, religious, and sociopolitical attitudes. The work of Hippocrates, about 400 B.C., began the movement away from belief in the supernatural. Hippocrates associated insanity and mental illness with an irregularity in the interaction of the four body fluids—blood, black bile, yellow bile, and phlegm. He called these body fluids **humors,** and associated each with a particular disposition. Disequilibrium among these four humors was thought to cause mental illness, and it was often treated by inducing vomiting and diarrhea with potent cathartic drugs.

During the Middle Ages (A.D. 500 to 1500), the association of mental illness with witchcraft and the supernatural continued to prevail in Europe. During this period, many severely mentally ill people were sent out to sea on sailing boats with little guidance to search for their lost rationality. The expression **"ship of fools"** was derived from this operation.

During the same period in the Middle Eastern Islamic countries, however, a change in attitude began to occur, from the perception of mental illness as the result of witchcraft or the supernatural to the idea that these individuals were actually ill. This notion gave rise to the establishment of special units for the mentally ill within general hospitals, as well as institutions specifically designed to house the insane. They can likely be considered the first asylums for the mentally ill.

Colonial Americans tended to reflect the attitudes of the European communities from which they had immigrated. Particularly in the New England area, individuals were punished for behavior attributed to witchcraft. In the 16th and 17th centuries, institutions for the mentally ill did not exist in the United States, and care of these individuals became a family responsibility. Those without family or other resources became the responsibility of the communities in which they lived and were incarcerated in places where they could do no harm to themselves or others.

The first hospital in America to admit mentally ill clients was established in Philadelphia in the middle of the 18th century. Benjamin Rush, often called the father of American psychiatry, was a physician at the hospital. He initiated the provision of humanistic treatment and care for the mentally ill. Although he included kindness, exercise, and socialization, he also employed harsher methods such as bloodletting, purging, various types of physical restraints, and extremes of temperatures, reflecting the medical therapies of that era.

The 19th century brought the establishment of a system of state asylums, largely the result of the work of Dorothea Dix, a former New England schoolteacher, who lobbied tirelessly on behalf of the mentally ill population. She was unfaltering in her belief that mental illness was curable and that state hospitals should provide humanistic therapeutic care. This system of hospital care for the mentally ill grew, but the mentally ill population grew faster. The institutions became overcrowded and understaffed, and conditions deteriorated. Therapeutic care reverted to custodial care. These state hospitals provided the largest resource for the mentally ill until the initiation of the community health movement of the 1960s (see Chapter 37).

The emergence of psychiatric nursing began in 1873 with the graduation of Linda Richards from the nursing program at the New England Hospital for Women and Children in Boston. She has come to be known as the first American psychiatric nurse. During her career, Richards was instrumental in the establishment of a number of psychiatric hospitals and the first school of psychiatric nursing at the McLean Asylum in Waverly, Massachusetts, in 1882. The focus in this school, and those that followed, was "training" in how to provide custodial care for clients in psychiatric asylums—training that did not include the study of psychological concepts. Significant change did not occur until 1955, when incorporation of psychiatric nursing into their curricula became a requirement for all undergraduate schools of nursing.

Nursing curricula emphasized the importance of the nurse-patient relationship and therapeutic communication techniques. Nursing intervention in the somatic therapies (e.g., insulin and electroconvulsive therapy) provided impetus for the incorporation of these concepts into nursing's body of knowledge.

With the apparently increasing need for psychiatric care in the aftermath of World War II, the government passed the National Mental Health Act of 1946. This legislation provided funds for the education of psychiatrists, psychologists, social workers, and psychiatric nurses. Graduate-level education in psychiatric nursing was established during this period. Also significant at this time was the introduction of antipsychotic medications, which made it possible for psychotic clients to more readily participate in their treatment, including nursing therapies.

Knowledge of the history of psychiatric/mental health care contributes to the understanding of the concepts presented in this chapter and those in Chapter 3, which describe the theories of personality development according to various 19th-century and 20th-century leaders in the psychiatric/mental health movement. Modern American psychiatric care has its roots in ancient times. A great deal of opportunity exists for continued advancement of this specialty within the practice of nursing.

Mental Health

A number of theorists have attempted to define the concept of mental health. Many of these concepts deal with various aspects of individual functioning. Maslow (1970) emphasized an individual's motivation in the continuous quest for self-actualization. He identified a "hierarchy of needs," the lower ones requiring fulfillment before those at higher levels can be achieved, with self-actualization being fulfillment of one's highest potential. An individual's position within the hierarchy may reverse from a higher level to a lower level based on life circumstances. For example, an individual

facing major surgery who has been working on tasks to achieve self-actualization may become preoccupied, if only temporarily, with the need for physiological safety. A representation of this needs hierarchy is presented in Figure 2–1.

Maslow described self-actualization as being "psychologically healthy, fully human, highly evolved, and fully mature." He believed that "healthy," or "self-actualized," individuals possessed the following characteristics:

■ An appropriate perception of reality
■ The ability to accept oneself, others, and human nature
■ The ability to manifest spontaneity
■ The capacity for focusing concentration on problem solving
■ A need for detachment and desire for privacy
■ Independence, autonomy, and a resistance to enculturation
■ An intensity of emotional reaction
■ A frequency of "peak" experiences that validates the worthwhileness, richness, and beauty of life
■ An identification with humankind
■ The ability to achieve satisfactory interpersonal relationships
■ A democratic character structure and strong sense of ethics
■ Creativeness
■ A degree of nonconformance

Jahoda (1958) has identified a list of six indicators that she suggests are a reflection of mental health:

1. **A Positive Attitude Toward Self.** This includes an objective view of self, including knowledge and acceptance of strengths and limitations. The individual feels a strong sense of personal identity and a security within the environment.

2. **Growth, Development, and the Ability to Achieve Self-actualization.** This indicator correlates with whether the individual successfully achieves the tasks associated with each level of development (see Erikson, Chapter 3). With successful achievement in each level, the individual gains motivation for advancement to his or her highest potential.

3. **Integration.** The focus here is on maintaining an equilibrium or balance among various life processes. Integration includes the ability to adaptively respond to the environment and the

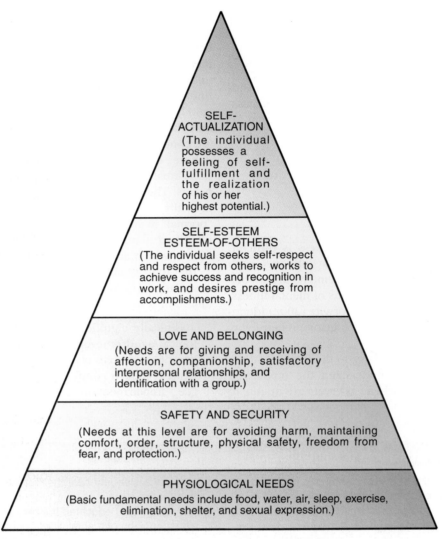

FIGURE 2–1   Maslow's hierarchy of needs.

development of a philosophy of life, both of which help the individual maintain anxiety at a manageable level in response to stressful situations.

4. **Autonomy.** This refers to the individual's ability to perform in an independent, self-directed manner. The individual makes choices and accepts responsibility for the outcomes.

5. **Perception of Reality.** Accurate reality perception is a positive indicator of mental health. This includes perception of the environment without distortion, as well as the capacity for empathy and social sensitivity—a respect and concern for the wants and needs of others.

6. **Environmental Mastery.** This indicator suggests that the individual has achieved a satisfactory role within the group, society, or environment. It suggests that he or she is able

to love and accept the love of others. When faced with life situations, the individual is able to strategize, make decisions, change, adjust, and adapt. Life offers satisfaction to the individual who has achieved environmental mastery.

The American Psychiatric Association (APA) (2003) defines mental health as:

A state of being that is relative rather than absolute. The successful performance of mental functions shown by productive activities, fulfilling relationships with other people, and the ability to adapt to change and to cope with adversity.

Robinson (1983) has offered the following definition of mental health:

a dynamic state in which thought, feeling, and behavior that is age-appropriate and congruent with the local and cultural norms is demonstrated. (p. 74)

For purposes of this text, and in keeping with the framework of stress/adaptation, a modification of Robinson's definition of mental health is considered. Thus, *mental health* is viewed as "the successful adaptation to stressors from the internal or external environment, evidenced by thoughts, feelings, and behaviors that are age-appropriate and congruent with local and cultural norms."

Mental Illness

A universal concept of mental illness is difficult, because of the cultural factors that influence such a definition. However, certain elements are associated with individuals' perceptions of mental illness, regardless of cultural origin. Horwitz (2002) identified two of these elements as (1) incomprehensibility and (2) cultural relativity.

Incomprehensibility relates to the inability of the general population to understand the motivation behind the behavior. When observers are unable to find meaning or comprehensibility in behavior, they are likely to label that behavior as mental illness. Horwitz stated, "Observers attribute labels of mental illness when the rules, conventions, and understandings they use to interpret behavior fail to find any intelligible motivation behind an action" (p. 17). The element of *cultural relativity* considers that these rules, conventions, and understandings are conceived within an individual's own particular culture. Behavior that is considered "normal" and "abnormal" is defined by one's cultural or societal norms. Therefore, a behavior that is recognized as mentally ill in one society may be viewed as "normal" in another society, and vice versa. Horwitz identified a number of cultural aspects of mental illness, which are presented in Box 2-1.

In the *DSM-IV-TR* (American Psychiatric Association [APA], 2000), the APA defines mental illness or a mental disorder as:

a clinically significant behavioral or psychological syndrome or pattern that occurs in a person and that is associated with present distress (e.g., a painful symptom) or disability (i.e., impairment in one or more important

---

BOX 2-1 Cultural Aspects of Mental Illness

1. Usually members of the lay community, rather than a psychiatric professional, initially recognize that an individual's behavior deviates from the societal norms.
2. People who are related to an individual or who are of the same cultural or social group are less likely to label an individual's behavior as mentally ill than someone who is relationally or culturally distant. Relatives (or people of the same cultural or social group) try to "normalize" the behavior; that is, they try to find an explanation for the behavior.
3. Psychiatrists see a person with mental illness most often when the family members can no longer deny the illness and often when the behavior is at its worst. The local or cultural norms define pathological behavior.
4. Individuals in the lowest social class usually display the highest amount of mental illness symptoms. However, they tend to tolerate a wider range of behaviors that deviate from societal norms and are less likely to consider these behaviors as indicative of mental illness. Mental illness labels are most often applied by psychiatric professionals.
5. The higher the social class, the greater the recognition of mental illness behaviors. Members of the higher social classes are likely to be self-labeled or labeled by family members or friends. Psychiatric

assistance is sought near the first signs of emotional disturbance.
6. The more highly educated the person, the greater the recognition of mental illness behaviors. However, even more relevant than the *amount* of education is the *type* of education. Individuals in the more humanistic types of professions (lawyers, social workers, artists, teachers, nurses) are more likely to seek psychiatric assistance than professionals such as business executives, computer specialists, accountants, and engineers.
7. In terms of religion, Jewish people are more likely to seek psychiatric assistance than are Catholics or Protestants.
8. Women are more likely than men to recognize the symptoms of mental illness and seek assistance.
9. The greater the cultural distance from the *mainstream* of society (i.e., the fewer the ties with *conventional* society), the greater the likelihood of negative response by society to mental illness. For example, immigrants have a greater distance from the mainstream than the native born, ethnic minorities greater than the dominant culture, and "bohemians" greater than the bourgeoisie. They are more likely to be subjected to coercive treatment, and involuntary psychiatric commitments are more common.

Adapted from Horwitz, A. V. (2002). The social control of mental illness. Clinton Corners, NY: Percheron Press.

areas of functioning), or with a significantly increased risk of suffering death, pain, disability, or an important loss of freedom . . . and is not merely an expectable and culturally sanctioned response to a particular event (e.g., the death of a loved one). (p. xxxi)

For purposes of this text, and in keeping with the framework of stress/adaptation, *mental illness* will be characterized as "maladaptive responses to stressors from the internal or external environment, evidenced by thoughts, feelings, and behaviors that are incongruent with the local and cultural norms, and interfere with the individual's social, occupational, and/or physical functioning."

Psychological Adaptation to Stress

All individuals exhibit some characteristics associated with both mental health and mental illness at any given point in time. Chapter 1 described how an individual's response to stressful situations was influenced by his or her personal perception of the event and a variety of predisposing factors, such as heredity, temperament, learned response patterns, developmental maturity, existing coping strategies, and support systems of caring others.

Anxiety and grief have been described as two major, primary psychological response patterns to stress. A variety of thoughts, feelings, and behaviors are associated with each of these response patterns. Adaptation is determined by the degree to which the thoughts, feelings, and behaviors interfere with an individual's functioning.

CORE CONCEPT

Anxiety

A diffuse apprehension that is vague in nature and is associated with feelings of uncertainty and helplessness.

Anxiety

Feelings of anxiety are so common in our society that they are almost considered universal. Anxiety arises from the chaos and confusion that exists in the world today. Fears of the unknown and conditions of ambiguity offer a perfect breeding ground for anxiety to take root and grow. Low levels of anxiety are adaptive and can provide the motivation required for survival. Anxiety becomes problematic

when the individual is unable to prevent the anxiety from escalating to a level that interferes with the ability to meet basic needs.

Peplau (1963) described four levels of anxiety: mild, moderate, severe, and panic. It is important for nurses to be able to recognize the symptoms associated with each level to plan for appropriate intervention with anxious individuals.

■ **Mild Anxiety.** This level of anxiety is seldom a problem for the individual. It is associated with the tension experienced in response to the events of day-to-day living. Mild anxiety prepares people for action. It sharpens the senses, increases motivation for productivity, increases the perceptual field, and results in a heightened awareness of the environment. Learning is enhanced and the individual is able to function at his or her optimal level.

■ **Moderate Anxiety.** As the level of anxiety increases, the extent of the perceptual field diminishes. The moderately anxious individual is less alert to events occurring in the environment. The individual's attention span and ability to concentrate decrease, although he or she may still attend to needs with direction. Assistance with problem solving may be required. Increased muscular tension and restlessness are evident.

■ **Severe Anxiety.** The perceptual field of the severely anxious individual is so greatly diminished that concentration centers on one particular detail only or on many extraneous details. Attention span is extremely limited, and the individual has much difficulty completing even the simplest task. Physical symptoms (e.g., headaches, palpitations, insomnia) and emotional symptoms (e.g., confusion, dread, horror) may be evident. Discomfort is experienced to the degree that virtually all overt behavior is aimed at relieving the anxiety.

■ **Panic Anxiety.** In this most intense state of anxiety, the individual is unable to focus on even one detail in the environment. Misperceptions are common, and a loss of contact with reality may occur. The individual may experience hallucinations or delusions. Behavior may be characterized by wild and desperate actions or extreme withdrawal. Human functioning and communication with others is ineffective. Panic anxiety is associated with a feeling of terror, and individuals may be convinced that they have a life-threatening illness or fear that they are "going crazy" or losing control (APA, 2000). Prolonged panic anxiety can lead to physical and emotional exhaustion and can be a life-threatening situation.

A synopsis of the characteristics associated with each of the four levels of anxiety is presented in Table 2-1.

Behavioral Adaptation Responses to Anxiety

A variety of behavioral adaptation responses occur at each level of anxiety. Figure 2–2 depicts these behavioral responses on a continuum of anxiety ranging from mild to panic.

Mild Anxiety

At the mild level, individuals employ any of a number of coping behaviors that satisfy their needs for comfort. Menninger (1963) described the following types of coping mechanisms that individuals use to relieve anxiety in stressful situations:

- Sleeping
- Eating
- Yawning
- Drinking
- Physical exercise
- Smoking
- Crying
- Pacing
- Foot swinging
- Fidgeting
- Daydreaming
- Laughing
- Cursing
- Nail biting
- Finger tapping
- Talking to someone with whom one feels comfortable

Undoubtedly there are many more responses too numerous to mention here, considering that each individual develops his or her own unique ways to relieve anxiety at the mild level. Some of these behaviors are more adaptive than others.

Mild-to-Moderate Anxiety

Sigmund Freud (1961) identified the ego as the reality component of the personality that governs problem solving and rational thinking. As the level of anxiety increases, the strength of the ego is

TABLE 2-1 Levels of Anxiety

LEVEL	PERCEPTUAL FIELD	ABILITY TO LEARN	PHYSICAL CHARACTERISTICS	EMOTIONAL/BEHAVIORAL CHARACTERISTICS
Mild	Heightened perception (e.g., noises may seem louder; details within the environment are clearer). Increased awareness Increased alertness.	Learning is enhanced.	Restlessness. Irritability.	May remain superficial with others. Rarely experienced as distressful. Motivation is increased.
Moderate	Reduction in perceptual field. Reduced alertness to environmental events (e.g., someone talking may not be heard; part of the room may not be noticed).	Learning still occurs, but not at optimal ability. Decreased attention span. Decreased ability to concentrate.	Increased restlessness. Increased heart and respiration rate. Increased perspiration. Gastric discomfort. Increased muscular tension. Increase in speech rate, volume, and pitch.	A feeling of discontent. May lead to a degree of impairment in interpersonal relationships as individual begins to focus on self and the need to relieve personal discomfort.
Severe	Greatly diminished; only extraneous details are perceived, or fixation on a single detail may occur. May not take notice of an event even when attention is directed by another.	Extremely limited attention span. Unable to concentrate or problem-solve. Effective learning cannot occur.	Headaches. Dizziness. Nausea. Trembling. Insomnia. Palpitations. Tachycardia. Hyperventilation. Urinary frequency. Diarrhea.	Feelings of dread, loathing, horror. Total focus on self and intense desire to relieve the anxiety.

TABLE 2-1 Levels of Anxiety—cont'd

LEVEL	PERCEPTUAL FIELD	ABILITY TO LEARN	PHYSICAL CHARACTERISTICS	EMOTIONAL/BEHAVIORAL CHARACTERISTICS
Panic	Unable to focus on even one detail within the environment. Misperceptions of the environment common (e.g., a perceived detail may be elabo-rated and out of proportion).	Learning cannot occur. Unable to concentrate. Unable to com-prehend even simple direc-tions.	Dilated pupils. Labored breathing. Severe trembling. Sleeplessness. Palpitations. Diaphoresis and pallor. Muscular incoordination. Immobility or purpose-less hyperactivity. Incoherence or inability to verbalize.	Sense of impending doom. Terror. Bizarre behavior, including shouting, screaming, running about wildly, clinging to anyone or anything from which a sense of safety and security is derived. Hallucinations; delusions. Extreme withdrawal into self.

FIGURE 2–2   Adaptation responses on a continuum of anxiety

tested, and energy is mobilized to confront the threat. Anna Freud (1953) identified a number of **defense mechanisms** employed by the ego in the face of threat to biological or psychological integri-ty. Some of these ego defense mechanisms are more adaptive than others, but all are used either con-sciously or unconsciously as a protective device for the ego in an effort to relieve mild to moderate anx-iety. They become maladaptive when they are used by an individual to such a degree that there is inter-ference with the ability to deal with reality, with effective interpersonal relations, or with occupation-al performance. Maladaptive use of defense mecha-nisms promotes disintegration of the ego. The major ego defense mechanisms identified by Anna Freud are discussed here and summarized in Table 2-2.

1. **Compensation** is the covering up of a real or perceived weakness by emphasizing a trait one considers more desirable.

EXAMPLES

(a) A handicapped boy who is unable to partici-pate in sports compensates by becoming a great scholar. (b) A young man who is the shortest among members of his peer group views this as a deficiency and compensates by being overly aggressive and daring.

2. **Denial** is the refusal to acknowledge the exis-tence of a real situation or the feelings associ-ated with it.

EXAMPLES

(a) A woman has been told by family doctor that she has a lump in her breast. An appointment is made for her with a surgeon; however, she does not keep the appointment and goes about her activities of daily living with no evidence of con-cern. (b) Individuals continue to smoke cigarettes even though they have been told of the health risk involved.

3. **Displacement** is the transferring of feelings from one target to another that is considered less threatening or neutral.

EXAMPLES

(a) A man who is passed over for promotion on his job says nothing to his boss but later belittles his son for not making the basketball team. (b) A boy who is teased and hit by the class bully on the playground comes home after school and kicks his dog.

4. **Identification** is an attempt to increase self-worth by acquiring certain attributes and characteristics of an individual one admires.

EXAMPLES

(a) A teenage girl emulates the mannerisms and style of dress of a popular female rock star. (b) The young son of a famous civil rights work-er adopts his father's attitudes and behaviors with the intent of pursuing similar aspirations.

TABLE 2-2 Ego Defense Mechanisms

DEFENSE MECHANISM	EXAMPLE	DEFENSE MECHANISM	EXAMPLE
Compensation Covering up a real or perceived weakness by emphasizing a trait one considers more desirable.	A physically handicapped boy is unable to participate in football, so he compensates by becoming a great scholar.	**Rationalization** Attempting to make excuses or formulate logical reasons to justify unacceptable feelings or behaviors.	John tells the rehab nurse, "I drink because it's the only way I can deal with my bad marriage and my worse job."
Denial Refusing to acknowledge the existence of a real situation or the feelings associated with it.	A woman drinks alcohol every day and cannot stop, failing to acknowledge that she has a problem.	**Reaction Formation** Preventing unacceptable or undesirable thoughts or behaviors from being expressed by exaggerating opposite thoughts or types of behaviors	Jane hates nursing. She attended nursing school to please her parents. During career day, she speaks to prospective students about the excellence of nursing as a career.
Displacement The transfer of feelings from one target to another that is considered less threatening or that is neutral.	A client is angry with his physician, does not express it, but becomes verbally abusive with the nurse.	**Regression** Retreating in response to stress to an earlier level of development and the comfort measures associated with that level of functioning.	When 2-year-old Jay is hospitalized for tonsillitis he will drink only from a bottle, even though his mom states he has been drinking from a cup for 6 months.
Identification An attempt to increase self-worth by acquiring certain attributes and characteristics of an individual one admires	A teenager who required lengthy rehabilitation after an accident decides to become a physical therapist as a result of his experiences.	**Repression** Involuntarily blocking unpleasant feelings and experiences from one's awareness	An accident victim can remember nothing about his accident.
Intellectualization An attempt to avoid expressing actual emotions associated with a stressful situation by using the intellectual processes of logic, reasoning, and analysis	S's husband is being transferred with his job to a city far away from her parents. She hides anxiety by explaining to her parents the advantages associated with the move.	**Sublimation** Rechanneling of drives or impulses that are personally or socially unacceptable into activities that are constructive	A mother whose son was killed by a drunk driver channels her anger and energy into being the president of the local chapter of Mothers Against Drunk Drivers.
Introjection Integrating the beliefs and values of another individual into one's own ego structure	Children integrate their parents' value system into the process of conscience formation. A child says to friend, "Don't cheat. It's wrong."	**Suppression** The voluntary blocking of unpleasant feelings and experiences from one's awareness	Scarlett O'Hara says, "I don't want to think about that now. I'll think about that tomorrow."

TABLE 2-2 Ego Defense Mechanisms—cont'd			
DEFENSE MECHANISM	**EXAMPLE**	**DEFENSE MECHANISM**	**EXAMPLE**
Isolation		Undoing	
Separating a thought or memory from the feeling tone, or emotion associated with it.	A young woman describes being attacked and raped, without showing any emotion.	Symbolically negating or canceling out an experience that one finds intolerable	Joe is nervous about his new job and yells at his wife. On his way home he stops and buys her some flowers.
Projection			
Attributing feelings or impulses unacceptable to one's self to another person	Sue feels a strong sexual attraction to her track coach and tells her friend, "He's coming on to me!"		

5. **Intellectualization** is an attempt to avoid expressing actual emotions associated with a stressful situation by using the intellectual processes of logic, reasoning, and analysis.

EXAMPLES

(a) A man whose brother is in a cardiac intensive care unit following a severe myocardial infarction (MI) spends his allotted visiting time in discussion with the nurse, analyzing test results and making a reasonable determination about the pathophysiology that may have occurred to induce the MI. (b) A young psychology professor receives a letter from his fiancée breaking off their engagement. He shows no emotion when discussing this with his best friend. Instead he analyzes his fiancée's behavior and tries to reason why the relationship failed.

6. **Introjection** is the internalization of the beliefs and values of another individual such that they symbolically become a part of the self to the extent that the feeling of separateness or distinctness is lost.

EXAMPLES

(a) A small child develops her conscience by internalizing what the parents believe is right and wrong. The parents literally become a part of the child. The child says to a friend while playing, "Don't hit people. It's not nice!" (b) A psychiatric client claims to be the Son of God, drapes himself in sheet and blanket, "performs miracles" on other clients, and refuses to respond unless addressed as Jesus Christ.

7. **Isolation** is the separation of a thought or a memory from the feeling tone or emotions

associated with it (sometimes called emotional isolation).

EXAMPLES

(a) A young woman describes being attacked and raped by a street gang. She displays an apathetic expression and no emotional tone. (b) A physician is able to isolate her feelings about the eventual death of a terminally ill cancer client by focusing her attention instead on the chemotherapy that will be given.

8. **Projection** is the attribution of feelings or impulses unacceptable to one's self to another person. The individual "passes the blame" for these undesirable feelings or impulses to another, thereby providing relief from the anxiety associated with them.

EXAMPLES

(a) A young soldier who has an extreme fear of participating in military combat tells his sergeant that the others in his unit are "a bunch of cowards." (b) A businessperson who values punctuality is late for a meeting and states, "Sorry I'm late. My assistant forgot to remind me of the time. It's so hard to find good help these days."

9. **Rationalization** is the attempt to make excuses or formulate logical reasons to justify unacceptable feelings or behaviors.

EXAMPLES

(a) A self-employed person deliberately neglects to report part of her income to the Internal Revenue Service, and justifies it to herself by saying, "It's okay. Everybody does it." (b) A young man is unable to afford the sports car he wants so desperately. He tells the salesperson, "I'd buy this car but I'll be getting married soon. This is really not the car for a family man."

10. **Reaction formation** is the prevention of unacceptable or undesirable thoughts or behaviors from being expressed by exaggerating opposite thoughts or types of behaviors.

EXAMPLES

(a) The young soldier who has an extreme fear of participating in military combat volunteers for dangerous front-line duty. (b) A secretary is sexually attracted to her boss and feels an intense dislike toward his wife. She treats her boss with detachment and aloofness while performing her secretarial duties and is overly courteous, polite, and flattering to his wife when she comes to the office.

11. **Regression** is the retreating to an earlier level of development and the comfort measures associated with that level of functioning.

EXAMPLES

(a) When his mother brings his new baby sister home from the hospital, 4-year-old Tommy, who had been toilet trained for more than a year, begins to wet his pants, cry to be held, and suck his thumb. (b) A person who is depressed may withdraw to his or her room, curl up in a fetal position on the bed, and sleep for long periods of time.

12. **Repression** is the involuntary blocking of unpleasant feelings and experiences from one's awareness.

EXAMPLES

(a) A woman cannot remember being sexually assaulted when she was 15 years old. (b) A teenage boy cannot remember driving the car that was involved in an accident in which his best friend was killed.

13. **Sublimation** is the rechanneling of drives or impulses that are personally or socially unacceptable (e.g., aggressiveness, anger, sexual drives) into activities that are more tolerable and constructive.

EXAMPLES

(a) A teenage boy with strong competitive and aggressive drives becomes the star football player on his high school team. (b) A young unmarried woman with a strong desire for marriage and a

family achieves satisfaction and success in establishing and operating a day-care center for preschool children.

14. **Suppression** is the voluntarily blocking of unpleasant feelings and experiences from one's awareness.

EXAMPLES

(a) Scarlett O'Hara says, "I'll think about that tomorrow." (b) A young woman who is depressed about a pending divorce proceeding tells the nurse, "I just don't want to talk about the divorce. There's nothing I can do about it anyway."

15. **Undoing** is the act of symbolically negating or canceling out a previous action or experience that one finds intolerable.

EXAMPLES

(a) A man spills some salt on the table, then sprinkles some over his left shoulder to "prevent bad luck." (b) A man who is anxious about giving a presentation at work yells at his wife during breakfast. He stops on his way home from work that evening to buy her a dozen red roses.

Moderate-to-Severe Anxiety

Anxiety at the moderate to severe level that remains unresolved over an extended period of time can contribute to a number of physiological disorders. The *DSM-IV-TR* (APA, 2000) describes these disorders as "the presence of one or more specific psychological or behavioral factors that adversely affect a general medical condition." The psychological factors may exacerbate symptoms of, delay recovery from, or interfere with treatment of the medical condition. The condition may be initiated or exacerbated by an environmental situation that the individual perceives as stressful. Measurable pathophysiology can be demonstrated.

The *DSM-IV-TR* states:

> Psychological and behavioral factors may affect the course of almost every major category of disease, including cardiovascular conditions, dermatological conditions, endocrinological conditions, gastrointestinal conditions, neoplastic conditions, neurological conditions, pulmonary conditions, renal conditions, and rheumatological conditions." (p. 732)

Severe Anxiety

Extended periods of repressed severe anxiety can result in psychoneurotic patterns of behaving. **Neurosis** is no longer a separate category of disorders in the *DSM-IV-TR* (APA, 2000). However, the term is still used in the literature to further describe the symptomatology of certain disorders. Neuroses are psychiatric disturbances characterized by excessive anxiety that is expressed directly or altered through defense mechanisms. A neurosis appears as a symptom, such as an obsession, a compulsion, a phobia, or a sexual dysfunction (Sadock & Sadock, 2007). The following are common characteristics of people with neuroses:

■ They are aware that they are experiencing distress.

■ They are aware that their behaviors are maladaptive.

■ They are unaware of any possible psychological causes of the distress.

■ They feel helpless to change their situation.

■ They experience no loss of contact with reality.

The following disorders are examples of psychoneurotic responses to anxiety as they appear in the *DSM-IV-TR*. They are discussed in this text in Chapters 29 and 30.

1. **Anxiety Disorders.** Disorders in which the characteristic features are symptoms of anxiety and avoidance behavior (e.g., phobias, obsessive-compulsive disorder, panic disorder, generalized anxiety disorder, and posttraumatic stress disorder).

2. **Somatoform Disorders.** Disorders in which the characteristic features are physical symptoms for which there is no demonstrable organic pathology. Psychological factors are judged to play a significant role in the onset, severity, exacerbation, or maintenance of the symptoms (e.g., hypochondriasis, conversion disorder, somatization disorder, pain disorder).

3. **Dissociative Disorders.** Disorders in which the characteristic feature is a disruption in the usually integrated functions of consciousness, memory, identity, or perception of the environment (e.g., dissociative amnesia, dissociative fugue, dissociative identity disorder, and depersonalization disorder).

Panic Anxiety

At this extreme level of anxiety, an individual is not capable of processing what is happening in the environment, and may lose contact with reality. **Psychosis** is defined as a loss of ego boundaries or a gross impairment in reality testing (APA, 2000). Psychoses are serious psychiatric disturbances characterized by the presence of delusions or hallucinations and the impairment of interpersonal functioning and relationship to the external world. The following are common characteristics of people with psychoses:

■ They experience minimal distress (emotional tone is flat, bland, or inappropriate).

■ They are unaware that their behavior is maladaptive.

■ They are unaware of any psychological problems.

■ They are exhibiting a flight from reality into a less stressful world or into one in which they are attempting to adapt.

Examples of psychotic responses to anxiety include the schizophrenic, schizoaffective, and delusional disorders. They are discussed at length in Chapter 26.

CORE CONCEPT

Grief

Grief is a subjective state of emotional, physical, and social responses to the loss of a valued entity.

Grief

Most individuals experience intense emotional anguish in response to a significant personal loss. A loss is anything that is perceived as such by the individual. Losses may be real, in which case they can be substantiated by others (e.g., death of a loved one, loss of personal possessions), or they may be perceived by the individual alone, unable to be shared or identified by others (e.g., loss of the feeling of femininity following mastectomy). Any situation that creates change for an individual can be identified as a loss. Failure (either real or perceived) also can be viewed as a loss.

The loss, or anticipated loss, of anything of value to an individual can trigger the grief response. This period of characteristic emotions and behaviors is called *mourning*. The "normal" mourning process is adaptive and is characterized by feelings of sadness, guilt, anger, helplessness, hopelessness, and despair. Indeed, an absence of mourning after a loss may be considered maladaptive.

Stages of Grief

Kübler-Ross (1969), in extensive research with terminally ill patients, identified five stages of feelings and behaviors that individuals experience in response to a real, perceived, or anticipated loss:

Stage 1—Denial. This is a stage of shock and disbelief. The response may be one of "No, it can't be true!" The reality of the loss is not acknowledged. Denial is a protective mechanism that allows the individual to cope in an immediate time frame while organizing more effective defense strategies.

Stage 2—Anger. "Why me?" and "It's not fair!" are comments often expressed during the anger stage. Envy and resentment toward individuals not affected by the loss are common. Anger may be directed at the self or displaced on loved ones, caregivers, and even God. There may be a preoccupation with an idealized image of the lost entity.

Stage 3—Bargaining. During this stage, which is usually not visible or evident to others, a "bargain" is made with God in an attempt to reverse or postpone the loss: "If God will help me through this, I promise I will go to church every Sunday and volunteer my time to help others." Sometimes the promise is associated with feelings of guilt for not having performed satisfactorily, appropriately, or sufficiently.

Stage 4—Depression. During this stage, the full impact of the loss is experienced. The sense of loss is intense, and feelings of sadness and depression prevail. This is a time of quiet desperation and disengagement from all association with the lost entity. It differs from *pathological* depression, which occurs when an individual becomes fixed in an earlier stage of the grief process. Rather, stage 4 of the grief response represents advancement toward resolution.

Stage 5—Acceptance. The final stage brings a feeling of peace regarding the loss that has occurred. It is a time of quiet expectation and resignation. The focus is on the reality of the loss and its meaning for the individuals affected by it.

All individuals do not experience each of these stages in response to a loss, nor do they necessarily experience them in this order. Some individuals' grieving behaviors may fluctuate, and even overlap, between stages.

Anticipatory Grief

When a loss is anticipated, individuals often begin the work of grieving before the actual loss occurs. Most people re-experience the grieving behaviors once the loss occurs, but having this time to prepare for the loss can facilitate the process of mourning, actually decreasing the length and intensity of the response. Problems arise, particularly in anticipating the death of a loved one, when family members experience **anticipatory grieving** and the mourning process is completed prematurely. They disengage emotionally from the dying person, who may then experience feelings of rejection by loved ones at a time when this psychological support is so necessary.

Resolution

The grief response can last from weeks to years. It cannot be hurried, and individuals must be allowed to progress at their own pace. In the loss of a loved one, grief work usually lasts for at least a year, during which the grieving person experiences each significant "anniversary" date for the first time without the loved one present.

Length of the grief process may be prolonged by a number of factors. If the relationship with the lost entity had been marked by ambivalence or if there had been an enduring "love-hate" association, reaction to the loss may be burdened with guilt. Guilt lengthens the grief reaction by promoting feelings of anger toward the self for having committed a wrongdoing or behaved in an unacceptable manner toward that which is now lost, and perhaps the grieving person may even feel that his or her behavior has contributed to the loss.

Anticipatory grieving is thought to shorten the grief response in some individuals who are able to work through some of the feelings before the loss occurs. If the loss is sudden and unexpected, mourning may take longer than it would if individuals were able to grieve in anticipation of the loss.

Length of the grieving process is also affected by the number of recent losses experienced by an individual and whether he or she is able to complete one grieving process before another loss occurs. This is particularly true for elderly individuals who may be experiencing numerous losses, such as spouse, friends, other relatives, independent functioning, home, personal possessions, and pets, in a relatively short time. Grief accumulates, and this represents a type of **bereavement overload,** which for some individuals presents an impossible task of grief work.

Resolution of the process of mourning is thought to have occurred when an individual can look back on the relationship with the lost entity and accept both the pleasures and the disappointments (both the positive and the negative aspects) of the association (Bowlby & Parkes, 1970). Disorganization and emotional pain have been experienced and tolerated. Preoccupation with the lost entity has been replaced with energy and the desire to pursue new situations and relationships.

Maladaptive Grief Responses

Maladaptive responses to loss occur when an individual is not able to satisfactorily progress through the stages of grieving to achieve resolution. These responses usually occur when an individual becomes fixed in the denial or anger stage of the grief process. Several types of grief responses have been identified as pathological. They include responses that are prolonged, delayed or inhibited, or distorted. The *prolonged* response is characterized by an intense preoccupation with memories of the lost entity for *many years after the loss has occurred*. Behaviors associated with the stages of denial or anger are manifested, and disorganization of functioning and intense emotional pain related to the lost entity are evidenced.

In the *delayed or inhibited* response, the individual becomes fixed in the denial stage of the grieving process. The emotional pain associated with the loss is not experienced, but anxiety disorders (e.g., phobias, hypochondriasis) or sleeping and eating disorders (e.g., insomnia, anorexia) may be evident. The individual may remain in denial for many years until the grief response is triggered by a reminder of the loss or even by another, unrelated loss.

The individual who experiences a *distorted* response is fixed in the anger stage of grieving. In the distorted response, all the normal behaviors associated with grieving, such as helplessness, hopelessness, sadness, anger, and guilt, are exaggerated out of proportion to the situation. The individual turns the anger inward on the self, is consumed with overwhelming despair, and is unable to function in normal activities of daily living. Pathological depression is a distorted grief response (see Chapter 27).

Mental Health/Mental Illness Continuum

Anxiety and grief have been described as two major, primary responses to stress. In Figure 2–3, both of

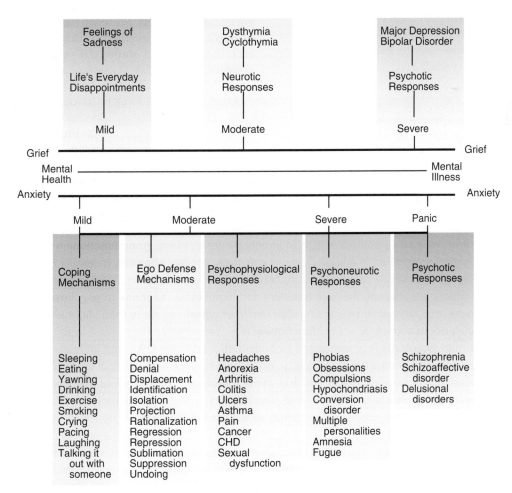

FIGURE 2–3 Conceptualization of anxiety and grief responses along the mental health/mental illness continuum.

these responses are presented on a continuum according to degree of symptom severity. Disorders as they appear in the *DSM-IV-TR* are identified at their appropriate placement along the continuum.

The DSM-IV-TR Multiaxial Evaluation System

The APA endorses case evaluation on a multiaxial system, "to facilitate comprehensive and systematic evaluation with attention to the various mental disorders and general medical conditions, psychosocial and environmental problems, and level of functioning that might be overlooked if the focus were on assessing a single presenting problem" (p. 27). Each individual is evaluated on five axes. They are defined by the *DSM-IV-TR* in the following manner:

Axis I—Clinical Disorders and Other Conditions That May Be a Focus of Clinical Attention. This includes all mental disorders (except personality disorders and mental retardation).

Axis II—Personality Disorders and Mental Retardation. These disorders usually begin in childhood or adolescence and persist in a stable form into adult life.

Axis III—General Medical Conditions. These include any current general medical condition that is potentially relevant to the understanding or management of the individual's mental disorder.

Axis IV—Psychosocial and Environmental Problems. These are problems that may affect the diagnosis, treatment, and prognosis of mental disorders named on axes I and II. These include problems related to primary support group, social environment, education, occupation, housing, economics, access to health care services, interaction with the legal system or crime, and other types of psychosocial and environmental problems.

Axis V—Global Assessment of Functioning. This allows the clinician to rate the individual's overall functioning on the Global Assessment of Functioning (GAF) Scale. This scale represents in global terms a single measure of the individual's psychological, social, and occupational functioning. A copy of the GAF Scale appears in Box 2-2.

The *DSM-IV-TR* outline of axes I and II categories and codes is presented in Appendix C. An example of a psychiatric diagnosis presented according to the multiaxial evaluation system appears in Table 2-3.

BOX 2-2 Global Assessment of Functioning (GAF) Scale

Consider psychological, social, and occupational functioning on a hypothetical continuum of mental health-illness. Do not include impairment in functioning due to physical (or environmental) limitations.

Code	(Note: Use intermediate codes when appropriate, e.g., 45, 68, 72)
100 | 91	**Superior functioning in a wide range of activities, life's problems never seem to get out of hand, is sought out by others because of his or her many positive qualities. No symptoms.**
90 | 81	**Absent or minimal symptoms** (e.g., mild anxiety before an exam), **good functioning in all areas, interested and involved in a wide range of activities, socially effective, generally satisfied with life, no more than everyday problems or concerns** (e.g., an occasional argument with family members).
80 | 71	**If symptoms are present, they are transient and expectable reactions to psychosocial stressors** (e.g., difficulty concentrating after family argument); **no more than slight impairment in social, occupational, or school functioning** (e.g., temporarily falling behind in schoolwork).
70 | 61	**Some mild symptoms** (e.g., depressed mood and mild insomnia) **OR some difficulty in social, occupational, or school functioning** (e.g., occasional truancy, or theft within the household), **but generally functioning pretty well, has some meaningful interpersonal relationships.**
60 | 51	**Moderate symptoms** (e.g., flat affect and circumstantial speech, occasional panic attacks) **OR moderate difficulty in social, occupational, or school functioning** (e.g., few friends, conflicts with peers or co-workers).
50 | 41	**Serious symptoms** (e.g., suicidal ideation, severe obsessional rituals, frequent shoplifting) **OR any serious impairment in social, occupational, or school functioning** (e.g., no friends, unable to keep a job).

BOX 2-2 Global Assessment of Functioning (GAF) Scale—cont'd

40 | | 31	**Some impairment in reality testing or communication** (e.g., speech is at times illogical, obscure, or irrelevant) **OR major impairment in several areas, such as work or school, family relations, judgment, thinking, or mood** (e.g., depressed man avoids friends, neglects family, and is unable to work; child frequently beats up younger children, is defiant at home, and is failing at school).
30 | | 21	**Behavior is considerably influenced by delusions or hallucinations OR serious impairment in communication or judgment** (e.g., sometimes incoherent, acts grossly inappropriately, suicidal preoccupation) **OR inability to function in almost all areas** (e.g., stays in bed all day; no job, home, or friends).
20 | | 11	**Some degree of hurting self or others** (e.g., suicide attempts without clear expectation of death; frequently violent; manic excitement) **OR occasionally fails to maintain minimal personal hygiene** (e.g., smears feces) **OR gross impairment in communication** (e.g., largely incoherent or mute).
10 | | 1	**Persistent danger of severely hurting self or others** (e.g., recurrent violence) **OR persistent inability to maintain minimal personal hygiene OR serious suicidal act with clear expectation of death.**
0	**Inadequate information.**

From American Psychiatric Association. (2000). *Diagnostic and statistical manual of mental disorders (4th ed.). Text revision.* Washington, DC: American Psychiatric Publishing, with permission.

TABLE 2-3 Example of a Psychiatric Diagnosis		
Axis I	300.4	Dysthymic Disorder
Axis II	301.6	Dependent Personality Disorder
Axis III	244.9	Hypothyroidism
Axis IV		Unemployed
Axis V	GAF = 65 (current)	

Summary and Key Points

■ Psychiatric care has its roots in ancient times, when etiology was based in superstition and ideas related to the supernatural.

■ Treatments were often inhumane and included brutal beatings, starvation, or other torturous means.

■ Hippocrates associated insanity and mental illness with an irregularity in the interaction of the four body fluids (humors)—blood, black bile, yellow bile, and phlegm.

■ Conditions for care of the mentally ill have improved, largely because of the influence of leaders such as Benjamin Rush, Dorothea Dix, and Linda Richards, whose endeavors provided a model for more humanistic treatment.

■ Maslow identified a "hierarchy of needs" that individuals seek to fulfill on their quest to self-actualization (one's highest potential).

■ For purposes of this text, the definition of *mental health* is viewed as "the successful adaptation to stressors from the internal or external environment, evidenced by thoughts, feelings, and behaviors that are age-appropriate and congruent with local and cultural norms."

■ In determining mental illness, individuals are influenced by *incomprehensibility* of the person's behavior; that is, whether or not they are able to understand the motivation behind the behavior.

■ Another consideration is *cultural relativity.* The "normality" of behavior is determined by cultural and societal norms.

■ For purposes of this text, the definition of *mental illness* is viewed as "maladaptive responses to stressors from the internal or external environment, evidenced by thoughts, feelings, and behaviors that are incongruent with the local and cultural norms, and interfere with the individual's social, occupational, and/or physical functioning."

■ Anxiety and grief have been described as two major, primary psychological response patterns to stress.

■ Peplau defined anxiety by levels of symptom severity: mild, moderate, severe, and panic.

■ Behaviors associated with levels of anxiety include coping mechanisms, ego defense mechanisms, psychophysiological responses, psychoneurotic responses, and psychotic reponses.

■ Grief is described as a response to loss of a valued entity. Loss is anything that is perceived as such by the individual.

■ Kübler-Ross, in extensive research with terminally ill patients, identified five stages of feelings and behaviors that individuals experience in response to a real, perceived, or anticipated loss: denial, anger, bargaining, depression, and acceptance.

■ Anticipatory grief is grief work that is begun, and sometimes completed, before the loss occurs.

■ Resolution is thought to occur when an individual is able to remember and accept both the positive and negative aspects associated with the lost entity.

■ Grieving is thought to be maladaptive when the mourning process is prolonged, delayed or inhibited, or becomes distorted and exaggerated out of proportion to the situation. Pathological depression is considered to be a distorted reaction.

■ Psychiatric diagnoses are presented by the American Psychiatric Association on a multi-axial evaluation system. Individuals are evaluated on five axes: major mental disorders, personality disorders/developmental level, general medical conditions, psychosocial and environmental problems, and level of functioning.

DavisPlus   Additional info available @ davisplus.fadavis.com

Review Questions
Self-Examination/Learning Exercise

*Select the answer that is **most** appropriate for each of the following questions:*

1. Three years ago, Anna's dog Lucky, whom she had had for 16 years, was run over by a car and killed. Anna's daughter reports that since that time Anna doesn't do a thing for herself anymore. She has lost weight, rarely leaves her home, and just sits and talks about Lucky. Anna's behavior would be considered maladaptive because:
   a. It has been more than 3 years since Lucky died.
   b. Her grief is too intense just over the loss of a dog.
   c. Her grief is interfering with her functioning.
   d. People in this culture would not comprehend such behavior over loss of a pet.

2. Based on the information in Question 1, Anna's grieving behavior would most likely be considered to be:
   a. Delayed.
   b. Inhibited.
   c. Prolonged.
   d. Distorted.

3. Anna is diagnosed with Major Depression. She is most likely fixed in which stage of the grief process?
   a. Denial.
   b. Anger.
   c. Depression.
   d. Acceptance.

Review Questions—cont'd
Self-Examination/Learning Exercise

4. Anna, who is 72 years old, is of the age when she may have experienced many losses coming close together. What is this called?
   a. Bereavement overload.
   b. Normal mourning.
   c. Isolation.
   d. Cultural relativity.

5. Anna is not able to take care of her activities of daily living, and wants only to make daily visits to Lucky's grave. Her daughter has likely put off seeking help for Anna because:
   a. Women are less likely to seek help for emotional problems than men.
   b. Relatives often try to "normalize" the behavior, rather than label it mental illness.
   c. She knows that all older people are expected to be a little depressed.
   d. She is afraid that the neighbors "will think her mother is crazy."

6. Anna's dog Lucky got away from her while they were taking a walk. He ran into the street and was hit by a car. Anna cannot remember any of these circumstances of his death. This is an example of what defense mechanism?
   a. Rationalization.
   b. Suppression.
   c. Denial.
   d. Repression.

7. Lucky sometimes refused to obey Anna, and indeed did not come back to her when she called to him on the day he was killed. But Anna continues to insist, "He was the very best dog. He always minded me. He always did everything I told him to do." This represents the defense mechanism of:
   a. Sublimation.
   b. Compensation.
   c. Reaction formation.
   d. Undoing.

8. Anna has been a widow for 20 years. Her maladaptive grief response to the loss of her dog may be attributed to which of the following? (Select all that apply.)
   a. Unresolved grief over loss of her husband.
   b. Loss of several relatives and friends over the last few years.
   c. Repressed feelings of guilt over the way in which Lucky died.
   d. Inability to prepare in advance for the loss.

9. For what reason would Anna's illness be considered a neurosis rather than a psychosis?
   a. She is unaware that her behavior is maladaptive.
   b. She exhibits inappropriate affect (emotional tone).
   c. She experiences no loss of contact with reality.
   d. She tells the nurse, "There is nothing wrong with me!"

10. Which of the following statements by Anna might suggest that she is achieving resolution of her grief over Lucky's death?
    a. "I don't cry anymore when I think about Lucky."
    b. "It's true. Lucky didn't always mind me. Sometimes he ignored my commands."
    c. "I remember how it happened now. I should have held tighter to his leash!"
    d. "I won't ever have another dog. It's just too painful to lose them."

References

American Psychiatric Association. (2003). *American psychiatric glossary* (8th ed.). Washington, DC: American Psychiatric Publishing.

American Psychiatric Association. (2000). *Diagnostic and statistical manual of mental disorders* (4th ed.). *Text revision.* Washington, DC: Author.

Horwitz, A. V. (2002). *The social control of mental illness.* Clinton Corners, NY: Percheron Press.

Sadock, B. J., & Sadock, V. A. (2007). *Synopsis of psychiatry: Behavioral sciences/clinical psychiatry* (10th ed.). Baltimore: Lippincott Williams & Wilkins.

Robinson, L. (1983). *Psychiatric nursing as a human experience* (3rd ed.). Philadelphia: W.B. Saunders.

Classical References

Bowlby, J., & Parkes, C. M. (1970). Separation and loss. In E. J. Anthony & C. Koupernik (Eds.), *International yearbook for child psychiatry and allied disciplines: The child and his family* (Vol. 1). New York: John Wiley & Sons.

Freud, A. (1953). *The ego and mechanisms of defense.* New York: International Universities Press.

Freud, S. (1961). The ego and the id. In *Standard edition of the complete psychological works of Freud* (Vol. XIX). London: Hogarth Press.

Jahoda, M. (1958). *Current concepts of positive mental health.* New York: Basic Books.

Kübler-Ross, E. (1969). *On death and dying.* New York: Macmillan.

Maslow, A. (1970). *Motivation and personality* (2nd ed.). New York: Harper & Row.

Menninger, K. (1963). *The vital balance.* New York: Viking Press.

Peplau, H. (1963). A working definition of anxiety. In S. Burd & M. Marshall (Eds.), *Some clinical approaches to psychiatric nursing.* New York: Macmillan.

Foundations for Psychiatric/Mental Health Nursing

Theoretical Models of Personality Development

KEY TERMS

cognitive development	id	surrogate
cognitive maturity	libido	symbiosis
counselor	psychodynamic nursing	technical expert
ego	superego	temperament

OBJECTIVES
After reading this chapter, the student will be able to:

1. Define *personality*.
2. Identify the relevance of knowledge associated with personality development to nursing in the psychiatric/mental health setting.
3. Discuss the major components of the following developmental theories:
   a. Psychoanalytic theory—Freud
   b. Interpersonal theory—Sullivan

   c. Theory of psychosocial development—Erikson
   d. Theory of object relations development—Mahler
   e. Cognitive development theory—Piaget
   f. Theory of moral development—Kohlberg
   g. A nursing model of interpersonal development—Peplau

HOMEWORK ASSIGNMENT
Please read the chapter and answer the following questions:

1. Which part of the personality as described by Freud is developed as the child internalizes the values and morals set forth by primary caregivers?
2. According to Erikson, what happens when the adolescent does not master the tasks of *identity vs. role confusion*?
3. According to Mahler's theory, the individual with borderline personality disorder harbors fears of abandonment and underlying rage based on fixation in what stage of development?
4. When Joey sees an old woman struggling with a heavy bag of groceries, he runs to help her carry them to her car. This describes behavior at which stage of moral development?

The *Diagnostic and Statistical Manual of Mental Disorders, Fourth Edition, Text Revision (DSM-IV-TR)* (American Psychiatric Association [APA], 2000) defines personality *traits* as "enduring patterns of perceiving, relating to, and thinking about the environment and oneself that are exhibited in a wide range of social and personal contexts" (p. 686).

Nurses must have a basic knowledge of human personality development to understand maladaptive behavioral responses commonly seen in psychiatric clients. Developmental theories identify behaviors associated with various *stages* through which individuals pass, thereby specifying what is appropriate or inappropriate at each developmental level.

Specialists in child development believe that infancy and early childhood are the major life periods for the origination and occurrence of developmental change. Specialists in life-cycle development believe that people continue to develop and change throughout life, thereby suggesting the possibility for renewal and growth in adults.

Developmental stages are identified by age. Behaviors can then be evaluated by whether or not they are recognized as age-appropriate. Ideally, an individual successfully fulfills all the tasks associated with one stage before moving on to the next stage (at the appropriate age). Realistically, however, this seldom happens. One reason is related to **temperament,** or the inborn personality characteristics that influence an individual's manner of reacting to the environment, and ultimately his or her developmental progression (Chess & Thomas, 1986). The environment may also influence one's developmental pattern. Individuals who are reared in a dysfunctional family system often have retarded ego development. According to specialists in life-cycle development, behaviors from an unsuccessfully completed stage can be modified and corrected in a later stage.

Stages overlap, and an individual may be working on tasks associated with several stages at one time. When an individual becomes fixed in a lower level of development, with age-inappropriate behaviors focused on fulfillment of those tasks, psychopathology may become evident. Only when personality traits are inflexible and maladaptive and cause either significant functional impairment or subjective distress do they constitute "personality disorders" (APA, 2000). These disorders are discussed in Chapter 34.

CORE CONCEPT

Personality
The combination of character, behavioral, temperamental, emotional, and mental traits that are unique to each specific individual.

Psychoanalytic Theory

Sigmund Freud (1961), who has been called the father of psychiatry, is credited as the first to identify development by stages. He considered the first 5 years of a child's life to be the most important, because he believed that an individual's basic character had been formed by the age of 5.

Freud's personality theory can be conceptualized according to structure and dynamics of the personality, topography of the mind, and stages of personality development.

Structure of the Personality

Freud organized the structure of the personality into three major components: the **id, ego,** and **superego.** They are distinguished by their unique functions and different characteristics.

Id

The *id* is the locus of instinctual drives—the "pleasure principle." Present at birth, it endows the infant with instinctual drives that seek to satisfy needs and achieve immediate gratification. Id-driven behaviors are impulsive and may be irrational.

Ego

The *ego,* also called the *rational self* or the "reality principle," begins to develop between the ages of 4 and 6 months. The ego experiences the reality of the external world, adapts to it, and responds to it. As the ego develops and gains strength, it seeks to bring the influences of the external world to bear upon the id, to substitute the reality principle for the pleasure principle (Marmer, 2003). A primary function of the ego is one of mediator; that is, it maintains harmony among the external world, the id, and the superego.

Superego

If the id is identified as the pleasure principle, and the ego the reality principle, the *superego* might be referred to as the "perfection principle." The superego, which develops between ages 3 and 6 years, internalizes the values and morals set forth by primary caregivers. Derived out of a system of rewards and punishments, the superego is composed of two major components: the *ego-ideal* and the *conscience.* When a child is consistently rewarded for "good" behavior, the self-esteem is enhanced, and the behavior becomes part of the ego-ideal; that is, it is internalized as part of his or her value system. The conscience is formed when the child is punished consistently for "bad" behavior. The child learns what is considered morally right or wrong from feedback received from parental figures and from society or culture. When moral and ethical principles or even internalized ideals and values are disregarded, the conscience generates a feeling of guilt within the individual. The superego is important in the socialization of the individual because it assists the ego in the control of id impulses. When the superego becomes rigid and punitive, problems with low self-confidence and low self-esteem arise. Examples of behaviors associated with these components of the personality are presented in Box 3-1.

Topography of the Mind

Freud classified all mental contents and operations into three categories: the conscious, the preconscious, and the unconscious.

■ The *conscious* includes all memories that remain within an individual's awareness. It is the smallest of the three categories. Events and experiences that are easily remembered or retrieved are considered to be within one's conscious awareness. Examples include telephone numbers, birthdays of self and significant others, the dates of special holidays, and what one had for lunch today. The conscious mind is thought to be under the control of the ego, the rational and logical structure of the personality.

■ The *preconscious* includes all memories that may have been forgotten or are not in present awareness but with attention can be readily recalled into consciousness. Examples include telephone numbers or addresses once known but little used and feelings associated with significant life events that may have occurred at sometime in the past. The preconscious enhances awareness by helping to *suppress* unpleasant or nonessential memories from consciousness. It is thought to be partially under the control of the superego, which helps to suppress unacceptable thoughts and behaviors.

■ The *unconscious* includes all memories that one is unable to bring to conscious awareness.

It is the largest of the three topographical levels. Unconscious material consists of unpleasant or nonessential memories that have been *repressed* and can be retrieved only through therapy or hypnosis, and with certain substances that alter awareness and have the capacity to restructure repressed memories. Unconscious material may also emerge in dreams and in seemingly incomprehensible behavior.

Dynamics of the Personality

Freud believed that *psychic energy* is the force or impetus required for mental functioning. Originating in the id, it instinctually fulfills basic physiological needs. Freud called this psychic energy (or the drive to fulfill basic physiological needs such as hunger, thirst, and sex) the **libido.** As the child matures, psychic energy is diverted from the id to form the ego and then from the ego to form the superego. Psychic energy is distributed within these three components, with the ego retaining the largest share to maintain a balance between the impulsive behaviors of the id and the idealistic behaviors of the superego. If an excessive amount of psychic energy is stored in one of these personality components, behavior will reflect that part of the personality. For instance, impulsive behavior prevails when excessive psychic energy is stored in the id. Overinvestment in the ego reflects self-absorbed, or narcissistic, behaviors; an excess within the superego results in rigid, self-deprecating behaviors.

Freud used the terms *cathexis* and *anticathexis* to describe the forces within the id, ego, and superego that are used to invest psychic energy in external sources to satisfy needs. Cathexis is the process by which the id invests energy into an object in an attempt to achieve gratification. An

---

BOX 3-1 Structure of the Personality

BEHAVIORAL EXAMPLES

Id	*Ego*	*Superego*
"I found this wallet; I will keep the money."	"I already have money. This money doesn't belong to me. Maybe the person who owns this wallet doesn't have any money."	"It is never right to take something that doesn't belong to you."
"Mom and Dad are gone. Let's party!!!!!"	"Mom and Dad said no friends over while they are away. Too risky."	"Never disobey your parents."
"I'll have sex with whomever I please, whenever I please."	"Promiscuity can be very dangerous."	"Sex outside of marriage is always wrong."

example is the individual who instinctively turns to alcohol to relieve stress. Anticathexis is the use of psychic energy by the ego and the superego to control id impulses. In the example cited, the ego would attempt to control the use of alcohol with rational thinking, such as, "I already have ulcers from drinking too much. I will call my AA counselor for support. I will not drink." The superego would exert control with thinking such as "I shouldn't drink. If I drink, my family will be hurt and angry. I should think of how it affects them. I'm such a weak person." Freud believed that an imbalance between cathexis and anticathexis resulted in internal conflicts, producing tension and anxiety within the individual. Freud's daughter Anna devised a comprehensive list of defense mechanisms believed to be used by the ego as a protective device against anxiety in mediating between the excessive demands of the id and the excessive restrictions of the superego (see Chapter 2).

Freud's Stages of Personality Development

Freud described formation of the personality through five stages of *psychosexual* development. He placed much emphasis on the first 5 years of life and believed that characteristics developed during these early years bore heavily on one's adaptation patterns and personality traits in adulthood. Fixation in an early stage of development will almost certainly result in psychopathology. An outline of these five stages is presented in Table 3-1.

Oral Stage: Birth to 18 Months

During the oral stage, behavior is directed by the id, and the goal is immediate gratification of needs. The focus of energy is the mouth, with behaviors that include sucking, chewing, and biting. The infant feels a sense of attachment and is unable to differentiate the self from the person who is providing the mothering. This includes feelings such as anxiety. Because of this lack of differentiation, a pervasive feeling of anxiety on the part of the mother may be passed on to her infant, leaving the child vulnerable to similar feelings of insecurity. With the beginning of development of the ego at age 4 to 6 months, the infant starts to view the self as separate from the mothering figure. A sense of security and the ability to trust others is derived from the gratification of fulfilling basic needs during this stage.

Anal Stage: 18 Months to 3 Years

The major tasks in the anal stage are gaining independence and control, with particular focus on the excretory function. Freud believed that the manner in which the parents and other primary caregivers approach the task of toilet training may have far-reaching effects on the child in terms of values and personality characteristics. When toilet training is strict and rigid, the child may choose to retain the feces, becoming constipated. Adult retentive personality traits influenced by this type of training include stubbornness, stinginess, and miserliness. An alternate reaction to strict toilet training is for the child to expel feces in an unacceptable manner or at inappropriate times. Far-reaching effects of this behavior pattern include malevolence, cruelty to others, destructiveness, disorganization, and untidiness.

Toilet training that is more permissive and accepting attaches the feeling of importance and desirability to feces production. The child becomes extroverted, productive, and altruistic.

TABLE 3-1 Freud's Stages of Psychosexual Development		
AGE	**STAGE**	**MAJOR DEVELOPMENTAL TASKS**
Birth–18 months	Oral	Relief from anxiety through oral gratification of needs
18 months–3 years	Anal	Learning independence and control, with focus on the excretory function
3–6 years	Phallic	Identification with parent of same gender; development of sexual identity; focus on genital organs
6–12 years	Latency	Sexuality repressed; focus on relationships with same-gender peers
13–20 years	Genital	Libido reawakened as genital organs mature; focus on relationships with members of the opposite gender

Phallic Stage: 3 to 6 Years

In the phallic stage, the focus of energy shifts to the genital area. Discovery of differences between genders results in a heightened interest in the sexuality of self and others. This interest may be manifested in sexual self-exploratory or group-exploratory play. Freud proposed that the development of the *Oedipus complex* (males) or *Electra complex* (females) occurred during this stage of development. He described this as the child's unconscious desire to eliminate the parent of the same gender and to possess the parent of the opposite gender for him- or herself. Guilt feelings result with the emergence of the superego during these years. Resolution of this internal conflict occurs when the child develops a strong identification with the parent of the same gender, and that parent's attitudes, beliefs, and value systems are subsumed by the child.

Latency Stage: 6 to 12 Years

During the elementary school years, the focus changes from egocentrism to more interest in group activities, learning, and socialization with peers. Sexuality is not absent during this period but remains obscure and imperceptible to others. The preference is for same-gender relationships, even rejecting members of the opposite gender.

Genital Stage: 13 to 20 Years

In the genital stage, the maturing of the genital organs results in a reawakening of the libidinal drive. The focus is on relationships with members of the opposite gender and preparations for selecting a mate. The development of sexual maturity evolves from self-gratification to behaviors deemed acceptable by societal norms. Interpersonal relationships are based on genuine pleasure derived from the interaction rather than from the more self-serving implications of childhood associations.

Relevance of Psychoanalytic Theory to Nursing Practice

Knowledge of the structure of the personality can assist nurses who work in the mental health setting. The ability to recognize behaviors associated with the id, the ego, and the superego assists in the assessment of developmental level. Understanding the use of ego defense mechanisms is important in making determinations about maladaptive behaviors, in planning care for clients to assist in creating change (if desired), or in helping clients accept themselves as unique individuals.

CLINICAL PEARL: Assessing Patient Behaviors

ID BEHAVIORS

Those behaviors that follow the principle of "if it feels good, do it." Social and cultural acceptability are not considered. It reflects a need for immediate gratification. Individuals with a strong id show little if any remorse for their unacceptable behavior.

EGO BEHAVIORS

Behaviors that reflect the rational part of the personality. An effort is made to delay gratification and to satisfy societal expectations. The ego uses defense mechanisms to cope and regain control over id impulses.

SUPEREGO BEHAVIORS

Behaviors that are somewhat uncompromising and rigid. Based on morality and society's values, behaviors of the superego strive for perfection. Violation of the superego's standards generates guilt and anxiety in an individual who has a strong superego.

Interpersonal Theory

Harry Stack Sullivan (1953) believed that individual behavior and personality development are the direct result of interpersonal relationships. Before the development of his own theoretical framework, Sullivan embraced the concepts of Freud. Later, he changed the focus of his work from the *intrapersonal* view of Freud to one with more *interpersonal* flavor in which human behavior could be observed in social interactions with others. His ideas, which were not universally accepted at the time, have been integrated into the practice of psychiatry through publication only since his death in 1949. Sullivan's major concepts include the following:

■ *Anxiety* is a feeling of emotional discomfort, toward the relief or prevention of which all behavior is aimed. Sullivan believed that anxiety is the "chief disruptive force in interpersonal relations and the main factor in the development of serious difficulties in living." It arises out of one's inability to satisfy needs or to achieve interpersonal security.

■ *Satisfaction of needs* is the fulfillment of all requirements associated with an individual's physiochemical environment. Sullivan identified examples of these requirements as oxygen, food, water, warmth, tenderness, rest, activity, sexual expression—virtually anything that, when absent, produces discomfort in the individual.

■ *Interpersonal security* is the feeling associated with relief from anxiety. When all needs have been met, one experiences a sense of total well-being, which Sullivan termed *interpersonal security.* He believed individuals have an innate need for interpersonal security.

■ *Self-system* is a collection of experiences, or security measures, adopted by the individual to protect against anxiety. Sullivan identified three components of the self-system, which are based on interpersonal experiences early in life:

• The "*good me*" is the part of the personality that develops in response to positive feedback from the primary caregiver. Feelings of pleasure, contentment, and gratification are experienced. The child learns which behaviors elicit this positive response as it becomes incorporated into the self-system.

• The "*bad me*" is the part of the personality that develops in response to negative feedback from the primary caregiver. Anxiety is experienced, eliciting feelings of discomfort, displeasure, and distress. The child learns to avoid these negative feelings by altering certain behaviors.

• The "*not me*" is the part of the personality that develops in response to situations that produce intense anxiety in the child. Feelings of horror, awe, dread, and loathing are experienced in response to these situations, leading the child to deny these feelings in an effort to relieve anxiety. These feelings, having then been denied, become "not me," but someone else. This withdrawal from emotions has serious implications for mental disorders in adult life.

Sullivan's Stages of Personality Development

Infancy: Birth to 18 Months

During the beginning stage, the major developmental task for the child is the gratification of needs. This is accomplished through activity associated with the mouth, such as crying, nursing, and thumb sucking.

Childhood: 18 Months to 6 Years

At ages 18 months to 6 years, the child learns that interference with fulfillment of personal wishes and desires may result in delayed gratification. He or she learns to accept this and feel comfortable with it, recognizing that delayed gratification often results in parental approval, a more lasting type of reward. Tools of this stage include the mouth, the anus, language, experimentation, manipulation, and identification.

Juvenile: 6 to 9 Years

The major task of the juvenile stage is formation of satisfactory relationships within peer groups. This is accomplished through the use of competition, cooperation, and compromise.

Preadolescence: 9 to 12 Years

The tasks at the preadolescence stage focus on developing relationships with persons of the same gender. One's ability to collaborate with and show love and affection for another person begins at this stage.

Early Adolescence: 12 to 14 Years

During early adolescence, the child is struggling with developing a sense of identity that is separate and independent from the parents. The major task is formation of satisfactory relationships with members of the opposite gender. Sullivan saw the emergence of lust in response to biological changes as a major force occurring during this period.

Late Adolescence: 14 to 21 Years

The late adolescent period is characterized by tasks associated with the attempt to achieve interdependence within the society and the formation of a lasting, intimate relationship with a selected member of the opposite gender. The genital organs are the major developmental focus of this stage.

An outline of the stages of personality development according to Sullivan's interpersonal theory is presented in Table 3-2.

Relevance of Interpersonal Theory to Nursing Practice

The interpersonal theory has significant relevance to nursing practice. Relationship development, which is a major concept of this theory, is a major psychiatric nursing intervention. Nurses develop therapeutic relationships with clients in an effort to help them generalize this ability to interact successfully with others.

Knowledge about the behaviors associated with all levels of anxiety and methods for alleviating anxiety helps nurses to assist clients in achieving interpersonal security and a sense of well-being. Nurses use the concepts of Sullivan's theory to help clients achieve a higher degree of independent and interpersonal functioning.

Theory of Psychosocial Development

Erik Erikson (1963) studied the influence of social processes on the development of the personality.

TABLE 3-2 Stages of Development in Sullivan's Interpersonal Theory

AGE	STAGE	MAJOR DEVELOPMENTAL TASKS
Birth–18 months	Infancy	Relief from anxiety through oral gratification of needs
18 months–6 years	Childhood	Learning to experience a delay in personal gratification without undue anxiety
6–9 years	Juvenile	Learning to form satisfactory peer relationships
9–12 years	Preadolescence	Learning to form satisfactory relationships with persons of the same gender; initiating feelings of affection for another person
12–14 years	Early adolescence	Learning to form satisfactory relationships with persons of the opposite gender; developing a sense of identity
14–21 years	Late adolescence	Establishing self-identity; experiencing satisfying relationships; working to develop a lasting, intimate opposite-gender relationship

He described eight stages of the life cycle during which individuals struggle with developmental "crises." Specific tasks associated with each stage must be completed for resolution of the crisis and for emotional growth to occur. An outline of Erikson's stages of psychosocial development is presented in Table 3-3.

Erikson's Stages of Personality Development

Trust Versus Mistrust: Birth to 18 Months

Major Developmental Task From birth to 18 months, the major task is to develop a basic trust in the mothering figure and learn to generalize it to others.

■ Achievement of the task results in self-confidence, optimism, faith in the gratification of needs and desires, and hope for the future. The infant learns to trust when basic needs are met consistently.

■ Nonachievement results in emotional dissatisfaction with the self and others, suspiciousness, and difficulty with interpersonal relationships. The task remains unresolved when primary caregivers fail to respond to the infant's distress signal promptly and consistently.

Autonomy Versus Shame and Doubt: 18 Months to 3 Years

Major Developmental Task The major task during the ages of 18 months to 3 years is to gain some self-control and independence within the environment.

■ Achievement of the task results in a sense of self-control and the ability to delay gratification, and a feeling of self-confidence in one's ability to perform. Autonomy is achieved when parents encourage and provide opportunities for independent activities.

■ Nonachievement results in a lack of self-confidence, a lack of pride in the ability to perform, a sense of being controlled by others, and a rage against the self. The task remains unresolved when primary caregivers restrict independent behaviors, both physically and verbally, or set the child up for failure with unrealistic expectations.

Initiative Versus Guilt: 3 to 6 Years

Major Developmental Task During the ages of 3 to 6 years, the goal is to develop a sense of purpose and the ability to initiate and direct one's own activities.

■ Achievement of the task results in the ability to exercise restraint and self-control of inappropriate social behaviors. Assertiveness and dependability increase, and the child enjoys learning and personal achievement. The conscience develops, thereby controlling the impulsive behaviors of the id. Initiative is achieved when creativity is encouraged and performance is recognized and positively reinforced.

■ Nonachievement results in feelings of inadequacy and a sense of defeat. Guilt is experienced to an excessive degree, even to the point of accepting liability in situations for which one is not responsible. The child may view him- or herself as evil and deserving of punishment. The task remains unresolved when creativity is stifled and parents continually expect a higher level of achievement than the child produces.

TABLE 3-3 Stages of Development in Erikson's Psychosocial Theory		
AGE	**STAGE**	**MAJOR DEVELOPMENTAL TASKS**
Infancy (Birth–18 months)	Trust vs. mistrust	To develop a basic trust in the mothering figure and learn to generalize it to others
Early childhood (18 months–3 years)	Autonomy vs. shame and doubt	To gain some self-control and independence within the environment
Late childhood (3–6 years)	Initiative vs. guilt	To develop a sense of purpose and the ability to initiate and direct own activities
School age (6–12 years)	Industry vs. inferiority	To achieve a sense of self-confidence by learning, competing, performing successfully, and receiving recognition from significant others, peers, and acquaintances
Adolescence (12–20 years)	Identity vs. role confusion	To integrate the tasks mastered in the previous stages into a secure sense of self
Young adulthood (20–30 years)	Intimacy vs. isolation	To form an intense, lasting relationship or a commitment to another person, cause, institution, or creative effort
Adulthood (30–65 years)	Generativity vs. stagnation	To achieve the life goals established for oneself, while also considering the welfare of future generations
Old age (65 years–death)	Ego integrity vs. despair	To review one's life and derive meaning from both positive and negative events, while achieving a positive sense of self-worth

Industry Versus Inferiority: 6 to 12 Years

Major Developmental Task The major task for 6- to 12-year-olds is to achieve a sense of self-confidence by learning, competing, performing successfully, and receiving recognition from significant others, peers, and acquaintances.

■ Achievement of the task results in a sense of satisfaction and pleasure in the interaction and involvement with others. The individual masters reliable work habits and develops attitudes of trustworthiness. He or she is conscientious, feels pride in achievement, and enjoys play but desires a balance between fantasy and "real-world" activities. Industry is achieved when encouragement is given to activities and responsibilities in the school and community, as well as those within the home, and recognition is given for accomplishments.

■ Nonachievement results in difficulty in interpersonal relationships because of feelings of personal inadequacy. The individual can neither cooperate and compromise with others in group activities nor problem-solve or complete tasks successfully. He or she may become either passive and meek or overly aggressive to cover up for feelings of inadequacy. If this occurs, the individual may manipulate or violate the rights of others to satisfy his or her

own needs or desires; he or she may become a workaholic with unrealistic expectations for personal achievement. This task remains unresolved when parents set unrealistic expectations for the child, when discipline is harsh and tends to impair self-esteem, and when accomplishments are consistently met with negative feedback.

Identity Versus Role Confusion: 12 to 20 Years

Major Developmental Task At 12 to 20 years, the goal is to integrate the tasks mastered in the previous stages into a secure sense of self.

■ Achievement of the task results in a sense of confidence, emotional stability, and a view of the self as a unique individual. Commitments are made to a value system, to the choice of a career, and to relationships with members of both genders. Identity is achieved when adolescents are allowed to experience independence by making decisions that influence their lives. Parents should be available to offer support when needed but should gradually relinquish control to the maturing individual in an effort to encourage the development of an independent sense of self.

■ Nonachievement results in a sense of self-consciousness, doubt, and confusion about one's role in life. Personal values or goals for one's life are absent. Long-term commitments to relationships with others are non-existent. A lack of self-confidence is often expressed by delinquent and rebellious behavior. Entering adulthood, with its accompanying responsibilities, may be an underlying fear. This task can remain unresolved for many reasons. Examples include the following:

• When independence is discouraged by the parents, and the adolescent is nurtured in the dependent family position
• When discipline within the home has been overly harsh, inconsistent, or absent
• When there has been parental rejection or frequent shifting of parental figures

Intimacy Versus Isolation: 20 to 30 Years

Major Developmental Task   The objective for 20- to 30-year-olds is to form an intense, lasting relationship or a commitment to another person, a cause, an institution, or a creative effort (Murray, Zentner, & Yakimo, 2008).

■ Achievement of the task results in the capacity for mutual love and respect between two people and the ability of an individual to pledge a total commitment to another. The intimacy goes far beyond the sexual contact between two people. It describes a commitment in which personal sacrifices are made for another, whether it be another person or, if one chooses, a career or other type of cause or endeavor to which an individual elects to devote his or her life. Intimacy is achieved when an individual has developed the capacity for giving of oneself to another. This is learned when one has been the recipient of this type of giving within the family unit.

■ Nonachievement results in withdrawal, social isolation, and aloneness. The individual is unable to form lasting, intimate relationships, often seeking intimacy through numerous superficial sexual contacts. No career is established; he or she may have a history of occupational changes (or may fear change and thus remain in an undesirable job situation). The task remains unresolved when love in the home has been deprived or distorted through the younger years (Murray et al., 2008). One fails to achieve the ability to give of the self without having been the recipient of such giving early on from primary caregivers.

Generativity Versus Stagnation or Self-Absorption: 30 to 65 Years

Major Developmental Task   The major task at this stage is to achieve the life goals established for oneself while also considering the welfare of future generations.

■ Achievement of the task results in a sense of gratification from personal and professional achievements, and from meaningful contributions to others. The individual is active in the service of and to society. Generativity is achieved when the individual expresses satisfaction with this stage in life and demonstrates responsibility for leaving the world a better place in which to live.

■ Nonachievement results in lack of concern for the welfare of others and total preoccupation with the self. He or she becomes withdrawn, isolated, and highly self-indulgent, with no capacity for giving of the self to others. The task remains unresolved when earlier developmental tasks are not fulfilled and the individual does not achieve the degree of maturity required to derive gratification out of a personal concern for the welfare of others.

Ego Integrity Versus Despair: 65 Years to Death

Major Developmental Task   Between the age of 65 years and death, the goal is to review one's life and derive meaning from both positive and negative events, while achieving a positive sense of self.

■ Achievement of the task results in a sense of self-worth and self-acceptance as one reviews life goals, accepting that some were achieved and some were not. The individual derives a sense of dignity from his or her life experiences and does not fear death, viewing it instead as another phase of development. Ego integrity is achieved when individuals have successfully completed the developmental tasks of the other stages and have little desire to make major changes in how their lives have progressed.

■ Nonachievement results in a sense of self-contempt and disgust with how life has progressed. The individual would like to start over and have a second chance at life. He or she feels worthless and helpless to change. Anger, depression, and loneliness are evident. The focus may be on past failures or perceived failures. Impending death is feared or denied, or ideas of suicide may prevail. The task remains unresolved when earlier tasks are not fulfilled: self-confidence, a concern for others, and a strong sense of self-identity were never achieved.

Relevance of Psychosocial Development Theory to Nursing Practice

Erikson's theory is particularly relevant to nursing practice in that it incorporates sociocultural concepts into the development of personality. Erikson provides a systematic, stepwise approach and outlines specific tasks that should be completed during each stage. This information can be used quite readily in psychiatric/mental health nursing. Many individuals with mental health problems are still struggling to achieve tasks from a number of developmental stages. Nurses can plan care to assist these individuals to fulfill these tasks and move on to a higher developmental level.

> **CLINICAL PEARL:** During assessment, nurses can determine if a client is experiencing difficulties associated with specific life tasks as described by Erikson. Knowledge about a client's developmental level, along with other assessment data, can help to identify accurate nursing interventions.

Theory of Object Relations

Margaret Mahler (Mahler, Pine, & Bergman, 1975) formulated a theory that describes the separation-individuation process of the infant from the maternal figure (primary caregiver). She described this process as progressing through three major phases. She further delineated phase III, the separation-individuation phase, into four subphases. Mahler's developmental theory is outlined in Table 3-4.

Phase I: The Autistic Phase (Birth to 1 Month)

In the autistic phase, also called *normal autism*, the infant exists in a half-sleeping, half-waking state and does not perceive the existence of other people or an external environment. The fulfillment of basic needs for survival and comfort is the focus and is merely accepted as it occurs.

Phase II: The Symbiotic Phase (1 to 5 Months)

Symbiosis is a type of "psychic fusion" of mother and child. The child views the self as an extension of the mother, but with a developing awareness that it is she who fulfills his or her every need. Mahler suggested that absence of, or rejection by, the maternal figure at this phase can lead to symbiotic psychosis.

Phase III: Separation-Individuation (5 to 36 Months)

This third phase represents what Mahler called the "psychological birth" of the child. *Separation* is defined as the physical and psychological attainment

TABLE 3-4 Stages of Development in Mahler's Theory of Object Relations		
AGE	**PHASE/SUBPHASE**	**MAJOR DEVELOPMENTAL TASKS**
Birth–1 month	I. Normal autism	Fulfillment of basic needs for survival and comfort
1–5 months	II. Symbiosis	Development of awareness of external source of need fulfillment
	III. Separation-Individuation	
5–10 months	a. Differentiation	Commencement of a primary recognition of separateness from the mothering figure
10–16 months	b. Practicing	Increased independence through locomotor functioning; increased sense of separateness of self
16–24 months	c. Rapprochement	Acute awareness of separateness of self; learning to seek "emotional refueling" from mothering figure to maintain feeling of security
24–36 months	d. Consolidation	Sense of separateness established; on the way to object constancy (i.e., able to internalize a sustained image of loved object/person when it is out of sight); resolution of separation anxiety

of a sense of personal distinction from the mothering figure. *Individuation* occurs with a strengthening of the ego and an acceptance of a sense of "self," with independent ego boundaries. Four subphases through which the child evolves in his or her progression from a symbiotic extension of the mothering figure to a distinct and separate being are described.

Subphase 1: Differentiation (5 to 10 Months)

The differentiation phase begins with the child's initial physical movements away from the mothering figure. A primary recognition of separateness commences.

Subphase 2: Practicing (10 to 16 Months)

With advanced locomotor functioning, the child experiences feelings of exhilaration from increased independence. He or she is now able to move away from, and return to, the mothering figure. A sense of omnipotence is manifested.

Subphase 3: Rapprochement (16 to 24 Months)

This third subphase, rapprochement, is extremely critical to the child's healthy ego development. During this time, the child becomes increasingly aware of his or her separateness from the mothering figure, while the sense of fearlessness and omnipotence diminishes. The child, now recognizing the mother as a separate individual, wishes to reestablish closeness with her but shuns the total re-engulfment of the symbiotic stage. The need is for the mothering figure to be available to provide "emotional refueling" on demand.

Critical to this subphase is the mothering figure's response to the child. If she is available to fulfill emotional needs as they arise, the child develops a sense of security in the knowledge that he or she is loved and will not be abandoned. However, if emotional needs are inconsistently met or if the mother rewards clinging, dependent behaviors and withholds nurturing when the child demonstrates independence, feelings of rage and a fear of abandonment develop and often persist into adulthood.

Subphase 4: Consolidation (24 to 36 Months)

With achievement of the consolidation subphase, a definite individuality and sense of separateness of self are established. Objects are represented as whole, with the child having the ability to integrate both "good" and "bad." A degree of object constancy is established as the child is able to internalize a sustained image of the mothering figure as enduring and loving, while maintaining the perception of her as a separate person in the outside world.

Relevance of Object Relations Theory to Nursing Practice

Understanding of the concepts of Mahler's theory of object relations assists the nurse to assess the client's level of individuation from primary caregivers. The emotional problems of many individuals can be traced to lack of fulfillment of the tasks of separation/individuation. Examples include problems related to dependency and excessive anxiety. The individual with borderline personality disorder is thought to be fixed in the rapprochement phase of development, harboring fears of abandonment and underlying rage. This knowledge is important in the provision of nursing care to these individuals.

Cognitive Development Theory

Jean Piaget (Piaget & Inhelder, 1969) has been called the father of child psychology. His work concerning **cognitive development** in children is based on the premise that human intelligence is an extension of biological adaptation, or one's ability to adapt psychologically to the environment. He believed that human intelligence progresses through a series of stages that are related to age, demonstrating at each successive stage a higher level of logical organization than at the previous stages.

From his extensive studies of cognitive development in children, Piaget discovered four major stages, each of which he believed to be a necessary prerequisite for the one that follows. An outline is presented in Table 3-5.

Stage 1: Sensorimotor (Birth to 2 Years)

At the beginning of his or her life, the child is concerned only with satisfying basic needs and comforts. The self is not differentiated from the external environment. As the sense of differentiation occurs, with increasing mobility and awareness, the mental system is expanded. The child develops a greater understanding regarding objects within the external environment and their effects upon him or her. Knowledge is gained regarding the ability to manipulate objects and experiences within the environment. The sense of *object permanence*—the notion that an object will continue to exist when it is no longer present to the senses—is initiated.

Stage 2: Preoperational (2 to 6 Years)

Piaget believed that preoperational thought is characterized by egocentrism. Personal experiences are thought to be universal, and the child is unable to

TABLE 3-5 Piaget's Stages of Cognitive Development		
AGE	**STAGE**	**MAJOR DEVELOPMENTAL TASKS**
Birth–2 years	Sensorimotor	With increased mobility and awareness, development of a sense of self as separate from the external environment; the concept of object permanence emerges as the ability to form mental images evolves
2–6 years	Preoperational	Learning to express self with language; development of understanding of symbolic gestures; achievement of object permanence
6–12 years	Concrete operations	Learning to apply logic to thinking; development of understanding of reversibility and spatiality; learning to differentiate and classify; increased socialization and application of rules
12–15+ years	Formal operations	Learning to think and reason in abstract terms; making and testing hypotheses; capability of logical thinking and reasoning expand and are refined; cognitive maturity achieved

accept the differing viewpoints of others. Language development progresses, as does the ability to attribute special meaning to symbolic gestures (e.g., bringing a story book to mother is a symbolic invitation to have a story read). Reality is often given to inanimate objects. Object permanence culminates in the ability to conjure up mental representations of objects or people.

Stage 3: Concrete Operations (6 to 12 Years)

The ability to apply logic to thinking begins in this stage; however, "concreteness" still predominates. An understanding of the concepts of reversibility and spatiality is developed. For example, the child recognizes that changing the shape of objects does not necessarily change the amount, weight, or volume, or the ability of the object to return to its original form. Another achievement of this stage is the ability to classify objects by any of their several characteristics. For example, he or she can classify all poodles as dogs but recognizes that all dogs are not poodles.

The concept of a lawful self is developed at this stage as the child becomes more socialized and rule conscious. Egocentrism decreases, the ability to cooperate in interactions with other children increases, and understanding and acceptance of established rules grow.

Stage 4: Formal Operations (12 to 15+ Years)

At this stage, the individual is able to think and reason in abstract terms. He or she can make and test hypotheses using logical and orderly problem solving. Current situations and reflections of the future are idealized, and a degree of egocentrism returns during this stage. There may be some diffi-

culty reconciling idealistic hopes with more rational prospects. Formal operations, however, enable individuals to distinguish between the ideal and the real. Piaget's theory suggests that most individuals achieve **cognitive maturity**, the capability to perform all mental operations needed for adulthood, in middle to late adolescence.

Relevance of Cognitive Development Theory to Nursing Practice

Nurses who work in psychiatry are likely to be involved in helping clients, particularly depressed clients, with techniques of cognitive therapy. In cognitive therapy, the individual is taught to control thought distortions that are considered to be a factor in the development and maintenance of mood disorders. In the cognitive model, depression is characterized by a triad of negative distortions related to expectations of the environment, self, and future. In this model, depression is viewed as a distortion in cognitive development, the self is unrealistically devalued, and the future is perceived as hopeless. Therapy focuses on changing "automatic thoughts" that occur spontaneously and contribute to the distorted affect. Nurses who assist with this type of therapy must have knowledge of how cognition develops in order to help clients identify the distorted thought patterns and make the changes required for improvement in affective functioning (see Chapter 20).

Theory of Moral Development

Lawrence Kohlberg's (1968) stages of moral development are not closely tied to specific age groups. Research was conducted with males ranging in age from 10 to 28 years. Kohlberg believed that each stage is necessary and basic to the next stage and that all individuals must progress through each stage sequentially. He defined three major levels of moral development, each of which is further subdivided into two stages each. An outline of Kohlberg's developmental stages is presented in Table 3-6. Most people do not progress through all six stages.

Level I: Preconventional Level (Prominent From Ages 4 to 10 Years)

Stage 1: Punishment and Obedience Orientation

At the punishment and obedience orientation stage, the individual is responsive to cultural guidelines of good or bad and right or wrong, but primarily in terms of the known related consequences. Fear of punishment is likely to be the incentive for conformity (e.g., "I'll do it, because if I don't I can't watch TV for a week.")

Stage 2: Instrumental Relativist Orientation

Behaviors at the instrumental relativist orientation stage are guided by egocentrism and concern for self. There is an intense desire to satisfy one's own needs, but occasionally the needs of others are considered. For the most part, decisions are based on personal benefits derived (e.g., "I'll do it if I get something in return," or occasionally, ". . . because you asked me to").

Level II: Conventional Level (Prominent From Ages 10 to 13 Years and Into Adulthood)*

Stage 3: Interpersonal Concordance Orientation

Behavior at the interpersonal concordance orientation stage is guided by the expectations of others. Approval and acceptance within one's societal group provide the incentive to conform (e.g., "I'll do it because you asked me to," ". . . because it will help you," or ". . . because it will please you").

Stage 4: Law and Order Orientation

In the law and order orientation stage, there is a personal respect for authority. Rules and laws are required and override personal principles and group mores. The belief is that all individuals and groups are subject to the same code of order, and no one shall be exempt (e.g., "I'll do it because it is the law").

Level III: Postconventional Level (Can Occur From Adolescence Onward)

Stage 5: Social Contract Legalistic Orientation

Individuals who reach stage 5 have developed a system of values and principles that determine for

---

*Eighty percent of adults are fixed in level II, with a majority of women in stage 3 and a majority of men in stage 4.

TABLE 3-6 Kohlberg's Stages of Moral Development		
LEVEL/AGE*	**STAGE**	**DEVELOPMENTAL FOCUS**
I. Preconventional (common from ages 4–10 years)	1. Punishment and obedience orientation	Behavior motivated by fear of punishment
	2. Instrumental relativist orientation	Behavior motivated by egocentrism and concern for self
II. Conventional (common from ages 10–13 years, and into adulthood)	3. Interpersonal concordance orientation	Behavior motivated by expectations of others; strong desire for approval and acceptance
	4. Law and order orientation	Behavior motivated by respect for authority
III. Postconventional (can occur from adolescence on)	5. Social contract legalistic orientation	Behavior motivated by respect for universal laws and moral principles; guided by internal set of values
	6. Universal ethical principle orientation	Behavior motivated by internalized principles of honor, justice, and respect for human dignity; guided by the conscience

*Ages in Kohlberg's theory are not well defined. The stage of development is determined by the motivation behind the individual's behavior.

them what is right or wrong; behaviors are acceptably guided by this value system, provided they do not violate the human rights of others. They believe that all individuals are entitled to certain inherent human rights, and they live according to universal laws and principles. However, they hold the idea that the laws are subject to scrutiny and change as needs within society evolve and change (e.g., "I'll do it because it is the moral and legal thing to do, even though it is not my personal choice").

Stage 6: Universal Ethical Principle Orientation

Behavior at stage 6 is directed by internalized principles of honor, justice, and respect for human dignity. Laws are abstract and unwritten, such as the "Golden Rule," "equality of human rights," and "justice for all." They are not the concrete rules established by society. The conscience is the guide, and when one fails to meet the self-expected behaviors, the personal consequence is intense guilt. The allegiance to these ethical principles is so strong that the individual will stand by them even knowing that negative consequences will result (e.g., "I'll do it because I believe it is the right thing to do, even though it is illegal and I will be imprisoned for doing it").

Relevance of Moral Development Theory to Nursing Practice

Moral development has relevance to psychiatric nursing in that it affects critical thinking about how individuals ought to behave and treat others. Moral behavior reflects the way a person interprets basic respect for other persons, such as the respect for human life, freedom, justice, or confidentiality. Psychiatric nurses must be able to assess the level of moral development of their clients in order to be able to help them in their effort to advance in their progression toward a higher level of developmental maturity.

A Nursing Model—Hildegard E. Peplau

Peplau (1991) applied interpersonal theory to nursing practice and, most specifically, to nurse-client relationship development. She provided a framework for "psychodynamic nursing," the interpersonal involvement of the nurse with a client in a given nursing situation. Peplau stated, "Nursing is helpful when both the patient and the nurse grow as a result of the learning that occurs in the nursing situation." (p. ix)

Peplau correlated the stages of personality development in childhood to stages through which clients advance during the progression of an illness. She also viewed these interpersonal experiences as learning situations for nurses to facilitate forward movement in the development of personality. She believed that, when there is fulfillment of psychological tasks associated with the nurse-client relationship, the personalities of both can be strengthened. Key concepts include the following:

■ *Nursing* is a human relationship between an individual who is sick, or in need of health services, and a nurse especially educated to recognize and to respond to the need for help.

■ **Psychodynamic nursing** is being able to understand one's own behavior, to help others identify felt difficulties, and to apply principles of human relations to the problems that arise at all levels of experience.

■ *Roles* are sets of values and behaviors that are specific to functional positions within social structures. Peplau identified the following *nursing roles:*

• A *resource person* provides specific, needed information that helps the client understand his or her problem and the new situation.

• A **counselor** listens as the client reviews feelings related to difficulties he or she is experiencing in any aspect of life. "Interpersonal techniques" have been identified to facilitate the nurse's interaction in the process of helping the client solve problems and make decisions concerning these difficulties.

• A *teacher* identifies learning needs and provides information to the client or family that may aid in improvement of the life situation.

• A *leader* directs the nurse-client interaction and ensures that appropriate actions are undertaken to facilitate achievement of the designated goals.

• A **technical expert** understands various professional devices and possesses the clinical skills necessary to perform the interventions that are in the best interest of the client.

• A **surrogate** serves as a substitute figure for another.

Phases of the nurse-client relationship are stages of overlapping roles or functions in relation to health problems, during which the nurse and client learn to work cooperatively to resolve difficulties. Peplau identified four phases:

■ *Orientation* is the phase during which the client, nurse, and family work together to recognize, clarify, and define the existing problem.

■ *Identification* is the phase after which the client's initial impression has been clarified and when he or she begins to respond selectively to those who seem to offer the help that is needed. Clients may respond in one of three ways: (1) on the basis of participation or interdependent relations with the nurse; (2) on the basis of independence or isolation from the nurse; or (3) on the basis of helplessness or dependence on the nurse (Peplau, 1991).

■ *Exploitation* is the phase during which the client proceeds to take full advantage of the services offered to him or her. Having learned which services are available, feeling comfortable within the setting, and serving as an active participant in his or her own health care, the client exploits the services available and explores all possibilities of the changing situation.

■ *Resolution* occurs when the client is freed from identification with helping persons and gathers strength to assume independence. Resolution is the direct result of successful completion of the other three phases.

Peplau's Stages of Personality Development

Psychological tasks are developmental lessons that must be learned on the way to achieving maturity of the personality. Peplau identified four psychological tasks that she associated with the stages of infancy and childhood described by Freud and Sullivan. She stated:

When psychological tasks are successfully learned at each era of development, biological capacities are used productively and relations with people lead to productive living. When they are not successfully learned they carry over into adulthood and attempts at learning continue in devious ways, more or less impeded by conventional adaptations that provide a superstructure over the baseline of actual learning. (Peplau, 1991, p. 166)

In the context of nursing, Peplau (1991) related these four psychological tasks to the demands made on nurses in their relations with clients. She maintained the following:

Nursing can function as a maturing force in society. Since illness is an event that is experienced along with feelings that derive from older experiences but are reenacted in the relationship of nurse to patient, the nurse-patient relationship is seen as an opportunity for nurses to help patients to complete the unfinished psychological tasks of childhood in some degree. (p. 159)

Peplau's psychological tasks of personality development include the four stages outlined in the following paragraphs. An outline of the stages of personality development according to Peplau's theory is presented in Table 3-7.

Learning to Count on Others

Nurses and clients first come together as strangers. Both bring to the relationship certain "raw materials," such as inherited biological components, personality characteristics (*temperament*), individual intellectual capacity, and specific cultural or environmental influences. Peplau related these to the same "raw materials" with which an infant comes into this world. The newborn is capable of experiencing *comfort* and *discomfort*. He or she soon learns to communicate feelings in a way that results in the fulfillment of comfort needs by the mothering figure who provides love and care

TABLE 3-7 Stages of Development in Peplau's Interpersonal Theory		
AGE	STAGE	MAJOR DEVELOPMENTAL TASKS
Infancy	Learning to count on others	Learning to communicate in various ways with the primary caregiver in order to have comfort needs fulfilled
Toddlerhood	Learning to delay satisfaction	Learning the satisfaction of pleasing others by delaying self-gratification in small ways
Early childhood	Identifying oneself	Learning appropriate roles and behaviors by acquiring the ability to perceive the expectations of others
Late childhood	Developing skills in participation	Learning the skills of compromise, competition, and cooperation with others; establishment of a more realistic view of the world and a feeling of one's place in it

unconditionally. However, fulfillment of these dependency needs is inhibited when goals of the mothering figure become the focus, and love and care are contingent on meeting the needs of the caregiver rather than the infant.

Clients with unmet dependency needs regress during illness and demonstrate behaviors that relate to this stage of development. Other clients regress to this level because of physical disabilities associated with their illness. Peplau believed that, when nurses provide unconditional care, they help these clients progress toward more mature levels of functioning. This may involve the role of "surrogate mother," in which the nurse fulfills needs for the client with the intent of helping him or her grow, mature, and become more independent.

Learning to Delay Satisfaction

Peplau related this stage to that of toddlerhood, or the first step in the development of interdependent social relations. Psychosexually, it is compared to the anal stage of development, when a child learns that, because of cultural mores, he or she cannot empty the bowels for relief of discomfort at will, but must delay to use the toilet, which is considered more culturally acceptable. When toilet training occurs too early or is very rigid, or when appropriate behavior is set forth as a condition for love and caring, tasks associated with this stage remain unfulfilled. The child feels powerless and fails to learn the satisfaction of pleasing others by delaying self-gratification in small ways. He or she may also exhibit rebellious behavior by failing to comply with demands of the mothering figure in an effort to counter the feelings of powerlessness. The child may accomplish this by withholding the fecal product or failing to deposit it in the culturally acceptable manner.

Peplau cited Fromm (1949) in describing the following potential behaviors of individuals who have failed to complete the tasks of the second stage of development:

- Exploitation and manipulation of others to satisfy their own desires because they are unable to do so independently

- Suspiciousness and envy of others, directing hostility toward others in an effort to enhance their own self-image

- Hoarding and withholding possessions from others; miserliness

- Inordinate neatness and punctuality

- Inability to relate to others through sharing of feelings, ideas, or experiences

- Ability to vary the personality characteristics to those required to satisfy personal desires at any given time

When nurses observe these types of behaviors in clients, it is important to encourage full expression and to convey unconditional acceptance. When the client learns to feel safe and unconditionally accepted, he or she is more likely to let go of the oppositional behavior and advance in the developmental progression. Peplau (1991) stated:

> Nurses who aid patients to feel safe and secure, so that wants can be expressed and satisfaction eventually achieved, also help them to strengthen personal power that is needed for productive social activities. (p. 207)

Identifying Oneself

"A concept of self develops as a product of interaction with adults" (Peplau, 1991, p. 211). A child learns to structure self-concept by observing how others interact with him or her. Roles and behaviors are established out of the child's perception of the expectations of others. When children perceive that adults expect them to maintain more-or-less permanent roles as infants, they perceive themselves as helpless and dependent. When the perceived expectation is that the child must behave in a manner beyond his or her maturational level, the child is deprived of the fulfillment of emotional and growth needs at the lower levels of development. Children who are given freedom to respond to situations and experiences unconditionally (i.e., with behaviors that are appropriate to their feelings) learn to improve on and reconstruct behavioral responses at their own individual pace. Peplau (1991) stated, "The ways in which adults appraise the child and the way he functions in relation to his experiences and perceptions are taken in or introjected and become the child's view of himself" (p. 213).

In nursing, it is important for the nurse to recognize cues that communicate how the client feels about him- or herself and about the presenting medical problem. In the initial interaction, it is difficult for the nurse to perceive the "wholeness" of the client, because the focus is on the condition that has caused him or her to seek help. Likewise, it is difficult for the client to perceive the nurse as a "mother (or father)" or "somebody's wife (or husband)" or as having a life aside from being there to offer assistance with the immediate presenting problem. As the relationship develops, nurses must be able to recognize client behaviors that indicate unfulfilled needs and provide experiences that promote growth. For example, the client who very proudly announces that she has completed activities of daily living independently and wants the nurse to come and inspect her room may still be craving the positive reinforcement associated with lower levels of development.

Nurses must also be aware of the predisposing factors that they bring to the relationship. Attitudes and beliefs about certain issues can have a deleterious effect on the client and interfere not only with the therapeutic relationship but also with the client's ability for growth and development. For example, a nurse who has strong beliefs against abortion may treat a client who has just undergone an abortion with disapproval and disrespect. The nurse may respond in this manner without even realizing he or she is doing so. Attitudes and values are introjected during early development and can be integrated so completely as to become a part of the self-system. Nurses must have knowledge and appreciation of their own concept of self in order to develop the flexibility required to accept all clients as they are, unconditionally. Effective resolution of problems that arise in the interdependent relationship can be the means for both client and nurse to reinforce positive personality traits and modify those more negative views of self.

Developing Skills in Participation

Peplau cited Sullivan's (1953) description of the "juvenile" stage of personality development (ages 6 through 9). During this stage, the child develops the capacity to "compromise, compete, and cooperate" with others. These skills are considered basic to one's ability to participate collaboratively with others. If a child tries to use the skills of an earlier level of development (e.g., crying, whining, demanding), he or she may be rejected by peers of this juvenile stage. As this stage progresses, children begin to view themselves through the eyes of their peers. Sullivan (1953) called this "consensual validation." Preadolescents take on a more realistic view of the world and a feeling of their place in it. The capacity to love others (besides the mother figure) develops at this time and is expressed in relation to one's self-acceptance.

Failure to develop appropriate skills at any point along the developmental progression results in an individual's difficulty with participation in confronting the recurring problems of life. It is not the responsibility of the nurse to teach solutions to problems, but rather to help clients improve their problem-solving skills so that they may achieve their own resolution. This is accomplished through development of the skills of competition, compromise, cooperation, consensual validation, and love of self

and others. Nurses can assist clients to develop or refine these skills by helping them to identify the problem, define a goal, and take the responsibility for performing the actions necessary to reach that goal. Peplau (1991) stated:

> Participation is required by a democratic society. When it has not been learned in earlier experiences, nurses have an opportunity to facilitate learning in the present and thus to aid in the promotion of a democratic society. (p. 259)

Relevance of Peplau's Model to Nursing Practice

Peplau's model provides nurses with a framework to interact with clients, many of whom are fixed in—or because of illness have regressed to—an earlier level of development. She suggested roles that nurses may assume to assist clients to progress, thereby achieving or resuming their appropriate developmental level. Appropriate developmental progression arms the individual with the ability to confront the recurring problems of life. Nurses serve to facilitate learning of that which has not been learned in earlier experiences.

Summary and Key Points

- Growth and development are unique with each individual and continue throughout the life span.

- Personality is defined as the combination of character, behavioral, temperamental, emotional, and mental traits that are unique to each specific individual.

- Sigmund Freud, who has been called the father of psychiatry, believed the basic character has been formed by the age of 5.

- Freud's personality theory can be conceptualized according to structure and dynamics of the personality, topography of the mind, and stages of personality development.

- Freud's structure of the personality includes the id, ego, and superego.

- Freud classified all mental contents and operations into three categories: the conscious, the preconscious, and the unconscious.

- Harry Stack Sullivan, author of the Interpersonal Theory of Psychiatry, believed that individual behavior and personality development are the direct result of interpersonal relationships. Major concepts include *anxiety, satisfaction of needs, interpersonal security,* and *self-system.*

■ Erik Erikson studied the influence of social processes on the development of the personality.

■ Erikson described eight stages of the life cycle from birth to death. He believed that individuals struggled with developmental "crises," and that each must be resolved for emotional growth to occur.

■ Margaret Mahler formulated a theory that describes the separation-individuation process of the infant from the maternal figure (primary caregiver). Stages of development describe the progression of the child from birth to object constancy at age 36 months.

■ Jean Piaget has been called the father of child psychology. He believed that human intelligence progresses through a series of stages that are related to age, demonstrating at each successive stage a higher level of logical organization than at the previous stages.

■ Lawrence Kohlberg outlined stages of moral development. His stages are not closely tied to specific age groups or the maturational process. He believed that moral stages emerge out of our own thinking and the stimulation of our mental processes.

■ Hildegard Peplau provided a framework for "psychodynamic nursing," the interpersonal involvement of the nurse with a client in a given nursing situation.

■ Peplau identified the nursing roles of resource person, counselor, teacher, leader, technical expert, and surrogate.

■ Peplau described four psychological tasks that she associated with the stages of infancy and childhood as identified by Freud and Sullivan.

■ Peplau believed that nursing is helpful when both the patient and the nurse grow as a result of the learning that occurs in the nursing situation.

 DavisPlus.   Additional info available @ davisplus.fadavis.com

Review Questions
Self-Examination/Learning Exercise

*Select the answer that is **most** appropriate for each of the following questions:*

1. Mr. J. is a new client on the psychiatric unit. He is 35 years old. Theoretically, in which level of psychosocial development (according to Erikson) would you place Mr. J.?
   a. Intimacy vs. isolation.
   b. Generativity vs. self-absorption.
   c. Trust vs. mistrust.
   d. Autonomy vs. shame and doubt.

2. Mr. J. has been diagnosed with Paranoid Schizophrenia. He refuses to eat, and told the nurse he knew he was "being poisoned." According to Erikson's theory, in what developmental stage would you place Mr. J.?
   a. Intimacy vs. isolation.
   b. Generativity vs. self-absorption.
   c. Trust vs. mistrust.
   d. Autonomy vs. shame and doubt.

3. Janet, a psychiatric client diagnosed with Borderline Personality Disorder, has just been hospitalized for threatening suicide. According to Mahler's theory, Janet did not receive the critical "emotional refueling" required during the rapprochement phase of development. What are the consequences of this deficiency?
   a. She has not yet learned to delay gratification.
   b. She does not feel guilt about wrongdoings to others.
   c. She is unable to trust others.
   d. She has internalized rage and fears of abandonment.

Continued

4. John is on the Alcohol Treatment Unit. He walks into the dayroom where other clients are watching a program on TV. He picks up the remote and changes the channel, saying, "That's a stupid program! I want to watch something else!" In what stage of development is John fixed according to Sullivan's interpersonal theory?
   a. Juvenile. He is learning to form satisfactory peer relationships.
   b. Childhood. He has not learned to delay gratification.
   c. Early adolescence. He is struggling to form an identity.
   d. Late adolescence. He is working to develop a lasting relationship.

5. Adam has Antisocial Personality Disorder. He says to the nurse, "I'm not crazy. I'm just fun-loving. I believe in looking out for myself. Who cares what anyone thinks? If it feels good, do it!" Which of the following describes the psychoanalytic structure of Adam's personality?
   a. Weak id, strong ego, weak superego.
   b. Strong id, weak ego, weak superego.
   c. Weak id, weak ego, punitive superego.
   d. Strong id, weak ego, punitive superego.

6. Larry, who has Antisocial Personality Disorder, feels no guilt about violating the rights of others. He does as he pleases without thought to possible consequences. In which of Peplau's stages of development would you place Larry?
   a. Learning to count on others.
   b. Learning to delay gratification.
   c. Identifying oneself.
   d. Developing skills in participation.

7. Danny, has been diagnosed with Paranoid Schizophrenia. On the unit, he appears very anxious, paces back and forth, and darts his head from side to side in a continuous scanning of the area. He has refused to eat, making some barely audible comment related to "being poisoned." In planning care for Danny, which of the following would be the primary focus for nursing?
   a. To decrease anxiety and develop trust.
   b. To set limits on his behavior.
   c. To ensure that he gets to group therapy.
   d. To attend to his hygiene needs.

8. The nurse has just admitted Nancy to the psychiatric unit. The psychiatrist has diagnosed Nancy with Major Depression. The nurse says to Nancy, "Please tell me what it was like when you were growing up." Which nursing role described by Peplau is the nurse fulfilling in this instance?
   a. Surrogate.
   b. Resource person.
   c. Counselor.
   d. Technical expert.

9. The nurse has just admitted Nancy to the psychiatric unit. The psychiatrist has diagnosed Nancy with Major Depression. The nurse asks Nancy, "What questions do you have about being here on the unit?" Which nursing role described by Peplau is the nurse fulfilling in this instance?
   a. Resource person.
   b. Counselor.
   c. Surrogate.
   d. Technical expert.

Review Questions—cont'd
Self-Examination/Learning Exercise

10. The nurse has just admitted Nancy to the psychiatric unit. The psychiatrist has diagnosed Nancy with Major Depression. The nurse says to Nancy, "Some changes will have to be made in your behavior. I care about what happens to you." Which nursing role described by Peplau is the nurse fulfilling in this instance?
    a. Counselor.
    b. Surrogate.
    c. Technical expert.
    d. Resource person.

References

American Psychiatric Association. (2000). *Diagnostic and statistical manual of mental disorders* (4th ed.). *Text revision.* Washington, DC: American Psychiatric Publishing.

Marmer, S. S. (2003). Theories of the mind and psychopathology. In R. E. Hales & S. C. Yudofsky (Eds.), *Textbook of clinical psychiatry* (4th ed., pp. 107–154). Washington, DC: American Psychiatric Publishing.

Murray, R. B., Zentner, J. P., & Yakimo, R. (2008). *Health promotion strategies through the life span* (8th ed.). Upper Saddle River, NJ: Prentice Hall.

Peplau, H. E. (1991). *Interpersonal relations in nursing.* New York: Springer.

Classical References

Chess, S., & Thomas, A. (1986). *Temperament in clinical practice.* New York: Guilford Press.

Erikson, E. (1963). *Childhood and society* (2nd ed.). New York: W.W. Norton.

Freud, S. (1961). The ego and the id. *Standard edition of the complete psychological works of Freud* (Vol. XIX). London: Hogarth Press.

Fromm, E. (1949). *Man for himself.* New York: Farrar & Rinehart.

Kohlberg, L. (1968). Moral development. In *International encyclopedia of social science.* New York: Macmillan.

Mahler, M., Pine, F., & Bergman, A. (1975). *The psychological birth of the human infant.* New York: Basic Books.

Piaget, J., & Inhelder, B. (1969). *The psychology of the child.* New York: Basic Books.

Sullivan, H. S. (1953). *The interpersonal theory of psychiatry.* New York: W.W. Norton.

Concepts of Psychobiology

CORE CONCEPTS

genetics
neuroendocrinology
psychobiology
psychoimmunology
psychotropic
    medication

KEY TERMS

axon
cell body
circadian rhythms
dendrites
genotype
limbic system

neuron
neurotransmitter
phenotype
receptor sites
synapse

OBJECTIVES
After reading this chapter, the student will be able to:

1. Identify gross anatomical structures of the brain and describe their functions.
2. Discuss the physiology of neurotransmission in the central nervous system.
3. Describe the role of neurotransmitters in human behavior.
4. Discuss the association of endocrine functioning to the development of psychiatric disorders.
5. Describe the role of genetics in the development of psychiatric disorders.
6. Discuss the correlation of alteration in brain functioning to various psychiatric disorders.
7. Identify various diagnostic procedures used to detect alteration in biological functioning that may be contributing to psychiatric disorders.
8. Discuss the influence of psychological factors on the immune system.
9. Discuss historical perspectives related to psychopharmacology.
10. Describe the physiological mechanism by which various psychotropic medications exert their effects.
11. Discuss the implications of psychobiological concepts to the practice of psychiatric/mental health nursing.

HOMEWORK ASSIGNMENT
Please read the chapter and answer the following questions:

1. A dramatic reduction in which neurotransmitter is most closely associated with Alzheimer's disease?
2. Anorexia nervosa has been associated with a primary dysfunction of which structure of the brain?
3. Many psychotropics work by blocking the reuptake of neurotransmitters. Describe the process of *reuptake*.
4. What psychiatric disorder may be linked to chronic hypothyroidism?

In recent years, a greater emphasis has been placed on the study of the organic basis for psychiatric illness. This "neuroscientific revolution" began in earnest when the 101st legislature of the United States designated the 1990s as the "decade of the brain." With this legislation came the challenge for studying the biological basis of behavior. Several mental illnesses are now being considered as physical disorders that are the result of malfunctions and/or malformations of the brain.

This is not to imply that psychosocial and sociocultural influences are totally discounted. Such a notion would negate the transactional model of stress/adaptation on which the framework of this textbook is conceptualized.

The systems of biology, psychology, and sociology are not mutually exclusive—they are interacting systems. This is clearly indicated by the fact that individuals experience biological changes in response to various environmental events. Indeed, each of these disciplines may be, at various times, most appropriate for explaining behavioral phenomena.

This chapter focuses on the role of neurophysiological, neurochemical, genetic, and endocrine influences on psychiatric illness. A discussion of psychopharmacology is included, and various diagnostic procedures used to detect alteration in biological function that may contribute to psychiatric illness are identified. The implications for psychiatric/mental health nursing are discussed.

CORE CONCEPT
Psychobiology
The study of the biological foundations of cognitive, emotional, and behavioral processes.

The Nervous System: An Anatomical Review

The Brain

The brain has three major divisions, subdivided into six major parts:

1. Forebrain
   a. Cerebrum
   b. Diencephalon
2. Midbrain
   a. Mesencephalon
3. Hindbrain
   a. Pons
   b. Medulla
   c. Cerebellum

Each of these structures is discussed individually. A summary is presented in Table 4-1.

Cerebrum

The cerebrum consists of a right and left hemisphere and constitutes the largest part of the human brain. The right and left hemispheres are

TABLE 4-1 Structure and Function of the Brain	
STRUCTURE	**PRIMARY FUNCTION**
I. The Forebrain	
A. Cerebrum	Composed of two hemispheres separated by a deep groove that houses a band of 200 million neurons called the corpus callosum. The outer shell is called the cortex. It is extensively folded and consists of billions of neurons. The left hemisphere appears to deal with logic and solving problems. The right hemisphere may be called the "creative" brain and is associated with affect, behavior, and spatial-perceptual functions. Each hemisphere is divided into four lobes.
1. Frontal lobes	Voluntary body movement, including movements that permit speaking, thinking and judgment formation, and expression of feelings.
2. Parietal lobes	Perception and interpretation of most sensory information (including touch, pain, taste, and body position).
3. Temporal lobes	Hearing, short-term memory, and sense of smell; expression of emotions through connection with limbic system.
4. Occipital lobes	Visual reception and interpretation.

Continued

TABLE 4-1 Structure and Function of the Brain—cont'd

STRUCTURE	PRIMARY FUNCTION
B. Diencephalon	Connects cerebrum with lower brain structures.
1. Thalamus	Integrates all sensory input (except smell) on way to cortex; some involvement with emotions and mood.
2. Hypothalamus	Regulates anterior and posterior lobes of pituitary gland; exerts control over actions of the autonomic nervous system; regulates appetite and temperature.
3. Limbic system	Consists of medially placed cortical and subcortical structures and the fiber tracts connecting them with one another and with the hypothalamus. It is sometimes called the "emotional brain"—associated with feelings of fear and anxiety; anger and aggression; love, joy, and hope; and with sexuality and social behavior.
II. The Midbrain A. Mesencephalon	Responsible for visual, auditory, and balance ("righting") reflexes.
III. The Hindbrain A. Pons	Regulation of respiration and skeletal muscle tone; ascending and descending tracts connect brainstem with cerebellum and cortex.
B. Medulla	Pathway for all ascending and descending fiber tracts; contains vital centers that regulate heart rate, blood pressure, and respiration; reflex centers for swallowing, sneezing, coughing, and vomiting.
C. Cerebellum	Regulates muscle tone and coordination and maintains posture and equilibrium.

connected by a deep groove, which houses a band of 200 million **neurons** (nerve cells) called the *corpus callosum*. Because each hemisphere controls different functions, information is processed through the corpus callosum so that each hemisphere is aware of the activity of the other.

The surface of the cerebrum consists of gray matter and is called the cerebral cortex. The gray matter is so called because the neuron cell bodies of which it is composed look gray to the eye. These gray matter cell bodies are thought to be the actual thinking structures of the brain. Another pair of masses of gray matter called *basal ganglia* is found deep within the cerebral hemispheres. They are responsible for certain subconscious aspects of voluntary movement, such as swinging the arms when walking, gesturing while speaking, and regulating muscle tone (Scanlon & Sanders, 2011).

The cerebral cortex is identified by numerous folds, called *gyri,* and deep grooves between the folds, called *sulci.* This extensive folding extends the surface area of the cerebral cortex, and thus permits the presence of millions more neurons than would be possible without it (as is the case in the brains of some animals, such as dogs and cats). Each hemisphere of the cerebral cortex is divided into the frontal lobe, parietal lobe, temporal lobe, and occipital lobe. These lobes, which are named

for the overlying bones in the cranium, are identified in Figure 4–1.

The Frontal Lobes

Voluntary body movement is controlled by the impulses through the frontal lobes. The right frontal lobe controls motor activity on the left side of the body and the left frontal lobe controls motor activity on the right side of the body. Movements that permit speaking are also controlled by the frontal lobe, usually only on the left side (Scanlon & Sanders, 2011). The frontal lobe may also play a role in the emotional experience, as evidenced by changes in mood and character after damage to this area. The alterations include fear, aggressiveness, depression, rage, euphoria, irritability, and apathy and are likely related to a frontal lobe connection to the **limbic system.** The frontal lobe may also be involved (indirectly through association fibers linked to primary sensory areas) in thinking and perceptual interpretation of information.

The Parietal Lobes

Somatosensory input occurs in the parietal lobe area of the brain. This input includes touch, pain and pressure, taste, temperature, perception of joint and body position, and visceral sensations. The parietal lobes also contain association fibers linked to the primary sensory areas through which

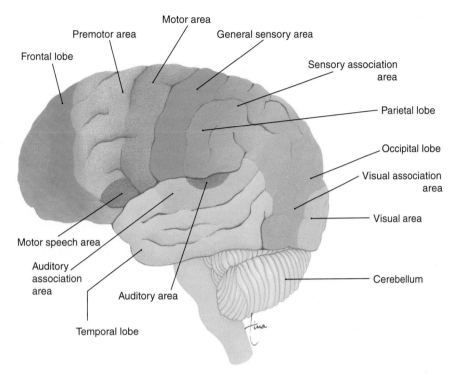

FIGURE 4–1   Left cerebral hemisphere showing some of the functional areas that have been mapped. (From Scanlon, V. C., & Sanders, T. [2011]. *Essentials of anatomy and physiology* [6th ed.]. Philadelphia: F.A. Davis, with permission.)

interpretation of sensory-perceptual information is made. Language interpretation is associated with the left hemisphere of the parietal lobe.

The Temporal Lobes

The upper anterior temporal lobe is concerned with auditory functions, while the lower part is dedicated to short-term memory. The sense of smell has a connection to the temporal lobes, as the impulses carried by the olfactory nerves end in this area of the brain (Scanlon & Sanders, 2011). The temporal lobes also play a role in the expression of emotions through an interconnection with the limbic system. The left temporal lobe, along with the left parietal lobe, is involved in language interpretation.

The Occipital Lobes

The occipital lobes are the primary area of visual reception and interpretation. Visual perception, which gives individuals the ability to judge spatial relationships such as distance and to see in three dimensions, is also processed in this area. Language interpretation is influenced by the occipital lobes through an association with the visual experience.

Diencephalon

The second part of the forebrain is the diencephalon, which connects the cerebrum with lower structures of the brain. The major components of

the diencephalon include the thalamus, the hypothalamus, and the limbic system. These structures are identified in Figures 4–2 and 4–3.

Thalamus

The thalamus integrates all sensory input (except smell) on its way to the cortex. This helps the cerebral cortex interpret the whole picture very rapidly, rather than experiencing each sensation individually. The thalamus is also involved in temporarily blocking minor sensations, so that an individual can concentrate on one important event when necessary. For example, an individual who is studying for an examination may be unaware of the clock ticking in the room, or even of another person walking into the room, because the thalamus has temporarily blocked these incoming sensations from the cortex.

Hypothalamus

The hypothalamus is located just below the thalamus and just above the pituitary gland and has a number of diverse functions.

1. **Regulation of the Pituitary Gland.** The pituitary gland consists of two lobes: the posterior lobe and the anterior lobe.
   a. *The posterior lobe* of the pituitary gland is actually extended tissue from the hypothalamus. The posterior lobe stores antidiuretic hormone (which helps to

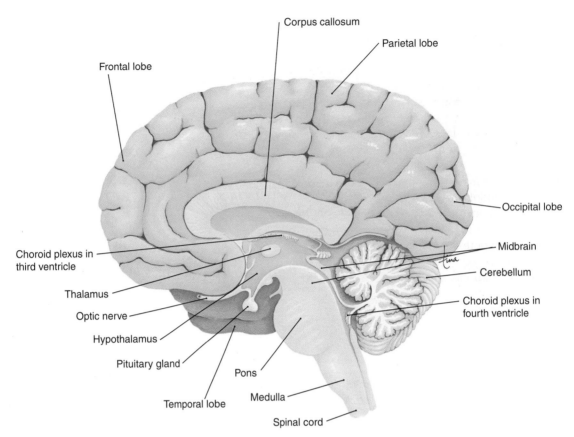

FIGURE 4–2   Midsagittal section of the brain as seen from the left side. This medial plane shows internal anatomy as well as the lobes of the cerebrum. (From Scanlon, V. C., & Sanders, T. [2011]. *Essentials of anatomy and physiology* [6th ed.]. Philadelphia: F.A. Davis, with permission.)

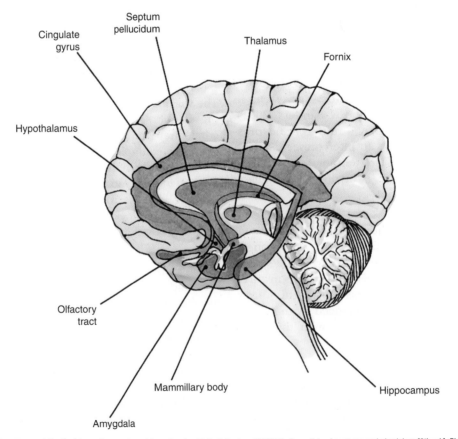

FIGURE 4–3   Structures of the limbic system. (Adapted from Scanlon, V. C., & Sanders, T. [2011]. *Essentials of anatomy and physiology* [6th ed.]. Philadelphia: F.A. Davis.)

maintain blood pressure through regulation of water retention) and oxytocin (the hormone responsible for stimulation of the uterus during labor, and the release of milk from the mammary glands). Both of these hormones are produced in the hypothalamus. When the hypothalamus detects the body's need for these hormones, it sends nerve impulses to the posterior pituitary for their release.

  b. *The anterior lobe* of the pituitary gland consists of glandular tissue that produces a number of hormones used by the body. These hormones are regulated by "releasing factors" from the hypothalamus. When one of these hormones is required by the body, the releasing factor stimulates the release of the hormone from the anterior pituitary and the hormone in turn stimulates its target organ to carry out its specific functions.

2. **Direct Neural Control Over the Actions of the Autonomic Nervous System.** The hypothalamus regulates the appropriate visceral responses during various emotional states. The actions of the autonomic nervous system are described later in this chapter.

3. **Regulation of Appetite.** Appetite is regulated through response to blood nutrient levels.

4. **Regulation of Temperature.** The hypothalamus senses internal temperature changes in the blood that flows through the brain. It receives information through sensory input from the skin about external temperature changes. The hypothalamus then uses this information to promote certain types of responses (e.g., sweating or shivering) that help to maintain body temperature within the normal range.

Limbic System

The part of the brain known as the limbic system consists of portions of the cerebrum and the diencephalon. The major components include the medially placed cortical and subcortical structures and the fiber tracts connecting them with one another and with the hypothalamus. The system is composed of the amygdala, mammillary body, olfactory tract, hypothalamus, cingulate gyrus, septum pellucidum, thalamus, hippocampus, and neuronal connecting pathways, such as the fornix and others. This system has been called "the emotional brain" and is associated with feelings of fear and anxiety; anger, rage, and aggression; love, joy, and hope; and with sexuality and social behavior.

Mesencephalon

Structures of major importance in the mesencephalon, or midbrain, include nuclei and fiber tracts. The mesencephalon extends from the pons to the hypothalamus and is responsible for integration of various reflexes, including visual reflexes (e.g., automatically turning away from a dangerous object when it comes into view), auditory reflexes (e.g., automatically turning toward a sound that is heard), and righting reflexes (e.g., automatically keeping the head upright and maintaining balance). The mesencephalon is identified in Figure 4–2.

Pons

The pons is a bulbous structure that lies between the midbrain and the medulla (Fig. 4–2). It is composed of large bundles of fibers and forms a major connection between the cerebellum and the brainstem. It also contains the central connections of cranial nerves V through VIII and centers for respiration and skeletal muscle tone.

Medulla

The medulla is the connecting structure between the spinal cord and the pons, and all of the ascending and descending fiber tracts pass through it. The vital centers are contained in the medulla, and it is responsible for regulation of heart rate, blood pressure, and respiration. Also in the medulla are reflex centers for swallowing, sneezing, coughing, and vomiting. It also contains nuclei for cranial nerves IX through XII. The medulla, pons, and midbrain form the structure known as the brainstem. These structures are identified in Figure 4–2.

Cerebellum

The cerebellum is separated from the brainstem by the fourth ventricle but has connections to the brainstem through bundles of fiber tracts. It is situated just below the occipital lobes of the cerebrum (Figs. 4–1 and 4–2). The functions of the cerebellum are concerned with involuntary movement, such as muscular tone and coordination and the maintenance of posture and equilibrium.

Nerve Tissue

The tissue of the central nervous system (CNS) consists of nerve cells called *neurons* that generate and transmit electrochemical impulses. The structure of a neuron is composed of a cell body, an axon, and dendrites. The **cell body** contains the nucleus and is essential for the continued life of the neuron. The **dendrites** are processes that transmit impulses toward the cell body, and the **axon** transmits impulses away from the cell body. The axons and dendrites are covered by layers of cells called *neuroglia* that form a coating, or "sheath," of myelin. *Myelin* is a phospholipid that provides insulation against short-circuiting of the neurons during their electrical activity and increases the velocity of the impulse. The white matter of the brain and spinal cord is so called because of the whitish appearance of the myelin sheath over the axons and dendrites. The gray matter is composed of cell bodies that contain no myelin.

The three classes of neurons include afferent (sensory), efferent (motor), and interneurons. The *afferent neurons* carry impulses from receptors in the internal and external periphery to the CNS, where they are then interpreted into various sensations. The *efferent neurons* carry impulses from the CNS to *effectors* in the periphery, such as muscles (that respond by contracting) and glands (that respond by secreting). A schematic of afferent and efferent neurons is presented in Figure 4–4.

Interneurons exist entirely within the CNS, and 99 percent of all nerve cells belong to this group. They may carry only sensory or motor impulses, or they may serve as integrators in the pathways between afferent and efferent neurons. They account in large part for thinking, feelings, learning,

Afferent (sensory) neuron

Efferent (motor) neuron

Dendrites

Axon terminal

Axon

Cell body

Nucleus

Nucleus

Axon

Schwann cell nucleus

Myelin sheath

Node of Ranvier

Cell body

Schwann cell

Dendrite

Axon

Myelin sheath

Neurolemma

Layers of myelin sheath

Receptors

C

Axon terminal

A

B

FIGURE 4–4 Neuron structure. **(A)** A typical sensory neuron. **(B)** A typical motor neuron. The *arrows* indicate the direction of impulse transmission. **(C)** Details of the myelin sheath and neurolemma formed by Schwann cells. (From Scanlon, V. C., & Sanders, T. [2011]. *Essentials of anatomy and physiology* [6th ed.]. Philadelphia: F.A. Davis, with permission.)

language, and memory. The directional pathways of afferent, efferent, and interneurons are presented in Figure 4–5.

Synapses

Information is transmitted through the body from one neuron to another. Some messages may be processed through only a few neurons, while others may require thousands of neuronal connections. The neurons that transmit the impulses do not actually touch each other. The junction between two neurons is called a **synapse.** The small space between the axon terminals of one neuron and the cell body or dendrites of another is called the *synaptic cleft.* Neurons conducting impulses toward the synapse are called *presynaptic neurons* and those conducting impulses away are called *postsynaptic neurons.*

A chemical, called a **neurotransmitter,** is stored in the axon terminals of the presynaptic neuron. An electrical impulse through the neuron causes the release of this neurotransmitter into the synaptic cleft. The neurotransmitter then diffuses across the synaptic cleft and combines with **receptor sites** that are situated on the cell membrane of the postsynaptic neuron. The result of the combination of neurotransmitter-receptor site is the determination of whether or not another electrical impulse is generated. If one is generated, the result is called an *excitatory response* and the electrical impulse moves on to the next synapse, where the same process recurs. If another electrical impulse is not generated by the neurotransmitter-receptor site combination, the result is called an *inhibitory response,* and synaptic transmission is terminated.

The cell body or dendrite of the postsynaptic neuron also contains a chemical *inactivator* that is specific to the neurotransmitter that has been released by the presynaptic neuron. When the synaptic transmission has been completed, the chemical inactivator quickly inactivates the neurotransmitter to prevent unwanted, continuous

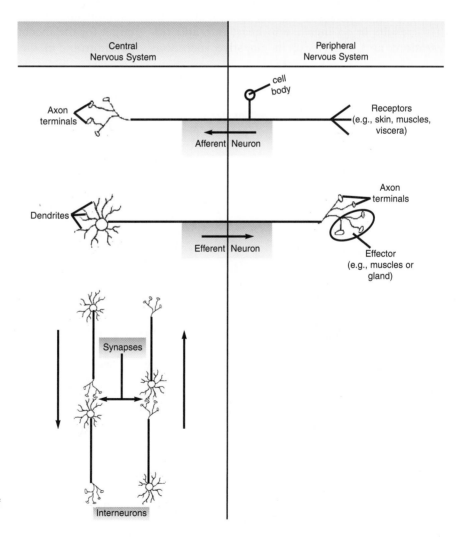

FIGURE 4–5   Directional pathways of neurons.

impulses, until a new impulse from the presynaptic neuron releases more neurotransmitter. A schematic representation of a synapse is presented in Figure 4–6.

Autonomic Nervous System

The autonomic nervous system (ANS) is actually considered part of the peripheral nervous system. Its regulation is integrated by the hypothalamus, however, and therefore the emotions exert a great deal of influence over its functioning. For this reason, the ANS has been implicated in the etiology of a number of psychophysiological disorders.

The ANS has two divisions: the sympathetic and the parasympathetic. The sympathetic division is dominant in stressful situations and prepares the body for the "fight or flight" response that was discussed in Chapter 1. The neuronal cell bodies of the sympathetic division originate in the thoracolumbar region of the spinal cord. Their axons extend to the chains of sympathetic ganglia, where they synapse with other neurons that subsequently innervate the visceral effectors. This results in an increase in heart rate and respirations and a decrease in digestive secretions and peristalsis. Blood is shunted to the vital organs and to skeletal muscles to ensure adequate oxygenation.

The neuronal cell bodies of the parasympathetic division originate in the brainstem and the sacral segments of the spinal cord, and extend to the parasympathetic ganglia, where the synapse takes place either very close to or actually in the visceral organ being innervated. In this way, a very localized response is possible. The parasympathetic division dominates when an individual is in a relaxed, nonstressful condition. The heart and respirations are maintained at a normal rate and secretions and peristalsis increase for normal digestion. Elimination functions are promoted. A schematic representation of the autonomic nervous system is presented in Figure 4–7.

Neurotransmitters

Neurotransmitters were described during the explanation of synaptic activity. They are discussed here separately and in detail because of the essential function they play in the role of human emotion and behavior and because they are the target for the mechanism of action of many of the psychotropic medications.

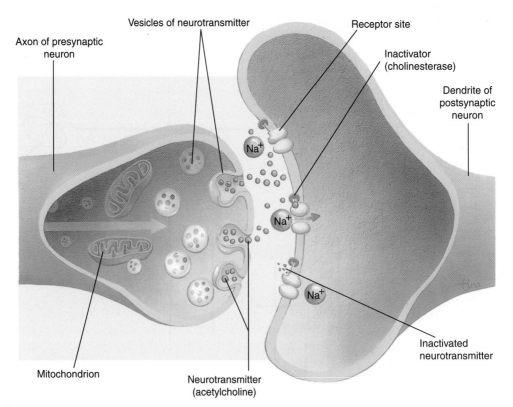

FIGURE 4–6 Impulse transmission at a synapse. The *arrow* indicates the direction of electrical impulses. (From Scanlon, V. C., & Sanders, T. [2011]. *Essentials of anatomy and physiology* [6th ed.]. Philadelphia: F.A. Davis, with permission.)

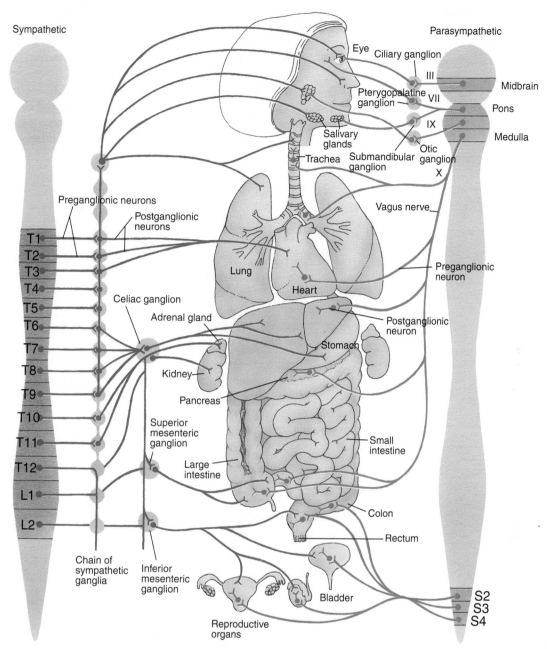

FIGURE 4–7 The autonomic nervous system. The sympathetic division is shown on the left, and the parasympathetic division is shown on the right (both divisions are bilateral). (From Scanlon, V. C., & Sanders, T. [2011]. *Essentials of anatomy and physiology* [6th ed.]. Philadelphia: F.A. Davis, with permission.)

Neurotransmitters are chemicals that convey information across synaptic clefts to neighboring target cells. They are stored in small vesicles in the axon terminals of neurons. When the action potential, or electrical impulse, reaches this point, the neurotransmitters are released from the vesicles. They cross the synaptic cleft and bind with receptor sites on the cell body or dendrites of the adjacent neuron to allow the impulse to continue its course or to prevent the impulse from continuing. After the neurotransmitter has performed its function in the synapse,

it either returns to the vesicles to be stored and used again, or it is inactivated and dissolved by enzymes. The process of being stored for reuse is called *reuptake,* a function that holds significance for understanding the mechanism of action of certain psychotropic medications.

Many neurotransmitters exist in the central and peripheral nervous systems, but only a limited number have implications for psychiatry. Major categories include cholinergics, monoamines, amino acids, and neuropeptides. Each of these is discussed separately and summarized in Table 4-2.

TABLE 4-2 Neurotransmitters in the Central Nervous System

NEUROTRANSMITTER	LOCATION/FUNCTION	POSSIBLE IMPLICATIONS FOR MENTAL ILLNESS
I. Cholinergics		
A. Acetylcholine	*ANS:* Sympathetic and parasympathetic presynaptic nerve terminals; parasympathetic postsynaptic nerve terminals *CNS:* Cerebral cortex, hippocampus, limbic structures, and basal ganglia *Functions:* Sleep, arousal, pain perception, movement, memory	*Increased levels:* depression *Decreased levels:* Alzheimer's disease, Huntington's disease, and Parkinson's disease
II. Monoamines		
A. Norepinephrine	*ANS:* Sympathetic postsynaptic nerve terminals *CNS:* Thalamus, hypothalamus, limbic system, hippocampus, cerebellum, cerebral cortex *Functions:* Mood, cognition,perception, locomotion, cardiovascular functioning, and sleep and arousal	*Decreased levels:* depression *Increased levels:* mania, anxiety states, and schizophrenia
B. Dopamine	Frontal cortex, limbic system, basal ganglia, thalamus, posterior pituitary, and spinal cord *Functions:* Movement and coordination, emotions, voluntary judgment, release of prolactin	*Decreased levels:* Parkinson's disease and depression *Increased levels:* mania and schizophrenia
C. Serotonin	Hypothalamus, thalamus, limbic system, cerebral cortex, cerebellum, spinal cord *Functions:* Sleep and arousal, libido, appetite, mood, aggression, pain perception, coordination, judgment	*Decreased levels:* depression *Increased levels:* anxiety states
D. Histamine	Hypothalamus *Functions:* Wakefulness; pain sensation and inflammatory response	*Decreased levels:* depression
III. Amino Acids		
A. Gamma-aminobutyric acid (GABA)	Hypothalamus, hippocampus, cortex, cerebellum, basal ganglia, spinal cord, retina *Functions:* Slowdown of body activity	*Decreased levels:* Huntington's disease, anxiety disorders, schizophrenia, and various forms of epilepsy
B. Glycine	Spinal cord and brainstem *Functions:* Recurrent inhibition of motor neurons	*Toxic levels:* "glycine encephalopathy," decreased levels are correlated with spastic motor movements
C. Glutamate and aspartate	Pyramidal cells of the cortex, cerebellum, and the primary sensory afferent systems; hippocampus, thalamus, hypothalamus, spinal cord *Functions:* Relay of sensory information and in the regulation of various motor and spinal reflexes	*Increased levels:* Huntington's disease, temporal lobe epilepsy, and spinal cerebellar degeneration

TABLE 4-2 Neurotransmitters in the Central Nervous System—cont'd		
NEUROTRANSMITTER	**LOCATION/FUNCTION**	**POSSIBLE IMPLICATIONS FOR MENTAL ILLNESS**
IV. Neuropeptides		
A. Endorphins and enkephalins	Hypothalamus, thalamus, limbic structures, midbrain, and brainstem; enkephalins are also found in the gastrointestinal tract *Functions:* Modulation of pain and reduced peristalsis (enkephalins)	Modulation of dopamine activity by opioid peptides may indicate some link to the symptoms of schizophrenia
B. Substance P	Hypothalamus, limbic structures, midbrain, brainstem, thalamus, basal ganglia, and spinal cord; also found in gastrointestinal tract and salivary glands *Function:* Regulation of pain	*Decreased levels:* Huntington's disease and Alzheimer's disease *Increased levels:* depression
C. Somatostatin	Cerebral cortex, hippocampus, thalamus, basal ganglia, brainstem, and spinal cord *Function:* Depending on part of the brain being affected, stimulates release of dopamine, serotonin, norepinephrine, and acetylcholine, and inhibits release of norepinephrine, histamine, and glutamate. Also acts as a neuromodulator for serotonin in the hypothalamus	*Decreased levels:* Alzheimer's disease *Increased levels:* Huntington's disease

Cholinergics

Acetylcholine

Acetylcholine was the first chemical to be identified and proven as a neurotransmitter. It is a major effector chemical in the ANS, producing activity at all sympathetic and parasympathetic presynaptic nerve terminals and all parasympathetic postsynaptic nerve terminals. It is highly significant in the neurotransmission that occurs at the junctions of nerve and muscles. Acetylcholinesterase is the enzyme that destroys acetylcholine or inhibits its activity.

In the CNS, acetylcholine neurons innervate the cerebral cortex, hippocampus, and limbic structures. The pathways are especially dense through the area of the basal ganglia in the brain.

Functions of acetylcholine are manifold and include sleep, arousal, pain perception, the modulation and coordination of movement, and memory acquisition and retention (Gilman & Newman, 2003). Cholinergic mechanisms may have some role in certain disorders of motor behavior and memory, such as Parkinson's disease, Huntington's disease, and Alzheimer's disease.

Monoamines

Norepinephrine

Norepinephrine is the neurotransmitter that produces activity at the sympathetic postsynaptic nerve terminals in the ANS resulting in the "fight or flight" responses in the effector organs. In the CNS, norepinephrine pathways originate in the pons and medulla and innervate the thalamus, dorsal hypothalamus, limbic system, hippocampus, cerebellum, and cerebral cortex. When norepinephrine is not returned for storage in the vesicles of the axon terminals, it is metabolized and inactivated by the enzymes monoamine oxidase (MAO) and catechol-*O*-methyltransferase (COMT).

The functions of norepinephrine include the regulation of mood, cognition, perception, locomotion, cardiovascular functioning, and sleep and arousal (Gilman & Newman, 2003). The activity of norepinephrine also has been implicated in certain mood disorders such as depression and mania, in anxiety states, and in schizophrenia (Sadock & Sadock, 2007).

Dopamine

Dopamine pathways arise from the midbrain and hypothalamus and terminate in the frontal cortex, limbic system, basal ganglia, and thalamus. Dopamine neurons in the hypothalamus innervate the posterior pituitary, and those from the posterior hypothalamus project to the spinal cord. As with norepinephrine, the inactivating enzymes for dopamine are MAO and COMT.

Dopamine functions include regulation of movements and coordination, emotions, and voluntary decision-making ability, and because of its influence on the pituitary gland, it inhibits the release of prolactin (Sadock & Sadock, 2007). Increased levels of dopamine are associated with mania (Dubovsky, Davies, & Dubovsky, 2003) and schizophrenia (Black & Andreasen, 2011).

Serotonin

Serotonin pathways originate from cell bodies located in the pons and medulla and project to areas including the hypothalamus, thalamus, limbic system, cerebral cortex, cerebellum, and spinal cord. Serotonin that is not returned to be stored in the axon terminal vesicles is catabolized by the enzyme MAO.

Serotonin may play a role in sleep and arousal, libido, appetite, mood, aggression, and pain perception. The serotoninergic system has been implicated in the etiology of certain psychopathological conditions, including anxiety states, mood disorders, and schizophrenia (Sadock & Sadock, 2007).

Histamine

The role of histamine in mediating allergic and inflammatory reactions has been well documented. Its role in the CNS as a neurotransmitter has only recently been confirmed, and the availability of information is limited. The highest concentrations of histamine are found within various regions of the hypothalamus. Histaminic neurons in the posterior hypothalamus are associated with sustaining wakefulness (Gilman & Newman, 2003). The enzyme that catabolizes histamine is MAO. Although the exact processes mediated by histamine within the CNS are uncertain, some data suggest that histamine may play a role in depressive illness.

Amino Acids

Inhibitory Amino Acids

Gamma-Aminobutyric Acid Gamma-aminobutyric acid (GABA) has a widespread distribution in the CNS, with high concentrations in the hypothalamus, hippocampus, cortex, cerebellum, and basal ganglia of the brain, in the gray matter of the dorsal horn of the spinal cord, and in the retina. Most GABA is associated with short inhibitory interneurons, although some long-axon

pathways within the brain also have been identified. GABA is catabolized by the enzyme GABA transaminase.

Inhibitory neurotransmitters, such as GABA, prevent postsynaptic excitation, interrupting the progression of the electrical impulse at the synaptic junction. This function is significant when slowdown of body activity is advantageous. Enhancement of the GABA system is the mechanism of action by which the benzodiazepines produce their calming effect.

Alterations in the GABA system have been implicated in the etiology of anxiety disorders, movement disorders (e.g., Huntington's disease), and various forms of epilepsy.

Glycine The highest concentrations of glycine in the CNS are found in the spinal cord and brainstem. Little is known about the possible enzymatic metabolism of glycine.

Glycine appears to be the neurotransmitter of recurrent inhibition of motor neurons within the spinal cord, and is possibly involved in the regulation of spinal and brainstem reflexes. It has been implicated in the pathogenesis of certain types of spastic disorders and in "glycine encephalopathy," which is known to occur with toxic accumulation of the neurotransmitter in the brain and cerebrospinal fluid (Hamosh, Scharer, & Van Hove, 2009).

Excitatory Amino Acids

Glutamate and Aspartate Glutamate and aspartate appear to be primary excitatory neurotransmitters in the pyramidal cells of the cortex, the cerebellum, and the primary sensory afferent systems. They are also found in the hippocamus, thalamus, hypothalamus, and spinal cord. Glutamate and aspartate are inactivated by uptake into the tissues and through assimilation in various metabolic pathways.

Glutamate and aspartate function in the relay of sensory information and in the regulation of various motor and spinal reflexes. Alteration in these systems has been implicated in the etiology of certain neurodegenerative disorders, such as Huntington's disease, temporal lobe epilepsy, and spinal cerebellar degeneration.

Neuropeptides

Numerous neuropeptides have been identified and studied. They are classified by the area of the body in which they are located or by their pharmacological or functional properties. Although their role as neurotransmitters has not been clearly established, it is known that they often coexist with the classic neurotransmitters within a neuron; however, the functional significansce of this coexistence still requires further study. Hormonal neuropeptides are discussed in the section of this chapter on neuroendocrinology.

Opioid Peptides

Opioid peptides, which include the endorphins and enkephalins, have been widely studied. Opioid peptides are found in various concentrations in the hypothalamus, thalamus, limbic structures, midbrain, and brainstem. Enkephalins are also found in the gastrointestinal (GI) tract. Opioid peptides are thought to have a role in pain modulation, with their natural morphine-like properties. They are released in response to painful stimuli, and may be responsible for producing the analgesic effect following acupuncture. Opioid peptides alter the release of dopamine and affect the spontaneous activity of the dopaminergic neurons. These findings may have some implication for opioid peptide–dopamine interaction in the etiology of schizophrenia.

Substance P

Substance P was the first neuropeptide to be discovered. It is present in high concentrations in the hypothalamus, limbic structures, midbrain, and brainstem, and is also found in the thalamus, basal ganglia, and spinal cord. Substance P has been found to be highly concentrated in sensory fibers, and for this reason is thought to play a role in sensory transmission, and particularly in the regulation of pain. Substance P abnormalities have been associated with Huntington's disease, dementia of the Alzheimer's type, and mood disorders (Sadock & Sadock, 2007).

Somatostatin

Somatostatin (also called growth hormone–inhibiting hormone) is found in the cerebral cortex, hippocampus, thalamus, basal ganglia, brainstem, and spinal cord, and has multiple effects on the CNS. In its function as a neurotransmitter, somatostatin exerts both stimulatory and inhibitory effects. Depending on the part of the brain being affected, it has been shown to stimulate dopamine, serotonin, norepinephrine, and acetylcholine, and inhibit norepinephrine, histamine, and glutamate. It also acts as a neuromodulator for serotonin in the hypothalamus, thereby regulating its release (i.e., determining whether it is stimulated or inhibited). It is possible that somatostatin may serve this function for other neurotransmitters as well. High concentrations of somatostatin have been reported in brain specimens of clients with Huntington's disease, and low concentrations in those with Alzheimer's disease.

> **CORE CONCEPT**
> *Neuroendocrinology*
> Study of the interaction between the nervous system and the endocrine system, and the effects of various hormones on cognitive, emotional, and behavioral functioning.

Neuroendocrinology

Human endocrine functioning has a strong foundation in the CNS, under the direction of the hypothalamus, which has direct control over the pituitary gland. The pituitary gland has two major lobes—the anterior lobe (also called the *adenohypophysis*) and the posterior lobe (also called the *neurohypophysis*). The pituitary gland is only about the size of a pea, but despite its size and because of the powerful control it exerts over endocrine functioning in humans, it is sometimes called the "master gland." (Figure 4–8 shows the hormones of the pituitary gland and their target organs.) Many of the hormones subject to hypothalamus-pituitary regulation may have implications for behavioral functioning. Discussion of these hormones is summarized in Table 4-3.

Pituitary Gland

The Posterior Pituitary (Neurohypophysis)

The hypothalamus has direct control over the posterior pituitary through efferent neural pathways. Two hormones are found in the posterior pituitary: vasopressin (antidiuretic hormone) and oxytocin. They are actually produced by the hypothalamus and stored in the posterior pituitary. Their release is mediated by neural impulses from the hypothalamus (Fig. 4–9).

Antidiuretic Hormone

The main function of antidiuretic hormone (ADH) is to conserve body water and maintain normal blood pressure. The release of ADH is stimulated by pain, emotional stress, dehydration, increased plasma concentration, and decreases in blood volume. An alteration in the secretion of this hormone may be a factor in the polydipsia observed in about 10 to 15 percent of hospitalized psychiatric patients. Other factors correlated with this behavior include adverse effects of psychotropic medications and features of the behavioral disorder itself. ADH also may play a role in learning and memory, in alteration of the pain response, and in the modification of sleep patterns.

Anterior pituitary hormones

Posterior pituitary hormones

FIGURE 4–8 Hormones of the pituitary gland and their target organs. (From Scanlon, V. C., & Sanders, T. [2011]. *Essentials of anatomy and physiology* [6th ed.]. Philadelphia: F.A. Davis, with permission.)

TABLE 4-3 Hormones of the Neuroendocrine System				
HORMONE	**LOCATION AND STIMULATION OF RELEASE**	**TARGET ORGAN**	**FUNCTION**	**POSSIBLE BEHAVIORAL CORRELATION TO ALTERED SECRETION**
Antidiuretic hormone (ADH)	Posterior pituitary; release stimulated by dehydration, pain, stress	Kidney (causes increased reabsorption)	Conservation of body water and maintenance of blood pressure	Polydipsia; altered pain response; modified sleep pattern
Oxytocin	Posterior pituitary; release stimulated by end of pregnancy; stress; during sexual arousal	Uterus; breasts	Contraction of the uterus for labor; release of breast milk	May play role in stress response by stimulation of ACTH

TABLE 4-3 Hormones of the Neuroendocrine System—cont'd

HORMONE	LOCATION AND STIMULATION OF RELEASE	TARGET ORGAN	FUNCTION	POSSIBLE BEHAVIORAL CORRELATION TO ALTERED SECRETION
Growth hormone (GH)	Anterior pituitary; release stimulated by growth hormone–releasing hormone from hypothalamus	Bones and tissues	Growth in children; protein synthesis in adults	Anorexia nervosa
Thyroid-stimulating hormone (TSH)	Anterior pituitary; release stimulated by thyrotropin-releasing hormone from hypothalamus	Thyroid gland	Stimulation of secretion of needed thyroid hormones for metabolism of food and regulation of temperature	*Increased levels:* insomnia, anxiety, emotional lability *Decreased levels:* fatigue, depression
Adrenocorticotropic hormone (ACTH)	Anterior pituitary; release stimulated by corticotropin-releasing hormone from hypothalamus	Adrenal cortex	Stimulation of secretion of cortisol, which plays a role in response to stress	*Increased levels:* mood disorders, psychosis *Decreased levels:* depression, apathy, fatigue
Prolactin	Anterior pituitary; release stimulated by prolactin-releasing hormone from hypothalamus	Breasts	Stimulation of milk production	*Increased levels:* depression, anxiety, decreased libido, irritability
Gonadotropic hormones	Anterior pituitary; release stimulated by gonadotropin-releasing hormone from hypothalamus	Ovaries and testes	Stimulation of secretion of estrogen, progesterone, and testosterone; role in ovulation and sperm production	*Decreased levels:* depression and anorexia nervosa *Increased testosterone:* increased sexual behavior and aggressiveness
Melanocyte-stimulating hormone (MSH)	Anterior pituitary; release stimulated by onset of darkness	Pineal gland	Stimulation of secretion of melatonin	*Increased levels:* depression

Oxytocin

Oxytocin stimulates contraction of the uterus at the end of pregnancy and stimulates release of milk from the mammary glands (Scanlon & Sanders, 2011). It is also released in response to stress and during sexual arousal. Its role in behavioral functioning is unclear, although it is possible that oxytocin may act in certain situations to stimulate the release of adrenocorticotropic hormone (ACTH), thereby playing a key role in the overall hormonal response to stress.

The Anterior Pituitary (Adenohypophysis)

The hypothalamus produces *releasing hormones* that pass through capillaries and veins of the hypophyseal portal system to capillaries in the anterior pituitary, where they stimulate secretion of specialized hormones. This pathway is presented in Figure 4–9. The hormones of the anterior pituitary gland regulate multiple body functions and include growth hormone, thyroid-stimulating hormone, ACTH, prolactin, gonadotropin-releasing hormone, and melanocyte-stimulating hormone. Most of these hormones are regulated by a *negative feedback mechanism*. Once the hormone has exerted its effects, this information is "fed back" to the anterior pituitary, which inhibits the release, and ultimately decreases the effects, of the stimulating hormones.

A

B

FIGURE 4–9 Structural relationships of hypothalamus and pituitary gland. **(A)** Posterior pituitary stores hormones produced in the hypothalamus. **(B)** Releasing hormones of the hypothalamus circulate directly to the anterior pituitary and influence its secretions. Notice the two networks of capillaries. (From Scanlon, V. C., & Sanders, T. [2011]. *Essentials of anatomy and physiology* [6th ed.]. Philadelphia: F.A. Davis, with permission.)

Growth Hormone

The release of growth hormone (GH), also called somatotropin, is stimulated by growth hormone–releasing hormone (GHRH) from the hypothalamus. Its release is inhibited by growth hormone–inhibiting hormone (GHIH), or somatostatin, also from the hypothalamus. It is responsible for growth in children, as well as continued protein synthesis throughout life. During periods of fasting, it stimulates the release of fat from the adipose tissue to be used for increased energy. The release of GHIH is stimulated in response to periods of hyperglycemia. GHRH is stimulated in response to hypoglycemia and to stressful situations. During prolonged stress, GH has a direct effect on protein, carbohydrate, and lipid metabolism, resulting in increased serum glucose and free fatty acids to be used for increased energy. There has been some indication of a possible correlation between abnormal secretion of growth hormone and anorexia nervosa.

Thyroid-Stimulating Hormone

Thyrotropin-releasing hormone (TRH) from the hypothalamus stimulates the release of thyroid-stimulating hormone (TSH), or thyrotropin, from the anterior pituitary. TSH stimulates the thyroid gland to secrete triiodothyronine (T_3) and thyroxine (T_4). Thyroid hormones are integral to the metabolism of food and the regulation of temperature.

A correlation between thyroid dysfunction and altered behavioral functioning has been studied. Early reports in the medical literature associated hyperthyroidism with irritability, insomnia, anxiety, restlessness, weight loss, and emotional lability, and in some instances with progressing to delirium or psychosis. Symptoms of fatigue, decreased libido, memory impairment, depression, and suicidal ideations have been associated with chronic hypothyroidism. Studies have correlated various forms of thyroid dysfunction with mood disorders, anxiety, eating disorders, schizophrenia, and dementia.

Adrenocorticotropic Hormone

Corticotropin-releasing hormone (CRH) from the hypothalamus stimulates the release of ACTH from the anterior pituitary. ACTH stimulates the adrenal cortex to secrete cortisol. The role of cortisol in human behaviors is not well understood, although it seems to be secreted under stressful situations. Disorders of the adrenal cortex can result in hyposecretion or hypersecretion of cortisol.

Addison's disease is the result of hyposecretion of the hormones of the adrenal cortex. Behavioral symptoms of hyposecretion include mood changes with apathy, social withdrawal, impaired sleep, decreased concentration, and fatigue. Hypersecretion of cortisol results in Cushing's disease and is associated with behaviors that include depression, mania, psychosis, and suicidal ideation. Cognitive impairments also have been commonly observed.

Prolactin

Serum prolactin levels are regulated by prolactin-releasing hormone (PRH) and prolactin-inhibiting hormone (PIH) from the hypothalamus. Prolactin stimulates milk production by the mammary glands in the presence of high levels of estrogen and progesterone during pregnancy. Behavioral symptoms associated with hypersecretion of prolactin include depression, decreased libido, stress intolerance, anxiety, and increased irritability.

Gonadotropic Hormones

The gonadotropic hormones are so called because they produce an effect on the gonads—the ovaries and the testes. The gonadotropins include follicle-stimulating hormone (FSH) and luteinizing hormone (LH), and their release from the anterior pituitary is stimulated by gonadotropin-releasing hormone (GnRH) from the hypothalamus. In women, FSH initiates maturation of ovarian follicles into the ova and stimulates their secretion of estrogen. LH is responsible for ovulation and the secretion of progesterone from the corpus luteum. In men, FSH initiates sperm production in the testes, and LH increases secretion of testosterone by the interstitial cells of the testes (Scanlon & Sanders, 2011). The gonadotropins are regulated by a negative feedback of gonadal hormones at the hypothalamic or pituitary level.

Limited evidence exists to correlate gonadotropins to behavioral functioning, although some observations have been made to warrant hypothetical consideration. Studies have indicated decreased levels of testosterone, LH, and FSH in depressed men. Increased sexual behavior and aggressiveness have been linked to elevated testosterone levels in both men and women. Decreased plasma levels of LH and FSH commonly occur in patients with anorexia nervosa. Supplemental estrogen therapy has resulted in improved mentation and mood in some depressed women.

Melanocyte-Stimulating Hormone

Melanocyte-stimulating hormone (MSH) from the hypothalamus stimulates the pineal gland to secrete melatonin. The release of melatonin appears to depend on the onset of darkness and is suppressed by light. Studies of this hormone have indicated that environmental light can affect neuronal activity and influence *circadian rhythms*. Correlation between abnormal secretion of melatonin and symptoms of depression has led to the implication of melatonin in the etiology of seasonal affective disorder (SAD), in which individuals become depressed only during the fall and winter months when the amount of daylight decreases.

Circadian Rhythms

Human biological rhythms are largely determined by genetic coding, with input from the external environment influencing the cyclic effects. **Circadian rhythms** in humans follow a near-24-hour cycle and may influence a variety of regulatory functions, including the sleep-wakefulness cycle, body temperature regulation, patterns of activity such as eating and drinking, and hormone secretion. The 24-hour rhythms in humans are affected to a large degree by the cycles of lightness and darkness. This occurs because of a "pacemaker" in the brain that sends messages to other systems in the body and maintains the 24-hour rhythm. This endogenous pacemaker appears to be the suprachiasmatic nuclei of the hypothalamus. These nuclei receive projections of light through the retina, and in turn stimulate electrical impulses to various other systems in the body, mediating the release of neurotransmitters or hormones that regulate bodily functioning.

Most of the biological rhythms of the body operate over a period of about 24 hours, but cycles of longer lengths have been studied. For example, women of menstruating age show monthly cycles of progesterone levels in the saliva, of skin temperature over the breasts, and of prolactin levels in the plasma of the blood (Hughes, 1989).

Some rhythms may even last as long as a year. These circannual rhythms are particularly relevant to certain medications, such as cyclosporine, that appear to be more effective at some times than others during the period of about a year (Hughes, 1989). One clinical study showed that administration of chemotherapy during the appropriate circadian phase can significantly increase the efficacy and decrease the toxic effects of certain cytotoxic agents (Lis et al., 2003).

The Role of Circadian Rhythms in Psychopathology

Circadian rhythms may play a role in psychopathology. Because many hormones have been implicated in behavioral functioning, it is reasonable to believe that peak secretion times could be influential in predicting certain behaviors. The association of depression with increased secretion of melatonin during darkness hours has already been discussed. External manipulation of the light-dark cycle and removal of external time cues often have beneficial effects on mood disorders.

Symptoms that occur in the premenstrual cycle have also been linked to disruptions in biological rhythms. A number of the symptoms associated with premenstrual dysphoric disorder (PMDD) strongly resemble those attributed to depression, and hormonal changes have been implicated in the etiology. Some of these changes include progesterone-estrogen imbalance, increase in prolactin and mineralocorticoids, high level of prostaglandins, decrease in endogenous opiates, changes in metabolism of biogenic amines (serotonin, dopamine, norepinephrine, acetylcholine), and variations in secretion of glucocorticoids or melatonin.

Sleep disturbances are common in both depression and PMDD. Because the sleep-wakefulness cycle is probably the most fundamental of biological rhythms, it will be discussed in greater detail. A representation of bodily functions affected by 24-hour biological rhythms is presented in Figure 4–10.

Sleep

The sleep-wakefulness cycle is genetically determined rather than learned and is established some time after birth. Even when environmental cues

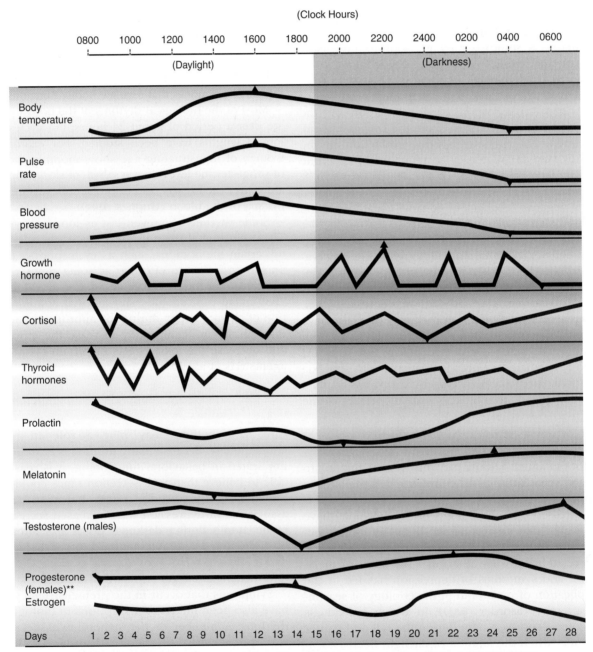

* ▼ indicates low point and ▲ indicates peak time of these biological factors within a 24-hour circadian rhythm.
** The female hormones are presented on a monthly rhythm because of their influence on the reproductive cycle. Daily rhythms of female gonadotropins are difficult to assay and are probably less significant than monthly.

FIGURE 4–10 Circadian biological rhythms

such as the ability to detect light and darkness are removed, the human sleep-wakefulness cycle generally develops about a 25-hour periodicity, which is close to the 24-hour normal circadian rhythm.

Sleep can be measured by the types of brain waves that occur during various stages of sleep activity. Dreaming episodes are characterized by rapid eye movement and are called REM sleep. The sleep-wakefulness cycle is represented by six distinct stages:

1. **Stage 0—Alpha Rhythm.** This stage of the sleep-wakefulness cycle is characterized by a relaxed, waking state with eyes closed. The alpha brain wave rhythm has a frequency of 8 to 12 cycles per second.

2. **Stage 1—Beta Rhythm.** Stage 1 characterizes the "transition" into sleep, or a period of dozing. Thoughts wander, and there is a drifting in and out of sleep. Beta brain wave rhythm has a frequency of 18 to 25 cycles per second.

3. **Stage 2—Theta Rhythm.** This stage characterizes the manner in which about half of sleep time is spent. Eye movement and muscular activity are minimal. Theta brain wave rhythm has a frequency of 4 to 7 cycles per second.

4. **Stage 3—Delta Rhythm.** This is a period of deep and restful sleep. Muscles are relaxed, heart rate and blood pressure fall, and breathing slows. No eye movement occurs. Delta brain wave rhythm has a frequency of 1.5 to 3 cycles per second.

5. **Stage 4—Delta Rhythm.** This is the stage of deepest sleep. Individuals who suffer from insomnia or other sleep disorders often do not experience this stage of sleep. Eye movement and muscular activity are minimal. Delta waves predominate.

6. **REM Sleep—Beta Rhythm.** This is the dream cycle. Eyes dart about beneath closed eyelids, moving more rapidly than when awake. The brain wave pattern is similar to that of stage 1 sleep. Heart and respiration rates increase, and blood pressure may increase or decrease. Muscles are hypotonic during REM sleep.

Stages 2 through REM repeat themselves throughout the cycle of sleep. One is more likely to experience longer periods of stages 3 and 4 sleep early in the cycle and longer periods of REM sleep later in the sleep cycle. Most people experience REM sleep about four to five times during the night. The amount of REM sleep and deep sleep decreases with age, while the time spent in drowsy wakefulness and dozing increases.

Neurochemical Influences

A number of neurochemicals have been shown to influence the sleep-wakefulness cycle. Several studies have revealed information about the sleep-inducing characteristics of serotonin. L-Tryptophan, the amino acid precursor to serotonin, has been used for many years as an effective sedative-hypnotic to induce sleep in individuals with sleep-onset disorder. Serotonin and norepinephrine both appear to be most active during non-REM sleep, whereas the neurotransmitter acetylcholine is activated during REM sleep (Skudaev, 2010). The exact role of GABA in sleep facilitation is unclear, although the sedative effects of drugs that enhance GABA transmission, such as the benzodiazepines, suggest that this neurotransmitter plays an important role in regulation of sleep and arousal. Some studies have suggested that acetylcholine induces and prolongs REM sleep, whereas histamine appears to have an inhibitory effect. Neuroendocrine mechanisms seem to be more closely tied to circadian rhythms than to the sleep-wakefulness cycle. One exception is growth hormone secretion, which exhibits increases during the early sleep period and may be associated with slow-wave sleep (Van Cauter et al., 1992).

CORE CONCEPT

Genetics
Study of the biological transmission of certain characteristics (physical and/or behavioral) from parent to offspring.

Genetics

Human behavioral genetics seeks to understand both the genetic and environmental contributions to individual variations in human behavior (McInerney, 2008). This type of study is complicated by the fact that behaviors, like all complex traits, involve *multiple genes.*

The term **genotype** refers to the total set of genes present in an individual at the time of conception, and coded in the DNA. The physical manifestations of a particular genotype are designated by characteristics that specify a specific **phenotype.** Examples of phenotypes include eye color, height, blood type, language, and hair type. As evident by the examples presented, phenotypes are not *only* genetic, but may also be acquired (i.e., influenced by the environment) or a combination of both. It is likely that many psychiatric disorders are the result of a combination of genetics and environmental influences.

Investigators who study the etiological implications for psychiatric illness may explore several risk factors. Studies to determine if an illness is *familial* compare the percentages of family members with the illness to those in the general population or within a control group of unrelated individuals. These studies estimate the prevalence of psychopathology among relatives, and make predictions about the predisposition to an illness based on familial risk factors. Schizophrenia, bipolar disorder, major depression, anorexia nervosa, panic disorder, somatization disorder, antisocial personality disorder, and alcoholism are examples of psychiatric illness in which familial tendencies have been indicated.

Studies that are purely genetic in nature search for a specific gene that is responsible for an individual having a particular illness. A number of disorders exist in which the mutation of a specific gene or change in the number or structure of a chromosome has been associated with the etiology. Examples include Huntington's disease, cystic fibrosis, phenylketonuria, Duchenne's muscular dystrophy, and Down syndrome.

The search for genetic links to certain psychiatric disorders continues. Risk factors for early-onset Alzheimer's disease have been linked to mutations on chromosomes 21, 14, and 1 (National Institute on Aging, 2009). Other studies have linked a gene in the region of chromosome 19 that produces apolipoprotein E (ApoE) with late-onset Alzheimer's disease. Additional research is required before definitive confirmation can be made.

In addition to familial and purely genetic investigations, other types of studies have been conducted to estimate the existence and degree of genetic and environmental contributions to the etiology of certain psychiatric disorders. Twin studies and adoption studies have been successfully employed for this purpose.

Twin studies examine the frequency of a disorder in monozygotic (genetically identical) and dizygotic (fraternal; not genetically identical) twins. Twins are called *concordant* when both members suffer from the same disorder in question. Concordance in monozygotic twins is considered stronger evidence of genetic involvement than it is in dizygotic twins. Disorders in which twin studies have suggested a possible genetic link include alcoholism, schizophrenia, major depression, bipolar disorder, anorexia nervosa, panic disorder, and obsessive-compulsive disorder (Baker, 2004; Gill, 2004).

Adoption studies allow comparisons to be made of the influences of genetics versus environment on the development of a psychiatric disorder. Knowles (2003) describes the following four types of adoption studies that have been conducted:

1. The study of adopted children whose biological parent(s) had a psychiatric disorder but whose adoptive parent(s) did not.
2. The study of adopted children whose adoptive parent(s) had a psychiatric disorder but whose biological parent(s) did not.
3. The study of adoptive and biological relatives of adopted children who developed a psychiatric disorder.
4. The study of monozygotic twins reared apart by different adoptive parents.

Disorders in which adoption studies have suggested a possible genetic link include alcoholism, schizophrenia, major depression, bipolar disorder, attention-deficit/hyperactivity disorder, and antisocial personality disorder (Knowles, 2003).

A summary of various psychiatric disorders and the possible biological influences discussed in this chapter is presented in Table 4-4. Various diagnostic procedures used to detect alteration in biological functioning that may contribute to psychiatric disorders are presented in Table 4-5.

CORE CONCEPT

Psychoimmunology

The branch of medicine that studies the effects of psychological and social factors on the functioning of the immune system.

Psychoimmunology

Normal Immune Response

Cells responsible for *nonspecific* immune reactions include neutrophils, monocytes, and macrophages. They work to destroy the invasive organism and initiate and facilitate damaged tissue. If these cells are not effective in accomplishing a satisfactory healing response, *specific* immune mechanisms take over.

Specific immune mechanisms are divided into two major types: the cellular response and the humoral response. The controlling elements of the cellular response are the T lymphocytes (T cells); those of the humoral response are called B lymphocytes

TABLE 4-4 Biological Implications of Psychiatric Disorders

ANATOMICAL BRAIN STRUCTURES INVOLVED	NEUROTRANSMITTER HYPOTHESIS	POSSIBLE ENDOCRINE CORRELATION	IMPLICATIONS OF CIRCADIAN RHYTHMS	POSSIBLE GENETIC LINK
Schizophrenia				
Frontal cortex, temporal lobes, limbic system	Dopamine hyperactivity	Decreased prolactin levels	May correlate antipsychotic medication administration to times of lowest level	Twin, familial, and adoption studies suggest genetic link
Depressive Disorders				
Frontal lobes, limbic system, temporal lobes	Decreased levels of norepinephrine, dopamine, and serotonin	Increased cortisol levels; thyroid hormone hyposecretion; increased melatonin	DST* used to predict effectiveness of antidepressants; melatonin linked to depression during periods of darkness	Twin, familial, and adoption studies suggest a genetic link
Bipolar Disorder				
Frontal lobes, limbic system, temporal lobes	Increased levels of norepinephrine and dopamine in acute mania	Some indication of elevated thyroid hormones in acute mania		Twin, familial, and adoption studies suggest a genetic link
Panic Disorder				
Limbic system, midbrain	Increased levels of norepinephrine; decreased GABA activity	Elevated levels of thyroid hormones	May have some application for times of medication administration	Twin and familial studies suggest a genetic link
Anorexia Nervosa				
Limbic system, particularly the hypothalamus	Decreased levels of norepinephrine, serotonin, and dopamine	Decreased levels of gonadotropins and growth hormone; increased cortisol levels	DST* often shows same results as in depression	Twin and familial studies suggest a genetic link
Obsessive-Compulsive Disorder				
Limbic system, basal ganglia (specifically caudate nucleus)	Decreased levels of serotonin	Increased cortisol levels	DST* often shows same results as in depression	Twin studies suggest a possible genetic link
Alzheimer's Disease				
Temporal, parietal, and occipital regions of cerebral cortex; hippocampus	Decreased levels of acetylcholine, norepinephrine, serotonin, and somatostatin	Decreased corticotropin-releasing hormone	Decreased levels of acetylcholine and serotonin may inhibit hypothalamic-pituitary axis and interfere with hormonal releasing factors	Familial studies suggest a genetic predisposition; late-onset disorder linked to marker on chromosome 19; early-onset to chromosomes 21, 14, and 1

*DST = dexamethasone suppression test. Dexamethasone is a synthetic glucocorticoid that suppresses cortisol secretion via the feedback mechanism. In this test, 1 mg of dexamethasone is administered at 11:30 p.m. and blood samples are drawn at 8:00 a.m., 4:00 p.m., and 11:00 p.m. on the following day. A plasma value greater than 5 μg/dl suggests that the individual is not suppressing cortisol in response to the dose of dexamethasone. This is a positive result for depression and may have implications for other disorders as well.

TABLE 4-5 Diagnostic Procedures Used to Detect Altered Brain Functioning

EXAM	TECHNIQUE USED	PURPOSE OF THE EXAM AND POSSIBLE FINDINGS
Electroencephalography (EEG)	Electrodes are placed on the scalp in a standardized position. Amplitude and frequency of beta, alpha, theta, and delta brain waves are graphically recorded on paper by ink markers for multiple areas of the brain surface.	Measures brain electrical activity; identifies dysrhythmias, asymmetries, or suppression of brain rhythms; used in the diagnosis of epilepsy, neoplasm, stroke, and metabolic or degenerative disease.
Computerized EEG mapping	EEG tracings are summarized by computer-assisted systems in which various regions of the brain are identified and functioning is interpreted by color coding or gray shading.	Measures brain electrical activity; used largely in research to represent statistical relationships between individuals and groups or between two populations of subjects (e.g., patients with schizophrenia vs. control subjects).
Computed tomographic (CT) scanning	CT scanning may be used with or without contrast medium. X-rays are taken of various transverse planes of the brain while a computerized analysis produces a precise reconstructed image of each segment.	Measures accuracy of brain structure to detect possible lesions, abscesses, areas of infarction, or aneurysm. CT has also identified various anatomical differences in patients with schizophrenia, organic mental disorders, and bipolar disorder.
Magnetic resonance imaging (MRI)	Within a strong magnetic field, the nuclei of hydrogen atoms absorb and re-emit electromagnetic energy that is computerized and transformed into image information. No radiation or contrast medium is used.	Measures anatomical and biochemical status of various segments of the brain; detects brain edema, ischemia, infection, neoplasm, trauma, and other changes such as demyelination. Morphological differences have been noted in brains of patients with schizophrenia as compared with control subjects.
Positron emission tomography (PET)	The patient receives an intravenous (IV) injection of a radioactive substance (type depends on brain activity to be visualized). The head is surrounded by detectors that relay data to a computer that interprets the signals and produces the image.	Measures specific brain functioning, such as glucose metabolism, oxygen utilization, blood flow, and, of particular interest in psychiatry, neurotransmitter-receptor interaction.
Single-photon emission computed tomography (SPECT)	The technique is similar to PET, but longer-acting radioactive substance must be used to allow time for a gamma-camera to rotate about the head and gather the data, which are then computer assembled into a brain image.	Measures various aspects of brain functioning, as with PET; has also been used to image activity of cerebrospinal fluid circulation.

(B cells). When the body is invaded by a specific antigen, the T cells, and particularly the CD4 T lymphocytes (also called *helper T cells*), become sensitized to and specific for the foreign antigen. These antigen-specific CD 4 T cells divide many times, producing antigen-specific CD4 T cells with other functions. One of these, the *killer T cell*, destroys viruses that reproduce inside other cells by puncturing the cell membrane of the host cell and allowing the contents of the cell, including viruses, to spill out into the bloodstream, where they can be engulfed by macrophages. Another cell produced through division of the CD4 T cells is the suppressor T cell, which serves to stop the immune response once the foreign antigen has been destroyed (Scanlon & Sanders, 2011).

The humoral response is activated when antigen-specific CD4 T cells communicate with the B cells in the spleen and lymph nodes. The B cells in turn produce the antibodies specific to the foreign antigen. Antibodies attach themselves to foreign antigens so that they are unable to invade body cells. These invader cells are then destroyed without being able to multiply.

Implications of the Immune System in Psychiatric Illness

In studies of the biological response to stress, it has been hypothesized that individuals become more susceptible to physical illness following exposure to a stressful stimulus or life event (see Chapter 1). This response is thought to be due to the effect of increased glucocorticoid release from the adrenal cortex following stimulation from the hypothalamic-pituitary-adrenal axis during stressful situations. The result is a suppression of lymphocyte proliferation and function.

Studies have shown that nerve endings exist in tissues of the immune system. The CNS has connections both in bone marrow and the thymus, where immune system cells are produced, and in the spleen and lymph nodes, where those cells are stored.

Growth hormone, which may be released in response to certain stressors, may enhance immune functioning, whereas testosterone is thought to inhibit immune functioning. Increased production of epinephrine and norepinephrine occurs in response to stress, and may decrease immunity. Serotonin has demonstrated both enhancing and inhibitory effects on immunity (Irwin, 2000).

Studies have correlated a decrease in lymphocyte functioning with periods of grief, bereavement, and depression, associating the degree of altered immunity with severity of the depression. A number of research studies have been conducted attempting to correlate the onset of schizophrenia to abnormalities of the immune system. These studies have considered autoimmune responses, viral infections, and immunogenetics (Sadock & Sadock, 2007). The role of these factors in the onset and course of schizophrenia remains unclear. Immunological abnormalities have also been investigated in a number of other psychiatric illnesses, including alcoholism, autism, and dementia.

Evidence exists to support a correlation between psychosocial stress and the onset of illness. Research is still required to determine the specific processes involved in stress-induced modulation of the immune system.

Psychopharmacology

The middle of the 20th century was a pivotal period in the treatment of the mentally ill. It was during this time that the phenothiazine class of antipsychotics was introduced into the United States. Before that time they had been used in France as preoperative medications. As Dr. Henri Laborit of the Hospital Boucicaut in Paris stated,

> It was our aim to decrease the anxiety of the patients to prepare them in advance for their postoperative recovery. With these new drugs, the phenothiazines, we were seeing a profound psychic and physical relaxation. . . a real indifference to the environment and to the upcoming operation. It seemed to me these drugs must have an application in psychiatry. (Sage, 1984)

Indeed they have had a significant application in psychiatry. Not only have they helped many individuals to function effectively, but they have also provided researchers and clinicians with information to study the origins and etiologies of mental illness. Knowledge gained from learning how these drugs work has promoted advancement in understanding how behavioral disorders develop. Dr. Arnold Scheibel, Director of the UCLA Brain Research Institute, stated,

> [When these drugs came out] there was a sense of disbelief that we could actually do something substantive for the patients . . . see them for the first time as sick individuals and not as something bizarre that we could literally not talk to. (Sage, 1984)

> ## CORE CONCEPT
> ### *Psychotropic Medication*
> Medication that affects psychic function, behavior, or experience.

Historical Perspectives

Historically, reaction to and treatment of the mentally ill ranged from benign involvement to intervention some would consider inhumane. Individuals with mental illness were feared because of common beliefs associating them with demons or the supernatural. They were looked upon as loathsome and often were mistreated.

Beginning in the late 18th century, a type of "moral reform" in the treatment of persons with mental illness began to occur. Community and state hospitals concerned with the needs of persons with mental illness were established. Considered a breakthrough in the humanization of care, these institutions, however well intentioned, fostered the concept of custodial care. Clients were ensured the provision of food and shelter but received little or no hope of change for the future. As they became increasingly dependent on the institution to fill their needs, the likelihood of their return to the family or community diminished.

The early part of the 20th century saw the advent of the somatic therapies in psychiatry. Individuals with mental illness were treated with insulin shock therapy, wet sheet packs, ice baths, electroconvulsive therapy, and psychosurgery. Before 1950, sedatives and amphetamines were the only significant psychotropic medications available. Even these had limited use because of their toxicity and addicting effects. Since the 1950s, the development of psychopharmacology has expanded to include widespread use of antipsychotic, antidepressant, and antianxiety medications. Research into how these drugs work has provided an understanding of the etiology of many psychiatric disorders.

Psychotropic medications are not intended to "cure" the mental illness. Most mental health practitioners who prescribe these medications for their clients use them as an adjunct to individual or group psychotherapy. Although their contribution to psychiatric care cannot be minimized, it must be emphasized that psychotropic medications relieve physical and behavioral symptoms. They do not resolve emotional problems.

Role of the Nurse
Ethical and Legal Implications

Nurses must understand the ethical and legal implications associated with the administration of psychotropic medications. Laws differ from state to state, but most adhere to the client's right to refuse treatment. Exceptions exist in emergency situations when it has been determined that clients are likely to harm themselves or others.

Assessment

A thorough baseline assessment must be conducted before a client is placed on a regimen of psychopharmacological therapy. A history and physical examination (see Chapter 9), an ethnocultural assessment (see Chapter 6), and a comprehensive medication assessment (see Box 4-1) are all essential components of this database.

Medication Administration and Evaluation

For the client in an inpatient setting, as well as for many others in partial hospitalization programs, day treatment centers, home health care, and other settings, the nurse is the key health-care professional in direct contact with the individual receiving the chemotherapy. Medication administration is followed by a careful evaluation, including continuous monitoring for side effects and adverse reactions. The nurse also evaluates the therapeutic effectiveness of the medication. It is essential for the nurse to have a thorough knowledge of psychotropic medications to be able to anticipate potential problems and outcomes associated with their administration.

Client Education

The information associated with psychotropic medications is copious and complex. An important role of the nurse is to translate that complex information into terms that can be easily understood by the client. Clients must understand why the medication has been prescribed, when it should be taken, and what they may expect in terms of side effects and possible adverse reactions. They must know whom to contact when they have a question and when it is important to report to their physician. Medication education encourages client cooperation and promotes accurate and effective management of the treatment regimen.

How Do Psychotropics Work?

Most of the medications have their effects at the neuronal synapse, producing changes in neurotransmitter release and the receptors to which they

BOX 4-1 **Medication Assessment Tool**

Date _____ Client's Name _____ Age _____

Marital Status _____ Children _____ Occupation _____

Presenting Symptoms (subjective & objective) _____

_____

Diagnosis (DSM-IV-TR) _____

Current Vital Signs: Blood Pressure: Sitting _____/_____; Standing _____/_____; Pulse _____;

Respirations _____ Height _____ Weight _____

CURRENT/PAST USE OF PRESCRIPTION DRUGS (Indicate with "c" or "p" beside name of drug whether current or past use):

Name	Dosage	How Long Used	Why Prescribed	By Whom	Side Effects/Results
____	____	____	____	____	____
____	____	____	____	____	____
____	____	____	____	____	____

CURRENT/PAST USE OF OVER-THE-COUNTER DRUGS (Indicate with "c" or "p" beside name of drug whether current or past use):

Name	Dosage	How Long Used	Why Prescribed	By Whom	Side Effects/Results
____	____	____	____	____	____
____	____	____	____	____	____
____	____	____	____	____	____

CURRENT/PAST USE OF STREET DRUGS, ALCOHOL, NICOTINE, AND/OR CAFFEINE (Indicate with "c" or "p" beside name of drug):

Name	Amount Used	How Often Used	When Last Used	Effects Produced
____	____	____	____	____
____	____	____	____	____
____	____	____	____	____

Any allergies to food or drugs? _____

Any special diet considerations? _____

Do you have (or have you ever had) any of the following? If yes, provide explanation on the back of this sheet.

	Yes	No			Yes	No			Yes	No
1. Difficulty swallowing	—	—	12. Chest pain	—	—		23. Sexual dysfunction	—	—	
2. Delayed wound healing	—	—	13. Blood clots/pain in legs	—	—		24. Lumps in your breasts	—	—	
3. Constipation problems	—	—	14. Fainting spells	—	—		25. Blurred or double vision	—	—	
4. Urination problems	—	—	15. Swollen ankles/legs/hands	—	—		26. Ringing in the ears	—	—	
5. Recent change in elimination patterns	—	—	16. Asthma	—	—		27. Insomnia	—	—	
			17. Varicose veins	—	—		28. Skin rashes	—	—	
6. Weakness or tremors	—	—	18. Numbness/tingling (location?)	—	—		29. Diabetes	—	—	
7. Seizures	—	—	19. Ulcers	—	—		30. Hepatitis (or other liver disease)	—	—	
8. Headaches	—	—	20. Nausea/vomiting	—	—					
9. Dizziness	—	—	21. Problems with diarrhea	—	—		31. Kidney disease	—	—	
10. High blood pressure	—	—	22. Shortness of breath	—	—		32. Glaucoma	—	—	
11. Palpitations	—	—								

Are you pregnant or breast feeding? _____ Date of last menses _____ Type of contraception used _____

Describe any restrictions/limitations that might interfere with your use of medication for your current problem. _____

_____

Prescription orders: Patient teaching related to medications prescribed:

Lab work or referrals prescribed:

Nurse's signature _____ **Client's signature** _____

bind (see Figure 4–11). Researchers hypothesize that most antidepressants work by blocking the reuptake of neurotransmitters, specifically, serotonin and norepinephrine. *Reuptake* is the process of neurotransmitter inactivation by which the neurotransmitter is reabsorbed into the presynaptic neuron from which it had been released. Blocking the reuptake process allows more of the neurotransmitter to be available for neuronal transmission. This mechanism of action may also result in undesirable side effects (see Table 4-6). Some antidepressants also block receptor sites that are unrelated to their mechanisms of action. These include alpha-adrenergic, histaminergic, and muscarinic cholinergic receptors. Blocking these receptors is also associated with the development of certain side effects.

Antipsychotic medications block dopamine receptors, and some affect muscarinic cholinergic, histaminergic, and alpha-adrenergic receptors. The "atypical" antipsychotics block a specific serotonin receptor. Benzodiazepines facilitate the transmission of the inhibitory neurotransmitter GABA. The psychostimulants work by increasing norepinephrine, serotonin, and dopamine release.

Although each psychotropic medication affects neurotransmission, the specific drugs within each class have varying neuronal effects. Their exact mechanisms of action are unknown. Many of the neuronal effects occur acutely; however, the therapeutic effects may take weeks to occur for some medications such as antidepressants and antipsychotics. Acute alterations in neuronal function do

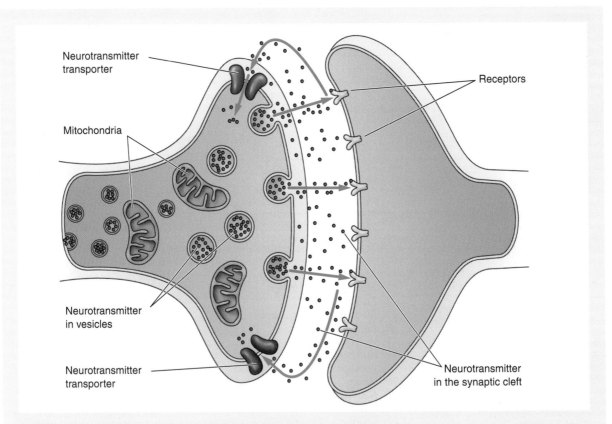

FIGURE 4–11 Area of synaptic transmission that is altered by drugs.
The transmission of electrical impulses from the axon terminal of one neuron to the dendrite of another is achieved by the controlled release of neurotransmitters into the synaptic cleft. Neurotransmitters include serotonin, norepinephrine, acetylcholine, dopamine, glutamate, gamma-aminobutyric acid (GABA), and histamine, among others. Prior to its release, the neurotransmitter is concentrated into specialized synaptic vesicles. Once fired, the neurotransmitter is released into the synaptic cleft, where it encounters receptors on the postsynaptic membrane. Each neurotransmitter has receptors specific to it alone. Some neurotransmitters are considered to be *excitatory*, whereas others are *inhibitory*, a feature that determines whether another action potential will occur. In the synaptic cleft, the neurotransmitter rapidly diffuses, is catabolized by enzymatic action, or is taken up by the neurotransmitter transporters and returned to vesicles inside the axon terminal to await another action potential.

Psychotropic medications exert their effects in various ways in this area of synaptic transmission. Reuptake inhibitors block reuptake of the neurotransmitters by the transporter proteins, thus resulting in elevated levels of extracellular neurotransmitter. Drugs that inhibit catabolic enzymes promote excess buildup of the neurotransmitter at the synaptic site.

Some drugs cause receptor blockade, thereby resulting in a reduction in transmission and decreased neurotransmitter activity. These drugs are called *antagonists*. Drugs that increase neurotransmitter activity by direct stimulation of the specific receptors are called *agonists*.

TABLE 4-6 Effects of Psychotropic Medications on Neurotransmitters

EXAMPLE OF MEDICATION	ACTION ON NEUROTRANSMITTER AND/OR RECEPTOR	PHYSIOLOGICAL EFFECTS	SIDE EFFECTS
SSRIs	Inhibit reuptake of serotonin (5-HT)	Reduces depression Controls anxiety Controls obsessions	Nausea, agitation, headache, sexual dysfunction
Tricyclic antidepressants	Inhibit reuptake of 5-HT Inhibit reuptake of NE Block NE (α_1) receptor Block ACh receptor Block H_1 receptor	Reduces depression Relief of severe pain Prevent panic attacks	Sexual dysfunction (NE & 5-HT) Sedation, weight gain (H_1) Dry mouth, constipation, blurred vision, urinary retention (ACh) Postural hypotension and tachycardia (α_1)
MAO inhibitors	Increase NE and 5-HT by inhibiting the enzyme that degrades them (MAO-A)	Reduces depression Controls anxiety	Sedation, dizziness Sexual dysfunction Hypertensive crisis (interaction with tyramine)
Trazodone and nefazodone	5-HT reuptake block $5-HT_2$ receptor antagonism Adrenergic receptor blockade	Reduces depression Reduces anxiety	Nausea (5-HT) Sedation ($5-HT_2$) Orthostasis (α_1) Priapism (α_2)
SNRIs: venlafaxine, desvenlafaxine, and duloxetine	Potent inhibitor of serotonin and NE reuptake Weak inhibitor of D reuptake	Reduces depression Relieves pain of neuropathy (duloxetine) Relieves anxiety (venlafaxine)	Nausea (5-HT) ↑ sweating (NE) Insomnia (NE) Tremors (NE) Sexual dysfunction (5-HT)
Bupropion	Inhibits reuptake of NE and D	Reduces depression Aid in smoking cessation ↓ symptoms of ADHD	Insomnia, dry mouth, tremor, seizures
Antipsychotics: phenothiazines and haloperidol	Strong D_2 receptor blockade Weaker blockade of ACh, H_1, α_1-adrenergic, and $5-HT_2$ receptors	Relief of psychosis Relief of anxiety (Some) provide relief from nausea and vomiting and intractable hiccoughs	Blurred vision, dry mouth, decreased sweating, constipation, urinary retention, tachycardia (ACh) EPS (D_2) ↑ plasma prolactin (D_2) Sedation; weight gain (H_1) Ejaculatory difficulty ($5-HT_2$) Postural hypotension (α; H_1)
Antipsychotics (Novel): aripiprazole, asenapine, clozapine, iloperidone, lurasidone, olanzapine, paliperidone, quetiapine, risperidone, ziprasidone	Receptor antagonism of: $5-HT_1$ and $5-HT_2$ $D_1 – D_5$ (varies with drug) H_1 α_1-adrenergic muscarinic (ACh)	Relief of psychosis (with minimal or no EPS) Relief of anxiety Relief of acute mania	Potential with some of the drugs for mild EPS (D_2) Sedation, weight gain (H_1) Orthostasis and dizziness (α-adrenergic) Blurred vision, dry mouth, decreased sweating, constipation, urinary retention, tachycardia (ACh)

Continued

TABLE 4-6 Effects of Psychotropic Medications on Neurotransmitters—cont'd			
EXAMPLE OF MEDICATION	**ACTION ON NEUROTRANSMITTER AND/OR RECEPTOR**	**PHYSIOLOGICAL EFFECTS**	**SIDE EFFECTS**
Antianxiety: benzodiazepines	Binds to BZ receptor sites on the $GABA_A$ receptor complex; increases receptor affinity for GABA	Relief of anxiety Sedation	Dependence (with long-term use) Confusion; memory impairment; motor incoordination
Antianxiety: Buspirone	$5\text{-}HT_{1A}$ agonist D_2 agonist D_2 antagonist	Relief of anxiety	Nausea, headache, dizziness Restlessness

ACh, acetylcholine; ADHD, attention-deficit/hyperactivity disorder; BZ, benzodiazepine; D, dopamine; EPS, extrapyramidal symptoms; GABA, gamma-aminobutyric acid; H, histamine; 5-HT, 5-hydroxytryptamine (serotonin); MAO, monoamine oxidase; NE, norepinephrine; SNRI, serotonin-norepinephrine reuptake inhibitor; SSRI, selective serotonin reuptake inhibitor.

not fully explain how these medications work. Long-term neuropharmacological reactions to increased norepinephrine and serotonin levels relate more to their mechanisms of action. Recent research suggests that the therapeutic effects are related to the nervous system's adaptation to increased levels of neurotransmitters. These adaptive changes result from a homeostatic mechanism, much like a thermostat, that regulates the cell and maintains equilibrium.

Implications for Nursing

The discipline of psychiatric/mental health nursing has always spoken of its role in holistic health care, but historical review reveals that emphasis has been placed on treatment approaches that focus on psychological and social factors. Psychiatric nurses must integrate knowledge of the biological sciences into their practices if they are to ensure safe and effective care to people with mental illness. In the Surgeon General's Report on Mental Health (U.S. Department of Health and Human Services, 1999), Dr. David Satcher wrote:

> The mental health field is far from a complete understanding of the biological, psychological, and sociocultural bases of development, but development clearly involves interplay among these influences. Understanding the process of development requires knowledge, ranging from the most fundamental level—that of gene expression and interactions between molecules and cells—all the way up to the highest levels of cognition, memory, emotion, and language.

The challenge requires integration of concepts from many different disciplines. A fuller understanding of development is not only important in its own right, but it is expected to pave the way for our ultimate understanding of mental health and mental illness and how different factors shape their expression at different stages of the life span. (pp. 61–62)

To ensure a smooth transition from a psychosocial focus to one of biopsychosocial emphasis, nurses must have a clear understanding of the following:

- *Neuroanatomy and neurophysiology:* the structure and functioning of the various parts of the brain and their correlation to human behavior and psychopathology.
- *Neuronal processes:* the various functions of the nerve cells, including the role of neurotransmitters, receptors, synaptic activity, and informational pathways.
- *Neuroendocrinology:* the interaction of the endocrine and nervous systems, and the role that the endocrine glands and their respective hormones play in behavioral functioning.
- *Circadian rhythms:* the regulation of biochemical functioning over periods of rhythmic cycles and its influence in predicting certain behaviors.
- *Genetic influences:* the hereditary factors that predispose individuals to certain psychiatric disorders.
- *Psychoimmunology:* the influence of stress on the immune system and its role in the susceptibility to illness.

■ *Psychopharmacology:* the increasing use of psychotropic drugs in the treatment of mental illness, demanding greater knowledge of psychopharmacological principles and nursing interventions necessary for safe and effective management.

■ *Diagnostic technology:* the importance of keeping informed about the latest in technological procedures for diagnosing alterations in brain structure and function.

Why are these concepts important to the practice of psychiatric/mental health nursing? The interrelationship between psychosocial adaptation and physical functioning has been established. Integrating biological and behavioral concepts into psychiatric nursing practice is essential for nurses to meet the complex needs of clients with mental illness. Psychobiological perspectives must be incorporated into nursing practice, education, and research to attain the evidence-based outcomes necessary for the delivery of competent care.

Summary and Key Points

■ It is important for nurses to understand the interaction between biological and behavioral factors in the development and management of mental illness.

■ Psychobiology is the study of the biological foundations of cognitive, emotional, and behavioral processes.

■ The limbic system has been called "the emotional brain." It is associated with feelings of fear and anxiety; anger, rage, and aggression; love, joy, and hope; and with sexuality and social behavior.

■ The three classes of neurons include afferent (sensory), efferent (motor), and interneurons. The junction between two neurons is called a synapse.

■ Neurotransmitters are chemicals that convey information across synaptic clefts to neighboring target cells. Many neurotransmitters have implications in the etiology of emotional disorders and in the pharmacological treatment of those disorders.

■ Major categories of neurotransmitters include cholinergics, monoamines, amino acids, and neuropeptides.

■ The endocrine system plays an important role in human behavior through the hypothalamic-pituitary axis.

■ Hormones and their circadian rhythm of regulation significantly influence a number of physiological and psychological life cycle phenomena, such as moods, sleep and arousal, stress response, appetite, libido, and fertility.

■ Research continues to validate the role of genetics in psychiatric illness.

■ Familial, twin, and adoption studies suggest that genetics may be implicated in the etiology of schizophrenia, bipolar disorder, depression, panic disorder, anorexia nervosa, alcoholism, and obsessive-compulsive disorder.

■ Psychoimmunology examines the impact of psychological factors on the immune system.

■ Evidence exists to support a link between psychosocial stressors and suppression of the immune response.

■ Technologies such as magnetic resonance imaging (MRI), computed tomography (CT) scanning, positron emission tomography (PET), and electroencephalography (EEG) are used as diagnostic tools for detecting alterations in psychobiological functioning.

■ Psychotropic medications have given many individuals a chance to function effectively.

■ Nurses must understand the ethical and legal implications associated with the administration of psychotropic medications, and have knowledge of the physiological mechanisms by which psychotropic medications exert their effects.

■ Integrating knowledge of the expanding biological focus into psychiatric nursing is essential if nurses are to meet the changing needs of today's psychiatric clients.

 Davis*Plus*   Additional info available @ davisplus.fadavis.com

Review Questions
Self-Examination/Learning Exercise

*Select the answer that is **most** appropriate for each of the following questions:*

1. Which of the following parts of the brain is associated with multiple feelings and behaviors and is sometimes referred to as the "emotional brain?"
   a. Frontal lobe.
   b. Thalamus.
   c. Hypothalamus.
   d. Limbic system.

2. Which of the following parts of the brain is concerned with visual reception and interpretation?
   a. Frontal lobe.
   b. Parietal lobe.
   c. Temporal lobe.
   d. Occipital lobe.

3. Which of the following parts of the brain is associated with voluntary body movement, thinking and judgment, and expression of feeling?
   a. Frontal lobe.
   b. Parietal lobe.
   c. Temporal lobe.
   d. Occipital lobe.

4. Which of the following parts of the brain integrates all sensory input (except smell) on the way to the cortex?
   a. Temporal lobe.
   b. Thalamus.
   c. Limbic system.
   d. Hypothalamus.

5. Which of the following parts of the brain deals with sensory perception and interpretation?
   a. Hypothalamus.
   b. Cerebellum.
   c. Parietal lobe.
   d. Hippocampus.

6. Which of the following parts of the brain is concerned with hearing, short-term memory, and sense of smell?
   a. Temporal lobe.
   b. Parietal lobe.
   c. Cerebellum.
   d. Hypothalamus.

7. Which of the following parts of the brain has control over the pituitary gland and autonomic nervous system, as well as regulating appetite and temperature?
   a. Temporal lobe.
   b. Parietal lobe.
   c. Cerebellum.
   d. Hypothalamus.

Review Questions—cont'd
Self-Examination/Learning Exercise

8. At a synapse, the determination of further impulse transmission is accomplished by means of which of the following?
   a. Potassium ions.
   b. Interneurons.
   c. Neurotransmitters.
   d. The myelin sheath.

9. A decrease in which of the following neurotransmitters has been implicated in depression?
   a. GABA, acetylcholine, and aspartate.
   b. Norepinephrine, serotonin, and dopamine.
   c. Somatostatin, substance P, and glycine.
   d. Glutamate, histamine, and opioid peptides.

10. Which of the following hormones has been implicated in the etiology of mood disorder with seasonal pattern?
    a. Increased levels of melatonin.
    b. Decreased levels of oxytocin.
    c. Decreased levels of prolactin.
    d. Increased levels of thyrotropin.

11. Psychotropic medications that block the reuptake of serotonin may result in which of the following side effects?
    a. Dry mouth.
    b. Constipation.
    c. Blurred vision.
    d. Sexual dysfunction.

12. Psychotropic medications that block the acetylcholine receptor may result in which of the following side effects?
    a. Dry mouth.
    b. Sexual dysfunction.
    c. Nausea.
    d. Priapism.

13. Psychotropic medications that are strong blockers of the D_2 receptor are more likely to result in which of the following side effects?
    a. Sedation.
    b. Urinary retention.
    c. Extrapyramidal symptoms.
    d. Hypertensive crisis.

References

Baker, C. (2004). *Behavioral genetics*. Washington, DC: American Association for the Advancement of Science.

Black, D. W., & Andreasen, N. C. (2011). Introductory textbook of psychiatry (5th ed.). Washington, DC: American Psychiatric Publishing.

Dubovsky, S. L., Davies, R., & Dubovsky, A. N. (2003). Mood disorders. In R. E. Hales & S. C. Yudofsky (Eds.), *Textbook of clinical psychiatry* (4th ed., pp. 439–542). Washington, DC: American Psychiatric Publishing.

Gill, M. (2004). Genetic approaches to the understanding of mental illness. *Genes and Mental Health*. Public symposium, October 9, 2004, Department of Psychiatry. Dublin: Trinity College.

Gilman, S., & Newman, S. W. (2003). *Essentials of clinical neuroanatomy and neurophysiology* (10th ed.). Philadelphia: F.A. Davis.

Hamosh, A., Scharer, G., & Van Hove, J. (2009). Glycine encephalopathy. *GeneReviews*. National Library of

Medicine. Retrieved April 30, 2010, from http://www.ncbi.nlm.nih.gov/bookshelf/br.fcgi?book=gene&part=nkh

Hughes, M. (1989). *Body clock: The effects of time on human health*. New York: Andromeda Oxford Ltd.

Irwin, M. (2000). Psychoneuroimmunology of depression. In F.E. Bloom & D.J. Kupfer (Eds.), *Psychopharmacology—the fourth generation of progress*. Nashville, TN: American College of Neuropsychopharmacology.

Knowles, J. A. (2003). Genetics. In R. E. Hales & S. C. Yudofsky (Eds.), *Textbook of psychiatry* (4th ed., pp. 3–66). Washington, DC: American Psychiatric Publishing.

Lis, C. G., Grutsch, J. F., Wood, P., You, M., Rich, I., & Hrushesky, W. J. (2003). Circadian timing in cancer treatment: The biological foundation for an integrative approach. *Integrative Cancer Therapies, 2*(2), 105–111.

McInerney, J. (2008). Behavioral genetics. *The Human Genome Project*. Retrieved May 2, 2010, from http://www.ornl.gov/sci/techresources/HumanGenome/elsi/behavior.shtml

National Institute on Aging. (2009). The Alzheimer's Disease Education and Referral Center. *Alzheimer's disease genetics.* Retrieved May 2, 2010, from http://www.nia.nih.gov/Alzheimers/Publications/geneticsfs.htm

Sadock, B. J., & Sadock, V. A. (2007). *Synopsis of psychiatry: Behavioral sciences/clinical psychiatry* (10th ed.). Philadelphia: Lippincott Williams & Wilkins.

Sage, D.L. (Producer). (1984). *The brain: Madness* [Television broadcast]. Washington, DC: Public Broadcasting Company.

Scanlon, V. C., & Sanders, T. (2011). *Essentials of anatomy and physiology* (6th ed.). Philadelphia: F.A. Davis.

Skudaev, S. (2010). The neurophysiology and neurochemistry of sleep. Retrieved May 2, 2010, from http://www.healthstairs.com/sleep3.php

U.S. Department of Health and Human Services. (1999). *Mental health: A report of the Surgeon General—executive summary.* Rockville, MD: U.S. Department of Health and Human Services.

Van Cauter, E., Kerkhofs, M., Caufriez, A., Van Onderbergen, A., Thorner, M. O., & Copinschi, G. (1992). A quantitative estimation of growth hormone secretion in normal man: Reproducibility and relation to sleep and time of day. *Journal of Clinical Endocrinology and Metabolism, 74,* 1441–1450.

Ethical and Legal Issues in Psychiatric/Mental Health Nursing

CHAPTER 5

KARYN I. MORGAN AND MARY C. TOWNSEND

CORE CONCEPTS

bioethics

ethics

moral behavior

right

values

values clarification

KEY TERMS

assault	ethical dilemma	negligence
autonomy	ethical egoism	nonmaleficence
battery	false imprisonment	privileged communication
beneficence	informed consent	slander
Christian ethics	justice	statutory law
civil law	Kantianism	tort
common law	libel	utilitarianism
criminal law	malpractice	veracity
defamation of character	natural law	

OBJECTIVES

After reading this chapter, the student will be able to:

1. Differentiate among *ethics, morals, values,* and *rights.*
2. Discuss ethical theories including utilitarianism, Kantianism, Christian ethics, natural law theories, and ethical egoism.
3. Define *ethical dilemma.*
4. Discuss the ethical principles of autonomy, beneficence, nonmaleficence, justice, and veracity.
5. Use an ethical decision-making model to make an ethical decision.
6. Describe ethical issues relevant to psychiatric/mental health nursing.
7. Define *statutory law* and *common law.*
8. Differentiate between civil and criminal law.
9. Discuss legal issues relevant to psychiatric/mental health nursing.
10. Differentiate between *malpractice* and *negligence.*
11. Identify behaviors relevant to the psychiatric/mental health setting for which specific malpractice action could be taken.

HOMEWORK ASSIGNMENT

Please read the chapter and answer the following questions:

1. Malpractice and negligence are examples of what kind of law?
2. What charges may be brought against a nurse for confining a client against his or her wishes (outside of an emergency situation)?
3. Which ethical theory espouses that what is right and good is what is best for the individual making the decision?
4. Name the three major elements of informed consent.

Nurses are constantly faced with the challenge of making difficult decisions regarding good and evil or life and death. Complex situations frequently arise in caring for individuals with mental illness, and nurses are held to the highest level of legal and ethical accountability in their professional practice. This chapter presents basic ethical and legal concepts and their relationship to psychiatric/mental health nursing. A discussion of ethical theory is presented as a foundation upon which ethical decisions may be made. The American Nurses Association (ANA) (2001) has established a code of ethics for nurses to use as a framework within which to make ethical choices and decisions (Box 5-1).

Because legislation determines what is *right* or *good* within a society, legal issues pertaining to psychiatric/mental health nursing are also discussed in this chapter. Definitions are presented, along with rights of psychiatric clients of which nurses must be aware. Nursing competency and client care accountability are compromised when the nurse has inadequate knowledge about the laws that regulate the practice of nursing.

Knowledge of the legal and ethical concepts presented in this chapter will enhance the quality of care the nurse provides in his or her psychiatric/mental health nursing practice and will also protect the nurse within the parameters of legal accountability. Indeed, the very right to practice nursing carries with it the responsibility to maintain a specific level of competency and to practice in accordance with certain ethical and legal standards of care.

CORE CONCEPTS

Ethics is a branch of philosophy that deals with systematic approaches to distinguishing right from wrong behavior (Butts & Rich, 2008). **Bioethics** is the term applied to these principles when they refer to concepts within the scope of medicine, nursing, and allied health.

Moral behavior is defined as conduct that results from serious critical thinking about how individuals ought to treat others. Moral behavior reflects the way a person interprets basic respect for other persons, such as the respect for autonomy, freedom, justice, honesty, and confidentiality (Pappas, 2006).

Values are personal beliefs about what is important and desirable (Butts & Rich, 2008). **Values clarification** is a process of self-exploration through which individuals identify and rank their own personal values. This process increases awareness about why individuals behave in certain ways. Values clarification is important in nursing to increase understanding about why certain choices and decisions are made over others and how values affect nursing outcomes.

A **right** is defined as, "a valid, legally recognized claim or entitlement, encompassing both freedom from government interference or discriminatory treatment and an entitlement to a benefit or service" (Levy & Rubenstein, 1996). A right is *absolute* when there is no restriction whatsoever on the individual's entitlement. A *legal right* is one on which the society has agreed and formalized into law. Both the National League for Nursing (NLN) and the American Hospital Association (AHA) have established guidelines of patients' rights. Although these are not considered legal documents, nurses and hospitals are considered responsible for upholding these rights of patients.

BOX 5-1 American Nurses' Association Code of Ethics for Nurses

1. The nurse, in all professional relationships, practices with compassion and respect for the inherent dignity, worth and uniqueness of every individual, unrestricted by consideration of social or economic status, personal attributes, or the nature of health problems.
2. The nurse's primary commitment is to the patient whether an individual, family, group or community.
3. The nurse promotes, advocates for and strives to protect the health, safety, and rights of the patient.
4. The nurse is responsible and accountable for individual nursing practice and determines the appropriate delegation of tasks consistent with the nurse's obligation to provide optimum patient care.
5. The nurse owes the same duties to self as to others, including the responsibility to preserve integrity and safety, to maintain competence, and to continue personal and professional growth.
6. The nurse participates in establishing, maintaining, and improving healthcare environments and conditions of employment conducive to the provision of quality healthcare and consistent with the values of the profession through individual and collective action.
7. The nurse participates in the advancement of the profession through contributions to practice, education, administration, and knowledge development.
8. The nurse collaborates with other health professionals and the public in promoting community, national, and international efforts to meet health needs.
9. The profession of nursing, as represented by associations and their members, is responsible for articulating nursing values, for maintaining the integrity of the profession and its practice, and for shaping social policy.

Ethical Considerations

Theoretical Perspectives

An *ethical theory* is a moral principle or a set of moral principles that can be used in assessing what is morally right or morally wrong (Ellis & Hartley, 2008). These principles provide guidelines for ethical decision making.

Utilitarianism

The basis of **utilitarianism** is "the greatest-happiness principle." This principle holds that actions are right to the degree that they tend to promote happiness and wrong as they tend to produce the reverse of happiness. Thus, the good is happiness and the right is that which promotes the good. Conversely, the wrongness of an action is determined by its tendency to bring about unhappiness. An ethical decision based on the utilitarian view looks at the end results of the decision. Action is taken based on the end results that produced the most good (happiness) for the most people.

Kantianism

Named for philosopher Immanuel Kant, **Kantianism** is directly opposed to utilitarianism. Kant argued that it is not the consequences or end results that make an action right or wrong; rather it is the principle or motivation on which the action is based that is the morally decisive factor. Kantianism suggests that our actions are bound by a sense of duty. This theory is often called *deontology* (from the Greek word *deon,* which means "that which is binding; duty"). Kantian-directed ethical decisions are made out of respect for moral law. For example, "I make this choice because it is morally right and my duty to do so" (not because of consideration for a possible outcome).

Christian Ethics

This approach to ethical decision making is focused on the way of life and teachings of Jesus Christ. It advances the importance of virtues such as love, forgiveness, and honesty. One basic principle often associated with Christian ethics is known as the golden rule: "Do unto others as you would have them do unto you." The imperative demand of **Christian ethics** is that all decisions about right and wrong should be centered in love for God and in treating others with the same respect and dignity with which we would expect to be treated.

Natural Law Theory

Natural law theory is based on the writings of St. Thomas Aquinas. It advances the idea that decisions about right versus wrong are self-evident and determined by human nature. The theory espouses that, as rational human beings, we inherently know the difference between good and evil (believed to be knowledge that is given to man from God), and this knowledge directs our decision making.

Ethical Egoism

Ethical egoism espouses that what is right and good is what is best for the individual making the decision. An individual's actions are determined by what is to his or her own advantage. The action may not be best for anyone else involved, but consideration is only for the individual making the decision.

Ethical Dilemmas

An **ethical dilemma** is a situation that requires an individual to make a choice between two equally unfavorable alternatives (Catalano, 2009). Evidence exists to support both moral "rightness" and moral "wrongness" related to a certain action. The individual who must make the choice experiences conscious conflict regarding the decision.

Not all ethical issues are dilemmas. An ethical dilemma arises when there is no clear reason to choose one action over another. Ethical dilemmas generally create a great deal of emotion. Often the reasons supporting each side of the argument for action are logical and appropriate. The actions associated with both sides are desirable in some respects and undesirable in others. In most situations, taking no action is considered an action taken.

Ethical Principles

Ethical principles are fundamental guidelines that influence decision making. The ethical principles of autonomy, beneficence, nonmaleficence, veracity, and justice are helpful and used frequently by health-care workers to assist with ethical decision making.

Autonomy

The principle of **autonomy** arises from the Kantian duty of respect for persons as rational agents. This viewpoint emphasizes the status of persons as autonomous moral agents whose right to determine their destinies should always be respected. This presumes that individuals are always capable of making independent choices for themselves. Health-care workers know this is not always the case. Children, comatose individuals, and the seriously mentally ill are examples of clients who are incapable of making informed choices. In these instances, a representative of the individual is usually asked to intervene and give consent. However, health-care workers must ensure that respect for an individual's autonomy is not disregarded in favor of what another person may view as best for the client.

Beneficence

Beneficence refers to one's duty to benefit or promote the good of others. Health-care workers who act in their clients' interests are beneficent, provided their actions really do serve the client's best interest. In fact, some duties do seem to take preference over other duties. For example, the duty to respect the autonomy of an individual may be overridden when that individual has been deemed harmful to self or others. Aiken (2004) stated, "The difficulty that sometimes arises in implementing the principle of beneficence lies in determining what exactly is good for another and who can best make that decision."

Peplau (1991) recognized client advocacy as an essential role for the psychiatric nurse. The term *advocacy* means acting in another's behalf—being a supporter or defender. Being a client advocate in psychiatric nursing means helping clients fulfill needs that, without assistance and because of their illness, may go unfulfilled. Individuals with mental illness are not always able to speak for themselves. Nurses serve in this manner to protect their clients' rights and interests. Strategies include educating clients and their families about their legal rights, ensuring that clients have sufficient information to make informed decisions or to give informed consent, and assisting clients to consider alternatives and supporting them in the decisions they make. Additionally, nurses may act as advocates by speaking on behalf of individuals with mental illness to secure essential mental health services.

Nonmaleficence

Nonmaleficence is the requirement that health-care providers do no harm to their clients, either intentionally or unintentionally (Aiken, 2004). Some philosophers suggest that this principle is more important than beneficence; that is, they support the notion that it is more important to avoid doing harm than it is to do good. In any event, ethical dilemmas often arise when a conflict exists between an individual's rights and what is thought to best represent the welfare of the individual. An example of this conflict might occur when a psychiatric client refuses antipsychotic medication (consistent with his or her rights), and the nurse must then decide how to maintain client safety while psychotic symptoms continue.

Justice

The principle of **justice** has been referred to as the "justice as fairness" principle. It is sometimes referred to as *distributive justice,* and its basic premise lies with the right of individuals to be treated equally regardless of race, sex, marital status, medical diagnosis, social standing, economic level, or religious belief (Aiken, 2004). The concept of justice reflects a duty to treat all individuals equally and fairly. When applied to health care, this principle suggests that all resources within the society (including health-care services) ought to be distributed evenly without respect to socioeconomic status. Thus, according to this principle, the vast disparity in the quality of care dispensed to the various classes within our society would be considered unjust. A more equitable distribution of care for all individuals would be favored.

Veracity

The principle of **veracity** refers to one's duty to always be truthful. Aiken (2004) stated, "Veracity requires that the health care provider tell the truth and not intentionally deceive or mislead clients." There are times when limitations must be placed on this principle, such as when the truth would knowingly produce harm or interfere with the recovery process. Being honest is not always easy, but rarely is lying justified. Clients have the right to know about their diagnosis, treatment, and prognosis.

A Model for Making Ethical Decisions

The following is a set of steps that may be used in making an ethical decision. These steps closely resemble the steps of the nursing process.

1. **Assessment:** Gather the subjective and objective data about a situation. Consider personal values as well as values of others involved in the ethical dilemma.

2. **Problem Identification:** Identify the conflict between two or more alternative actions.

3. **Planning:**
   a. Explore the benefits and consequences of each alternative.
   b. Consider principles of ethical theories.
   c. Select an alternative.

4. **Implementation:** Act on the decision made and communicate the decision to others.

5. **Evaluation:** Evaluate outcomes.

A schematic of this model is presented in Figure 5–1. A case study using this decision-making model is presented in Box 5-2. If the outcome is acceptable, action continues in the manner selected.

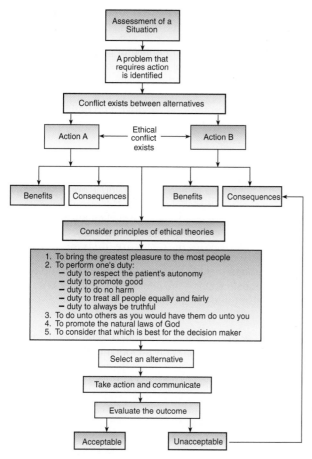

FIGURE 5–1   Ethical decision-making model.

If the outcome is unacceptable, benefits and consequences of the remaining alternatives are reexamined, and steps 3 through 7 in Box 5-2 are repeated.

Ethical Issues in Psychiatric/Mental Health Nursing

The Right to Refuse Medication

The AHA's (1992) Patient's Bill of Rights states: "The patient has the right to refuse treatment to the extent permitted by law, and to be informed of the medical consequences of his action." In psychiatry, refusal of treatment primarily concerns the administration of psychotropic medications. "To the extent permitted by law" may be defined within the U.S. Constitution and several of its amendments (e.g., the First Amendment, which addresses the rights of speech, thought, and expression; the Eighth Amendment, which grants the right to freedom from cruel and unusual punishment; and the Fifth and Fourteenth Amendments, which grant due process of law and equal protection for all). In psychiatry, "the medical consequences of his action" may include such steps as involuntary commitment, legal competency hearing, or client discharge from the hospital.

Although many courts are supporting a client's right to refuse medications in the psychiatric area,

---

BOX 5-2 Ethical Decision Making—A Case Study

STEP 1. ASSESSMENT

Tonja is a 17-year-old girl who is currently on the psychiatric unit with a diagnosis of conduct disorder. Tonja reports that she has been sexually active since she was 14. She had an abortion when she was 15 and a second one just 6 weeks ago. She states that her mother told her she has "had her last abortion," and that she has to start taking birth control pills. She asks her nurse, Kimberly, to give her some information about the pills and to tell her how to go about getting some. Kimberly believes Tonja desperately needs information about birth control pills, as well as other types of contraceptives, but the psychiatric unit is part of a Catholic hospital, and hospital policy prohibits distributing this type of information.

STEP 2. PROBLEM IDENTIFICATION

A conflict exists between the client's need for information, the nurse's desire to provide that information, and the institution's policy prohibiting the provision of that information.

STEP 3. ALTERNATIVES—BENEFITS AND CONSEQUENCES

1. Alternative 1: Give the client information and risk losing job.
2. Alternative 2: Do not give client information and compromise own values of holistic nursing.
3. Alternative 3: Refer client to another source outside the hospital and risk reprimand from supervisor.

STEP 4. CONSIDER PRINCIPLES OF ETHICAL THEORIES

1. Alternative 1: Giving the client information would certainly respect the client's autonomy and would benefit the client by decreasing her chances of becoming pregnant again. It would not be to the best advantage of Kimberly, in that she would likely lose her job. And according to the beliefs of the Catholic hospital, the natural laws of God would be violated.

Continued

BOX 5-2 Ethical Decision Making—A Case Study—cont'd

2. Alternative 2: Withholding information restricts the client's autonomy. It has the potential for doing harm, in that without the use of contraceptives, the client may become pregnant again (and she implies that this is not what she wants). Kimberly's Christian ethic is violated in that this action is not what she would want "done unto her."

3. Alternative 3: A referral would respect the client's autonomy, would promote good, would do no harm (except perhaps to Kimberly's ego from the possible reprimand), and this decision would comply with Kimberly's Christian ethic.

STEP 5. SELECT AN ALTERNATIVE

Alternative 3 is selected based on the ethical theories of utilitarianism (does the most good for the greatest number), Christian ethics (Kimberly's belief of "Do unto others as you would have others do unto you"), and Kantianism (to perform one's duty), and the ethical principles of autonomy, beneficence, and nonmaleficence. The success of this decision depends on the client's follow-through with the referral and compliance with use of the contraceptives.

STEP 6. TAKE ACTION AND COMMUNICATE

Taking action involves providing information in writing for Tonja, perhaps making a phone call and setting up an appointment for her with Planned Parenthood. Communicating suggests sharing the information with Tonja's mother. Communication also includes documentation of the referral in the client's chart.

STEP 7. EVALUATE THE OUTCOME

An acceptable outcome might indicate that Tonja did indeed keep her appointment at Planned Parenthood and is complying with the prescribed contraceptive regimen. It might also include Kimberly's input into the change process in her institution to implement these types of referrals to other clients who request them.

An unacceptable outcome might be indicated by Tonja's lack of follow-through with the appointment at Planned Parenthood or lack of compliance in using the contraceptives, resulting in another pregnancy. Kimberly may also view a reprimand from her supervisor as an unacceptable outcome, particularly if she is told that she must select other alternatives should this situation arise in the future. This may motivate Kimberly to make another decision–that of seeking employment in an institution that supports a philosophy more consistent with her own.

---

some limitations do exist. Weiss-Kaffie and Purtell (2001) stated:

> The treatment team must determine that three criteria be met to force medication without client consent. The client must exhibit behavior that is dangerous to self or others; the medication ordered by the physician must have a reasonable chance of providing help to the client; and clients who refuse medication must be judged incompetent to evaluate the benefits of the treatment in question. (p. 361)

The Right to the Least-Restrictive Treatment Alternative

Health-care personnel must attempt to provide treatment in a manner that least restricts the freedom of clients. The "restrictiveness" of psychiatric therapy can be described in the context of a continuum, based on severity of illness. Clients may be treated on an outpatient basis, in day hospitals, or through voluntary or involuntary hospitalization. Symptoms may be treated with verbal rehabilitative techniques and move successively to behavioral techniques, chemical interventions, seclusion, mechanical restraints, or electroconvulsive therapy. The problem appears to arise in selecting the least restrictive means among involuntary chemical intervention, seclusion, and mechanical restraints. Sadock and Sadock (2007) stated:

> Distinguishing among these interventions on the basis of restrictiveness proves to be a purely subjective exercise fraught with personal bias. Moreover, each of these three interventions is both more and less restrictive than each of the other two. Nevertheless, the effort should be made to think in terms of restrictiveness when deciding how to treat patients. (p. 1376)

Legal Considerations

In 1980, the 96th Congress of the United States passed the Mental Health Systems Act, which includes a Patient's Bill of Rights, for recommendation to the States. An adaptation of these rights is presented in Box 5-3.

Nurse Practice Acts

The legal parameters of professional and practical nursing are defined within each state by the state's nurse practice act. These documents are passed by the state legislature and in general are concerned with such provisions as the following:

- The definition of important terms, including the definition of nursing and the various types of nurses recognized

- A statement of the education and other training or requirements for licensure and reciprocity

- Broad statements that describe the scope of practice for various levels of nursing (APN, RN, LPN)

- Conditions under which a nurse's license may be suspended or revoked, and instructions for appeal

- The general authority and powers of the state board of nursing (Fedorka & Resnick, 2001).

Most nurse practice acts are general in their terminology, and do not provide specific guidelines for practice. Nurses must understand the scope of practice that is protected by their license, and should seek assistance from legal counsel if they are unsure about the proper interpretation of a nurse practice act.

Types of Law

There are two general categories or types of law that are of most concern to nurses: statutory law and common law. These laws are identified by their source or origin.

Statutory Law

A **statutory law** is a law that has been enacted by a legislative body, such as a county or city council, state legislature, or the U.S. Congress. An example of statutory law is the nurse practice acts.

Common Law

Common laws are derived from decisions made in previous cases. These laws apply to a body of principles that evolve from court decisions resolving various controversies. Because common law in the United States has been developed on a state basis, the law on specific subjects may differ from state to state. An example of a common law might be how different states deal with a nurse's refusal to provide care for a specific client.

Classifications Within Statutory and Common Law

Broadly speaking, there are two kinds of unlawful acts: civil and criminal. Both statutory

---

BOX 5-3 **Bill of Rights for Psychiatric Patients**

1. The right to appropriate treatment and related services in the setting that is most supportive and least restrictive to personal freedom.
2. The right to an individualized, written treatment or service plan; the right to treatment based on such a plan; and the right to periodic review and revision of the plan based on treatment needs.
3. The right, consistent with one's capabilities, to participate in and receive a reasonable explanation of the care and treatment process.
4. The right to refuse treatment except in an emergency situation or as permitted by law.
5. The right not to participate in experimentation in the absence of informed, voluntary, written consent.
6. The right to freedom from restraint or seclusion except in an emergency situation.
7. The right to a humane treatment environment that affords reasonable protection from harm and appropriate privacy.
8. The right to confidentiality of medical records (also applicable following patient's discharge).
9. The right of access to medical records except information received from third parties under promise of confidentiality, and when access would be detrimental to the patient's health (also applicable following patient's discharge).
10. The right of access to use of the telephone, personal mail, and visitors, unless deemed inappropriate for treatment purposes.
11. The right to be informed of these rights in comprehensible language.
12. The right to assert grievances if rights are infringed.
13. The right to referral as appropriate to other providers of mental health services upon discharge.

Adapted from Mental Health Systems Act, Pub. L. No. 96-398, Title V, § 501.94, Stat. 1598 (1980).

law and common law have civil and criminal components.

Civil Law

Civil law protects the private and property rights of individuals and businesses. Private individuals or groups may bring a legal action to court for breach of civil law. These legal actions are of two basic types: torts and contracts.

Torts

A **tort** is a violation of a civil law in which an individual has been wronged. In a tort action, one party asserts that wrongful conduct on the part of the other has caused harm, and seeks compensation for harm suffered. A tort may be *intentional* or *unintentional*. Examples of unintentional torts are malpractice and negligence actions. An example of an intentional tort is the touching of another person without that person's consent. Intentional touching (e.g., a medical treatment) without the client's consent can result in a charge of battery, an intentional tort.

Contracts

In a contract action, one party asserts that the other party, in failing to fulfill an obligation, has breached the contract, and either compensation or performance of the obligation is sought as remedy. An example is an action by a mental health professional whose clinical privileges have been reduced or terminated in violation of an implied contract between the professional and a hospital.

Criminal Law

Criminal law provides protection from conduct deemed injurious to the public welfare. It provides for punishment of those found to have engaged in such conduct, which commonly includes imprisonment, parole conditions, a loss of privilege (such as a license), a fine, or any combination of these (Ellis & Hartley, 2008). An example of a violation of criminal law is the theft by a hospital employee of supplies or drugs.

Legal Issues in Psychiatric/Mental Health Nursing

Confidentiality and Right to Privacy

The Fourth, Fifth, and Fourteenth Amendments to the U.S. Constitution protect an individual's privacy. Most states have statutes protecting the confidentiality of client records and communications. The only individuals who have a right to observe a client or have access to medical information are those involved in his or her medical care.

HIPPA

Until 1996, client confidentiality in medical records was not protected by federal law. In August 1996, President Clinton signed the Health Insurance Portability and Accountability Act (HIPAA) into law. Under this law, individuals have the rights to access their medical records, to have corrections made to their medical records, and to decide with whom their medical information may be shared. The actual document belongs to the facility or the therapist, but the information contained therein belongs to the client.

This federal privacy rule pertains to data that is called *protected health information* (PHI) and applies to most individuals and institutions involved in health care. Notice of privacy policies must be provided to clients upon entry into the health-care system. PHI is individually identifiable health information indicators that "relate to past, present, or future physical or mental health or condition of the individual, or the past, present, or future payment for the provision of health care to an individual; and (1) that identifies the individual; or (2) with respect to which there is a reasonable basis to believe the information can be used to identify the individual" (U.S. Department of Health and Human Services, 2003). These specific identifiers are listed in Box 5-4.

Pertinent medical information may be released without consent in a life-threatening situation. If information is released in an emergency, the following information must be recorded in the client's record: date of disclosure, person to whom information was disclosed, reason for disclosure, reason written consent could not be obtained, and the specific information disclosed.

Most states have statutes that pertain to the doctrine of **privileged communication.** Although the codes differ markedly from state to state, most grant certain professionals privileges under which they may refuse to reveal information about, and communications with, clients. In most states, the doctrine of privileged communication applies to psychiatrists and attorneys; in some instances, psychologists, clergy, and nurses are also included.

In certain instances nurses may be called on to testify in cases in which the medical record is used as evidence. In most states, the right to privacy of these records is exempted in civil or criminal proceedings. Therefore, it is important that nurses document with these possibilities in mind. Strict record-keeping using statements that are objective and nonjudgmental, having care plans that are specific in their prescriptive interventions, and keeping documentation that describes those interventions

BOX 5-4 **Protected Health Information (PIH): Individually Identifiable Indicators**

1. Names
2. Postal address information, (except state), including street address, city, county, precinct, and zip code
3. All elements of dates (except year) for dates directly related to an individual, including birth date, admission date, discharge date, date of death; and all ages over 89 and all elements of dates (including year) indicative of such age, except that such ages and elements may be aggregated into a single category of age 90 or older
4. Telephone numbers
5. Fax numbers
6. Electronic mail addresses
7. Social Security numbers
8. Medical record numbers
9. Health plan beneficiary numbers
10. Account numbers
11. Certificate/license numbers
12. Vehicle identifiers and serial numbers, including license plate numbers
13. Device identifiers and serial numbers
14. Web Universal Resource Locators (URLs)
15. Internet protocol (IP) address numbers
16. Biometric identifiers, including finger and voice prints
17. Full face photographic images and any comparable images
18. Any other unique identifying number, characteristic, or code

From U.S. Department of Health and Human Services. (2003). Standards for privacy of individually identifiable health information. Washington, DC: Author.

and their subsequent evaluation all serve the best interests of the client, the nurse, and the institution should questions regarding care arise. Documentation very often weighs heavily in malpractice case decisions.

The right to confidentiality is a basic one, and especially so in psychiatry. Although societal attitudes are improving, individuals have experienced discrimination in the past for no other reason than for having a history of emotional illness. Nurses working in psychiatry must guard the privacy of their clients with great diligence.

Exception: A Duty to Warn (Protection of a Third Party)

There are exceptions to the laws of privacy and confidentiality. One of these exceptions stems from the 1974 case of *Tarasoff v. Regents of the University of California*. The incident from which this case evolved came about in the late 1960s. A young man from Bengal, India (Mr. P.), who was a graduate student at the University of California (UC), Berkeley, fell in love with another university student (Ms. Tarasoff). Because she was not interested in an exclusive relationship with Mr. P., he became very resentful and angry. He began to stalk her and to record some of their conversations in an effort to determine why she didn't love him. He

soon became very depressed and neglected his health, appearance, and studies.

Ms. Tarasoff spent the summer of 1969 in South America. During this time Mr. P. entered therapy with a psychologist at UC. He confided in the psychologist that he intended to kill his former girlfriend (identifying her by name) when she returned from vacation. The psychologist recommended civil commitment for Mr. P., claiming he was suffering from acute and severe paranoid schizophrenia. Mr. P. was picked up by the campus police but released a short time later because he appeared rational and promised to stay away from Ms. Tarasoff. Neither Ms. Tarasoff nor her parents received any warning of the threat of Mr. P.'s intention to kill her.

When Ms. Tarasoff returned to campus in October 1969, Mr. P. resumed his stalking behavior and eventually stabbed her to death. Ms. Tarasoff's parents sued the psychologist, several psychiatrists, and the university for failure to warn. The case was referred to the California Supreme Court, which ruled that a mental health professional has a duty not only to a client, but also to individuals who are being threatened by that client. The Court stated:

Once a therapist does in fact determine, or under applicable professional standards should have determined, that a patient poses a serious danger of violence to others, he bears a duty to exercise reasonable care to protect the foreseeable victim of that danger. While the discharge of this duty of due care will necessarily vary with the facts of each case, in each instance the adequacy of the therapist's conduct must be measured against the traditional negligence standard of reasonable care under the circumstances. (*Tarasoff v. Regents of University of California,* 1974a)

The defendants argued that warning the woman or her family would have breached professional ethics and violated the client's right to privacy. But the court ruled that "the confidential character of patient-psychotherapist communications must yield to the extent that disclosure is essential to avert danger to others. The protective privilege ends where the public peril begins" (*Tarasoff v. Regents of University of California,* 1974b).

In 1976, the California Supreme Court expanded the original case ruling (now referred to as *Tarasoff I*). The second ruling (known as *Tarasoff II*) broadened the ruling of "duty to warn" to include "duty to protect." They stated that, under certain circumstances, a therapist might be required to warn an individual, notify police, or take whatever steps are necessary to protect the intended victim from harm. This duty to protect can also "occur in instances when patients, because of their vulnerable state and their inability to distinguish potentially harmful situations, must be protected by healthcare providers" (Guido, 2006, p. 383).

The Tarasoff rulings created a great deal of controversy in the psychiatric community regarding breach of confidentiality and the subsequent negative impact on the client-therapist relationship. However, most states now recognize that therapists have ethical and legal obligations to prevent their clients from harming themselves or others. Many states have passed their own variations on the original "protect and warn" legislation, but in most cases, courts have outlined the following guidelines for therapists to follow in determining their obligation to take protective measures:

1. Assessment of a threat of violence by a client toward another individual

2. Identification of the intended victim

3. Ability to intervene in a feasible, meaningful way to protect the intended victim

When these guidelines apply to a specific situation, it is reasonable for the therapist to notify the victim, law enforcement authorities, and/or relatives of the intended victim, and/or to initiate voluntary or involuntary commitment of the client in an effort to prevent potential violence.

Implications for Nursing Advanced practice psychiatric nurses who are licensed to practice independently would be held to the same duty as other therapists. Generalist psychiatric nurses who are not acting independently, but rather under the supervision of a psychiatrist, nevertheless have a responsibility to protect a third party who is being threatened by the client. If a client confides in the nurse the potential for harm to an intended victim, it is the duty of the nurse to report this information to the psychiatrist or to other team members. This is not a breach of confidentiality, and the nurse may be considered negligent for failure to do so. All members of the treatment team must be made aware of the potential danger that the client poses to self or others. Detailed written documentation of the situation is also essential.

Informed Consent

According to law, all individuals have the right to decide whether to accept or reject treatment. A health-care provider can be charged with assault and battery for providing life-sustaining treatment to a client when the client has not agreed to it. The rationale for the doctrine of **informed consent** is the preservation and protection of individual autonomy in determining what will and will not happen to the person's body (Guido, 2006).

Informed consent is a client's permission granted to a physician to perform a therapeutic procedure, before which information about the procedure has been presented to the client with adequate time given for consideration about the pros and cons. The client should receive information such as what treatment alternatives are available; why the physician believes this treatment is most appropriate; the possible outcomes, risks, and adverse effects; the possible outcome should the client select another treatment alternative; and the possible outcome should the client choose to have no treatment. An example of a treatment in the psychiatric area that requires informed consent is electroconvulsive therapy.

There are some conditions under which treatment may be performed without obtaining informed consent. A client's refusal to accept treatment may be challenged under the following circumstances (Aiken, 2004; Guido, 2006; Levy & Rubenstein, 1996; Mackay, 2001):

1. When a client is mentally incompetent to make a decision and treatment is necessary to preserve life or avoid serious harm

2. When refusing treatment endangers the life or health of another

3. During an emergency, in which a client is in no condition to exercise judgment

4. When the client is a child (consent is obtained from parent or surrogate)

5. In the case of therapeutic privilege: Information about a treatment may be withheld if the physician can show that full disclosure would
   a. hinder or complicate necessary treatment
   b. cause severe psychological harm, or
   c. be so upsetting as to render a rational decision by the client impossible.

Although most clients in psychiatric/mental health facilities are competent and capable of giving informed consent, those with severe psychiatric illness do not possess the cognitive ability to do so. If an individual has been legally determined to be mentally incompetent, consent is obtained from the legal guardian. Difficulty arises when no legal determination has been made, but the individual's current mental state prohibits informed decision making (e.g., the person who is psychotic, unconscious, or inebriated). In these instances, informed consent is usually obtained from the individual's nearest relative, or if none exists and time permits, the physician may ask the court to appoint a conservator or guardian. When time does not permit court intervention, permission may be sought from the hospital administrator.

A client or guardian always has the right to withdraw consent after it has been given. When this occurs, the physician should inform (or reinform) the client about the consequences of refusing treatment. If treatment has already been initiated, the physician should terminate treatment in a way least likely to cause injury to the client and inform the client or guardian of the risks associated with interrupted treatment (Guido, 2006).

The nurse's role in obtaining informed consent is usually defined by agency policy. A nurse may sign the consent form as witness for the client's signature. However, legal liability for informed consent lies with the physician. The nurse acts as client advocate to ensure that the following three major elements of informed consent have been addressed:

1. **Knowledge:** The client has received adequate information on which to base his or her decision.

2. **Competency:** The individual's cognition is not impaired to an extent that would interfere with decision making or, if so, the individual has a legal representative.

3. **Free Will:** The individual has given consent voluntarily without pressure or coercion from others.

Restraints and Seclusion

An individual's privacy and personal security are protected by the U.S. Constitution and supported by the Mental Health Systems Act of 1980, out of which was conceived a Bill of Rights for psychiatric patients. These include "the right to freedom from restraint or seclusion except in an emergency situation." The use of seclusion and restraint as a therapeutic intervention for psychiatric patients has been controversial, and many efforts have been made through federal and state regulations and through standards set forth by accrediting bodies to minimize or eliminate its use. Because there have been injuries and deaths associated with restraint and seclusion, this treatment requires careful attention when it is used. Further, the laws, regulations, accreditation standards, and hospital policies are frequently being revised, so it is important for anyone practicing in inpatient psychiatric settings to be well informed in each of these areas.

In psychiatry, the term *restraints* generally refers to a set of leather straps that are used to restrain the extremities of an individual whose behavior is out of control and who poses an immediate risk to the physical safety and psychological well-being of the individual and staff. It is important to note that the current, generally accepted definition of restraint refers not to only leather restraints but rather to any manual method or medication used to restrict a person's freedom of movement (The Joint Commission, 2010). Restraints are never to be used as punishment or for the convenience of staff. Other measures to decrease agitation, such as "talking down" (verbal intervention) and chemical restraints (tranquilizing medication), are usually tried first. If these interventions are ineffective, mechanical restraints may be instituted (although some controversy exists as to whether chemical restraints are indeed less restrictive than mechanical restraints). *Seclusion* is another type of physical restraint in which the client is confined alone in a room from which he or she is unable to leave. The room is usually minimally furnished with items to promote the client's comfort and safety.

The Joint Commission, an association that accredits health-care organizations, has established specific standards regarding the use of seclusion and restraint. Some examples of current standards include the following (The Joint Commission, 2010):

1. Seclusion or restraint is discontinued at the earliest possible time regardless of when the order is scheduled to expire.

2. Unless state law is more restrictive, orders for restraint or seclusion must be renewed every 4 hours for adults 18 and older, every 2 hours for children and adolescents ages 9 to 17, and every hour for children younger than 9 years. Orders may be renewed according to these time limits for a maximum of 24 consecutive hours.

3. An in-person evaluation (by a physician, clinical psychologist, or other licensed independent practitioner responsible for the care of the patient) must be conducted within 1 hour of initiating restraint or seclusion. Appropriately trained registered nurses and physician assistants may also conduct this assessment, but they must consult with the physician.

4. Patients who are simultaneously restrained and secluded must be continuously monitored by trained staff, either in person or through audio or video equipment positioned near the patient.

5. Staff who are involved in restraining and secluding patients must be trained to monitor the physical and psychological well-being of the patient, including (but not limited to) respiratory and circulatory status, skin integrity, and vital signs.

The laws, regulations, accreditation standards, and hospital policies pertaining to restraint and seclusion share a common priority of maintaining patient safety for a procedure that has the potential to incur injury or death. The importance of close and careful monitoring cannot be overstated.

False imprisonment is the deliberate and unauthorized confinement of a person within fixed limits by the use of verbal or physical means (Ellis & Hartley, 2008). Health-care workers may be charged with false imprisonment for restraining or secluding—against the wishes of the client—anyone having been admitted to the hospital voluntarily. Should a voluntarily admitted client decompensate to a point that restraint or seclusion for protection of self or others is necessary, court intervention to determine competency and involuntary commitment is required to preserve the client's rights to privacy and freedom.

Commitment Issues

Voluntary Admissions

Each year, more than 1 million persons are admitted to health-care facilities for psychiatric treatment; of these admissions, approximately two thirds are considered voluntary. To be admitted voluntarily, an individual makes direct application to the institution for services and may stay as long as treatment is deemed necessary. He or she may sign out of the hospital at any time unless, following a mental status examination, the health-care professional determines that the client may be harmful to self or others and recommends that the admission status be changed from voluntary to involuntary. Although these types of admissions are considered voluntary, it is important to ensure that the individual comprehends the meaning of his or her actions, has not been coerced in any manner, and is willing to proceed with admission.

Involuntary Commitment

Because involuntary hospitalization results in substantial restrictions of the rights of an individual, the admission process is subject to the guarantee of the Fourteenth Amendment to the U.S. Constitution that provides citizens protection against loss of liberty and ensures due process rights (Weiss-Kaffie & Purtell, 2001). Involuntary commitments are made for various reasons. Most states commonly cite the following criteria:

■ In an emergency situation (for the client who is dangerous to self or others)

■ For observation and treatment of mentally ill persons

■ When an individual is unable to take care of basic personal needs (the "gravely disabled")

Under the Fourth Amendment, individuals are protected from unlawful searches and seizures without probable cause. Therefore, the individual seeking the involuntary commitment must show probable cause why the client should be hospitalized against his or her wishes; that is, the person must show that there is cause to believe that the client would be dangerous to self or others, is mentally ill and in need of treatment, or is gravely disabled.

Emergency Commitments

Emergency commitments are sought when an individual manifests behavior that is clearly and imminently dangerous to self or others. These admissions are usually instigated by relatives or friends of the individual, police officers, the court, or health-care professionals. Emergency commitments are time limited, and a court hearing for the individual is scheduled, usually within 72 hours. At that time the court may decide that the client may be discharged; or, if deemed necessary, and voluntary admission is refused by the client, an additional period of involuntary commitment may be ordered. In most instances, another hearing is scheduled for a specified time (usually in 7 to 21 days).

The Mentally Ill Person in Need of Treatment

A second type of involuntary commitment is for the observation and treatment of mentally ill persons in need of treatment. Most states have established definitions of what constitutes "mentally ill" for purposes of state involuntary admission statutes. Some examples include individuals who, because of severe mental illness, are:

■ Unable to make informed decisions concerning treatment

■ Likely to cause harm to self or others

■ Unable to fulfill basic personal needs necessary for health and safety

In determining whether commitment is required, the court looks for substantial evidence of abnormal conduct—evidence that cannot be explained as the result of a physical cause. There must be "clear and convincing evidence" as well as "probable cause" to substantiate the need for involuntary commitment to ensure that an individual's rights under the Constitution are protected. The U.S. Supreme Court, in *O'Connor v. Donaldson,* held that the existence of mental illness alone does not justify involuntary hospitalization. State standards require a specific impact or consequence to flow from the mental illness that involves danger or an inability to care for one's own needs. These clients are entitled to court hearings with representation, at which time determination of commitment and length of stay are considered. Legislative statutes governing involuntary commitments vary from state to state.

Involuntary Outpatient Commitment

Involuntary outpatient commitment (IOC) is a court-ordered mechanism used to compel a person with mental illness to submit to treatment on an outpatient basis. A number of eligibility criteria for commitment to outpatient treatment have been cited (Appelbaum, 2001; Maloy, 1996; Torrey & Zdanowicz, 2001). Some of these include:

■ A history of repeated decompensation requiring involuntary hospitalization

■ Likelihood that without treatment the individual will deteriorate to the point of requiring inpatient commitment

■ Presence of severe and persistent mental illness (e.g., schizophrenia or bipolar disorder) and limited awareness of the illness or need for treatment

■ The presence of severe and persistent mental illness contributing to a risk of becoming homeless, incarcerated, or violent, or of committing suicide

■ The existence of an individualized treatment plan likely to be effective and a service provider who has agreed to provide the treatment

Most states have already enacted IOC legislation or currently have resolutions that speak to this topic on their agendas. Most commonly, clients who are committed into the IOC programs are those with severe and persistent mental illness, such as schizophrenia. The rationale behind the legislation is to improve preventive care and reduce the number of readmissions and lengths of hospital stays of these clients. The need for this kind of legislation arose after it was recognized that patients with schizophrenia who did not meet criteria for involuntary hospital treatment were, in some cases, ultimately dangerous to themselves or others. In New York, public attention to this need arose after a man with schizophrenia who had stopped taking his medication pushed a young woman into the path of a subway train. He would not have met criteria for involuntary hospitalization until he was deemed dangerous to others, but advocates for this legislation argued that there should be provisions to prevent violence rather than waiting until it happens. The subsequent law governing IOC in New York became known as Kendra's Law in reference to the woman who was pushed to her death. Opponents of this legislation fear that it may violate the individual rights of psychiatric clients without significant improvement in outcomes.

Some research studies have attempted to evaluate whether IOC improves care, reduces lengths of stay in the hospital, and/or reduces episodes of violence. One study at Bellevue Hospital in New York found no difference in treatment outcomes between court-ordered outpatient treatment and voluntary outpatient treatment (Steadman et al., 2001). Other studies have shown positive outcomes, including a decrease in hospital readmissions, with IOC (Ridgely, Borum, & Petrila, 2001; Swartz et al., 2001). Continuing research is required to determine if IOC will improve treatment compliance and enhance quality of life in the community for individuals with severe and persistent mental illness.

The Gravely Disabled Client

A number of states have statutes that specifically define the "gravely disabled" client. For those that do not use this label, the description of the individual who, because of mental illness, is unable to take care of basic personal needs is very similar.

Gravely disabled is generally defined as a condition in which an individual, as a result of mental illness, is in danger of serious physical harm resulting from inability to provide for basic needs such as food, clothing, shelter, medical care, and personal safety. Inability to care for oneself cannot be established by showing that an individual lacks the resources to provide the necessities of life. Rather, it is the inability to make use of available resources.

Should it be determined that an individual is gravely disabled, a guardian, conservator, or committee will be appointed by the court to ensure the management of the person and his or her estate. To legally restore competency then requires another court hearing to reverse the previous ruling. The individual whose competency is being determined has the right to be represented by an attorney.

Nursing Liability

Mental health practitioners—psychiatrists, psychologists, psychiatric nurses, and social workers—have a duty to provide appropriate care based on the standards of their professions and the standards set by law. The standards of care for psychiatric/mental health nursing are presented in Chapter 9.

Malpractice and Negligence

The terms **malpractice** and **negligence** are often used interchangeably. Negligence has been defined as:

> The failure to exercise the standard of care that a reasonably prudent person would have exercised in a similar situation; any conduct that falls below the legal standard established to protect others against unreasonable risk of harm, except for conduct that is intentionally, wantonly, or willfully disregardful of others' rights. (Garner, 1999)

Any person may be negligent. In contrast, malpractice is a specialized form of negligence applicable only to professionals.

Black's Law Dictionary defines malpractice as:

> An instance of negligence or incompetence on the part of a professional. To succeed in a malpractice claim, a plaintiff must also prove proximate cause and damages. (Garner, 1999)

In the absence of any state statutes, common law is the basis of liability for injuries to clients caused by acts of malpractice and negligence of individual practitioners. In other words, most decisions of negligence in the professional setting are based on legal precedent (decisions that have previously been made about similar cases) rather than any specific action taken by the legislature.

To summarize, when the breach of duty is characterized as malpractice, the action is weighed against the professional standard. When it is brought forth as negligence, action is contrasted with what a reasonably prudent professional would have done in the same or similar circumstances.

Marchand (2001) cited the following basic elements of a nursing malpractice lawsuit:

1. The existence of a duty, owed by the nurse to a patient, to conform to a recognized standard of care
2. A failure to conform to the required nursing standard of care
3. Actual injury
4. A reasonably close causal connection between the nurse's conduct and the patient's injury

For the client to prevail in a malpractice claim, each of these elements must be proved. Juries' decisions are generally based on the testimony of expert witnesses, because members of the jury are laypeople and cannot be expected to know what nursing interventions should have been carried out. Without the testimony of expert witnesses, a favorable verdict usually goes to the defendant nurse.

Types of Lawsuits That Occur in Psychiatric Nursing

Most malpractice suits against nurses are civil actions; that is, they are considered breach of conduct actions on the part of the professional, for which compensation is being sought. The nurse in the psychiatric setting should be aware of the types of behaviors that may result in charges of malpractice.

Basic to the psychiatric client's hospitalization is his or her right to confidentiality and privacy. A nurse may be charged with *breach of confidentiality* for revealing aspects about a client's case, or even for revealing that an individual has been hospitalized, if that person can show that making this information known resulted in harm.

When shared information is detrimental to the client's reputation, the person sharing the information may be liable for **defamation of character.** When the information is in writing, the action is called **libel.** Oral defamation is called **slander.** Defamation of character involves communication that is malicious and false (Ellis & Hartley, 2008). Occasionally, libel arises out of critical, judgmental statements written in the client's medical record. Nurses need to be very objective in their charting, backing up all statements with factual evidence.

Invasion of privacy is a charge that may result when a client is searched without probable cause. Many institutions conduct body searches on mentally ill clients as a routine intervention. In these cases, there should be a physician's order and written rationale showing probable cause for the intervention. Many institutions are reexamining their policies regarding this procedure.

Assault is an act that results in a person's genuine fear and apprehension that he or she will be touched without consent. **Battery** is the unconsented touching of another person. These charges can result when a treatment is administered to a client against his or her wishes and outside of an emergency situation. Harm or injury need not have occurred for these charges to be legitimate.

For confining a client against his or her wishes, and outside of an emergency situation, the nurse may be charged with false imprisonment. Examples of actions that may invoke these charges include locking an individual in a room; taking a client's clothes for purposes of detainment against his or her will; and retaining in mechanical restraints a competent voluntary client who demands to be released.

Avoiding Liability

Hall and Hall (2001) suggested the following proactive nursing actions in an effort to avoid nursing malpractice:

1. Responding to the patient
2. Educating the patient
3. Complying with the standard of care
4. Supervising care
5. Adhering to the nursing process
6. Documentation
7. Follow-up

In addition, it is a positive practice to develop and maintain a good interpersonal relationship with the client and his or her family. Some clients appear to be more "suit prone" than others. Suit-prone clients are often very critical, complaining, uncooperative, and even hostile. A natural response by the staff to these clients is to become defensive or withdrawn. Either of these behaviors increases the likelihood of a lawsuit should an unfavorable event occur (Ellis & Hartley, 2008). No matter how high the degree of technical competence and skill of the nurse, his or her insensitivity to a client's complaints and failure to meet the client's

emotional needs often influence whether or not a lawsuit is generated. A great deal depends on the psychosocial skills of the health-care professional.

> **CLINICAL PEARLS**
> • Always put the client's rights and welfare first.
> • Develop and maintain a good interpersonal relationship with each client and his or her family.

Summary and Key Points

■ *Ethics* is a branch of philosophy that addresses methods for determining the rightness or wrongness of one's actions

■ *Bioethics* is the term applied to these principles when they refer to concepts within the scope of medicine, nursing, and allied health.

■ *Moral behavior* is defined as conduct that results from serious critical thinking about how individuals ought to treat others.

■ *Values* are personal beliefs about what is important or desirable.

■ A *right* is defined as, "a valid, legally recognized claim or entitlement, encompassing both freedom from government interference or discriminatory treatment and an entitlement to a benefit or service."

■ The ethical theory of utilitarianism is based on the premise that what is right and good is that which produces the most happiness for the most people.

■ The ethical theory of Kantianism suggests that actions are bound by a sense of duty, and that ethical decisions are made out of respect for moral law.

■ The code of Christian ethics is that all decisions about right and wrong should be centered in love for God and in treating others with the same respect and dignity with which we would expect to be treated.

■ The moral precept of the natural law theory is "do good and avoid evil." Good is viewed as that which is inscribed by God into the nature of things. Evil acts are never condoned, even if they are intended to advance the noblest of ends.

■ Ethical egoism espouses that what is right and good is what is best for the individual making the decision.

■ Ethical principles include autonomy, beneficence, nonmaleficence, veracity, and justice.

■ An ethical dilemma is a situation that requires an individual to make a choice between two equally unfavorable alternatives.

■ Ethical issues may arise in psychiatric/mental health nursing around the right to refuse medication and the right to the least-restrictive treatment alternative.

■ Statutory laws are those that have been enacted by legislative bodies, and common laws are derived from decisions made in previous cases. Both types of laws have civil and criminal components.

■ Civil law protects the private and property rights of individuals and businesses, and criminal law provides protection from conduct deemed injurious to the public welfare.

■ Legal issues in psychiatric/mental health nursing center around confidentiality and the right to privacy, informed consent, restraints and seclusion, and commitment issues.

■ Nurses are accountable for their own actions in relation to legal issues, and violation can result in malpractice lawsuits against the physician, the hospital, and the nurse.

■ Developing and maintaining a good interpersonal relationship with the client and his or her family appears to be a positive factor when the question of malpractice is being considered.

 DavisPlus Additional info available @ davisplus.fadavis.com

Review Questions
Self-Examination/Learning Exercise

*Select the answer that is **most** appropriate for each of the following questions:*

1. Nurse Jones decides to go against family wishes and tell the client of his terminal status because that is what she would want if she were the client. Which of the following ethical theories is considered in this decision?
   a. Kantianism.
   b. Christian ethics.
   c. Natural law theories.
   d. Ethical egoism.

2. Nurse Jones decides to respect family wishes and not tell the client of his terminal status because that would bring the most happiness to the most people. Which of the following ethical theories is considered in this decision?
   a. Utilitarianism.
   b. Kantianism.
   c. Christian ethics.
   d. Ethical egoism.

3. Nurse Jones decides to tell the client of his terminal status because she believes it is her duty to do so. Which of the following ethical theories is considered in this decision?
   a. Natural law theories.
   b. Ethical egoism.
   c. Kantianism.
   d. Utilitarianism.

4. The nurse assists the physician with electroconvulsive therapy on his client who has refused to give consent. With which of the following legal actions might the nurse be charged because of this nursing action?
   a. Assault.
   b. Battery.
   c. False imprisonment.
   d. Breach of confidentiality.

Review Questions—cont'd
Self-Examination/Learning Exercise

5. A competent, voluntary client has stated he wants to leave the hospital. The nurse hides his clothes in an effort to keep him from leaving. With which of the following legal actions might the nurse be charged because of this nursing action?
   a. Assault.
   b. Battery.
   c. False imprisonment.
   d. Breach of confidentiality.

6. Joe is very restless and is pacing a lot. The nurse says to Joe, "If you don't sit down in the chair and be still, I'm going to put you in restraints!" With which of the following legal actions might the nurse be charged because of this nursing action?
   a. Defamation of character.
   b. Battery.
   c. Breach of confidentiality.
   d. Assault.

7. An individual may be considered *gravely disabled* for which of the following reasons? (Select all that apply.)
   a. A person, because of mental illness, cannot fulfill basic needs.
   b. A mentally ill person is in danger of physical harm based on inability to care for self.
   c. A mentally ill person lacks the resources to provide the necessities of life.
   d. A mentally ill person is unable to make use of available resources to meet daily living requirements.

8. Which of the following statements is (are) correct regarding the use of restraints? (Select all that apply.)
   a. Restraints may never be initiated without a physician's order.
   b. Orders for restraints must be reissued by a physician every 2 hours for children and adolescents.
   c. Clients in restraints must be observed and assessed every hour for issues regarding circulation, nutrition, respiration, hydration, and elimination.
   d. An in-person evaluation must be conducted within 1 hour of initiating restraints.

9. Guidelines relating to "duty to warn" state that a therapist should consider taking action to warn a third party when his or her client: (Select all that apply.)
   a. Threatens violence toward another individual.
   b. Identifies a specific intended victim.
   c. Is having command hallucinations.
   d. Reveals paranoid delusions about another individual.

10. Attempting to calm an angry client by using "talk therapy" is an example of which of the following clients' rights?
    a. The right to privacy.
    b. The right to refuse medication.
    c. The right to the least-restrictive treatment alternative.
    d. The right to confidentiality.

References

Aiken, T. D. (2004). *Legal, ethical, and political issues in nursing* (2nd ed.). Philadelphia: F.A. Davis.

American Hospital Association. (1992). *A Patient's Bill of Rights.* Chicago: Author.

American Nurses Association. (2001). *Code of ethics for nurses with interpretive statements.* Washington, DC: Author.

Appelbaum, P. S. (2001, March). Thinking carefully about outpatient commitment. *Psychiatric Services, 52*(3), 347–350.

Butts, J., & Rich, K. (2008). *Nursing ethics: Across the curriculum and into practice* (2nd ed). Sudbury, MA: Jones and Bartlett.

Catalano, J. T. (2009). *Nursing now! Today's issues, tomorrow's trends* (5th ed.). Philadelphia: F.A. Davis.

Ellis, J. R., & Hartley, C. L. (2008). *Nursing in today's world: Challenges, issues, and trends* (9th ed.). Philadelphia: Lippincott Williams & Wilkins.

Fedorka, P., & Resnick, L. K. (2001). Defining nursing practice. In M. E. O'Keefe (Ed.), *Nursing practice and the law: Avoiding malpractice and other legal rights* (pp. 97–117). Philadelphia: F.A. Davis.

Garner, B. A. (Ed.). (1999). *Black's law dictionary.* St. Paul, MN: West Group.

Guido, G. W. (2006). *Legal and ethical issues in nursing* (4th ed.). Upper Saddle River, NJ: Prentice Hall.

Hall, J. K., & Hall, D. (2001). Negligence specific to nursing. In M. E. O'Keefe (Ed.), *Nursing practice and the law: Avoiding malpractice and other legal risks* (pp. 132–149). Philadelphia: F.A. Davis.

Levy, R. M., & Rubenstein, L. S. (1996). *The rights of people with mental disabilities.* Carbondale, IL: Southern Illinois University Press.

Mackay, T. R. (2001). Informed consent. In M. E. O'Keefe (Ed.), *Nursing practice and the law: Avoiding malpractice and other legal risks* (pp. 199–213). Philadelphia: F.A. Davis.

Maloy, K. A. (1996). Does involuntary outpatient commitment work? In B. D. Sales & S. A. Shah (Eds.), *Mental health and law: Research, policy and services* (pp. 41–74). Durham, NC: Carolina Academic Press.

Marchand, L. (2001). Legal terminology. In M. E. O'Keefe (Ed.), *Nursing practice and the law: Avoiding malpractice and other legal risks* (pp. 23–41). Philadelphia: F.A. Davis.

Mental Health Systems Act, Pub. L. No. 96-398, Title V, § 501.94, Stat. 1598 (1980).

Pappas, A. (2006). Ethical issues. In J. Zerwekh & J. C. Claborn (Eds.), *Nursing today: Transition and trends* (5th ed., pp. 425–453). New York: Elsevier.

Peplau, H. E. (1991). *Interpersonal relations in nursing: A conceptual frame of reference for psychodynamic nursing.* New York: Springer.

Ridgely, M. S., Borum, R., & Petrila, J. (2001). *The effectiveness of involuntary outpatient treatment: Empirical evidence and the experience of eight states.* Santa Monica, CA: Rand Publications.

Sadock, B. J., & Sadock, V. A. (2007). *Synopsis of psychiatry: Behavioral sciences/clinical psychiatry* (10th ed.). Philadelphia: Lippincott Williams & Wilkins.

Steadman, H., Gounis, K., Dennis, D., Hopper, K., Roche, B., Swartz, M., et al. (2001). Assessing the New York City involuntary outpatient commitment pilot program. *Psychiatric Services, 52*(3), 330–336.

Swartz, M., Swanson, J., Hiday, V., Wagner, H. R., Burns, B., & Borum, R. (2001). A randomized controlled trial of outpatient commitment in North Carolina. *Psychiatric Services, 52*(3), 325–329.

Tarasoff v. Regents of University of California et al., 551 P.d 345 (1974a).

Tarasoff v. Regents of University of California et al., 554 P.d 347 (1974b).

The Joint Commission. (2010). *The comprehensive accreditation manual for hospitals: The official handbook* (January, 2010). Oakbrook Terrace, IL: Joint Commission Resources.

Torrey, E.F., & Zdanowicz, M. (2001). Outpatient commitment: What, why, and for whom. *Psychiatric Services 52*(3), 337–341.

U.S. Department of Health and Human Services. (2003). *Standards for privacy of individually identifiable health information.* Washington, DC: Author.

Weiss-Kaffie, C. J., & Purtell, N. E. (2001). Psychiatric nursing. In M. E. O'Keefe (Ed.), *Nursing Practice and the law: Avoiding malpractice and other legal risks* (pp. 352–371). Philadelphia: F.A. Davis.

Cultural and Spiritual Concepts Relevant to Psychiatric/Mental Health Nursing

KARYN I. MORGAN AND MARY C. TOWNSEND

CHAPTER

6

CORE CONCEPTS

culture
ethnicity
religion
spirituality

CHAPTER OUTLINE

Objectives

Homework Assignment

Cultural Concepts

How Do Cultures Differ?

Application of the Nursing Process

Spiritual Concepts

Assessment of Spiritual and Religious Needs

Summary and Key Points

Review Questions

KEY TERMS

culture-bound syndromes

curandera

curandero

density

distance

folk medicine

shaman

stereotyping

territoriality

yin and yang

OBJECTIVES

After reading this chapter, the student will be able to:

1. Define and differentiate between *culture* and *ethnicity*.
2. Identify cultural differences based on six characteristic phenomena.
3. Describe cultural variances, based on the six phenomena, for:
   a. Northern European Americans
   b. African Americans
   c. Native Americans
   d. Asian/Pacific Islander Americans
   e. Latino Americans

f. Western European Americans
g. Arab Americans
h. Jewish Americans

4. Apply the nursing process in the care of individuals from various cultural groups.
5. Define and differentiate between *spirituality* and *religion*.
6. Identify clients' spiritual and religious needs.
7. Apply the six steps of the nursing process to individuals with spiritual and religious needs.

HOMEWORK ASSIGNMENT

Please read the chapter and answer the following questions:

1. Which cultural group may use a medicine man (or woman) called a *shaman?*
2. Restoring a balance between opposite forces is a fundamental concept of Asian health practices. What is this called?
3. Name five types of human spiritual needs.

4. What is the largest ethnic minority group in the United States?
5. What is the perception of mental illness in the Arab culture?

103

CULTURAL CONCEPTS

What is culture? How does it differ from ethnicity? Why are these questions important? The answers lie in the changing face of America. Immigration is not new in the United States. Indeed, most U.S. citizens are either immigrants or descendants of immigrants, and the numbers of foreign-born residents in this country continue to grow on a yearly basis. This pattern continues because of the many individuals who want to take advantage of the technological growth and upward mobility that exists in this country. A breakdown of cultural groups in the United States is presented in Figure 6–1.

CORE CONCEPTS

Culture describes a particular society's entire way of living, encompassing shared patterns of belief, feeling, and knowledge that guide people's conduct and are passed down from generation to generation.
Ethnicity is a somewhat narrower term and relates to people who identify with each other because of a shared heritage (Griffith, Gonzalez, & Blue, 2003).

Knowledge related to culture and ethnicity is important because these influences affect human behavior, its interpretation, and the response to it. Therefore, it is essential for nurses to understand the effects of these cultural influences if they are to work effectively with the diverse population. Caution must be taken, however, not to assume that all individuals who share a culture or ethnic group are identical or exhibit behaviors perceived as characteristic of the group. This constitutes **stereotyping** and must be avoided. Many variations and subcultures occur within a culture. These differences may be related to status, ethnic background, residence, religion, education, or other factors (Purnell & Paulanka, 2008). Every individual must be appreciated for his or her uniqueness.

This chapter explores the ways in which various cultures differ. The nursing process is applied to the delivery of psychiatric/mental health nursing care for individuals from the following cultural groups: Northern European Americans, African Americans, Native Americans, Asian/Pacific Islander Americans, Latino Americans, Western European Americans, Arab Americans, and Jewish Americans.

HOW DO CULTURES DIFFER?

It is difficult to generalize about any one specific group in a country that is known for its heterogeneity. Within our American "melting pot," any or all characteristics could apply to individuals within any or all of the cultural groups represented. As these differences continue to be integrated, one American culture will eventually emerge. This is already evident in certain regions of the country today, particularly in the urban coastal areas. However, some differences still do exist, and it is important for nurses to be aware of certain cultural influences that may affect individuals' behaviors and beliefs, particularly as they apply to health care.

Giger and Davidhizar (2008) suggested six cultural phenomena that vary with application and use yet are evidenced among all cultural groups: (1) communication, (2) space, (3) social organization, (4) time, (5) environmental control, and (6) biological variations.

Communication

All verbal and nonverbal behavior in connection with another individual is communication. Therapeutic communication has always been considered an essential part of the nursing process and represents a critical element in the curricula of most schools of nursing. Communication has its roots in culture. Cultural mores, norms, ideas, and customs provide the basis for our way of thinking. Cultural values are learned and differ from society to society. Communication is expressed through language (the spoken and written word), paralanguage (the voice quality, intonation, rhythm, and speed of the spoken word), and gestures (touch,

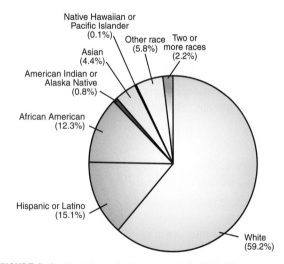

FIGURE 6–1 Breakdown of cultural groups in the United States. (From U.S. Census Bureau. [2009]. *2006–2008 American Community Survey.* Retrieved July 9, 2010, from http://factfinder.census.gov/.)

facial expression, eye movements, body posture, and physical appearance). The nurse who is planning care must have an understanding of the client's needs and expectations as they are being communicated. As a third party, an interpreter often complicates matters, but one may be necessary when the client does not speak the same language as the nurse. Interpreting is a very complex process, however, that requires a keen sensitivity to cultural nuances, and not just the translating of words into another language. Tips for facilitating the communication process when using an interpreter are presented in Box 6-1.

Space

Spatial determinants relate to the place where the communication occurs and encompass the concepts of *territoriality, density,* and *distance.* **Territoriality** refers to the innate tendency to own space. The need for territoriality is met only if the individual has control of a space, can establish rules for that space, and is able to defend the space against invasion or misuse by others. **Density,** which refers to the number of people within a given environmental space, can influence interpersonal interaction. **Distance** is the means by which various cultures use space to communicate. Hall (1966) identified three primary dimensions of space in interpersonal interactions in the Western culture: the intimate zone (0 to 18 inches), the personal zone (18 inches to 3 feet), and the social zone (3 to 6 feet).

Social Organization

Cultural behavior is socially acquired through a process called *enculturation,* which involves acquiring knowledge and internalizing values (Giger & Davidhizar, 2008). Children are acculturated by observing adults within their social organizations. Social organizations include families, religious groups, and ethnic groups.

Time

An awareness of the concept of time is a gradual learning process. Some cultures place great importance on values that are measured by clock time. Punctuality and efficiency are highly valued in the United States, whereas some cultures are actually scornful of clock time. For example, some rural people in Algeria label the clock as the "devil's mill" and therefore have no notion of scheduled appointment times or mealtimes (Giger & Davidhizar, 2008). They are totally indifferent to the passage of clock time, and they despise haste in all human endeavors. Other cultural implications regarding time have to do with perception of time orientation. Whether individuals are present oriented or future oriented in their perception of time influences many aspects of their lives.

BOX 6-1 Using an Interpreter

When using an interpreter, keep the following points in mind:

- Address the client directly rather than speaking to the interpreter. Maintain eye contact with the client to ensure the client's involvement.
- Do not interrupt the client and the interpreter. At times their interaction may take longer because of the need to clarify, and descriptions may require more time because of dialect differences or the interpreter's awareness that the client needs more preparation before being asked a particular question.
- Ask the interpreter to give you verbatim translations so that you can assess what the client is thinking and understanding.
- Avoid using medical jargon that the interpreter or client may not understand.
- Avoid talking or commenting to the interpreter at length; the client may feel left out and distrustful.
- Be aware that asking intimate or emotionally laden questions may be difficult for both the client and the interpreter. Lead up to these questions slowly. Always ask permission to discuss these topics first, and prepare the interpreter for the content of the interview.
- When possible, allow the client and the interpreter to meet each other ahead of time to establish some rapport. If possible, try to use the same interpreter for succeeding interviews with the client.
- If possible, request an interpreter of the same gender as the client and of similar age. To make good use of the interpreter's time, decide beforehand which questions you will ask. Meet with the interpreter briefly before going to see the client so that you can let the interpreter know what you are planning to ask. During the session, face the client and direct your questions to the client, not the interpreter.

From Gorman, L. M., & Sultan, D. F. (2008). Psychosocial nursing for general patient care (3rd ed.). Philadelphia: F.A. Davis, with permission.

Environmental Control

The variable of environmental control has to do with the degree to which individuals perceive that they have control over their environment. Cultural beliefs and practices influence how an individual responds to his or her environment during periods of wellness and illness. To provide culturally appropriate care, the nurse should not only respect the individual's unique beliefs, but should also have an understanding of how these beliefs can be used to promote optimal health in the client's environment.

Biological Variations

Biological differences exist among people in various racial groups. Giger and Davidhizar (2008) stated:

> The strongest argument for including concepts on biological variations in nursing education and subsequently nursing practice is that scientific facts about biological variations can aid the nurse in giving culturally appropriate health care. (p. 145)

These differences include body structure (both size and shape), skin color, physiological responses to medication, electrocardiographic patterns, susceptibility to disease, and nutritional preferences and deficiencies.

Application of the Nursing Process

Background Assessment Data

A cultural assessment tool for gathering information related to culture and ethnicity that is important in the planning of client care is provided in Box 6-2.

BOX 6-2 Cultural Assessment Tool

Client's name _____ Ethnic origin _____
Address _____ Birthdate _____
Name of significant other _____ Relationship _____
Primary language spoken _____ Second language spoken _____
How does client usually communicate with people who speak a different language? _____
Is an interpreter required? _____ Available? _____
Highest level of education achieved: _____ Occupation: _____
Presenting problem: _____
Has this problem ever occurred before? _____
    If so, in what manner was it handled previously? _____
What is the client's usual manner of coping with stress? _____
Who is (are) the client's main support system(s)? _____
Describe the family living arrangements: _____
Who is the major decision maker in the family? _____
Describe client's/family members' roles within the family. _____
_____
Describe religious beliefs and practices: _____
    Are there any religious requirements or restrictions that place limitations on the client's care? _____
    If so, describe: _____
Who in the family takes responsibility for health concerns? _____
Describe any special health beliefs and practices: _____
_____
From whom does family usually seek medical assistance in time of need? _____
Describe client's usual emotional/behavioral response to:
    Anxiety: _____
    Anger: _____
    Loss/change/failure: _____
    Pain: _____
    Fear: _____
Describe any topics that are particularly sensitive or that the client is unwilling to discuss (because of cultural taboos):
_____
Describe any activities in which the client is unwilling to participate (because of cultural customs or taboos):
_____
What are the client's personal feelings regarding touch? _____
What are the client's personal feelings regarding eye contact? _____
What is the client's personal orientation to time? (past, present, future) _____

BOX 6-2 Cultural Assessment Tool—cont'd

Describe any particular illnesses to which the client may be bioculturally susceptible (e.g., hypertension and sickle cell anemia in African Americans):
_____

Describe any nutritional deficiencies to which the client may be bioculturally susceptible (e.g., lactose intolerance in Native and Asian Americans) _____
Describe client's favorite foods: _____
Are there any foods the client requests or refuses because of cultural beliefs related to this illness (e.g., "hot" and "cold" foods for Latino Americans and Asian Americans)? If so, please describe: _____
_____

Describe client's perception of the problem and expectations of health care: _____
_____
_____

Northern European Americans

Northern European Americans have their origins in England, Ireland, Wales, Finland, Sweden, Norway, Germany, Poland, and the Baltic states of Estonia, Latvia, and Lithuania. English is their primary language. Their language may also include words and phrases that reflect the influence of the languages spoken in the countries of their heritage. The descendants of these immigrants now make up what is considered the dominant cultural group in the United States today. Specific dialects and rate of speech are common to various regions of the country. Northern European Americans value territory. Personal space preference is about 18 inches to 3 feet.

With the advent of technology and widespread mobility, less emphasis has been placed on the cohesiveness of the family. Data on marriage, divorce, and remarriage in the United States show that approximately one third of first marriages end in separation or divorce within 10 years (Centers for Disease Control and Prevention [CDC], 2010). The value that was once placed on religion also seems to be diminishing in the American culture. With the exception of a few months following the terrorist attacks of September 11, 2001, when attendance increased, a steady decline was reported in church attendance from 1992 to 2008 (Gallup, 2008). The number of Americans reporting affiliation with Christianity declined from 91 percent in the first 1948 Gallup Poll to 77 percent in 2008. The number of Americans reporting no religious affiliation rose from 2 percent to 12 percent during the same period (Gallup, 2009). Punctuality and efficiency are highly valued in the culture that promoted the work ethic, and most within this cultural group tend to be future oriented (Murray, Zentner, & Yakimo, 2009).

Northern European Americans, particularly those who achieve middle-class socioeconomic status, value preventive medicine and primary health care. This value follows along with the socioeconomic group's educational level, successful achievement, and financial capability to maintain a healthy lifestyle. Most recognize the importance of regular physical exercise.

A typical diet for many Northern European Americans is high in fats and cholesterol and low in fiber. Americans, in general, are learning about the health benefits of reducing fats and increasing nutrients in their diet. However, they still enjoy fast food, which conforms to their fast-paced lifestyles.

The United States, viewed as a "melting pot" of multiple worldwide ethnic groups, has its own unique culture that impacts the health and care of individuals. It is important that the nurse is self-aware of these conscious/unconscious attitudes and values within the U.S. culture when caring for clients, and also how these characteristics can impact mental health/illness. Characteristics common to the U.S. culture are presented in Box 6-3.

African Americans

The language dialect of some African Americans is different from what is considered standard English. The origin of the black dialect is not clearly understood but is thought to be a combination of various African languages and the languages of other cultural groups (e.g., Dutch, French, English, and Spanish) present in the United States at the time of its settlement. Personal space tends to be smaller than that of the dominant culture.

Patterns of discrimination date back to the days of slavery, and evidence of segregation still exists, usually in the form of predominantly black neighborhoods, churches, and schools, which are still visible in some U.S. cities. Some African Americans

---

BOX 6-3 Characteristics Common to the Culture of the United States

1. **Individuality**—independence, self reliance, "do it yourself," determining one's life, aspire for internal control of self vs. external control, desire for choice in health care provider/practices
2. **Perfectionism**—strong emphasis on achievement in jobs, sports, physical beauty and home construction
3. **Direct Communication**—display of emotions is proper, within limits. Constructive criticism is considered helpful for others.
4. **Time Adherence**—activities organized around schedules, hurried, active lifestyles causing difficulty with relaxation. Punctuality is important.
5. **Informality/Friendliness**—of general behaviors, speech and relationship with others. There is common use of first name when addressing others. Many friendly expressions, such as "let's get together soon" and "drop by any time," are sincere at the time, but because of busy lifestyles are not meant literally.
6. **Consumerism**—mass luxuries, need for material goods, standardized "high end" designer homes/clothing/automobiles; widespread attempts for mass accumulation of goods leading to economic stress and increased unemployment; overconsumption in food practices leading to increased obesity and decreased health
7. **Social Challenges**—suburban tract housing, widespread drive-through dining, frequent relocations, solo car travel, decreased family connections, increased mall shopping vs. local shopping, loss of amusement areas/parks, etc.

Contributed by Lois Angelo, Assistant Professor, Massachusetts College of Pharmacy and Health Sciences, Boston, MA.

---

find it difficult to assimilate into the mainstream culture and choose to remain within their own social organization.

The most recent survey by the U.S. Census Bureau revealed that 45 percent of African American family households were headed by a woman (U.S. Census Bureau, 2009b). Social support systems may be large and include sisters, brothers, aunts, uncles, cousins, boyfriends, girlfriends, neighbors, and friends. Many African Americans have a strong religious orientation, with the vast majority practicing some form of Protestantism (Pew Forum on Religion and Public Life, 2009).

African Americans who have assimilated into the dominant culture are likely to be well educated, professional, and future oriented. Some who have not become assimilated may believe that planning for the future is hopeless, a belief based on their previous experiences and encounters with racism and discrimination (Cherry & Giger, 2008). Among this group, some may be unemployed or have low-paying jobs, with little expectation for improvement. They are unlikely to value time or punctuality to the same degree as the dominant cultural group, which may result in their being labeled as irresponsible.

Some African Americans, particularly those from the rural South, may reach adulthood never having encountered a physician. They receive their medical care from the local folk practitioner, known as "granny" or "the old lady," or a "spiritualist." Incorporated into the system of **folk medicine** is the belief that health is a gift from God, whereas illness is a punishment from God or a retribution for sin and evil. Historically, African Americans

have turned to folk medicine either because they could not afford the cost of mainstream medical treatment or because of the insensitive treatment by caregivers in the health-care delivery system.

Hypertension occurs more frequently, and sickle cell disease occurs predominantly, in African Americans. Hypertension carries a strong hereditary risk factor, whereas sickle cell disease is genetically derived. Alcoholism is a serious problem among members of the black community, leading to a high incidence of alcohol-related illness and death (Cherry & Giger, 2008).

The diet of most African Americans differs little from that of the mainstream culture. However, some African Americans follow their heritage and still enjoy what has come to be known as "soul" food, which includes poke salad, collard greens, beans, corn, fried chicken, black-eyed peas, grits, okra, and cornbread. These foods are now considered typical Southern fare and are regularly consumed and enjoyed by most individuals who inhabit the southern region of the United States.

Native Americans

The federal government currently recognizes 564 American Indian tribes and Alaska Native groups. Approximately 200 tribal languages are still spoken, some by only a few individuals and others by many (Bureau of Indian Affairs [BIA], 2010). Fewer than half of these individuals still live on reservations, but many return regularly to participate in family and tribal life and sometimes to retire.

Touch is an aspect of communication that is not the same among Native Americans as in the dominant

American culture. Some Native Americans view the traditional handshake as somewhat aggressive. Instead, if a hand is offered to another, it may be accepted with a light touch or just a passing of hands. Some Native Americans will not touch a dead person (Hanley, 2008).

Native Americans may appear silent and reserved. They may be uncomfortable expressing emotions because the culture encourages keeping private thoughts to oneself. Eye contact is avoided and considered rude (Hodgins & Hodgins, 2008).

The concept of space is very concrete to Native Americans. Living space is often crowded with members of both nuclear and extended families. A large network of kin is very important to Native Americans. However, a need for extended space exists, as demonstrated by a distance of many miles between individual homes or camps.

The primary social organizations of Native Americans are the family and the tribe. From infancy, Native American children are taught the importance of these units. Traditions are passed down by the elderly, and children are taught to respect tradition and to honor wisdom.

Most Native Americans are very present-time oriented. The concept of time is very casual, and tasks are accomplished not with the notion of a particular time in mind, but merely in a present-oriented time frame. Not only are Native Americans not ruled by the clock, some do not even own clocks.

Religion and health practices are intertwined in the Native American culture. The medicine man (or woman) is called the **shaman** and may use a variety of methods in his or her practice. Some use crystals to diagnose illness, some sing and perform healing ceremonies, and some use herbs and other plants or roots to create remedies with healing properties. The Native American healers and U.S. Indian Health Service (IHS) have worked together with mutual respect for many years. Hanley (2008) related that a Native American healer may confer with a physician regarding the care of a client in the hospital. Research studies have continued to show the importance of each of these health-care approaches in the overall wellness of Native American people.

The risks of illness and premature death from alcoholism, diabetes, tuberculosis, heart disease, accidents, homicide, suicide, pneumonia, and influenza are dramatically higher for Native Americans than for the U.S. population as a whole. The risks of illness and premature death from alcoholism alone are reported as 519 percent higher (Indian Health Service, 2009). Alcoholism is not only

a significant problem among Native Americans but it may also be related to a number of other serious problems, such as depression, automobile accidents, homicides, spouse and child abuse, and suicides.

Nutritional deficiencies are not uncommon among tribal Native Americans. Fruits and green vegetables are often scarce in many of the federally defined Indian geographical regions. Meat and corn products are identified as preferred foods. Fiber intake is relatively low, while fat intake is often of the saturated variety. A large number of Native Americans living on or near reservations recognized by the federal or state government receive commodity foods supplied by the U.S. Department of Agriculture's food distribution program (U.S. Department of Agriculture, 2009).

Asian/Pacific Islander Americans

Asian Americans comprise 4.4 percent of the U.S. population. The Asian American culture includes peoples (and their descendants) from Japan, China, Vietnam, the Philippines, Thailand, Cambodia, Korea, Laos, India, and the Pacific Islands. Although this discussion relates to these peoples as a single culture, it is important to keep in mind that a multiplicity of differences regarding attitudes, beliefs, values, religious practices, and language exist among these subcultures.

Many Asian Americans, particularly Japanese, are third- and even fourth-generation Americans. These individuals are likely to be acculturated to the U.S. culture. Kuo and Roysircar-Sodowsky (2000) described three patterns common to Asian Americans in their attempt to adjust to the American culture:

1. **The traditionalists:** These individuals tend to be the older-generation Asians who hold on to the traditional values and practices of their native culture. They have strong internalized Asian values. Primary allegiance is to the biological family.

2. **The marginal people:** These individuals reject the traditional values and totally embrace Western culture. Often they are members of the younger generations.

3. **Asian Americans:** These individuals incorporate traditional values and beliefs with Western values and beliefs. They become integrated into the American culture, while maintaining a connection with their ancestral culture.

The languages and dialects of Asian Americans are very diverse. In general, they do share a similar belief in harmonious interaction. To raise one's voice is likely to be interpreted as a sign of loss of control. The English language is very difficult to master, and even bilingual Asian Americans may encounter communication problems because of the differences in meaning assigned to nonverbal cues, such as facial gestures, verbal intonation and speed, and body movements. In Asian cultures, touching during communication has historically been considered unacceptable. However, with the advent of Western acculturation, younger generations of Asian Americans accept touching as more appropriate than did their ancestors. Eye contact is often avoided as it connotes rudeness and lack of respect in some Asian cultures. Acceptable personal and social spaces are larger than in the dominant American culture. Some Asian Americans have a great deal of difficulty expressing emotions. Because of their reserved public demeanor, Asian Americans may be perceived as shy, cold, or uninterested.

The family is the ultimate social organization in traditional Asian American culture, and loyalty to family is emphasized above all else. Children are expected to obey and honor their parents. Misbehavior is perceived as bringing dishonor to the entire family. Filial piety (one's social obligation or duty to one's parents) is held in high regard. Failure to fulfill these obligations can create a great deal of guilt and shame in an individual. A chronological hierarchy exists, with the elderly maintaining positions of authority. Several generations, or even extended families, may share a single household.

Although education is highly valued among Asian Americans, many remain undereducated. Religious beliefs and practices are diverse and exhibit influences of Taoism, Buddhism, Confucianism, Islam, Hinduism, and Christianity.

Many Asian Americans value both a past and a present orientation. Emphasis is placed on the wishes of one's ancestors, while adjusting to demands of the present. Little value is given to prompt adherence to schedules or rigid standards of activities.

Restoring the balance of **yin and yang** is the fundamental concept of Asian health practices. Yin and yang represent opposite forces of energy, such as negative/positive, dark/light, cold/hot, hard/soft, and feminine/masculine. The belief is that illness occurs when there is a disruption in the balance of these energy forces. In medicine, the opposites are expressed as "hot" and "cold," and health is the result of a balance between hot and cold elements (Wang & Purnell, 2008). Food, medicines, and herbs are classified according to their hot and cold properties and are used to restore balance between yin and yang (cold and hot), thereby restoring health.

Rice, vegetables, and fish are the main staple foods of Asian Americans. Milk is seldom consumed because a large majority of Asian Americans experience lactose intolerance. With Western acculturation, their diet is changing, and unfortunately, with more meat being consumed, the percentage of fat in the diet is increasing.

Many Asian Americans believe that psychiatric illness is merely behavior that is out of control. They view this as a great shame to the individual and the family. They often attempt to manage the ill person on their own until they can no longer handle the situation. It is not uncommon for Asian Americans to somaticize. Expressing mental distress through various physical ailments may be viewed as more acceptable than expressing true emotions (Xu & Chang, 2008).

The incidence of alcohol dependence is low among Asians. This may be a result of a possible genetic intolerance of the substance. Some Asians develop unpleasant symptoms, such as flushing, headaches, and palpitations, on drinking alcohol. Research indicates that this is due to an isoenzyme variant that quickly converts alcohol to acetaldehyde and the absence of an isoenzyme that is needed to oxidize acetaldehyde. This results in a rapid accumulation of acetaldehyde that produces the unpleasant symptoms (Wall et al., 1997).

Latino Americans

Latino Americans are the fastest growing group of people in the United States, comprising 15.1 percent of the population (U.S. Census Bureau, 2009a). They represent the largest ethnic minority group.

Latino Americans trace their ancestry to countries such as Mexico, Spain, Puerto Rico, Cuba, and other countries of Central and South America. The common language is Spanish, spoken with a number of dialects by the various peoples. Touch is a common form of communication among Latinos; however, they are very modest and are likely to withdraw from any infringement on their modesty.

Traditional Latino Americans are very group-oriented and often interact with large groups of relatives. Touching and embracing are common modes of communication. The family is the primary social organization and includes nuclear family members as well as numerous extended family members. The traditional nuclear family is male dominated, and the father possesses ultimate authority.

Latino Americans tend to be focused on the present time. The concept of being punctual and giving attention to activities that concern the future are perceived as less important than activities in the present time.

Roman Catholicism is the predominant religion among Latino Americans. Most Latinos identify with the Roman Catholic Church, even if they do not attend services. Religious beliefs and practices are likely to be strong influences in their lives. Especially in times of crisis, such as in cases of illness and hospitalization, Latino Americans rely on priests and the family to carry out important religious rituals, such as promise making, offering candles, visiting shrines, and offering prayers (Spector, 2009).

Folk beliefs regarding health are a combination of elements incorporating views of Roman Catholicism and Indian and Spanish beliefs. The folk healer is called a **curandero** (male) or **curandera** (female). Among traditional Latino Americans, the *curandero* is believed to have a gift from God for healing the sick and is often the first contact made when illness is encountered. Treatments used include massage, diet, rest, suggestions, practical advice, indigenous herbs, prayers, magic, and supernatural rituals (Gonzalez, Owen, & Esperat, 2008). Many Latino Americans still subscribe to the "hot and cold theory" of disease. This concept is similar to the Asian perception of yin and yang discussed earlier in this chapter. Diseases and the foods and medicines used to treat them are classified as "hot" or "cold," and the intention is to restore the body to a balanced state.

A recent national study reported that the lifetime prevalence for selected psychiatric disorders is 36.8 percent for U.S.-born Latinos, which is higher than the prevalence for immigrants from the same cultural group (Alegria et al., 2007). The authors theorized that this may be related to stress experienced as they attempt to assimilate to the economic and cultural ideals in the United States while still maintaining minority group status. They also noted that the Puerto Rican subgroup manifests a higher incidence of depression, substance abuse, and anxiety disorders (particularly posttraumatic stress disorder) when compared to Cuban, Mexican, or other Latino groups. These prevalence rates may even be conservative, because "certain symptoms of psychiatric disorders among immigrant populations (e.g., *ataque de nervios*) would not be represented in the diagnostic batteries used with the general population" (Kaplan, 2007, p. 2). As this cultural group, and particularly U.S.-born Latino Americans, continues to grow in number, mental health professionals will need to develop awareness of this increased risk for illness and sensitivity to the cultural values that may impact seeking treatment.

Western European Americans

Western European Americans have their origin in France, Italy, and Greece. Each of these cultures possesses its own language, in which a number of dialects are noticeable. Western Europeans are considered to be very warm and affectionate people. They tend to be physically expressive, using a lot of body language, including hugging and kissing.

Like Latino Americans, Western European Americans are very family oriented. They interact in large groups, and it is not uncommon for several generations to live together or in close proximity. A strong allegiance to the cultural heritage exists, and it is not uncommon, particularly among Italians, to find settlements of immigrants clustering together.

Roles within the family are clearly defined, with the man as the head of the household. Traditional Western European women view their role as mother and homemaker, and children are prized and cherished. The elderly are held in positions of respect and often are cared for in the home rather than placed in nursing homes.

Roman Catholicism is the predominant religion for French and Italian people, Greek Orthodox for the Greek community. A number of religious traditions are observed surrounding rites of passage. Masses and rituals are observed for births, first communions, marriages, anniversaries, and deaths.

Western Europeans tend to be present-time oriented, with a somewhat fatalistic view of the future. A priority is placed on the here and now, and whatever happens in the future is perceived as God's will.

Most Western European Americans follow health beliefs and practices of the dominant American culture, but some folk beliefs and superstitions still endure. Spector (2009) reported the following superstitions and practices of Italians as they relate to health and illness:

1. Congenital abnormalities can be attributed to the unsatisfied desire for food during pregnancy.

2. If a woman is not given food that she craves or smells, the fetus will move inside, and a miscarriage can result.

3. If a pregnant woman bends or turns or moves in a certain way, the fetus may not develop normally.

4. A woman must not reach during pregnancy because reaching can harm the fetus.

5. Sitting in a draft can cause a cold that can lead to pneumonia.

Food is very important in the Western European American culture. Italian, Greek, and French cuisine is world famous, and food is used in a social manner, as well as for nutritional purposes. Wine is consumed by all (even the children, who are given a mixture of water and wine) and is the beverage of choice with meals. However, among Greek Americans, drunkenness engenders social disgrace on the individual and the family (Papadopoulos & Purnell, 2008).

Arab Americans*

Arab Americans trace their ancestry and traditions to the nomadic desert tribes of the Arabian Peninsula. The Arab countries include Algeria, Bahrain, Comoros, Djibouti, Egypt, Iraq, Jordan, Kuwait, Lebanon, Libya, Mauritania, Morocco, Oman, Palestine, Qatar, Saudi Arabia, Somalia, Sudan, Syria, Tunisia, United Arab Emirates, and Yemen. First-wave immigrants, primarily Christians, came to the United States between 1887 and 1913 seeking economic opportunity. First-wave immigrants and their descendants typically resided in urban centers of the Northeast. Second-wave immigrants entered the United States after World War II. Most are refugees from nations beset by war and political instability. This group includes a large number of professionals and individuals seeking educational degrees who have subsequently remained in the United States. Most are Muslims and favor professional occupations.

Arabic is the official language of the Arab world. Although English is a common second language, language and communication can pose formidable problems in health-care settings. Communication is highly contextual, where unspoken expectations are more important than the actual spoken words. While conversing, individuals stand close together, maintain steady eye contact, and touch (only between members of the same gender) the other's hand or shoulder.

Speech may be loud and expressive and characterized by repetition and gesturing, particularly when involved in serious discussions. Observers witnessing impassioned communication may incorrectly assume that members of this culture are argumentative, confrontational, or aggressive. Privacy is valued, and many resist disclosure of personal information to strangers, especially when it relates to familial disease conditions. Among friends and relatives, Arabs express feelings freely. Devout Muslim men may not shake hands with women. When an Arab man is introduced to an Arab woman, the man waits for the woman to extend her hand.

Punctuality is not taken seriously except in cases of business or professional meetings. Social events and appointments tend not to have a fixed beginning or end.

Gender roles are clearly defined. The man is the head of the household and women are subordinate to men. Men are breadwinners, protectors, and decision makers. Women are responsible for the care and education of children and for the maintenance of a successful marriage by tending to their husbands' needs.

The family is the primary social organization, and children are loved and indulged. The father is the disciplinarian and the mother is an ally and mediator. Loyalty to one's family takes precedence over personal needs. Sons are responsible for supporting elderly parents.

Women value modesty, especially devout Muslims, for whom modesty is expressed with their attire. Many Muslim women view the practice of *hijab,* covering the body except for one's face and hands, as offering them protection in situations in which the genders mix.

Sickle cell disease and the thalassemias are common in the eastern Mediterranean. Sedentary lifestyle and high fat intake among Arab Americans place them at higher risk for cardiovascular diseases. The rates of cholesterol testing, colorectal cancer screening, and uterine cancer screening are low; however, in recent years, the rate of mammography screening has increased.

Arab cooking shares many general characteristics. Spices and herbs include cinnamon, allspice, cloves, ginger, cumin, mint, parsley, bay leaves, garlic, and onions. Bread accompanies every meal and is viewed as a gift from God. Lamb and chicken are the most popular meats. Muslims are prohibited from eating pork and pork products. Food is eaten with the right hand because it is regarded as clean. Eating and drinking at the same time is viewed as unhealthy. Eating properly, consuming nutritious foods, and fasting are believed to cure disease. Gastrointestinal complaints are the most frequent reason for seeking health care. Lactose intolerance is common.

Most Arabs are Muslims. Islam is the religion of most Arab countries, and in Islam there is no

---

*This section on Arab Americans is taken from Kulwicki, A. D. (2008). People of Arab heritage. In L. D. Purnell & B. J. Paulanka (Eds.), *Transcultural health care: A culturally competent approach* (3rd ed.). © F.A. Davis. Used with permission.

separation of church and state; a certain amount of religious participation is obligatory. Many Muslims believe in combining spiritual medicine, performing daily prayers, and reading or listening to the Qur'an with conventional medical treatment. The devout client may request that his or her chair or bed be turned to face Mecca and that a basin of water be provided for ritual washing or ablution before praying. Sometimes illness is considered punishment for one's sins.

Mental illness is a major social stigma. Psychiatric symptoms may be denied or attributed to "bad nerves" or evil spirits. When individuals suffering from mental distress seek medical care, they are likely to present with a variety of vague complaints such as abdominal pain, lassitude, anorexia, and shortness of breath. Clients often expect and may insist on somatic treatment, at least vitamins and tonics. When mental illness is accepted as a diagnosis, treatment with medications, rather than counseling, is preferred.

Jewish Americans

To be Jewish is to belong to a specific group of people and a specific religion. The term *Jewish* does not refer to a race. The Jewish people came to the United States mostly from Spain, Portugal, Germany, and Eastern Europe (Schwartz, 2008). There are more than 5 million Jewish Americans living in the United States, and they live primarily in the larger urban areas.

Four main Jewish religious groups exist today: Orthodox, Reform, Conservative, and Reconstructionist. Orthodox Jews adhere to strict interpretation and application of Jewish laws and ethics. They believe that the laws outlined in the Torah (the five books of Moses) are divine, eternal, and unalterable. Reform Judaism is the largest Jewish religious group in the United States. The Reform group believes in the autonomy of the individual in interpreting the Jewish code of law, and a more liberal interpretation is followed. Conservative Jews also accept a less strict interpretation. They believe that the code of laws comes from God, but accept flexibility and adaptation of those laws to absorb aspects of the culture while remaining true to Judaism's values. The Reconstructionists have modern views that generally override traditional Jewish laws. They do not believe that Jews are God's chosen people and they reject the notion of divine intervention. Reconstructionists are generally accepting of interfaith marriage.

The primary language of Jewish Americans is English. Hebrew, the official language of Israel and the Torah, is used for prayers and is taught in Jewish religious education. Early Jewish immigrants spoke a Judeo-German dialect called Yiddish, and some of those words have become part of American English (e.g., *klutz, kosher, tush*).

Although traditional Jewish law is clearly male oriented, with acculturation little difference is seen today with regard to gender roles. Formal education is a highly respected value among the Jewish people. Over one third of Jewish Americans hold advanced degrees and are employed as professionals (e.g., science, medicine, law, education), more than any other group within the U.S. white population.

While most Jewish people live for today and plan for and worry about tomorrow, they are raised with stories of their past, especially of the Holocaust. They are warned to "never forget," lest history be repeated. Therefore, their time orientation is simultaneously to the past, the present, and the future (Purnell & Selekman, 2008).

Children are considered blessings and valued treasures, treated with respect, and deeply loved. They play an active role in most holiday celebrations and services. Respecting and honoring one's parents is one of the Ten Commandments. Children are expected to be forever grateful to their parents for giving them the gift of life (Purnell & Selekman, 2008). The rite of passage into adulthood occurs during a religious ceremony called a *bar* or *bat mitzvah* (son or daughter of the commandment) and is usually commemorated by a family celebration.

Because of the respect afforded physicians and the emphasis on keeping the body and mind healthy, Jewish Americans tend to be health conscious. In general, they practice preventive health care, with routine physical, dental, and vision screening. Circumcision for male infants is both a medical procedure and a religious rite and is performed on the eighth day of life. The procedure is usually performed at home and is considered a family festivity.

A number of genetic diseases are more common in the Jewish population, including Tay-Sachs disease, Gaucher's disease, and familial dysautonomia. Other conditions that occur with increased incidence in the Jewish population include inflammatory bowel disease (ulcerative colitis and Crohn's disease), colorectal cancer, and breast and ovarian cancer. Jewish people have a higher rate of side effects from the antipsychotic clozapine. About 20 percent develop agranulocytosis, which has been attributed to a specific gene that was recently identified (Purnell & Selekman, 2008).

Alcohol, especially wine, is an essential part of religious holidays and festive occasions. It is viewed as appropriate and acceptable as long as it is used in moderation. For Jewish people who follow the dietary laws, a tremendous amount of attention is given to the slaughter of livestock and the preparation and consumption of food. Religious laws dictate which foods are permissible. The term *kosher* means "fit to eat," and following these guidelines is considered a commandment of God. Meat may be eaten only if the permitted animal has been slaughtered, cooked, or served following kosher guidelines. Pigs are considered unclean, and pork and pork products are forbidden. Dairy products and meat may not be mixed together in cooking, serving, or eating.

Judaism opposes discrimination against people with physical, mental, and developmental conditions. The maintenance of one's mental health is considered just as important as the maintenance of one's physical health. Mental incapacity has always been recognized as grounds for exemption from all obligations under Jewish law (Purnell & Selekman, 2008).

A summary of information related to the six cultural phenomena as they apply to the cultural groups discussed here is presented in Table 6-1.

Culture-Bound Syndromes

The *Diagnostic and Statistical Manual of Mental Disorders, 4th Edition, Text Revision* (*DSM-IV-TR*) (American Psychiatric Association [APA], 2000) recognizes various symptoms that are associated with specific cultures and that may be expressed differently from those of the dominant American culture. Although presentations associated with the major *DSM-IV-TR* categories can be found throughout the world, many of the responses are influenced by local cultural factors (APA, 2000). The *DSM-IV-TR* defines **culture-bound syndromes** as follows:

> Recurrent, locality-specific patterns of aberrant behavior and troubling experience that may or may not be linked to a particular DSM-IV diagnostic category. Many of these patterns are indigenously considered to be "illnesses," or at least afflictions, and most have local names. (p. 898)

It is important for nurses to understand that individuals from diverse cultural groups may exhibit these physical and behavioral manifestations. The syndromes are viewed within these cultural groups

as folk, diagnostic categories with specific sets of experiences and observations (APA, 2000). Examples of culture-bound syndromes are presented in Table 6-2.

Diagnosis/Outcome Identification

Nursing diagnoses are selected based on the information gathered during the assessment process. With background knowledge of cultural variables and information uniquely related to the individual, the following nursing diagnoses may be appropriate:

- Impaired verbal communication related to cultural differences evidenced by inability to speak the dominant language
- Anxiety (moderate to severe) related to entry into an unfamiliar health-care system and separation from support systems evidenced by apprehension and suspicion, restlessness, and trembling
- Imbalanced nutrition, less than body requirements, related to refusal to eat unfamiliar foods provided in the health-care setting, evidenced by loss of weight
- Spiritual distress related to inability to participate in usual religious practices because of hospitalization, evidenced by alterations in mood (e.g., anger, crying, withdrawal, preoccupation, anxiety, hostility, apathy)

Outcome criteria related to these nursing diagnoses may include the following:

The client has:

1. Had all basic needs fulfilled.
2. Communicated with staff through an interpreter.
3. Maintained anxiety at a manageable level by having family members stay with him or her during hospitalization.
4. Maintained weight by eating foods that he or she likes brought to the hospital by family members.
5. Restored spiritual strength through use of cultural rituals and beliefs and visits from a spiritual leader.

Planning/Implementation

The following interventions have special cultural implications for nursing:

1. Use an interpreter if necessary to ensure that there are no barriers to communication. Be careful with nonverbal communication because it may be interpreted differently by different cultures (e.g., Asians and Native

TABLE 6-1 Summary of Six Cultural Phenomena in Comparison of Various Cultural Groups

CULTURAL GROUP AND COUNTRIES OF ORIGIN	COMMUNICATION	SPACE	SOCIAL ORGANIZATION	TIME	ENVIRONMENTAL CONTROL	BIOLOGICAL VARIATIONS
Northern European Americans (England, Ireland, Germany, others)	National languages (although many learn English very quickly) Dialects (often regional) English More verbal than nonverbal	Territory valued Personal space: 18 inches to 3 feet Uncomfortable with personal contact and touch	Families: nuclear and extended Religions: Jewish and Christian Organizations: social community	Future-oriented	Most value preventive medicine and primary health care through traditional health-care delivery system Alternative methods on the increase	Health concerns: Cardiovascular disease Cancer Diabetes mellitus
African Americans (Africa, West Indian Islands, Dominican Republic, Haiti, Jamaica)	National languages Dialects (pidgin, Creole, Gullah, French, Spanish) Highly verbal and nonverbal	Close personal space Comfortable with touch	Large, extended families Many female-headed households Strong religious orientation, mostly Protestant Community social organizations	Present-time oriented	Traditional health-care delivery system Some individuals prefer to use folk practitioner ("granny" or voodoo healer) Home remedies	Health concerns: Cardiovascular disease Hypertension Sickle cell disease Diabetes mellitus Lactose intolerance
Native Americans (North America, Alaska, Aleutian Islands)	200 tribal languages recognized Comfortable with silence Direct eye contact considered rude	Large, extended space important Uncomfortable with touch	Families: nuclear and extended Children taught importance of tradition Social organizations: tribe and family most important	Present-time oriented	Religion and health practices intertwined Non-traditional healer (shaman) uses folk practices to heal Shaman may work with modern medical practitioner	Health concerns: Alcoholism Tuberculosis Accidents Diabetes mellitus Heart disease

Continued

TABLE 6-1 Summary of Six Cultural Phenomena in Comparison of Various Cultural Groups—cont'd

CULTURAL GROUP AND COUNTRIES OF ORIGIN	COMMUNICATION	SPACE	SOCIAL ORGANIZATION	TIME	ENVIRONMENTAL CONTROL	BIOLOGICAL VARIATIONS
Asian/Pacific Islander Americans (Japan, China, Korea, Vietnam, Philippines, Thailand, Cambodia, Laos, Pacific Islands, others)	More than 30 different languages spoken Comfortable with silence Uncomfortable with eye-to-eye contact Nonverbal connotations may be misunderstood	Large personal space Uncomfortable with touch	Families: nuclear and extended Children taught importance of family loyalty and tradition Many religions: Taoism, Buddhism, Islam, Hinduism, Christianity Community social organizations	Present-time oriented Past is important and valued	Traditional health care delivery system Some prefer to use folk practices (e.g., yin and yang, herbal medicine, and moxibustion)	Health concerns: Hypertension Cancer Diabetes mellitus Thalassemia Lactose intolerance
Latino Americans (Mexico, Spain, Cuba, Puerto Rico, other countries of Central and South America)	Spanish, with many dialects	Close personal space Lots of touching and embracing Very group oriented	Families: nuclear and large extended families Strong ties to Roman Catholicism Community social organizations	Present-time oriented	Traditional health-care delivery system Some prefer to use folk practitioner, called *curandero* or *curandera* Folk practices include "hot and cold" herbal remedies	Health concerns: Heart disease Cancer Diabetes mellitus Accidents Lactose intolerance
Western European Americans (France, Italy, Greece)	National languages Dialects	Close personal space Lots of touching and embracing Very group oriented	Families: nuclear and large extended families France and Italy: Roman Catholic Greece: Greek Orthodox	Present-time oriented	Traditional health-care delivery system Lots of home remedies and practices based on superstition	Health concerns: Heart disease Cancer Diabetes mellitus Thalassemia

Group (Origin)	Language	Personal space/touch	Family/Religion	Time orientation	Health-care beliefs	Health concerns
Arab Americans (Algeria, Bahrain, Comoros, Djibouti, Egypt, Iraq, Jordan, Kuwait, Lebanon, Libya, Mauritania, Morocco, Oman, Palestine, Qatar, Saudi Arabia, Somalia, Sudan, Syria, Tunisia, United Arab Emirates, Yemen)	Arabic English	Large personal space between members of the opposite gender outside of the family. Touching common between members of same gender	Families: nuclear and extended. Religion: Muslim and Christianity	Past and present-time oriented	Traditional health-care delivery system. Some superstitious beliefs. Authority of physician is seldom challenged or questioned. Adverse outcomes are attributed to God's will. Mental illness viewed as a social stigma	Health concerns: Sickle cell disease Thalassemia Cardiovascular disease Cancer
Jewish Americans (Spain, Portugal, Germany, Eastern Europe)	English, Hebrew, Yiddish	Touch forbidden between opposite genders in the Orthodox tradition. Closer personal space common among non-orthodox Jews	Families: nuclear and extended. Community social organizations	Past, present-time, and future oriented.	Great respect for physicians. Emphasis on keeping body and mind healthy. Practice preventive health care	Health concerns: Tay-Sachs disease Gaucher's disease Familial dysautonomia Ulcerative colitis Crohn's disease Colorectal cancer Breast cancer Ovarian cancer

SOURCES: Giger and & Davidhizar (2008); Murray, Zentner, and & Yakimo (2009); Purnell and & Paulanka (2008); and Spector (2009).

TABLE 6-2 Culture-Bound Syndromes

SYNDROME	CULTURE	SYMPTOMS
Amok	Malaysia, Laos, Philippines, Polynesia, Papua New Guinea, Puerto Rico	A dissociative episode followed by an outburst of violent, aggressive, or homicidal behavior directed at people and objects. May be associated with psychotic episode.
Ataque de nervios	Latin American and Latin Mediterranean groups	Uncontrollable shouting, crying, trembling, verbal or physical aggression, sometimes accompanied by dissociative experiences, seizure-like or fainting episodes, and suicidal gestures. Often occurs in response to stressful family event.
Bilis and colera *(muina)*	Latin American	Acute nervous tension, headache, trembling, screaming, stomach disturbances, and sometimes loss of consciousness. Thought to occur in response to intense anger or rage.
Boufee delirante	West Africa and Haiti	Sudden outburst of agitated and aggressive behavior, confusion, and psychomotor excitement. May be accompanied by hallucinations or paranoia.
Brain fag	West Africa	Difficulty concentrating, remembering, and thinking. Pain and pressure around head and neck; blurred vision. Associated with challenges of schooling.
Dhat	India	Severe anxiety and hypochondriasis associated with the discharge of semen, whitish discoloration of the urine, and feelings of weakness and exhaustion.
Falling out or blacking out	Southern United States and the Caribbean	Sudden collapse. May or may not be preceded by dizziness. Person can hear but cannot move. Eyes are open, but individual claims inability to see.
Ghost sickness	American Indian tribes	Preoccupation with death and the deceased. Bad dreams, weakness, feelings of danger, loss of appetite, fainting, dizziness, fear, anxiety, hallucinations, loss of consciousness, confusion, feelings of futility, and a sense of suffocation.
Hwa-byung (anger syndrome)	Korea	Insomnia, fatigue, panic, fear of impending death, dysphoric affect, indigestion, anorexia, dyspnea, palpitations, and generalized aches and pains. Attributed to the suppression of anger.
Koro	Southern and Eastern Asia	Sudden and intense anxiety that the penis (in males) or the vulva and nipples (in females) will recede into the body and cause death.
Latah	Malaysia, Indonesia	Hypersensitivity to sudden fright, often with echopraxia, echolalia, and dissociative or trancelike behavior.
Locura	Latinos in the U.S. and Latin America	Incoherence, agitation, hallucinations, ineffective social interaction, unpredictability, and possible violence. Attributed to genetics or environmental stress, or a combination of both.

TABLE 6-2 Culture-Bound Syndromes—cont'd		
SYNDROME	**CULTURE**	**SYMPTOMS**
Mal de ojo (evil eye)	Mediterranean cultures	Occurs primarily in children. Fitful sleep, crying, diarrhea, vomiting, and fever.
Nervios	Latinos in the U.S. and Latin America	Headaches, irritability, stomach disturbances, sleep difficulties, nervousness, easy tearfulness, inability to concentrate, trembling, tingling sensations, and dizziness. Occurs in response to stressful life experiences.
Pibloktoq	Eskimo cultures	Abrupt dissociative episode accompanied by extreme excitement and sometimes followed by convulsions and coma lasting up to 12 hours.
Qi-gong psychotic reaction	China	Dissociative, paranoid, or other psychotic or nonpsychotic symptoms that occur in individuals who become overly involved in the Chinese health-enhancing practice of qi-gong ("exercise of vital energy")
Rootwork	African Americans, European Americans, Caribbean cultures	Anxiety, gastrointestinal complaints, weakness, dizziness, fear of being poisoned or killed. Symptoms are ascribed to hexing, witchcraft, sorcery, or the evil influence of another person.
Sangue dormido ("sleeping blood")	Portuguese Cape Verde Islanders	Pain, numbness, tremor, paralysis, convulsions, stroke, blindness, heart attack, infection, and miscarriage.
Shenjing shuairuo ("neurasthenia")	China	Physical and mental fatigue, dizziness, headaches, other pains, concentration difficulties, sleep disturbance, memory loss, gastrointestinal problems, sexual dysfunction, irritability, excitability, and various signs suggesting disturbance of the autonomic nervous system.
Shenkui (Shenkuei)	China (Taiwan)	Anxiety or panic, with dizziness, backache, fatigability, general weakness, insomnia, frequent dreams, and sexual dysfunction. Attributed to excessive semen loss.

Adapted from Diagnostic and Statistical Manual of Mental Disorders, 4th Edition, Text Revision. © 2000, American Psychiatric Association. With permission.

Americans may be uncomfortable with touch and direct eye contact, whereas Latinos and Western Europeans perceive touch as a sign of caring).

2. Make allowances for individuals from other cultures to have family members around them and even participate in their care. Large numbers of extended family members are very important to African Americans, Native Americans, Asian Americans, Latino Americans, and Western European Americans. To deny

access to these family support systems could interfere with the healing process.

3. Ensure that the individual's spiritual needs are being met. Religion is an important source of support for many individuals, and the nurse must be tolerant of various rituals that may be connected with different cultural beliefs about health and illness.

4. Be aware of the differences in concept of time among the various cultures. Most members of the dominant American culture are

future oriented and place a high value on punctuality and efficiency. Other cultures such as African Americans, Native Americans, Asian Americans, Latino Americans, Arab Americans and Western European Americans are more present-time oriented. Nurses must be aware that such individuals may not share the value of punctuality. They may be late to appointments and appear to be indifferent to some aspects of their therapy. Nurses must be accepting of these differences and refrain from allowing existing attitudes to interfere with delivery of care.

5. Be aware of different beliefs about health care among the various cultures, and recognize the importance of these beliefs to the healing process. If an individual from another culture has been receiving health care from a spiritualist, granny, curandero, or other nontraditional healer, it is important for the nurse to listen to what has been done in the past and even to consult with these cultural healers about the care being given to the client.

6. Follow the health-care practices that the client views as essential, provided they do no harm or do not interfere with the healing process of the client. For example, the concepts of yin and yang and the "hot and cold" theory of disease are very important to the well-being of some Asians and Latinos, respectively. Try to ensure that a balance of these foods is included in the diet as an important reinforcement for traditional medical care.

7. Be aware of favorite foods of individuals from different cultures. The health-care setting may seem strange and somewhat isolated, and for some individuals it feels good to have anything around them that is familiar. They may even refuse to eat foods that are unfamiliar to them. If it does not interfere with his or her care, allow family members to provide favorite foods for the client.

8. The nurse working in psychiatry must realize that psychiatric illness is stigmatized in some cultures. Individuals who believe that expressing emotions is unacceptable (e.g., Asian Americans and Native Americans) will present unique problems when they are clients in a psychiatric setting. Nurses must have patience and work slowly to establish trust in order to provide these individuals with the assistance they require.

Evaluation

Evaluation of nursing actions is directed at achievement of the established outcomes. Part of the evaluation process is continuous reassessment to ensure that the selected actions are appropriate and the goals and outcomes are realistic. Including the family and extended support systems in the evaluation process is essential if cultural implications of nursing care are to be measured. Modifications to the plan of care are made as the need is determined.

SPIRITUAL CONCEPTS

CORE CONCEPT

Spirituality
The human quality that gives meaning and sense of purpose to an individual's existence. Spirituality exists within each individual regardless of belief system and serves as a force for interconnectedness between the self and others, the environment, and a higher power.

Spirituality is difficult to describe. Historically, it has had distinctly religious connections, with a spiritual person being described as "someone with whom the Spirit of God dwelt." More recently, however, it has been considered "something people define for themselves that is largely free of the rules, regulations and responsibilities associated with religion" (Koenig, 2009).

In the treatment of mental illness, some of the earliest practices focused on including spiritual treatment, because insanity was considered a disruption of mind and spirit (Reeves & Reynolds, 2009). However, Freud (often described as a forefather of psychiatric treatment) believed that religion had a negative effect on mental health, and that it was linked to a host of psychiatric symptoms. Thus religion and spiritually have been avoided rather than embraced as a valuable aspect of treatment. More recently, the focus is changing once again. Reeves and Reynolds (2009) noted that the large volume of contemporary research (more than 60 studies) demonstrating the value of spirituality for both medical and psychiatric patients is influencing this change. Nursing has embraced this new focus by the inclusion of nursing responsibility for spiritual care in the International Council of Nurses *Code of Ethics* and in the American Holistic Nurses Association *Standards for Holistic Nursing*

Practice. The inclusion of spiritual care is also evidenced by the development of the nursing diagnosis category of Spiritual Distress by NANDA International (Wright, 2005).

Smucker (2001) stated:

> Spirituality is the recognition or experience of a dimension of life that is invisible, and both within us and yet beyond our material world, providing a sense of connectedness and interrelatedness with the universe. (p. 5)

Smucker (2001) identified the following factors as types of spiritual needs associated with human beings:

1. Meaning and purpose in life
2. Faith or trust in someone or something beyond ourselves
3. Hope
4. Love
5. Forgiveness

Spiritual Needs

Meaning and Purpose in Life

Humans by nature appreciate order and structure in their lives. Having a purpose in life gives one a sense of control and the feeling that life is worth living. Indeed, Burkhardt and Nagai-Jacobson (2002) described the essence of spirituality as the developing awareness of who we are, what is our purpose in being, and the understanding of our connectedness with ourselves as well as beyond ourselves. Each nurse's exploration of his or her own spirituality and efforts to grow spiritually are foundational to being responsive to those needs in others. Walsh (1999) described "seven perennial practices" that he believes promote enlightenment, aid in transformation, and encourage spiritual growth. He identified the seven perennial practices as follows:

1. **Transform your motivation:** Reduce craving and find your soul's desire.
2. **Cultivate emotional wisdom:** Heal your heart and learn to love.
3. **Live ethically:** Feel good by doing good.
4. **Concentrate and calm your mind:** Accept the challenge of mastering attention and mindfulness.
5. **Awaken your spiritual vision:** See clearly and recognize the sacred in all things.
6. **Cultivate spiritual intelligence:** Develop wisdom and understand life.

7. **Express spirit in action:** Embrace generosity and the joy of service. (p. 14)

In the final analysis, each individual must determine his or her own perception of what is important and what gives meaning to life. Throughout one's existence, the meaning of life will undoubtedly be challenged many times. A solid spiritual foundation may help an individual confront the challenges that result from life's experiences.

Faith

Faith is often thought of as the acceptance of a belief in the absence of physical or empirical evidence. Smucker (2001) stated:

> For all people, faith is an important concept. From childhood on, our psychological health depends on having faith or trust in something or someone to help meet our needs. (p. 7)

Having faith requires that individuals rise above that which they can only experience through the five senses. Indeed, faith transcends the appearance of the physical world. An increasing amount of medical and scientific research is showing that what individuals believe exists can have as powerful an impact as what actually exists. Karren, Hafen, Smith, and Frandsen (2006) stated:

> Personal belief gives us an unseen power that enables us to do the impossible, to perform miracles—even to heal ourselves. It has been found that patients who exhibit faith become less concerned about their symptoms, have less-severe symptoms, and have less-frequent symptoms with longer periods of relief between them than patients who lack faith. (p. 473)

Evidence suggests that faith, combined with conventional treatment and an optimistic attitude, can be a very powerful element in the healing process.

Hope

Hope has been defined as a special kind of positive expectation (Karren et al., 2006). With hope, individuals look at a situation, and no matter how negative, find something positive on which to focus. Hope functions as an energizing force. In addition, research indicates that hope may promote healing, facilitate coping, and enhance quality of life (Nekolaichuk, Jevne, & Maguire, 1999).

Kübler-Ross (1969), in her classic study of dying patients, stressed the importance of hope. She suggested that, even though these patients could not hope for a cure, they could hope for additional time to live, to be with loved ones, for freedom from pain, or for a peaceful death with dignity. She found hope to be a satisfaction unto itself, whether or not it was fulfilled. She stated, "If a patient stops expressing hope, it is usually a sign of imminent death" (p. 140).

Researchers in the field of psychoneuroimmunology have found that the attitudes we have and the emotions we experience have a definite effect on the body. An optimistic feeling of hope is not just a mental state. Hope and optimism produce positive physical changes in the body that can influence the immune system and the functioning of specific body organs. The medical literature abounds with countless examples of individuals with terminal conditions who suddenly improve when they find something to live for. Conversely, there are also many accounts of patients whose conditions deteriorate when they lose hope.

Love

Love may be identified as a projection of one's own good feelings onto others. To love others, one must first experience love of self, and then be able and willing to project that warmth and affectionate concern for others (Karren et al., 2006). Smucker (2001) stated:

> Love, in its purest unconditional form, is probably life's most powerful force and our greatest spiritual need. Not only is it important to receive love, but equally important to give love to others. Thinking about and caring for the needs of others keeps us from being too absorbed with ourselves and our needs to the exclusion of others. We all have experienced the good feelings that come from caring for and loving others. (p. 10)

Love may be a very important key in the healing process. Karren and associates (2006) stated:

> People who become more loving and less fearful, who replace negative thoughts with the emotion of love, are often able to achieve physical healing. Most of us are familiar with the emotional effects of love, the way love makes us feel inside. But . . . true love—a love that is patient, trusting, protecting, optimistic, and kind—has actual physical effects on the body, too. (p. 466)

Some researchers suggest that love has a positive effect on the immune system. This has been shown to be true in adults and children, and also in animals (Fox & Fox, 1988; Ornish, 1998). The giving and receiving of love may also result in

higher levels of endorphins, thereby contributing to a sense of euphoria and helping to reduce pain.

In one long-term study, researchers Werner and Smith (1992) studied children who were reared in impoverished environments. Their homes were troubled by discord, desertion, or divorce, or marred by parental alcoholism or mental illness. The subjects were studied at birth, childhood, adolescence, and adulthood. Two out of three of these high-risk children had developed serious learning and/or behavioral problems by age 10, or had a record of delinquencies, mental health problems, or pregnancies by age 18. One fourth of them had developed "very serious" physical and psychosocial problems. By the time they reached adulthood, more than three fourths of them suffered from profound psychological and behavioral problems and even more were in poor physical health. But of particular interest to the researchers were the 15 to 20 percent who remained resilient and well despite their impoverished and difficult existence. The children who remained resilient and well had experienced a warm and loving relationship with another person during their first year of life, whereas the children who developed serious psychological and physical problems did not. This research indicates that the earlier people have the benefit of a strong, loving relationship, the better they seem able to resist the effects of a deleterious lifestyle.

Forgiveness

Karren and associates (2006) stated, "Essential to a spiritual nature is forgiveness—the ability to release from the mind all the past hurts and failures, all sense of guilt and loss" (p. 434). Feelings of bitterness and resentment take a physical toll on an individual by generating stress hormones, which, when maintained for long periods, can have a detrimental effect on a person's health. Forgiveness enables a person to cast off resentment and begin the pathway to healing.

Forgiveness is not easy. Individuals often have great difficulty when called upon to forgive others and even greater difficulty in attempting to forgive themselves. Many people carry throughout their lives a sense of guilt for having committed a mistake for which they do not believe they have been forgiven or for which they have not forgiven themselves.

To forgive is not necessarily to condone or excuse one's own or someone else's inappropriate behavior. Karren and associates (2006) suggested that forgiveness is:

> . . . an attitude that implies that you are willing to accept responsibility for your perceptions,

realizing that your perceptions are a choice and not an objective fact; a decision to see beyond the limits of another's personality, and to gradually transform yourself from being a helpless victim of your circumstances to being a powerful and loving co-creator of your reality. (pp. 434–435)

Holding on to grievances causes pain, suffering, and conflict. Forgiveness (of self and others) is a gift to oneself. It offers freedom and peace of mind.

It is important for nurses to be able to assess the spiritual needs of their clients. Nurses need not serve the role of professional counselor or spiritual guide, but because of the closeness of their relationship with clients, nurses may be the part of the health-care team to whom clients may reveal the most intimate details of their lives. Smucker (2001) stated:

Just as answering a patient's question honestly and with accurate information and responding to his needs in a timely and sensitive manner communicates caring, so also does high-quality professional nursing care reach beyond the physical body or the illness to that part of the person where identity, self-worth, and spirit lie. In this sense, good nursing care is also good spiritual care. (pp. 11–12)

Religion

> ### CORE CONCEPT
>
> #### Religion
> A set of beliefs, values, rites, and rituals adopted by a group of people. The practices are usually grounded in the teachings of a spiritual leader.

Religion is one way in which an individual's spirituality may be expressed. There are more than 6500 religions in the world (Bronson, 2005). Some individuals seek out various religions in an attempt to find answers to fundamental questions that they have about life, and indeed, about their very existence. Others, although they may regard themselves as spiritual, choose not to affiliate with an organized religious group. In either situation, however, it is inevitable that questions related to life and the human condition arise during the progression of spiritual maturation.

Brodd (2003) suggested that all religious traditions manifest seven dimensions: experiential,

mythic, doctrinal, ethical, ritual, social, and material. He explained that these seven dimensions are intertwined and complementary and, depending on the particular religion, certain dimensions are emphasized more than others. For example, Zen Buddhism has a strong experiential dimension, but says little about doctrines. Roman Catholicism is strong in both ritual and doctrine. The social dimension is a significant aspect of religion, as it provides a sense of community, of belonging to a group such as a parish or a congregation, which is empowering for some individuals.

Affiliation with a religious group has been shown to be a health-enhancing endeavor (Karren et al., 2006). A number of studies have been conducted that indicate a correlation between religious faith/church attendance and increased chance of survival following serious illness, less depression and other mental illness, longer life, and overall better physical and mental health. In an extensive review of the literature, Maryland psychologist John Gartner (1998) found that individuals with a religious commitment had lower suicide rates, lower drug use and abuse, less juvenile delinquency, lower divorce rates, and improved mental illness outcomes.

It is not known how religious participation protects health and promotes well-being. Some churches actively promote healthy lifestyles and discourage behavior that would be harmful to health or interfere with treatment of disease. But some researchers believe that the strong social support network found in churches may be the most important force in boosting the health and well-being of their members. More so than merely an affiliation, however, it is regular church attendance and participation that appear to be the key factors.

Addressing Spiritual and Religious Needs Through the Nursing Process

Assessment

It is important for nurses to consider spiritual and religious needs when planning care for their clients. The Joint Commission requires that nurses address the psychosocial, spiritual, and cultural variables that influence the perception of illness. Dossey (1998) has developed a spiritual assessment tool (Box 6-4) about which she stated,

The Spiritual Assessment Tool provides reflective questions for assessing, evaluating, and increasing awareness of spirituality in patients and their significant others. The

BOX 6-4 **Spiritual Assessment Tool**

The following reflective questions may assist you in assessing, evaluating, and increasing awareness of spirituality in yourself and others.

MEANING AND PURPOSE

These questions assess a person's ability to seek meaning and fulfillment in life, manifest hope, and accept ambiguity and uncertainty.

- What gives your life meaning?
- Do you have a sense of purpose in life?
- Does your illness interfere with your life goals?
- Why do you want to get well?
- How hopeful are you about obtaining a better degree of health?
- Do you feel that you have a responsibility in maintaining your health?
- Will you be able to make changes in your life to maintain your health?
- Are you motivated to get well?
- What is the most important or powerful thing your life?

INNER STRENGTHS

These questions assess a person's ability to manifest joy and recognize strengths, choices, goals, and faith.

- What brings you joy and peace in your life?
- What can you do to feel alive and full of spirit?
- What traits do you like about yourself?
- What are your personal strengths?
- What choices are available to you to enhance your healing?
- What life goals have you set for yourself?
- Do you think that stress in any way caused your illness?
- How aware were you of your body before you became sick?
- What do you believe in?
- Is faith important in your life?
- How has your illness influenced your faith?
- Does faith play a role in recognizing your health?

INTERCONNECTIONS

These questions assess a person's positive self-concept, self-esteem, and sense of self; sense of belonging in the world with others; capacity to pursue personal interests; and ability to demonstrate love of self and self-forgiveness.

- How do you feel about yourself right now?
- How do you feel when you have a true sense of yourself?
- Do you pursue things of personal interest?
- What do you do to show love for yourself?
- Can you forgive yourself?
- What do you do to heal your spirit?

These questions assess a person's ability to connect in life-giving ways with family, friends, and social groups and to engage in the forgiveness of others.

- Who are the significant people in your life?
- Do you have friends or family in town who are available to help you?
- Who are the people to whom you are closest?
- Do you belong to any groups?
- Can you ask people for help when you need it?
- Can you share your feelings with others?
- What are some of the most loving things that others have done for you?
- What are the loving things that you do for other people?
- Are you able to forgive others?

These questions assess a person's capacity for finding meaning in worship or religious activities, and a connectedness with a divinity.

- Is worship important to you?
- What do you consider the most significant act of worship in your life?
- Do you participate in any religious activities?
- Do you believe in God or a higher power?
- Do you think that prayer is powerful?
- Have you ever tried to empty your mind of all thoughts to see what the experience might be?
- Do you use relaxation or imagery skills?
- Do you meditate?
- Do you pray?
- What is your prayer?
- How are your prayers answered?
- Do you have a sense of belonging in this world?

These questions assess a person's ability to experience a sense of connection with life and nature, an awareness of the effects of the environment on life and well-being, and a capacity or concern for the health of the environment.

- Do you ever feel a connection with the world or universe?
- How does your environment have an impact on your state of well-being?
- What are your environmental stressors at work and at home?
- What strategies reduce your environmental stressors?
- Do you have any concerns for the state of your immediate environment?
- Are you involved with environmental issues such as recycling environmental resources at home, work, or in your community?
- Are you concerned about the survival of the planet?

SOURCES: Burkhardt, M. A. (1989). Spirituality: An analysis of the concept. *Holistic Nursing Practice, 3(3),* 69–77; Dossey, B. M., et al. (Eds.). (1995). *Holistic nursing: A handbook for practice (2nd ed.).* Gaithersburg, MD: Aspen.
From Dossey, B. M. (1998). Holistic modalities and healing moments. *American Journal of Nursing, 98(6),* 44–47, with permission.

tool's reflective questions can facilitate healing because they stimulate spontaneous, independent, meaningful initiatives to improve the patient's capacity for recovery and healing (p. 45)

Assessing the spiritual needs of a client with a psychotic disorder can pose some additional challenges. Approximately 25 percent of people with schizophrenia and 15 to 22 percent of people with bipolar disorder have religious delusions (Koenig, 2009). Sometimes these delusions can be difficult to differentiate from general religious or cultural beliefs, but "longitudinal studies suggest that nonpsychotic religious activity may actually improve long-term prognosis in patients with psychotic disorders" (Koenig, 2009, p. 288). Engaging family members and significant others in the assessment process can be a great help in determining which religious beliefs and activities have been beneficial to the patient versus those that have been detrimental to their progress.

Diagnoses/Outcome Identification

Nursing diagnoses that may be used when addressing spiritual and religious needs of clients include:

- Risk for Spiritual Distress
- Spiritual Distress
- Readiness for Enhanced Spiritual Well-being
- Risk for Impaired Religiosity
- Impaired Religiosity
- Readiness for Enhanced Religiosity

The following outcomes may be used as guidelines for care and to evaluate effectiveness of the nursing interventions.

The client will:

1. Identify meaning and purpose in life that reinforce hope, peace, and contentment.
2. Verbalize acceptance of self as a worthwhile human being.
3. Accept and incorporate change into life in a healthy manner.
4. Express understanding of relationship between difficulties in current life situation and interruption in previous religious beliefs and activities.
5. Discuss beliefs and values about spiritual and religious issues.
6. Express desire and ability to participate in beliefs and activities of desired religion.

Planning/Implementation

NANDA International (2009) information related to the diagnoses Risk for Spiritual Distress and Risk for Impaired Religiosity is as follows:

Risk for Spiritual Distress

Definition: At risk for an impaired ability to experience and integrate meaning and purpose in life through a person's connectedness with self, other persons, art, music, literature, nature, and/or a power greater than oneself.

Risk Factors

Physical: Physical/chronic illness; substance abuse

Psychosocial: Low self-esteem; depression; anxiety; stress; poor relationships; separate from support systems; blocks to experiencing love; inability to forgive; loss; racial/cultural conflict; change in religious rituals; change in spiritual practices

Developmental: Life change; developmental life changes

Environmental: Environmental changes; natural disasters

Risk for Impaired Religiosity

Definition: At risk for an impaired ability to exercise reliance on religious beliefs and/or participate in rituals of a particular faith tradition.

Risk Factors

Physical: Illness/hospitalization; pain

Psychological: Ineffective support/coping/caregiving; depression; lack of security

Sociocultural: Lack of social interaction; cultural barrier to practicing religion; social isolation

Spiritual: Suffering

Environmental: Lack of transportation; environmental barriers to practicing religion

Developmental: Life transitions

A plan of care addressing the client's spiritual/religious needs is presented in Table 6-3. Selected nursing diagnoses are presented, along with appropriate nursing interventions and rationales for each.

Evaluation

Evaluation of nursing actions is directed at achievement of the established outcomes. Part of the evaluation process is continuous reassessment to ensure that the selected actions are appropriate

Table 6-3 CARE PLAN FOR THE CLIENT WITH SPIRITUAL AND RELIGIOUS NEEDS*

NURSING DIAGNOSIS: RISK FOR SPIRITUAL DISTRESS
RELATED TO: Life changes; environmental changes; stress; anxiety; depression
EVIDENCED BY: Questioning meaning of life and own existence; inner conflict about personal beliefs and values

OUTCOME CRITERIA	NURSING INTERVENTIONS	RATIONALE
Client will identify meaning and purpose in life that reinforce hope, peace, contentment, and self-satisfaction.	1. Assess current situation.	1–8. Thorough assessment is necessary to develop an accurate care plan for the client.
	2. Listen to client's expressions of anger, concern, self-blame.	
	3. Note reason for living and whether it is directly related to situation.	
	4. Determine client's religious/spiritual orientation, current involvement, and presence of conflicts, especially in current circumstances.	
	5. Assess sense of self-concept, worth, ability to enter into loving relationships.	
	6. Observe behavior indicative of poor relationships with others.	
	7. Determine support systems available to and used by client and significant others.	
	8. Assess substance use/abuse.	
	9. Establish an environment that promotes free expression of feelings and concerns.	9. Trust is the basis of a therapeutic nurse-client relationship.
	10. Have client identify and prioritize current/immediate needs.	10. Helps client focus on what needs to be done and identify manageable steps to take.
	11. Discuss philosophical issues related to impact of current situation on spiritual beliefs and values.	11. Helps client to understand that certain life experiences can cause individuals to question personal values and that this response is not uncommon.
	12. Use therapeutic communication skills of reflection and active listening.	12. Helps client find own solutions to concerns.
	13. Review coping skills used and their effectiveness in current situation.	13. Identifies strengths to incorporate into plan and techniques that need revision.
	14. Provide a role model (e.g., nurse, individual experiencing similar situation).	14. Sharing of experiences and hope assists client to deal with reality.
	15. Suggest use of journaling.	15. Journaling can assist in clarifying beliefs and values and in recognizing and resolving feelings about current life situation.
	16. Discuss client's interest in the arts, music, literature.	16. Provides insight into meaning of these issues and how they are integrated into an individual's life.
	17. Role-play new coping techniques. Discuss possibilities of taking classes, becoming involved in discussion groups, cultural activities of client's choice.	17. These activities will help to enhance integration of new skills and necessary changes in client's lifestyle.
	18. Refer client to appropriate resources for help.	18. Client may require additional assistance with an individual who specializes in these types of concerns.

Table 6-3 CARE PLAN FOR THE CLIENT WITH SPIRITUAL AND RELIGIOUS NEEDS*—cont'd

NURSING DIAGNOSIS: RISK FOR IMPAIRED RELIGIOSITY

RELATED TO: Suffering; depression; illness; life transitions

EVIDENCED BY: Concerns about relationship with deity; unable to participate in usual religious practices; anger toward God

OUTCOME CRITERIA	NURSING INTERVENTIONS	RATIONALE
Client will express achievement of support and personal satisfaction from spiritual/religious practices.	1. Assess current situation (e.g., illness, hospitalization, prognosis of death, presence of support systems, financial concerns).	1. This information identifies problems client is dealing with in the moment that are affecting desire to be involved with religious activities.
	2. Listen nonjudgmentally to client's expressions of anger and possible belief that illness/condition may be a result of lack of faith.	2. Individuals often blame themselves for what has happened and reject previous religious beliefs and/or God.
	3. Determine client's usual religious/spiritual beliefs, current involvement in specific church activities.	3. This is important background for establishing a database.
	4. Note quality of relationships with significant others and friends.	4. Individual may withdraw from others in relation to the stress of illness, pain, and suffering.
	5. Assess substance use/abuse.	5. When in distress, individuals often turn to use of various substances, and this can affect the ability to deal with problems in a positive manner.
	6. Develop nurse-client relationship in which individual can express feelings and concerns freely.	6. Trust is the basis for a therapeutic nurse-client relationship.
	7. Use therapeutic communication skills of active listening, reflection, and "I" messages.	7. Helps client to find own solutions to problems and concerns and promotes sense of control.
	8. Be accepting and nonjudgmental when client expresses anger and bitterness toward God. Stay with the client.	8. The nurse's presence and nonjudgmental attitude increase the client's feelings of self-worth and promote trust in the relationship.
	9. Encourage client to discuss previous religious practices and how these practices provided support in the past.	9. A nonjudgmental discussion of previous sources of support may help the client work through current rejection of them as potential sources of support.
	10. Allow the client to take the lead in initiating participation in religious activities, such as prayer.	10. Client may be vulnerable in current situation and needs to be allowed to decide own resumption of these actions.
	11. Contact spiritual leader of client's choice, if he or she requests.	11. These individuals serve to provide relief from spiritual distress and often can do so when other support persons cannot.

*The interventions for this care plan were adapted from Doenges, Moorhouse, and Murr (2010).

and the goals and outcomes are realistic. Including the family and extended support systems in the evaluation process is essential if spiritual and religious implications of nursing care are to be measured. Modifications to the plan of care are made as the need is determined.

Summary and Key Points

■ Culture encompasses shared patterns of belief, feeling, and knowledge that guide people's conduct and are passed down from generation to generation.

■ Ethnic groups are tied together by a shared heritage.

■ Cultural groups differ in terms of communication, space, social organization, time, environmental control, and biological variations.

■ Northern European Americans are the descendants of the first immigrants to the United States and make up the current dominant cultural group. They value punctuality, work responsibility, and a healthy lifestyle.

■ African Americans trace their roots in the United States to the days of slavery. Most have large support systems and a strong religious orientation. Many have assimilated into and have many of the same characteristics as the dominant culture. Some African Americans from the rural South may receive health care from a folk practitioner.

■ Many Native Americans still live on reservations. They speak many different languages and dialects. They often appear silent and reserved, and many are uncomfortable with touch and expressing emotions. Health care may be delivered by a healer called a *shaman.*

■ Asian American languages are very diverse. Touching during communication has historically been considered unacceptable. Asian Americans may have difficulty expressing emotions and appear cold and aloof. Family loyalty is emphasized. Psychiatric illness is viewed as behavior that is out of control and brings shame on the family.

■ The common language of Latino Americans is Spanish. Large family groups are important, and touch is a common form of communication. The predominant religion is Roman Catholicism and the church is often a source of strength in times of crisis. Health care may be delivered by a folk healer called a *curandero,*

who uses various forms of treatment to restore the body to a balanced state.

■ Western European Americans have their origins in Italy, France, and Greece. They are warm and expressive and use touch as a common form of communication. The dominant religion is Roman Catholicism for the Italians and French and Greek Orthodoxy for the Greeks. Most Western European Americans follow the health practices of the dominant culture, but some folk beliefs and superstitions endure.

■ Arab Americans trace their ancestry and traditions to the nomadic desert tribes of the Arabian Peninsula. Arabic is the official language of the Arab world, and the dominant religion is Islam. Mental illness is considered a social stigma, and symptoms are often somaticized.

■ The Jewish people came to the United States predominantly from Spain, Portugal, Germany, and Eastern Europe. Four main Jewish religious groups exist today: Orthodox, Reform, Conservative, and Reconstructionist. The primary language is English. A high value is placed on education. Jewish Americans are very health conscious and practice preventive health care. The maintenance of one's mental health is considered just as important as the maintenance of one's physical health.

■ Culture-bound syndromes are clusters of physical and behavioral symptoms that are considered as illnesses or "afflictions" by specific cultures and recognized as such by the *DSM-IV-TR.*

■ Spirituality is the human quality that gives meaning and sense of purpose to an individual's existence.

■ Individuals possess a number of spiritual needs that include meaning and purpose in life, faith or trust in someone or something beyond themselves, hope, love, and forgiveness.

■ Religion is a set of beliefs, values, rites, and rituals adopted by a group of people.

■ Religion is one way in which an individual's spirituality may be expressed.

■ Affiliation with a religious group has been shown to be a health-enhancing endeavor.

■ Nurses must consider cultural, spiritual, and religious needs when planning care for their clients.

Davis*Plus* Additional info available @ davisplus.fadavis.com

Review Questions
Self-Examination/Learning Exercise

*Select the answer that is **most** appropriate for each of the following questions:*

1. Miss Lee is an Asian American on the psychiatric unit. She tells the nurse, "I must have the hot ginger root for my headache. It is the only thing that will help." What meaning does the nurse attach to this statement by Miss Lee?
   a. She is being obstinate and wants control over her care.
   b. She believes that ginger root has magical qualities.
   c. She subscribes to the restoration of health through the balance of yin and yang.
   d. Asian Americans refuse to take traditional medicine for pain.

2. Miss Lee, an Asian American on the psychiatric unit, says she is afraid that no one from her family will visit her. On what belief does Miss Lee base her statement?
   a. Many Asian Americans do not believe in hospitals.
   b. Many Asian Americans do not have close family support systems.
   c. Many Asian Americans believe the body will heal itself if left alone.
   d. Many Asian Americans view psychiatric problems as bringing shame to the family.

3. Joe, a Native American, appears at the community health clinic with an oozing stasis ulcer on his lower right leg. It is obviously infected, and he tells the nurse that the shaman has been treating it with herbs. The nurse determines that Joe needs emergency care, but Joe states he will not go to the emergency department (ED) unless the shaman is allowed to help treat him. How should the nurse handle this situation?
   a. Contact the shaman and have him meet them at the ED to consult with the attending physician.
   b. Tell Joe that the shaman is not allowed in the ED.
   c. Explain to Joe that the shaman is at fault for his leg being in the condition it is in now.
   d. Have the shaman try to talk Joe into going to the ED without him.

4. Joe, a Native American, goes to the emergency department (ED) because he has an oozing stasis ulcer on his leg. He is accompanied by the tribal shaman, who has been treating Joe on the reservation. As a greeting, the physician extends his hand to the shaman, who lightly touches the physician's hand, then quickly moves away. How should the physician interpret this gesture?
   a. The shaman is snubbing the physician.
   b. The shaman is angry at Joe for wanting to go to the ED.
   c. The shaman does not believe in traditional medicine.
   d. The shaman does not feel comfortable with touch.

5. Sarah is an African American woman who receives a visit from the psychiatric home health nurse. A referral for a mental health assessment was made by the public health nurse, who noticed that Sarah was becoming exceedingly withdrawn. When the psychiatric nurse arrives, Sarah says to her, "No one can help me. I was an evil person in my youth, and now I must pay." How might the nurse assess this statement?
   a. Sarah is having delusions of persecution.
   b. Some African Americans believe illness is God's punishment for their sins.
   c. Sarah is depressed and just wants to be left alone.
   d. African Americans do not believe in psychiatric help.

Continued

Review Questions—cont'd
Self-Examination/Learning Exercise

6. Sarah is an African American woman who lives in the rural South. She receives a visit from the public health nurse. Sarah says to the nurse, "Granny told me to eat a lot of poke greens and I would feel better." How should the nurse interpret this statement?
   a. Sarah's grandmother believes in the healing power of poke greens.
   b. Sarah believes everything her grandmother tells her.
   c. Sarah has been receiving health care from a "folk practitioner."
   d. Sarah is trying to determine if the nurse agrees with her grandmother.

7. Frank is a Latino American who has an appointment at the community health center for 1:00 p.m. The nurse is angry when Frank shows up at 3:30 p.m. stating, "I was visiting with my brother." How must the nurse interpret this behavior?
   a. Frank is being passive-aggressive by showing up late.
   b. This is Frank's way of defying authority.
   c. Frank is a member of a cultural group that is present-time oriented.
   d. Frank is a member of a cultural group that rejects traditional medicine.

8. The nurse must give Frank, a Latino American, a physical examination. She tells him to remove his clothing and put on an examination gown. Frank refuses. How should the nurse interpret this behavior?
   a. Frank does not believe in taking orders from a woman.
   b. Frank is modest and embarrassed to remove his clothes.
   c. Frank doesn't understand why he must remove his clothes.
   d. Frank does not think he needs a physical examination.

9. Maria is an Italian American who is in the hospital after having suffered a miscarriage at 5 months' gestation. Her room is filled with relatives who have brought a variety of foods and gifts for Maria. They are all talking, seemingly at the same time, and some, including Maria, are crying. They repeatedly touch and hug Maria and each other. How should the nurse handle this situation?
   a. Explain to the family that Maria needs her rest and they must all leave.
   b. Allow the family to remain and continue their activity as described, as long as they do not disturb other clients.
   c. Explain that Maria will not get over her loss if they keep bringing it up and causing her to cry so much.
   d. Call the family priest to come and take charge of this family situation.

10. Maria is an Italian American who is in the hospital after having suffered a miscarriage at 5 months' gestation. Maria's mother says to the nurse, "If only Maria had told me she wanted the biscotti. I would have made them for her." What is the meaning behind Maria's mother's statement?
    a. Some Italian Americans believe a miscarriage can occur if a woman does not eat a food she craves.
    b. Some Italian Americans think biscotti can prevent miscarriage.
    c. Maria's mother is taking the blame for Maria's miscarriage.
    d. Maria's mother believes the physician should have told Maria to eat biscotti.

Review Questions—cont'd
Self-Examination/Learning Exercise

11. Joe, who has come to the mental health clinic with symptoms of depression, says to the nurse, "My father is dying. I have always hated my father. He physically abused me when I was a child. We haven't spoken for many years. He wants to see me now, but I don't know if I want to see him." With which spiritual need is Joe struggling?
    a. Forgiveness.
    b. Faith.
    c. Hope.
    d. Meaning and purpose in life.

12. As a child, Joe was physically abused by his father. The father is now dying and has expressed a desire to see his son before he dies. Joe is depressed and says to the mental health nurse, "I'm so angry! Why did God have to give me a father like this? I feel cheated of a father! I've always been a good person. I deserved better. I hate God!" From this subjective data, which nursing diagnosis might the nurse apply to Joe?
    a. Readiness for enhanced religiosity.
    b. Risk for impaired religiosity.
    c. Readiness for enhanced spiritual well-being.
    d. Spiritual distress.

References

Alegria, M., Mulvaney-Day, N., Torres, M., Polo, A., Cao, Z., & Canino, G. (2007). Prevalence of psychiatric disorders across Latino subgroups in the United States. *American Journal of Public Health, 97*(1), 68–75.

American Psychiatric Association. (2000). *Diagnostic and statistical manual of mental disorders* (4th ed.). *Text revision*. Washington, DC: Author.

Brodd, J. (2003). *World religions: A voyage of discovery* (2nd ed.). Winona, MN: Saint Mary's Press.

Bronson, M. (2005). *Why are there so many religions?* Retrieved May 13, 2010, from http://www.biblehelp.org/relig.htm

Bureau of Indian Affairs (BIA). (2010). *Frequently asked questions.* Retrieved May 13, 2010, from http://www.bia.gov/FAQs/index.htm

Burkhardt, M., & Nagai-Jacobson, M. G. (2002). *Spirituality: Living our connectedness.* Albany, NY: Delmar Thomson Learning.

Centers for Disease Control and Prevention (CDC). (2010). Marriage and cohabitation in the United States: A statistical portrait based on Cycle 6 (2002) of the National Survey of Family Growth. National Center for Health Statistics. *Vital and Health Statistics, 23*(28).

Cherry, B., & Giger, J. N. (2008). African-Americans. In J. N. Giger & R. E. Davidhizar (Eds.), *Transcultural nursing: Assessment and intervention* (5th ed., pp. 190–238). St. Louis: Elsevier.

Doenges, M. E., Moorhouse, M. F., & Murr, A. C. (2010). *Nursing diagnosis manual: Planning, individualizing, and documenting client care* (3rd ed.). Philadelphia: F.A. Davis.

Dossey, B. M. (1998). Holistic modalities and healing moments. *American Journal of Nursing, 98*(6), 44–47.

Fox, A., & Fox, B. (1988). *Wake up! You're alive.* Deerfield Beach, FL: Health Communications.

Gallup. (2008). *No evidence bad times are boosting church attendance.* Retrieved January 28, 2010, from http://www.gallup.com/poll/113452/evidence-bad-times-boosting-church-attendance.aspx

Gallup. (2009). *This Easter a smaller percentage of Americans are Christians.* Retrieved May 13, 2010, from http://www.gallup.com/poll/117409/Easter-Smaller-Percentage-Americans-Christians.aspx

Gartner, J. (1998). Religious commitment, mental health, and prosocial behavior: A review of the empirical literature. In E. Shafranske (Ed.), *Religion and the clinical practice of psychology.* Washington, DC: American Psychological Association.

Giger, J. N., & Davidhizar, R. E. (2008). *Transcultural nursing: Assessment and intervention* (5th ed.). St. Louis: Elsevier.

Gonzalez, E. W., Owen, D. C., & Esperat, M. C. (2008). Mexican Americans. In J. N. Giger & R. E. Davidhizar, (Eds.), *Transcultural nursing: Assessment and intervention* (5th ed., pp. 239–275). St. Louis: Elsevier.

Griffith, E. E. H., Gonzalez, C. A., & Blue, H. C. (2003). Introduction to cultural psychiatry. In R. E. Hales & S. C. Yudofsky (Eds.), *Textbook of clinical psychiatry* (4th ed., pp. 1551–1583). Washington, DC: American Psychiatric Publishing.

Hanley, C. E. (2008). Navajos. In J. N. Giger & R. E. Davidhizar (Eds.), *Transcultural nursing: Assessment and intervention* (5th ed., pp. 276–299). St. Louis: Elsevier.

Hodgins, O., & Hodgins, D. (2008). Navajo Indians. In L. D. Purnell & B. J. Paulanka (Eds.), *Transcultural health care: A culturally competent approach* (3rd ed., pp. 397–398). Philadelphia: F.A. Davis.

Indian Health Service. (2009). *Indian health disparities.* Retrieved May 19, 2010, from http://info.ihs.gov/Disparities.asp

Kaplan, A. (2007). Mental illness in U.S. Latinos addressed in survey, outreach efforts. *Psychiatric Times, 24*(3), 1–2.

Karren, K. J., Hafen, B. Q., Smith, N. L., & Frandsen, K. J. (2006). *Mind/body health: The effects of attitudes, emotions, and relationships* (3rd ed.). San Francisco: Benjamin Cummings.

Koenig, H. G. (2009). Research on religion, spirituality, and mental health: A review. *The Canadian Journal of Psychiatry, 54*(5), 283–291.

Kulwicki, A. D. (2008). People of Arab heritage. In L. D. Purnell & B. J. Paulanka (Eds.), *Transcultural health care: A culturally competent approach* (3rd ed., pp. 113–128). Philadelphia: F.A. Davis.

Kuo, P. Y. & Roysircar-Sodowsky, G. (2000). Political ethnic identity versus cultural ethnic identity: An understanding of research on Asian Americans. In D. S. Sandhu (Ed.), *Asian and Pacific Islander Americans: Issues and concerns for counseling and psychotherapy.* Hauppauge, NY: Nova Science Publishers.

Murray, R. B., Zentner, J. P., & Yakimo, R. (2009). *Health promotion strategies through the life span* (8th ed.). Upper Saddle River, NJ: Prentice Hall.

NANDA International. (2009). *Nursing diagnoses: Definitions & classification 2009–2011.* Hoboken, NJ: Wiley-Blackwell.

Nekolaichuk, C. L., Jevne, R. F., & Maguire, T. O. (1999). Structuring the meaning of hope in health and illness. *Social Science and Medicine, 48*(5), 591–605.

Ornish, D. (1998). *Love and survival: Eight pathways to intimacy and health.* New York: Harper Perennial.

Papadopoulos, I., & Purnell, L. D. (2008). People of Greek heritage. In L. D. Purnell & B. J. Paulanka (Eds.), *Transcultural health care: A culturally competent approach* (3rd ed.). Available from *DavisPlus* at http://davisplus.fadavis.com/purnell/Bonus_Chapters/Ch25.pdf

Pew Forum on Religion and Public Life. (2009). *A religious portrait of African Americans.* Retrieved May 19, 2010, from http://pewforum.org/docs/?DocID=389

Purnell, L. D. & Paulanka, B. J. (2008). *Transcultural health care: A culturally competent approach* (3rd ed.). Philadelphia: F.A. Davis.

Purnell, L. D., & Selekman, J. (2008). People of Jewish heritage. In L. D. Purnell & B. J. Paulanka (Eds.), *Transcultural health care: A culturally competent approach* (3rd ed., pp. 278–292). Philadelphia: F.A. Davis.

Reeves, R., & Reynolds, M. (2009). What is the role of spirituality in mental health treatment? *Journal of Psychosocial Nursing, 54*(5), 8–9.

Schwartz, E. A. (2008). Jewish Americans. In J. N. Giger & R. E. Davidhizar (Eds.), *Transcultural nursing: Assessment & intervention* (5th ed., pp. 592–618). St. Louis: Elsevier.

Smucker, C. J. (2001). Overview of nursing the spirit. In D. L. Wilt & C. J. Smucker (Eds.), *Nursing the spirit: The art and science of applying spiritual care* (pp. 1–18). Washington, DC: American Nurses Publishing.

Spector, R. E. (2009). *Cultural diversity in health and illness* (7th ed.). Upper Saddle River, NJ: Pearson Prentice Hall.

U.S. Census Bureau. (2009a). *2006–2008 American Community Survey.* Retrieved July 9, 2010, from http://factfinder.census.gov

U.S. Census Bureau. (2009b). *2006—2008 American Community Survey* (Table B11001B). Retrieved July 9, 2010, from http://factfinder.census.gov/servlet/DatasetTableListServlet?_ds_name=ACS_2008_3YR_G00_&_type=table&_program=ACS&_lang=en&_ts=296737332578

U.S. Department of Agriculture. (2009). *Food, nutrition, and consumer services.* Retrieved May 13, 2010, from http://www.aphis.usda.gov/anawg/Bluebook/guidefive.html

Wall, T. L., Peterson, C. M., Peterson, K. P., Johnson, M. L., Thomasson, H. R., Cole, M., et al. (1997). Alcohol metabolism in Asian-American men with genetic polymorphisms of aldehyde dehydrogenase. *Annals of Internal Medicine, 127,* 376–379.

Walsh, R. (1999). *Essential spirituality.* New York: John Wiley & Sons.

Wang, Y., & Purnell, L. D. (2008). People of Chinese heritage. In L. D. Purnell & B. J. Paulanka (Eds.), *Transcultural health care: A culturally competent approach* (3rd ed., pp. 129–144). Philadelphia: F.A. Davis.

Werner, E. E., & Smith, R. S. (1992). *Overcoming the odds: High risk children from birth to adulthood.* Ithaca, NY: Cornell University Press.

Wright, L. M. (2005). *Spirituality, suffering, and illness.* Philadelphia: F.A. Davis.

Xu, Y., & Chang, K. (2008). Chinese Americans. In J. N. Giger & R. E. Davidhizar (Eds.), *Transcultural nursing: Assessment and intervention* (5th ed., pp. 442–466). St. Louis: Elsevier.

Classical References

Hall, E. T. (1966). *The hidden dimension.* Garden City, NY: Doubleday.

Kübler-Ross, E. (1969). *On death and dying.* New York: Macmillan.

Therapeutic Approaches in Psychiatric Nursing Care

CORE CONCEPT

therapeutic
relationship

KEY TERMS

attitude	countertransference	sympathy
belief	empathy	transference
concrete thinking	genuineness	unconditional positive regard
confidentiality	rapport	values

OBJECTIVES
After reading this chapter, the student will be able to:

1. Describe the relevance of a therapeutic nurse-client relationship.
2. Discuss the dynamics of a therapeutic nurse-client relationship.
3. Discuss the importance of self-awareness in the nurse-client relationship.
4. Identify goals of the nurse-client relationship.
5. Identify and discuss essential conditions for a therapeutic relationship to occur.
6. Describe the phases of relationship development and the tasks associated with each phase.

HOMEWORK ASSIGNMENT
Please read the chapter and answer the following questions:

1. When the nurse's verbal and nonverbal interactions are congruent, he or she is thought to be expressing which characteristic of therapeutic communication?
2. During which phase of the nurse-client relationship do each of the following occur:
   a. The nurse may become angry and anxious in the presence of the client.
   b. A plan of action for dealing with stress is established.
   c. The nurse examines personal feelings about working with client.
   d. Nurse and client establish goals of care.
3. What is the goal of using the Johari Window?
4. How do sympathy and empathy differ?

The nurse-client relationship is the foundation on which psychiatric nursing is established. It is a relationship in which both participants must recognize each other as unique and important human beings. It is also a relationship in which mutual learning occurs. Peplau (1991) stated:

> Shall a nurse do things *for* a patient or can participant relationships be emphasized so that a

nurse comes to do things *with* a patient as her share of an agenda of work to be accomplished in reaching a goal—health. It is likely that the nursing process is educative and therapeutic when nurse and patient can come to know and to respect each other, as persons who are alike, and yet, different, as persons who share in the solution of problems. (p. 9)

This chapter examines the role of the psychiatric nurse and the use of self as the therapeutic tool in the nursing of clients with emotional illness. Phases of the therapeutic relationship are explored and conditions essential to the development of a therapeutic relationship are discussed. The importance of values clarification in the development of self-awareness is emphasized.

CORE CONCEPT

Therapeutic Relationship

An interaction between two people (usually a caregiver and a care receiver) in which input from both participants contributes to a climate of healing, growth promotion, and/or illness prevention.

Role of the Psychiatric Nurse

What is a nurse? Undoubtedly, this question would elicit as many different answers as the number of people to whom it was presented. Nursing as a *concept* has probably existed since the beginning of the civilized world, with the provision of "care" to the ill or infirm by anyone in the environment who took the time to administer to those in need. However, the emergence of nursing as a *profession* only began in the late 1800s with the graduation of Linda Richards from the New England Hospital for Women and Children in Boston upon achievement of the diploma in nursing. Since that time, the nurse's role has evolved from that of custodial caregiver and physician's handmaiden to recognition as a unique, independent member of the professional health-care team.

Peplau (1991) identified several subroles within the role of the nurse:

1. **The Stranger.** A nurse is at first a stranger to the client. The client is also a stranger to the nurse. Peplau (1991) stated:

   Respect and positive interest accorded a stranger is at first nonpersonal and includes the same ordinary courtesies that are accorded to a new guest who has been brought into any situation. This principle implies: (1) accepting the patient as he is; (2) treating the patient as an emotionally able stranger and relating to him on this basis until evidence shows him to be otherwise. (p. 44)

2. **The Resource Person.** According to Peplau, "a resource person provides specific answers to questions usually formulated with relation to a larger problem" (1991, p. 47). In the role of resource person, the nurse explains, in language that the client can understand, information related to the client's health care.

3. **The Teacher.** In this subrole the nurse identifies learning needs and provides information required by the client or family to improve the health situation.

4. **The Leader.** According to Peplau, "democratic leadership in nursing situations implies that the patient will be permitted to be an active participant in designing nursing plans for him" (1991, p. 49). Autocratic leadership promotes overvaluation of the nurse and clients' substitution of the nurse's goals for their own. Laissez-faire leaders convey a lack of personal interest in the client.

5. **The Surrogate.** Outside of their awareness, clients often perceive nurses as symbols of other individuals. They may view the nurse as a mother figure, a sibling, a former teacher, or another nurse who has provided care in the past. This occurs when a client is placed in a situation that generates feelings similar to ones he or she has experienced previously. Peplau (1991) explained that the nurse-client relationship progresses along a continuum. When a client is acutely ill, he or she may incur the role of infant or child, while the nurse is perceived as the mother surrogate. Peplau (1991) stated, "Each nurse has the responsibility for exercising her professional skill in aiding the relationship to move forward on the continuum, so that person to person relations compatible with chronological age levels can develop" (p. 55).

6. **The Counselor.** The nurse uses "interpersonal techniques" to assist clients to learn to adapt to difficulties or changes in life experiences. Peplau stated, "Counseling in nursing has to do with helping the patient to remember and to understand fully what is happening to him in the present situation, so that the experience can be integrated with, rather than dissociated from, other experiences in life" (1991, p. 64).

Peplau (1962) believed that the emphasis in psychiatric nursing is on the counseling subrole. How then does this emphasis influence the role of the nurse in the psychiatric setting? Many sources define the *nurse therapist* as having graduate preparation in psychiatric/mental health nursing. He or she has developed skills through intensive supervised educational experiences to provide helpful individual, group, or family therapy.

Peplau suggested that it is essential for the *staff nurse working in psychiatry* to have a general knowledge of basic counseling techniques. A therapeutic or "helping" relationship is established through use of these interpersonal techniques and is based on a sound knowledge of theories of personality development and human behavior.

Sullivan (1953) believed that emotional problems stem from difficulties with interpersonal relationships. Interpersonal theorists, such as Peplau and Sullivan, emphasize the importance of relationship development in the provision of emotional care. Through establishment of a satisfactory nurse-client relationship, individuals learn to generalize the ability to achieve satisfactory interpersonal relationships to other aspects of their lives.

Dynamics of a Therapeutic Nurse-Client Relationship

Travelbee (1971), who expanded on Peplau's theory of interpersonal relations in nursing, has stated that it is only when each individual in the interaction perceives the other as a unique human being that a relationship is possible. She refers not to a nurse-client relationship, but rather to a human-to-human relationship, which she describes as a "mutually significant experience." That is, both the nurse and the recipient of care have needs met when each views the other as a unique human being, not as "an illness," as "a room number, " or as "all nurses" in general.

Therapeutic relationships are goal oriented. Ideally, the nurse and client decide together what the goal of the relationship will be. Most often the goal is directed at learning and growth promotion, in an effort to bring about some type of change in the client's life. In general, the goal of a therapeutic relationship may be based on a problem-solving model.

EXAMPLE

Goal
The client will demonstrate more adaptive coping strategies for dealing with (specific life situation).
Interventions

- Identify what is troubling the client at the present time.

- Encourage the client to discuss changes he or she would like to make.

- Discuss with the client which changes are possible and which are not possible.

- Have the client explore feelings about aspects that cannot be changed and alternative ways of coping more adaptively.

- Discuss alternative strategies for creating changes the client desires to make.

- Weigh the benefits and consequences of each alternative.

- Assist the client to select an alternative.

- Encourage the client to implement the change.

- Provide positive feedback for the client's attempts to create change.

- Assist the client to evaluate outcomes of the change and make modifications as required.

Therapeutic Use of Self

Travelbee (1971) described the instrument for delivery of the process of interpersonal nursing as the *therapeutic use of self,* which she defined as "the ability to use one's personality consciously and in full awareness in an attempt to establish relatedness and to structure nursing intervention" (p. 19).

Use of the self in a therapeutic manner requires that the nurse have a great deal of self-awareness and self-understanding, having arrived at a philosophical belief about life, death, and the overall human condition. The nurse must understand that the ability and extent to which one can effectively help others in time of need is strongly influenced by this internal value system—a combination of intellect and emotions.

Gaining Self-Awareness

Values Clarification

Knowing and understanding oneself enhances the ability to form satisfactory interpersonal relationships. Self-awareness requires that an individual recognize and accept what he or she values and learn to accept the uniqueness and differences in others. This concept is important in everyday life and in the nursing profession in general; it is *essential* in psychiatric nursing.

An individual's value system is established very early in life and has its foundations in the value system held by the primary caregivers. It is culturally oriented; it may change many times over the course of a lifetime; and it consists of beliefs, attitudes, and values. Values clarification is one process by which an individual may gain self-awareness.

Beliefs
A **belief** is an idea that one holds to be true, and it can take any of several forms:

- *Rational beliefs.* Ideas for which objective evidence exists to substantiate their truth.

EXAMPLE

Alcoholism is a disease.

■ *Irrational beliefs.* Ideas that an individual holds as true despite the existence of objective contradictory evidence. Delusions can be a form of irrational beliefs.

EXAMPLE

Once an alcoholic has been through detox and rehab, he or she can drink socially if desired.

■ *Faith (sometimes called "blind beliefs").* An ideal that an individual holds as true for which no objective evidence exists.

EXAMPLE

Belief in a higher power can help an alcoholic stop drinking.

■ *Stereotype.* A socially shared belief that describes a concept in an oversimplified or undifferentiated matter.

EXAMPLE

All alcoholics are skid-row bums.

Attitudes

An **attitude** is a frame of reference around which an individual organizes knowledge about his or her world. An attitude also has an emotional component. It can be a prejudgment and may be selective and biased. Attitudes fulfill the need to find meaning in life and to provide clarity and consistency for the individual. The prevailing stigma attached to mental illness is an example of a negative attitude. An associated belief might be that "all people with mental illness are dangerous."

Values

Values are abstract standards, positive or negative, that represent an individual's ideal mode of conduct and ideal goals. Some examples of ideal mode of conduct include seeking truth and beauty; being clean and orderly; and behaving with sincerity, justice, reason, compassion, humility, respect, honor, and loyalty. Examples of ideal goals are security, happiness, freedom, equality, ecstasy, fame, and power.

Values differ from attitudes and beliefs in that they are action oriented or action producing. One may hold many attitudes and beliefs without behaving in a way that shows one holds those attitudes and beliefs. For example, a nurse may believe that all clients have the right to be told the truth about their diagnosis; however, he or she may not always act on the belief and tell all clients the complete truth about their condition. Only when the belief is acted on does it become a value.

Attitudes and beliefs flow out of one's set of values. An individual may have thousands of beliefs and hundreds of attitudes, but his or her values probably only number in the dozens. Values may be viewed as a kind of core concept or basic standards that determine one's attitudes and beliefs, and ultimately, one's behavior. Raths, Merril, and Simon (1966) identified a seven-step process of valuing that can be used to help clarify personal values. This process is presented in Table 7-1. The process can be used by applying these seven steps to an attitude or belief that one holds. When

TABLE 7-1 The Process of Values Clarification

LEVEL OF OPERATIONS	CATEGORY	CRITERIA	EXPLANATION
Cognitive	Choosing	1. Freely 2. From alternatives 3. After careful consideration of the consequences	"This value is mine. No one forced me to choose it. I understand and accept the consequences of holding this value."
Emotional	Prizing	4. Satisfied; pleased with the choice 5. Making public affirmation of the choice, if necessary	"I am proud that I hold this value, and I am willing to tell others about it."
Behavioral	Acting	6. Taking action to demonstrate the value behaviorally 7. Demonstrating this pattern of behavior consistently and repeatedly	The value is reflected in the individual's behavior for as long as he or she holds it.

an attitude or belief has met each of the seven criteria, it can be considered a value.

The Johari Window

The self arises out of self-appraisal and the appraisal of others and represents each individual's unique pattern of values, attitudes, beliefs, behaviors, emotions, and needs. Self-awareness is the recognition of these aspects and understanding about their impact on the self and others. The Johari Window is a representation of the self and a tool that can be used to increase self-awareness (Luft, 1970). The Johari Window is presented in Figure 7–1 and is divided into four quadrants.

The Open or Public Self

The upper left quadrant of the window represents the part of the self that is public; that is, aspects of the self about which both the individual and others are aware.

EXAMPLE

Susan, a nurse who is the adult child of an alcoholic, has strong feelings about helping alcoholics to achieve sobriety. She volunteers her time to be a support person on call to help recovering alcoholics. She is aware of her feelings and her desire to help others. Members of the Alcoholics Anonymous group in which she volunteers her time are also aware of Susan's feelings and they feel comfortable calling her when they need help refraining from drinking.

The Unknowing Self

The upper right quadrant of the window represents the part of the self that is known to others but remains hidden from the awareness of the individual.

EXAMPLE

When Susan takes care of patients in detox, she does so without emotion, tending to the technical aspects of the task in a way that the clients perceive as cold and judgmental. She is unaware that she comes across to the clients in this way.

The Private Self

The lower left quadrant of the window represents the part of the self that is known to the individual, but which the individual deliberately and consciously conceals from others.

EXAMPLE

Susan would prefer not to take care of the clients in detox because doing so provokes painful memories from her childhood. However, because she does not want the other staff members to know about these feelings, she volunteers to take care of the detox clients whenever they are assigned to her unit.

The Unknown Self

The lower right quadrant of the window represents the part of the self that is unknown both to the individual and to others.

EXAMPLE

Susan felt very powerless as a child growing up with an alcoholic father. She seldom knew in what condition she would find her father or what his behavior would be. She learned over the years to find small ways to maintain control over her

	Known to self	Unknown to self
Known to Others	The open or public self	The unknowing self
Unknown to Others	The private self	The unknown self

FIGURE 7–1 The Johari Window. (From Luft, J. [1970]. *Group processes: An introduction to group dynamics.* Palo Alto, CA: National Press Books, with permission.)

life situation, and left home as soon as she graduated from high school. The need to stay in control has always been very important to Susan, and she is unaware that working with recovering alcoholics helps to fulfill this need in her. The people she is helping are also unaware that Susan is satisfying an unfulfilled personal need as she provides them with assistance.

The goal of increasing self-awareness by using the Johari Window is to increase the size of the quadrant that represents the open or public self. The individual who is open to self and others has the ability to be spontaneous and to share emotions and experiences with others. This individual also has a greater understanding of personal behavior and of others' responses to him or her. Increased self-awareness allows an individual to interact with others comfortably, to accept the differences in others, and to observe each person's right to respect and dignity.

Conditions Essential to Development of a Therapeutic Relationship

Several characteristics that enhance the achievement of a therapeutic relationship have been identified. These concepts are highly significant to the use of self as the therapeutic tool in interpersonal relationship development.

Rapport

Getting acquainted and establishing **rapport** is the primary task in relationship development. Rapport implies special feelings on the part of both the client and the nurse based on acceptance, warmth, friendliness, common interest, a sense of trust, and a nonjudgmental attitude. Establishing rapport may be accomplished by discussing non–health-related topics. Travelbee (1971) stated:

> [To establish rapport] is to create a sense of harmony based on knowledge and appreciation of each individual's uniqueness. It is the ability to be still and experience the other as a human being—to appreciate the unfolding of each personality one to the other. The ability to truly care for and about others is the core of rapport. (pp. 152, 155)

Trust

To trust another, one must feel confidence in that person's presence, reliability, integrity, veracity, and sincere desire to provide assistance when requested. As discussed in Chapter 3, trust is the initial

developmental task described by Erikson. If the task has not been achieved, this component of relationship development becomes more difficult. That is not to say that trust cannot be established, but only that additional time and patience may be required on the part of the nurse.

> **CLINICAL PEARL** The nurse must convey an aura of trustworthiness, which requires that he or she possess a sense of self-confidence. Confidence in the self is derived out of knowledge gained through achievement of personal and professional goals, as well as the ability to integrate these roles and to function as a unified whole.

Trust cannot be presumed; it must be earned. Trustworthiness is demonstrated through nursing interventions that convey a sense of warmth and caring to the client. These interventions are initiated simply and concretely and directed toward activities that address the client's basic needs for physiological and psychological safety and security. Many psychiatric clients experience **concrete thinking,** which focuses their thought processes on specifics rather than generalities, and immediate issues rather than eventual outcomes. Examples of nursing interventions that would promote trust in an individual who is thinking concretely include the following:

- Providing a blanket when the client is cold
- Providing food when the client is hungry
- Keeping promises
- Being honest (e.g., saying "I don't know the answer to your question, but I'll try to find out") and then following through
- Simply and clearly providing reasons for certain policies, procedures, and rules
- Providing a written, structured schedule of activities
- Attending activities with the client if he or she is reluctant to go alone
- Being consistent in adhering to unit guidelines
- Taking the client's preferences, requests, and opinions into consideration when possible in decisions concerning his or her care
- Ensuring **confidentiality;** providing reassurance that what is discussed will not be repeated outside the boundaries of the health care team

Trust is the basis of a therapeutic relationship. The nurse working in psychiatry must perfect the skills that foster the development of trust. Trust must be established in order for the nurse-client relationship to progress beyond the superficial level of tending to the client's immediate needs.

Respect

To show respect is to believe in the dignity and worth of an individual regardless of his or her unacceptable behavior. The psychologist Carl Rogers called this **unconditional positive regard** (Raskin, Rogers, & Witty, 2011). The attitude is nonjudgmental, and the respect is unconditional in that it does not depend on the behavior of the client to meet certain standards. The nurse, in fact, may not approve of the client's lifestyle or pattern of behaving. However, with unconditional positive regard, the client is accepted and respected for no other reason than that he or she is considered to be a worthwhile and unique human being.

Many psychiatric clients have very little self-respect because, as a result of their behavior, they have been rejected by others in the past. Recognition that they are being accepted and respected as unique individuals on an unconditional basis can serve to elevate feelings of self-worth and self-respect. The nurse can convey an attitude of respect by:

■ Calling the client by name (and title, if he or she prefers)

■ Spending time with the client

■ Allowing for sufficient time to answer the client's questions and concerns

■ Promoting an atmosphere of privacy during therapeutic interactions with the client or when the client may be undergoing physical examination or therapy

■ Always being open and honest with the client, even when the truth may be difficult to discuss

■ Taking the client's ideas, preferences, and opinions into consideration when planning care

■ Striving to understand the motivation behind the client's behavior, regardless of how unacceptable it may seem

Genuineness

The concept of **genuineness** refers to the nurse's ability to be open, honest, and "real" in interactions with the client. To be "real" is to be aware of what one is experiencing internally and to allow the quality of this inner experiencing to be apparent in the therapeutic relationship. When one is genuine, there is *congruence* between what is felt and what is being expressed (Raskin et al., 2011). The nurse who possesses the quality of genuineness responds to the client with truth and honesty, rather than with responses he or she may consider more "professional" or ones that merely reflect the "nursing role."

Genuineness may call for a degree of *self-disclosure* on the part of the nurse. This is not to say that the nurse must disclose to the client *everything* he or she is feeling or *all* personal experiences that may relate to what the client is going through. Indeed, care must be taken when using self-disclosure, to avoid reversing the roles of nurse and client.

When the nurse uses self-disclosure, a quality of "humanness" is revealed to the client, creating a role for the client to model in similar situations. The client may then feel more comfortable revealing personal information to the nurse.

Most individuals have an uncanny ability to detect other people's artificiality. When the nurse does not bring the quality of genuineness to the relationship, a reality base for trust cannot be established. These qualities are essential if the actualizing potential of the client is to be released and for change and growth to occur (Raskin et al., 2011).

Empathy

Empathy is the ability to see beyond outward behavior and to understand the situation from the client's point of view. With empathy, the nurse can accurately perceive and comprehend the meaning and relevance of the client's thoughts and feelings. The nurse must also be able to communicate this perception to the client by attempting to translate words and behaviors into feelings.

It is not uncommon for the concept of empathy to be confused with that of **sympathy**. The major difference is that, with *empathy*, the nurse "accurately perceives or understands" what the client is feeling and encourages the client to explore these feelings. With *sympathy*, the nurse actually "shares" what the client is feeling, and experiences a need to alleviate distress. Schuster (2000) stated:

> Empathy means that you remain emotionally separate from the other person, even though you can see the patient's viewpoint clearly. This is different from sympathy. Sympathy implies taking on the other's needs and problems as if they were your own and becoming emotionally involved to the point of losing your objectivity. To empathize rather than sympathize, you must show feelings but not get caught up in feelings or overly identify with the patient's and family's concerns. (p. 102)

Empathy is considered to be one of the most important characteristics of a therapeutic relationship. Accurate empathetic perceptions on the part of the nurse assist the client to identify feelings that may have been suppressed or denied. Positive emotions are generated as the client realizes that he or she is truly understood by another. As the feelings surface and are explored, the client learns aspects about self of which he or she may have been unaware. This contributes to the process of personal identification and the promotion of positive self-concept.

With empathy, while understanding the client's thoughts and feelings, the nurse is able to maintain sufficient objectivity to allow the client to achieve problem resolution with minimal assistance. With sympathy, the nurse actually feels what the client is feeling, objectivity is lost, and the nurse may become focused on relief of personal distress rather than on helping the client resolve the problem at hand. The following is an example of an empathetic and sympathetic response to the same situation.

EXAMPLE

Situation: BJ is a client on the psychiatric unit with a diagnosis of dysthymic disorder. She is 5'5" tall and weighs 295 lb. BJ has been overweight all her life. She is single, has no close friends, and has never had an intimate relationship with another person. It is her first day on the unit, and she is refusing to come out of her room. When she appeared for lunch in the dining room following admission, she was embarrassed when several of the other clients laughed out loud and called her "fatso."

Sympathetic response: Nurse: "I can certainly identify with what you are feeling. I've been overweight most of my life, too. I just get so angry when people act like that. They are so insensitive! It's just so typical of skinny people to act that way. You have a right to want to stay away from them. We'll just see how loud they laugh when *you* get to choose what movie is shown on the unit after dinner tonight."

Empathetic response: Nurse: "You feel angry and embarrassed by what happened at lunch today." As tears fill BJ's eyes, the nurse encourages her to cry if she feels like it and to express her anger at the situation. She stays with BJ but does not dwell on her *own* feelings about what happened. Instead she focuses on BJ and what the client perceives are her most immediate needs at this time.

Phases of a Therapeutic Nurse-Client Relationship

Psychiatric nurses use interpersonal relationship development as the primary intervention with clients in various psychiatric/mental health settings. This is congruent with Peplau's (1962) identification of *counseling* as the major subrole of nursing in psychiatry. Sullivan (1953), from whom Peplau patterned her own interpersonal theory of nursing, strongly believed that many emotional problems were closely related to difficulties with interpersonal relationships. With this concept in mind, this role of the nurse in psychiatry becomes especially meaningful and purposeful. It becomes an integral part of the total therapeutic regimen.

The therapeutic interpersonal relationship is the means by which the nursing process is implemented. Through the relationship, problems are identified and resolution is sought. Tasks of the relationship have been categorized into four phases: (1) the preinteraction phase, (2) the orientation (introductory) phase, (3) the working phase, and (4) the termination phase. Although each phase is presented as specific and distinct from the others, there may be some overlapping of tasks, particularly when the interaction is limited. The major nursing goals during each phase of the nurse-client relationship are listed in Table 7-2.

The Preinteraction Phase

The preinteraction phase involves preparation for the first encounter with the client. Tasks include the following:

■ Obtaining available information about the client from his or her chart, significant others, or other health team members. From this information, the initial assessment is begun. This

TABLE 7-2 Phases of Relationship Development and Major Nursing Goals

PHASE	GOALS
1. Preinteraction	Explore self-perceptions
2. Orientation (introductory)	Establish trust Formulate contract for intervention
3. Working	Promote client change
4. Termination	Evaluate goal attainment Ensure therapeutic closure

initial information may also allow the nurse to become aware of personal responses to knowledge about the client.

■ Examining one's feelings, fears, and anxieties about working with a particular client. For example, the nurse may have been reared in an alcoholic family and have ambivalent feelings about caring for a client who is alcohol dependent. All individuals bring attitudes and feelings from prior experiences to the clinical setting. The nurse needs to be aware of how these preconceptions may affect his or her ability to care for individual clients.

The Orientation (Introductory) Phase

During the orientation phase, the nurse and client become acquainted. Tasks include:

■ Creating an environment for the establishment of trust and rapport

■ Establishing a contract for intervention that details the expectations and responsibilities of both nurse and client.

■ Gathering assessment information to build a strong client database

■ Identifying the client's strengths and limitations

■ Formulating nursing diagnoses

■ Setting goals that are mutually agreeable to the nurse and client

■ Developing a plan of action that is realistic for meeting the established goals

■ Exploring feelings of both the client and nurse in terms of the introductory phase

Introductions are often uncomfortable, and the participants may experience some anxiety until a degree of rapport has been established. Interactions may remain on a superficial level until anxiety subsides. Several interactions may be required to fulfill the tasks associated with this phase.

The Working Phase

The therapeutic work of the relationship is accomplished during this phase. Tasks include:

■ Maintaining the trust and rapport that was established during the orientation phase

■ Promoting the client's insight and perception of reality

■ Problem solving using the model presented earlier in this chapter

■ Overcoming resistance behaviors on the part of the client as the level of anxiety rises in response to discussion of painful issues

■ Continuously evaluating progress toward goal attainment

Transference and Countertransference

Transference and countertransference are common phenomena that often arise during the course of a therapeutic relationship.

Transference

Transference occurs when the client unconsciously displaces (or "transfers") to the nurse feelings formed toward a person from his or her past (Sadock & Sadock, 2007). These feelings toward the nurse may be triggered by something about the nurse's appearance or personality characteristics that reminds the client of the person. Transference can interfere with the therapeutic interaction when the feelings being expressed include anger and hostility. Anger toward the nurse can be manifested by uncooperativeness and resistance to the therapy.

Transference can also take the form of overwhelming affection for the nurse or excessive dependency on the nurse. The nurse is overvalued and the client forms unrealistic expectations of the nurse. When the nurse is unable to fulfill those expectations or meet the excessive dependency needs, the client becomes angry and hostile.

Interventions for Transference Hilz (2008) stated:

In cases of transference, the relationship does not usually need to be terminated, except when the transference poses a serious barrier to therapy or safety. The nurse should work with the patient in sorting out the past from the present, and assist the patient into identifying the transference and reassign a new and more appropriate meaning to the current nurse-patient relationship. The goal is to guide patients toward independence by teaching them to assume responsibility for their own behaviors, feelings, and thoughts, and to assign the correct meanings to the relationships based on present circumstances instead of the past.

Countertransference

Countertransference refers to the nurse's behavioral and emotional response to the client. These responses may be related to unresolved feelings toward significant others from the nurse's past, or they may be generated in response to transference feelings on the part of the client. It is not easy to refrain from becoming angry when the client is consistently antagonistic, to feel flattered when showered with affection and attention by the client, or even to feel quite powerful when the client exhibits excessive dependency on the nurse. These feelings can interfere with the therapeutic relationship when they initiate the following types of behaviors:

■ The nurse overidentifies with the client's feelings, as they remind him or her of problems from the nurse's past or present.

■ The nurse and client develop a social or personal relationship.

■ The nurse begins to give advice or attempts to "rescue" the client.

■ The nurse encourages and promotes the client's dependence.

■ The nurse's anger engenders feelings of disgust toward the client.

■ The nurse feels anxious and uneasy in the presence of the client.

■ The nurse is bored and apathetic in sessions with the client.

■ The nurse has difficulty setting limits on the client's behavior.

■ The nurse defends the client's behavior to other staff members.

The nurse may be completely unaware or only minimally aware of the countertransference as it is occurring (Hilz, 2008).

Interventions for Countertransference Hilz (2008) stated:

> The relationship usually should not be terminated in the presence of countertransference. Rather, the nurse or staff member experiencing the countertransference should be supportively assisted by other staff members to identify his or her feelings and behaviors and recognize the occurrence of the phenomenon. It may be helpful to have evaluative sessions with the nurse after his or her encounter with the patient, in which both the nurse and other staff members (who are observing the interactions) discuss and compare the exhibited behaviors in the relationship.

The Termination Phase

Termination of the relationship may occur for a variety of reasons: the mutually agreed-on goals may have been reached; the client may be discharged from the hospital; or, in the case of a student nurse, it may be the end of a clinical rotation. Termination can be a difficult phase for both the client and nurse. The main task involves bringing a therapeutic conclusion to the relationship. This occurs when:

■ Progress has been made toward attainment of mutually set goals.

■ A plan for continuing care or for assistance during stressful life experiences is mutually established by the nurse and client.

■ Feelings about termination of the relationship are recognized and explored. Both the nurse and client may experience feelings of sadness and loss. The nurse should share his or her feelings with the client. Through these interactions, the client learns that it is acceptable to have these kinds of feelings at a time of separation. Through this knowledge, the client experiences growth during the process of termination.

> **CLINICAL PEARL** When the client feels sadness and loss, behaviors to delay termination may become evident. If the nurse experiences the same feelings, he or she may allow the client's behaviors to delay termination. For therapeutic closure, the nurse must establish the reality of the separation and resist being manipulated into repeated delays by the client.

Boundaries in the Nurse-Client Relationship

A boundary indicates a border or a limit. It determines the extent of acceptable limits. Many types of boundaries exist. Examples include the following:

■ **Material boundaries.** These are physical property that can be seen, such as fences that border land.

■ **Social boundaries.** These are established within a culture and define how individuals are expected to behave in social situations

■ **Personal boundaries.** These are boundaries that individuals define for themselves. These include *physical distance boundaries,* or just how close individuals will allow others to invade their physical space; and *emotional boundaries,* or how much individuals choose to disclose of their most private and intimate selves to others.

■ **Professional boundaries.** These boundaries limit and outline expectations for appropriate professional relationships with clients. They separate therapeutic behavior from any other behavior that, well intentioned or not, could lessen the benefit of care to clients (College and Association of Registered Nurses of Alberta [CARNA], 2005).

Concerns regarding professional boundaries are commonly related to the following issues:

■ **Self-disclosure.** Self-disclosure on the part of the nurse may be appropriate when it is judged that the information may therapeutically benefit the client. It should never be undertaken for the purpose of meeting the nurse's needs.

■ **Gift-giving.** Individuals who are receiving care often feel indebted toward health-care providers. And, indeed, gift giving may be part of the therapeutic process for people who receive care (CARNA, 2005). Cultural beliefs and values may also enter into the decision of whether to accept a gift from a client. In some cultures, failure to do so would be interpreted as an insult. Accepting financial gifts is never appropriate, but in some instances nurses may be permitted to suggest instead a donation to a charity of the client's choice. If acceptance of a small gift of gratitude is deemed appropriate, the nurse may choose to share it with other staff members who have been involved in the client's care. In all instances, nurses should exercise professional judgment when deciding whether to accept a gift from a client. Attention should be given to what the gift-giving means to the client, as well as to institutional policy, the American Nurses Association (ANA) *Code of Ethics for Nurses,* and the ANA *Scope and Standards of Practice.*

■ **Touch.** Nursing by its very nature involves touching clients. Touching is required to perform the many therapeutic procedures involved in the physical care of clients. Caring touch is the touching of clients when there is no physical need (Registered Nurses Association of British Columbia [RNABC], 2003). Caring touch often provides comfort or encouragement and, when it is used appropriately, it can have a therapeutic effect on the client. However, certain vulnerable clients may misinterpret the meaning of touch. Certain cultures, such as Native Americans and Asian Americans, are often uncomfortable with touch. The nurse must be sensitive to these cultural nuances and aware when touch is crossing a personal boundary. Additionally, clients who are experiencing high levels of anxiety or suspicious or psychotic behaviors may interpret touch as aggressive. These are times when touch should be avoided or considered with extreme caution.

■ **Friendship or Romantic Association.** When a nurse is acquainted with a client, the relationship must move from one of a personal nature to professional. If the nurse is unable to accomplish this separation, he or she should withdraw from the nurse-client relationship. Likewise, nurses must guard against personal relationships developing as a result of the nurse-client relationship. Romantic, sexual, or similar personal relationships are never appropriate between nurse and client.

Certain warning signs exist that indicate that professional boundaries of the nurse-client relationship may be in jeopardy. Some of these include the following (Coltrane & Pugh, 1978):

■ Favoring one client's care over that of another

■ Keeping secrets with a client

■ Changing dress style for working with a particular client

■ Swapping client assignments to care for a particular client

■ Giving special attention or treatment to one client over others

■ Spending free time with a client

■ Frequently thinking about the client when away from work

■ Sharing personal information or work concerns with the client

■ Receiving of gifts or continued contact/communication with the client after discharge

Boundary crossings can threaten the integrity of the nurse-client relationship. Nurses must gain self-awareness and insight to be able to recognize when professional integrity is being compromised. Peternelj-Taylor and Yonge (2003) stated:

> The nursing profession needs nurses who have the ability to make decisions about boundaries based on the best interests of the clients in their care. This requires nurses to reflect on their knowledge and experiences, on how they think and how they feel, and not simply to buy blindly into a framework that says, "do this," "don't do that." (p. 65)

Summary and Key Points

■ Nurses who work in the psychiatric/mental health field use special skills, or "interpersonal techniques," to assist clients in adapting to difficulties or changes in life experiences.

■ Therapeutic nurse-client relationships are goal oriented, and the problem-solving model is used to try to bring about some type of change in the client's life.

■ The instrument for delivery of the process of interpersonal nursing is the therapeutic use of self, which requires that the nurse possess a strong sense of self-awareness and self-understanding.

■ Hildegard Peplau identified six subroles within the role of nurse: stranger, resource person, teacher, leader, surrogate, and counselor.

■ Characteristics that enhance the achievement of a therapeutic relationship include rapport, trust, respect, genuineness, and empathy.

■ Phases of a therapeutic nurse-client relationship include the preinteraction phase, the orientation (introductory) phase, the working phase, and the termination phase.

■ Transference occurs when the client unconsciously displaces (or "transfers") to the nurse feelings formed toward a person from the past.

■ Countertransference refers to the nurse's behavioral and emotional response to the client. These responses may be related to unresolved feelings toward significant others from the nurse's past, or they may be generated in response to transference feelings on the part of the client.

■ Types of boundaries include material, social, personal, and professional.

■ Concerns associated with professional boundaries include self-disclosure, gift-giving, touch, and developing a friendship or romantic association.

■ Boundary crossings can threaten the integrity of the nurse-client relationship.

DavisPlus   Additional info available @ davisplus.fadavis.com

Review Questions
Self-Examination/Learning Exercise

*Select the answer that is **most** appropriate for each of the following questions:*

1. Nurse Mary has been providing care for Tom during his hospital stay. On Tom's day of discharge, his wife brings a bouquet of flowers and box of chocolates to his room. He presents these gifts to Nurse Mary saying, "Thank you for taking care of me." What is a correct response by the nurse?
   a. "I don't accept gifts from patients."
   b. "Thank you so much! It is so nice to be appreciated."
   c. "Thank you. I will share these with the rest of the staff."
   d. "Hospital policy forbids me to accept gifts from patients."

2. Nancy says to the nurse, "I worked as a secretary to put my husband through college, and as soon as he graduated, he left me. I hate him! I hate all men!" Which is an empathetic response by the nurse?
   a. "You are very angry now. This is a normal response to your loss."
   b. "I know what you mean. Men can be very insensitive."
   c. "I understand completely. My husband divorced me, too."
   d. "You are depressed now, but you will feel better in time."

3. Which of the following behaviors suggest a possible breach of professional boundaries? (Select all that apply.)
   a. The nurse repeatedly requests to be assigned to a specific client.
   b. The nurse shares the details of her divorce with the client.
   c. The nurse makes arrangements to meet the client outside of the therapeutic environment.
   d. The nurse shares how she dealt with a similar difficult situation.

Continued

Review Questions—cont'd
Self-Examination/Learning Exercise

4. Which of the following tasks are associated with the orientation phase of relationship development? (Select all that apply.)
   a. Promoting the client's insight and perception of reality.
   b. Creating an environment for the establishment of trust and rapport.
   c. Using the problem-solving model toward goal fulfillment.
   d. Obtaining available information about the client from various sources.
   e. Formulating nursing diagnoses and setting goals.

5. Nurse Carol, who is the adult child of an alcoholic, is working with John, a client who abuses alcohol. John has experienced a successful detoxification process and is beginning a program of rehabilitation. He says to Carol, "I'm not going to go to those stupid AA meetings. They don't help anything." Carol, whose father died of complications from alcoholism, responds with anger: "Don't you even care what happens to your children?" Carol's response is an example of which of the following?
   a. Transference.
   b. Countertransference.
   c. Self-disclosure.
   d. A breach of professional boundaries.

6. Nurse Jones is working with Kim, a client in the anger-management program. Which of the following identifies actions associated with the working phase of the therapeutic relationship?
   a. Kim tells Nurse Jones she wants to learn more adaptive ways to handle her anger. Together, they set some goals.
   b. The goals of therapy have been met, but Kim cries and says she has to keep coming to therapy in order to be able to handle her anger appropriately.
   c. Nurse Jones reads Kim's previous medical records. She explores her feelings about working with a woman who has abused her child.
   d. Nurse Jones helps Kim practice various techniques to control her angry outbursts. She gives Kim positive feedback for attempting to improve maladaptive behaviors.

7. When there is congruence between what is felt and what is being expressed, the nurse is exhibiting which of the following characteristics?
   a. Trust.
   b. Respect.
   c. Genuineness.
   d. Empathy.

8. When the nurse shows unconditional acceptance of an individual as a worthwhile and unique human being, he or she is exhibiting which of the following characteristics?
   a. Trust.
   b. Respect.
   c. Genuineness.
   d. Empathy.

9. Hildegard Peplau identified six subroles within the role of the nurse. She believed the emphasis in psychiatric nursing was on which of the subroles?
   a. The resource person.
   b. The teacher.
   c. The surrogate.
   d. The counselor.

Review Questions—cont'd
Self-Examination/Learning Exercise

10. Which of the following behaviors are associated with the phenomenon of *transference?* (Select all that apply.)
    a. The client attributes toward the nurse feelings associated with a person from the client's past.
    b. The nurse attributes toward the client feelings associated with a person from the nurse's past.
    c. The client forms an overwhelming affection for the nurse.
    d. The client becomes excessively dependent on the nurse and forms unrealistic expectations of him or her.

References

College and Association of Registered Nurses of Alberta. (2005). *Professional boundaries for registered nurses: Guidelines for the nurse-client relationship.* Edmonton, AB: Author.

Hilz, L. M. (2008). Transference and countertransference. *Kathi's mental health review.* Retrieved July 12, 2010, at http://www.toddlertime.com/mh/terms/countertransference-transference-3.htm

Peplau, H. E. (1991). *Interpersonal relations in nursing.* New York: Springer.

Peternelj-Taylor, C. A., & Yonge, O. (2003). Exploring boundaries in the nurse-client relationship: Professional roles and responsibilities. *Perspectives in Psychiatric Care, 39*(2), 55–66.

Raskin, N. J., Rogers, C. R., & Witty, M. C. (2011). Client-centered therapy. In R. J. Corsini & D. Wedding (Eds.), *Current psychotherapies* (9th ed., pp. 148–195). Belmont, CA: Brooks/Cole.

Registered Nurses' Association of British Columbia. (2003). *Nurse-client relationships.* Vancouver, BC: Author.

Sadock, B. J., & Sadock, V. A. (2007). *Synopsis of psychiatry: Behavioral sciences/clinical psychiatry* (10th ed.). Philadelphia: Lippincott Williams & Wilkins.

Schuster, P. M. (2000). *Communication: The key to the therapeutic relationship.* Philadelphia: F.A. Davis.

Classical References

Coltrane, F., & Pugh, C. (1978). Danger signals in staff/patient relationships. *Journal of Psychiatric Nursing & Mental Health Services, 16*(6), 34–36.

Luft, J. (1970). *Group processes: An introduction to group dynamics.* Palo Alto, CA: National Press Books.

Peplau, H. E. (1962). Interpersonal techniques: The crux of psychiatric nursing. *American Journal of Nursing, 62*(6): 50–54.

Raths, L., Merril, H., & Simon, S. (1966). *Values and teaching.* Columbus, OH: Merrill.

Sullivan, H. S. (1953). *The interpersonal theory of psychiatry.* New York: W.W. Norton.

Travelbee, J. (1971). *Interpersonal aspects of nursing* (2nd ed.). Philadelphia: F.A. Davis.

Therapeutic Communication

8

KEY TERMS

density	personal distance
distance	public distance
intimate distance	social distance
paralanguage	territoriality

OBJECTIVES

After reading this chapter, the student will be able to:

1. Discuss the transactional model of communication.
2. Identify types of preexisting conditions that influence the outcome of the communication process.
3. Define *territoriality, density,* and *distance* as components of the environment.
4. Identify components of nonverbal expression.
5. Describe therapeutic and nontherapeutic verbal communication techniques.
6. Describe active listening.
7. Discuss therapeutic feedback.

HOMEWORK ASSIGNMENT
Please read the chapter and answer the following questions:

1. "What do *you* think you should do?" If the nurse makes this statement to a client, it is an example of what technique? Is it therapeutic or nontherapeutic?
2. "Just hang in there. Everything will be all right." If the nurse makes this statement to a client, it is an example of what technique? Is it therapeutic or nontherapeutic?
3. Why might it be more appropriate to conduct a client interview in a conference room or interview room rather than in the client's room or nurse's office?
4. Name the five elements of constructive feedback.

Development of the *therapeutic interpersonal relationship* was described in Chapter 7 as the process by which nurses provide care for clients in need of psychosocial intervention. *Therapeutic use of self* was identified as the instrument for delivery of care. The focus of this chapter is on

techniques—or, more specifically, *interpersonal communication techniques*—to facilitate the delivery of that care.

Hays and Larson (1963) stated, "To relate therapeutically with a patient it is necessary for the nurse to understand his or her role and its relationship to the patient's illness." (p. 1) They describe the role of the nurse as providing the client with the opportunity to accomplish the following:

1. Identify and explore problems in relating to others.

2. Discover healthy ways of meeting emotional needs.

3. Experience a satisfying interpersonal relationship.

These goals are achieved through use of interpersonal communication techniques (both verbal and nonverbal). The nurse must be aware of the therapeutic or nontherapeutic value of the communication techniques used with the client because they are the "tools" of psychosocial intervention.

> ### CORE CONCEPT
> *Communication*
> An interactive process of transmitting information between two or more entities.

What Is Communication?

It has been said that individuals "cannot *not* communicate." Every word that is spoken, every movement that is made, and every action that is taken or failed to be taken gives a message to someone. Interpersonal communication is a *transaction* between the sender and the receiver. In the transactional model of communication, both participants simultaneously perceive each other, listen to each other, and are mutually involved in creating meaning in a relationship. The transactional model is illustrated in Figure 8–1.

FIGURE 8–1   The Transactional Model of Communication.

The Impact of Preexisting Conditions

In all interpersonal transactions, both the sender and receiver bring certain preexisting conditions to the exchange that influence both the intended message and the way in which it is interpreted. Examples of these conditions include one's value system, internalized attitudes and beliefs, culture or religion, social status, gender, background knowledge and experience, and age or developmental level. The type of environment in which the communication takes place may also influence the outcome of the transaction. Figure 8–2 shows how these influencing factors are positioned on the transactional model.

Values, Attitudes, and Beliefs

Values, attitudes, and beliefs are learned ways of thinking. Children generally adopt the value systems and internalize the attitudes and beliefs of their parents. Children may retain this way of thinking into adulthood or develop a different set of attitudes and values as they mature.

Values, attitudes, and beliefs can influence communication in numerous ways. For example, prejudice is expressed verbally through negative stereotyping.

One's value system may be communicated with behaviors that are more symbolic in nature. For example, an individual who values youth may dress and behave in a manner that is characteristic

FIGURE 8–2   Factors influencing the Transactional Model of Communication.

of one who is much younger. Persons who value freedom and the American way of life may fly the U.S. flag in front of their homes each day. In each of these situations, a message is being communicated.

Culture or Religion

Communication has its roots in culture. Cultural mores, norms, ideas, and customs provide the basis for our way of thinking. Cultural values are learned and differ from society to society. For example, in some European countries (e.g., Italy, Spain, and France), men may greet each other with hugs and kisses. These behaviors are appropriate in those cultures but would communicate a different message in the United States or England.

Religion can influence communication as well. Priests and ministers who wear clerical collars publicly communicate their mission in life. The collar may also influence the way in which others relate to them, either positively or negatively. Other symbolic gestures, such as wearing a cross around the neck or hanging a crucifix on the wall, also communicate an individual's religious beliefs.

Social Status

Studies of nonverbal indicators of social status or power have suggested that high-status persons are associated with gestures that communicate their higher-power position. For example, they use less eye contact, have a more relaxed posture, use louder voice pitch, place hands on hips more frequently, are "power dressers," have greater height, and maintain more distance when communicating with individuals considered to be of lower social status.

Gender

Gender influences the manner in which individuals communicate. Most cultures have *gender signals* that are recognized as either masculine or feminine and provide a basis for distinguishing between members of each gender. Examples include differences in posture, both standing and sitting, between many men and women in the United States. Men usually stand with thighs 10 to 15 degrees apart, the pelvis rolled back, and the arms slightly away from the body. Women often are seen with legs close together, the pelvis tipped forward, and the arms close to the body. When sitting, men may lean back in the chair with legs apart or may rest the ankle of one leg over the knee of the other. Women tend to sit more upright in the chair with legs together, perhaps crossed at the ankles, or one leg crossed over the other at thigh level.

Roles have historically been identified as either male or female. For example, in the United States masculinity typically was communicated through such roles as husband, father, breadwinner, doctor, lawyer, or engineer. Traditional female roles included those of wife, mother, homemaker, nurse, teacher, or secretary.

Gender signals are changing in U.S. society as sexual roles become less distinct. Behaviors that had been considered typically masculine or feminine in the past may now be generally accepted in members of both genders. Words such as "unisex" communicate a desire by some individuals to diminish the distinction between genders and minimize the discrimination of either. Gender roles are changing as both women and men enter professions that were once dominated by members of the opposite gender.

Age or Developmental Level

Age influences communication, and this is never more evident than during adolescence. In their struggle to separate from parental confines and establish their own identity, adolescents generate a unique pattern of communication that changes from generation to generation. Words such as "dude," "groovy," "clueless," "awesome," "cool," and "wasted" have had special meaning for certain generations of adolescents.

Developmental influences on communication may relate to physiological alterations. One example is American Sign Language, the system of unique gestures used by many people who are deaf or hearing impaired. Individuals who are blind at birth never learn the subtle nonverbal gesticulations that accompany language and can totally change the meaning of the spoken word.

Environment in Which the Transaction Takes Place

The place where the communication occurs influences the outcome of the interaction. Some individuals who feel uncomfortable and refuse to speak during a group therapy session may be open and willing to discuss problems privately on a one-to-one basis with the nurse.

Territoriality, density, and **distance** are aspects of environment that communicate messages. *Territoriality* is the innate tendency to own space. Individuals lay claim to areas around them as their own. This influences communication when an interaction takes place in the territory "owned" by one or the other. Interpersonal communication can be more successful if the interaction takes place in a "neutral" area. For example, with the concept of territoriality in mind, the nurse may choose to conduct the psychosocial assessment in an interview room rather than in his or her office or in the client's room.

Density refers to the number of people within a given environmental space. It has been shown to influence interpersonal interaction. Some studies indicate that a correlation exists between prolonged high-density situations and certain behaviors, such as aggression, stress, criminal activity, hostility toward others, and a deterioration of mental and physical health.

Distance is the means by which various cultures use space to communicate. Hall (1966) identified four kinds of spatial interaction, or distances, that people maintain from each other in their interpersonal interactions and the kinds of activities in which people engage at these various distances. **Intimate distance** is the closest distance that individuals will allow between themselves and others. In the United States, this distance, which is restricted to interactions of an intimate nature, is 0 to 18 inches. **Personal distance** is approximately 18 to 40 inches and reserved for interactions that are personal in nature, such as close conversations with friends or colleagues. **Social distance** is about 4 to 12 feet away from the body. Interactions at this distance include conversations with strangers or acquaintances, such as at a cocktail party or in a public building. A **public distance** is one that exceeds 12 feet. Examples include speaking in public or yelling to someone some distance away. This distance is considered public space, and communicants are free to move about in it during the interaction.

Nonverbal Communication

It has been estimated that about 70 to 80 percent of all effective communication is nonverbal (Khan, 2009). Some aspects of nonverbal expression have been discussed in the previous section on preexisting conditions that influence communication. Other components of nonverbal communication include physical appearance and dress, body movement and posture, touch, facial expressions, eye behavior, and vocal cues or paralanguage. These nonverbal messages vary from culture to culture.

Physical Appearance and Dress

Physical appearance and dress are part of the total nonverbal stimuli that influence interpersonal responses and, under some conditions, they are the primary determinants of such responses. Body coverings—both dress and hair—are manipulated by the wearer in a manner that conveys a distinct message to the receiver. Dress can be formal or casual, stylish or unkempt. Hair can be long or short, and even the presence or absence of hair conveys a message about the person. Other body adornments that are also considered potential communicative stimuli include tattoos, masks, cosmetics, badges, jewelry, and eyeglasses. Some jewelry worn in specific ways can give special messages (e.g., a gold band or diamond ring worn on the third finger of the left hand, a pin bearing Greek letters worn on the lapel, or the wearing of a ring that is inscribed with the insignia of a college or university). Some individuals convey a specific message with the total absence of any type of body adornment.

Body Movement and Posture

The way in which an individual positions his or her body communicates messages regarding self-esteem, gender identity, status, and interpersonal warmth or coldness. The individual whose posture is slumped, with head and eyes pointed downward, conveys a message of low self-esteem. Specific ways of standing or sitting are considered to be either feminine or masculine within a defined culture. In the United States, to stand straight and tall with head high and hands on hips indicates a superior status over the person being addressed.

Reece and Whitman (1962) identified response behaviors that were used to designate individuals as either "warm" or "cold" persons. Individuals who were perceived as warm responded to others with a shift of posture toward the other person, a smile, direct eye contact, and hands that remained still. Individuals who responded to others with a slumped posture, by looking around the room, drumming fingers on the desk, and not smiling were perceived as cold.

Touch

Touch is a powerful communication tool. It can elicit both negative and positive reactions, depending on the people involved and the circumstances of the interaction. It is a very basic and primitive form of communication, and the appropriateness of its use is culturally determined.

Touch can be categorized according to the message communicated (Knapp & Hall, 2001):

■ **Functional-Professional.** This type of touch is impersonal and businesslike. It is used to accomplish a task.

EXAMPLE

A tailor measuring a customer for a suit or a physician examining a client.

■ **Social-Polite.** This type of touch is still rather impersonal, but it conveys an affirmation or acceptance of the other person.

EXAMPLE

A handshake.

■ **Friendship-Warmth.** Touch at this level indicates a strong liking for the other person, a feeling that he or she is a friend.

EXAMPLE

Laying one's hand on the shoulder of another.

■ **Love-Intimacy.** This type of touch conveys an emotional attachment or attraction for another person.

EXAMPLE

Engaging in a strong, mutual embrace.

■ **Sexual Arousal.** Touch at this level is an expression of physical attraction only.

EXAMPLE

Touching another in the genital region.

Some cultures encourage more touching of various types than others. "Contact cultures" (e.g., France, Latin America, Italy) use a greater frequency of touch cues than do those in "non-contact cultures" (e.g., Germany, United States, Canada) (Givens, 2010a). The nurse should understand the cultural meaning of touch before using this method of communication in specific situations.

Facial Expressions

Next to human speech, facial expression is the primary source of communication. Facial expressions primarily reveal an individual's emotional states, such as happiness, sadness, anger, surprise, and fear. The face is a complex multimessage system. Facial expressions serve to complement and qualify other communication behaviors, and at times even take the place of verbal messages. A summary of feelings associated with various facial expressions is presented in Table 8-1.

Eye Behavior

Eyes have been called the "windows of the soul." It is through eye contact that individuals view and are viewed by others in a revealing way. An interpersonal connectedness occurs through eye contact. In American culture, eye contact conveys a personal

TABLE 8-1 Summary of Facial Expressions	
FACIAL EXPRESSION	**ASSOCIATED FEELINGS**
Nose:	
Nostril flare	Anger; arousal
Wrinkling up	Dislike; disgust
Lips:	
Grin; smile	Happiness; contentment
Grimace	Fear; pain
Compressed	Anger; frustration
Canine-type snarl	Disgust
Pouted; frown	Unhappiness; discontented; disapproval
Pursing	Disagreement
Sneer	Contempt; disdain
Brows:	
Frown	Anger; unhappiness; concentration
Raised	Surprise; enthusiasm
Tongue:	
Stick out	Dislike; disagree
Eyes:	
Widened	Surprise; excitement
Narrowed; lids squeezed shut	Threat; fear
Stare	Threat
Stare/blink/look away	Dislike; disinterest
Eyes downcast; lack of eye contact	Submission; low self-esteem
Eye contact (generally intermittent, as opposed to a stare)	Self-confidence; interest

SOURCES: Adapted from Givens (2010b); Hughey (1990); and Simon (2005).

interest in the other person. Eye contact indicates that the communication channel is open, and it is often the initiating factor in verbal interaction between two people.

Eye behavior is regulated by social rules. These rules dictate where, when, for how long, and at whom we can look. Staring is often used to register disapproval of the behavior of another. People are extremely sensitive to being looked at, and if the gazing or staring behavior violates social rules, they often assign meaning to it, such as the following statement implies: "He kept staring at me, and I began to wonder if I was dressed inappropriately or had mustard on my face!"

Gazing at another's eyes arouses strong emotions. Thus, eye contact rarely lasts longer than 3 seconds before one or both viewers experience a powerful urge to glance away. Breaking eye contact lowers stress levels (Givens, 2010c).

Vocal Cues, or Paralanguage

Paralanguage is the gestural component of the spoken word. It consists of pitch, tone, and loudness of spoken messages; the rate of speaking; expressively placed pauses; and emphasis assigned to certain words. These vocal cues greatly influence the way individuals interpret verbal messages. A normally soft-spoken individual whose pitch and rate of speaking increases may be perceived as being anxious or tense.

Different vocal emphases can alter interpretation of the message. Three examples follow:

1. "I felt **SURE** you would notice the change." *Interpretation:* I was **SURE** you would, but you didn't.
2. "I felt sure **YOU** would notice the change." *Interpretation:* I thought **YOU** would, even if nobody else did.
3. "I felt sure you would notice the **CHANGE.**" *Interpretation:* Even if you didn't notice anything else, I thought you would notice the **CHANGE.**

Verbal cues play a major role in determining responses in human communication situations. *How* a message is verbalized can be as important as *what* is verbalized.

CORE CONCEPT

Therapeutic Communication
Caregiver verbal and nonverbal techniques that focus on the care receiver's needs and advance the promotion of healing and change. Therapeutic communication encourages exploration of feelings and fosters understanding of behavioral motivation. It is nonjudgmental, discourages defensiveness, and promotes trust.

Therapeutic Communication Techniques

Hays and Larson (1963) identified a number of techniques to assist the nurse in interacting more therapeutically with clients. These are the "technical procedures" carried out by the nurse working in psychiatry, and they should serve to enhance development of a therapeutic nurse-client relationship. Table 8-2 includes a list of these techniques, a short explanation of their usefulness, and examples of each.

Nontherapeutic Communication Techniques

Several approaches are considered to be barriers to open communication between the nurse and client. Hays and Larson (1963) identified a number of these techniques, which are presented in

TABLE 8-2 Therapeutic Communication Techniques		
TECHNIQUE	**EXPLANATION/RATIONALE**	**EXAMPLES**
Using silence	Gives the client the opportunity to collect and organize thoughts, to think through a point, or to consider introducing a topic of greater concern than the one being discussed.	
Accepting	Conveys an attitude of reception and regard.	"Yes, I understand what you said." Eye contact; nodding.
Giving recognition	Acknowledging and indicating awareness; better than complimenting, which reflects the nurse's judgment.	"Hello, Mr. J. I notice that you made a ceramic ashtray in OT." "I see you made your bed."
Offering self	Making oneself available on an unconditional basis, increasing client's feelings of self-worth.	"I'll stay with you awhile." "We can eat our lunch together." "I'm interested in you."

Continued

TABLE 8-2 Therapeutic Communication Techniques—cont'd

TECHNIQUE	EXPLANATION/RATIONALE	EXAMPLES
Giving broad openings	Allows the client to take the initiative in introducing the topic; emphasizes the importance of the client's role in the interaction.	"What would you like to talk about today?" "Tell me what you are thinking."
Offering general leads	Offers the client encouragement to continue.	"Yes, I see." "Go on." "And after that?"
Placing the event in time or sequence	Clarifies the relationship of events in time so that the nurse and client can view them in perspective.	"What seemed to lead up to . . .?" "Was this before or after . . .?" "When did this happen?"
Making observations	Verbalizing what is observed or perceived. This encourages the client to recognize specific behaviors and compare perceptions with the nurse.	"You seem tense." "I notice you are pacing a lot." "You seem uncomfortable when you . . ."
Encouraging description of perceptions	Asking the client to verbalize what is being perceived; often used with clients experiencing hallucinations.	"Tell me what is happening now." "Are you hearing the voices again?" "What do the voices seem to be saying?"
Encouraging comparison	Asking the client to compare similarities and differences in ideas, experiences, or interpersonal relationships. This helps the client recognize life experiences that tend to recur as well as those aspects of life that are changeable.	"Was this something like . . .?" "How does this compare with the time when . . .?" "What was your response the last time this situation occurred?"
Restating	The main idea of what the client has said is repeated. This lets the client know whether or not an expressed statement has been understood and gives him or her the chance to continue, or to clarify if necessary.	Cl: "I can't study. My mind keeps wandering." Ns: "You have difficulty concentrating." Cl: "I can't take that new job. What if I can't do it?" Ns: "You're afraid you will fail in this new position."
Reflecting	Questions and feelings are referred back to the client so that they may be recognized and accepted, and so that the client may recognize that his or her point of view has value—a good technique to use when the client asks the nurse for advice.	Cl: "What do you think I should do about my wife's drinking problem?" Ns: "What do you think you should do?" Cl: "My sister won't help a bit toward my mother's care. I have to do it all!" Ns: "You feel angry when she doesn't help."
Focusing	Taking notice of a single idea or even a single word; works especially well with a client who is moving rapidly from one thought to another. This technique is not therapeutic, however, with the client who is very anxious. Focusing should not be pursued until the anxiety level has subsided.	"This point seems worth looking at more closely. Perhaps you and I can discuss it together."

TABLE 8-2 Therapeutic Communication Techniques—cont'd

TECHNIQUE	EXPLANATION/RATIONALE	EXAMPLES
Exploring	Delving further into a subject, idea, experience, or relationship; especially helpful with clients who tend to remain on a superficial level of communication. However, if the client chooses not to disclose further information, the nurse should refrain from pushing or probing in an area that obviously creates discomfort.	"Please explain that situation in more detail." "Tell me more about that particular situation."
Seeking clarification and validation	Striving to explain that which is vague or incomprehensible and searching for mutual understanding. Clarifying the meaning of what has been said facilitates and increases understanding for both client and nurse.	"I'm not sure that I understand. Would you please explain?" "Tell me if my understanding agrees with yours." "Do I understand correctly that you said . . .?"
Presenting reality	When the client has a misperception of the environment, the nurse defines reality or indicates his or her perception of the situation for the client.	"I understand that the voices seem real to you, but I do not hear any voices." "There is no one else in the room but you and me."
Voicing doubt	Expressing uncertainty as to the reality of the client's perceptions; often used with clients experiencing delusional thinking.	"I find that hard to believe." "That seems rather doubtful to me." "I understand that you believe this to be true, but I see this situation differently than you."
Verbalizing the implied	Putting into words what the client has only implied or said indirectly; it can also be used with the client who is mute or is otherwise experiencing impaired verbal communication. This clarifies that which is *implicit* rather than *explicit*.	Cl: "It's a waste of time to be here. I can't talk to you or anyone." Ns: "Are you feeling that no one understands?" Cl: (Mute) Ns: "It must have been very difficult for you when your husband died in the fire."
Attempting to translate words into feelings	When feelings are expressed indirectly, the nurse tries to "desymbolize" what has been said and to find clues to the underlying true feelings.	Cl: "I'm way out in the ocean." Ns: "You must be feeling very lonely now."
Formulating a plan of action	When a client has a plan in mind for dealing with what is considered to be a stressful situation, it may serve to prevent anger or anxiety from escalating to an unmanageable level.	"What could you do to let your anger out harmlessly?" "Next time this comes up, what might you do to handle it more appropriately?"

Adapted from Hays, J. S., & Larson, K. H. (1963). Interacting with patients. New York: Macmillan.

Table 8-3. Nurses should recognize and eliminate the use of these patterns in their relationships with clients. Avoiding these communication barriers will maximize the effectiveness of communication and enhance the nurse-client relationship.

Active Listening

To listen actively is to be attentive to what the client is saying, both verbally and nonverbally. Attentive listening creates a climate in which the client can communicate. With active listening the nurse communicates acceptance and respect for the client, and trust is enhanced. A climate is established within the relationship that promotes openness and honest expression.

Several nonverbal behaviors have been designated as facilitative skills for attentive listening. Those listed here can be identified by the acronym SOLER:

S—Sit squarely facing the client. This gives the message that the nurse is there to listen and is interested in what the client has to say.

O—Observe an open posture. Posture is considered "open" when arms and legs remain uncrossed. This suggests that the nurse is

TABLE 8-3 Nontherapeutic Communication Techniques		
TECHNIQUE	**EXPLANATION/RATIONALE**	**EXAMPLES**
Giving reassurance	Indicates to the client that there is no cause for anxiety, thereby devaluing the client's feelings; may discourage the client from further expression of feelings if he or she believes they will only be downplayed or ridiculed.	"I wouldn't worry about that if I were you." "Everything will be all right." **Better to say:** "We will work on that together."
Rejecting	Refusing to consider or showing contempt for the client's ideas or behavior. This may cause the client to discontinue interaction with the nurse for fear of further rejection.	"Let's not discuss . . ." "I don't want to hear about . . ." **Better to say:** "Let's look at that a little closer."
Approving or disapproving	Sanctioning or denouncing the client's ideas or behavior; implies that the nurse has the right to pass judgment on whether the client's ideas or behaviors are "good" or "bad," and that the client is expected to please the nurse. The nurse's acceptance of the client is then seen as conditional depending on the client's behavior.	"That's good. I'm glad that you . . ." "That's bad. I'd rather you wouldn't . . ." **Better to say:** "Let's talk about how your behavior invoked anger in the other clients at dinner."
Agreeing or disagreeing	Indicating accord with or opposition to the client's ideas or opinions; implies that the nurse has the right to pass judgment on whether the client's ideas or opinions are "right" or "wrong." Agreement prevents the client from later modifying his or her point of view without admitting error. Disagreement implies inaccuracy, provoking the need for defensiveness on the part of the client.	"That's right. I agree." "That's wrong. I disagree." "I don't believe that." **Better to say:** "Let's discuss what you feel is unfair about the new community rules."
Giving advice	Telling the client what to do or how to behave implies that the nurse knows what is best, and that the client is incapable of any self-direction. It nurtures the client in the dependent role by discouraging independent thinking.	"I think you should . . ." "Why don't you . . ." **Better to say:** "What do you think you should do?" or "What do you think would be the best way to solve this problem?"

TABLE 8-3 Nontherapeutic Communication Techniques—cont'd		
TECHNIQUE	**EXPLANATION/RATIONALE**	**EXAMPLES**
Probing	Persistent questioning of the client; pushing for answers to issues the client does not wish to discuss. This causes the client to feel used and valued only for what is shared with the nurse and places the client on the defensive.	"Tell me how your mother abused you when you were a child." "Tell me how you feel toward your mother now that she is dead." "Now tell me about . . ." **Better technique:** The nurse should be aware of the client's response and discontinue the interaction at the first sign of discomfort.
Defending	Attempting to protect someone or something from verbal attack. To defend what the client has criticized is to imply that he or she has no right to express ideas, opinions, or feelings. Defending does not change the client's feelings and may cause the client to think the nurse is taking sides against the client.	"No one here would lie to you." "You have a very capable physician. I'm sure he only has your best interests in mind." **Better to say:** "I will try to answer your questions and clarify some issues regarding your treatment.
Requesting an explanation	Asking the client to provide the reasons for thoughts, feelings, behavior, and events. Asking "why" a client did something or feels a certain way can be very intimidating, and implies that the client must defend his or her behavior or feelings.	"Why do you think that?" "Why do you feel this way?" "Why did you do that?" **Better to say:** "Describe what you were feeling just before that happened."
Indicating the existence of an external source of power	Attributing the source of thoughts, feelings, and behavior to others or to outside influences. This encourages the client to project blame for his or her thoughts or behaviors on others rather than accepting the responsibility personally.	"What makes you say that?" "What made you do that?" "What made you so angry last night?" **Better to say:** "You became angry when your brother insulted your wife."
Belittling feelings expressed	When the nurse misjudges the degree of the client's discomfort, a lack of empathy and understanding may be conveyed. The nurse may tell the client to "perk up" or "snap out of it." This causes the client to feel insignificant or unimportant. When one is experiencing discomfort, it is no relief to hear that others are or have been in similar situations.	Cl: "I have nothing to live for. I wish I were dead." Ns: "Everybody gets down in the dumps at times. I feel that way myself sometimes." **Better to say:** "You must be very upset. Tell me what you are feeling right now."
Making stereotyped comments	Clichés and trite expressions are meaningless in a nurse-client relationship. When the nurse makes empty conversation, it encourages a like response from the client.	"I'm fine, and how are you?" "Hang in there. It's for your own good." "Keep your chin up." **Better to say:** "The therapy must be difficult for you at times. How do you feel about your progress at this point?"

Continued

TABLE 8-3 Nontherapeutic Communication Techniques—cont'd

TECHNIQUE	EXPLANATION/RATIONALE	EXAMPLES
Using denial	When the nurse denies that a problem exists, he or she blocks discussion with the client and avoids helping the client identify and explore areas of difficulty.	Cl: "I'm nothing." Ns: "Of course you're something. Everybody is somebody. **Better to say:** "You're feeling like no one cares about you right now."
Interpreting	With this technique the therapist seeks to make conscious that which is unconscious, to tell the client the meaning of his or her experience.	"What you really mean is . . ." "Unconsciously you're saying . . ." **Better technique:** The nurse must leave interpretation of the client's behavior to the psychiatrist. The nurse has not been prepared to perform this technique, and in attempting to do so, may endanger other nursing roles with the client.
Introducing an unrelated topic	Changing the subject causes the nurse to take over the direction of the discussion. This may occur in order to get to something that the nurse wants to discuss with the client or to get away from a topic that he or she would prefer not to discuss.	Cl: "I don't have anything to live for." Ns: "Did you have visitors this weekend?" **Better technique:** The nurse must remain open and free to hear the client, to take in all that is being conveyed, both verbally and nonverbally.

Adapted from Hays, J. S., & Larson, K. H. (1963). *Interacting with patients.* New York: Macmillan.

"open" to what the client has to say. With a "closed" position, the nurse can convey a somewhat defensive stance, possibly invoking a similar response in the client.

L—Lean forward toward the client. This conveys to the client that you are involved in the interaction, interested in what is being said, and making a sincere effort to be attentive.

E—Establish eye contact. Eye contact, intermittently directed, is another behavior that conveys the nurse's involvement and willingness to listen to what the client has to say. The absence of eye contact or the constant shifting of eye contact elsewhere in the environment gives the message that the nurse is not really interested in what is being said.

> **CLINICAL PEARL** Ensure that eye contact conveys warmth and is accompanied by smiling and intermittent nodding of the head, and does not come across as staring or glaring, which can create intense discomfort in the client.

R—Relax. Whether sitting or standing during the interaction, the nurse should communicate a sense of being relaxed and comfortable with the client. Restlessness and fidgetiness communicate a lack of interest and may convey a feeling of discomfort that is likely to be transferred to the client.

Process Recordings

Process recordings are written reports of verbal interactions with clients. They are verbatim (to the extent that this is possible) accounts, written by the nurse or student as a tool for improving interpersonal communication techniques. The process recording can take many forms, but usually includes the verbal and nonverbal communication of both nurse and client. The exercise provides a means for the nurse to analyze both the content and the pattern of the interaction. The process recording, which is not considered documentation, is intended to be used as a learning tool for professional development. An example of one type of process recording is presented in Table 8-4.

TABLE 8-4 Sample Process Recording

NURSE VERBAL (NONVERBAL)	CLIENT VERBAL (NONVERBAL)	NURSE'S THOUGHTS AND FEELINGS CONCERNING THE INTERACTION	ANALYSIS OF THE INTERACTION
Do you still have thoughts about harming yourself? (Sitting facing the client; looking directly at client.)	Not really. I still feel sad, but I don't want to die. (Looking at hands in lap.)	Felt a little uncomfortable. Always a hard question to ask.	**Therapeutic.** Asking a direct question about suicidal intent.
Tell me what you were feeling before you took all the pills the other night. (Still using SOLER techniques of active listening.)	I was just so angry! To think that my husband wants a divorce now that he has a good job. I worked hard to put him through college. (Fists clenched. Face and neck reddened.)	Beginning to feel more comfortable. Client seems willing to talk and I think she trusts me.	**Therapeutic.** Exploring. Delving further into the experience.
You wanted to hurt him because you felt betrayed. (SOLER)	Yes! If I died, maybe he'd realize that he loved me more than that other woman. (Tears starting to well up in her eyes.)	Starting to feel sorry for her.	**Therapeutic.** Attempting to translate words into feelings.
Seems like a pretty drastic way to get your point across. (Small frown.)	I know. It was a stupid thing to do. (Wiping eyes.)	Trying hard to remain objective.	**Nontherapeutic.** Sounds disapproving. Better to have pursued her feelings.
How are you feeling about the situation now? (SOLER)	I don't know. I still love him. I want him to come home. I don't want him to marry her. (Starting to cry again.)	Wishing there was an easy way to help relieve some of her pain.	**Therapeutic.** Focusing on her feelings.
Yes, I can understand that you would like things to be the way they were before. (Offer client a tissue.)	(Silence. Continues to cry softly.)	I'm starting to feel some anger toward her husband. Sometimes it's so hard to remain objective!	**Therapeutic.** Conveying empathy.
What do you think are the chances of your getting back together? (SOLER)	None. He's refused marriage counseling. He's already moved in with her. He says it's over. (Wipes tears. Looks directly at nurse.)	Relieved to know that she isn't using denial about the reality of the situation.	**Therapeutic.** Reflecting. Seeking client's perception of the situation.
So how are you preparing to deal with this inevitable outcome? (SOLER)	I'm going to do the things we talked about: join a divorced women's support group, increase my job hours to full-time, do some volunteer work, and call the suicide hot line if I feel like taking pills again. (Looks directly at nurse. Smiles.)	Positive feeling to know that she remembers what we discussed earlier and plans to follow through.	**Therapeutic.** Formulating a plan of action.

Continued

TABLE 8-4 Sample Process Recording—cont'd

NURSE VERBAL (NONVERBAL)	CLIENT VERBAL (NONVERBAL)	NURSE'S THOUGHTS AND FEELINGS CONCERNING THE INTERACTION	ANALYSIS OF THE INTERACTION
It won't be easy. But you have come a long way, and I feel you have gained strength in your ability to cope. (Standing. Looking at client. Smiling.)	Yes, I know I will have hard times. But I also know I have support, and I want to go on with my life and be happy again. (Standing, smiling at nurse.)	Feeling confident that the session has gone well; hopeful that the client will succeed in what she wants to do with her life.	**Therapeutic.** Presenting reality.

Feedback

Feedback is a method of communication for helping the client consider a modification of behavior. Feedback gives information to clients about how they are being perceived by others. It should be presented in a manner that discourages defensiveness on the part of the client. Feedback can be useful to the client if presented with objectivity by a trusted individual.

Some criteria about useful feedback include the following:

■ Feedback is descriptive rather than evaluative and focuses on the behavior rather than on the client. Avoiding evaluative language reduces the need for the client to react defensively. Objective descriptions allow clients to take the information and use it in whatever way they choose. When the focus is on the client, the nurse makes judgments about the client.

EXAMPLE

Descriptive and focused on behavior	"Jane was very upset in group today when you called her 'fatty' and laughed at her in front of the others."
Evaluative	"You were very rude and inconsiderate to Jane in group today."
Focus on client	"You are a very insensitive person."

■ Feedback should be specific rather than general. Information that gives details about the client's behavior can be used more easily than a generalized description for modifying the behavior.

EXAMPLE

| Specific | "You were talking to Joe when we were deciding on the issue. Now you want to argue about the outcome." |
| General | "You just don't pay attention." |

■ Feedback should be directed toward behavior that the client has the capacity to modify. To provide feedback about a characteristic or situation that the client cannot change only provokes frustration.

EXAMPLE

| Can modify | "I noticed that you did not want to hold your baby when the nurse brought her to you." |
| Cannot modify | "Your baby daughter is mentally retarded because you took drugs when you were pregnant." |

■ Feedback should impart information rather than offer advice. Giving advice fosters dependence and may convey the message to the client that he or she is not capable of making decisions and solving problems independently. It is the client's right and privilege to be as self-sufficient as possible.

EXAMPLE

| Imparting information | "There are various methods of assistance for people who want to lose weight, such as Overeaters Anonymous, Weight Watchers, regular visits to a dietitian, and the Physician's Weight Loss Program. You can decide what is best for you." |
| Giving advice | "You obviously need to lose a great deal of weight. I think the Physician's Weight Loss Program would be best for you." |

■ Feedback should be well timed. Feedback is most useful when given at the earliest appropriate opportunity following the specific behavior.

EXAMPLE

| Prompt response | "I saw you hit the wall with your fist just now when you hung up the phone after talking to your mother." |
| Delayed | "You need to learn some more appropriate ways of dealing with your anger. Last week after group I saw you pounding your fist against the wall." |

Summary and Key Points

■ Interpersonal communication is a transaction between the sender and the receiver.

■ In all interpersonal transactions, both the sender and receiver bring certain preexisting conditions to the exchange that influences both the intended message and the way in which it is interpreted.

■ Examples of these preexisting conditions include one's value system, internalized attitudes and beliefs, culture or religion, social status, gender, background knowledge and experience, age or developmental level, and the type of environment in which the communication takes place.

■ Nonverbal expression is a primary communication system in which meaning is assigned to various gestures and patterns of behavior.

■ Some components of nonverbal communication include physical appearance and dress, body movement and posture, touch, facial expressions, eye behavior, and vocal cues or paralanguage.

■ Meaning of the nonverbal components of communication is culturally determined.

■ Therapeutic communication includes verbal and nonverbal techniques that focus on the care receiver's needs and advance the promotion of healing and change.

■ Nurses must also be aware of and avoid a number of techniques that are considered to be barriers to effective communication.

■ Active listening is described as being attentive to what the client is saying, through both verbal and nonverbal cues. Skills associated with active listening include sitting squarely facing the client, observing an open posture, leaning forward toward the client, establishing eye contact, and being relaxed.

■ Process recordings are written reports of verbal interactions with clients. They are used as learning tools for professional development.

■ Feedback is a method of communication for helping the client consider a modification of behavior.

■ The nurse must be aware of the therapeutic or nontherapeutic value of the communication techniques used with the client because they are the "tools" of psychosocial intervention.

 DavisPlus Additional info available @ davisplus.fadavis.com

Review Questions
Self-Examination/Learning Exercise

*Select the answer that is **most** appropriate for each of the following questions:*

1. A client states: "I refuse to shower in this room. I must be very cautious. The FBI has placed a camera in here to monitor my every move." Which of the following is the therapeutic response?
   a. "That's not true."
   b. "I have a hard time believing that is true."
   c. "Surely you don't really believe that."
   d. "I will help you search this room so that you can see there is no camera."

Continued

Review Questions—cont'd
Self-Examination/Learning Exercise

2. Nancy, a depressed client who has been unkept and untidy for weeks, today comes to group therapy wearing makeup and a clean dress and having washed and combed her hair. Which of the following responses by the nurse is most appropriate?
   a. "Nancy, I see you have put on a clean dress and combed your hair."
   b. "Nancy, you look wonderful today!"
   c. "Nancy, I'm sure everyone will appreciate that you have cleaned up for the group today."
   d. "Now that you see how important it is, I hope you will do this every day."

3. Dorothy was involved in an automobile accident while under the influence of alcohol. She swerved her car into a tree and narrowly missed hitting a child on a bicycle. She is in the hospital with multiple abrasions and contusions. She is talking about the accident with the nurse. Which of the following statements by the nurse is most appropriate?
   a. "Now that you know what can happen when you drink and drive, I'm sure you won't let it happen again."
   b. "You know that was a terrible thing you did. That child could have been killed."
   c. "I'm sure everything is going to be okay now that you understand the possible consequence of such behavior."
   d. "How are you feeling about what happened?"

4. Judy has been in the hospital for 3 weeks. She has used Valium "to settle my nerves" for the past 15 years. She was admitted by her psychiatrist for safe withdrawal from the drug. She has passed the physical symptoms of withdrawal at this time, but states to the nurse, "I don't know if I will be able to make it without Valium after I go home. I'm already starting to feel nervous. I have so many personal problems." Which is the most appropriate response by the nurse?
   a. "Why do you think you have to have drugs to deal with your problems?"
   b. "Everybody has problems, but not everybody uses drugs to deal with them. You'll just have to do the best that you can."
   c. "We will just have to think about some things that you can do to decrease your anxiety without resorting to drugs."
   d. "Just hang in there. I'm sure everything is going to be okay."

5. Mrs. S. asks the nurse, "Do you think I should tell my husband about my affair with my boss?" Which is the most appropriate response by the nurse?
   a. "What do you think would be best for you to do?"
   b. "Of course you should. Marriage has to be based on truth."
   c. "Of course not. That would only make things worse."
   d. "I can't tell you what to do. You have to decide for yourself."

6. Carol, an adolescent, just returned from group therapy and is crying. She says to the nurse, "All the other kids laughed at me! I try to fit in, but I always seem to say the wrong thing. I've never had a close friend. I guess I never will." Which is the most appropriate response by the nurse?
   a. "What makes you think you will never have any friends?"
   b. "You're feeling pretty down on yourself right now."
   c. "I'm sure they didn't mean to hurt your feelings."
   d. "Why do you feel this way about yourself?"

Review Questions—cont'd
Self-Examination/Learning Exercise

7. Walter is angry with his psychiatrist and says to the nurse, "He doesn't know what he is doing. That medication isn't helping a thing!" The nurse responds, "He has been a doctor for many years and has helped many people." This is an example of what nontheraputic technique?
   a. Rejecting.
   b. Disapproving.
   c. Probing.
   d. Defending.

8. The client says to the nurse, "I've been offered a promotion, but I don't know if I can handle it." The nurse replies, "You're afraid you may fail in the new position." This is an example of which therapeutic technique?
   a. Restating.
   b. Making observations.
   c. Focusing.
   d. Verbalizing the implied.

9. The environment in which the communication takes place influences the outcome of the interaction. Which of the following are aspects of the environment that influence communication? (Select all that apply.)
   a. Territoriality.
   b. Density.
   c. Dimension.
   d. Distance.
   e. Intensity.

10. The nurse says to a client, "You are being readmitted to the hospital. Why did you stop taking your medication?" What communication technique does this represent?
   a. Disapproving.
   b. Requesting an explanation.
   c. Disagreeing.
   d. Probing.

References

Givens, D. B. (2010a). The nonverbal dictionary. Center for Nonverbal Studies. Retrieved July 13, 2010, at http://web.archive.org/web/20060627081330/members.aol.com/doder1/touch1.htm

Givens, D. B. (2010b). The nonverbal dictionary. Center for Nonverbal Studies. Retrieved July 13, 2010, at http://web.archive.org/web/20060617171011/members.aol.com/nonverbal3/facialx.htm

Givens, D. B. (2010c). The nonverbal dictionary. Center for Nonverbal Studies. Retrieved July 13, 2010, at http://web.archive.org/web/20060619132216/members.aol.com/nonverbal3/eyecon.htm

Hughey, J. D. (1990). *Speech communication*. Stillwater, OK: Oklahoma State University.

Khan, A. (2009). *Principles for personal growth*. Bellevue, WA: YouMe Works.

Knapp, M. L., & Hall, J. A. (2001). *Nonverbal communication in human interaction* (5th ed.). Belmont, CA: Wadsworth.

Simon, M. (2005). *Facial expressions: A visual reference for artists*. New York: Watson-Guptill.

Classical References

Hall, E. T. (1966). *The hidden dimension*. Garden City, NY: Doubleday.

Hays, J. S., & Larson, K. H. (1963). *Interacting with patients*. New York: Macmillan.

Reece, M., & Whitman, R. (1962). Expressive movements, warmth, and verbal reinforcement. *Journal of Abnormal and Social Psychology, 64,* 234–236.

9

The Nursing Process in Psychiatric/Mental Health Nursing

KEY TERMS

case management
case manager
concept mapping
critical pathways of care
Focus Charting®
interdisciplinary

managed care
Nursing Interventions Classification (NIC)
Nursing Outcomes Classification (NOC)
nursing process
PIE charting
problem-oriented recording

OBJECTIVES

After reading this chapter, the student will be able to:

1. Define *nursing process.*
2. Identify six steps of the nursing process and describe nursing actions associated with each.
3. Describe the benefits of using nursing diagnosis.
4. Discuss the list of nursing diagnoses approved by NANDA International for clinical use and testing.

5. Define and discuss the use of case management and critical pathways of care in the clinical setting.
6. Apply the six steps of the nursing process in the care of a client within the psychiatric setting.
7. Document client care that validates use of the nursing process.

HOMEWORK ASSIGNMENT

Please read the chapter and answer the following questions:

1. Nursing outcomes (sometimes referred to as goals) are derived from the nursing diagnosis. Name two essential aspects of an acceptable outcome or goal.
2. Define *managed care.*
3. The ANA identifies certain interventions that may only be performed by psychiatric nurses in advanced practice. What are they?
4. In Focus Charting®, one item cannot be used as the focus for documentation. What is this item?

For many years the **nursing process** has provided a systematic framework for the delivery of nursing care. It is nursing's means of fulfilling the requirement for a *scientific methodology* in order to be considered a profession.

This chapter examines the steps of the nursing process as they are set forth by the American Nurses Association (ANA) in *Nursing: Scope and Standards of Practice* (ANA, 2010a). An explanation is provided for the implementation of case management and the tool used in the delivery of care with this methodology, critical pathways of care. A description of concept mapping is included, and documentation that validates the use of the nursing process is discussed.

The Nursing Process

Definition

The nursing process consists of six steps and uses a problem-solving approach that has come to be accepted as nursing's scientific methodology. It is goal directed, with the objective being delivery of quality client care.

The nursing process is dynamic, not static. It is an ongoing process that continues for as long as the nurse and client have interactions directed toward change in the client's physical or behavioral responses. Figure 9–1 presents a schematic of the ongoing nursing process.

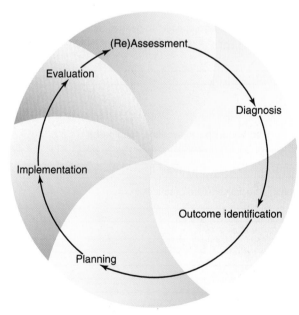

FIGURE 9–1   The ongoing nursing process.

Standards of Practice

The ANA, in collaboration with the American Psychiatric Nurses Association (APNA) and the International Society of Psychiatric-Mental Health Nurses (ISPN), has delineated a set of standards that psychiatric nurses are expected to follow as they provide care for their clients. The ANA (2010a) stated,

> The Standards of Practice describe a competent level of nursing care as demonstrated by the critical thinking model known as the nursing process. The nursing process includes the components of assessment, diagnosis, outcomes identification, planning, implementation, and evaluation. Accordingly, the nursing process encompasses significant actions taken by registered nurses, and forms the foundation of the nurse's decision-making. (p. 9)

Following are the standards of practice for psychiatric/mental health nurses as set forth by the ANA, APNA, and ISPN (2007).

CORE CONCEPT

Assessment

A systematic, dynamic process by which the registered nurse, through interaction with the patient, family, groups, communities, populations, and health-care providers, collects and analyzes data. Assessment may include the following dimensions: physical, psychological, sociocultural, spiritual, cognitive, functional abilities, developmental, economic, and lifestyle (ANA, 2010a).

Standard 1: Assessment

The Psychiatric-Mental Health Registered Nurse collects comprehensive health data that is pertinent to the patient's health or situation.

In this first step, information is gathered from which to establish a database for determining the best possible care for the client. Information for this database is gathered from a variety of sources, including interviews with the client or family, observation of the client and his or her environment, consultation with other health team members, review of the client's records, and a nursing physical examination. A biopsychosocial assessment tool based on the stress-adaptation framework is included in Box 9-1.

(text continues on page 171)

BOX 9-1 **Nursing History and Assessment Tool**

I. General Information

Client name: _____ Allergies: _____

Room number: _____ Diet: _____

Doctor: _____ Height/weight: _____

Age: _____ Vital signs: TPR/BP _____

Sex: _____ Name and phone no. of significant other: _____

Race: _____

Dominant language: _____ City of residence: _____

Marital status: _____ Diagnosis (admitting & current): _____

Chief complaint: _____

_____

Conditions of admission:

Date: _____ Time: _____

Accompanied by: _____

Route of admission (wheelchair; ambulatory; cart): _____

Admitted from: _____

II. Predisposing Factors

A. *Genetic Influences*

1. Family configuration (use genograms):

Family of origin: Present family:

Family dynamics (describe significant relationships between family members): _____

_____

_____

_____

2. Medical/psychiatric history:

a. Client: _____

_____

_____

b. Family members: _____

_____

_____

3. Other genetic influences affecting present adaptation. This might include effects specific to gender, race, appearance, such as genetic physical defects, or any other factor related to genetics that is affecting the client's adaptation that has not been mentioned elsewhere in this assessment.

_____

_____

B. *Past Experiences*

1. Cultural and social history:

a. Environmental factors (family living arrangements, type of neighborhood, special working conditions):

_____

_____

b. Health beliefs and practices (personal responsibility for health; special self-care practices):

_____

_____

c. Religious beliefs and practices: _____

_____

d. Educational background: _____

_____

e. Significant losses/changes (include dates): _____

_____

BOX 9-1 **Nursing History and Assessment Tool—cont'd**

    f. Peer/friendship relationships: _____

    _____

    _____

    g. Occupational history: _____

    _____

    _____

    h. Previous pattern of coping with stress: _____

    _____

    _____

    i. Other lifestyle factors contributing to present adaptation: _____

    _____

    _____

C *Existing Conditions*
  1. Stage of development (Erikson):
    a. Theoretically: _____
    b. Behaviorally: _____
    c. Rationale: _____

    _____

    _____

  2. Support systems: _____

    _____

  3. Economic security: _____

    _____

  4. Avenues of productivity/contribution:
    a. Current job status: _____

    b. Role contributions and responsibility for others: _____

    _____

III. Precipitating Event
Describe the situation or events that precipitated this illness/hospitalization: _____

_____

_____

IV. Client's Perception of the Stressor
Client's or family member's understanding or description of stressor/illness and expectations of hospitalization:

_____

_____

_____

_____

V. Adaptation Responses
  A. *Psychosocial*
  1. Anxiety level (circle level and check the behaviors that apply):   mild   moderate   severe   panic
    calm _____ friendly _____ passive _____ alert _____ perceives environment correctly _____ cooperative _____
    impaired attention _____ "jittery" _____ unable to concentrate _____ hypervigilant _____ tremors _____ rapid
    speech _____ withdrawn _____ confused _____ disoriented _____ fearful _____ hyperventilating _____ misinterpreting
    the environment (hallucinations or delusions) _____ depersonalization _____ obsessions _____ compulsions _____
    somatic complaints _____ excessive hyperactivity _____ other _____

  2. Mood/affect (circle as many as apply):   happiness   sadness   dejection   despair   elation   euphoria
    suspiciousness   apathy (little emotional tone)   anger/hostility

  3. Ego defense mechanisms (describe how used by client):
    Projection _____
    Suppression _____
    Undoing _____

Continued

BOX 9-1 Nursing History and Assessment Tool—cont'd

Displacement _____
Intellectualization _____
Rationalization _____
Denial _____
Repression _____
Isolation _____
Regression _____
Reaction Formation _____
Splitting _____
Religiosity _____
Sublimation _____
Compensation _____

4. Level of self-esteem (circle one):   low   moderate   high
   Things client likes about self _____
   _____
   Things client would like to change about self _____

   Objective assessment of self-esteem:
   Eye contact _____
   General appearance _____
   _____
   Personal hygiene _____
   Participation in group activities and interactions with others _____
   _____

5. Stage and manifestations of grief (circle one):
   denial   anger   bargaining   depression   acceptance
   Describe the client's behaviors that are associated with this stage of grieving in response to loss or change.
   _____
   _____
   _____

6. Thought processes (circle as many as apply): clear logical easy to follow relevant confused blocking delusional
   rapid flow of thoughts slowness in thought association suspicious Recent memory: loss intact Remote
   memory: loss intact
   Other: _____
   _____

7. Communication patterns (circle as many as apply): clear coherent slurred speech incoherent neologisms loose
   associations flight of ideas aphasic perseveration rumination tangential speech loquaciousness slow,
   impoverished speech   speech impediment (describe) _____
   Other _____
   _____

8. Interaction patterns (describe client's pattern of interpersonal interactions with staff and peers on the unit, e.g.,
   manipulative, withdrawn, isolated, verbally or physically hostile, argumentative, passive, assertive, aggressive,
   passive-aggressive, other): _____
   _____
   _____
   _____

9. Reality orientation (check those that apply):
   Oriented to: Time _____   Person _____
                 Place _____   Situation _____

10. Ideas of destruction to self/others?   Yes   No
    If yes, consider plan; available means _____
    _____
    _____
    _____

BOX 9-1 Nursing History and Assessment Tool—cont'd

B. *Physiological*

  1. Psychosomatic manifestations (describe any somatic complaints that may be stress-related): _____
_____
_____
_____

  2. Drug history and assessment:
Use of prescribed drugs:

Name	Dosage	Prescribed For	Results

Use of over-the-counter drugs:

Name	Dosage	Used For	Results

Use of street drugs or alcohol:

Name	Amount Used	How Often Used	When Last Used	Effects Produced

  3. Pertinent physical assessments:
a. Respirations: normal _____ labored _____
Rate _____ Rhythm _____

b. Skin: warm _____ dry _____ moist _____ cool _____ clammy _____ pink_____
cyanotic _____ poor turgor _____ edematous _____
Evidence of: rash _____ bruising _____ needle tracks _____ hirsutism _____
loss of hair _____ other _____
_____

c. Musculoskeletal status: weakness _____ tremors _____
Degree of range of motion (describe limitations) _____
_____
Pain (describe) _____
_____
Skeletal deformities (describe) _____
Coordination (describe limitations) _____

d. Neurological status:
History of (check all that apply): seizures _____ (describe method of control) _____
_____
headaches (describe location and frequency) _____
fainting spells _____ dizziness _____
tingling/numbness (describe location) _____

e. Cardiovascular: B/P _____ Pulse _____
History of (check all that apply):
hypertension _____ palpitations _____
heart murmur _____ chest pain _____
shortness of breath _____ pain in legs _____
phlebitis _____ ankle/leg edema _____
numbness/tingling in extremities _____
varicose veins _____

Continued

BOX 9-1 Nursing History and Assessment Tool—cont'd

f. Gastrointestinal:
  Usual diet pattern: _____
  Food allergies: _____
  Dentures? Upper _____ Lower _____
  Any problems with chewing or swallowing? _____
  Any recent change in weight? _____
  Any problems with:
    Indigestion/heartburn? _____
    Relieved by _____
    Nausea/vomiting? _____
    Relieved by _____
    History of ulcers? _____
    Usual bowel pattern _____
      Constipation? _____ Diarrhea? _____
      Type of self-care assistance provided for either of the above problems _____
      _____

g. Genitourinary/Reproductive:
  Usual voiding pattern _____
  Urinary hesitancy? _____ Frequency? _____
  Nocturia? _____ Pain/burning? _____
  Incontinence? _____
  Any genital lesions? _____
    Discharge? _____ Odor? _____
  History of sexually transmitted disease? _____
    If yes, please explain: _____
    _____
  Any concerns about sexuality/sexual activity? _____
    _____
  Method of birth control used _____
  Females:
    Date of last menstrual cycle _____
    Length of cycle _____
    Problems associated with menstruation? _____
    _____
  Breasts: Pain/tenderness? _____
    Swelling? _____ Discharge? _____
    Lumps? _____ Dimpling? _____
  Practice breast self-examination? _____
    Frequency? _____
  Males:
    Penile discharge? _____
    Prostate problems? _____

h. Eyes:

	Yes	No	Explain
Glasses?	_____	_____	_____
Contacts?	_____	_____	_____
Swelling?	_____	_____	_____
Discharge?	_____	_____	_____
Itching?	_____	_____	_____
Blurring?	_____	_____	_____
Double vision?	_____	_____	_____

i. Ears

	Yes	No	Explain
Pain?	_____	_____	_____
Drainage?	_____	_____	_____
Difficulty hearing?	_____	_____	_____
Hearing aid?	_____	_____	_____
Tinnitus?	_____	_____	_____

j. Medication side effects:
  What symptoms is the client experiencing that may be attributed to current medication usage?
  _____
  _____

BOX 9-1 Nursing History and Assessment Tool—cont'd

    k. Altered lab values and possible significance: _____

_____

_____

    l. Activity/rest patterns:

        Exercise (amount, type, frequency) _____

_____

        Leisure time activities: _____

_____

        Patterns of sleep: Number of hours per night _____

        Use of sleep aids? _____

        Pattern of awakening during the night? _____

_____

        Feel rested upon awakening? _____

    m. Personal hygiene/activities of daily living:

        Patterns of self-care: independent _____

        Requires assistance with: mobility _____

                            hygiene _____

                              toileting _____

                              feeding _____

                              dressing _____

                              other _____

        Statement describing personal hygiene and general appearance _____

_____

_____

    n. Other pertinent physical assessments: _____

_____

_____

  VI. Summary of Initial Psychosocial/Physical Assessment:

    Knowledge Deficits Identified:

    Nursing Diagnoses Indicated:

An example of a simple and quick mental status evaluation is presented in Table 9-1. Its focus is on the cognitive aspects of mental functioning. Areas such as mood, affect, thought content, judgment, and insight are not evaluated. A number of these types of tests are available, but they must be considered only a part of the comprehensive diagnostic assessment. A mental status assessment guide, with explanations and selected sample interview questions, is provided in Appendix B.

CORE CONCEPT

Nursing Diagnosis

Clinical judgments about individual, family, or community responses to actual or potential health problems/life processes. A nursing diagnosis provides the basis for selection of nursing interventions to achieve outcomes for which the nurse is accountable (NANDA International, 2009).

TABLE 9-1 Brief Mental Status Evaluation

AREA OF MENTAL FUNCTION EVALUATED	EVALUATION ACTIVITY
Orientation to time	"What year is it? What month is it? What day is it?" (3 points)
Orientation to place	"Where are you now?" (1 point)
Attention and immediate recall	"Repeat these words now: bell, book, & candle." (3 points) "Remember these words and I will ask you to repeat them in a few minutes."
Abstract thinking	"What does this mean: No use crying over spilled milk." (3 points)
Recent memory	"Say the 3 words I asked you to remember earlier." (3 points)
Naming objects	Point to eyeglasses and ask, "What is this?" Repeat with 1 other item (e.g., calendar, watch, pencil). (2 points possible)
Ability to follow simple verbal command	"Tear this piece of paper in half and put it in the trash container." (2 points)
Ability to follow simple written command	Write a command on a piece of paper (e.g., TOUCH YOUR NOSE), give the paper to the patient and say, "Do what it says on this paper." (1 point for correct action)
Ability to use language correctly	Ask the patient to write a sentence. (3 points if sentence has a subject, a verb, and has valid meaning).
Ability to concentrate	"Say the months of the year in reverse, starting with December." (1 point each for correct answers from November through August. 4 points possible.)
Understanding spatial relationships	"Draw a clock; put in all the numbers; and set the hands on 3 o'clock." (clock circle = 1 point; numbers in correct sequence = 1 point; numbers placed on clock correctly = 1 point; two hands on the clock = 1 point; hands set at correct time = 1 point. (5 points possible)

Scoring: 30–21 = normal; 20–11 = mild cognitive impairment; 10–0 = severe cognitive impairment. (Scores are not absolute and must be considered within the comprehensive diagnostic assessment.)
SOURCES: Merck Manual of Health & Aging (2005); Folstein, Folstein, and McHugh (1975); Kaufman and Zun (1995); Kokman, Smith, Petersen, Tangalos, and Ivnik (1991); and Pfeiffer (1975).

Standard 2: Diagnosis

The Psychiatric-Mental Health Registered Nurse analyzes the assessment data to determine diagnoses or problems, including level of risk.

In the second step, data gathered during the assessment are analyzed. Diagnoses and potential problem statements are formulated and prioritized. Diagnoses conform to accepted classification systems, such as the NANDA International Nursing Diagnosis Classification (see Appendix D); International Classification of Diseases (World Health Organization [WHO], 1993); and *Diagnostic and Statistical Manual of Mental Disorders, Fourth Edition, Text Revision* (DSM-IV-TR) (APA, 2000) (see Appendix C).

CORE CONCEPT

Outcomes
End results that are measurable, desirable, and observable, and translate into observable behaviors (ANA, 2010a).

Standard 3: Outcomes Identification

The Psychiatric-Mental Health Registered Nurse identifies expected outcomes for a plan individualized to the patient or to the situation.

Expected outcomes are derived from the diagnosis. They must be measurable and include a time estimate for attainment. They must be realistic for the client's capabilities, and are most effective when formulated cooperatively by the interdisciplinary team members, the client, and significant others.

Nursing Outcomes Classification (NOC)

The **Nursing Outcomes Classification (NOC)** is a comprehensive, standardized classification of patient/client outcomes developed to evaluate the effects of nursing interventions (Moorhead, Johnson, Maas, & Swanson, 2008). The outcomes have been linked to North American Nursing Diagnosis Association (NANDA) diagnoses and to the **Nursing Interventions Classification (NIC).** NANDA, NIC, and NOC represent all domains of nursing and can be used together or separately (Moorhead & Dochterman, 2012). Each of the 385 NOC outcomes has a label name, a definition, a list of indicators to evaluate client status in relation to the outcome, and a 5-point Likert scale to measure client status (Moorhead et al., 2008).

Standard 4: Planning

The Psychiatric-Mental Health Registered Nurse develops a plan that prescribes strategies and alternatives to attain expected outcomes.

The care plan is individualized to the client's mental health problems, condition, or needs and is developed in collaboration with the client, significant others, and interdisciplinary team members, if possible. For each diagnosis identified, the most appropriate interventions, based on current psychiatric/mental health nursing practice and research, are selected. Client education and necessary referrals are included. Priorities for delivery of nursing care are determined.

Nursing Interventions Classification (NIC)

NIC is a comprehensive, standardized language describing treatments that nurses perform in all settings and in all specialties. NIC includes both physiological and psychosocial interventions, as well as those for illness treatment, illness prevention, and health promotion. NIC interventions are comprehensive, based on research, and reflect current clinical practice. They were developed inductively based on existing practice.

NIC contains 542 interventions each with a definition and a detailed set of activities that describe what a nurse does to implement the intervention (Bulechek, Butcher, & Dochterman, 2008). The use of a standardized language is thought to enhance continuity of care and facilitate communication among nurses and between nurses and other providers.

Standard 5: Implementation

The Psychiatric-Mental Health Registered Nurse implements the identified plan.

Interventions selected during the planning stage are executed, taking into consideration the nurse's level of practice, education, and certification. The care plan serves as a blueprint for delivery of safe, ethical, and appropriate interventions. Documentation of interventions also occurs at this step in the nursing process.

Several specific interventions are included among the standards of psychiatric/mental health clinical nursing practice (ANA, APNA, & ISPN, 2007).

Standard 5A: Coordination of Care

The Psychiatric-Mental Health Registered Nurse coordinates care delivery.

Standard 5B: Health Teaching and Health Promotion

The Psychiatric-Mental Health Registered Nurse employs strategies to promote health and a safe environment.

Standard 5C: Milieu Therapy

The Psychiatric-Mental Health Registered Nurse provides, structures, and maintains a safe and therapeutic environment in collaboration with patients, families, and other healthcare clinicians.

Standard 5D: Pharmacological, Biological, and Integrative Therapies

The Psychiatric-Mental Health Registered Nurse incorporates knowledge of pharmacological, biological, and complementary interventions with applied clinical skills to restore the patient's health and prevent further disability.

Standard 5E: Prescriptive Authority and Treatment

The Psychiatric-Mental Health Advanced Practice Registered Nurse uses prescriptive authority, procedures, referrals, treatments, and therapies in accordance with state and federal laws and regulations.

Standard 5F: Psychotherapy

The Psychiatric-Mental Health Advanced Practice Registered Nurse conducts individual, couples, group, and family psychotherapy using evidence-based psychotherapeutic frameworks and nurse-patient therapeutic relationships.

Standard 5G: Consultation

The Psychiatric-Mental Health Advanced Practice Registered Nurse provides consultation to influence the identified plan, enhance the abilities of other clinicians to provide services for patients, and effect change.

CORE CONCEPT

Evaluation

The process of determining the progress toward attainment of expected outcomes, including the effectiveness of care (ANA, 2010a).

Standard 6: Evaluation

The Psychiatric-Mental Health Registered Nurse evaluates progress toward attainment of expected outcomes.

During the evaluation step, the nurse measures the success of the interventions in meeting the outcome criteria. The client's response to treatment is documented, validating use of the nursing process in the delivery of care. The diagnoses, outcomes, and plan of care are reviewed and revised as need is determined by the evaluation.

Why Nursing Diagnosis?

The concept of nursing diagnosis is not new. For centuries, nurses have identified specific client responses for which nursing interventions were used in an effort to improve quality of life. Historically, however, the autonomy of practice to which nurses were entitled by virtue of their licensure was lacking in the provision of nursing care. Nurses assisted physicians as required, and performed a group of specific tasks that were considered within their scope of responsibility.

The term *diagnosis* in relation to nursing first began to appear in the literature in the early 1950s. The formalized organization of the concept, however, was initiated only in 1973 with the convening of the First Task Force to Name and Classify Nursing Diagnoses. The Task Force of the National Conference Group on the Classification of Nursing Diagnoses was developed during this conference (NANDA International, 2010b). These individuals were charged with the task of identifying and classifying nursing diagnoses.

Also in the 1970s, the ANA began to write standards of practice around the steps of the nursing process, of which nursing diagnosis is an inherent part. This format encompassed both the general and specialty standards outlined by the ANA. The standards of psychiatric/mental health nursing practice are summarized in Box 9-2.

From this progression a statement of policy was published in 1980 and included a definition of nursing. The ANA defined nursing as "the diagnosis and treatment of human responses to actual or potential health problems" (ANA, 2010b). This definition has been expanded to describe more appropriately nursing's commitment to society and to the profession itself. The ANA (2010b) defines nursing as follows:

> Nursing is the protection, promotion, and optimization of health and abilities, prevention of illness and injury, alleviation of suffering through the diagnosis and treatment of human response, and advocacy in the care of individuals, families, communities, and populations. (p. 10)

Nursing diagnosis is an inherent component of both the original and expanded definitions.

Decisions regarding professional negligence are made based on the standards of practice defined by the ANA and the individual state nurse practice acts. A number of states have incorporated the steps of the nursing process, including nursing diagnosis, into the scope of nursing practice described in their nurse practice acts. When this is the case, it is the legal duty of the nurse to show that nursing process and nursing diagnosis were accurately implemented in the delivery of nursing care.

NANDA International (NANDA-I) evolved from the original task force that was convened in 1973 to name and classify nursing diagnoses. The major purpose of NANDA-I is to "to develop, refine and promote terminology that accurately reflects nurses' clinical judgments. NANDA-I will be a global force for the development and use of nursing's standardized terminology to ensure patient safety through evidence-based care, thereby improving the health care of all people" (NANDA-I, 2010a). A list of nursing diagnoses approved by NANDA-I for use and testing is presented in Appendix D. This list is by no means exhaustive or all-inclusive. For purposes of this text, however, the existing list will be used in an effort to maintain a common language within nursing and to encourage clinical testing of what is available.

The use of nursing diagnosis affords a degree of autonomy that historically has been lacking in the practice of nursing. Nursing diagnosis describes

BOX 9-2 Standards of Psychiatric-Mental Health Clinical Nursing Practice

Standard 1. Assessment
The Psychiatric-Mental Health Registered Nurse collects comprehensive health data that is pertinent to the patient's health or situation.

Standard 2. Diagnosis
The Psychiatric-Mental Health Registered Nurse analyzes the assessment data to determine diagnoses or problems, including level of risk.

Standard 3. Outcomes Identification
The Psychiatric-Mental Health Registered Nurse identifies expected outcomes for a plan individualized to the patient or to the situation.

Standard 4. Planning
The Psychiatric-Mental Health Registered Nurse develops a plan that prescribes strategies and alternatives to attain expected outcomes.

Standard 5. Implementation
The Psychiatric-Mental Health Registered Nurse implements the identified plan.

Standard 5A. Coordination of Care
The Psychiatric-Mental Health Registered Nurse coordinates care delivery.

Standard 5B. Health Teaching and Health Promotion
The Psychiatric-Mental Health Registered Nurse employs strategies to promote health and a safe environment.

Standard 5C. Milieu Therapy
The Psychiatric-Mental Health Registered Nurse provides, structures, and maintains a safe and therapeutic environment in collaboration with patients, families, and other healthcare clinicians.

Standard 5D. Pharmacological, Biological, and Integrative Therapies
The Psychiatric-Mental Health Registered Nurse incorporates knowledge of pharmacological, biological, and complementary interventions with applied clinical skills to restore the patient's health and prevent further disability.

Standard 5E. Prescriptive Authority and Treatment
The Psychiatric-Mental Health *Advanced Practice* Registered Nurse uses prescriptive authority, procedures, referrals, treatments, and therapies in accordance with state and federal laws and regulations.

Standard 5F. Psychotherapy
The Psychiatric-Mental Health *Advanced Practice* Registered Nurse conducts individual, couples, group, and family psychotherapy using evidence-based psychotherapeutic frameworks and nurse-patient therapeutic relationships.

Standard 5G. Consultation
The Psychiatric-Mental Health *Advanced Practice* Registered Nurse provides consultation to influence the identified plan, enhance the abilities of other clinicians to provide services for patients, and effect change.

Standard 6. Evaluation
The Psychiatric-Mental Health Registered Nurse evaluates progress toward attainment of expected outcomes.

From ANA, APNA, & ISPN. (2007). *Psychiatric-mental health nursing: Scope and standards of practice.* Silver Spring, MD: American Nurses Association, with permission.

the client's condition, facilitating the prescription of interventions and establishment of parameters for outcome criteria based on what is uniquely nursing. The ultimate benefit is to the client, who receives effective and consistent nursing care based on knowledge of the problems that he or she is experiencing and of the most beneficial nursing interventions to resolve them.

Nursing Case Management

The concept of **case management** evolved with the advent of diagnosis-related groups (DRGs) and shorter hospital stays. Case management is an innovative model of care delivery than can result in improved client care. Within this model, clients are assigned a manager who negotiates with multiple providers to obtain diverse services. This type of health-care delivery process serves to decrease fragmentation of care while striving to contain cost of services.

Case management in the acute care setting strives to organize client care through an episode of illness so that specific clinical and financial outcomes are achieved within an allotted time frame. Commonly, the allotted time frame is determined by the established protocols for length of stay as defined by the DRGs.

Case management has been shown to be an effective method of treatment for individuals with a severe and persistent mental illness. This type of care strives to improve functioning by assisting the individual to solve problems, improve work and socialization skills, promote leisure-time activities, and enhance overall independence.

Ideally, case management incorporates concepts of care at the primary, secondary, and tertiary levels of prevention. Various definitions have emerged and should be clarified, as follows.

Managed care refers to a strategy employed by purchasers of health services who make determinations about various types of services in order to maintain quality and control costs. In a managed care program, individuals receive health care based on need, as assessed by coordinators of the providership. Managed care exists in many settings, including (but not limited to) the following:

■ Insurance-based programs

■ Employer-based medical providerships

■ Social service programs

■ The public health sector

Managed care may exist in virtually any setting in which medical providership is a part of the service, that is, in any setting in which an organization (whether private or government based) is responsible for payment of health-care services for a group of people. Examples of managed care are health maintenance organizations (HMOs) and preferred provider organizations (PPOs).

Case management is the method used to achieve managed care. It is the actual coordination of services required to meet the needs of a client within the fragmented health-care system. Case management strives to help at-risk clients prevent avoidable episodes of illness. Its goal is to provide these services while attempting to control health-care costs to the consumer and third-party payers.

Types of clients who benefit from case management include (but are not limited to) the following:

■ The frail elderly

■ The developmentally disabled

■ The physically handicapped

■ The mentally handicapped

■ Individuals with long-term medically complex problems that require multifaceted, costly care (e.g., high-risk infants, those with human immunodeficiency virus [HIV] or acquired immunodeficiency syndrome [AIDS], and transplant clients)

■ Individuals who are severely compromised by an acute episode of illness or an acute exacerbation of a chronic illness (e.g., schizophrenia)

The **case manager** is responsible for negotiating with multiple health-care providers to obtain a variety of services for the client. Nurses are exceptionally qualified to serve as case managers. The very nature of nursing, which incorporates knowledge about the biological, psychological, and sociocultural aspects related to human functioning, makes nurses highly appropriate as case managers. Several years of experience as a registered nurse is usually required for employment as a case manager. Some case management programs prefer master's-prepared clinical nurse specialists who have experience working with the specific populations for whom the case management service will be rendered. The American Nurses Credentialing Center (ANCC) offers an examination for nurses to become board certified in nursing case management.

Critical Pathways of Care

Critical pathways of care (CPCs) have emerged as the tools for provision of care in a case management system. A critical pathway is a type of abbreviated plan of care that provides outcome-based guidelines for goal achievement within a designated length of stay. A sample CPC is presented in Table 9-2. Only one nursing diagnosis is used in this sample. A CPC may have nursing diagnoses for several individual problems.

CPCs are intended to be used by the entire interdisciplinary team, which may include a nurse case manager, clinical nurse specialist, social worker, psychiatrist, psychologist, dietitian, occupational therapist, recreational therapist, chaplain, and others. The team decides what categories of care are to be performed, by what date, and by whom. Each member of the team is then expected to carry out his or her functions according to the timeline designated on the CPC. The nurse, as case manager, is ultimately responsible for ensuring that each of the assignments is carried out. If variations occur at any time in any of the categories of care, a rationale must be documented in the progress notes.

For example, with the sample CPC presented, the nurse case manager may admit the client into the detoxification center. The nurse contacts the psychiatrist to inform him or her of the admission. The psychiatrist performs additional assessments to determine if other consultations are required. The psychiatrist also writes the orders for the initial diagnostic work-up and medication regimen. Within 24 hours, the interdisciplinary team meets to decide on other categories of care, to complete the CPC, and to make individual care assignments from the CPC. This particular sample CPC relies heavily on nursing care of the client through the critical withdrawal period. However, other problems for the same client, such as imbalanced nutrition, impaired physical mobility, or spiritual distress, may involve other members of the team to a greater degree. Each member of the team stays in contact with the nurse case manager regarding individual assignments. Ideally, team meetings are

TABLE 9-2 Sample Critical Pathway of Care for Client in Alcohol Withdrawal

Estimated Length of Stay: 7 Days—Variations From Designated Pathway Should Be Documented in Progress Notes

NURSING DIAGNOSES AND CATEGORIES OF CARE	TIME DIMENSION	GOALS AND/OR ACTIONS	TIME DIMENSION	GOALS AND/OR ACTIONS	TIME DIMENSION	DISCHARGE OUTCOME
Risk for injury related to CNS agitation					Day 7	Client shows no evidence of injury obtained during ETOH withdrawal
Referrals	Day 1	Psychiatrist Assess need for: Neurologist Cardiologist Internist			Day 7	Discharge with follow-up appointments as required.
Diagnostic studies	Day 1	Blood alcohol level Drug screen (urine and blood) Chemistry Profile Urinalysis Chest X-ray ECG	Day 4	Repeat of selected diagnostic studies as necessary.		
Additional assessments	Day 1 Day 1–5 Ongoing Ongoing	VS q4h I&O Restraints p.r.n. for client safety Assess withdrawal symptoms: tremors, nausea/vomiting, tachycardia, sweating, high blood pressure, seizures, insomnia, hallucinations	Day 2–3 Day 6 Day 4	VS q8h if stable DC I&O Marked decrease in objective withdrawal symptoms	Day 4–7 Day 7	VS bid; remain stable Discharge; absence of objective withdrawal symptoms
Medications	Day 1 Day 2 Day 1–6 Day 1–7	Librium* 200 mg in divided doses Librium 160 mg in divided doses Librium p.r.n. Maalox ac & hs	Day 3 Day 4	Librium 120 mg in divided doses Librium 80 mg in divided doses	Day 5 Day 6 Day 7	Librium 40 mg Discontinue librium Discharge; no withdrawal symptoms
Client education			Day 5	Discuss goals of AA and need for outpatient therapy	Day 7	Discharge with information regarding AA attendance or outpatient treatment

*Note: Some physicians may elect to use Serax or Tegretol in the detoxification process.

held daily or every other day to review progress and modify the plan as required.

CPCs can be standardized, as they are intended to be used with uncomplicated cases. A CPC can be viewed as protocol for various clients with problems for which a designated outcome can be predicted.

Applying the Nursing Process in the Psychiatric Setting

Based on the definition of *mental health* set forth in Chapter 2, the role of the nurse in psychiatry focuses on helping the client successfully adapt to stressors within the environment. Goals are directed toward changes in thoughts, feelings, and behaviors that are age appropriate and congruent with local and cultural norms.

Therapy within the psychiatric setting is very often team, or **interdisciplinary,** oriented. Therefore, it is important to delineate nursing's involvement in the treatment regimen. Nurses are indeed valuable members of the team. Having progressed beyond the role of custodial caregiver in the psychiatric setting, nurses now provide services that are defined within the scope of nursing practice. Nursing diagnosis is helping to define these nursing boundaries, providing the degree of autonomy and professionalism that has for so long been unrealized.

For example, a newly admitted client with the medical diagnosis of schizophrenia may be demonstrating the following behaviors:

■ Inability to trust others

■ Verbalizing hearing voices

■ Refusing to interact with staff and peers

■ Expressing a fear of failure

■ Poor personal hygiene

From these assessments, the treatment team may determine that the client has the following problems:

■ Paranoid delusions

■ Auditory hallucinations

■ Social withdrawal

■ Developmental regression

Team goals would be directed toward the following:

■ Reducing suspiciousness

■ Terminating auditory hallucinations

■ Increasing feelings of self-worth

From this team treatment plan, nursing may identify the following nursing diagnoses:

■ Disturbed sensory perception, auditory (evidenced by hearing voices)

■ Disturbed thought processes (evidenced by delusions)

■ Low self-esteem (evidenced by fear of failure and social withdrawal)

■ Self-care deficit (evidenced by poor personal hygiene)

Nursing diagnoses are prioritized according to life-threatening potential. Maslow's hierarchy of needs is a good model to follow in prioritizing nursing diagnoses. In this instance, disturbed sensory perception (auditory) is identified as the priority nursing diagnosis, because the client may be hearing voices that command him or her to harm self or others. Psychiatric nursing, regardless of the setting—hospital (inpatient or outpatient), office, home, community—is goal-directed care. The goals (or expected outcomes) are client oriented, are measurable, and focus on resolution of the problem (if this is realistic) or on a more short-term outcome (if resolution is unrealistic). For example, in the previous situation, expected outcomes for the identified nursing diagnoses might be as follows:

The client will:

■ Demonstrate trust in one staff member within 3 days.

■ Verbalize understanding that the voices are not real (not heard by others) within 5 days.

■ Complete one simple craft project within 5 days.

■ Take responsibility for own self-care and perform activities of daily living independently by time of discharge.

Nursing's contribution to the interdisciplinary treatment regimen will focus on establishing trust on a one-to-one basis (thus reducing the level of anxiety that is promoting hallucinations), giving positive feedback for small day-to-day accomplishments in an effort to build self-esteem, and assisting with and encouraging independent self-care. These interventions describe *independent nursing* actions and goals that are evaluated apart from, while also being directed toward achievement of, the *team's* treatment goals.

In this manner of collaboration with other team members, nursing provides a service that is unique and based on sound knowledge of psychopathology, scope of practice, and legal implications of the role. Although there is no dispute that "following doctor's orders" continues to be accepted as a priority of care, nursing intervention that enhances achievement of the overall goals of treatment is being recognized for its important contribution. The nurse who administers a medication prescribed by the physician to decrease anxiety may also choose to stay with the anxious client and offer reassurance of safety and security, thereby providing an independent nursing action that is distinct from, yet complementary to, the medical treatment.

Concept Mapping*

Concept mapping is a diagrammatic teaching and learning strategy that allows students and faculty to visualize interrelationships between medical diagnoses, nursing diagnoses, assessment data, and treatments. The concept map care plan is an innovative approach to planning and organizing nursing care. Basically, it is a diagram of client problems and interventions. Compared to the commonly used column-format care plans, concept map care plans are more succinct. They are practical, realistic, and time saving, and they serve to enhance critical thinking skills and clinical reasoning ability.

The nursing process is foundational to developing and using the concept map care plan, just as it is with all types of nursing care plans. Client data are collected and analyzed, nursing diagnoses are formulated, outcome criteria are identified, nursing actions are planned and implemented, and the success of the interventions in meeting the outcome criteria is evaluated.

The concept map care plan may be presented in its entirety on one page, or the assessment data and nursing diagnoses may appear in diagram format on one page, with outcomes, interventions, and evaluation written on a second page. Alternatively, the diagram may appear in circular format, with nursing diagnoses and interventions branching off the "client" in the center of the diagram. Or, it may begin with the "client" at the top of the diagram, with branches emanating in a linear fashion downward.

As stated previously, the concept map care plan is based on the components of the nursing process. Accordingly, the diagram is assembled in the nursing process stepwise fashion, beginning with the client and his or her reason for needing care, nursing diagnoses with subjective and objective clinical evidence for each, nursing interventions, and outcome criteria for evaluation.

Figure 9–2 presents one example of a concept map care plan. It is assembled for the hypothetical client with schizophrenia discussed in the previous section, "Applying the Nursing Process in the Psychiatric Setting." Different colors may be used in the diagram to designate various components of the care plan. Connecting lines are drawn between

components to indicate any relationships that exist. For example, there may be a relationship between two nursing diagnoses (e.g., between the nursing diagnoses of pain or anxiety and disturbed sleep pattern). A line between these nursing diagnoses should be drawn to show the relationship.

Concept map care plans allow for a great deal of creativity on the part of the user, and permit viewing the "whole picture" without generating a great deal of paperwork. Because they reflect the steps of the nursing process, concept map care plans also are valuable guides for documentation of client care. Doenges, Moorhouse, and Murr (2010) stated,

> As students, you are asked to develop plans of care that often contain more detail than what you see in the hospital plans of care. This is to help you learn how to apply the nursing process and create individualized client care plans. However, even though much time and energy may be spent focusing on filling the columns of traditional clinical care plan forms, some students never develop a holistic view of their clients and fail to visualize how each client need interacts with other identified needs. A new technique or learning tool [concept mapping] has been developed to assist you in visualizing the linkages, to enhance your critical thinking skills, and to facilitate the creative process of planning client care. (p. 32)

Documentation of the Nursing Process

Equally important as using the nursing process in the delivery of care is the written documentation that it has been used. Some contemporary nursing leaders are advocating that with solid standards of practice and procedures in place within the institution, nurses need only chart when there has been a deviation in the care as outlined by that standard. This method of documentation, known as charting by exception, is not widely accepted, as many legal decisions are still based on the precept that "if it was not charted, it was not done."

Because nursing process and nursing diagnosis are mandated by nurse practice acts in some states, documentation of their use is being considered in those states as evidence in determining certain cases of negligence by nurses. Some health-care organization accrediting agencies also require that nursing process be reflected in the delivery of care. Therefore, documentation must bear written testimony to the use of the nursing process.

A variety of documentation methods can be used to reflect use of the nursing process in the

---

*Content in this section is adapted from Doenges, Moorhouse, and Murr (2010) and Schuster (2008).

Clinical Vignette: Harry has been admitted to the psychiatric unit with a diagnosis of Paranoid Schizophrenia. He is socially isolated and stays in his room unless strongly encouraged by the nurse to come out. He says to the nurse, "You have to be your own boss. You can't trust anybody." He is refusing to eat any food from his tray, telling the nurse that the voice of his deceased grandfather is telling him it is poisoned. His clothes are dirty, and he has an objectionable body order. The nurse develops the following concept map care plan for Harry.

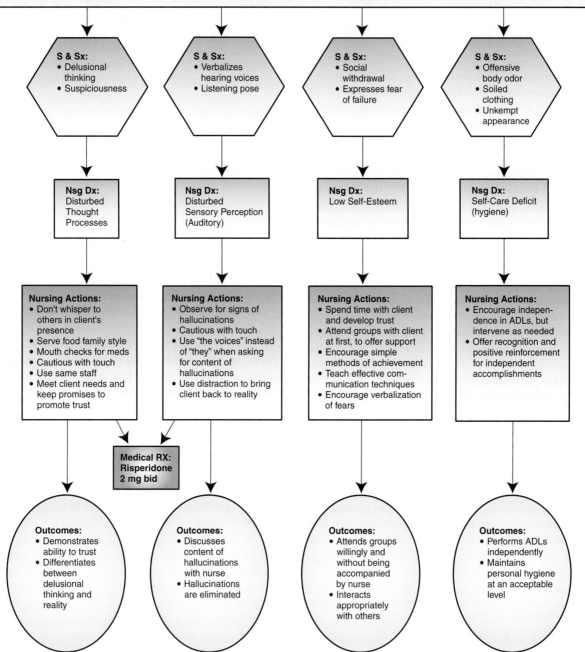

S & Sx:
• Delusional thinking
• Suspiciousness

S & Sx:
• Verbalizes hearing voices
• Listening pose

S & Sx:
• Social withdrawal
• Expresses fear of failure

S & Sx:
• Offensive body odor
• Soiled clothing
• Unkempt appearance

Nsg Dx:
Disturbed Thought Processes

Nsg Dx:
Disturbed Sensory Perception (Auditory)

Nsg Dx:
Low Self-Esteem

Nsg Dx:
Self-Care Deficit (hygiene)

Nursing Actions:
• Don't whisper to others in client's presence
• Serve food family style
• Mouth checks for meds
• Cautious with touch
• Use same staff
• Meet client needs and keep promises to promote trust

Nursing Actions:
• Observe for signs of hallucinations
• Cautious with touch
• Use "the voices" instead of "they" when asking for content of hallucinations
• Use distraction to bring client back to reality

Nursing Actions:
• Spend time with client and develop trust
• Attend groups with client at first, to offer support
• Encourage simple methods of achievement
• Teach effective communication techniques
• Encourage verbalization of fears

Nursing Actions:
• Encourage independence in ADLs, but intervene as needed
• Offer recognition and positive reinforcement for independent accomplishments

Medical RX:
Risperidone 2 mg bid

Outcomes:
• Demonstrates ability to trust
• Differentiates between delusional thinking and reality

Outcomes:
• Discusses content of hallucinations with nurse
• Hallucinations are eliminated

Outcomes:
• Attends groups willingly and without being accompanied by nurse
• Interacts appropriately with others

Outcomes:
• Performs ADLs independently
• Maintains personal hygiene at an acceptable level

FIGURE 9–2 Example: Concept map care plan for client with schizophrenia.

delivery of nursing care. Three examples are presented here: problem-oriented recording (POR); Focus Charting®; and the problem, intervention, evaluation (PIE) system of documentation.

Problem-Oriented Recording

Problem-oriented recording follows the subjective, objective, assessment, plan, implementation, and evaluation (SOAPIE) format. It has as its basis a list of problems. When it is used in nursing, the problems (nursing diagnoses) are identified on a written plan of care, with appropriate nursing interventions described for each. Documentation written in the SOAPIE format includes the following:

S = Subjective data: Information gathered from what the client, family, or other source has said or reported.

O = Objective data: Information gathered by direct observation by the person performing the assessment; may include a physiological measurement such as blood pressure or a behavioral response such as affect.

A = Assessment: The nurse's interpretation of the subjective and objective data.

P = Plan: The actions or treatments to be carried out (may be omitted in daily charting if the plan is clearly explained in the written nursing care plan and no changes are expected).

I = Intervention: Those nursing actions that were actually carried out.

E = Evaluation of the problem following nursing intervention (some nursing interventions cannot be evaluated immediately, so this section may be optional).

Table 9-3 shows how POR corresponds to the steps of the nursing process. Following is an example of a three-column documentation in the POR format.

EXAMPLE

DATE/TIME	PROBLEM	PROGRESS NOTES
9-12-10 1000	Social isolation	**S:** States he does not want to sit with or talk to others; "they frighten me." **O:** Stays in room alone unless strongly encouraged to come out; no group involvement; at times listens to group conversations from a distance but does not interact; some hypervigilance and scanning noted. **A:** Inability to trust; panic level of anxiety; delusional thinking **I:** Initiated trusting relationship by spending time alone with the client; discussed his feelings regarding interactions with others; accompanied client to group activities; provided positive feedback for voluntarily participating in assertiveness training.

TABLE 9-3 Validation of the Nursing Process With Problem-Oriented Recording

PROBLEM-ORIENTED RECORDING	WHAT IS RECORDED	NURSING PROCESS
S and O (Subjective and Objective data)	Verbal reports to, and direct observation and examination by, the nurse	Assessment
A (Assessment)	Nurse's interpretation of S and O	Diagnosis and outcome identification
P (Plan) (Omitted in charting if written plan describes care to be given)	Description of appropriate nursing actions to resolve the identified problem	Planning
I (Intervention)	Description of nursing actions actually carried out	Implementation
E (Evaluation)	A reassessment of the situation to determine results of nursing actions implemented	Evaluation

Focus Charting

Another type of documentation that reflects use of the nursing process is **Focus Charting**®. Focus Charting differs from POR in that the main perspective has been changed from "problem" to "focus," and a data, action, and response (DAR) format has replaced SOAPIE.

Lampe (1985) suggested that a focus for documentation can be any of the following:

1. Nursing diagnosis
2. Current client concern or behavior
3. Significant change in the client status or behavior
4. Significant event in the client's therapy

The focus cannot be a medical diagnosis. The documentation is organized in the format of DAR. These categories are defined as follows:

D = Data: Information that supports the stated focus or describes pertinent observations about the client

A = Action: Immediate or future nursing actions that address the focus, and evaluation of the present care plan along with any changes required

R = Response: Description of client's responses to any part of the medical or nursing care.

Table 9-4 shows how Focus Charting corresponds to the steps of the nursing process. Following is an example of a three-column documentation in the DAR format.

EXAMPLE

DATE/TIME	FOCUS	PROGRESS NOTES
9-12-10 1000	Social isolation related to mistrust, panic anxiety, delusions	**D:** States he does not want to sit with or talk to others; they "frighten" him; stays in room alone unless strongly encouraged to come out; no group involvement; at times listens to group conversations from a distance, but does not interact; some hypervigilance and scanning noted. **A:** Initiated trusting relationship by spending time alone with client; discussed his feelings regarding interactions with others; accompanied client to group activities; provided positive feedback for voluntarily participating in assertiveness training. **R:** Cooperative with therapy; still acts uncomfortable in the presence of a group of people; accepted positive feedback from nurse.

TABLE 9-4 Validation of the Nursing Process With Focus Charting		
FOCUS CHARTING	**WHAT IS RECORDED**	**NURSING PROCESS**
D (Data)	Information that supports the stated focus or describes pertinent observations about the client.	Assessment
Focus	A nursing diagnosis; current client concern or behavior; significant change in client status; significant event in the client's therapy. **NOTE:** If outcome appears on written care plan, it need not be repeated in daily documentation unless a change occurs.	Diagnosis and outcome identification
A (Action)	Immediate or future nursing actions that address the focus; appraisal of the care plan along with any changes required.	Plan and implementation
R (Response)	Description of client responses to any part of the medical or nursing care.	Evaluation

The PIE Method

The PIE method, or more specifically "APIE" (assessment, problem, intervention, evaluation), is a systematic approach of documenting to nursing process and nursing diagnosis. A problem-oriented system, **PIE charting** uses accompanying flow sheets that are individualized by each institution. Criteria for documentation are organized in the following manner:

A = Assessment: A complete client assessment is conducted at the beginning of each shift. Results are documented under this section in the progress notes. Some institutions elect instead to use a daily client assessment sheet designed to meet specific needs of the unit. Explanation of any deviation from the norm is included in the progress notes.

P = Problem: A problem list, or list of nursing diagnoses, is an important part of the APIE method of charting. The name or number of the problem being addressed is documented in this section.

I = Intervention: Nursing actions are performed, directed at resolution of the problem.

E = Evaluation: Outcomes of the implemented interventions are documented, including an evaluation of client responses to determine the effectiveness of nursing interventions and the presence or absence of progress toward resolution of a problem.

Table 9-5 shows how APIE charting corresponds to the steps of the nursing process. Following is an example of a three-column documentation in the APIE format.

EXAMPLE

DATE/TIME	PROBLEM	PROGRESS NOTES
9-12-10 1000	Social Isolation	**A:** States he does not want to sit with or talk to others; they "frighten" him; stays in room alone unless strongly encouraged to come out; no group involvement; at times listens to group conversations from a distance but does not interact; some hypervigilance and scanning noted. **P:** Social isolation related to inability to trust, panic level of anxiety, and delusional thinking. **I:** Initiated trusting relationship by spending time alone with client; discussed his feelings regarding interactions with others; accompanied client to group activities; provided positive feedback for voluntarily participating in assertiveness training. **E:** Cooperative with therapy; still uncomfortable in the presence of a group of people; accepted positive feedback from nurse.

TABLE 9-5 Validation of the Nursing Process With APIE Method

APIE CHARTING	WHAT IS RECORDED	NURSING PROCESS
A (Assessment)	Subjective and objective data about the client that are gathered at the beginning of each shift	Assessment
P (Problem)	Name (or number) of nursing diagnosis being addressed from written problem list, and identified outcome for that problem. **NOTE:** If outcome appears on written care plan, it need not be repeated in daily documentation unless a change occurs.	Diagnosis and outcome identification
I (Intervention)	Nursing actions performed, directed at problem resolution	Plan and implementation
E (Evaluation)	Appraisal of client responses to determine effectiveness of nursing interventions	Evaluation

Electronic Documentation

Most health-care facilities have implemented—or are in the process of implementing—some type of electronic health records (EHRs) or electronic documentation system. EHRs have been shown to improve both the quality of client care and the efficiency of the health-care system (Hopper & Ames, 2004). In 2003, the U.S. Department of Health and Human Services commissioned the Institute of Medicine (IOM) to study the capabilities of an EHR system. The IOM identified a set of eight core functions that EHR systems should perform in the delivery of safer, higher quality, and more efficient health care. These eight core capabilities include the following (Tang, 2003):

■ **Health Information and Data.** EHRs would provide more rapid access to important patient information (e.g., allergies, laboratory test results, a medication list, demographic information, and clinical narratives), thereby improving care providers' ability to make sound clinical decisions in a timely manner.

■ **Results Management.** Computerized results of all types (e.g., laboratory test results, radiology procedure result reports) can be accessed more easily by the provider at the time and place they are needed.

■ **Order Entry/Order Management.** Computer-based order entries improve workflow processes by eliminating lost orders and ambiguities caused by illegible handwriting, generating related orders automatically, monitoring for duplicate orders, and improving the speed with which orders are executed.

■ **Decision Support.** Computerized decision support systems enhance clinical performance for many aspects of health care. Using reminders and prompts, improvement in regular screenings and other preventive practices can be accomplished. Other aspects of health-care support include identifying possible drug interactions and facilitating diagnosis and treatment.

■ **Electronic Communication and Connectivity.** Improved communication among care associates, such as medicine, nursing, laboratory, pharmacy, and radiology, can enhance client safety and quality of care. Efficient communication among providers improves continuity of care, allows for more timely interventions, and reduces the risk of adverse events.

■ **Patient Support.** Computer-based interactive client education, self-testing, and self-monitoring have been shown to improve control of chronic illnesses.

■ **Administrative Processes.** Electronic scheduling systems (e.g., for hospital admissions and outpatient procedures) increase the efficiency of health-care organizations and provide more timely service to patients.

■ **Reporting and Population Health Management.** Health-care organizations are required to report health-care data to government and private sectors for patient safety and public health. Uniform electronic data standards facilitate this process at the provider level, reduce the associated costs, and increase the speed and accuracy of the data reported.

Table 9-6 lists some of the advantages and disadvantages of paper records and EHRs.

TABLE 9-6 Advantages and Disadvantages of Paper Records and EHRs	
PAPER*	**EHR**
Advantages	Advantages
■ People know how to use it.	■ Can be accessed by multiple providers from remote sites.
■ It is fast for current practice.	■ Facilitates communication between disciplines.
■ It is portable.	■ Provides reminders about completing information.
■ It is nonbreakable.	■ Provides warnings about incompatibilities of medications or variances from normal standards.
■ It accepts multiple data types, such as graphs, photographs, drawings, and text.	■ Reduces redundancy of information.
■ Legal issues and costs are understood.	■ Requires less storage space and more difficult to lose.
Disadvantages	■ Easier to research for audits, quality assurance, and epidemiological surveillance.
■ It can be lost.	
■ It is often illegible and incomplete.	

TABLE 9-6 Advantages and Disadvantages of Paper Records and EHRs—cont'd	
PAPER*	**EHR**
■ It has no remote access. ■ It can be accessed by only one person at a time. ■ It is often disorganized. ■ Information is duplicated. ■ It is hard to store. ■ It is difficult to research, and continuous quality improvement is laborious. ■ Same client has separate records at each facility (physician's office, hospital, home care). ■ Records are shared only through hard copy.	■ Provides immediate retrieval of information (e.g., test results). ■ Provides links to multiple databases of health-care knowledge, thus providing diagnostic support. ■ Decreases charting time. ■ Reduces errors due to illegible handwriting. ■ Facilitates billing and claims procedures. **Disadvantages** ■ Excessive expense to initiate the system. ■ Substantial learning curve involved for new users; training and retraining required. ■ Stringent requirements to maintain security and confidentiality. ■ Technical difficulties are possible. ■ Legal and ethical issues involving privacy and access to client information. ■ Requires consistent use of standardized terminology to support information sharing across wide networks.

From Young, K. M. (2009). Nursing informatics. In J. T. Catalano (Ed.), Nursing now! Today's issues, tomorrow's trends (5th ed., pp. 357–377). Philadelphia: F.A. Davis, with permission.

Summary and Key Points

■ The nursing process provides a methodology by which nurses may deliver care using a systematic, scientific approach.

■ The focus of the nursing process is goal directed and based on a decision-making or problem-solving model, consisting of six steps: assessment, diagnosis, outcome identification, planning, implementation, and evaluation.

■ Assessment is a systematic, dynamic process by which the nurse, through interaction with the client, significant others, and health-care providers, collects and analyzes data about the client.

■ Nursing diagnoses are clinical judgments about individual, family, or community responses to actual or potential health problems/life processes.

■ Outcomes are measurable, expected, patient-focused goals that translate into observable behaviors.

■ Evaluation is the process of determining both the client's progress toward the attainment of expected outcomes and the effectiveness of nursing care.

■ The psychiatric nurse uses the nursing process to assist clients to adapt successfully to stressors within the environment.

■ The nurse serves as a valuable member of the interdisciplinary treatment team, working both independently and cooperatively with other team members.

■ Case management is an innovative model of care delivery that serves to provide quality client care while controlling health-care costs. Critical pathways of care (CPCs) serve as the tools for provision of care in a case management system.

■ Nurses may serve as case managers, who are responsible for negotiating with multiple health-care providers to obtain a variety of services for the client.

■ Concept mapping is a diagrammatic teaching and learning strategy that allows students and faculty to visualize interrelationships between medical diagnoses, nursing diagnoses, assessment data, and treatments. The concept map care plan is an innovative approach to planning and organizing nursing care.

■ Nurses must document that the nursing process has been used in the delivery of care. Three methods of documentation that reflect use of the nursing process include POR, Focus Charting, and the PIE method.

■ Many health-care facilities have implemented the use of electronic health records (EHRs) or electronic documentation systems. EHRs have been shown to improve both the quality of

client care and the efficiency of the health-care system.

Additional info available @
davisplus.fadavis.com

Review Questions
Self-Examination/Learning Exercise

*Select the answer that is **most** appropriate for each of the following questions:*

1. The nurse is using the nursing process to care for a suicidal client. Which of the following nursing actions is a part of the assessment step of the nursing process?
   a. Identifies nursing diagnosis: Risk for suicide.
   b. Notes client's family reports recent suicide attempt.
   c. Prioritizes the necessity for maintaining a safe environment for the client.
   d. Obtains a short-term contract from the client to seek out staff if feeling suicidal.

2. The nurse is using the nursing process to care for a suicidal client. Which of the following nursing actions is a part of the diagnosis step of the nursing process?
   a. Identifies nursing diagnosis: Risk for suicide.
   b. Notes client's family reports recent suicide attempt.
   c. Prioritizes the necessity for maintaining a safe environment for the client.
   d. Obtains a short-term contract from the client to seek out staff if feeling suicidal.

3. The nurse is using the nursing process to care for a suicidal client. Which of the following nursing actions is a part of the outcome identification step of the nursing process?
   a. Prioritizes the necessity for maintaining a safe environment for the client.
   b. Determines if nursing interventions have been appropriate to achieve desired results.
   c. Obtains a short-term contract from the client to seek out staff if feeling suicidal.
   d. Establishes goal of care: Client will not harm self during hospitalization.

4. The nurse is using the nursing process to care for a suicidal client. Which of the following nursing actions is a part of the planning step of the nursing process?
   a. Prioritizes the necessity for maintaining a safe environment for the client.
   b. Determines if nursing interventions have been appropriate to achieve desired results.
   c. Obtains a short-term contract from the client to seek out staff if feeling suicidal.
   d. Establishes goal of care: Client will not harm self during hospitalization.

5. The nurse is using the nursing process to care for a suicidal client. Which of the following nursing actions is a part of the implementation step of the nursing process?
   a. Prioritizes the necessity for maintaining a safe environment for the client.
   b. Determines if nursing interventions have been appropriate to achieve desired results.
   c. Obtains a short-term contract from the client to seek out staff if feeling suicidal.
   d. Establishes goal of care: Client will not harm self during hospitalization.

Review Questions—cont'd
Self-Examination/Learning Exercise

6. The nurse is using the nursing process to care for a suicidal client. Which of the following nursing actions is a part of the evaluation step of the nursing process?
   a. Prioritizes the necessity for maintaining a safe environment for the client.
   b. Determines if nursing interventions have been appropriate to achieve desired results.
   c. Obtains a short-term contract from the client to seek out staff if feeling suicidal.
   d. Establishes goal of care: Client will not harm self during hospitalization.

7. S.T. is a 15-year-old girl who has just been admitted to the adolescent psychiatric unit with a diagnosis of anorexia nervosa. She is 5′5″ tall and weighs 82 lb. She was elected to the cheer-leading squad for the fall but states that she is not as good as the others on the squad. The treatment team has identified the following problems: refusal to eat, occasional purging, refusing to interact with staff and peers, and fear of failure. Which of the following nursing diagnoses would be appropriate for S.T.? (Select all that apply.)
   a. Social Isolation.
   b. Disturbed Body Image.
   c. Low Self-Esteem.
   d. Imbalanced Nutrition: Less than body requirements.

8. S.T. is a 15-year-old girl who has just been admitted to the adolescent psychiatric unit with a diagnosis of anorexia nervosa. She is 5′5″ tall and weighs 82 lb. She was elected to the cheer-leading squad for the fall but states that she is not as good as the others on the squad. The treatment team has identified the following problems: refusal to eat, occasional purging, refusing to interact with staff and peers, and fear of failure. Which of the following nursing diagnoses would be the priority diagnosis for S.T.?
   a. Social Isolation.
   b. Disturbed Body Image.
   c. Low Self-Esteem.
   d. Imbalanced Nutrition: Less than body requirements.

9. Nursing diagnoses are prioritized according to:
   a. Degree of potential for resolution.
   b. Legal implications associated with nursing intervention.
   c. Life-threatening potential.
   d. Client and family requests.

10. Which of the following describe advantages to electronic health records (EHRs)? (Select all that apply.)
    a. They reduce redundancy of information.
    b. They reduce issues regarding privacy.
    c. They decrease charting time.
    d. They facilitate communication between disciplines.

References

American Nurses Association. (2010a). *Nursing: Scope and standards of practice* (2nd ed.). Silver Spring, MD: Author.

American Nurses Association. (2010b). *Nursing's social policy statement: The essence of the profession.* Silver Spring, MD: Author.

American Nurses Association, American Psychiatric Nurses Association, & International Society of Psychiatric-Mental Health Nurses. (2007). *Psychiatric-mental health nursing: Scope and standards of practice.* Silver Spring, MD: American Nurses Association.

American Psychiatric Association. (2000). *Diagnosis and statistical manual of mental disorders* (4th ed.). *Text revision.* Washington, DC: American Psychiatric Publishing.

Bulechek, G. M., Butcher, H. K., & Dochterman, J. M. (2008). *Nursing interventions classification (NIC)* (5th ed.). St. Louis: Mosby Elsevier.

Doenges, M. E., Moorhouse, M. F. & Murr, A. C. (2010). *Nursing diagnosis manual: Planning, individualizing, and documenting client care* (3rd ed.). Philadelphia: F.A. Davis.

Folstein, M. F., Folstein, S. E., & McHugh, P. R. (1975). Mini-mental state: A practical method for grading the cognitive state of patients for the clinician. *Journal of Psychiatric Research, 12,* 189–198.

Hopper, K., & Ames, K. J. (2004). *Health policy analysis: Standardized EMRs.* Durham, NC: Duke University.

Kaufman, D. M., & Zun, L. (1995). A quantifiable, brief mental status examination for emergency patients. *Journal of Emergency Medicine, 13,* 440–456.

Kokman, E., Smith, G. E., Petersen, R. C., Tangalos, E., & Ivnik, R. C. (1991). The short test of mental status: Correlations with standardized psychometric testing. *Archives of Neurology, 48,* 725–728.

Lampe, S. S. (1985). Focus charting: Streamlining documentation. *Nursing Management, 16*(7), 43–46.

Merck Manual of Health & Aging. (2005). New York: Random House.

Moorhead, S., & Dochterman, J. M. (2012). Languages and development of the linkages. In M. Johnson, S. Moorhead, G. Bulechek, M. Butcher, M. Maas & E. Swanson, *NOC and NIC linkages to NANDA-I and clinical conditions: Supporting critical reasoning and quality care* (3rd ed., pp. 1–10). Maryland Heights, MO: Mosby.

Moorhead, S., Johnson, M., Maas, M., & Swanson, E. (2008). *Nursing outcomes classification (NOC)* (4th ed.). St. Louis: Mosby Elsevier.

NANDA International. (2009). *Nursing diagnoses: Definitions and classification, 2009–2011.* Hoboken, NJ: Wiley-Blackwell.

NANDA International. (2010a). *About NANDA International.* Retrieved September 10, 2010, from http://www.nanda.org/AboutUs.aspx

NANDA International. (2010b). *NANDA-I history: 1973–1979.* Retrieved September 10, 2010, from http://www.nanda.org/AboutUs/History/1973to1979.aspx

Pfeiffer, E. (1975). A short portable mental status questionnaire for the assessment of organic brain deficit in elderly patients. *Journal of the American Geriatric Society, 23,* 433–441.

Schuster, P. M. (2008). *Concept mapping: A critical-thinking approach to care planning* (2nd ed.). Philadelphia: F.A. Davis.

Tang, P. (2003). *Key capabilities of an electronic health record system.* Institute of Medicine Committee on Data Standards for Patient Safety. Board on Health Care Services. Washington, DC: National Academies Press.

World Health Organization. (1993). *International classification of diseases* (10th ed.). Geneva: Author.

Young, K. M. (2009). Nursing informatics. In J. T. Catalano (Ed.), *Nursing now! Today's issues, tomorrow's trends* (5th ed., pp. 357–377). Philadelphia: F.A. Davis.

Therapeutic Groups

CORE CONCEPTS

group
group therapy

KEY TERMS

altruism
autocratic
catharsis

democratic
laissez-faire

psychodrama
universality

OBJECTIVES

After reading this chapter, the student will be able to:

1. Define a *group.*
2. Discuss eight functions of a group.
3. Identify various types of groups.
4. Describe physical conditions that influence groups.
5. Discuss "curative factors" that occur in groups.
6. Describe the phases of group development.
7. Identify various leadership styles in groups.
8. Identify various roles that members assume within a group.
9. Discuss psychodrama as a specialized form of group therapy.
10. Describe the role of the nurse in group therapy.

HOMEWORK ASSIGNMENT

Please read the chapter and answer the following questions:

1. What is the difference between therapeutic groups and group therapy?
2. What are the expectations of the leader in the initial or orientation phase of group development?
3. How does an autocratic leadership style affect member enthusiasm and morale?
4. How does size of the group influence group dynamics?

Human beings are complex creatures who share their activities of daily living with various *groups* of people. Sampson and Marthas (1990) have stated:

> We are *biological* organisms possessing qualities shared with all living systems and with others of our species. We are *psychological* beings with distinctly human capabilities for

thought, feeling, and action. We are also *social* beings, who function as part of the complex webs that link us with other people. (p. 3.)

Health-care professionals not only share their personal lives with groups of people but also encounter multiple group situations in their professional operations. Team conferences, committee meetings, grand rounds, and in-service sessions are but a few. In psychiatry, work with clients and families often takes the form of groups. With group work, not only does the nurse have the opportunity to reach out to a greater number of people at one time, but those individuals also assist each other by bringing to the group and sharing their feelings, opinions, ideas, and behaviors. Clients learn from each other in a group setting.

This chapter explores various types and methods of therapeutic groups that can be used with psychiatric clients, and the role of the nurse in group intervention.

CORE CONCEPT

Group

A *group* is a collection of individuals whose association is founded on shared commonalities of interest, values, norms, or purpose. Membership in a group is generally by chance (born into the group), by choice (voluntary affiliation), or by circumstance (the result of life-cycle events over which an individual may or may not have control).

Functions of a Group

Sampson and Marthas (1990) outlined eight functions that groups serve for their members. They contend that groups may serve more than one function and usually serve different functions for different members of the group. The eight functions are as follows:

1. **Socialization.** The cultural group into which we are born begins the process of teaching social norms. This is continued throughout our lives by members of other groups with which we become affiliated.

2. **Support.** One's fellow group members are available in time of need. Individuals derive a feeling of security from group involvement.

3. **Task completion.** Group members provide assistance in endeavors that are beyond the capacity of one individual alone or when results can be achieved more effectively as a team.

4. **Camaraderie.** Members of a group provide the joy and pleasure that individuals seek from interactions with significant others.

5. **Informational.** Learning takes place within groups. Knowledge is gained when individual members learn how others in the group have resolved situations similar to those with which they are currently struggling.

6. **Normative.** This function relates to the ways in which groups enforce the established norms.

7. **Empowerment.** Groups help to bring about improvement in existing conditions by providing support to individual members who seek to bring about change. Groups have power that individuals alone do not.

8. **Governance.** An example of the governing function is that of rules being made by committees within a larger organization.

Types of Groups

The functions of a group vary depending on the reason the group was formed. Clark (2003) identified three types of groups in which nurses most often participate: task, teaching, and supportive/therapeutic groups.

Task Groups

The function of a task group is to accomplish a specific outcome or task. The focus is on solving problems and making decisions to achieve this outcome. Often a deadline is placed on completion of the task, and such importance is placed on a satisfactory outcome that conflict in the group may be smoothed over or ignored in order to focus on the priority at hand.

Teaching Groups

Teaching, or educational, groups exist to convey knowledge and information to a number of individuals. Nurses can be involved in teaching groups of many varieties, such as medication education, childbirth education, breast self-examination, and effective parenting classes. These groups usually have a set time frame or a set number of meetings. Members learn from each other as well as from the designated instructor. The objective of teaching groups is verbalization or demonstration by the learner of the material presented by the end of the designated period.

Supportive/Therapeutic Groups

The primary concern of support groups is to prevent future upsets by teaching participants effective ways of dealing with emotional stress arising from situational or developmental crises.

CORE CONCEPT

Group Therapy

A form of psychosocial treatment in which a number of clients meet together with a therapist for purposes of sharing, gaining personal insight, and improving interpersonal coping strategies.

For the purposes of this text, it is important to differentiate between *therapeutic groups* and *group therapy.* Leaders of group therapy generally have advanced degrees in psychology, social work, nursing, or medicine. They often have additional training or experience under the supervision of an accomplished professional in conducting group psychotherapy based on various theoretical frameworks such as psychoanalytic, psychodynamic, interpersonal, or family dynamics. Approaches based on these theories are used by the group therapy leaders to encourage improvement in the ability of group members to function on an interpersonal level.

Therapeutic groups, on the other hand, are based to a lesser degree in theory. Focus is more on group relations, interactions among group members, and the consideration of a selected issue. Like group therapists, individuals who lead therapeutic groups must be knowledgeable in *group process,* that is, the *way* in which group members interact with each other. Interruptions, silences, judgments, glares, and scapegoating are examples of group processes (Clark, 2003). They must also have a thorough knowledge of *group content,* the topic or issue being discussed within the group, and the ability to present the topic in language that can be understood by all group members. Many nurses who work in psychiatry lead supportive/therapeutic groups.

Self-Help Groups

An additional type of group, in which nurses may or may not be involved, is the self-help group. Self-help groups have grown in numbers and in credibility in recent years. They allow clients to talk about their fears and relieve feelings of isolation, while receiving comfort and advice from others undergoing similar experiences. Examples of self-help groups are Alzheimer's Disease and Related Disorders, Anorexia Nervosa and Associated Disorders, Weight Watchers, Alcoholics Anonymous, Reach to Recovery, Parents Without Partners, Overeaters Anonymous, Adult Children of Alcoholics, and many others related to specific needs or illnesses. These groups may or may not have a professional leader or consultant. They are run by the members, and leadership often rotates from member to member.

Nurses may become involved with self-help groups either voluntarily or because their advice or participation has been requested by the members. The nurse may function as a referral agent, resource person, member of an advisory board, or leader of the group. Self-help groups are a valuable source of referral for clients with specific problems. However, nurses must be knowledgeable about the purposes of the group, membership, leadership, benefits, and problems that might threaten the success of the group before making referrals to their clients for a specific self-help group. The nurse may find it necessary to attend several meetings of a particular group, if possible, to assess its effectiveness of purpose and appropriateness for client referral.

Physical Conditions That Influence Group Dynamics

Seating

The physical conditions for the group should be set up so that there is no barrier between the members. For example, a circle of chairs is better than chairs set around a table. Members should be encouraged to sit in different chairs each meeting. This openness and change creates an uncomfortableness that encourages anxious and unsettled behaviors that can then be explored within the group.

Size

Various authors have suggested different ranges of size as ideal for group interaction: 5 to 10 (Yalom & Leszcz, 2005), 2 to 15 (Sampson & Marthas, 1990), and 4 to 12 (Clark, 2003). Group size does make a difference in the interaction among members. The larger the group, the less time is available to devote to individual members. In fact, in larger groups, those more aggressive individuals are most likely to be heard, whereas quieter members may be left out of the discussions altogether. On the other hand, larger groups provide more opportunities for individuals to learn from other members. The wider range of life experiences and knowledge provides a greater potential for effective group problem solving. Studies have indicated that a composition of 7 or 8 members provides a favorable climate for optimal group interaction and relationship development.

Membership

Whether the group is open or closed ended is another condition that influences the dynamics of group process. Open-ended groups are those in which members leave and others join at any time while the group is active. The continuous movement of members in and out of the group creates the type of discomfort described previously that encourages unsettled behaviors in individual members and fosters the exploration of feelings. These are the most common types of groups held on short-term inpatient units, although they are used in outpatient and long-term care facilities as well. Closed-ended groups usually have a predetermined, fixed time frame. All members join at the time the group is organized and terminate at the end of the designated time period. Closed-ended groups are often composed of individuals with common issues or problems they wish to address.

Curative Factors

Why are therapeutic groups helpful? Yalom and Leszcz (2005) described 11 curative factors that individuals can achieve through interpersonal interactions within the group, some of which are present in most groups in varying degrees.

1. **The Instillation of Hope.** By observing the progress of others in the group with similar problems, a group member garners hope that his or her problems can also be resolved.

2. **Universality.** Through **universality,** individuals come to realize that they are not alone in the problems, thoughts, and feelings they are experiencing. Anxiety is relieved by the support and understanding of others in the group who share similar (universal) experiences.

3. **The Imparting of Information.** Knowledge is gained through formal instruction as well as the sharing of advice and suggestions among group members.

4. **Altruism. Altruism** is assimilated by group members through mutual sharing and concern for each other. Providing assistance and support to others creates a positive self-image and promotes self-growth.

5. **The Corrective Recapitulation of the Primary Family Group.** Group members are able to re-experience early family conflicts that remain unresolved. Attempts at resolution are promoted through feedback and exploration.

6. **The Development of Socializing Techniques.** Through interaction with and feedback from other members within the group, individuals are able to correct maladaptive social behaviors and learn and develop new social skills.

7. **Imitative Behavior.** In this setting, one who has mastered a particular psychosocial skill or developmental task can be a valuable role model for others. Individuals may imitate selected behaviors that they wish to develop in themselves.

8. **Interpersonal Learning.** The group offers many and varied opportunities for interacting with other people. Insight is gained regarding how one perceives and is being perceived by others.

9. **Group Cohesiveness.** Members develop a sense of belonging that separates the individual ("I am") from the group ("we are"). Out of this alliance emerges a common feeling that both individual members and the total group are of value to each other.

10. **Catharsis.** Within the group, members are able to express both positive and negative feelings—perhaps feelings that have never been expressed before—in a nonthreatening atmosphere. This **catharsis,** or open expression of feelings, is beneficial for the individual within the group.

11. **Existential Factors.** The group is able to help individual members take direction of their own lives and to accept responsibility for the quality of their existence.

It may be helpful for a group leader to explain these curative factors to members of the group. Positive responses are experienced by individuals who understand and are able to recognize curative factors as they occur within the group.

Phases of Group Development

Groups, like individuals, move through phases of life-cycle development. Ideally, groups will progress from the phase of infancy to advanced maturity in an effort to fulfill the objectives set forth by the membership. Unfortunately, as with individuals, some groups become fixed in early developmental levels and never progress, or experience periods of regression in the developmental process. Three phases of group development are discussed here.

Phase I: Initial or Orientation Phase

Group Activities

Leader and members work together to establish the rules that will govern the group (e.g., when and where meetings will occur, the importance of confidentiality, how meetings will be structured). Goals of the group are established. Members are introduced to each other.

Leader Expectations

The leader is expected to orient members to specific group processes, encourage members to participate without disclosing too much too soon, promote an environment of trust, and ensure that rules established by the group do not interfere with fulfillment of the goals.

Member Behaviors

In phase I, members have not yet established trust and will respond to this lack of trust by being overly polite. There is a fear of not being accepted by the group. They may try to "get on the good side" of the leader with compliments and conforming behaviors. A power struggle may ensue as members compete for their position in the "pecking order" of the group.

Phase II: Middle or Working Phase

Group Activities

Ideally, during the working phase, cohesiveness has been established within the group. This is when the productive work toward completion of the task is undertaken. Problem solving and decision making occur within the group. In the mature group, cooperation prevails, and differences and disagreements are confronted and resolved.

Leader Expectations

The role of leader diminishes and becomes more one of facilitator during the working phase. Some leadership functions are shared by certain members of the group as they progress toward resolution. The leader helps to resolve conflict and continues to foster cohesiveness among the members while ensuring that they do not deviate from the intended task or purpose for which the group was organized.

Member Behaviors

At this point trust has been established among the members. They turn more often to each other and less often to the leader for guidance. They accept criticism from each other, using it in a constructive manner to create change. Occasionally, subgroups will form in which two or more members conspire with each other to the exclusion of the rest of the group. To maintain group cohesion, these subgroups must be confronted and discussed by the entire membership. Conflict is managed by the group with minimal assistance from the leader.

Phase III: Final or Termination Phase

Group Activities

The longer a group has been in existence, the more difficult termination is likely to be for the members. Termination should be mentioned from the outset of group formation. It should be discussed in depth for several meetings prior to the final session. A sense of loss that precipitates the grief process may be in evidence, particularly in groups that have been successful in their stated purpose.

Leader Expectations

In the termination phase, the leader encourages the group members to reminisce about what has occurred within the group, to review the goals and discuss the actual outcomes, and to encourage members to provide feedback to each other about individual progress within the group. The leader encourages members to discuss feelings of loss associated with termination of the group.

Member Behaviors

Members may express surprise over the actual materialization of the end. This represents the grief response of denial, which may then progress to anger. Anger toward other group members or toward the leader may reflect feelings of abandonment (Sampson & Marthas, 1990). These feelings may lead to individual members' discussions of previous losses for which similar emotions were experienced. Successful termination of the group may help members develop the skills needed when losses occur in other dimensions of their lives.

Leadership Styles

Lippitt and White (1958) identified three of the most common group leadership styles: autocratic, democratic, and laissez-faire. Table 10-1 shows an outline of various similarities and differences among the three leadership styles.

Autocratic

Autocratic leaders have personal goals for the group. They withhold information from group members, particularly issues that may interfere with

TABLE 10-1 Leadership Styles—Similarities and Differences

CHARACTERISTICS	AUTOCRATIC	DEMOCRATIC	LAISSEZ-FAIRE
1. Focus	Leader	Members	Undetermined
2. Task strategy	Members are persuaded to adopt leader ideas	Members engage in group problem solving	No defined strategy exists
3. Member participation	Limited	Unlimited	Inconsistent
4. Individual creativity	Stifled	Encouraged	Not addressed
5. Member enthusiasm and morale	Low	High	Low
6. Group cohesiveness	Low	High	Low
7. Productivity	High	High (may not be as high as autocratic)	Low
8. Individual motivation and commitment	Low (tend to work only when leader is present to urge them to do so)	High (satisfaction derived from personal input and participation)	Low (feelings of frustration from lack of direction or guidance)

achievement of their own objectives. The message that is conveyed to the group is: "We will do it my way. My way is best." The focus in this style of leadership is on the leader. Members are dependent on the leader for problem solving, decision making, and permission to perform. The approach of the autocratic leader is one of persuasion, striving to persuade others in the group that his or her ideas and methods are superior. Productivity is high with this type of leadership, but often morale within the group is low because of lack of member input and creativity.

Democratic

The **democratic** leadership style focuses on the members of the group. Information is shared with members in an effort to allow them to make decisions regarding achieving the goals for the group. Members are encouraged to participate fully in problem solving of issues that relate to the group, including taking action to effect change. The message that is conveyed to the group is: "Decide what must be done, consider the alternatives, make a selection, and proceed with the actions required to complete the task." The leader provides guidance and expertise as needed. Productivity is lower than it is with autocratic leadership, but morale is much higher because of the extent of input allowed all members of the group and the potential for individual creativity.

Laissez-Faire

This leadership style allows people to do as they please. There is no direction from the leader. In fact, the **laissez-faire** leader's approach is noninvolvement. Goals for the group are undefined. No decisions are made, no problems are solved, and no action is taken. Members become frustrated and confused, and productivity and morale are low.

Member Roles

Benne and Sheats (1948) identified three major types of roles that individuals play within the membership of the group. These are roles that serve to:

1. Complete the task of the group.
2. Maintain or enhance group processes.
3. Fulfill personal or individual needs.

Task roles and maintenance roles contribute to the success or effectiveness of the group. Personal roles satisfy needs of the individual members, sometimes to the extent of interfering with the effectiveness of the group.

Table 10-2 presents an outline of specific roles within these three major types and the behaviors associated with each.

Psychodrama

A specialized type of therapeutic group, called **psychodrama,** was introduced by J. L. Moreno, a Viennese psychiatrist. Moreno's method employs a dramatic approach in which clients become "actors" in life-situation scenarios.

TABLE 10-2 Member Roles Within Groups

ROLE	BEHAVIORS
Task Roles	
Coordinator	Clarifies ideas and suggestions that have been made within the group; brings relationships together to pursue common goals
Evaluator	Examines group plans and performance, measuring against group standards and goals
Elaborator	Explains and expands upon group plans and ideas
Energizer	Encourages and motivates group to perform at its maximum potential
Initiator	Outlines the task at hand for the group and proposes methods for solution
Orienter	Maintains direction within the group
Maintenance Roles	
Compromiser	Relieves conflict within the group by assisting members to reach a compromise agreeable to all
Encourager	Offers recognition and acceptance of others' ideas and contributions
Follower	Listens attentively to group interaction; is passive participant
Gatekeeper	Encourages acceptance of and participation by all members of the group
Harmonizer	Minimizes tension within the group by intervening when disagreements produce conflict
Individual (Personal) Roles	
Aggressor	Expresses negativism and hostility toward other members; may use sarcasm in effort to degrade the status of others
Blocker	Resists group efforts; demonstrates rigid and sometimes irrational behaviors that impede group progress
Dominator	Manipulates others to gain control; behaves in authoritarian manner
Help-seeker	Uses the group to gain sympathy from others; seeks to increase self-confidence from group feedback; lacks concern for others or for the group as a whole
Monopolizer	Maintains control of the group by dominating the conversation
Mute or silent member	Does not participate verbally; remains silent for a variety of reasons—may feel uncomfortable with self-disclosure or may be seeking attention through silence
Recognition seeker	Talks about personal accomplishments in an effort to gain attention for self
Seducer	Shares intimate details about self with group; is the least reluctant of the group to do so; may frighten others in the group and inhibit group progress with excessive premature self-disclosure

Adapted from Benne, K. B., & and Sheats, P. (1948, Spring). Functional roles of group members. Journal of Social Issues, 4(2), 42–49.

The group leader is called the *director,* group members are the *audience,* and the *set,* or *stage,* may be specially designed or may just be any room or part of a room selected for this purpose. Actors are members from the audience who agree to take part in the "drama" by role-playing a situation about which they have been informed by the director. Usually the situation is an issue with which one individual client has been struggling. The client plays the role of himself or herself and is called the *protagonist.* In this role, the client is able to express true feelings toward individuals (represented by group members) with whom he or she has unresolved conflicts.

In some instances, the group leader may ask for a client to volunteer to be the protagonist for that session. The client may chose a situation he or she wishes to enact and select the audience members to portray the roles of others in the life situation. The psychodrama setting provides the client with a safer and less threatening atmosphere than the real situation in which to express true feelings. Resolution of interpersonal conflicts is facilitated.

When the drama has been completed, group members from the audience discuss the situation they have observed, offer feedback, express their feelings, and relate their own similar experiences. In this way, all group members benefit from the session, either directly or indirectly.

Nurses often serve as actors, or role-players, in psychodrama sessions. Leaders of psychodrama have graduate degrees in psychology, social work, nursing, or medicine with additional training in group therapy and specialty preparation to become a psychodramatist.

The Role of the Nurse in Group Therapy

Nurses participate in group situations on a daily basis. In health-care settings, nurses serve on or lead task groups that create policy, describe procedures, and plan client care. They are also involved in a variety of other groups aimed at the institutional effort of serving the consumer. Nurses are encouraged to use the steps of the nursing process as a framework for task-group leadership.

In psychiatry, nurses may lead various types of therapeutic groups, such as client education, assertiveness training, support, parent, and transition to discharge groups, among others. To function effectively in the leadership capacity for these groups, nurses need to be able to recognize various processes that occur in groups (such as the phases of group development, the various roles that people play within group situations, and the motivation behind the behavior). They also need to be able to select the most appropriate leadership style for the type of group being led. Generalist nurses may develop these skills as part of their undergraduate education, or they may pursue additional study while serving and learning as the co-leader of a group with a more experienced nurse leader.

Generalist nurses in psychiatry rarely serve as leaders of psychotherapy groups. The *Psychiatric-Mental Health Nursing: Scope and Standards of Practice* (American Nurses Association, 2007)

specifies that nurses who serve as group psychotherapists should have a minimum of a master's degree in psychiatric nursing. Other criteria that have been suggested are educational preparation in group theory, extended practice as a group co-leader or leader under the supervision of an experienced psychotherapist, and participation in group therapy on an experiential level. Additional specialist training is required beyond the master's level to prepare nurses to become family therapists or psychodramatists.

Leading therapeutic groups is within the realm of nursing practice. Because group work is such a common therapeutic approach in the discipline of psychiatry, nurses working in this field must continually strive to expand their knowledge and use of group process as a significant psychiatric nursing intervention.

> **CLINICAL PEARL** Knowledge of human behavior in general and the group process in particular is essential to effective group leadership.

Summary and Key Points

- A *group* has been defined as a collection of individuals whose association is founded on shared commonalities of interest, values, norms, or purpose.

- Eight group functions have been identified: socialization, support, task completion, camaraderie, informational, normative, empowerment, and governance.

- There are three major types of groups: task groups, teaching groups, and supportive/therapeutic groups.

- The function of task groups is to solve problems, make decisions, and achieve a specific outcome.

- In teaching groups, knowledge and information are conveyed to a number of individuals.

- The function of supportive/therapeutic groups is to educate people to deal effectively with emotional stress in their lives.

- In self-help groups, members share the same type of problem and help each other to prevent decompensation related to that problem.

- Therapeutic groups differ from group therapy in that group therapy is more theory based and the leaders generally have advanced degrees in psychology, social work, nursing, or medicine.

■ Placement of the seating and size of the group can influence group interaction.

■ Groups can be open-ended (when members leave and others join at any time while the group is active) or closed-ended (when groups have a predetermined, fixed time frame and all members join at the same time and leave when the group disbands).

■ Yalom and Leszcz (2005) describe the following curative factors that individuals derive from participation in therapeutic groups: the instillation of hope, universality, the imparting of information, altruism, the corrective recapitulation of the primary family group, the development of socializing techniques, imitative behavior, interpersonal learning, group cohesiveness, catharsis, and existential factors.

■ Groups progress through three phases: the initial (orientation) phase, the working phase, and the termination phase.

■ Group leadership styles include autocratic, democratic, and laissez-faire.

■ Members play various roles within groups. These roles are categorized according to task roles, maintenance roles, and personal roles.

■ Psychodrama is a specialized type of group therapy that uses a dramatic approach in which clients become "actors" in life-situation scenarios.

■ The psychodrama setting provides the client with a safer and less threatening atmosphere than the real situation in which to express and work through unresolved conflicts.

■ Nurses lead various types of therapeutic groups in the psychiatric setting. Knowledge of human behavior in general and the group process in particular is essential to effective group leadership.

DavisPlus   Additional info available @ davisplus.fadavis.com

Review Questions
Self-Examination/Learning Exercise

*Select the answer that is **most** appropriate for each of the following questions:*

1. N.J. is the nurse leader of a childbirth preparation group. Each week she shows various films and sets out various reading materials. She expects the participants to utilize their time on a topic of their choice or practice skills they have observed on the films. Two couples have dropped out of the group, stating, "This is a big waste of time." Which type of group and style of leadership is described in this situation?
   a. Task, democratic.
   b. Teaching, laissez-faire.
   c. Self-help, democratic.
   d. Supportive/therapeutic, autocratic.

2. M.K. is a psychiatric nurse who has been selected to lead a group for women who desire to lose weight. The criterion for membership is that they must be at least 20 pounds overweight. All have tried to lose weight on their own many times in the past without success. At their first meeting, M.K. provides suggestions as the members determine what their goals will be and how they plan to go about achieving those goals. They decided how often they wanted to meet, and what they planned to do at each meeting. Which type of group and style of leadership is described in this situation?
   a. Task, autocratic.
   b. Teaching, democratic.
   c. Self-help, laissez-faire.
   d. Supportive/therapeutic, democratic.

Continued

Review Questions—cont'd
Self-Examination/Learning Exercise

3. J.J. is a staff nurse on a surgical unit. He has been selected as leader of a newly established group of staff nurses organized to determine ways to decrease the number of medication errors occurring on the unit. J.J. has definite ideas about how to bring this about. He has also applied for the position of Head Nurse on the unit and believes that, if he is successful in leading the group toward achievement of its goals, he can also facilitate his chances for promotion. At each meeting he addresses the group in an effort to convince the members to adopt his ideas. Which type of group and style of leadership is described in this situation?
   a. Task, autocratic.
   b. Teaching, autocratic.
   c. Self-help, democratic.
   d. Supportive/therapeutic, laissez-faire.

4. The nurse leader is explaining about group "curative factors" to members of the group. She tells the group that group situations are beneficial because members can see that they are not alone in their experiences. This is an example of which curative factor?
   a. Altruism.
   b. Imitative behavior.
   c. Universality.
   d. Imparting of information.

5. Nurse Jones is the leader of a bereavement group for widows. Nancy is a new member. She listens to the group and sees that Jane has been a widow for 5 years now. Jane has adjusted well and Nancy thinks maybe she can too. This is an example of which curative factor?
   a. Universality.
   b. Imitative behavior.
   c. Installation of hope.
   d. Imparting of information.

6. Paul is a member of an anger management group. He knew that people did not want to be his friend because of his violent temper. In the group, he has learned to control his temper and form satisfactory interpersonal relationships with others. This is an example of which curative factor?
   a. Catharsis.
   b. Altruism.
   c. Imparting of information.
   d. Development of socializing techniques.

7. Henry is a member of an Alcoholics Anonymous group. He learned about the effects of alcohol on the body when a nurse from the chemical dependency unit spoke to the group. This is an example of which curative factor?
   a. Catharsis.
   b. Altruism.
   c. Imparting of information.
   d. Universality.

8. Sandra is the nurse leader of a supportive/therapeutic group for individuals with anxiety disorders. In this group, Nancy talks incessantly. When someone else tries to make a comment, she refuses to allow him or her to speak. What type of member role is Nancy assuming in this group?
   a. Aggressor.
   b. Monopolizer.
   c. Blocker.
   d. Seducer.

Review Questions—cont'd
Self-Examination/Learning Exercise

9. Sandra is the nurse leader of a supportive/therapeutic group for individuals with anxiety disorders. On the first day the group meets, Valerie speaks first and begins by sharing the intimate details of her incestuous relationship with her father. What type of member role is Nancy assuming in this group?
   a. Aggressor.
   b. Monopolizer.
   c. Blocker.
   d. Seducer.

10. Sandra is the nurse leader of a supportive/therapeutic group for individuals with anxiety disorders. Violet, who is beautiful but lacks self-confidence, states to the group, "Maybe if I became a blond my boyfriend would love me more." Larry responds, "Listen, dummy, you need more than blond hair to keep the guy around. A bit more in the brains department would help!" What type of member role is Larry assuming in this group?
    a. Aggressor.
    b. Monopolizer.
    c. Blocker.
    d. Seducer.

References

American Nurses Association. (2007). *Psychiatric-mental health nursing: Scope and standards of practice.* Silver Spring, MD: Author.

Clark, C. C. (2003). *Group leadership skills* (4th ed.). New York: Springer.

Sampson, E. E., & Marthas, M. (1990). *Group process for the health professions* (3rd ed.). Albany, NY: Delmar Publishers.

Yalom, I. D., & Leszcz, M. (2005). *The theory and practice of group psychotherapy* (5th ed.). New York: Basic Books.

Classical References

Benne, K. B., & Sheats, P. (1948, Spring). Functional roles of group members. *Journal of Social Issues, 4*(2), 42–49.

Lippitt, R., & White, R. K. (1958). An experimental study of leadership and group life. In E. E. Maccoby, T. M. Newcomb, & E. L. Hartley (Eds.), *Readings in social psychology* (3rd ed.). New York: Holt, Rinehart, & Winston.

CHAPTER 11

Intervention With Families

CORE CONCEPTS

family

family therapy

KEY TERMS

boundaries

disengagement

double-bind communication

enmeshment

family structure

family system

genogram

marital schism

marital skew

paradoxical intervention

pseudohostility

pseudomutuality

reframing

scapegoating

subsystems

triangles

OBJECTIVES

After reading this chapter, the student will be able to:

1. Define the term *family.*
2. Identify stages of family development.
3. Describe major variations to the American middle-class family life cycle.
4. Discuss characteristics of adaptive family functioning.
5. Describe behaviors that interfere with adaptive family functioning.
6. Discuss the essential components of family systems, structural, and strategic therapies.
7. Construct a family genogram.
8. Apply the steps of the nursing process in therapeutic intervention with families.

HOMEWORK ASSIGNMENT
Please read the chapter and answer the following questions:

1. Describe the concept of "reframing."
2. Describe the process of triangulation in a dysfunctional family pattern.
3. How are genograms helpful in family therapy?
4. What behaviors are indicative of a positive family climate?

What is a family? Wright and Leahey (2009) proposed the following definition: a family is who they say they are. Many family forms exist within society today, such as the biological family of procreation, the nuclear family that incorporates one or more members of the extended family (family of origin), the sole-parent family, the stepfamily, the communal family, and the homosexual couple or family. Labeling individuals as "families" based on their group composition may not be the best way, however. Instead, family consideration may be more appropriately determined based on attributes of affection, strong emotional ties, a sense of belonging, and durability of membership (Wright & Leahey, 2009).

Many nurses have interactions with family members on a daily basis. A client's illness or hospitalization affects all members of the family, and nurses must understand how to work with the family as a unit, knowing that family members can have a profound effect on the client's healing process.

Nurse generalists should be familiar with the tasks associated with adaptive family functioning. With this knowledge, they are able to assess family interaction and recognize problems when they arise. They can provide support to families with an ill member and make referrals to other professionals when assistance is required to restore adaptive functioning.

Nurse specialists usually possess an advanced degree in nursing. Some nurse specialists have education or experience that qualifies them to perform family therapy. Family therapy is broadly defined as "a form of intervention in which members of a family are assisted in identifying and changing problematic, maladaptive, repetitive relationship patterns, as well as self-defeating or self-limiting belief systems" (Goldenberg, Goldenberg, & Pelavin, 2011, p. 417). Family therapy has a strong theoretical focus, and a number of conceptual approaches have been introduced and suggested as frameworks for this intervention.

This chapter explores the stages of family development and compares the "typical" family within various subcultures. Characteristics of adaptive family functioning and behaviors that interfere with this adaptation are discussed. Theoretical components of selected therapeutic approaches are described. Instructions for construction of a family genogram are included. Nursing process provides the framework for nursing intervention with families.

> ## CORE CONCEPT
>
> ### *Family*
>
> Two or more individuals who depend on one another for emotional, physical, and economical support. The members of the family are self-defined (Kaakinen, Hanson, & Denham, 2010).

Stages of Family Development

McGoldrick, Carter, and Garcia-Preto (2011) identified stages and developmental tasks that describe the family life cycle. It is acknowledged that these tasks would vary greatly among diverse cultural groups, as well as the various forms of families previously described. These stages, however, provide a valuable framework from which the nurse may study families, emphasizing expansion (the addition of members), contraction (the loss of members), and realignment of relationships as members experience developmental changes. These stages of family development are described in the following paragraphs, and are summarized in Table 11-1.

The Single Young Adult

This model begins with the launching of the young adult from the family of origin. This is a difficult stage because young adults must decide what social standards from the family of origin will be preserved and what they will change for themselves to be incorporated into a new family. Tasks of this stage include forming an identity separate from the parents, establishing intimate peer relationships, and advancing toward financial independence. Problems can arise when either the

FAMILY LIFE CYCLE STAGES	EMOTIONAL PROCESS OF TRANSITION: KEY PRINCIPLES	CHANGES REQUIRED IN FAMILY STATUS TO PROCEED DEVELOPMENTALLY
The Single Young Adult	Accepting separation from parents and emotional and financial responsibility for self	■ Differentiation of self in relation to family of origin ■ Development of intimate peer relationships ■ Establishment of self in respect to work and financial independence ■ Establishment of self in community and larger society
The Family Joined Through Marriage/ Union	Commitment to new system	■ Formation of partner systems ■ Realignment of relationships with extended family, friends, and larger community and social system to include new partners

TABLE 11-1 Stages of the Family Life Cycle

Continued

TABLE 11-1 Stages of the Family Life Cycle—cont'd

FAMILY LIFE CYCLE STAGES	EMOTIONAL PROCESS OF TRANSITION: KEY PRINCIPLES	CHANGES REQUIRED IN FAMILY STATUS TO PROCEED DEVELOPMENTALLY
The Family With Young Children	Accepting new members into the system	■ Adjustment of couple system to make space for children ■ Collaboration in child rearing, financial and housekeeping tasks ■ Realignment of relationships with extended family to include parenting and grandparenting roles ■ Realignment of relationships with community and larger social system to include new family structure and relationships
The Family With Adolescents	Increasing flexibility of family boundaries to permit children's independence and grandparents' frailties	■ Shifting of parent/child relationships to permit adolescents to move in and out of system ■ Refocus on midlife couple and career issues ■ Beginning shift toward caring for older generation ■ Realignment with community and larger social system to include shifting family of emerging adolescent and parents in new formation patterns of relating
The Family Launching Children and Moving on in Midlife	Accepting a multitude of exits from and entries into the family system	■ Renegotiation of couple system as a dyad ■ Development of adult-to-adult relationships between parents and grown children ■ Realignment of relationships to include in-laws and grandchildren ■ Realignment of relationships with community and larger social system to include new structure and constellation of family relationships ■ Exploration of new interests/career given the freedom from childcare responsibilities ■ Dealing with care needs, disabilities and death of parents (grandparents)
The Family in Later Life (late middle age to end of life)	■ Accepting the shifting of generational roles ■ Accepting the realities of limitations and death	■ Maintaining own and/or couple functioning and interests in face of physiological decline; exploration of new familial and social role options ■ Supporting more central role of middle generations ■ Realignment of the system in relation to community and larger social system to acknowledge changed pattern of family relationships of this stage ■ Making room in the system for the wisdom and experience of the elders; supporting the older generation without overfunctioning for them ■ Dealing with loss of spouse, siblings, and other peers, and preparation for own death; life review and integration ■ Managing reversed roles in caretaking between middle and older generations

Adapted from McGoldrick, M., Carter, B., & Garcia-Preto, N. (2011). Overview: The life cycle in its changing context. In M. McGoldrick, B. Carter, & N. Garcia-Preto (Eds.), The expanded family life cycle (4th ed., pp.1-19). Boston: Allyn & Bacon. Reprinted by permission.

young adults or the parents encounter difficulty terminating the interdependent relationship that has existed in the family of origin.

The Family Joined Through Marriage/Union

Uniting as a couple is a difficult transition because renegotiation must include the integration of contrasting issues that each partner brings to the relationship and issues they may have redefined for themselves as a couple. In addition, the new couple must renegotiate relationships with parents, siblings, and other relatives in view of the new partnership. Tasks of this stage include establishing a new identity as a couple, realigning relationships with members of the extended family, and making decisions about having children. Problems can arise if either partner remains too enmeshed with their family of origin or when the couple chooses to cut themselves off completely from extended family.

The Family With Young Children

Adjustments in relationships must occur with the arrival of children. The entire family system is affected, and role realignments are necessary for both new parents and new grandparents. Tasks of this stage include making adjustments within the couple system to meet the responsibilities associated with parenthood while maintaining the integrity of the relationship, sharing equally in the tasks of childrearing, and integrating the roles of extended family members into the newly expanded family organization. Problems can arise when parents lack knowledge about normal childhood development and adequate patience to allow children to express themselves through behavior.

The Family With Adolescents

This stage of family development is characterized by a great deal of turmoil and transition. Parents are approaching a midlife stage and adolescents are undergoing biological, emotional, and sociocultural changes that place demands on each individual and on the family unit. Grandparents, too, may require assistance with the tasks of later life. These developments can create a "sandwich" effect for the parents, who must deal with issues confronting three generations. Tasks of this stage include redefining the level of dependence so that adolescents are provided with greater autonomy while parents remain responsive to the teenager's dependency needs. Midlife issues related to marriage, career, and aging parents must also be resolved during this period. Problems can arise when parents are unable to relinquish control and allow the adolescent greater autonomy and freedom to make independent decisions or when parents are unable to agree and support each other in this effort.

The Family Launching Children and Moving on in Midlife

A great deal of realignment of family roles occurs during this stage. This stage is characterized by the intermittent exiting and entering of various family members. Children leave home for further education and careers; marriages occur, and new spouses, in-laws, and children enter the system; and new grandparent roles are established. Adult-to-adult relationships among grown children and their parents are renegotiated. Tasks associated with this stage include reestablishing the bond of the dyadic couple relationship; realigning relationships to include grown children, in-laws, and new grandchildren; and accepting the additional caregiving responsibilities and eventual death of elderly parents. Problems can arise when feelings of loss and depression become overwhelming in response to the departure of children from the home, when parents are unable to accept their children as adults or cope with the disability or death of their own parents, and when the couple bond has deteriorated.

The Family in Later Life (Late Middle Age to End of Life)

This stage can begin with retirement and last until the death of both spouses (Wright & Leahey, 2009). However, many older people who have the opportunity to do so are choosing to retire early, while large numbers of those over age 65 are remaining in the work force and delaying their retirement. Thus, the beginning of this stage varies widely. Most adults in their later years are still a prominent part of the family system, and many are able to offer support to their grown children in the middle generation. Tasks associated with this stage include exploring new social roles related to retirement and possible change in socioeconomic status; accepting some decline in physiological functioning; dealing with the deaths of spouse, siblings, and friends; and confronting and preparing for one's own death. Problems may arise when older adults have failed to fulfill the tasks associated with earlier levels of development and are dissatisfied with the way their lives have gone. They are unable to find happiness in retirement or emotional satisfaction with children and grandchildren, and they are unable to accept the deaths of loved ones or to prepare for their own impending death.

Major Variations

Divorce

McGoldrick, Carter, and Garcia-Preto (2011) also discussed stages and tasks of families experiencing divorce and remarriage. Data on marriage, divorce, and remarriage in the United States show that approximately one third of first marriages end in separation or divorce within 10 years (Centers for Disease Control [CDC], 2010). Some statistics indicate that the divorce rate may be on the decline since the 1970s. In 2007, however, 25 percent of all families in the United States were headed by solo parents (Kreider & Elliott, 2009). Stages in the family life cycle of divorce include deciding to divorce, planning the break-up of the system, separation, and divorce. Tasks include accepting one's own part in the failure of the marriage, working cooperatively on problems related to custody and visitation of children and finances, realigning relationships with extended family, and mourning the loss of the marriage relationship and the intact family.

After the divorce, the custodial parent must adjust to functioning as the single leader of an ongoing family while working to rebuild a new social network. The noncustodial parent must find ways to continue to be an effective parent while remaining outside the normal parenting role.

Remarriage

About three fourths of people who divorce will eventually remarry (Kreider & Fields, 2002). In 2004, 17 percent (12.2 million) of all children in the United States lived in blended families (those that contain stepchildren and their stepparents, half-siblings, or stepsiblings) (Kreider, 2008). The challenges that face the joining of two established families are immense, and statistics reveal that the rate of divorce for remarried couples is even higher than the divorce rate following first marriages (Bramlett & Mosher, 2002). Stages in the remarried family life cycle include entering the new relationship, planning the new marriage and family, and remarriage and reestablishment of family. Tasks include making a firm commitment to confronting the complexities of combining two families, maintaining open communication, facing fears, realigning relationships with extended family to include new spouse and children, and encouraging healthy relationships with biological (noncustodial) parents and grandparents.

Problems can arise when there is a blurring of boundaries between the custodial and noncustodial families. Children may contemplate, "Who is the boss now? Who is most important, me or the new spouse?" "Mom loves her new husband more than she loves me." "Dad lets me do more than my new stepdad does. I don't have to mind him; he's not my real dad." Confusion and distress for both the children and the parents can be avoided with the establishment of clear boundaries.

Goldenberg and Goldenberg (2008) stated:

> Successful adaptation to stepfamily life calls for the ability to recognize and cope with a variety of problems: stepparents assuming a parental role, rule changes, jealousy and competition between stepsiblings as well as between birth parents and stepparents, loyalty conflicts in children between the absent parent and the stepparent, and financial obligations for child support while entering into a new marriage, to name but a few. Remarriage itself may resurrect old, unresolved feelings, such as anger and hurt left over from a previous marriage. (p. 400)

Cultural Variations

It is difficult to generalize about variations in family life-cycle development according to culture. Most families have become acculturated to the U.S. society and conform to the life-cycle stages previously described. However, cultural diversity does exist, and nurses must be aware of possible differences in family expectations related to sociocultural beliefs. They must also be aware of a great deal of variation within ethnic groups as well as among them. Some variations that may be considered follow.

Marriage

A number of U.S. subcultures maintain traditional values in terms of marriage. Traditional views about family life and Roman Catholicism exert important influences on attitudes toward marriage in many Italian American and Latino American families. Although the tradition of arranged marriages is disappearing in Asian American families, there is still frequently a much stronger influence by the family on mate selection than there is for other cultures in the United States (Earp, 2008). In these subcultures, the father is considered the authority figure and head of the household and the mother assumes the role of homemaker and caretaker. Family loyalty is intense, and a breach of this loyalty brings considerable shame to the family.

Valley (2005) made the following statement about Jewish families:

> The Jewish family today encompasses a wide variety of textures and forms. Decades of high intermarriage have diversified the customs and complexions of the family. High divorce rates, meanwhile, have altered the very definition of what is "normal." Whereas single-parent households were once a rare exception, they now account for an increasing proportion of American Jewish families. Some in the community have interpreted the changing family in strident and judgmental terms: it is a sign of rampant assimilation, loss of tradition or moral permissiveness. But such scolding does nothing to respond to the new realities and to the changing needs of Jews today. (p. 2)

Children

In traditional Latino American and Italian American cultures, children are central to the family system. Many of these individuals have strong ties to Roman Catholicism, which historically has promoted marital relations for procreation only, and encouraged families to have large numbers of children. Regarding birth control, the Catechism of the Catholic Church (U.S. Catholic Church, 2003) states:

> Every action which, whether in anticipation of the conjugal act, or in its accomplishment, or in the development of its natural consequences, proposes, whether as an end or as a means, to render procreation impossible is intrinsically evil. (p. 629)

In the traditional Jewish community, having children is seen as a scriptural and social obligation. "You shall be fruitful and multiply" is a commandment of the Torah.

In some traditional Asian American cultures, sons are more highly valued than are daughters, and there is a strong preference for sons over daughters (Earp, 2008; Xu & Chang, 2008). Younger siblings are expected to follow the guidance of the oldest son throughout their lives, and when the father dies, the oldest son takes over the leadership of the family.

In all of these cultures, children are expected to be respectful of their parents and not bring shame to the family. Especially in the Asian culture, children learn a sense of obligation to their parents for bringing them into this world and caring for them when they were helpless. This is viewed as a debt that can never be truly repaid, and no matter what the parents may do, the child is still obligated to give respect and obedience.

Extended Family

The concept of extended family varies among societies (Purnell, 2008). The extended family is extremely important in the Western European, Latino, and Asian cultures, playing a central role in all aspects of life, including decision making.

In some U.S. subcultures, such as Asian, Latino, Italian, and Iranian, it is not uncommon to find several generations living together. Older family members are valued for their experience and wisdom. Because extended families often share living quarters, or at least live nearby, tasks of childrearing may be shared by several generations.

Divorce

In the Jewish community, divorce is often seen as a violation of family togetherness. Some Jewish parents take their child's divorce personally, with the response, "How could you possibly do this to me?"

Because Roman Catholicism has traditionally opposed divorce, those cultures that are largely Catholic have followed this dictate. Historically, a low divorce rate has existed among Italian Americans, Irish Americans, and Latino Americans. The number of divorces among these subcultures is on the rise, however, particularly in successive generations that have become more acculturated into a society where divorce is more acceptable.

Family Functioning

Boyer and Jeffrey (1994) described six elements on which families are assessed to be either functional or dysfunctional. Each can be viewed on a continuum, although families rarely fall at extreme ends of the continuum. Rather, they tend to be dynamic and fluctuate from one point to another within the different areas. These six elements of assessment are described below and summarized in Table 11-2.

Communication

Functional communication patterns are those in which verbal and nonverbal messages are clear, direct, and congruent between sender and intended receiver. Family members are encouraged to express honest feelings and opinions, and all members participate in decisions that affect the family system. Each member is an active listener to the other members of the family.

Behaviors that interfere with functional communication include the following.

TABLE 11-2 Family Functioning: Elements of Assessment

ELEMENTS OF ASSESSMENT	CONTINUUM	
	Functional	Dysfunctional
Communication	Clear, direct, open, and honest, with congruence between verbal and nonverbal	Indirect, vague, controlled, with many double-bind messages
Self-concept reinforcement	Supportive, loving, praising, approving, with behaviors that instill confidence	Unsupportive, blaming, "put-downs," refusing to allow self-responsibility
Family members' expectations	Flexible, realistic, individualized	Judgmental, rigid, controlling, ignoring individuality
Handling differences	Tolerant, dynamic, negotiating	Attacking, avoiding, surrendering
Family interactional patterns	Workable, constructive, flexible, and promoting the needs of all members	Contradictory, rigid, self-defeating, and destructive
Family climate	Trusting, growth-promoting, caring, general feeling of well-being	Distrusting, emotionally painful, with absence of hope for improvement

Adapted from Boyer, P. A., & Jeffery, R. J. (1994). A guide for the family therapist. Northvale, NJ: Jason Aronson.

Making Assumptions

With this behavior, one assumes that others will know what is meant by an action or an expression (or sometimes even what one is thinking); or, on the other hand, one assumes to know what another member is thinking or feeling without checking to make certain.

EXAMPLE

A mother says to her teenaged daughter, "You should have known that I expected you to clean up the kitchen while I was gone!"

Belittling Feelings

This action involves ignoring or minimizing another's feelings when they are expressed. This encourages the individual to withhold honest feelings to avoid being hurt by the negative response.

EXAMPLE

When the young woman confides to her mother that she is angry because the grandfather has touched her breast, the mother responds, "Oh, don't be angry. He doesn't mean anything by that."

Failing to Listen

With this behavior, one does not hear what the other individual is saying. This can mean not hearing the words by "tuning out" what is being said, or it can be "selective" listening, in which a person hears only a selective part of the message or interprets it in a selective manner.

EXAMPLE

The father explains to Johnny, "If the contract comes through and I get this new job, we'll have a little extra money and we will consider sending you to State U." Johnny relays the message to his friend, "Dad says I can go to State U!"

Communicating Indirectly

This usually means that an individual does not or cannot present a message to a receiver directly, so seeks to communicate through a third person.

EXAMPLE

A father does not want his teenage daughter to see a certain boyfriend, but wants to avoid the angry response he expects from his daughter if he tells her so. He expresses his feelings to his wife, hoping she will share them with their daughter.

Presenting Double-Bind Messages

Double-bind communication conveys a "damned if I do and damned if I don't" message. A family member may respond to a direct request by another family member, only to be rebuked when the request is fulfilled.

EXAMPLE

The father tells his son that he is spending too much time playing football, and as a result, his grades are falling. He is expected to bring his grades up over the next 9 weeks or his car will be taken away. When the son tells the father he has quit the football team so he can study more, Dad responds angrily, "I won't allow any son of mine to be a quitter!"

Self-Concept Reinforcement

Functional families strive to reinforce and strengthen each member's self-concept, with the positive results being that family members feel loved and valued. Boyer and Jeffrey (1994) stated:

> The manner in which children see and value themselves is influenced most significantly by the messages they receive concerning their value to other members of the family. Messages that convey praise, approval, appreciation, trust, and confidence in decisions and that allow family members to pursue individual needs and ultimately to become independent are the foundation blocks of a child's feelings of self-worth. Adults also need and depend heavily on this kind of reinforcement for their own emotional well-being. (p. 27)

Behaviors that interfere with self-concept reinforcement follow.

Expressing Denigrating Remarks

These remarks are commonly called "put downs." Individuals receive messages that they are worthless or unloved.

EXAMPLE

A child spills a glass of milk at the table. The mother responds, "You are hopeless! How could anybody be so clumsy?!"

Withholding Supportive Messages

Some family members find it very difficult to provide others with reinforcing and supportive messages. This may be because they themselves have not been the recipients of reinforcement from significant others and have not learned how to provide support to others.

EXAMPLE

A 10-year-old boy playing Little League baseball retrieves the ball and throws it to second base for an out. After the game he says to his Dad, "Did you see my play on second base?" Dad responds, "Yes, I did, son, but if you had been paying better attention, you could have caught the ball for a direct and immediate out."

Taking Over

This occurs when one family member fails to permit another member to develop a sense of responsibility and self-worth, by doing things for the individual instead of allowing him or her to manage the situation independently.

EXAMPLE

Twelve-year-old Eric has a job delivering the evening paper, which he usually begins right after school. Today he must serve a 1-hour detention after school for being late to class yesterday. He tells his Mom, "Tommy said he would throw my papers for me today if I help him wash his Dad's car on Saturday." Mom responds, "Never mind. Tell Tommy to forget it. I'll take care of your paper route today."

Family Members' Expectations

All individuals have some expectations about the outcomes of the life situations they experience. These expectations are related to and significantly influenced by earlier life experiences. In functional families, expectations are realistic, thereby avoiding setting family members up for failure. In functional families, expectations are also flexible. Life situations are full of extraneous and unexpected interferences. Flexibility allows for changes and interruptions to occur without creating conflict. Finally, in functional families, expectations are individualized. Each family member is different, with different strengths and limitations. The outcome of a life situation for one family member may not be realistic for another. Each member must be valued independently, and comparison among members avoided.

Behaviors that interfere with adaptive functioning in terms of member expectations include the following.

Ignoring Individuality

This occurs when family members expect others to do things or behave in ways that do not fit with the latter's individuality or current life situation (Boyer & Jeffrey, 1994). This sometimes happens when parents expect their children to fulfill the hopes and dreams the parents have failed to achieve, yet the children have their own, different hopes and dreams.

EXAMPLE

Bob, an only child, leaves for college next year. Bob's father, Robert, inherited a hardware store that was founded by Bob's great-grandfather and has been in the family for three generations.

Robert expects Bob to major in business, work in the store after college, and take over the business when Robert retires. Bob, however, has a talent for writing, wants to major in communication, and wants to work in TV news when he graduates. Robert sees this as a betrayal of the family.

Demanding Proof of Love

Boyer and Jeffrey (1994) stated:

> Family members place expectations on others' behavior that are used as standards by which the expecting member determines how much the other members care for him or her. The message attached to these expectations is: "If you will not be as I wish you to be, you don't love me." (p. 32)

EXAMPLE

This is the message that Bob receives from his father in the example cited in the previous paragraph.

Handling Differences

It is difficult to conceive of two or more individuals living together who agree on everything all of the time. Serious problems in a family's functioning appear when differences become equated with "badness" or when disagreement is seen as "not caring" (Boyer & Jeffrey, 1994). Members of a functional family understand that it is acceptable to disagree and deal with differences in an open, nonattacking manner. Members are willing to hear the other person's position, respect the other person's right to hold an opposing position, and work to modify the expectations on both sides of the issue in order to negotiate a workable solution.

Behaviors that interfere with successful family negotiations follow.

Attacking

A difference of opinion can deteriorate into a direct personal attack and may be manifested by blaming another person, bringing up the past, making destructive comparisons, or lashing out with other expressions of anger and hurt (Boyer & Jeffrey, 1994).

EXAMPLE

When Nancy's husband, John, buys an expensive set of golf clubs, Nancy responds, "How could you do such a thing? You know we can't afford those! No wonder we don't have a nice house like all our friends. You spend all our money before we can save for a down payment. You're so selfish! We'll never have anything nice and it's all your fault!"

Avoiding

With this tactic, differences are never acknowledged openly. The individual who disagrees avoids discussing it for fear that the other person will withdraw love or approval or become angry in response to the disagreement. Avoidance also occurs when an individual fears loss of control of his or her temper if the disagreement is brought out into the open.

EXAMPLE

Vicki and Clint have been married 6 months. This is Vicki's second marriage and she has a 4-year-old son from her first marriage, Derek, who lives with her and Clint. Both Vicki and Clint work, and Derek goes to day care. Since the marriage 6 months ago, Derek cries every night continuously unless Vicki spends all her time with him, which she does in order to keep him quiet. Clint resents this but says nothing for fear he will come across as interfering; however, he has started going back to work in his office in the evenings to avoid the family situation.

Surrendering

The person who surrenders in the face of disagreement does so at the expense of denying his or her own needs or rights. The individual avoids expressing a difference of opinion for fear of angering another person or of losing approval and support.

EXAMPLE

Elaine is the only child of wealthy parents. She attends an exclusive private college in a small New England town, where she met Andrew, the son of a farming couple from the area. Andrew attended the local community college for 2 years but chose to work on his parents' farm rather than continue college. Elaine and Andrew love each other and want to be married, but Elaine's parents say they will disown her if she marries Andrew, who they believe is below her social status. Elaine breaks off her relationship with Andrew rather than challenge her parents' wishes.

Family Interactional Patterns

Interactional patterns have to do with the ways in which families "behave." All families develop recurring, predictable patterns of interaction over time. These are often thought of as "family rules." The mentality conveys, "This is the way we have always done it" and provides a sense of security and stability for family members that comes from predictability. These interactions may have to do with communication, self-concept reinforcement, expressing expectations, and handling differences (all of the behaviors that were discussed previously), but because they are repetitive, and recur over time, they become the "rules" that govern patterns of interaction among family members.

Family rules are functional when they are workable, are constructive, and promote the needs of all family members. They are dysfunctional when they become contradictory, self-defeating, and destructive. Family therapists often find that individuals are unaware that dysfunctional family rules exist and may vehemently deny their existence even when confronted with a specific behavioral interaction. The development of dysfunctional interactional patterns occurs through a habituation process and out of fear of change or reprisal or a lack of knowledge as to how a given situation might be handled differently (Boyer & Jeffrey, 1994). Many are derived out of the parents' own growing-up experiences.

Patterns of interaction that interfere with adaptive family functioning include the following.

Patterns That Cause Emotional Discomfort

Interactions can promote hurt and anger in family members. This is particularly true of emotions that individuals feel uncomfortable expressing or are not permitted (according to "family rules") to express openly. These interactional patterns include behaviors such as never apologizing or never admitting that one has made a mistake, forbidding flexibility in life situations ("you must do it my way, or you will not do it at all"), making statements that devalue the worth of others, or withholding statements that promote increased self-worth.

EXAMPLE

Priscilla and Bill had been discussing buying a new car but could not agree on the make or model to buy. One day, Bill appeared at Priscilla's office over the lunch hour and said, "Come outside and see our new car." In front of the building, Bill had parked a brand new sports car that he explained he had purchased with their combined savings. Priscilla was furious, but kept quiet and proceeded to finish her workday. At home, she expressed her anger to Bill for making the purchase without consulting her. Bill refused to apologize or admit to making a mistake. They both remained cool and hardly spoke to each other for weeks.

Patterns That Perpetuate or Intensify Problems Rather Than Solve Them

When problems go unresolved over a long period of time, it sometimes appears to be easier just to ignore them. If problems of the same nature occur, the tendency to ignore them then becomes the safe and predictable pattern of interaction for dealing with this type of situation. This may occur until the problem intensifies to a point when it can no longer be ignored.

EXAMPLE

Dan works hard in the automobile factory and demands peace and quiet from his family when he comes home from work. His children have learned over the years not to share their problems with him because they fear his explosive temper. Their mother attempts to handle unpleasant situations alone as best she can. When son Ron was expelled from school for being caught smoking pot for the third time, Dan yelled, "Why wasn't I told about this before?"

Patterns That Are in Conflict With Each Other

Some family rules may appear to be functional—very workable and constructive—on the surface, but in practice may serve to destroy healthy interactional patterns. Boyer and Jeffrey (1994) described the following scenario as an example.

EXAMPLE

Dad insists that all members of the family eat dinner together every evening. No one may leave the table until everyone is finished because dinnertime is one of the few times left when the family can be together. Yet Dad frequently uses the time to reprimand Bobby about his poor grades in math, to scold Ann for her sloppy room, or to make not-so-subtle gibes at Mom for "spending all day on the telephone and never getting anything accomplished."

Family Climate

The atmosphere or climate of a family is composed of a blend of the feelings and experiences that are the result of family members' verbal and nonverbal sharing and interacting. Boyer and Jeffrey (1994) suggested that a positive family climate is founded on trust and is reflected in openness, appropriate humor and laughter, expressions of caring, mutual respect, a valuing of the quality of each individual, and a general feeling of well-being. A dysfunctional family climate is evidenced by tension, pain, physical disabilities, frustration, guilt, persistent anger, and feelings of hopelessness.

> ### CORE CONCEPT
>
> ***Family Therapy***
> A type of therapeutic modality in which the focus of treatment is on the family as a unit. It represents a form of intervention in which members of a family are assisted to identify and change problematic, maladaptive, self-defeating, repetitive relationship patterns (Goldenberg et al., 2011).

Therapeutic Modalities With Families

The Family as a System

General systems theory is a way of organizing thought according to the holistic perspective. A system is considered greater than the sum of its parts. A system is considered dynamic and ever changing. A change in one part of the system causes a change in the other parts of the system and in the system as a whole. When studying families, it is helpful to conceptualize a hierarchy of systems.

The family can be viewed as a system composed of various subsystems, such as the marital subsystem, parent-child subsystems, and sibling subsystems. Each of these subsystems is further divided into subsystems of individuals. The family system is also a subsystem of a larger suprasystem, such as the neighborhood or community. A schematic of a hierarchy of systems is presented in Figure 11–1.

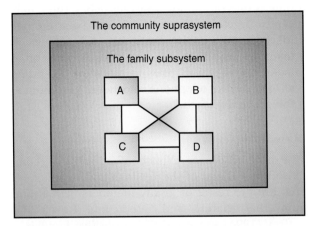

Key:

A = Father subsystem CD = Sibling subsystem
B = Mother subsystem AD = Parent-child subsystem
C = Child subsystem BC = Parent-child subsystem
D = Child subsystem AC = Parent-child subsystem
AB =Marital subsystem BD = Parent-child subsystem

FIGURE 11–1 A hierarchy of systems.

Major Concepts

Bowen (1978) did a great deal of work with families using a systems approach. Bowen's theoretical approach to family therapy is composed of eight major concepts: (1) differentiation of self, (2) triangles, (3) nuclear family emotional process, (4) family projection process, (5) multigenerational transmission process, (6) sibling position, (7) emotional cutoff, and (8) societal emotional process.

Differentiation of Self

Differentiation of self is the ability to define oneself as a separate being. The Bowen theory suggests that "a person with a well-differentiated self recognizes his [or her] realistic dependence on others, but can stay calm and clear headed enough in the face of conflict, criticism, and rejection to distinguish thinking rooted in a careful assessment of the facts from thinking clouded by emotionality" (Georgetown Family Center, 2010a).

The degree of differentiation of self can be viewed on a continuum from high levels, in which an individual manifests a clearly defined sense of self, to low levels, or undifferentiated, in which emotional fusion exists and the individual is unable to function separately from a relationship system. Healthy families encourage differentiation, and the process of separation from the family ego mass is most pronounced during the ages of 2 to 5 and again between the ages of 13 and 15. Families that do not understand the child's need to be different during these times may perceive the child's behavior as objectionable.

Bowen (1971) used the term *stuck-togetherness* to describe the family with the fused ego mass. When family fusion occurs, none of the members has a true sense of self as an independent individual. Boundaries between members are blurred, and the family becomes enmeshed without individual distinguishing characteristics. In this situation, family members can neither gain true intimacy nor separate and become individuals.

Triangles

The concept of **triangles** refers to a three-person emotional configuration that is considered the basic building block of the family system. Bowen (1978) offered the following description of triangles:

> The basic building block of any emotional system is the triangle. When emotional tension in a two-person system exceeds a certain level, it triangles in a third person, permitting the tension to shift about within the triangle. Any two in the original triangle can add a new triangle. An emotional system is composed of a series of interlocking triangles. (p. 306)

Triangles are dysfunctional in that they offer relief from anxiety through diversion rather than through resolution of the issue. When stress develops in a two-person relationship, "one or both partners will turn to someone else for sympathy or the conflict will draw in a third person to try to help" (Nichols, 2010, p. 115). When the dynamics within a triangle stabilize, a fourth person may be brought in to form additional triangles, in an effort to reduce tension. This triangulation can continue almost indefinitely as extended family and people outside the family, including the family therapist, can become entangled in the process. The therapist working with families must strive to remain "detriangled" from this emotional system.

Nuclear Family Emotional Process

The nuclear family emotional process describes the patterns of emotional functioning in a single generation. The nuclear family begins with a relationship between two people who form a couple. The most open relationship usually occurs during courtship, when most individuals chose partners with similar levels of differentiation. The lower the level of differentiation, the greater the possibility of problems in the future. A degree of fusion occurs with permanent commitment. This fusion results in anxiety and must be dealt with by each partner in an effort to maintain a healthy degree of differentiation.

Family Projection Process

Spouses who are unable to work through the undifferentiation or fusion that occurs with permanent commitment may, when they become parents, project the resulting anxiety onto the children. This occurrence is manifested as a father-mother-child triangle. These triangles are common and exist in various gradations of intensity in most families with children.

The child who becomes the target of the projection may be selected for various reasons:

■ A particular child reminds one of the parents of an unresolved childhood issue.

■ The child is of a particular gender or position in the family.

■ The child is born with special needs.

■ The parent has a negative attitude about the pregnancy.

This behavior is called **scapegoating.** It is harmful to both the child's emotional stability and his or her ability to function outside the family. Goldenberg and associates (2011) stated,

Scapegoated family members not only assume the role assigned them, but they may become so entrenched in that role that they are unable to act otherwise. Particularly in dysfunctional families, individuals may be repeatedly labeled as the "bad child"—incorrigible, destructive, unmanageable, troublesome—and they proceed to act accordingly. Scapegoated children are inducted into specific family roles, which over time become fixed and serve as the basis for chronic behavioral disturbance. (p. 432)

Multigenerational Transmission Process

Bowen (1978) described the multigenerational transmission process as the manner in which interactional patterns are transferred from one generation to another. Attitudes, values, beliefs, behaviors, and patterns of interaction are passed along from parents to children over many lifetimes, so that it becomes possible to show in a family assessment that a certain behavior has existed within a family through multiple generations.

Genograms A convenient way to plot a multigenerational assessment is with the use of **genograms.** Genograms offer the convenience of a great deal of information in a small amount of space. They can also be used as teaching tools with the family itself. An overall picture of the life of the family over several generations can be conveyed, including roles that various family members play as well as emotional distance between specific individuals. Areas for change can be easily identified. A sample genogram is presented in Figure 11–2.

Sibling Position

The thesis regarding sibling position profiles is that the position one holds in a family influences the development of predictable personality characteristics. For example, firstborn children are thought to be perfectionistic, reliable, and conscientious; middle children are described as independent, loyal, and intolerant of conflict; and youngest children tend to be charming, precocious, and gregarious (Leman, 2004). Bowen used this thesis to help determine level of differentiation within a family and the possible direction of the family projection process. For example, if an oldest child exhibits characteristics more representative of a youngest child, there is evidence that this child may be the product of triangulation. Sibling position profiles are also used when studying multigenerational transmission processes and verifiable data are missing for certain family members.

Emotional Cutoff

Emotional cutoff describes differentiation of self from the perception of the child. All individuals have some degree of unresolved emotional attachment

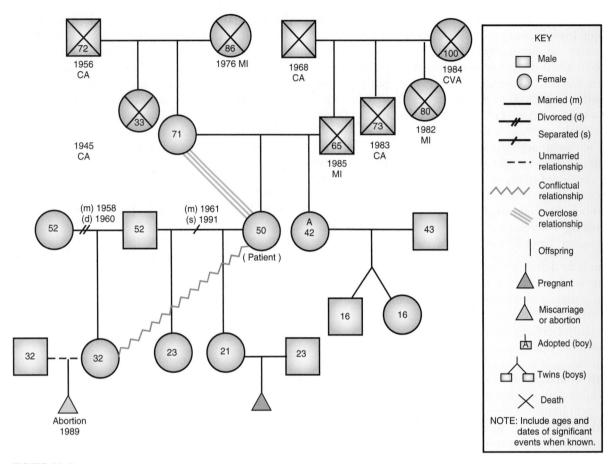

FIGURE 11–2 Sample genogram.

to their parents and the lower the level of differentiation, the greater the degree of unresolved emotional attachment.

Emotional cutoff has very little to do with how far away one lives from the family of origin. Individuals who live great distances from their parents can still be undifferentiated, whereas some individuals are emotionally cut off from their parents who live in the same town or even the same neighborhood.

Bowen (1976) suggested that emotional cutoff is the result of dysfunction within the family of origin in which fusion has occurred and that emotional cutoff promotes the same type of dysfunction in the new nuclear family. He contended that maintaining some emotional contact with the family of origin promotes healthy differentiation.

Societal Emotional Process

The Bowen theory views society as an emotional system. The concept of societal emotional process compares society's response to stress to the same type of response seen in individuals and families in response to emotional crisis: stress creates uncomfortable

levels of anxiety, which leads to hasty solutions, which add to the problems, and the cycle continues. This concept of Bowen's theory is explained as follows (Georgetown Family Center, 2010b):

> Human societies undergo periods of regression and progression in their history. The current regression seems related to factors such as the population explosion, a sense of diminishing frontiers, and the depletion of natural resources. The "symptoms" of societal regression include a growth of crime and violence, an increasing divorce rate, a more litigious attitude, a greater polarization between racial groups, less principled decision-making by leaders, the drug abuse epidemic, an increase in bankruptcy, and a focus on rights over responsibilities.

Goal and Techniques of Therapy

The goal of Bowen's systems approach to family therapy is to increase the level of differentiation of self, while remaining in touch with the family system. The premise is that intense emotional problems within the nuclear family can be resolved only by resolving undifferentiated relationships with the family of origin. Emphasis is given to the understanding of past relationships.

The therapeutic role is that of "coach" or supervisor, and emotional involvement with the family is minimized. Therapist techniques include:

1. Defining and clarifying the relationship between the family members.

2. Helping family members develop one-to-one relationships with each other and minimizing triangles within the system.

3. Teaching family members about the functioning of emotional systems.

4. Promoting differentiation by encouraging members to speak as individuals rather than as a family unit.

The Structural Model

Structural family therapy is associated with a model developed by Minuchin (1974). In this model, the family is viewed as a social system within which the individual lives and to which the individual must adapt. The individual both contributes and responds to stresses within the family.

Major Concepts

Systems

The structural model views the family as a system. The structure of the **family system** is founded on a set of invisible principles that influence the interaction among family members. These principles concern how, when, and with whom to relate, and are established over time and through repeated transactions, until they become rules that govern the conduct of various family members (Goldenberg & Goldenberg, 2008).

Transactional Patterns

Transactional patterns are the rules that have been established over time that organize the ways in which family members relate to one another. A hierarchy of authority is one example of a transactional pattern. Usually, parents have a higher level of authority in a family than the children, so parental behavior reflects this role. A balance of authority may exist between husband and wife, or one may reflect a higher level than the other. These patterns of behavioral expectations differ from family to family and may trace their origin over generations of family negotiations.

Subsystems

Minuchin (1974) described subsystems as smaller elements that make up the larger family system. Subsystems can be individuals or can consist of two or more persons united by gender, relationship, generation, interest, or purpose. A family member may belong to several subsystems at the same time, in which he or she may experience different levels of power and require different types of skills. For example, a young man has a different level of power and a different set of expectations in his father-son subsystem than in a subsystem with his younger brother.

Boundaries

Boundaries define the level of participation and interaction among subsystems. Boundaries are appropriate when they permit appropriate contact with others while preventing excessive interference. Clearly defined boundaries promote adaptive functioning. Maladaptive functioning can occur when boundaries are *rigid* or *diffuse.*

A rigid boundary is characterized by decreased communication and lack of support and responsiveness. Rigid boundaries prevent a subsystem (family member or subgroup) from achieving appropriate closeness or interaction with others in the system. Rigid boundaries promote **disengagement,** or extreme separateness, among family members.

A diffuse boundary is characterized by dependency and overinvolvement. Diffuse boundaries interfere with adaptive functioning because of the overinvestment, overinvolvement, and lack of differentiation between certain subsystems. Diffuse boundaries promote **enmeshment,** or exaggerated connectedness, among family members.

EXAMPLE

Sally and Jim have been married for 12 years, during which time they have tried without success to have children. Six months ago they were thrilled to have the opportunity to adopt a 5-year-old girl, Annie. Since both Sally and Jim have full-time teaching jobs, Annie stays with her maternal grandmother, Krista, during the day after she gets home from half-day kindergarten.

At first, Annie was a polite and obedient child. However, in the last few months, she has become insolent and oppositional, and has temper tantrums when she cannot have her way. Sally and Krista agree that Annie should have whatever she desires and should not be punished for her behavior. Jim believes that discipline is necessary, but Sally and Krista refuse to enforce any guidelines he tries to establish. Annie is aware of this discordance and manipulates it to her full advantage.

In this situation, diffuse boundaries exist among the Sally-Krista-Annie subsystems. They have become enmeshed. They have also established a rigid boundary against Jim, disengaging him from the system.

Goal and Techniques of Therapy

The goal of structural family therapy is to facilitate change in the **family structure.** Family structure is changed with modification of the family "principles" or transactional patterns that are contributing to dysfunction within the family. The family is viewed as the unit of therapy, and all members are counseled together. Little, if any, time is spent exploring past experiences. The focus of structural therapy is on the present. Therapist techniques include the following:

- **Joining the Family.** The therapist must become a part of the family if restructuring is to occur. The therapist joins the family but maintains a leadership position. He or she may at different times join various subsystems within the family, but ultimately includes the entire family system as the target of intervention.

- **Evaluating the Family Structure.** Even though a family may come for therapy because of the behavior of one family member (the identified patient), the family as a unit is considered problematic. The family structure is evaluated by assessing transactional patterns, system flexibility and potential for change, boundaries, family developmental stage, and role of the identified patient within the system.

- **Restructuring the Family.** An alliance or contract for therapy is established with the family. By becoming an actual part of the family, the therapist is able to manipulate the system and facilitate the circumstances and experiences that can lead to structural change.

The Strategic Model

The strategic model of family therapy uses the interactional or communications approach. Communication theory is viewed as the foundation for this model. Communication is the actual transmission of information among individuals. All behavior sends a message, so all behavior in the presence of two or more individuals is communication. In this model, families considered to be functional are open systems where clear and precise messages, congruent with the situation, are sent and received. Healthy communication patterns promote nurturance and individual self-worth. Dysfunctional families are viewed as partially closed systems in which communication is vague, and messages are often inconsistent and incongruent with the situation. Destructive patterns of communication tend to inhibit healthful nurturing and decrease individual feelings of self-worth.

Major Concepts

Double-Bind Communication

Double-bind communication occurs when a statement is made and succeeded by a contradictory statement. It also occurs when a statement is made accompanied by nonverbal expression that is inconsistent with the verbal communication. These incompatible communications can interfere with ego development in an individual and promote mistrust of all communications. Double-bind communication often results in a "damned if I do and damned if I don't" situation.

> **EXAMPLE**
>
> A mother freely gives and receives hugs and kisses from her 6-year-old son some of the time, while at other times she pushes him away saying, "Big boys don't act like that." The little boy receives a conflicting message and is presented with an impossible dilemma: "To please my mother I must not show her that I love her, but if I do not show her that I love her, I'm afraid I will lose her."

Pseudomutuality and Pseudohostility

A healthy functioning individual is able to relate to other people while still maintaining a sense of separate identity. In a dysfunctional family, patterns of interaction may be reflected in the remoteness or closeness of relationships. These relationships may reflect erratic interaction (i.e., sometimes remote and sometimes close), or inappropriate interaction (i.e., excessive closeness or remoteness).

Pseudomutuality and pseudohostility are seen as collective defenses against reality of the underlying meaning of the relationships in a dysfunctional family system. **Pseudomutuality** is characterized by a facade of mutual regard. Emotional investment is directed at maintaining outward representation of reciprocal fulfillment rather than in the relationship itself. The style of relating is fixed and rigid, and pseudomutuality allows family members to deny underlying fears of separation and hostility.

> **EXAMPLE**
>
> Janet, age 16, is the only child of State Senator J. and his wife. Janet was recently involved in a joyriding experience with a group of teenagers her parents call "the wrong crowd." In family therapy, Mrs. J. says, "We have always been a close family. I can't imagine why she is doing these things." Senator J. states, "I don't know another

colleague who has a family that is as close as mine." Janet responds, "Yes, we are close. I just don't see my parents very much. Dad has been in politics since I was a baby, and Mom is always with him. I wish I could spend more time with them. But we are a close family."

Pseudohostility is also a fixed and rigid style of relating, but the facade being maintained is that of a state of chronic conflict and alienation among family members. This relationship pattern allows family members to deny underlying fears of tenderness and intimacy.

EXAMPLE

Jack, 14, and his sister Jill, 15, will have nothing to do with each other. When they are together they can agree on nothing, and the barrage of "putdowns" is constant. This behavior reflects pseudohostility used by individuals who are afraid to reveal feelings of intimacy.

Schism and Skew

Lidz, Cornelison, Fleck, and Terry (1957) observed two patterns within families that relate to a dysfunctional marital dyad. A **marital schism** is defined as "a state of severe chronic disequilibrium and discord, with recurrent threats of separation." Each partner undermines the other, mutual trust is absent, and a competition exists for closeness with the children. Often a partner establishes an alliance with his or her parent against the spouse. Children lack appropriate role models. **Marital skew** describes a relationship in which there is lack of equal partnership. One partner dominates the relationship and the other partner. The marriage remains intact as long as the passive partner allows the domination to continue. Children also lack role models when a marital skew exists.

Goal and Techniques of Therapy

The goal of strategic family therapy is to create change in destructive behavior and communication patterns among family members. The identified family *problem* is the unit of therapy, and all family members need not be counseled together. In fact, strategic therapists may prefer to see subgroups or individuals separately in an effort to achieve problem resolution. Therapy is oriented in the present, and the therapist assumes full responsibility for devising an effective strategy for family change. Therapeutic techniques include the following:

■ **Paradoxical Intervention.** A paradox can be called a contradiction in therapy, or

"prescribing the symptom." With **paradoxical intervention,** the therapist requests that the family continue to engage in the behavior that they are trying to change. Alternatively, specific directions may be given for continuing the defeating behavior. For example, a couple that regularly engages in insulting shouting matches is instructed to have one of these encounters on Tuesdays and Thursdays from 8:30 to 9:00 p.m. Boyer and Jeffrey (1994) explained:

A family using its maladaptive behavior to control or punish other people loses control of the situation when it finds itself continuing the behavior under a therapist's direction and being praised for following instructions. If the family disobeys the therapist's instruction, the price it pays is sacrificing the old behavior pattern and experiencing more satisfying ways of interacting with one another. A family that maintains it has no control over its behavior, or whose members contend that others must change before they can themselves, suddenly finds itself unable to defend such statements. (p. 125)

■ **Reframing.** Goldenberg and associates (2011) describe **reframing** as "relabeling problematic behavior by viewing it in a new, more positive light that emphasizes its good intention." Therefore, with reframing, the *behavior* may not actually change, but the *consequences* of the behavior may change, because of a change in the meaning attached to the behavior. This technique is sometimes referred to as *positive reframing.*

EXAMPLE

Tom has a construction job and makes a comfortable living for his wife, Sue, and their two children. Tom and Sue have been arguing a lot and came to the therapist for counseling. Sue says Tom frequently drinks too much and is often late getting home from work. Tom counters, "I never used to drink on my way home from work, but Sue started complaining to me the minute I walked in the door about being so dirty and about tracking dirt and mud on 'her nice, clean floors.' It was the last straw when she made me undress before I came in the house and leave my dirty clothes and shoes in the garage. I thought a man's home was his castle. Well, I sure don't feel like a king. I need a few stiff drinks to face her nagging!"

The therapist used reframing to attempt change by helping Sue to view the situation in a more positive light. He suggested to Sue that she try to change her thinking by focusing on how much her husband must love her and her children to work as hard has he does. He asked her to focus on the dirty clothes and shoes as symbols of his love for them and to respond to his "dirty" arrivals home with greater affection. This positive reframing set the tone for healing and for increased intimacy within the marital relationship.

The Evolution of Family Therapy

Bowen's family theory and the structural and strategic models are sometimes referred to as basic models of family therapy. Goldenberg and Goldenberg (2008) stated:

> While noteworthy differences continue to exist in the theoretical assumptions each school of thought makes about the nature and origin of psychological dysfunction, in what precisely they look for in understanding family patterns, and in their strategies for therapeutic intervention, in practice the trend today is toward eclecticism and integration in family therapy. (p. 146)

Nichols (2010) suggested that contemporary family therapists "borrow from each other's arsenal of techniques." The basic models described here have provided a foundation for the progression and growth of the discipline of family therapy. Examples of newer models include the following:

- **Narrative therapy:** An approach to treatment that emphasizes the role of the stories people construct about their experience (Nichols, 2010, p. 463).

- **Feminist family therapy:** A form of collaborative, egalitarian, nonsexist intervention, applicable to both men and women, addressing family gender roles, patriarchal attitudes, and social and economic inequalities in male-female relationships (Goldenberg & Goldenberg, 2008, p. 468).

- **Social constructionist therapy:** Concerned with the assumptions or premises different family members hold about the problem. Efforts are focused on engaging families in conversations to solicit everyone's views, and not in imposing on families what is considered objectivity, truth, or "established knowledge" (Goldenberg & Goldenberg, 2008, p. 347).

- **Psychoeducational family therapy:** Therapy that emphasizes educating family members to help them understand and cope with a seriously disturbed family member (Nichols, 2010, p. 464).

The goal of most family therapy models is to provide the opportunity for change based on family members' perceptions of available options. The basic differences among models arise in how they go about achieving this goal. Goldenberg and Goldenberg (2008) stated:

> Regardless of procedures, all attempt to create a therapeutic environment conducive to self-examination, to reduce discomfort and conflict, to mobilize family resilience and empowerment, and to help the family members improve their overall functioning. (p. 440)

The Nursing Process—A Case Study

Assessment

Wright and Leahey (2009) have developed the Calgary Family Assessment Model (CFAM), a multidimensional model originally adapted from a framework developed by Tomm and Sanders (1983). The CFAM consists of three major categories: structural, developmental, and functional. Wright and Leahey (2009) stated:

> Each category contains several subcategories. It is important for each nurse to decide which subcategories are relevant and appropriate to explore and assess with each family at each point in time. That is, not all subcategories need to be assessed at a first meeting with a family, and some subcategories need never be assessed. If the nurse uses too many subcategories, he or she may become overwhelmed by all the data. If the nurse and the family discuss too few subcategories, each may have a distorted view of the family's strengths or problems and the family situation. (pp. 47–48)

A diagram of the CFAM is presented in Figure 11–3. The three major categories are listed, along with the subcategories for assessment under each. This diagram is used to assess the Marino family, a case study presented in Box 11-1.

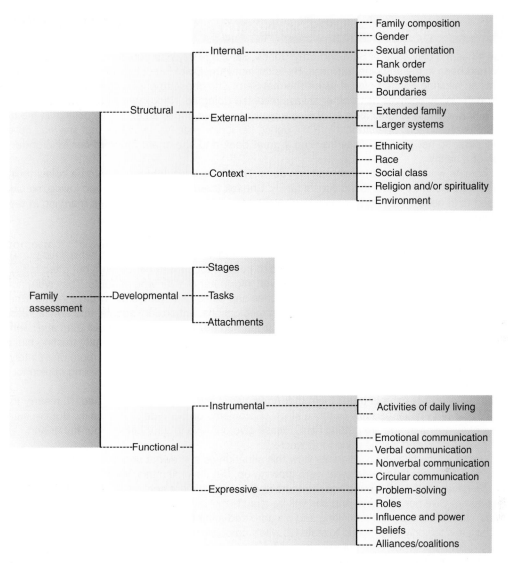

FIGURE 11–3 Branching diagram of the Calgary Family Assessment Model (CFAM). (From Wright, L. M., & Leahey, M. [2009]. *Nurses and families: A guide to family assessment and intervention* [5th ed.]. Philadelphia: F.A. Davis, with permission.)

BOX 11-1 The Marino Family—A Case Study

John and Nancy Marino have been married for 19 years. They have a 17-year-old son, Peter, and a 15-year-old daughter, Anna. Anna was recently hospitalized for taking an overdose of fluoxetine, her mother's prescription antidepressant. The family is attending family therapy sessions while Anna is in the hospital. Anna states, "I just couldn't take the fighting anymore! Our house is an awful place to be. Everyone hates each other, and everyone is unhappy. Dad drinks too much and Mom is always sick! Peter stays away as much as he can and I don't blame him. I would too if I had someplace to stay. I just thought I'd be better off dead."

John Marino, age 44, is the oldest of five children. His father, Paulo, age 66, is a first-generation Italian American whose parents emigrated from Italy in the early 1900s. Paulo retired last year after 32 years as a cutter in a meatpacking plant. His wife, Carla, age 64, has never worked outside the home. John and his siblings all worked at minimum-wage jobs during high school, and John and his two brothers worked their way through college. His two sisters married young, and both are housewives and mothers. John was able to go to law school with the help of loans, grants, and scholarships. He has held several positions since graduation and is currently employed as a corporate attorney for a large aircraft company.

Continued

BOX 11-1 The Marino Family—A Case Study—cont'd

Nancy, age 43, is the only child of Sam and Ethyl Jones. Sam, age 67, inherited a great deal of money from his family who had been in the shipping business. He is currently the Chief Executive Officer of this business. Ethyl, also 67, was an aspiring concert pianist when she met Sam. She chose to give up her career for marriage and family, although Nancy believes her mother always resented doing so. Nancy was reared in an affluent lifestyle. She attended private boarding schools as she was growing up and chose an exclusive college in the East to pursue her interest in art. She studied in Paris during her junior year. Nancy states that she was never emotionally close to her parents. They traveled a great deal, and she spent much of her time under the supervision of a nanny.

Nancy's parents were opposed to her marrying John. They perceived John's family to be below their social status. Nancy, on the other hand, loved John's family. She felt them to be very warm and loving, so unlike what she was used to in her own family. Her family is Protestant and also disapproved of her marrying in the Roman Catholic Church.

FAMILY DYNAMICS

As their marriage progressed, Nancy's health became very fragile. She had continued her artistic pursuits but seemed to achieve little satisfaction from it. She tried to keep in touch with her parents but often felt spurned by them. They traveled a great deal and often did not even inform her of their whereabouts. They were not present at the birth of her children. She experiences many aches and pains and spends many days in bed. She sees several physicians, who have prescribed various pain medications, antianxiety agents, and antidepressants but can find nothing organically wrong. Five years ago she learned that John had been having an affair with his secretary. He promised to break it off and fired the secretary, but Nancy has had difficulty trusting him since that time. She brings up his infidelity whenever they have an argument, which is more and more often lately. When he is home, John drinks, usually until he falls asleep. Peter frequently comes home smelling of alcohol and a number of times has been clearly intoxicated.

When Nancy called her parents to tell them that Anna was in the hospital, Ethyl replied, "I'm sorry to hear that, dear. We certainly never had any of those kinds of problems on our side of the family. But I'm sure everything will be okay now that you are getting help. Please give our love to your family. Your father and I are leaving for Europe on Saturday and will be gone for 6 weeks."

Although more supportive, John's parents view this situation as somewhat shameful for the family. John's dad responded, "We had hard times when you were growing up, but never like this. We always took care of our own problems. We never had to tell a bunch of strangers about them. It's not right to air your dirty laundry in public. Bring Anna home. Give her your love and she will be okay."

In therapy, Nancy blames John's drinking and his admitted affair for all their problems. John states that he drinks because it is the only way he can tolerate his wife's complaining about his behavior and her many illnesses. Peter is very quiet most of the time but says he will be glad when he graduates in 4 months and can leave "this looney bunch of people." Anna cries as she listens to her family in therapy and says, "Nothing's ever going to change."

Structural Assessment

A graphic representation of the Marino family structure is presented in the genogram in Figure 11–4.

Internal Structure

The Marino family consists of a husband, a wife, and their biological son and daughter who live together in the same home. They conform to the traditional gender roles. John is the eldest child from a rather large family, and Nancy has no siblings. In this family, their son, Peter, is the first-born and his sister, Anna, is 2 years younger. Neither spousal, sibling, nor spousal-sibling subsystems appear to be close in this family, and some are clearly conflictual. Problematic subsystems include John-Nancy, John-Nancy-children, and Nancy-Ethyl. The subsystem boundaries are quite rigid, and the family members appear to be emotionally disengaged from one another.

External Structure

This family has ties to extended family, although the availability of support is questionable. Nancy's parents offered little emotional support to her as a developing child. They never approved of her marriage to John and still remain distant and cold. John's family consists of a father, mother, two brothers, and two sisters. They are warm and supportive most of the time, but cultural influences interfere with their understanding of this current

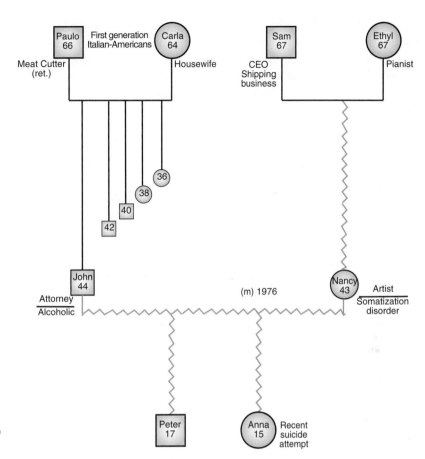

FIGURE 11–4 Genogram of the Marino family.

situation. At this time, the Marino family is probably receiving the most support from health-care professionals who have intervened during Anna's hospitalization.

Context

John is a second-generation Italian American. His family of origin is large, warm, and supportive. However, John's parents believe that family problems should be dealt with in the family, and disapprove of bringing "strangers" in to hear what they consider to be private information. They believe that Anna's physical condition should be stabilized, and then she should be discharged to deal with family problems at home.

John and Nancy were reared in different social classes. In John's family, money was not available to seek out professional help for every problem that arose. Italian cultural beliefs promote the provision of help within the nuclear and extended family network. If outside counseling is sought, it is often with the family priest. John and Nancy did not seek this type of counseling because they no longer attend church regularly.

In Nancy's family, money was available to obtain the very best professional help at the first sign of

trouble. However, Nancy's parents refused to acknowledge, both then and now, that any difficulty ever existed in their family situation.

The Marino family lives comfortably on John's salary as a corporate attorney. They have health insurance and access to any referrals that are deemed necessary. They are well educated but have been attempting to deny the dysfunctional dynamics that exist in their family.

Developmental Assessment

The Marino family falls within the "family with adolescents" stage of McGoldrick and associates' family life cycle. In this stage, parents are expected to respond to adolescents' requests for increasing independence, while being available to continue to fulfill dependency needs. They may also be required to provide additional support to aging grandparents. This may be a time when parents may also begin to reexamine their own marital and career issues.

The Marino family is not fulfilling the dependency needs of its adolescents; in fact, they may be establishing premature independence. The parents are absorbed in their own personal problems to the exclusion of their children. Peter responds to this neglect by staying away as much as possible, drinking with his friends, and planning to leave home at the first opportunity. Anna's attempted suicide is a cry for help. She has needs that are unfulfilled by her parents, and this crisis situation may be required for them to recognize that a problem exists. This may be the time when they begin to reexamine their unresolved marital issues. Extended family are still self-supporting and do not require assistance from John and Nancy at this time.

Functional Assessment

Instrumental Functioning

This family has managed to adjust to the maladaptive functioning in an effort to meet physical activities of daily living. They subsist on fast food, or sometimes Nancy or Anna will prepare a meal. Seldom do they sit down at the table to eat together. Nancy must take pain medication or sedatives to sleep. John usually drinks himself to sleep. Anna and Peter take care of their own needs independently. Often they do not even see their parents in the evenings. Each manages to do fairly well in school. Peter says, "I don't intend to ruin my chances of getting out of this hell hole as soon as I can!"

Expressive Functioning

John and Nancy Marino argue a great deal about many topics. This family seldom shows affection to one another. Nancy and Anna express sadness with tears, whereas John and Peter have a tendency to withdraw or turn to alcohol when experiencing unhappiness. Nancy somaticizes her internal pain, and numbs this pain with medication. Anna internalized her emotional pain until it became unbearable. A notable lack of constructive communication is evident.

This family is unable to solve its problems effectively. In fact, it is unlikely that it has even identified its problems, which undoubtedly have been in existence for a long while. These problems have only recently been revealed in light of Anna's suicide attempt.

Diagnosis

The following nursing diagnoses were identified for the Marino family:

■ **Interrupted family processes** related to unsuccessful achievement of family developmental tasks and dysfunctional coping strategies evidenced by inability of family members to relate to each other in an adaptive manner; adolescents' unmet dependency needs; inability of family members to express a wide range of feelings and to send and receive clear messages.

■ **Disabled family coping** related to highly ambivalent family relationships and lack of support evidenced by inability to problem-solve; each member copes in response to dysfunctional family processes with destructive behavior (John drinks, Nancy somaticizes, Peter drinks and withdraws; and Anna attempts suicide).

Outcome Identification

The following criteria were identified as measurement of outcomes in counseling of the Marino family:

■ Family members will demonstrate effective communication patterns.

■ Family members will express feelings openly and honestly.

■ Family members will establish more adaptive coping strategies.

■ Family members will be able to identify destructive patterns of functioning and problem-solve them effectively.

■ Boundaries between spousal subsystems and spousal-children subsystems will become more clearly defined.

■ Family members will establish stronger bonds with extended family.

Planning/Implementation

The Marino family will undoubtedly require many months of outpatient therapy. It is even likely that each member will need individual psychotherapy in addition to the family therapy. Once Anna has been stabilized physiologically and is discharged from the hospital, family/individual therapy will begin.

Several strategies for family therapy have been discussed in this chapter. As mentioned previously, family therapy has a strong theoretical framework and is performed by individuals with specialized education in family theory and process. Some advanced practice nurses possess the credentials required to perform family therapy. It is important, however, for all nurses to have some knowledge about working with families, to be able to assess family interaction, and to recognize when problems exist.

Some interventions with the Marino family might include the following:

1. Create a therapeutic environment that fosters trust, and in which the family members can feel safe and comfortable. The nurse can promote this type of environment by being empathetic, listening actively (see Chapter 8),

accepting feelings and attitudes, and being nonjudgmental.

2. Promote effective communication by
   a. Seeking clarification when vague and generalized statements are made (e.g., Anna states, "I just want my family to be like my friends' families." Nurse: "Anna, would you please explain to the group exactly what you mean by that?").
   b. Setting clear limits (e.g., "Peter, it is okay to state when you are angry about something that has been said. It is not okay to throw the chair against the wall.").
   c. Being consistent and fair (e.g., "I encourage each of you to contribute to the group process and to respect one another's opportunity to contribute equally.").
   d. Addressing each individual clearly and directly and encouraging family members to do the same (e.g., "Nancy, I think it would be more appropriate if you directed that statement to John instead of to me.").

3. Identify patterns of interaction that interfere with successful problem resolution. For example, John asks Nancy many "Why?" questions that keep her on the defensive. He criticizes her for "always being sick." Nancy responds by frequently reminding John of his infidelity. Peter and Anna interrupt each other and their parents when the level of conflict reaches a certain point. Provide examples of more appropriate ways to communicate that can improve interpersonal relations and lead to more effective patterns of interaction.

4. Help the Marino family to identify problems that may necessitate change. Encourage each member to discuss a family process that he or she would like to change. As a group, promote discussion of what must take place for change to occur and allow each member to explore whether he or she could realistically cooperate with the necessary requirements for change.

5. As the problem-solving process progresses, encourage all family members to express honest feelings. Address each one directly, "John (Nancy, Peter, Anna), how do you feel about what the others are suggesting?" Ensure that all participants understand that each member may express honest feelings (e.g., anger, sadness, fear, anxiety, guilt, disgust, helplessness) without criticism, judgment, or fear of personal reprisal.

6. Avoid becoming triangled in the family emotional system. Remain neutral and objective. Do not take sides in family disagreements; instead, provide alternative explanations and suggestions (e.g., "Perhaps we can look at that situation in a different light. . .").

7. Reframe vague problem descriptions into ones for which resolution is more realistic. For example, rather than defining the problem as "We don't love each other any more," the problem could be defined as, "We do not spend time together in family activities any more." This definition evolves from the family members' description of what they mean by the more general problem description.

8. Discuss present coping strategies. Encourage each family member to describe how he or she copes with stress and with the adversity within the family. Explore each member's possible contribution to the family's problems. Encourage family members to discuss possible solutions among themselves.

9. Identify community resources that may assist individual family members and provide support for establishing more adaptive coping mechanisms: for example, Alcoholics Anonymous for John; Al-Anon for Nancy; and Alateen for Peter and Anna. Other groups that may be of assistance to this family include Emotions Anonymous, Parent's Support Group, Families Helping Families, Marriage Enrichment, Parents of Teenagers, and We Saved Our Marriage (WESOM). Local self-help networks often provide a directory of resources within specific communities.

10. Discuss with the family the possible need for psychotherapy for individual members. Provide names of therapists who would perform assessments to determine individual needs. Encourage follow-through with appointments.

11. Assist family members in planning leisure-time activities together. This could include time to play together, exercise together, or engage in a shared project.

Evaluation

Evaluation is the final step in the nursing process. In this step, progress toward attainment of outcomes is measured.

1. Do family members demonstrate effective patterns of communication?

2. Can family members express feelings openly and honestly without fear of reprisal?

3. Can family members accept their own personal contribution to the family's problems?

4. Can individual members identify maladaptive coping methods and express a desire to improve?

5. Do family members work together to solve problems?

6. Can family members identify resources in the community from which they can seek assistance and support?

7. Do family members express a desire to form stronger bonds with the extended family?

8. Are family members willing to seek individual psychotherapy?

9. Are family members pursuing shared activities?

Summary and Key Points

■ Nurses must have sufficient knowledge of family functioning to assess family interaction and recognize when problems exist.

■ McGoldrick, Carter, and Garcia-Preto (2011) identified stages that describe the family life cycle. They include the following:
- The single young adult
- The family joined through marriage/union
- The family with young children
- The family with adolescents
- The family launching children and moving on in midlife
- The family in later life (late middle age to end of life)

■ Tasks of families experiencing divorce and remarriage, and those that vary according to cultural norms, were also presented.

■ Families are assessed as functional or dysfunctional based on the following six elements: communication, self-concept reinforcement, family members' expectations, handling differences, family interactional patterns, and family climate.

■ Bowen viewed the family as a system that was composed of various subsystems. His theoretical approach to family therapy includes eight major concepts: differentiation of self, triangles, nuclear family emotional process, family projection process, multigenerational transmission process, sibling position, emotional cutoff, and societal emotional process.

■ In the structural model of family therapy, the family is viewed as a social system within which the individual lives and to which the individual must adapt.

■ In the strategic model of family therapy, communication is viewed as the foundation of functioning. Functional families are open systems where clear and precise messages are sent and received. Dysfunctional families are viewed as partially closed systems in which communication is vague, and messages are often inconsistent and incongruent with the situation.

■ Many family therapists today follow an eclectic approach and incorporate concepts from several models into their practices.

■ The nursing process is used as a framework for assessing, diagnosing, planning, implementing, and evaluating care to families who require assistance to maintain or regain adaptive functioning.

 DavisPlus   Additional info available @ davisplus.fadavis.com

Review Questions
Self-Examination/Learning Exercise

*Select the answer that is **most** appropriate for each of the following questions:*

1. The nurse-therapist is counseling the Smith family: Mr. and Mrs. Smith, 10-year-old Rob, and 8-year-old Lisa. When Mr. and Mrs. Smith start to argue, Rob hits Lisa and Lisa starts to cry. The Smiths then turn their attention to comforting Lisa and scolding Rob, complaining that he is "out of control and we don't know what to do about his behavior." These dynamics are an example of
   a. Double-bind messages.
   b. Triangulation.
   c. Pseudohostility.
   d. Multigenerational transmission.

Review Questions—cont'd
Self-Examination/Learning Exercise

2. Using Bowen's systems approach with a family in therapy, the therapist would:
   a. Try to change family principles that may be promoting dysfunctional behavior patterns.
   b. Strive to create change in destructive behavior through improvement in communication and interaction patterns.
   c. Encourage increase in the differentiation of individual family members.
   d. Promote change in dysfunctional behavior by encouraging the formation of more diffuse boundaries between family members.

3. Using the structural approach with a family in therapy, the therapist would:
   a. Try to change family principles that may be promoting dysfunctional behavior patterns.
   b. Strive to create change in destructive behavior through improvement in communications and interaction patterns.
   c. Encourage increase in the differentiation of individual family members.
   d. Promote change in dysfunctional behavior by encouraging the formation of more diffuse boundaries between family members.

4. Using the strategic approach with a family in therapy, the therapist would:
   a. Try to change family principles that may be promoting dysfunctional behavior patterns.
   b. Strive to create change in destructive behavior through improvement in communication and interaction patterns.
   c. Encourage increase in the differentiation of individual family members.
   d. Promote change in dysfunctional behavior by encouraging the formation of more diffuse boundaries between family members.

5. Carol, a nurse in a family medicine outpatient clinic, conducts initial interviews when new families are referred. She has just finished interviewing a mother who has come to the clinic with her three children, ages 5, 7, and 11. The mother says to the oldest child, "You have been such a help to me, playing with your brothers while I talk to the nurse." In assessing family interaction, the nurse recognizes this statement as a direct indicator of
   a. Family climate.
   b. Family members' expectations.
   c. Handling differences.
   d. Self-concept reinforcement.

6. The intermittent exiting and entering of various family members and reestablishing of the bond of the dyadic couple relationship are characteristics associated with which stage of family development:
   a. The family joined through marriage/union.
   b. The family with adolescents.
   c. The family launching grown children.
   d. The family in later life.

7. The nurse psychotherapist is working with the Jones family in the outpatient mental health clinic. The husband says, "We can't agree on anything! And it seems like every time we disagree on something it ends up in a screaming match." Which of the following prescriptions by the nurse represents a paradoxical intervention for the Jones family?
   a. Mr. and Mrs. Jones must not have a disagreement for one full day.
   b. Mr. and Mrs. Jones will yell at each other on Tuesdays and Thursdays from 8:00 p.m. until 8:10 p.m.
   c. Mr. and Mrs. Jones must refrain from yelling at each other until the next counseling session.
   d. Mr. and Mrs. Jones must not discuss serious issues until they can do so without yelling at each other.

Continued

Review Questions—cont'd
Self-Examination/Learning Exercise

8. Mr. and Mrs. Jones have been married for 21 years. Mr. Jones is the family breadwinner, and Mrs. Jones has never worked outside the home. Mr. Jones has always made all the decisions for the family and Mrs. Jones has always been compliant. According to the strategic model of family therapy, this is an example of which of the following?
   a. Marital schism.
   b. Pseudomutuality.
   c. Marital skew.
   d. Pseudohostility.

9. Jack and Ann have come to the clinic for family therapy. They have been married for 18 years. Jack had an affair with his secretary 5 years ago. He fired the secretary and assures Ann and the nurse that he has been faithful ever since. Jack tells the nurse, "We have never been able to get along with each other. We can't talk about anything...all we do is shout at each other. And every time she gets angry with me, she brings up my infidelity. I can't even imagine how many times each of us has threatened divorce over the years. Our kids don't have any idea what it is like to have parents who get along with each other. I've really had enough!" The nurse would most likely document which of the following in her assessment of this couple?
   a. Marital skew.
   b. Pseudohostility.
   c. Double-bind communication.
   d. Marital schism.

10. Mr. and Mrs. Smith and their 3 children (ages 5, 8, and 10) are in therapy with the nurse psychotherapist. Mrs. Smith tells the nurse that their marriage has been "falling apart" since the birth of their youngest child, Tom. She explains that they "did not want a third child, and I became pregnant even after my husband had undergone a vasectomy. We were very angry, the pregnancy was a problematic one, and the child has been difficult since birth. We had problems before he was born, but since Tom was born, things have gone from bad to worse. No one can control him, and he is wrecking our family!" The nurse assesses that which of the following may be occurring in this family?
   a. Scapegoating.
   b. Triangling.
   c. Disengagement.
   d. Enmeshment.

References

Boyer, P. A., & Jeffrey, R. J. (1994). *A guide for the family therapist.* Northvale, NJ: Jason Aronson.

Bramlett, M. D., & Mosher, W. D. (2002). Cohabitation, marriage, divorce, and remarriage in the United States. National Center for Health Statistics. *Vital and Health Statistics, 23*(22).

Centers for Disease Control and Prevention. (2010). Marriage and cohabitation in the United States: A statistical portrait based on Cycle 6 (2002) of the National Survey of Family Growth. National Center for Health Statistics. *Vital and Health Statistics, 23*(28).

Earp, J. K. (2008). Korean Americans. In J. N. Giger & R. E. Davidhizar (Eds.), *Transcultural nursing: Assessment and Intervention* (5th ed., pp. 619–641). St. Louis: Mosby.

Georgetown Family Center. (2010a). *Bowen theory: Differentiation of self.* Retrieved July 18, 2010, from http://www.thebowencenter.org/pages/conceptds.html

Georgetown Family Center. (2010b). *Bowen theory: Societal emotional process.* Retrieved July 18, 2010, from http://www.thebowencenter.org/pages/conceptsep.html

Goldenberg, I., & Goldenberg. H. (2008). *Family therapy: An overview* (7th ed.). Belmont, CA: Brooks/Cole.

Goldenberg, I., Goldenberg, H., & Pelavin, E. G. (2011). Family therapy. In R. J. Corsini & D. Wedding (Eds.), *Current psychotherapies* (9th ed., pp. 417–453). Belmont, CA: Brooks/Cole.

Kaakinen, J. R., Hanson, S. M. H., & Denham, S. A. (2010). Family health care nursing: An introduction. In J. R. Kaakinen, V. Gedaly-Duff, D. P. Coehlo, & S. M. H. Hanson (Eds.), *Family health care nursing* (4th ed., pp. 3–33). Philadelphia: F.A. Davis.

Kreider, R. M. (2008). *Living arrangements of children: 2004.* Current Population Reports, P70-114. Washington, DC: U.S. Census Bureau.

Kreider, R. M., & Elliott, D. B. (2009). *America's families and living arrangements: 2007.* Current Population Reports, P20-561. Washington, DC: U.S. Census Bureau.

Kreider, R. M., & Fields, J. M. (2002). *Number, timing, and duration of marriages and divorces.* Current Population Reports, P70-80. Washington, DC: U.S. Census Bureau.

Leman, K. (2004). *The birth order book: Why you are the way you are.* Grand Rapids, MI: Baker Books.

McGoldrick, M., Carter, B., & Garcia-Preto, N. (2011). Overview: The life cycle in its changing context. In M. McGoldrick, B. Carter, & N. Garcia-Preto (Eds.), *The expanded family life cycle* (4th ed., pp.1-19). Boston: Allyn & Bacon.

Nichols, M. P. (2010). *Family therapy: Concepts and methods* (9th ed.). Boston: Allyn & Bacon.

Purnell, L. D. (2008). The Purnell model for cultural competence. In L. D. Purnell & B. J. Paulanka (Eds.), *Transcultural health care: A culturally competent approach* (3rd ed., pp. 19–55). Philadelphia: F.A. Davis.

Tomm, K., & Sanders, G. (1983). Family assessment in a problem oriented record. In J. C. Hansen & B. F. Keeney (Eds.), *Diagnosis and assessment in family therapy.* London: Aspen Systems.

U.S. Catholic Church. (2003). *Catechism of the Catholic Church* (2nd ed.). New York: Doubleday Religion.

Valley, E. (2005). The changing nature of the Jewish family. *Contact: The Journal of Jewish Life Network, 7*(3), 1–16.

Wright, L. M., & Leahey, M. (2009). *Nurses and families: A guide to family assessment and intervention* (5th ed.). Philadelphia: F.A. Davis.

Xu, Y., & Chang, K. (2008). Chinese Americans. In J. N. Giger & R. E. Davidhizar (Eds.), *Transcultural nursing: Assessment and intervention* (5th ed., pp. 442–466). St. Louis: Mosby.

Classical References

Bowen, M. (1971). The use of family theory in clinical practice. In J. Haley (Ed.), *Changing families.* New York: Grune & Stratton.

Bowen, M. (1976). Theory in the practice of psychotherapy. In P. Guerin (Ed.), *Family therapy: Theory and practice.* New York: Gardner Press.

Bowen, M. (1978). *Family therapy in clinical practice.* New York: Jason Aronson.

Lidz, T., Cornelison, A., Fleck, S., & Terry, D. (1957). The intrafamilial environment of schizophrenic patients: II. Marital schism and marital skew. *American Journal of Psychiatry, 114,* 241–248.

Minuchin, S. (1974). *Families and family therapy.* Cambridge, MA: Harvard University Press.

Milieu Therapy—The Therapeutic Community

CHAPTER OUTLINE

KEY TERMS

milieu

therapeutic community

OBJECTIVES
After reading this chapter, the student will be able to:

1. Define *milieu therapy.*
2. Explain the goal of therapeutic community/
   milieu therapy.
3. Identify seven basic assumptions of a
   therapeutic community.
4. Discuss conditions that characterize a
   therapeutic community.
5. Identify the various therapies that may be
   included within the program of the therapeutic community and the health-care
   workers who make up the interdisciplinary
   treatment team.
6. Describe the role of the nurse on the
   interdisciplinary treatment team.

HOMEWORK ASSIGNMENT
Please read the chapter and answer the following questions:

1. How are unit rules established in a therapeutic community setting?
2. Which member of the interdisciplinary
   treatment team has a focus on rehabilitation and vocational training?
3. How are client responsibilities assigned in
   the therapeutic community setting?
4. Which member of the interdisciplinary
   treatment team serves as leader?

Standard 5c of the *Psychiatric-Mental Health Nursing: Scope and Standards of Practice* (American Nurses Association [ANA], 2007) states that, "The psychiatric-mental health nurse provides, structures, and maintains a safe and therapeutic environment in collaboration with patients, families, and other health care clinicians" (p. 39).

This chapter defines and explains the goal of milieu therapy. The conditions necessary for a therapeutic environment are discussed, and the roles of the various health-care workers within the interdisciplinary team are delineated. An interpretation of the nurse's role in milieu therapy is included.

Milieu, Defined

The word **milieu** is French for "middle." The English translation of the word is "surroundings, or environment." In psychiatry, therapy involving the milieu, or environment, may be called milieu therapy, the **therapeutic community,** or the therapeutic environment. The goal of milieu therapy is to manipulate the environment so that all aspects of the client's hospital experience are considered therapeutic. Within this therapeutic community setting, the client is expected to learn adaptive coping, interaction, and relationship skills that can be generalized to other aspects of his or her life.

CORE CONCEPT

Milieu Therapy

A scientific structuring of the environment in order to effect behavioral changes and to improve the psychological health and functioning of the individual (Skinner, 1979).

Current Status of the Therapeutic Community

Milieu therapy came into its own during the 1960s through early 1980s. During this period, psychiatric inpatient treatment provided sufficient time to implement programs of therapy that were aimed at social rehabilitation. Nursing's focus of establishing interpersonal relationships with clients fit well within this concept of therapy. Patients were encouraged to be active participants in their therapy, and individual autonomy was emphasized.

The current focus of inpatient psychiatric care has changed. Hall (1995) stated:

> Care in inpatient psychiatric facilities can now be characterized as short and biologically based. By the time patients have stabilized enough to benefit from the socialization that would take place in a milieu as treatment program, they [often] have been discharged. (p. 51)

Although strategies for milieu therapy are still used, they have been modified to conform to the short-term approach to care or to outpatient treatment programs. Some programs (e.g., those for children and adolescents, clients with substance addictions, and geriatric clients) have successfully adapted the concepts of milieu treatment to their specialty needs (Bowler, 1991; DeSocio, Bowllan, & Staschak, 1997; Whall, 1991).

Echternacht (2001) suggested that more emphasis should be placed on unstructured components of milieu therapy. She described the unstructured components as a multitude of complex interactions between clients, staff, and visitors that occur around the clock. Echternacht called these interactions "fluid group work." They involve spontaneous opportunities within the milieu environment for the psychiatric nurse to provide "on-the-spot therapeutic interventions designed to enhance socialization competency and interpersonal relationship awareness. Emphasis is on social skills and activities in the context of interpersonal interactions." (p. 40). With fluid group work, the nurse applies psychotherapeutic knowledge and skills to brief clinical encounters that occur spontaneously in the therapeutic milieu setting. Echternacht (2001) believed that, by using these techniques, nurses can "reclaim their milieu therapy functions in the midst of a changing health care environment" (p. 40).

Many of the original concepts of milieu therapy are presented in this chapter. It is important to remember that a number of modifications to these concepts have been applied in practice for use in a variety of settings.

Basic Assumptions

Skinner (1979) outlined seven basic assumptions on which a therapeutic community is based:

1. **The Health in Each Individual Is to Be Realized and Encouraged to Grow.** All individuals are considered to have strengths as well as limitations. These healthy aspects of the individual are identified and serve as a foundation for growth in the personality and in the ability to function more adaptively and productively in all aspects of life.

2. **Every Interaction Is an Opportunity for Therapeutic Intervention.** Within this structured setting, it is virtually impossible to avoid interpersonal interaction. The ideal situation exists for clients to improve communication and relationship development skills. Learning occurs from immediate feedback of personal perceptions.

3. **The Client Owns His or Her Own Environment.** Clients make decisions and solve problems related to government of the unit. In this way, personal needs for autonomy as well as needs that pertain to the group as a whole are fulfilled.

4. **Each Client Owns His or Her Behavior.** Each individual within the therapeutic community is

expected to take responsibility for his or her own behavior.

5. **Peer Pressure Is a Useful and a Powerful Tool.** Behavioral group norms are established through peer pressure. Feedback is direct and frequent, so that behaving in a manner acceptable to the other members of the community becomes essential.

6. **Inappropriate Behaviors Are Dealt With as They Occur.** Individuals examine the significance of their behavior, look at how it affects other people, and discuss more appropriate ways of behaving in certain situations.

7. **Restrictions and Punishment Are to Be Avoided.** Destructive behaviors can usually be controlled with group discussion. However, if an individual requires external controls, temporary isolation is preferred over lengthy restriction or other harsh punishment.

Conditions That Promote a Therapeutic Community

In a therapeutic community setting, everything that happens to the client, or within the client's environment, is considered to be part of the treatment program. The community setting is the foundation for the program of treatment. Community factors—such as social interactions, the physical structure of the treatment setting, and schedule of activities—may generate negative responses from some clients. These stressful experiences are used as examples to help the client learn how to manage stress more adaptively in real-life situations.

Under what conditions, then, is a hospital environment considered therapeutic? A number of criteria have been identified:

1. **Basic Physiological Needs Are Fulfilled.** As Maslow (1968) suggested, individuals do not move to higher levels of functioning until the basic biological needs for food, water, air, sleep, exercise, elimination, shelter, and sexual expression have been met.

2. **The Physical Facilities Are Conducive to Achievement of the Goals of Therapy.** Space is provided so that each client has sufficient privacy, as well as physical space, for therapeutic interaction with others. Furnishings are arranged to present a home-like atmosphere—usually in spaces that accommodate communal living, dining, and activity areas—for facilitation of interpersonal interaction and communication.

3. **A Democratic Form of Self-Government Exists.** In the therapeutic community, clients participate in the decision making and problem solving that affect the management of the treatment setting. This is accomplished through regularly scheduled community meetings. These meetings are attended by staff and clients, and all individuals have equal input into the discussions. At these meetings, the norms and rules and behavioral limits of the treatment setting are set forth. This reinforces the democratic posture of the treatment setting, because these are expectations that affect all clients on an equal basis. An example might be the rule that no client may enter a room being occupied by a client of the opposite gender. Consequences of violating the rules are explained.

Other issues that may be discussed at the community meetings include those with which certain clients have some disagreements. A decision is then made by the entire group in a democratic manner. For example, several clients in an inpatient unit may disagree with the hours that have been designated for watching television on a weekend night. They may elect to bring up this issue at a community meeting and suggest an extension in television-viewing time. After discussion by the group, a vote will be taken, and clients and staff agree to abide by the expressed preference of the majority. Some therapeutic communities elect officers (usually a president and a secretary) who serve for a specified time. The president calls the meeting to order, conducts the business of discussing old and new issues, and asks for volunteers (or makes appointments, alternately, so that all clients have a turn) to accomplish the daily tasks associated with community living, for example, cleaning the tables after each meal and watering plants in the treatment facility. New assignments are made at each meeting. The secretary reads the minutes of the previous meeting and takes minutes of the current meeting. Minutes are important in the event that clients have a disagreement about issues that were discussed at various meetings. Minutes provide written evidence of decisions made by the group. In treatment settings where clients have short attention spans or disorganized thinking, meetings are brief. Business is generally limited to introductions and expectations of the here and now. Discussions also may include comments about a recent occurrence in the group or something that has been bothering a member and about which he or she has some questions. These meetings are usually conducted by staff, although all clients have equal input into the discussions.

All clients are expected to attend the meetings. Exceptions are made for times when aspects of therapy interfere (e.g., scheduled testing, x-ray examinations, electroencephalograms). An explanation is made to clients present so that false perceptions of danger are not generated by another person's absence. All staff members are expected to attend the meetings, unless client care precludes their attendance.

4. **Responsibilities Are Assigned According to Client Capabilities.** Increasing self-esteem is an ultimate goal of the therapeutic community. Therefore, a client should not be set up for failure by being assigned a responsibility that is beyond his or her level of ability. By assigning clients responsibilities that promote achievement, self-esteem is enhanced. Consideration must also be given to times during which the client will show some regression in the treatment regimen. Adjustments in assignments should be made in a way that preserves self-esteem and provides for progression to greater degrees of responsibility as the client returns to his or her previous level of functioning.

5. **A Structured Program of Social and Work-Related Activities Is Scheduled as Part of the Treatment Program.** Each client's therapeutic program consists of group activities in which interpersonal interaction and communication with other individuals are emphasized. Time is also devoted to personal problems. Various group activities may be selected for clients with specific needs (e.g., an exercise group for a person who expresses anger inappropriately, an assertiveness group for a person who is passive-aggressive, or a stress-management group for a person who is anxious). A structured schedule of activities is the major focus of a therapeutic community. Through these activities, change in the client's personality and behavior can be achieved. New coping strategies are learned and social skills are developed. In the group situation, the client is able to practice what he or she has learned to prepare for transition to the general community.

6. **Community and Family Are Included in the Program of Therapy in an Effort to Facilitate Discharge From Treatment.** An attempt is made to include family members, as well as certain aspects of the community that affect the client, in the treatment program. It is important to keep as many links to the client's life outside of therapy as possible. Family members are invited to participate in specific therapy groups and, in some instances, to share meals with the client in the communal dining room. Connection with community life may be maintained through client group activities, such as shopping, picnicking, attending movies, bowling, and visiting the zoo. Inpatient clients may be awarded passes to visit family or may participate in work-related activities, the length of time being determined by the activity and the client's condition. These connections with family and community facilitate the discharge process and may help to prevent the client from becoming too dependent on the therapy.

The Program of Therapeutic Community

Care for clients in the therapeutic community is directed by an interdisciplinary treatment (IDT) team. An initial assessment is made by the admitting psychiatrist, nurse, or other designated admitting agent who establishes a priority of care. The IDT team determines a comprehensive treatment plan and goals of therapy and assigns intervention responsibilities. All members sign the treatment plan and meet regularly to update the plan as needed. Depending on the size of the treatment facility and scope of the therapy program, members representing a variety of disciplines may participate in the promotion of a therapeutic community. For example, an IDT team may include a psychiatrist, clinical psychologist, psychiatric clinical nurse specialist, psychiatric nurse, mental health technician, psychiatric social worker, occupational therapist, recreational therapist, music therapist, art therapist, psychodramatist, dietitian, and chaplain. Table 12-1 provides an explanation of responsibilities and educational preparation required for these members of the IDT team.

The Role of the Nurse in Milieu Therapy

Milieu therapy can take place in a variety of inpatient and outpatient settings. In the hospital, nurses are generally the only members of the IDT team who spend time with the clients on a 24-hour basis, and they assume responsibility for management of the therapeutic milieu. In all settings, the nursing process is used for the delivery of nursing care. Ongoing assessment, diagnosis, outcome identification, planning, implementation, and evaluation of

TABLE 12-1 The Interdisciplinary Treatment Team in Psychiatry

TEAM MEMBER	RESPONSIBILITIES	CREDENTIALS
Psychiatrist	Serves as the leader of the team. Responsible for diagnosis and treatment of mental disorders. Performs psychotherapy; prescribes medication and other somatic therapies.	Medical degree with residency in psychiatry and license to practice medicine.
Clinical psychologist	Conducts individual, group, and family therapy. Administers, interprets, and evaluates psychological tests that assist in the diagnostic process.	Doctorate in clinical psychology with 2- to 3-year internship supervised by a licensed clinical psychologist. State license is required to practice.
Psychiatric clinical nurse specialist	Conducts individual, group, and family therapy. Presents educational programs for nursing staff. Provides consultation services to nurses who require assistance in the planning and implementation of care for individual clients.	Registered nurse with minimum of a master's degree in psychiatric nursing. Some institutions require certification by national credentialing association
Psychiatric nurse	Provides ongoing assessment of client condition, both mentally and physically. Manages the therapeutic milieu on a 24-hour basis. Administers medications. Assists clients with all therapeutic activities as required. Focus is on one-to-one relationship development.	Registered nurse with hospital diploma, associate degree, or baccalaureate degree. Some psychiatric nurses have national certification.
Mental health technician (also called psychiatric aide or assistant or psychiatric technician)	Functions under the supervision of the psychiatric nurse. Provides assistance to clients in the fulfillment of their activities of daily living. Assists activity therapists as required in conducting their groups. May also participate in one-to-one relationship development.	Varies from state to state. Requirements include high school education, with additional vocational education or on-the-job training. Some hospitals hire individuals with baccalaureate degree in psychology in this capacity. Some states require a licensure examination to practice.
Psychiatric social worker	Conducts individual, group, and family therapy. Is concerned with client's social needs, such as placement, financial support, and community requirements. Conducts in-depth psychosocial history on which the needs assessment is based. Works with client and family to ensure that requirements for discharge are fulfilled and needs can be met by appropriate community resources.	Minimum of a master's degree in social work. Some states require additional supervision and subsequent licensure by examination.
Occupational therapist	Works with clients to help develop (or redevelop) independence in performance of activities of daily living. Focus is on rehabilitation and vocational training in which clients learn to be productive, thereby enhancing self-esteem. Creative activities and therapeutic relationship skills are used.	Baccalaureate or master's degree in occupational therapy.

TABLE 12-1 The Interdisciplinary Treatment Team in Psychiatry—cont'd

TEAM MEMBER	RESPONSIBILITIES	CREDENTIALS
Recreational therapist	Uses recreational activities to promote clients to redirect their thinking or to rechannel destructive energy in an appropriate manner. Clients learn skills that can be used during leisure time and during times of stress following discharge from treatment. Examples include bowling, volleyball, exercises, and jogging. Some programs include activities such as picnics, swimming, and even group attendance at the state fair when it is in session.	Baccalaureate or master's degree in recreational therapy.
Music therapist	Encourages clients in self-expression through music. Clients listen to music, play instruments, sing, dance, and compose songs that help them get in touch with feelings and emotions that they may not be able to experience in any other way.	Graduate degree with specialty in music therapy.
Art therapist	Uses the client's creative abilities to encourage expression of emotions and feelings through artwork. Helps clients to analyze their own work in an effort to recognize and resolve underlying conflict.	Graduate degree with specialty in art therapy.
Psychodramatist	Directs clients in the creation of a "drama" that portrays real-life situations. Individuals select problems they wish to enact, and other clients play the roles of significant others in the situations. Some clients are able to "act out" problems that they are unable to work through in a more traditional manner. All members benefit through intensive discussion that follows.	Graduate degree in psychology, social work, nursing, or medicine with additional training in group therapy and specialty preparation to become a psychodramatist.
Dietitian	Plans nutritious meals for all clients. Works on consulting basis for clients with specific eating disorders, such as anorexia nervosa, bulimia nervosa, obesity, and pica.	Baccalaureate or master's degree with specialty in dietetics.
Chaplain	Assesses, identifies, and attends to the spiritual needs of clients and their family members. Provides spiritual support and comfort as requested by client or family. May provide counseling if educational background includes this type of preparation.	College degree with advanced education in theology, seminary, or rabbinical studies.

the environment are necessary for the successful management of a therapeutic milieu. Nurses are involved in all day-to-day activities that pertain to client care. Suggestions and opinions of nursing staff are given serious consideration in the planning of care for individual clients. Information from the initial nursing assessment is used to create the IDT plan. Nurses have input into therapy goals and participate in the regular updates and modification of treatment plans.

In some treatment facilities, a separate nursing care plan is required in addition to the IDT plan.

When this is the case, the nursing care plan must reflect diagnoses that are specific to nursing and include problems and interventions from the IDT plan that have been assigned specifically to the discipline of nursing.

In the therapeutic milieu, nurses are responsible for ensuring that clients' physiological needs are met. Clients must be encouraged to perform as independently as possible in fulfilling activities of daily living. However, the nurse must make ongoing assessments to provide assistance for those who require it. Assessing physical status is an important nursing responsibility that must not be overlooked in a psychiatric setting that emphasizes holistic care.

Reality orientation for clients who have disorganized thinking or who are disoriented or confused is important in the therapeutic milieu. Clocks with large hands and numbers, calendars that give the day and date in large print, and orientation boards that discuss daily activities and news happenings can help keep clients oriented to reality. Nurses should ensure that clients have written schedules of activities to which they are assigned and that they arrive at those activities on schedule. Some clients may require an identification sign on their door to remind them which room is theirs. On short-term units, nurses who are dealing with psychotic clients usually rely on a basic activity or topic that helps keep people oriented: for example, showing pictures of the hospital where they are housed, introducing people who were admitted during the night, and providing name badges with their first name.

Nurses are responsible for the management of medication administration on inpatient psychiatric units. In some treatment programs, clients are expected to accept the responsibility and request their medication at the appropriate time. Although ultimate responsibility lies with the nurse, he or she must encourage clients to be self-reliant. Nurses must work with the clients to determine methods that result in achievement and provide positive feedback for successes.

A major focus of nursing in the therapeutic milieu is the one-to-one relationship that grows out of a developing trust between client and nurse. Many clients with psychiatric disorders have never achieved the ability to trust. If this can be accomplished in a relationship with the nurse, the trust may be generalized to other relationships in the client's life. Within an atmosphere of trust, the client is encouraged to express feelings and emotions and to discuss unresolved issues that are creating problems in his or her life.

CLINICAL PEARL

Developing trust means keeping promises that have been made. It means total acceptance of the individual as a person, separate from behavior that is unacceptable. It means responding to the client with concrete behaviors that are understandable to him or her (e.g., "If you are frightened, I will stay with you"; "If you are cold, I will bring you a blanket"; "If you are thirsty, I will bring you a drink of water").

The nurse is responsible for setting limits on unacceptable behavior in the therapeutic milieu. This requires stating to the client in understandable terminology what behaviors are not acceptable and what the consequences will be should the limits be violated. These limits must be established, written, and carried out by all staff. Consistency in carrying out the consequences of violation of the established limits is essential if the learning is to be reinforced.

The role of client teacher is important in the psychiatric area, as it is in all areas of nursing. Nurses must be able to assess learning readiness in individual clients. Do they want to learn? What is their level of anxiety? What is their level of ability to understand the information being presented? Topics for client education in psychiatry include information about medical diagnoses, side effects of medications, the importance of continuing to take medications, and stress management, among others. Some topics must be individualized for specific clients, whereas others may be taught in group situations. Table 12-2 outlines various topics of nursing concern for client education in psychiatry. (Refer to Appendix G for sample client teaching guides.)

Echternacht (2001) stated:

Milieu therapy interventions are recognized as one of the basic-level functions of psychiatric-mental health nurses as addressed [in the *Psychiatric-Mental Health Nursing: Scope and Standards of Practice* (ANA, 2007)]. Milieu therapy has been described as an excellent framework for operationalizing [Hildegard] Peplau's interpretation and extension of Harry Stack Sullivan's Interpersonal Theory for use in nursing practice. (p. 39)

Now is the time to rekindle interest in the therapeutic milieu concept and to reclaim nursing's traditional milieu intervention functions. Nurses need to identify the number of registered nurses necessary to carry out structured and unstructured milieu functions consistent with their Standards of Practice. (p. 43)

TABLE 12-2 The Therapeutic Milieu—Topics for Client Education
1. Ways to increase self-esteem
2. Ways to deal with anger appropriately
3. Stress-management techniques
4. How to recognize signs of increasing anxiety and intervene to stop progression
5. Normal stages of grieving and behaviors associated with each stage
6. Assertiveness techniques
7. Relaxation techniques a. Progressive relaxation b. Tense and relax c. Deep breathing d. Autogenics
8. Medications (specify) a. Reason for taking b. Harmless side effects c. Side effects to report to physician d. Importance of taking regularly e. Importance of not stopping abruptly
9. Effects of (substance) on the body a. Alcohol b. Other depressants c. Stimulants d. Hallucinogens e. Narcotics f. Cannabinols
10. Problem-solving skills
11. Thought-stopping/thought-switching techniques
12. Sex education a. Structure and function of reproductive system b. Contraceptives c. Sexually transmitted diseases
13. The essentials of good nutrition
14. (For parents/guardians) a. Signs and symptoms of substance abuse b. Effective parenting techniques

Summary and Key Points

■ In psychiatry, milieu therapy (or a therapeutic community) constitutes a manipulation of the environment in an effort to create behavioral changes and to improve the psychological health and functioning of the individual.

■ The goal of therapeutic community is for the client to learn adaptive coping, interaction, and relationship skills that can be generalized to other aspects of his or her life.

■ The community environment itself serves as the primary tool of therapy.

■ According to Skinner (1979), a therapeutic community is based on seven basic assumptions:
• The health in each individual is to be realized and encouraged to grow.
• Every interaction is an opportunity for therapeutic intervention.
• The client owns his or her own environment.
• Each client owns his or her behavior.
• Peer pressure is a useful and a powerful tool.
• Inappropriate behaviors are dealt with as they occur.
• Restrictions and punishment are to be avoided.

■ Because the goals of milieu therapy relate to helping the client learn to generalize that which is learned to other aspects of his or her life, the conditions that promote a therapeutic community in the psychiatric setting are similar to the types of conditions that exist in real-life situations.

■ Conditions that promote a therapeutic community include the following:
• The fulfillment of basic physiological needs.
• Physical facilities that are conducive to achievement of the goals of therapy.
• The existence of a democratic form of self-government.
• The assignment of responsibilities according to client capabilities.
• A structured program of social and work-related activities.
• The inclusion of community and family in the program of therapy in an effort to facilitate discharge from treatment.

■ The program of therapy on the milieu unit is conducted by the IDT team.

■ The team includes some, or all, of the following disciplines and may include others that are not specified here: psychiatrist, clinical psychologist, psychiatric clinical nurse specialist, psychiatric nurse, mental health technician, psychiatric social worker, occupational therapist, recreational therapist, art therapist, music therapist, psychodramatist, dietitian, and chaplain.

■ Nurses play a crucial role in the management of a therapeutic milieu. They are involved in the assessment, diagnosis, outcome identification, planning, implementation, and evaluation of all treatment programs.

■ Nurses have significant input into the IDT plans, which are developed for all clients. They are responsible for ensuring that clients' basic needs are fulfilled; assessing physical and psychosocial status; administering medication; helping the client develop trusting relationships; setting limits on unacceptable behaviors; educating clients; and ultimately, helping clients, within the limits of their capability, to become productive members of society.

 Additional info available @ davisplus.fadavis.com

Review Questions
Self-Examination/Learning Exercise

*Select the answer that is **most** appropriate for each of the following questions:*

1. Which of the following are basic assumptions of milieu therapy? (Select all that apply.)
   a. The client owns his or her own environment.
   b. Each client owns his or her behavior.
   c. Peer pressure is a useful and powerful tool.
   d. Inappropriate behaviors are punished immediately.

2. John tells the nurse, "I think lights out at 10 o'clock on a weekend is stupid. We should be able to watch TV until midnight!" Which of the following is the most appropriate response from the nurse on the milieu unit?
   a. "John, you were told the rules when you were admitted."
   b. "You may bring it up before the others at the community meeting, John."
   c. "Some people want to go to bed early, John."
   d. "You are not the only person on this unit, John. You must think of the others."

3. In prioritizing care within the therapeutic environment, which of the following nursing interventions would receive the highest priority?
   a. Ensuring that the physical facilities are conducive to achievement of the goals of therapy.
   b. Scheduling a community meeting for 8:30 each morning.
   c. Attending to the nutritional and comfort needs of all clients.
   d. Establishing contacts with community resources.

4. In the community meeting, which of the following actions is most important for reinforcing the democratic posture of the therapy setting?
   a. Allowing each person a specific and equal amount of time to talk.
   b. Reviewing group rules and behavioral limits that apply to all clients.
   c. Reading the minutes from yesterday's meeting.
   d. Waiting until all clients are present before initiating the meeting.

5. One of the goals of a therapeutic community is for clients to become more independent and accept self-responsibility. Which of the following approaches by staff best encourages fulfillment of this goal?
   a. Including client input and decisions into the treatment plan.
   b. Insisting that each client take a turn as "president" of the community meeting.
   c. Making decisions for the client regarding plans for treatment.
   d. Requiring that the client be bathed, be dressed, and attend breakfast on time each morning.

Review Questions—cont'd
Self-Examination/Learning Exercise

6. Client teaching is an important nursing function in milieu therapy. Which of the following statements by the client indicates the need for knowledge and a readiness to learn?
   a. "Get away from me with that medicine! I'm not sick!"
   b. "I don't need psychiatric treatment. It's my migraine headaches that I need help with."
   c. "I've taken Valium every day of my life for the last 20 years. I'll stop when I'm good and ready!"
   d. "The doctor says I have bipolar disorder. What does that really mean?"

7. Which of the following activities would be a responsibility of the clinical psychologist member of the IDT team?
   a. Locates halfway house and arranges living conditions for client being discharged from the hospital.
   b. Manages the therapeutic milieu on a 24-hour basis.
   c. Administers and evaluates psychological tests that assist in diagnosis.
   d. Conducts psychotherapy and administers electroconvulsive therapy treatments.

8. Which of the following activities would be a responsibility of the psychiatric clinical nurse specialist on the IDT team?
   a. Manages the therapeutic milieu on a 24-hour basis.
   b. Conducts group therapies and provides consultation and education to staff nurses.
   c. Directs a group of clients in acting out a situation that is otherwise too painful for a client to discuss openly.
   d. Locates halfway house and arranges living conditions for client being discharged from the hospital.

9. On the milieu unit, duties of the staff psychiatric nurse include which of the following? (Select all that apply.)
   a. Medication administration.
   b. Client teaching.
   c. Medical diagnosis.
   d. Reality orientation.
   e. Relationship development.
   f. Group therapy.

10. Sally was sexually abused as a child. She is a client on the milieu unit with a diagnosis of Borderline Personality Disorder. She has refused to talk to anyone. Which of the following therapies might the IDT team choose for Sally? (Select all that apply.)
    a. Music therapy.
    b. Art therapy.
    c. Psychodrama.
    d. Electroconvulsive therapy.

References

American Nurses Association. (2007). *Psychiatric-mental health nursing: Scope and standards of practice.* Silver Spring, MD: Author.

Bowler, J. B. (1991). Transformation into a healing healthcare environment: Recovering the possibilities of psychiatric/mental health nursing. *Perspectives in Psychiatric Care, 27*(2), 21–25.

DeSocio, J., Bowllan, N., & Staschak, S. (1997). Lessons learned in creating a safe and therapeutic milieu for children, adolescents, and families: Developmental considerations. *Journal of Child and Adolescent Psychiatric Nursing 10*(4), 18–26.

Echternacht, M. R. (2001). Fluid group: Concept and clinical application in the therapeutic milieu. *Journal of the American Psychiatric Nurses Association, 7*(2), 39–44.

Hall, B. A. (1995). Use of milieu therapy: The context and environment as therapeutic practice for psychiatric-mental health nurses. In C. A. Anderson (Ed.), *Psychiatric nursing 1974 to 1994: A report on the state of the art* (pp. 46–56). St. Louis: Mosby-Year Book.

Whall, A. L. (1991). Using the environment to improve the mental health of the elderly. *Journal of Gerontological Nursing, 17*(7), 39.

Classical References

Maslow, A. (1968). *Towards a psychology of being* (2nd ed.). New York: D. Van Nostrand.

Skinner, K. (1979, August). The therapeutic milieu: Making it work. *Journal of Psychiatric Nursing and Mental Health Services,* 38–44.

Crisis Intervention

CORE CONCEPT

crisis

KEY TERMS

crisis intervention

disaster

OBJECTIVES

After reading this chapter, the student will be able to:

1. Define *crisis.*
2. Describe four phases in the development
   of a crisis.
3. Identify types of crises that occur in
   people's lives.
4. Discuss the goal of crisis intervention.
5. Describe the steps in crisis intervention.
6. Identify the role of the nurse in crisis
   intervention.
7. Apply the nursing process to care of
   victims of disasters

HOMEWORK ASSIGNMENT

Please read the chapter and answer the following questions:

1. Name the three factors that determine
   whether or not a person experiences a
   crisis in response to a stressful situation.
2. What is the goal of crisis intervention?
3. Individuals in crisis need to develop more
   adaptive coping strategies. How does the
   nurse provide assistance with this
   process?
4. Describe behaviors common to preschool
   children following a traumatic event.

Stressful situations are a part of everyday life. Any stressful situation can precipitate a crisis. Crises result in a disequilibrium from which many individuals require assistance to recover. **Crisis intervention** requires problem-solving skills that are often diminished by the level of anxiety accompanying disequilibrium. Assistance with problem solving during the crisis period preserves self-esteem and promotes growth with resolution.

In recent years, individuals in the United States have been faced with a number of catastrophic events, including natural disasters such as tornados, earthquakes, hurricanes, and floods. Also, man-made disasters, such as the Oklahoma City bombing and the attacks on the World Trade Center and the Pentagon, have created psychological stress of astronomical proportions in populations around the world.

This chapter examines the phases in the development of a crisis and the types of crises that occur in people's lives. The methodology of crisis intervention, including the role of the nurse, is explored. A discussion of disaster nursing is also presented.

FIGURE 13–1 Chinese symbol for crisis.

> ## CORE CONCEPT
> *Crisis*
> A sudden event in one's life that disturbs homeostasis, during which usual coping mechanisms cannot resolve the problem (Lagerquist, 2006, p. 393).

Characteristics of a Crisis

A number of characteristics have been identified that can be viewed as assumptions upon which the concept of crisis is based (Aguilera, 1998; Caplan, 1964; Winston, 2008). They include the following:

1. Crisis occurs in all individuals at one time or another and is not necessarily equated with psychopathology.

2. Crises are precipitated by specific identifiable events.

3. Crises are personal by nature. What may be considered a crisis situation by one individual may not be so for another.

4. Crises are acute, not chronic, and will be resolved in one way or another within a brief period.

5. A crisis situation contains the potential for psychological growth or deterioration.

Individuals who are in crisis feel helpless to change. They do not believe they have the resources to deal with the precipitating stressor. Levels of anxiety rise to the point that the individual becomes nonfunctional, thoughts become obsessional, and all behavior is aimed at relief of the anxiety being experienced. The feeling is overwhelming and may affect the individual physically as well as psychologically.

Bateman and Peternelj-Taylor (1998) stated:

> Outside Western culture, a crisis is often viewed as a time for movement and growth. The Chinese symbol for crisis consists of the characters for *danger* and *opportunity* [Figure 13–1]. When a crisis is viewed as an opportunity for growth, those involved are much more capable of resolving related issues and more able to move toward positive changes. When the crisis experience is overwhelming because of its scope and nature or when there has not been adequate preparation for the necessary changes, the dangers seem paramount and

overshadow any potential growth. The results are maladaptive coping and dysfunctional behavior. (pp. 144–145)

Phases in the Development of a Crisis

The development of a crisis situation follows a relatively predictable course. Caplan (1964) outlined four specific phases through which individuals progress in response to a precipitating stressor and that culminate in the state of acute crisis.

Phase 1. *The individual is exposed to a precipitating stressor.* Anxiety increases; previous problem-solving techniques are employed.

Phase 2. *When previous problem-solving techniques do not relieve the stressor, anxiety increases further.* The individual begins to feel a great deal of discomfort at this point. Coping techniques that have worked in the past are attempted, only to create feelings of helplessness when they are not successful. Feelings of confusion and disorganization prevail.

Phase 3. *All possible resources, both internal and external, are called on to resolve the problem and relieve the discomfort.* The individual may try to view the problem from a different perspective, or even to overlook certain aspects of it. New problem-solving techniques may be used, and, if effectual, resolution may occur at this phase, with the individual returning to a higher, a lower, or the previous level of premorbid functioning.

Phase 4. *If resolution does not occur in previous phases, Caplan stated that "the tension mounts beyond a further threshold or its burden increases over time to a breaking point. Major disorganization of the individual with drastic results often occurs."* Anxiety may reach panic levels. Cognitive functions are disordered, emotions are labile, and behavior may reflect the presence of psychotic thinking.

These phases are congruent with the Transactional Model of Stress/Adaptation outlined in Chapter 1. The relationship between the two perspectives is presented in Figure 13–2. Similarly, Aguilera (1998) spoke of "balancing factors" that affect the way in which an individual perceives and responds to a precipitating stressor. A schematic of these balancing factors is illustrated in Figure 13–3.

The paradigm set forth by Aguilera suggests that whether or not an individual experiences a crisis in response to a stressful situation depends upon the following three factors:

1. **The individual's perception of the event.** If the event is perceived realistically, the individual is more likely to draw upon adequate resources to restore equilibrium. If the perception of the event is distorted, attempts at problem solving are likely to be ineffective, and restoration of equilibrium goes unresolved.

2. **The availability of situational supports.** Aguilera stated, "Situational supports are those persons who are available in the environment and who can be depended on to help solve the problem" (p. 37). Without adequate situational supports during a stressful situation, an individual is most likely to feel overwhelmed and alone.

3. **The availability of adequate coping mechanisms.** When a stressful situation occurs, individuals draw upon behavioral strategies that have been successful for them in the past. If these coping strategies work, a crisis may be diverted. If not, disequilibrium may continue and tension and anxiety increase.

As previously set forth, it is assumed that crises are acute, not chronic, situations that will be resolved in one way or another within a brief period. Winston (2008) stated, "Crises tend to be time limited, generally lasting no more than a few months; the duration depends on the stressor and

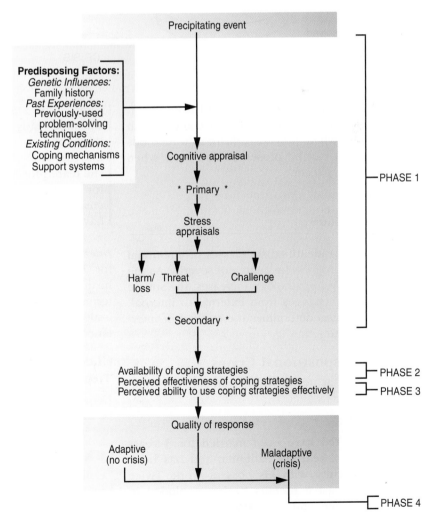

FIGURE 13–2 Relationship between Transactional Model of Stress/Adaptation and Caplan's phases in the development of a crisis.

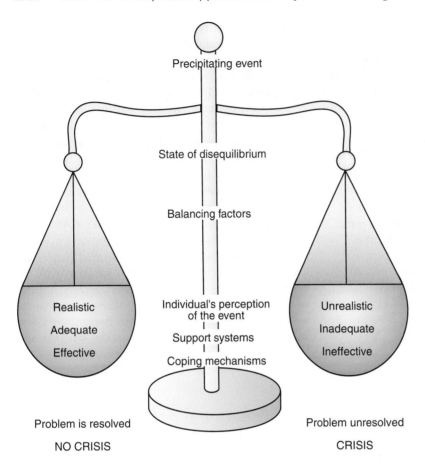

FIGURE 13–3 The effects of balancing factors in a stressful event.

on the individual's perception of and response to the stressor" (p. 1270). Crises can become growth opportunities when individuals learn new methods of coping that can be preserved and used when similar stressors recur.

Types of Crises

Baldwin (1978) identified six classes of emotional crises, which progress by degree of severity. As the measure of psychopathology increases, the source of the stressor changes from external to internal. The type of crisis determines the method of intervention selected.

Class 1: Dispositional Crises

Definition An acute response to an external situational stressor.

▍EXAMPLE

Nancy and Ted have been married for 3 years and have a 1-year-old daughter. Ted has been having difficulty with his boss at work. Twice during the past 6 months he has exploded in anger at home and has become abusive with Nancy. Last night he became angry that dinner was not ready when he expected. He grabbed the baby from Nancy and tossed her, screaming, into her crib. He hit and punched Nancy until she feared for her life. This morning when he left for work, she took the baby and went to the emergency department of the city hospital, not having anywhere else to go.

Intervention Nancy's physical wounds were cared for in the emergency department. The mental health counselor provided support and guidance in terms of presenting alternatives to her. Needs and issues were clarified, and referrals for agency assistance were made.

Class 2: Crises of Anticipated Life Transitions

Definition Normal life-cycle transitions that may be anticipated but over which the individual may feel a lack of control.

▍EXAMPLE

College student J.T. is placed on probationary status because of low grades this semester. His wife had a baby and had to quit her job. He increased his working hours from part time to full time to compensate, and therefore had little time for studies. He presents himself to the student-health nurse practitioner complaining of numerous vague physical complaints.

Intervention Physical examination should be performed (physical symptoms could be caused by depression) and ventilation of feelings encouraged. Reassurance and support should be provided as needed. J.T. should be referred to services that can provide financial and other types of needed assistance. Problematic areas should be identified and approaches to change discussed.

Class 3: Crises Resulting From Traumatic Stress

Definition Crises precipitated by unexpected external stresses over which the individual has little or no control and as a result of which he or she feels emotionally overwhelmed and defeated.

EXAMPLE

Sally is a waitress whose shift ends at midnight. Two weeks ago, while walking to her car in the deserted parking lot, she was abducted by two men with guns, taken to an abandoned building, and raped and beaten. Since that time, her physical wounds have nearly healed. However, Sally cannot be alone; is constantly fearful; relives the experience in flashbacks and dreams; and is unable to eat, sleep, or work at her job in the restaurant. Her friend offers to accompany her to the mental health clinic.

Intervention The nurse should encourage Sally to talk about the experience and to express her feelings associated with it. The nurse should offer reassurance and support; discuss stages of grief and how rape causes a loss of self-worth, triggering the grief response; identify support systems that can help Sally to resume her normal activities; and explore new methods of coping with emotions arising from a situation with which she has had no previous experience.

Class 4: Maturational/Developmental Crises

Definition Crises that occur in response to situations that trigger emotions related to unresolved conflicts in one's life. These crises are of internal origin and reflect underlying developmental issues that involve dependency, value conflicts, sexual identity, control, and capacity for emotional intimacy.

EXAMPLE

Bob is 40 years old. He has just been passed over for a job promotion for the third time. He has moved many times within the large company for which he works, usually after angering and alienating himself from the supervisor. His father was domineering and became abusive when Bob did not comply with his every command. Over the years, Bob's behavioral response became one of passive-aggressiveness—first with his father, then with his supervisors. This third rejection has created feelings of depression and intense anxiety in Bob. At his wife's insistence, he has sought help at the mental health clinic.

Intervention The primary intervention is to help Bob identify the unresolved developmental issue that is creating the conflict. Support and guidance are offered during the initial crisis period, then assistance is given to help Bob work through the underlying conflict in an effort to change response patterns that are creating problems in his current life situation.

Class 5: Crises Reflecting Psychopathology

Definition Emotional crises in which preexisting psychopathology has been instrumental in precipitating the crisis or in which psychopathology significantly impairs or complicates adaptive resolution. Examples of psychopathology that may precipitate crises include borderline personality, severe neuroses, characterological disorders, or schizophrenia.

EXAMPLE

Sonja, age 29, was diagnosed with borderline personality at age 18. She has been in therapy on a weekly basis for 10 years, with several hospitalizations for suicide attempts during that time. She has had the same therapist for the past 6 years. This therapist told Sonja today that she is to be married in 1 month and will be moving across the country with her new husband. Sonja is distraught and experiencing intense feelings of abandonment. She is found wandering in and out of traffic on a busy expressway, oblivious to her surroundings. Police bring her to the emergency department of the hospital.

Intervention The initial intervention is to help bring down the level of anxiety in Sonja that has created feelings of unreality in her. She requires that someone stay with her and reassure her of her safety and security. After the feelings of panic anxiety have subsided, she should be encouraged to verbalize her feelings of abandonment. Regressive behaviors should be discouraged. Positive reinforcement should be given for independent activities and accomplishments. The primary therapist will need to pursue this issue of termination with Sonja at length. Referral to a long-term care facility may be required.

Class 6: Psychiatric Emergencies

Definition Crisis situations in which general functioning has been severely impaired and the individual rendered incompetent or unable to assume personal responsibility. Examples include acutely suicidal individuals, drug overdoses, reactions to hallucinogenic drugs, acute psychoses, uncontrollable anger, and alcohol intoxication.

▌EXAMPLE

Jennifer, age 16, had been dating Joe, the star high school football player, for 6 months. After the game on Friday night, Jennifer and Joe went to Jackie's house, where a number of high school students had gathered for an after-game party. No adults were present. About midnight, Joe told Jennifer that he did not want to date her anymore. Jennifer became hysterical, and Jackie was frightened by her behavior. She took Jennifer to her parent's bedroom and gave her a Valium from a bottle in her mother's medicine cabinet. She left Jennifer lying on her parent's bed and returned to the party downstairs. About an hour later, she returned to her parent's bedroom and found that Jennifer had removed the bottle of Valium from the cabinet and swallowed all of the tablets. Jennifer was unconscious and Jackie could not awaken her. An ambulance was called and Jennifer was transported to the local hospital.

Intervention The crisis team monitored vital signs, ensured maintenance of adequate airway, initiated gastric lavage, and administered activated charcoal to minimize absorption. Jennifer's parents were notified and rushed to the hospital. The situation was explained to them, and they were encouraged to stay by her side. When the physical crisis was resolved, Jennifer was transferred to the psychiatric unit. In therapy, she was encouraged to ventilate her feelings regarding the rejection and subsequent overdose. Family therapy sessions were conducted in an effort to clarify interpersonal issues and to identify areas for change. On an individual level, Jennifer's therapist worked with her to establish more adaptive methods of coping with stressful situations.

Crisis Intervention

Individuals experiencing crises have an urgent need for assistance. In crisis intervention the therapist, or other intervener, becomes a part of the individual's life situation. Because of the individual's emotional state, he or she is unable to problem-solve, and so requires guidance and support from another to help mobilize the resources needed to resolve the crisis.

Lengthy psychological interpretations are not appropriate for crisis intervention. It is a time for doing what is needed to help the individual get relief and for calling into action all the people and other resources required to do so. Aguilera (1998) stated:

> The goal of crisis intervention is the resolution of an immediate crisis. Its focus is on the supportive, with the restoration of the individual to his precrisis level of functioning or possibly to a higher level of functioning. The therapist's role is direct, supportive, and that of an active participant. (p. 24)

Crisis intervention takes place in both inpatient and outpatient settings. The basic methodology relies heavily on orderly problem-solving techniques and structured activities that are focused on change. Through adaptive change, crises are resolved and growth occurs. Because of the time limitation of crisis intervention, the individual must experience some degree of relief almost from the first interaction. Crisis intervention, then, is not aimed at major personality change or reconstruction (as may be the case in long-term psychotherapy), but rather at using a given crisis situation, at the very least, to restore functioning and, at most, to enhance personal growth.

Phases of Crisis Intervention: The Role of the Nurse

Nurses respond to crisis situations on a daily basis. Crises can occur on every unit in the general hospital, in the home setting, in the community health care setting, in schools and offices, and in private practice. Indeed, nurses may be called on to function as crisis helpers in virtually any setting committed to the practice of nursing.

Roberts and Ottens (2005) provided a seven-stage model of crisis intervention. This model is summarized in Table 13-1. Aguilera (1998) described four specific phases in the technique of crisis intervention that are clearly comparable to

TABLE 13-1 Roberts' Seven-Stage Crisis Intervention Model	
STAGE	**INTERVENTIONS**
Stage I. Psychosocial and Lethality Assessment	■ Conduct a rapid but thorough biopsychosocial assessment
Stage II. Rapidly Establish Rapport	■ The counselor uses genuineness, respect, and unconditional acceptance to establish rapport with the client. ■ Skills such as good eye contact, a nonjudgmental attitude, flexibility, and maintaining a positive mental attitude are important.
Stage III. Identify the Major Problems or Crisis Precipitants	■ Identify the precipitating event that has led the client to seek help at the present time. ■ Identify other situations that led up to the precipitating event. ■ Prioritize major problems with which the client needs help. ■ Discuss client's current style of coping, and offer assistance in areas where modification would be helpful in resolving the present crisis and preventing future crises.
Stage IV. Deal with Feelings and Emotions	■ Encourage client to vent feelings. Provide validation. ■ Use therapeutic communication techniques to help client explain his or her story about the current crisis situation. ■ Eventually, and cautiously, begin to challenge maladaptive beliefs and behaviors, and help client adopt more rational and adaptive options.
Stage V. Generate and Explore Alternatives	■ Collaboratively explore options with client. ■ Identify coping strategies that have been successful for the client in the past ■ Help client problem-solve strategies for confronting current crisis adaptively.
Stage VI. Implement an Action Plan	■ There is a shift at this stage from crisis to resolution. ■ Develop a concrete plan of action to deal directly with the current crisis. ■ Having a concrete plan restores the client's equilibrium and psychological balance. ■ Work through the meaning of the event that precipitated the crisis. How could it have been prevented? What responses may have aggravated the situation?
Stage VII. Follow-Up	■ Plan a follow-up visit with the client to evaluate the post-crisis status of the client. ■ Beneficial scheduling of follow-up visits include 1-month and 1-year anniversaries of the crisis event.

Adapted from Roberts, A. R., & and Ottens, A. J. (2005). The seven-stage crisis intervention model: A road map to goal attainment, problem solving, and crisis resolution. Brief Treatment and Crisis Intervention, 5(4), 329–339.

the steps of the nursing process. These phases are discussed in the following paragraphs.

Phase 1: Assessment

In this phase, the crisis helper gathers information regarding the precipitating stressor and the resulting crisis that prompted the individual to seek professional help. A nurse in crisis intervention might perform some of the following assessments:

■ Ask the individual to describe the event that precipitated this crisis.

■ Determine when it occurred.

■ Assess the individual's physical and mental status.

■ Determine if the individual has experienced this stressor before. If so, what method of coping was used? Have these methods been tried this time?

• If previous coping methods were tried, what was the result?

• If new coping methods were tried, what was the result?

■ Assess suicide or homicide potential, plan, and means.

■ Assess the adequacy of support systems.

■ Determine level of precrisis functioning. Assess the usual coping methods, available support systems, and ability to problem-solve.

■ Assess the individual's perception of personal strengths and limitations.

■ Assess the individual's use of substances.

Information from the comprehensive assessment is then analyzed, and appropriate nursing diagnoses reflecting the immediacy of the crisis situation are identified. Some nursing diagnoses that may be relevant include:

■ Ineffective coping

■ Anxiety (severe to panic)

■ Disturbed thought processes

■ Risk for self- or other-directed violence

■ Rape-trauma syndrome

■ Post-trauma syndrome

■ Fear

Phase 2: Planning of Therapeutic Intervention

In the planning phase of the nursing process, the nurse selects the appropriate nursing actions for the identified nursing diagnoses. In planning the interventions, the type of crisis, as well as the individual's strengths and available resources for support, are taken into consideration. Goals are established for crisis resolution and a return to, or increase in, the precrisis level of functioning.

Phase 3: Intervention

During phase 3, the actions that were identified in phase 2 are implemented. The following interventions are the focus of nursing in crisis intervention:

■ Use a reality-oriented approach. The focus of the problem is on the here and now.

■ Remain with the individual who is experiencing panic anxiety.

■ Establish a rapid working relationship by showing unconditional acceptance, by active listening, and by attending to immediate needs.

■ Discourage lengthy explanations or rationalizations of the situation; promote an atmosphere for verbalization of true feelings.

■ Set firm limits on aggressive, destructive behaviors. At high levels of anxiety, behavior is likely to be impulsive and regressive. Establish at the

outset what is acceptable and what is not, and maintain consistency.

■ Clarify the problem that the individual is facing. The nurse does this by describing his or her perception of the problem and comparing it with the individual's perception of the problem.

■ Help the individual determine what he or she believes precipitated the crisis.

■ Acknowledge feelings of anger, guilt, helplessness, and powerlessness, while taking care not to provide positive feedback for these feelings.

■ Guide the individual through a problem-solving process by which he or she may move in the direction of positive life change:
  • Help the individual confront the source of the problem that is creating the crisis response.
  • Encourage the individual to discuss changes he or she would like to make. Jointly determine whether or not desired changes are realistic.
  • Encourage exploration of feelings about aspects that cannot be changed, and explore alternative ways of coping more adaptively in these situations.
  • Discuss alternative strategies for creating changes that are realistically possible.
  • Weigh benefits and consequences of each alternative.
  • Assist the individual to select alternative coping strategies that will help alleviate future crisis situations.

> **CLINICAL PEARL** Coping mechanisms are highly individual, and the choice ultimately must be made by the client. The nurse may offer suggestions and provide guidance to help the client identify coping mechanisms that are realistic for him or her, and that can promote positive outcomes in a crisis situation.

■ Identify external support systems and new social networks from which the individual may seek assistance in times of stress.

Phase 4: Evaluation of Crisis Resolution and Anticipatory Planning

To evaluate the outcome of crisis intervention, a reassessment is made to determine if the stated objective was achieved:

■ Have positive behavioral changes occurred?

■ Has the individual developed more adaptive coping strategies? Have they been effective?

■ Has the individual grown from the experience by gaining insight into his or her responses to crisis situations?

■ Does the individual believe that he or she could respond with healthy adaptation in future stressful situations to prevent crisis development?

■ Can the individual describe a plan of action for dealing with stressors similar to the one that precipitated this crisis?

During the evaluation period, the nurse and client summarize what has occurred during the intervention. They review what the individual has learned and "anticipate" how he or she will respond in the future. A determination is made regarding follow-up therapy; if needed, the nurse provides referral information.

Disaster Nursing

Although there are many definitions of **disaster,** a common feature is that the event overwhelms local resources and threatens the function and safety of the community (Norwood, Ursano, & Fullerton, 2000). A violent disaster, whether natural or man-made, may leave devastation of property or life. Such tragedies also leave victims with a damaged sense of safety and well-being, and varying degrees of emotional trauma (Oklahoma State Department of Health [OSDH], 2001). Children, who lack life experiences and coping skills, are particularly vulnerable. Their sense of order and security has been seriously disrupted, and they are unable to understand that the disruption is time limited and that their world will eventually return to normal.

Application of the Nursing Process to Disaster Nursing

Background Assessment Data

Individuals respond to traumatic events in many ways. Grieving is a natural response following any loss, and it may be more extreme if the disaster is directly experienced or witnessed (OSDH, 2001). The emotional effects of loss and disruption may show up immediately or may appear weeks or months later.

Psychological and behavioral responses common in adults following trauma and disaster include anger; disbelief; sadness; anxiety; fear; irritability; arousal; numbing; sleep disturbance; and

increases in alcohol, caffeine, and tobacco use (Norwood et al., 2000). Preschool children commonly experience separation anxiety, regressive behaviors, nightmares, and hyperactive or withdrawn behaviors. Older children may have difficulty concentrating, somatic complaints, sleep disturbances, and concerns about safety. Adolescents' responses are often similar to those of adults.

Norwood and associates (2000) stated:

Traumatic bereavement is recognized as posing special challenges to survivors. While the death of loved ones is always painful, an unexpected and violent death can be more difficult to assimilate. Family members may develop intrusive images of the death based on information gleaned from authorities or the media. Witnessing or learning of violence to a loved one also increases vulnerability to psychiatric disorders. The knowledge that one has been exposed to toxins is a potent traumatic stressor...and the focus of much concern in the medical community preparing for responses to terrorist attacks using biological, chemical, or nuclear agents. (p. 214)

Nursing Diagnoses/Outcome Identification

Information from the assessment is analyzed, and appropriate nursing diagnoses reflecting the immediacy of the situation are identified. Some nursing diagnoses that may be relevant include:

■ Risk for injury (trauma, suffocation, poisoning)

■ Risk for infection

■ Anxiety (panic)

■ Fear

■ Spiritual distress

■ Risk for post-trauma syndrome

■ Ineffective community coping

The following criteria may be used for measurement of outcomes in the care of the client having experienced a traumatic event. Timelines are individually determined.

The client:

■ Experiences minimal/no injury to self.

■ Demonstrates behaviors necessary to protect self from further injury.

■ Identifies interventions to prevent/reduce risk of infection.

■ Is free of infection.

■ Maintains anxiety at manageable level.

■ Expresses beliefs and values about spiritual issues.

■ Demonstrates ability to deal with emotional reactions in an individually appropriate manner.

■ Demonstrates an increase in activities to improve community functioning.

Planning/Implementation

Table 13-2 provides a plan of care for the client who has experienced a traumatic event. Selected nursing diagnoses are presented, along with outcome criteria, appropriate nursing interventions, and rationales for each.

Evaluation

In the final step of the nursing process, a reassessment is conducted to determine if the nursing actions have been successful in achieving the objectives of care. Evaluation of the nursing actions for the client who has experienced a traumatic event may be facilitated by gathering information utilizing the following types of questions:

■ Has the client escaped serious injury, or have injuries been resolved?

■ Have infections been prevented or resolved?

■ Is the client able to maintain anxiety at manageable level?

(text continues on page 251)

Table 13-2 CARE PLAN FOR THE CLIENT WHO HAS EXPERIENCED A TRAUMATIC EVENT

NURSING DIAGNOSIS: ANXIETY (PANIC)/FEAR

RELATED TO: Real or perceived threat to physical well-being; threat of death; situational crisis; exposure to toxins; unmet needs

EVIDENCED BY: Persistent feelings of apprehension and uneasiness; sense of impending doom; impaired functioning; verbal expressions of having no control or influence over situation, outcome, or self-care; sympathetic stimulation; extraneous physical movements

OUTCOME CRITERIA	NURSING INTERVENTIONS	RATIONALE
Client will maintain anxiety at manageable level.	1. Determine degree of anxiety/fear present, associated behaviors (e.g., laughter, crying, calm or agitation, excited/hysterical behavior, expressions of disbelief and/or self-blame), and reality of perceived threat.	1. Clearly understanding client's perception is pivotal to providing appropriate assistance in overcoming the fear. Individual may be agitated or totally overwhelmed. Panic state increases risk for client's own safety as well as the safety of others in the environment.
	2. Note degree of disorganization.	2. Client may be unable to handle ADLs or work requirements and need more intensive intervention.
	3. Create as quiet an area as possible. Maintain a calm confident manner. Speak in even tone using short simple sentences.	3. Decreases sense of confusion or overstimulation; enhances sense of safety. Helps client focus on what is said and reduces transmission of anxiety.
	4. Develop trusting relationship with the client.	4. Trust is the basis of a therapeutic nurse-client relationship and enables them to work effectively together.
	5. Identify whether incident has reactivated preexisting or coexisting situations (physical or psychological).	5. Concerns and psychological issues will be recycled every time trauma is re-experienced and affect how the client views the current situation.
	6. Determine presence of physical symptoms (e.g., numbness, headache, tightness in chest, nausea, and pounding heart).	6. Physical problems need to be differentiated from anxiety symptoms so appropriate treatment can be given.

Table 13-2 CARE PLAN FOR THE CLIENT WHO HAS EXPERIENCED A TRAUMATIC EVENT—cont'd

OUTCOME CRITERIA	NURSING INTERVENTIONS	RATIONALE
	7. Identify psychological responses (e.g., anger, shock, acute anxiety, panic, confusion, denial). Record emotional changes.	7. Although these are normal responses at the time of the trauma, they will recycle again and again until they are dealt with adequately.
	8. Discuss with client the perception of what is causing the anxiety.	8. Increases the ability to connect symptoms to subjective feeling of anxiety, providing opportunity to gain insight/control and make desired changes.
	9. Assist client to correct any distortions being experienced. Share perceptions with client.	9. Perceptions based on reality will help to decrease fearfulness. How the nurse views the situation may help client to see it differently.
	10. Explore with client or significant other the manner in which client has previously coped with anxiety-producing events.	10. May help client regain sense of control and recognize significance of trauma.
	11. Engage client in learning new coping behaviors (e.g., progressive muscle relaxation, thought-stopping).	11. Replacing maladaptive behaviors can enhance ability to manage and deal with stress. Interrupting obsessive thinking allows client to use energy to address underlying anxiety, whereas continued rumination about the incident can retard recovery.
	12. Encourage use of techniques to manage stress and vent emotions such as anger and hostility.	12. Reduces the likelihood of eruptions that can result in abusive behavior.
	13. Give positive feedback when client demonstrates better ways to manage anxiety and is able to calmly and realistically appraise the situation.	13. Provides acknowledgement and reinforcement, encouraging use of new coping strategies. Enhances ability to deal with fearful feelings and gain control over situation, promoting future successes.
	14. Administer medications as indicated: Antianxiety: diazepam, alprazolam, oxazepam; *or* Antidepressants: fluoxetine, paroxetine, bupropion	14. Provides temporary relief of anxiety symptoms, enhancing ability to cope with situation. To lift mood and help suppress intrusive thoughts and explosive anger.

NURSING DIAGNOSIS: SPIRITUAL DISTRESS

RELATED TO: Physical or psychological stress; energy-consuming anxiety; loss(es), intense suffering; separation from religious or cultural ties; challenged belief and value system

EVIDENCED BY: Expressions of concern about disaster and the meaning of life and death or belief systems; inner conflict about current loss of normality and effects of the disaster; anger directed at deity; engaging in self-blame; seeking spiritual assistance

OUTCOME CRITERIA	NURSING INTERVENTIONS	RATIONALE
Client expresses beliefs and values about spiritual issues	1. Determine client's religious/spiritual orientation, current involvement, and presence of conflicts.	1. Provides baseline for planning care and accessing appropriate resources.
	2. Establish environment that promotes free expression of feelings and concerns. Provide calm, peaceful setting when possible.	2. Promotes awareness and identification of feelings so they can be dealt with.

Continued

Table 13-2 CARE PLAN FOR THE CLIENT WHO HAS EXPERIENCED A TRAUMATIC EVENT—cont'd

OUTCOME CRITERIA	NURSING INTERVENTIONS	RATIONALE
	3. Listen to client's and significant others' expressions of anger, concern, alienation from God, belief that situation is a punishment for wrongdoing, etc.	3. It is helpful to understand the client's and significant others' points of view and how they are questioning their faith in the face of tragedy.
	4. Note sense of futility, feelings of hopelessness and helplessness, lack of motivation to help self.	4. These thoughts and feelings can result in the client feeling paralyzed and unable to move forward to resolve the situation.
	5. Listen to expressions of inability to find meaning in life and reason for living. Evaluate for suicidal ideation.	5. May indicate need for further intervention to prevent suicide attempt.
	6. Determine support systems available to client.	6. Presence or lack of support systems can affect client's recovery.
	7. Ask how you can be most helpful. Convey acceptance of client's spiritual beliefs and concerns.	7. Promotes trust and comfort, encouraging client to be open about sensitive matters.
	8. Make time for nonjudgmental discussion of philosophic issues and questions about spiritual impact of current situation.	8. Helps client to begin to look at basis for spiritual confusion. *Note:* There is a potential for care provider's belief system to interfere with client finding own way. Therefore, it is most beneficial to remain neutral and not espouse own beliefs.
	9. Discuss difference between grief and guilt and help client to identify and deal with each, assuming responsibility for own actions, expressing awareness of the consequences of acting out of false guilt.	9. Blaming self for what has happened impedes dealing with the grief process and needs to be discussed and dealt with.
	10. Use therapeutic communication skills of reflection and active listening.	10. Helps client find own solutions to concerns.
	11. Encourage client to experience meditation, prayer, and forgiveness. Provide information that anger with God is a normal part of the grieving process.	11. This can help to heal past and present pain.
	12. Assist client to develop goals for dealing with life situation.	12. Enhances commitment to goal, optimizing outcomes and promoting sense of hope.
	13. Identify and refer to resources that can be helpful, e.g., pastoral/parish nurse or religious counselor, crisis counselor, psychotherapy, Alcoholics/Narcotics Anonymous.	13. Specific assistance may be helpful to recovery (e.g., relationship problems, substance abuse, suicidal ideation).
	14. Encourage participation in support groups.	14. Discussing concerns and questions with others can help client resolve feelings.

Table 13-2 CARE PLAN FOR THE CLIENT WHO HAS EXPERIENCED A TRAUMATIC EVENT—cont'd

NURSING DIAGNOSIS: RISK FOR POST-TRAUMA SYNDROME

RELATED TO: Events outside the range of usual human experience; serious threat or injury to self or loved ones; witnessing horrors or tragic events; exaggerated sense of responsibility; survivor's guilt or role in the event; inadequate social support

OUTCOME CRITERIA	NURSING INTERVENTIONS	RATIONALE
Client demonstrates ability to deal with emotional reactions in an individually appropriate manner.	1. Determine involvement in event (e.g., survivor, significant other, rescue/aid worker, healthcare provider, family member).	1. All those concerned with a traumatic event are at risk for emotional trauma and have needs related to their involvement in the event. *Note:* Close involvement with victims affects individual responses and may prolong emotional suffering.
	2. Evaluate current factors associated with the event, such as displacement from home due to illness/injury, natural disaster, or terrorist attack. Identify how client's past experiences may affect current situation.	2. Affects client's reaction to current event and is basis for planning care and identifying appropriate support systems and resources.
	3. Listen for comments of taking on responsibility (e.g., "I should have been more careful or gone back to get her.")	3. Statements such as these are indicators of "survivor's guilt" and blaming self for actions.
	4. Identify client's current coping mechanisms.	4. Noting positive or negative coping skills provides direction for care.
	5. Determine availability and usefulness of client's support systems, family, social contacts, and community resources.	5. Family and others close to the client may also be at risk and require assistance to cope with the trauma.
	6. Provide information about signs and symptoms of post-trauma response, especially if individual is involved in a high-risk occupation.	6. Awareness of these factors helps individual identify need for assistance when signs and symptoms occur.
	7. Identify and discuss client's strengths as well as vulnerabilities.	7. Provides information to build on for coping with traumatic experience.
	8. Evaluate individual's perceptions of events and personal significance (e.g., rescue worker trained to provide lifesaving assistance but recovering only dead bodies).	8. Events that trigger feelings of despair and hopelessness may be more difficult to deal with, and require long-term interventions.
	9. Provide emotional and physical presence by sitting with client/significant other and offering solace.	9. Strengthens coping abilities.
	10. Encourage expression of feelings. Note whether feelings expressed appear congruent with events experienced.	10. It is important to talk about the incident repeatedly. Incongruencies may indicate deeper conflict and can impede resolution.
	11. Note presence of nightmares, reliving the incident, loss of appetite, irritability, numbness and crying, and family or relationship disruption.	11. These responses are normal in the early post-incident time frame. If prolonged and persistent, they may indicate need for more intensive therapy.

Continued

Table 13-2 CARE PLAN FOR THE CLIENT WHO HAS EXPERIENCED A TRAUMATIC EVENT—cont'd

OUTCOME CRITERIA	NURSING INTERVENTIONS	RATIONALE
	12. Provide a calm, safe environment.	12. Helps client deal with the disruption in life.
	13. Encourage and assist client in learning stress-management techniques.	13. Promotes relaxation and helps individual exercise control over self and what has happened.
	14. Recommend participation in debriefing sessions that may be provided following major disaster events.	14. Dealing with the stresses promptly may facilitate recovery from the event or prevent exacerbation.
	15. Identify employment, community resource groups.	15. Provides opportunity for ongoing support to deal with recurrent feelings related to the trauma.
	16. Administer medications as indicated, such as antipsychotics (e.g., chlorpromazine, haloperidol, olanzapine, or quetiapine) or carbamazepine (Tegretol).	16. Low doses may be used for reduction of psychotic symptoms when loss of contact with reality occurs, usually for clients with especially disturbing flashbacks. Carbamazepine may be used to alleviate intrusive recollections/flashbacks, impulsivity, and violent behavior.

NURSING DIAGNOSIS: INEFFECTIVE COMMUNITY COPING

RELATED TO: Natural or man-made disasters (earthquakes, tornados, floods, reemerging infectious agents, terrorist activity); ineffective or nonexistent community systems (e.g., lack of or inadequate emergency medical system, transportation system, or disaster planning systems)

EVIDENCED BY: Deficits of community participation; community does not meet its own expectations; expressed vulnerability; community powerlessness; stressors perceived as excessive; excessive community conflicts; high illness rates

OUTCOME CRITERIA	NURSING INTERVENTIONS	RATIONALE
Client demonstrates an increase in activities to improve community functioning.	1. Evaluate community activities that are related to meeting collective needs within the community itself and between the community and the larger society. Note immediate needs, such as healthcare, food, shelter, funds.	1. Provides a baseline to determine community needs in relation to current concerns or threats.
	2. Note community reports of functioning including areas of weakness or conflict.	2. Provides a view of how the community itself sees these areas.
	3. Identify effects of related factors on community activities.	3. In the face of a current threat, local or national, community resources need to be evaluated, updated, and given priority to meet the identified need.
	4. Determine availability and use of resources. Identify unmet demands or needs of the community.	4. Information necessary to identify what else is needed to meet the current situation.
	5. Determine community strengths.	5. Promotes understanding of the ways in which the community is already meeting the identified needs.
	6. Encourage community members/groups to engage in problem-solving activities.	6. Promotes a sense of working together to meet the needs.

Table 13-2 CARE PLAN FOR THE CLIENT WHO HAS EXPERIENCED A TRAUMATIC EVENT—cont'd

OUTCOME CRITERIA	NURSING INTERVENTIONS	RATIONALE
	7. Develop a plan jointly with the members of the community to address immediate needs.	7. Deals with deficits in support of identified goals.
	8. Create plans managing interactions within the community itself and between the community and the larger society.	8. Meets collective needs when the concerns/threats are shared beyond a local community.
	9. Make information accessible to the public. Provide channels for dissemination of information to the community as a whole (e.g., print media, radio/television reports and community bulletin boards, internet sites, speaker's bureau, reports to committees/councils/advisory boards).	9. Readily available accurate information can help citizens deal with the situation.
	10. Make information available in different modalities and geared to differing educational levels/cultures of the community.	10. Using languages other than English and making written materials accessible to all members of the community will promote understanding.
	11. Seek out and evaluate needs of underserved populations.	11. Homeless and those residing in lower income areas may have special requirements that need to be addressed with additional resources.

ADLs = activities of daily living.
From Doenges, M. E., Moorhouse, M. F., & Murr, A. C. (2010). Nursing care plans: Guidelines for individualizing client care across the life span (8th ed.). Philadelphia: F.A. Davis, with permission.

■ Does he or she demonstrate appropriate problem-solving skills?

■ Is the client able to discuss his or her beliefs about spiritual issues?

■ Does the client demonstrate the ability to deal with emotional reactions in an individually appropriate manner?

■ Does he or she verbalize a subsiding of the physical manifestations (e.g., pain, nightmares, flashbacks, fatigue) associated with the traumatic event?

■ Has there been recognition of factors affecting the community's ability to meet its own demands or needs?

■ Has there been a demonstration of increased activities to improve community functioning?

■ Has a plan been established and put in place to deal with future contingencies?

Summary and Key Points

■ A *crisis* is defined as "a sudden event in one's life that disturbs homeostasis, during which usual coping mechanisms cannot resolve the problem" (Lagerquist, 2006).

■ All individuals experience crises at one time or another. This does not necessarily indicate psychopathology.

■ Crises are precipitated by specific identifiable events and are determined by an individual's personal perception of the situation.

■ Crises are acute rather than chronic and generally last no more than a few weeks to a few months.

■ Crises occur when an individual is exposed to a stressor and previous problem-solving techniques are ineffective. This causes the level of anxiety to rise. Panic may ensue when new techniques are tried and resolution fails to occur.

■ Six types of crises have been identified. They include dispositional crises, crises of anticipated life transitions, crises resulting from traumatic stress, maturation/developmental crises, crises reflecting psychopathology, and psychiatric emergencies. The type of crisis determines the method of intervention selected.

■ Crisis intervention is designed to provide rapid assistance for individuals who have an urgent need.

■ The minimum therapeutic goal of crisis intervention is psychological resolution of the individual's immediate crisis and restoration to at least the level of functioning that existed before the crisis period. A maximum goal is improvement in functioning above the precrisis level.

■ Nurses regularly respond to individuals in crisis in all types of settings. Nursing process is the vehicle by which nurses assist individuals in crisis with a short-term problem-solving approach to change.

■ A four-phase technique of crisis intervention includes assessment/analysis, planning of therapeutic intervention, intervention, and evaluation of crisis resolution and anticipatory planning.

■ Through this structured method of assistance, nurses help individuals in crisis to develop more adaptive coping strategies for dealing with stressful situations in the future.

■ Nurses have many important skills that can assist individuals and communities in the wake of traumatic events. Nursing interventions presented in this chapter were developed for the nursing diagnoses of panic anxiety/fear, spiritual distress, risk for post-trauma syndrome, and ineffective community coping.

 Davis*Plus*. Additional info available @ davisplus.fadavis.com

Review Questions
Self-Examination/Learning Exercise

*Select the answer that is **most** appropriate for each of the following questions:*

1. Which of the following is a correct assumption regarding the concept of crisis?
   a. Crises occur only in individuals with psychopathology.
   b. The stressful event that precipitates crisis is seldom identifiable.
   c. A crisis situation contains the potential for psychological growth or deterioration.
   d. Crises are chronic situations that recur many times during an individual's life.

2. Crises occur when an individual:
   a. Is exposed to a precipitating stressor.
   b. Perceives a stressor to be threatening.
   c. Has no support systems.
   d. Experiences a stressor and perceives coping strategies to be ineffective.

3. Amanda's mobile home was destroyed by a tornado. Amanda received only minor injuries, but is experiencing disabling anxiety in the aftermath of the event. This type of crisis is called:
   a. Crisis resulting from traumatic stress.
   b. Maturational/developmental crisis.
   c. Dispositional crisis.
   d. Crisis of anticipated life transitions.

4. The most appropriate crisis intervention with Amanda (from question 3) would be to:
   a. Encourage her to recognize how lucky she is to be alive.
   b. Discuss stages of grief and feelings associated with each.
   c. Identify community resources that can help Amanda.
   d. Suggest that she find a place to live that provides a storm shelter.

Review Questions—cont'd
Self-Examination/Learning Exercise

5. Jenny reported to the high school nurse that her mother drinks too much. She is drunk every afternoon when Jenny gets home from school. Jenny is afraid to invite friends over because of her mother's behavior. This type of crisis is called:
   a. Crisis resulting from traumatic stress.
   b. Maturational/developmental crisis.
   c. Dispositional crisis.
   d. Crisis reflecting psychopathology.

6. The most appropriate nursing intervention with Jenny (from question 5) would be to:
   a. Make arrangements for her to start attending Alateen meetings.
   b. Help her identify the positive things in her life and recognize that her situation could be a lot worse than it is.
   c. Teach her about the effects of alcohol on the body and that it can be hereditary.
   d. Refer her to a psychiatrist for private therapy to learn to deal with her home situation.

7. Ginger, age 19 and an only child, left 3 months ago to attend a college of her choice 500 miles away from her parents. It is Ginger's first time away from home. She has difficulty making decisions and will not undertake anything new without first consulting her mother. They talk on the phone almost every day. Ginger has recently started having anxiety attacks. She consults the nurse practitioner in the student health center. This type of crisis is called:
   a. Crisis resulting from traumatic stress.
   b. Dispositional crisis.
   c. Psychiatric emergency.
   d. Maturational/developmental crisis.

8. The most appropriate nursing intervention with Ginger (from question 7) would be to:
   a. Suggest she move to a college closer to home.
   b. Work with Ginger on unresolved dependency issues.
   c. Help her find someone in the college town from whom she could seek assistance rather than calling her mother regularly.
   d. Recommend that the college physician prescribe an antianxiety medication for Ginger.

9. Marie, age 56, is the mother of five children. Her youngest child, who had been living at home and attending the local college, recently graduated and accepted a job in another state. Marie has never worked outside the home and has devoted her life to satisfying the needs of her husband and children. Since the departure of her last child from home, Marie has become more and more despondent. Her husband has become very concerned, and takes her to the local mental health center. This type of crisis is called:
   a. Dispositional crisis.
   b. Crisis of anticipated life transitions.
   c. Psychiatric emergency.
   d. Crisis resulting from traumatic stress.

10. The most appropriate nursing intervention with Marie (from question 9) would be to:
   a. Refer her to her family physician for a complete physical examination.
   b. Suggest she seek outside employment now that her children have left home.
   c. Identify convenient support systems for times when she is feeling particularly despondent.
   d. Begin grief work and assist her to recognize areas of self-worth separate and apart from her children.

Continued

Review Questions—cont'd
Self-Examination/Learning Exercise

11. The desired outcome of working with an individual who has witnessed a traumatic event and is now experiencing panic anxiety is:
    a. The individual will experience no anxiety.
    b. The individual will demonstrate hope for the future.
    c. The individual will maintain anxiety at a manageable level.
    d. The individual will verbalize acceptance of self as worthy.

12. Andrew, a New York City firefighter, and his entire unit responded to the terrorist attacks at the World Trade Center. Working as a team, he and his best friend, Carlo, entered the area together. Carlo was killed when the building collapsed. Andrew was injured, but survived. Since that time, Andrew has had frequent nightmares and anxiety attacks. He says to the mental health worker, "I don't know why Carlo had to die and I didn't!" This statement by Andrew suggests that he is experiencing:
    a. Spiritual distress.
    b. Night terrors.
    c. Survivor's guilt.
    d. Suicidal ideation.

13. Intervention with Andrew (from question 12) would include:
    a. Encouraging expression of feelings.
    b. Antianxiety medications.
    c. Participation in a support group.
    d. a and c.
    e. All of the above.

References

Aguilera, D. C. (1998). *Crisis intervention: Theory and methodology* (8th ed.). St. Louis: Mosby.

Bateman, A., & Peternelj-Taylor, C. (1998). Crisis intervention. In C. A. Glod (Ed.), *Contemporary psychiatric-mental health nursing: The brain-behavior connection* (pp. 142–156). Philadelphia: F.A. Davis.

Doenges, M. E., Moorhouse, M. F., & Murr, A. C. (2010). *Nursing care plans: Guidelines for individualizing client care across the life span* (8th ed.). Philadelphia: F.A. Davis.

Lagerquist, S. L. (2006). *Davis's NCLEX-RN Success* (2nd ed.). Philadelphia: F.A. Davis.

Norwood, A. E., Ursano, R. J., & Fullerton, C. S. (2000). Disaster psychiatry: Principles and practice. *Psychiatric Quarterly, 71*(3), 207–226.

Oklahoma State Department of Health. (2001). *After the storm: Helping families cope with disaster.* Oklahoma City, OK: Author.

Roberts, A. R., & Ottens, A. J. (2005). The seven-stage crisis intervention model: A road map to goal attainment, problem solving, and crisis resolution. *Brief Treatment and Crisis Intervention, 5*(4), 329–339.

Winston, A. (2008). Supportive psychotherapy. In R. E. Hales, S. C. Yudofsky, & G. O. Gabbard (Eds.), *Textbook of psychiatry* (5th ed., pp. 1257–1277). Washington, DC: American Psychiatric Publishing.

Classical References

Baldwin, B. A. (1978, July). A paradigm for the classification of emotional crises: Implications for crisis intervention. *American Journal of Orthopsychiatry, 48*, 538–551.

Caplan, G. (1964). *Principles of preventive psychiatry.* New York: Basic Books.

Relaxation Therapy CHAPTER

14

CORE CONCEPTS
relaxation

stress

KEY TERMS

biofeedback

meditation

mental imagery

progressive relaxation

stress management

OBJECTIVES
After reading this chapter, the student will be able to:

1. Identify conditions for which relaxation is appropriate therapy.
2. Describe physiological and behavioral manifestations of relaxation.
3. Discuss various methods of achieving relaxation.
4. Describe the role of the nurse in relaxation therapy.

HOMEWORK ASSIGNMENT
Please read the chapter and answer the following questions:

1. Describe the physiological manifestations of relaxation.
2. What is the major difference in the techniques of progressive relaxation and modified (or passive) progressive relaxation?
3. What is the goal of meditation?
4. How does physical exercise work to decrease anxiety and depression?

Researchers now know that stress has a definite effect on the body. They know that stress on the body can be caused by positive events as well as negative ones, and they know that prolonged stress can result in many physiological illnesses. Many times we hear "Relax, take it easy, don't work so hard, don't worry so much; you'll live longer that way." This is good advice no doubt, but it is easier to say than to do.

Nurses are in an ideal position to assist individuals in the management of stress in their lives. This chapter discusses the therapeutic benefits to the individual of regular participation in relaxation exercises. Various methods of achieving relaxation are described, and the nurse's role in helping individuals learn how to use relaxation techniques adaptively is explored.

CORE CONCEPT

Stress
A biological, psychological, social, or chemical factor that causes physical or emotional tension and may be a factor in the etiology of certain illnesses.

The Stress Epidemic

Individuals experience stress as a daily fact of life; it cannot be avoided. It is generated by both positive and negative experiences that require adjustment to various changes in one's current routine. Whether or not there is more stress today than in the past is unknown, but some experts have suggested that it has become more pervasive. Perhaps this is due to the many uncertainties and salient risks that challenge our most basic value systems on a day-to-day basis.

In Chapter 1, a lengthy discussion was presented regarding the "fight or flight" response of the human body to stressful situations. This response served our ancestors well. The extra burst of adrenaline primed their muscles and focused their attention on the danger at hand. Indeed, the response provided early *Homo sapiens* with the essentials to deal with life-and-death situations, such as an imminent attack by a saber-toothed tiger or grizzly bear.

Today, with stress rapidly permeating our society, large segments of the population experience the "fight or flight" response on a regular basis. However, the physiological reinforcements are not used in a manner by which the individual is returned to the homeostatic condition within a short period. The "fight or flight" emergency response is inappropriate to today's psychosocial stresses that persist over long periods. In fact, in today's society, rather than assisting with life-and-death situations, the response may actually be a contributing factor in some life-and-death situations. Stress is now known to be a major contributor, either directly or indirectly, to coronary heart disease, cancer, lung ailments, accidental injuries, cirrhosis of the liver, and suicide—six of the leading causes of death in the United States (Karren, Hafen, Smith, & Frandsen, 2009).

Stress management has become a multimillion-dollar business in the United States. Corporation managers have realized increases in production by providing employees with stress-reduction programs. Hospitals and clinics have responded to the need for services that offer stress management information to individuals and groups.

When, then, is relaxation therapy required? The answer to this question depends largely on *predisposing factors*—the genetic influences, past experiences, and existing conditions that influence how an individual perceives and responds to stress. For example, temperament (i.e., behavioral characteristics that are present at birth) often plays a determining role in the individual's manner of responding to stressful situations. Some individuals, by temperament, naturally respond with a greater degree of anxiety than others.

Past experiences are occurrences that result in learned patterns that can influence an individual's adaptation response. They include previous exposure to the stressor or other stressors, learned coping responses, and degree of adaptation to previous stressors.

Existing conditions are the individual vulnerabilities that can influence the adequacy of the physical, psychological, and social resources for dealing with stressful situations. Examples include current health status, motivation, developmental maturity, severity and duration of the stressor, financial and educational resources, age, existing coping strategies, and a support system of caring others.

All individuals react to stress with predictable physiological and psychosocial responses. These predisposing factors determine the degree of severity of the response. Undoubtedly, there are very few people who would not benefit from some form of relaxation therapy. Miller and Rahe (1997) developed the Recent Life Changes Questionnaire, which correlated an individual's susceptibility to physical or psychological illness with his or her level of stress (see Chapter 1). The lay literature now provides various self-tests that individuals may perform to determine their vulnerability to stress. Two of these are presented in Boxes 14-1 and 14-2.

BOX 14-1 How Vulnerable Are You to Stress?

Score each item from 1 (almost always) to 5 (never), according to how much of the time each statement applies to you.

_____ 1. I eat at least one hot, balanced meal a day.
_____ 2. I get 7 to 8 hours sleep at least four nights a week.
_____ 3. I give and receive affection regularly.
_____ 4. I have at least one relative within 50 miles on whom I can rely.
_____ 5. I exercise to the point of perspiration at least twice a week.
_____ 6. I smoke less than half a pack of cigarettes a day.
_____ 7. I take fewer than five alcoholic drinks a week.
_____ 8. I am the appropriate weight for my height.
_____ 9. I have an income adequate to meet basic expenses.
_____ 10. I get strength from my religious beliefs.

BOX 14-1 How Vulnerable Are You to Stress?—cont'd

_____ 11. I regularly attend club or social activities.

_____ 12. I have a network of friends and acquaintances.

_____ 13. I have one or more friends to confide in about personal matters.

_____ 14. I am in good health (including eyesight, hearing, and teeth).

_____ 15. I am able to speak openly about my feelings when angry or worried.

_____ 16. I have regular conversations with the people I live with about domestic problems (e.g., chores, money, and daily living issues).

_____ 17. I do something for fun at least once a week.

_____ 18. I am able to organize my time effectively.

_____ 19. I drink fewer than three cups of coffee (or tea or colas) a day.

_____ 20. I take quiet time for myself during the day.

_____ TOTAL

To get your score, add up the figures and subtract 20. Any number over 30 indicates a vulnerability to stress. You are seriously vulnerable if your score is between 50 and 75, and extremely vulnerable if it is over 75.

The above test was developed by psychologists Lyle H. Miller, Ph.D., and Alma Dell Smith, Ph.D., of Stress Directions, Inc., Boston, MA. Susceptibility Scale from the Personal Stress Navigator™ by Lyle Miller, Ph.D., and Alma Dell Smith, Ph.D., © 2003 Stress Directions, Inc., www.stressdirections.com. Used by permission of the author

BOX 14-2 Are You "Stressed Out?"

Check yes or no for each of the following questions.

	Yes	No
1. Do you have recurrent headaches, neck tension, or back pain?	____	____
2. Do you often have indigestion, nausea, or diarrhea?	____	____
3. Have you unintentionally gained or lost 5–10 lb in the last month?	____	____
4. Do you have difficulty falling or staying asleep?	____	____
5. Do you often feel restless?	____	____
6. Do you have difficulty concentrating?	____	____
7. Do you drink alcohol, smoke, or take drugs to relax?	____	____
8. Have you had a major illness, surgery or an accident in the past year?	____	____
9. Have you lost five or more days of work due to illness in the past 6 months?	____	____
10. Have you had a change in job status (been fired, laid off, promoted, demoted, and so on) in the past 6 months?	____	____
11. Do you work more than 48 hr a week?	____	____
12. Do you have serious financial problems?	____	____
13. Have you recently experienced family or marital problems?	____	____
14. Has a person of significance in your life died in the past year?	____	____
15. Have you been divorced or separated in the past year?	____	____
16. Do you find you've lost interest in hobbies, physical activity, and leisure time?	____	____
17. Have you lost interest in your relationship with your spouse, relative, or friend?	____	____
18. Do you find yourself watching more TV than you should?	____	____
19. Are you emotional or easily irritated lately?	____	____
20. Do you seem to experience more distress and discomfort than most people?	____	____

SCORING:

Each yes is worth 1 point; each no is worth 0.

Total your points:

0–3 = mildly stressed

4–6 = moderately stressed

7 or more = extremely vulnerable. You may be at risk for stress-related illness.

From The Department of Psychiatry, St. Joseph Medical Center, Wichita, KS. Printed in The Wichita Eagle, November 10, 1990. With permission.

CORE CONCEPT

Relaxation

A decrease in tension or intensity, resulting in refreshment of body and mind. A state of refreshing tranquility.

Physiological, Cognitive, and Behavioral Manifestations of Relaxation

The physiological, cognitive, and behavioral manifestations of stress are well documented (see Chapters 1 and 2). A review of these symptoms is presented in Table 14-1. The persistence of these symptoms over long periods can contribute to the development of numerous stress-related illnesses.

The achievement of relaxation can counteract many of these symptoms. In a state of deep relaxation, the respiration rate may slow to as few as four to six breaths per minute and the heart rate to as low as 24 beats per minute (Pelletier, 1992). Blood pressure decreases and the metabolic rate slows down. Muscle tension diminishes, pupils constrict, and blood vessels in the periphery dilate, leading to increased temperature and feeling of warmth in the extremities.

One's level of consciousness moves from beta activity, which occurs when one is mentally alert and actively thinking, to alpha activity, a state of altered consciousness (Davis, Eshelman, & McKay, 2008). Benefits associated with achievement of alpha consciousness include an increase in creativity, memory, and the ability to concentrate.

Ultimately, an improvement in adaptive functioning may be realized.

When deeply relaxed, individuals are less attentive to distracting stimuli in the external environment. They will respond to questions directed at them but do not initiate verbal interaction. Physical demeanor is very composed. Virtually no muscle activity is observed. Eyes are closed, jaws may be slightly parted, and palms are open with fingers curled, but not clenched. The head may be slightly tilted to the side.

A summary of the physiological, cognitive, and behavioral manifestations of relaxation is presented in Table 14-2.

Methods of Achieving Relaxation

Deep-Breathing Exercises

Deep breathing is a simple technique that is basic to most other relaxation skills. Tension is released when the lungs are allowed to breathe in as much oxygen as possible (Sobel & Ornstein, 1996). Breathing exercises have been found to be effective in reducing anxiety, depression, irritability, muscular tension, and fatigue (Davis et al., 2008; Sobel & Ornstein, 1996). An advantage of these exercises is that they may be accomplished anywhere and at any time. A good guideline is to practice deep breathing for a few minutes three or four times a day or whenever a feeling of tenseness occurs.

Technique

1. Sit, stand, or lie in a comfortable position, ensuring that the spine is straight.

TABLE 14-1 Physiological, Cognitive, and Behavioral Manifestations of Stress		
PHYSIOLOGICAL	**COGNITIVE**	**BEHAVIORAL**
Epinephrine and norepinephrine are released into the bloodstream.	Anxiety increases.	Restlessness
Pupils dilate.	Confusion and disorientation may be evident.	Irritability
Respiration rate increases.	The person is unable to problem solve.	Use or misuse of defense mechanisms
Heart rate increases.	The person is unable to concentrate.	Disorganized routine functioning
Blood pressure increases.		Insomnia and anorexia
Digestion subsides.	Cognitive processes focus on achieving relief from anxiety.	Compulsive or bizarre behaviors (depending on level of anxiety being experienced)
Blood sugar increases.	Learning is inhibited.	
Metabolism increases.		
Serum free fatty acids, cholesterol, and triglycerides increase.	Thoughts may reflect obsessions and ruminations	

TABLE 14-2 Physiological, Cognitive, and Behavioral Manifestations of Relaxation

PHYSIOLOGICAL	COGNITIVE	BEHAVIORAL
Lower levels of epinephrine and norepinephrine in the blood	Change from beta consciousness to alpha consciousness	Distractibility to environmental stimuli is decreased
Respiration rate decreases (sometimes as low as 4-6 breaths per minute)	Creativity and memory are enhanced	Will respond to questions but does not initiate verbal interaction
Heart rate decreases (sometimes as low as 24 beats per minute)	Increased ability to concentrate	Calm, tranquil demeanor; no evidence of restlessness
Blood pressure decreases		Common mannerisms include eyes closed, jaws parted, palms open, fingers curled, and head slightly tilted to the side
Metabolic rate slows down		
Muscle tension diminishes		
Pupils constrict		
Vasodilation and increased temperature in the extremities		

2. Place one hand on your abdomen and the other on your chest.

3. Inhale slowly and deeply through your nose. The abdomen should be expanding and pushing up on your hand. The chest should be moving only slightly.

4. When you have breathed in as much as possible, hold your breath for a few seconds before exhaling.

5. Begin exhaling slowly through the mouth, pursing your lips as if you were going to whistle. Pursing the lips helps to control how fast you exhale and keeps airways open as long as possible.

6. Feel the abdomen deflate as the lungs are emptied of air.

7. Begin the inhale-exhale cycle again. Focus on the sound and feeling of your breathing as you become more and more relaxed.

8. Continue the deep-breathing exercises for 5 to 10 minutes at a time. Once mastered, the technique may be used as often as required to relieve tension.

Progressive Relaxation

Progressive relaxation, a method of deep-muscle relaxation, was developed in 1929 by Chicago physician Edmond Jacobson. His technique is based on the premise that the body responds to anxiety-provoking thoughts and events with muscle tension. Excellent results have been observed with this method in the treatment of muscular tension, anxiety, insomnia, depression, fatigue,

irritable bowel, muscle spasms, neck and back pain, high blood pressure, mild phobias, and stuttering (Davis et al., 2008).

Technique

Each muscle group is tensed for 5 to 7 seconds and then relaxed for 20 to 30 seconds, during which time the individual concentrates on the difference in sensations between the two conditions. Soft, slow background music may facilitate relaxation.

1. Sit in a comfortable chair with your hands in your lap, your feet flat on the floor, and your eyes closed.

2. Begin by taking three deep, slow breaths, inhaling through the nose and releasing the air slowly through the mouth.

3. Now starting with the feet, pull the toes forward toward the knees, stiffen your calves, and hold for a count of 5.

4. Now release the hold. Let go of the tension. Feel the sensation of relaxation and warmth as the tension flows out of the muscles.

5. Next, tense the muscles of the thighs and buttocks, and hold for a count of 5.

6. Now release the hold. Feel the tension drain away, and be aware of the difference in sensation—perhaps a heaviness or feeling of warmth that you did not feel when the muscles were tensed. Concentrate on this feeling for a few seconds.

7. Next, tense the abdominal muscles. Hold for a count of 5.

8. Now release the hold. Concentrate on the feeling of relaxation in the muscles. You may feel a warming sensation. Hold on to that feeling for 15 to 20 seconds.

9. Next, tense the muscles in the back and hold for a count of 5.

10. Now release the hold. Feel the sensation of relaxation and warmth as the tension flows out of the muscles.

11. Next, tense the muscles of your hands, biceps, and forearms. Clench your hands into a tight fist. Hold for a count of 5.

12. Now release the hold. Notice the sensations. You may feel tingling, warmth, or a light, airy feeling. Recognize these sensations as tension leaves the muscles.

13. Next, tense the muscles of the shoulders and neck. Shrug the shoulders tightly and hold for a count of 5.

14. Now release the hold. Sense the tension as it leaves the muscles and experience the feeling of relaxation.

15. Next, tense the muscles of the face. Wrinkle the forehead, frown, squint the eyes, and purse the lips. Hold for a count of 5.

16. Now release the hold. Recognize a light, warm feeling flowing into the muscles.

17. Now feel the relaxation in your whole body. As the tension leaves your entire being, you feel completely relaxed.

18. Open your eyes and enjoy renewed energy.

Modified (or Passive) Progressive Relaxation

Technique

In this version of total-body relaxation the muscles are not tensed. The individual learns to relax muscles by concentrating on the feeling of relaxation within the muscle. These instructions may be presented by one person for another or they may be self-administered. Playing soft, slow background music during the activity may facilitate relaxation.

1. Assume a comfortable position. Some suggestions include the following:
   a. Sitting straight up in a chair with your hands in your lap or at your sides and your feet flat on the floor.
   b. Sitting in a reclining chair with your hands in your lap or at your sides and your legs up on an elevated surface.
   c. Lying flat with your head slightly elevated on a pillow and your arms at your sides.

2. Close your eyes and take three deep breaths through your nose, slowly releasing the air through your mouth.

3. Allow a feeling of peacefulness to descend over you—a pleasant, enjoyable sensation of being comfortable and at ease.

4. Remain in this state for several minutes.

5. It is now time to turn your attention to various parts of your body.

6. Begin with the muscles of the head, face, throat, and shoulders. Concentrate on these muscles, paying particular attention to those in the forehead and jaws. Feel the tension leave the area. The muscles start to feel relaxed, heavy, and warm. Concentrate on this feeling for a few minutes.

7. Now let the feeling of relaxation continue to spread downward to the muscles of your biceps, forearms, and hands. Concentrate on these muscles. Feel the tension dissolve, the muscles starting to feel relaxed and heavy. A feeling of warmth spreads through these muscles all the way to the fingertips. They are feeling very warm and very heavy. Concentrate on this feeling for a few minutes.

8. The tension is continuing to dissolve now, and you are feeling very relaxed. Turn your attention to the muscles in your chest, abdomen, and lower back. Feel the tension leave these areas. Allow these muscles to become very relaxed. They start to feel very warm and very heavy. Concentrate on this feeling for a few minutes.

9. The feeling of relaxation continues to move downward now as we move to the muscles of the thighs, buttocks, calves, and feet. Feel the tension moving down and out of your body. These muscles feel very relaxed now. Your legs are feeling very heavy and very limp. A feeling of warmth spreads over the area, all the way to the toes. You can feel that all the tension has been released.

10. Your whole body feels relaxed and warm. Listen to the music for a few moments and concentrate on this relaxed, warm feeling. Take several deep, slow breaths through your nose, releasing the air through your mouth. Continue to concentrate on how relaxed and warm you feel.

11. It is now time to refocus your concentration on the present and wake up your body to resume activity. Open your eyes and stretch

or massage your muscles. Wiggle your fingers and toes. Take another deep breath, arise, and enjoy the feeling of renewed energy.

Meditation

Records and phenomenological accounts of meditative practices date back more than 2000 years, but only recently have empirical studies revealed the psychophysiological benefits of regular use (Pelletier, 1992). The goal of **meditation** is to gain "mastery over attention." It brings on a special state of consciousness as attention is concentrated solely on one thought or object.

Historically, meditation has been associated with religious doctrines and disciplines by which individuals sought enlightenment with God or another higher power. However, meditation can be practiced independently from any religious philosophy and purely as a means of achieving inner harmony and increasing self-awareness.

During meditation, the respiration rate, heart rate, and blood pressure decrease. The overall metabolism declines, and the need for oxygen consumption is reduced. Alpha brain waves—those associated with brain activity during periods of relaxation—predominate (Pelletier, 1992).

Meditation has been used successfully in the prevention and treatment of various cardiovascular diseases. It has proved helpful in curtailing obsessive thinking, anxiety, depression, and hostility (Davis et al., 2008). Meditation improves concentration and attention.

Technique

1. Select a quiet place and a comfortable position. Various sitting positions are appropriate for meditation. Examples include:
   a. Sitting in a chair with your feet flat on the floor approximately 6 inches apart, arms resting comfortably in your lap.
   b. Cross-legged on the floor or on a cushion.
   c. In the Japanese fashion with your knees on the floor, great toes together, pointed backward, and your buttocks resting comfortably on the bottom of your feet.
   d. In the lotus yoga position, sitting on the floor with your legs flexed at the knees. The ankles are crossed and each foot rests on top of the opposite thigh.
2. Select an object, word, or thought on which to dwell. During meditation, the individual becomes preoccupied with the selected focus. This total preoccupation serves to prevent distractions from interrupting attention. Examples of foci include:
   a. *Counting One's Breaths.* All attention is focused on breathing in and out.
   b. *Mantras.* A *mantra* is a syllable, word, or name that is repeated many times as the mind is cleared of thoughts. Any mantra is appropriate if it works to focus attention and prevent distracting thoughts.
   c. *Objects for Contemplation.* Select an object, such as a rock, a marble, or anything that does not hold a symbolic meaning that might cause distraction. Contemplate the object both visually and tactilely. Focus total attention on the object.
   d. *A Thought That Has Special Meaning to You.* With eyes closed, focus total attention on a specific thought or idea.
3. Practice directing attention on your selected focus for 10 to 15 minutes a day for several weeks. It is essential that the individual does not become upset if intrusive thoughts find their way into the meditation practice. They should merely be dealt with and dismissed as the individual returns to the selected focus of attention. Worrying about one's progress in the ability to meditate is a self-inhibiting behavior.

Mental Imagery

Mental imagery uses the imagination in an effort to reduce the body's response to stress. The frame of reference is very personal, based on what each individual considers to be a relaxing environment. Some might select a scene at the seashore, some might choose a mountain atmosphere, and some might choose floating through the air on a fluffy white cloud. The choices are as limitless as one's imagination. Following is an example of how one individual uses imagery for relaxation. The information is most useful when taped and played back at a time when the individual wishes to achieve relaxation.

Technique

Sit or lie down in a comfortable position. Close your eyes. Imagine that you and someone you love are walking along the seashore. No other people are in sight in any direction. The sun is shining, the sky is blue, and a gentle breeze is blowing. You select a spot to stop and rest. You lie on the sand and close your eyes. You hear the sound of the waves as they splash against the shore. The sun feels warm on your face and body. The sand feels soft and warm against your back. An occasional wave splashes you with a cool mist that dries rapidly in the warm sun. The coconut fragrance of your suntan lotion wafts gently and pleasantly in the air. You lie in this quiet place for what seems like a very long time, taking in the sounds of the waves, the warmth of the sun, and the cooling sensations of the mist and ocean breeze. It is very quiet. It is very warm. You feel very relaxed, very contented. This is your special place. You may come to this special place whenever you want to relax.

Biofeedback

Biofeedback is the use of instrumentation to become aware of processes in your body that you usually do not notice and to help bring them under voluntary control. Biofeedback machines give immediate information about an individual's own biological conditions, such as muscle tension, skin surface temperature, brain-wave activity, skin conductivity, blood pressure, and heart rate (Sadock & Sadock, 2007). Some conditions that can be treated successfully with biofeedback include spastic colon, hypertension, tension and migraine headaches, muscle spasms/pain, anxiety, phobias, stuttering, and teeth grinding.

Technique

Biological conditions are monitored by the biofeedback equipment. Sensors relate muscle spasticity, body temperature, brain-wave activity, heart rate, and blood pressure. Each of these conditions will elicit a signal from the equipment, such as a blinking light, a measure on a meter, or an audible tone. The individual practices using relaxation and voluntary control to modify the signal, in turn indicating a modification of the autonomic function it represents.

Various types of biofeedback equipment have been developed for home use. Often they are less than effective, however, because they usually measure only one autonomic function. In fact, modification of several functions may be required to achieve the benefits of total relaxation.

Biofeedback can help monitor the progress an individual is making toward learning to relax. It is often used together with other relaxation techniques such as deep breathing, progressive relaxation, and mental imagery.

Special training is required to become a biofeedback practitioner. Nurses can support and encourage individuals learning to use this method of stress management. Nurses can also teach other techniques of relaxation that enhance the results of biofeedback training.

Physical Exercise

Regular exercise is viewed by many as one of the most effective methods for relieving stress. Physical exertion provides a natural outlet for the tension produced by the body in its state of arousal for "fight or flight." Following exercise, physiological equilibrium is restored, resulting in a feeling of relaxation and revitalization. Physical inactivity increases all causes of mortality and doubles the risk of cardiovascular disease, type 2 diabetes, and obesity. It also increases the risks of colon and breast cancer, high blood pressure, lipid disorders, osteoporosis, depression, and anxiety (World Health Organization [WHO], 2010).

Aerobic exercises strengthen the cardiovascular system and increase the body's ability to use oxygen more efficiently. Aerobic exercises include brisk walking, jogging, running, cycling, swimming, and dancing, among other activities. To achieve the benefits of aerobic exercises, they must be performed regularly—for at least 30 minutes, three times per week.

Individuals can also benefit from low-intensity physical exercise. Although there is little benefit to the cardiovascular system, low-intensity exercise can help prevent obesity, relieve muscular tension, prevent muscle spasms, and increase flexibility. Examples of low-intensity exercise include slow walking, housecleaning, shopping, light gardening, calisthenics, and weight lifting.

Studies indicate that physical exercise can be effective in reducing general anxiety and depression. Vigorous exercise has been shown to increase levels of beta-endorphins and monoamines (serotonin, norepinephrine, and dopamine), all of which have been implicated in mood regulation (Craft & Perna, 2004). Depressed people are often deficient in these monoamines. Endorphins act as natural narcotics and mood elevators.

The Role of the Nurse in Relaxation Therapy

Nurses work with anxious clients in all departments of the hospital and in community and home health services. Individuals experience stress daily; it cannot be eliminated. Stress is a response to both pleasant and unpleasant events, and usually requires some readjustment on the part of the individual to adapt to it.

> **CLINICAL PEARL** Management of stress must be considered a lifelong function. Nurses can help individuals recognize the sources of stress in their lives and identify methods of adaptive coping.

Assessment

Stress management requires a holistic approach. Physical and psychosocial dimensions are considered in determining the individual's adaptation to stress. Following are some examples of assessment data for collection. Other assessments may need to be made, depending on specific circumstances of each individual.

1. Genetic influences
   a. Identify medical/psychiatric history of client and biological family members.
2. Past experiences
   a. Describe your living/working conditions.
   b. When did you last have a physical examination?
   c. Do you have a spiritual or religious position from which you derive support?
   d. Do you have a job? Have you experienced any recent employment changes or other difficulties on your job?
   e. What significant changes have occurred in your life in the last year?
   f. What is your usual way of coping with stress?
   g. Do you have someone to whom you can go for support when you feel stressed?
3. Client's perception of the stressor
   a. What do you feel is the major source of stress in your life right now?
4. Adaptation responses
   a. Do you ever feel anxious? Confused? Unable to concentrate? Fearful?
   b. Do you have tremors? Stutter or stammer? Sweat profusely?
   c. Do you often feel angry? Irritable? Moody?
   d. Do you ever feel depressed? Do you ever feel like harming yourself or others?
   e. Do you have difficulty communicating with others?
   f. Do you experience pain? In what part of your body? When do you experience it? When does it worsen?
   g. Do you ever experience stomach upset? Constipation? Diarrhea? Nausea and vomiting?
   h. Do you ever feel your heart pounding in your chest?
   i. Do you take any drugs (prescription, over-the-counter, or street)?
   j. Do you drink alcohol? Smoke cigarettes? How much?
   k. Are you eating more/less than usual?
   l. Do you have difficulty sleeping?
   m. Do you have a significant other? Describe the relationship.
   n. Describe your relationship with other family members.
   o. Do you perceive any problems in your sexual lifestyle or behavior?

Diagnosis

Possible nursing diagnoses for individuals requiring assistance with stress management are listed here. Others may be appropriate for individuals with particular problems.

- Risk-prone health behavior
- Anxiety (specify level)
- Disturbed body image
- Coping, defensive
- Coping, ineffective
- Decisional conflict (specify)
- Denial, ineffective
- Fear
- Grieving
- Grieving, complicated
- Hopelessness
- Deficient knowledge (specify)
- Pain (acute or chronic)
- Parental role conflict
- Post-trauma syndrome
- Powerlessness
- Rape-trauma syndrome
- Role performance, ineffective
- Low self-esteem
- Sexual dysfunction
- Sexuality patterns, ineffective
- Sleep pattern, disturbed
- Social interaction, impaired
- Social isolation
- Spiritual distress
- Violence, risk for self-directed or other-directed

Outcome Identification/Implementation

The immediate goal for nurses working with individuals needing assistance with stress management is to help minimize current maladaptive symptoms. The long-term goal is to assist individuals toward achievement of their highest potential for wellness. Examples of outcome criteria may include:

- Client will verbalize a reduction in pain following progressive relaxation techniques.

■ Client will be able to voluntarily control a decrease in blood pressure following 3 weeks of biofeedback training.

■ Client will be able to maintain stress at a manageable level by performing deep-breathing exercises when feeling anxious.

Implementation of nursing actions has a strong focus on the role of client teacher. Relaxation therapy, as described in this chapter, is one way to help individuals manage stress. These techniques are well within the scope of nursing practice.

Evaluation

Evaluation requires that the nurse and client assess whether or not these techniques are achieving the desired outcomes. Various alternatives may be attempted and reevaluated.

Relaxation therapy provides alternatives to old, maladaptive methods of coping with stress. Lifestyle changes may be required, and change does not come easily. Nurses must help individuals analyze the usefulness of these techniques in the management of stress in their daily lives.

Summary and Key Points

■ Stress is part of our everyday lives. It can be positive or negative, but it cannot be eliminated.

■ Keeping stress at a manageable level is a lifelong process.

■ Individuals under stress respond with a physiological arousal that can be dangerous over long periods.

■ The stress response has been shown to be a major contributor, either directly or indirectly, to coronary heart disease, cancer, lung ailments, accidental injuries, cirrhosis of the liver, and suicide—six of the leading causes of death in the United States.

■ Relaxation therapy is an effective means of reducing the stress response in some individuals.

■ The degree of anxiety that an individual experiences in response to stress is related to certain predisposing factors, such as characteristics of temperament with which he or she was born, past experiences resulting in learned patterns of responding, and existing conditions, such as health status, coping strategies, and adequate support systems.

■ Deep relaxation can counteract the physiological and behavioral manifestations of stress.

■ Some examples of relaxation therapy include deep-breathing exercises, progressive relaxation, passive progressive relaxation, meditation, mental imagery, biofeedback, and physical exercise.

■ Nurses use the nursing process to assist individuals in the management of stress.

■ Assessment data are collected from which nursing diagnoses are derived.

■ Outcome criteria that help individuals reduce current maladaptive symptoms and ultimately achieve their highest potential for wellness are identified.

■ Implementation includes instructing clients and their families in the various techniques for achieving relaxation. Behavioral changes provide objective measurements for evaluation.

 DavisPlus. Additional info available @ davisplus.fadavis.com

Review Questions
Self-Examination/Learning Exercise

Select the answer that is most appropriate for each of the following questions:

1. Which of the following are considered good forms of aerobic exercise? (Select all that apply.)
   a. Swimming.
   b. Cycling.
   c. Shopping.
   d. Housecleaning.
   e. Running.

Review Questions—cont'd
Self-Examination/Learning Exercise

2. Which of the following are cognitive manifestations of stress? (Select all that apply.)
   a. Inability to concentrate.
   b. Obsessive thoughts.
   c. Alpha brain waves predominate.
   d. Anxiety increases.
   e. Creativity is enhanced.

3. John tells the nurse that he suffers from test anxiety, and gets very stressed prior to and during exams. The nurse suggests to John that he take short breaks during the exam to de-stress. Which of the following relaxation exercises would be *most* appropriate for the nurse to suggest to John under these circumstances?
   a. Deep-breathing exercises.
   b. Progressive relaxation exercises.
   c. Meditation.
   d. Mental imagery.

4. Linda has just been promoted from the typing pool to a position as personal secretary to the CEO of a large corporation. She is now expected to attend and take minutes of all board meetings, screen calls and visitors for her boss, keep track of his schedule and remind him of important appointments, and make decisions for him in his absence. She tells the nurse that she is fearful of making mistakes and is constantly "nervous." She is having trouble sleeping and has lost 10 pounds since taking over the job. Which of the following nursing diagnoses would be a priority for Linda?
   a. Decisional conflict.
   b. Powerlessness.
   c. Anxiety (severe).
   d. Low self-esteem.

5. Based on the answer in question 4, which of the following would be appropriate outcome criteria for Linda?
   a. Linda will verbalize choices in a plan to maintain control over her life.
   b. Linda verbalizes a positive perception about herself.
   c. Linda will make a decision about whether to stay in her current position.
   d. Linda will demonstrate ability to maintain anxiety at manageable level.

References

Craft, L. L., & Perna, F. M. (2004). The benefits of exercise for the clinically depressed. *Primary Care Companion Journal of Clinical Psychiatry, 6*(4), 104–111.

Davis, M. D., Eshelman, E. R., & McKay, M. (2008). *The relaxation and stress reduction workbook* (6th ed.) Oakland, CA: New Harbinger Publications.

Karren, K. J., Hafen, B. Q., Smith, N. L., & Frandsen, K. J. (2009). *Mind/body health: The effects of attitudes, emotions, and relationships* (4th ed.). San Francisco: Benjamin Cummings.

Miller, M. A., & Rahe, R. H. (1997). Life changes scaling for the 1990s. *Journal of Psychosomatic Research 43*(3), 279–292.

Pelletier, K. R. (1992). *Mind as healer, mind as slayer.* New York: Dell.

Sadock, B. J., & Sadock, V. A. (2007). *Synopsis of psychiatry: Behavioral sciences/clinical psychiatry* (10th ed.). Philadelphia: Lippincott Williams & Wilkins.

Sobel, D. S., & Ornstein, R. (1996). *The healthy mind, healthy body handbook.* Los Altos, CA: DR$_X$.

World Health Organization. (2010). *Global strategy on diet, physical activity, and health.* Retrieved August 2, 2010, from http://www.who.int/dietphysicalactivity/publications/en/

CHAPTER 15 Assertiveness Training

CORE CONCEPT
assertive behavior

KEY TERMS

aggressive
assertive
nonassertive

passive-aggressive
thought stopping

OBJECTIVES
After reading this chapter, the student will be able to:

1. Define *assertive behavior.*
2. Discuss basic human rights.
3. Differentiate among nonassertive, assertive, aggressive, and passive-aggressive behaviors.
4. Describe techniques that promote assertive behavior.
5. Demonstrate thought-stopping techniques.
6. Discuss the role of the nurse in assertiveness training

HOMEWORK ASSIGNMENT
Please read the chapter and answer the following questions:

1. What is the goal of assertive behavior?
2. Assertive individuals accept negative aspects about themselves, and admit when they have made a mistake. What is this technique called?
3. What technique may be used to rid the mind of negative thoughts with which an individual may be obsessed? Give an example.
4. Why are "I" statements an effective communication technique?

Alberti and Emmons (2008) have proposed the following questions:

Are you able to express warm, positive feelings to another person? Are you comfortable starting a conversation with strangers at a party? Do you sometimes feel ineffective in making your desires clear to others? Do you have difficulty saying no to persuasive people? Are you often at the bottom of the "pecking order," pushed around by others? Or maybe you're the one who pushes others around to get your way? (p. 5)

Assertive behavior promotes a feeling of personal power and self-confidence. These two components are commonly lacking in clients with emotional disorders. Becoming more assertive empowers individuals by promoting self-esteem, without diminishing the esteem of others.

This chapter describes a number of rights that are considered basic to human beings. Various kinds of behaviors are explored, including assertive, nonassertive, aggressive, and passive-aggressive. Techniques that promote assertive behavior and the nurse's role in assertiveness training are presented.

Assertive Communication

Assertive behavior helps us feel good about ourselves and increases our self-esteem. It helps us feel good about other people and increases our ability to develop satisfying relationships with others. This is accomplished out of honesty, directness, appropriateness, and respecting one's own basic rights as well as the rights of others.

Honesty is basic to assertive behavior. Assertive honesty is not an outspoken declaration of everything that is on one's mind. It is instead an accurate representation of feelings, opinions, or preferences expressed in a manner that promotes self-respect and respect for others.

Direct communication is stating what one wants to convey with clarity and candor. Hinting and "beating around the bush" are indirect forms of communication.

Communication must occur in an appropriate context to be considered assertive. The location and timing, as well as the manner (tone of voice, nonverbal gestures) in which the communication is presented, must be correct for the situation.

Basic Human Rights

A number of authors have identified a variety of "assertive rights" (Davis, McKay, & Eshelman, 2008; Lloyd, 2002; Powell & Enright, 1990; Schuster, 2000; Sobel & Ornstein, 1996). Following is a composite of 10 basic assertive human rights adapted from the aggregation of sources.

1. The right to be treated with respect.
2. The right to express feelings, opinions, and beliefs.
3. The right to say "no" without feeling guilty.
4. The right to make mistakes and accept the responsibility for them.
5. The right to be listened to and taken seriously.
6. The right to change your mind.
7. The right to ask for what you want.
8. The right to put yourself first, sometimes.
9. The right to set your own priorities.
10. The right to refuse justification for your feelings or behavior.

In accepting these rights, an individual also accepts the responsibilities that accompany them. Rights and responsibilities are reciprocal entities. To experience one without the other is inherently destructive to an individual. Some responsibilities associated with basic assertive human rights are presented in Table 15-1.

Response Patterns

Individuals develop patterns of responding to others. Some of the patterns that have been identified include:

1. Watching other people (role modeling).
2. Being positively reinforced or punished for a certain response.
3. Inventing a response.
4. Not being able to think of a better way to respond.
5. Not developing the proper skills for a better response.
6. Consciously choosing a response style.

The nurse should be able to recognize his or her own pattern of responding, as well as that of others. Four response patterns will be discussed here: nonassertive, assertive, aggressive, and passive-aggressive.

Nonassertive Behavior

Individuals who are **nonassertive** (sometimes called *passive*) seek to please others at the expense of denying their own basic human rights. They seldom let their true feelings show and often feel hurt and anxious because they allow others to choose for them. They seldom achieve their own desired goals (Alberti & Emmons, 2008). They come across as being very apologetic and tend to be self-deprecating. They use actions instead of words and hope someone will "guess" what they want. Their voices are hesitant, weak, and expressed in a monotone. Their eyes are usually downcast. They feel uncomfortable in interpersonal interactions. All they want is to please and to be liked by others. Their behavior helps them avoid

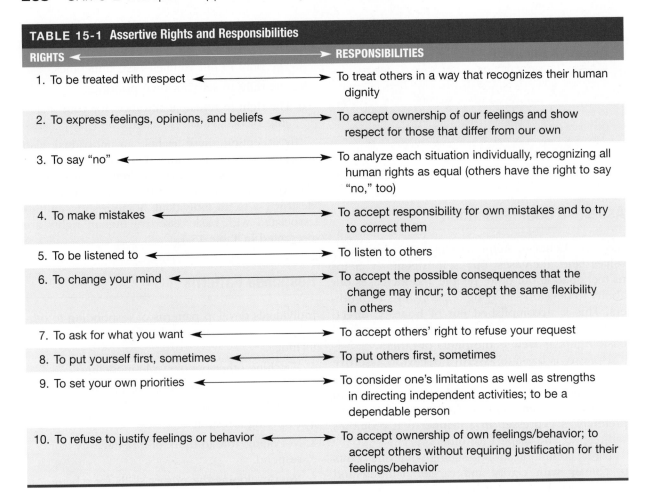

TABLE 15-1 Assertive Rights and Responsibilities

RIGHTS ⬅⎯⎯⎯⎯⎯⎯⎯⎯➡	RESPONSIBILITIES
1. To be treated with respect ⬅⎯⎯⎯➡	To treat others in a way that recognizes their human dignity
2. To express feelings, opinions, and beliefs ⬅⎯➡	To accept ownership of our feelings and show respect for those that differ from our own
3. To say "no" ⬅⎯⎯⎯⎯⎯⎯⎯➡	To analyze each situation individually, recognizing all human rights as equal (others have the right to say "no," too)
4. To make mistakes ⬅⎯⎯⎯⎯⎯➡	To accept responsibility for own mistakes and to try to correct them
5. To be listened to ⬅⎯⎯⎯⎯➡	To listen to others
6. To change your mind ⬅⎯⎯⎯➡	To accept the possible consequences that the change may incur; to accept the same flexibility in others
7. To ask for what you want ⬅⎯⎯➡	To accept others' right to refuse your request
8. To put yourself first, sometimes ⬅⎯➡	To put others first, sometimes
9. To set your own priorities ⬅⎯⎯➡	To consider one's limitations as well as strengths in directing independent activities; to be a dependable person
10. To refuse to justify feelings or behavior ⬅⎯➡	To accept ownership of own feelings/behavior; to accept others without requiring justification for their feelings/behavior

unpleasant situations and confrontations with others; however, they often harbor anger and resentment.

Assertive Behavior

Assertive individuals stand up for their own rights while protecting the rights of others. Feelings are expressed openly and honestly. They assume responsibility for their own choices and allow others to choose for themselves. They maintain self-respect and respect for others by treating everyone equally and with human dignity. They communicate tactfully, using lots of "I" statements. Their voices are warm and expressive, and eye contact is intermittent but direct. These individuals desire to communicate effectively with, and be respected by, others. They are self-confident and experience satisfactory and pleasurable relationships with others.

Aggressive Behavior

Individuals who are **aggressive** defend their own basic rights by violating the basic rights of others. Feelings are often expressed dishonestly and inappropriately. They say what is on their minds, often at the expense of others. Aggressive behavior commonly results in a *putdown* of the receiver. With his or her rights denied, the receiver feels hurt, defensive, and humiliated (Alberti & Emmons, 2008). Aggressive individuals devalue the self-worth of others on whom they impose their choices. They express an air of superiority, and their voices are often loud, demanding, angry, or cold, without emotion. Eye contact may be "to intimidate others by staring them down." They want to increase their feeling of power by dominating or humiliating others. Aggressive behavior hinders interpersonal relationships.

Passive-Aggressive Behavior

Passive-aggressive individuals defend their own rights by expressing resistance to social and occupational demands (American Psychiatric Association [APA], 2000). Sometimes called *indirect aggression,* this behavior takes the form of passive, nonconfrontive action (Alberti & Emmons, 2008). These individuals are devious, manipulative, and sly, and they undermine others with behavior that expresses the opposite of what they are feeling. They are highly critical and sarcastic. They allow others to make choices for them, then resist by using passive behaviors, such as procrastination, dawdling, stubbornness, and "forgetfulness." They use actions instead of words to convey their message, and the actions express covert aggression. They become sulky, irritable, or argumentative when asked to do something they do not want to do. They may protest to others about the demand but will not confront the person who is making the demand. Instead, they may deal with the demand by "forgetting" to do it. The goal is domination through retaliation. This behavior offers a feeling of control and power, although passive-aggressive individuals actually feel resentment and that they are being taken advantage of. They possess extremely low self-confidence.

A comparison of these four behavior patterns is presented in Table 15-2.

TABLE 15-2 Comparison of Behavioral Response Patterns

	NONASSERTIVE	ASSERTIVE	AGGRESSIVE	PASSIVE-AGGRESSIVE
Behavioral Characteristics	Passive, does not express true feelings, self-deprecating, denies own rights	Stands up for own rights, protects rights of others, honest, direct, appropriate	Violates rights of others, expresses feelings dishonestly and inappropriately	Defends own rights with passive resistance, is critical and sarcastic; often expresses opposite of true feelings
Examples	"Uh, well, uh, sure, I'll be glad to stay and work an extra shift."	"I don't want to stay and work an extra shift today. I stayed over yesterday. It's someone else's turn today."	"You've got to be kidding!"	"Okay, I'll stay and work an extra shift." (Then to peer: "How dare she ask me to work over again! Well, we'll just see how much work she gets out of me!")
Goals	To please others; to be liked by others	To communicate effectively; to be respected by others	To dominate or humiliate others	To dominate through retaliation
Feelings	Anxious, hurt, disappointed with self, angry, resentful	Confident, successful, proud, self-respecting	Self-righteous, controlling, superior	Angry, resentful, manipulated, controlled
Compensation	Is able to avoid unpleasant situations and confrontations with others	Increased self-confidence, self-respect, respect for others, satisfying interpersonal relationships	Anger is released, increasing feeling of power and superiority	Feels self-righteous and in control
Outcomes	Goals not met; others meet *their* goals at nonassertive person's expense; anger and resentment grow; feels violated and manipulated	Goals met; desires most often fulfilled while defending own rights as well as rights of others	Goals may be met but at the expense of others; they feel hurt and vengeful	Goals not met, nor are the goals of others met due to retaliatory nature of the interaction

SOURCES: *Alberti and Emmons (2008); Davis, McKay, and Eshelman (2008); Lloyd (2002); and Powell and Enright (1990).*

Behavioral Components of Assertive Behavior

Alberti and Emmons (2008) have identified several defining characteristics of assertive behavior:

- **Eye contact.** Eye contact is considered appropriate when it is intermittent (i.e., looking directly at the person to whom one is speaking but looking away now and then). Individuals feel uncomfortable when someone stares at them continuously and intently. Intermittent eye contact conveys the message that one is interested in what is being said.

- **Body posture.** Sitting and leaning slightly toward the other person in a conversation suggests an active interest in what is being said. Emphasis on an assertive stance can be achieved by standing with an erect posture, squarely facing the other person. A slumped posture conveys passivity or nonassertiveness.

- **Distance/physical contact.** The distance between two individuals in an interaction or the physical contact between them has a strong cultural influence. For example, in the United States, intimate distance is considered approximately 18 inches from the body. We are very careful about whom we allow to enter this intimate space. Invasion of this space may be interpreted by some individuals as very aggressive.

- **Gestures.** Nonverbal gestures may also be culturally related. Gesturing can add emphasis, warmth, depth, or power to the spoken word.

- **Facial expression.** Various facial expressions convey different messages (e.g., frown, smile, surprise, anger, fear). It is difficult to "fake" these messages. In assertive communication, the facial expression is congruent with the verbal message.

- **Voice.** The voice conveys a message by its loudness, softness, degree and placement of emphasis, and evidence of emotional tone.

- **Fluency.** Being able to discuss a subject with ease and with obvious knowledge conveys assertiveness and self-confidence. This message is impeded by numerous pauses or filler words such as "and, uh . . ." or "you know . . . .."

- **Timing.** Assertive responses are most effective when they are spontaneous and immediate. However, most people have experienced times when it was not appropriate to respond (e.g., in front of a group of people) or times when an appropriate response is generated only after the fact ("If only I had said . . ."). Alberti and Emmons (2008) stated that " . . . it is never too late to be assertive!" It is correct and worthwhile to seek out the individual at a later time and express the assertive response.

- **Listening.** Assertive listening means giving the other individual full attention by making eye contact, nodding to indicate acceptance of what is being said, and taking time to understand what is being said before giving a response.

- **Thoughts.** Cognitive processes affect one's assertive behavior. Two such processes are (1) an individual's attitudes about the appropriateness of assertive behavior in general and (2) the appropriateness of assertive behavior for himself or herself specifically.

- **Content.** Many times individuals do not respond to an unpleasant situation because "I just didn't know what to say." Perhaps *what* is being said is not as important as *how* it is said. Emotions should be expressed when they are experienced. It is also important to accept ownership of those emotions and not devalue the worth of another individual to assert oneself.

- **Persistence.** This element of assertive behavior speaks to not giving up; that is, to refrain from concluding that the individual is not worth whatever it is he or she is pursuing. Alberti and Emmons (2008) suggested that all of the components of assertive behavior are important; "the element of persistence simply means applying them again, and again, and again, as needed" (p. 81).

Techniques That Promote Assertive Behavior

The following techniques have been shown to be effective in responding to criticism and avoiding manipulation by others.

1. **Standing up for one's basic human rights.**

EXAMPLE

"I have the right to express my opinion."

2. **Assuming responsibility for one's own statements.**

EXAMPLE

"I *don't want* to go out with you tonight," instead of "I *can't* go out with you tonight." The latter implies a lack of power or ability.

3. **Responding as a "broken record."** Persistently repeating in a calm voice what is wanted.

EXAMPLE

Telephone salesperson: "I want to help you save money by changing long-distance services."

Assertive response: "I don't want to change my long-distance service."

Telephone salesperson: "I can't believe you don't want to save money!"

Assertive response: "I don't want to change my long-distance service."

4. **Agreeing assertively.** Assertively accepting negative aspects about oneself; admitting when an error has been made.

EXAMPLE

Ms. Jones: "You sure let that meeting get out of hand. What a waste of time."

Ms. Smith: "Yes, I didn't do a very good job of conducting the meeting today."

5. **Inquiring assertively.** Seeking additional information about critical statements.

EXAMPLE

Male board member: "You made a real fool of yourself at the board meeting last night."

Female board member: "Oh, really? Just what about my behavior offended you?"

Male board member: "You were so damned pushy!"

Female board member: "Were you offended that I spoke up for my beliefs, or was it because my beliefs are in direct opposition to yours?"

6. **Shifting from content to process.** Changing the focus of the communication from discussing the topic at hand to analyzing what is actually going on in the interaction.

EXAMPLE

Wife: "Would you please call me if you will be late for dinner?"

Husband: "Why don't you just get off my back! I always have to account for every minute of my time with you!"

Wife: "Sounds to me like we need to discuss some other things here. What are you *really* angry about?"

7. **Clouding/fogging.** Concurring with the critic's argument without becoming defensive and without agreeing to change.

EXAMPLE

Nurse 1: "You never come to the Nurses' Association meetings. I don't know why you even belong!"

Nurse 2: "You're right. I haven't attended very many of the meetings."

8. **Defusing.** Putting off further discussion with an angry individual until he or she is calmer.

EXAMPLE

"You are very angry right now. I don't want to discuss this matter with you while you are so upset. I will discuss it with you in my office at 3 o'clock this afternoon."

9. **Delaying assertively.** Putting off further discussion with another individual until one is calmer.

EXAMPLE

"That's a very challenging position you have taken, Mr. Brown. I'll need time to give it some thought. I'll call you later this afternoon."

10. **Responding assertively with irony.**

EXAMPLE

Man: "I bet you're one of them so-called 'women's libbers,' aren't you?"

Woman: "Why, yes. Thank you for noticing."

11. **Using "I" statements.** "I" statements allow an individual to take ownership for his or her feelings rather than saying they are caused by another person.

"I" statements are sometimes called "feeling" statements. They express directly what an individual is feeling. "You" statements are accusatory and put the receiver on the defensive. "I" statements have four parts:

1. How I feel: *these are my feelings and I accept ownership of them*
2. When: *describe in a neutral manner the behavior that is the problem*
3. Why: *describe what it is about the behavior that is objectionable*
4. Suggest change: *offering a preferred alternative to the behavior*

EXAMPLE

John has just returned from a hunting trip and walked into the living room in his muddy boots leaving a trail of mud on the carpet. His wife, Mary, may respond as follows:

With a "you" statement: "You are such a jerk! Can't you see the trail of mud you are leaving on the carpet? I just cleaned this carpet. You make me so angry!"

With an "I" statement: "I feel so angry when you walk on the carpet in your muddy boots. I just cleaned it, and now I will have to clean it again. I would appreciate it if you would remove your boots on the porch before you come in the house."

"You" statements are negative and focus on what the person has done wrong. They don't explain what is being requested of the person. "I" statements are more positive. They explain *how* one is feeling, *why* he or she is feeling that way, and *what* the individual wants instead. Hopkins (2010) stated the following about the importance of "I" statements:

Part of being assertive involves the ability to appropriately express your needs and feelings. You can accomplish this by using "I" statements. These [statements] indicate ownership, do not attribute blame, focus on behavior, identify the effect of the behavior, are direct and honest, and contribute to the growth of your relationship with each other. (p. 2)

Thought-Stopping Techniques

Assertive thinking is sometimes inhibited by repetitive, negative thoughts of which the mind refuses to let go. Individuals with low self-worth may be obsessed with thoughts such as, "I know he'd never want to go out with me. I'm too ugly (or plain, or fat, or dumb)" or "I just know I'll never be able to do this job well" or "I just can't seem to do anything right." This type of thinking fosters the belief that one's individual rights do not deserve the same consideration as those of others, and reflects nonassertive communication and behavioral response patterns.

Thought-stopping techniques, as described here, were developed by psychiatrist Joseph Wolpe (1990) and are intended to eliminate intrusive, unwanted thoughts.

Method

In a practice setting, with eyes closed, the individual concentrates on an unwanted recurring thought. Once the thought is clearly established in the mind, he or she shouts aloud: "STOP!" This action will interrupt the thought, and it is actually removed from one's awareness. The individual then immediately shifts his or her thoughts to one that is considered pleasant and desirable.

It is possible that the unwanted thought may soon recur, but with practice, the length of time between recurrences will increase until the unwanted thought is no longer intrusive.

Obviously, one cannot go about his or her daily life shouting, "STOP!" in public places. After a number of practice sessions, the technique is equally effective if the word "stop!" is used silently in the mind.

Role of the Nurse in Assertiveness Training

It is important for nurses to become aware of and recognize their own behavioral responses. Are they mostly nonassertive? Assertive? Aggressive? Passive-aggressive? Do they consider their behavioral responses effective? Do they wish to change? Remember, all individuals have the right to choose whether or not they want to be assertive. A self-assessment of assertiveness is found in Box 15-1.

The ability to respond assertively is especially important to nurses who are committed to further development of the profession. Assertive skills facilitate the implementation of change—change that is required if the image of nursing is to be upgraded to the level of professionalism that most nurses desire. Assertive communication is useful in the political arena for nurses who choose to become involved at both state and national levels in striving to influence legislation and, ultimately, to improve the system of health-care provision in our country.

Nurses who understand and use assertiveness skills themselves can in turn assist clients who wish to effect behavioral change in an effort to increase self-esteem and improve interpersonal relationships. The nursing process is a useful tool for nurses who are involved in helping clients increase their assertiveness.

Assessment

Nurses can help clients become more aware of their behavioral responses. Many tools for assessing the level of assertiveness have been developed over the years. None has been very effective. Perhaps this is because it is so difficult to *generalize* when attempting to measure

BOX 15-1 An Assertiveness Quiz

Assign a number to each item using the following scale: 1 = Never; 3 = Sometimes; 5 = Always

_____ 1. I ask others to do things without feeling guilty or anxious.

_____ 2. When someone asks me to do something I don't want to do, I say no without feeling guilty or anxious.

_____ 3. I am comfortable when speaking to a large group of people.

_____ 4. I confidently express my honest opinions to authority figures (such as my boss).

_____ 5. When I experience powerful feelings (anger, frustration, disappointment, and so on), I verbalize them easily.

_____ 6. When I express anger, I do so without blaming others for "making me mad."

_____ 7. I am comfortable speaking up in a group situation.

_____ 8. If I disagree with the majority opinion in a meeting, I can "stick to my guns" without feeling uncomfortable or being abrasive.

_____ 9. When I make a mistake, I acknowledge it.

_____10. I tell others when their behavior creates a problem for me.

_____11. Meeting new people in social situations is something I do with ease and comfort.

_____12. When discussing my beliefs, I do so without labeling the opinions of others as "crazy," "stupid," "ridiculous," or "irrational."

_____13. I assume that most people are competent and trustworthy and do not have difficulty delegating tasks to others.

_____14. When considering doing something I have never done, I feel confident I can learn to do it.

_____15. I believe that my needs are as important as those of others, and I am entitled to have my needs satisfied.

_____   TOTAL SCORE

SCORING:

If your total score is 60 or higher, you have a consistently assertive philosophy and probably handle most situations well.

   If your total score is 45–59, you have a fairly assertive outlook, but may benefit from some assertiveness training.

   If your total score is 30–44, you may be assertive in some situations, but your natural response is either nonassertive or aggressive. Assertiveness training is suggested.

   If your total score is 15–29, you have considerable difficulty being assertive. Assertiveness training is recommended.

From Lloyd, S. R. (2002). Developing positive assertiveness (3rd ed.). Menlo Park, CA: Crisp Publications, with permission.

assertive behaviors. Box 15-2 and Figure 15–1 represent examples of assertiveness inventories that could be personalized to describe life situations of individual clients more specifically. Obviously, "everyday situations that may require assertiveness" are not the same for all individuals.

Diagnosis

Possible nursing diagnoses for individuals needing assistance with assertiveness include:

1. Coping, defensive
2. Coping, ineffective
3. Decisional conflict
4. Denial, ineffective
5. Personal identity, disturbed
6. Powerlessness
7. Rape-trauma syndrome
8. Self-esteem, low
9. Social interaction, impaired
10. Social isolation

Outcome Identification/Implementation

The goal for nurses working with individuals needing assistance with assertiveness is to help them develop more satisfying interpersonal relationships. Individuals who do not feel good about themselves either allow others to violate their rights or cover up their low self-esteem by being overtly or covertly aggressive. Individuals should be given information regarding their individual human rights. They must know what these rights are before they can stand up for them.

   Outcome criteria would be derived from specific nursing diagnoses. Some examples include the following. Timelines are individually determined.

■ The client verbalizes and accepts responsibility for his or her own behavior.

BOX 15-2 Everyday Situations That May Require Assertiveness

AT WORK

How do you respond when:
1. You receive a compliment on your appearance or someone praises your work?
2. You are criticized unfairly?
3. You are criticized legitimately by a superior?
4. You have to confront a subordinate for continual lateness or sloppy work?
5. Your boss makes a sexual innuendo or makes a pass at you?

IN PUBLIC

How do you respond when:
1. In a restaurant, the food you ordered arrives cold or overcooked?
2. A fellow passenger in a no-smoking compartment lights a cigarette?
3. You are faced with an unhelpful shop assistant?
4. Somebody barges in front of you in a waiting line?
5. You take an inferior article back to a shop?

AMONG FRIENDS

How do you respond when:
1. You feel angry with the way a friend has treated you?
2. A friend makes what you consider to be an unreasonable request?
3. You want to ask a friend for a favor?
4. You ask a friend for repayment of a loan of money?
5. You have to negotiate with a friend on which film to see or where to meet?

AT HOME

How do you respond when:
1. One of your parents criticizes you?
2. You are irritated by a persistent habit in someone you love?
3. Everybody leaves the cleaning-up chores to you?
4. You want to say "no" to a proposed visit to a relative?
5. Your partner feels amorous but you are not in the mood?

From Powell, T. J., & Enright, S. J. (1990). Anxiety and stress management. London, Routledge, with permission.

■ The client is able to express opinions and disagree with the opinions of others in a socially acceptable manner and without feeling guilty.

■ The client is able to verbalize positive aspects about self.

■ The client verbalizes choices made in a plan to maintain control over his or her life situation.

■ The client approaches others in an appropriate manner for one-to-one interaction.

In a clinical setting, nurses can teach clients the techniques to use to increase their assertive responses. This can be done on a one-to-one basis or in group situations. Once these techniques have been discussed, nurses can assist clients to practice them through role-playing. Each client should compose a list of specific personal examples of situations that create difficulties for him or her. These situations will then be simulated in the therapy setting so that the client may practice assertive responses in a nonthreatening environment. In a group situation, feedback from peers can provide valuable insight about the effectiveness of the response.

CLINICAL PEARL An important part of this type of intervention is to ensure that clients are aware of the differences among assertive, nonassertive, aggressive, and passive-aggressive behaviors in the same situation. When discussion is held about what the best (assertive) response would be, it is also important to discuss the other types of responses as well, so that clients can begin to recognize their pattern of response and make changes accordingly.

CLINICAL EXAMPLE

Linda comes to day hospital once a week to attend group therapy and assertiveness training. She has had problems with depression and low self-esteem. She is married to a man who is

DIRECTIONS: Fill in each block with a rating of your assertiveness on a 5-point scale. A rating of 0 means you have no difficulty asserting yourself. A rating of 5 means that you are completely unable to assert yourself. Evaluation can be made by analyzing the scores:

1. totally by activity, including all of the different people categories
2. totally by people, including all of the different activity categories
3. on an individual basis, considering specific people and specific activities

PEOPLE / ACTIVITY	Friends of the same sex	Friends of the opposite sex	Intimate relations or spouse	Authority figures	Relatives/ family members	Colleagues and sub-ordinates	Strangers	Service workers; waiters; shop assistants, etc.
Giving and receiving compliments								
Asking for favors/help								
Initiating and maintaining conversation								
Refusing requests								
Expressing personal opinions								
Expressing anger/dis-pleasure								
Expressing liking, love, affection								
Stating your rights and needs								

FIGURE 15–1 Rating your assertiveness. (From Powell, T. J., & Enright, S. J. [1990]. *Anxiety and stress management.* London: Routledge, with permission.)

verbally abusive. He is highly critical, is seldom satisfied with anything Linda does, and blames her for negative consequences that occur in their lives, whether or not she is involved.

Since the group began, the nurse who leads the assertiveness training group has taught the participants about basic human rights and the various types of response patterns. When the nurse asks for client situations to be presented in group, Linda volunteers to discuss an incident that occurred in her home this week. She related that she had just put some chicken on the stove to cook for supper when her 7-year-old son came running in the house yelling that he had been hurt. Linda went to him and observed that he had blood dripping down the side of his head from his forehead. He said he and some friends had been playing on the jungle gym in the schoolyard down the street, and he had fallen and hit his head. Linda went with him to the bathroom to clean the wound and apply

some medication. Her husband, Joe, was reading the newspaper in the living room. By the time she got back to the chicken on the stove, it was burned and inedible. Her husband shouted, "You stupid woman! You can't do anything right!" Linda did not respond but burst into tears.

The nurse asked the other members in the group to present some ideas about how Linda could have responded to Joe's criticism. After some discussion, they agreed that Linda might have stated, "I made a mistake. I am not stupid and I do lots of things right." They also discussed other types of responses and why they were less acceptable. They recognized that Linda's lack of verbal response and bursting into tears was a nonassertive response. They also agreed on other examples, such as:

1. An aggressive response might be, "Cook your own supper!" and toss the skillet out the back door.

2. A passive-aggressive response might be to fix sandwiches for supper and not speak to Joe for 3 days.

Practice on the assertive response began, with the nurse and various members of the group playing the role of Joe so that Linda could practice until she felt comfortable with the response. She participated in the group for 6 months, regularly submitting situations with which she needed help. She also learned from the situations presented by other members of the group. These weekly sessions gave Linda the self-confidence that she needed to stand up to Joe's criticism. She was aware of her basic human rights and, with practice, was able to stand up for them in an assertive manner. She was happy to report to the group after a few months that Joe seemed to be less critical and that their relationship was improving.

Evaluation

Evaluation requires that the nurse and client assess whether or not these techniques are achieving the desired outcomes. Reassessment might include the following questions:

■ Is the client able to accept criticism without becoming defensive?

■ Can the client express true feelings to (spouse, friend, boss, and so on) when his or her basic human rights are violated?

■ Is the client able to decline a request without feeling guilty?

■ Can the client verbalize positive qualities about himself or herself?

■ Does the client verbalize improvement in interpersonal relationships?

Assertiveness training serves to extend and create more flexibility in an individual's communication style so that he or she has a greater choice of responses in various situations. Although change does not come easily, assertiveness training can be an effective way of changing behavior. Nurses can assist individuals to become more assertive, thereby encouraging them to become what they want to be, promoting an improvement in self-esteem, and fostering a respect for their own rights and the rights of others.

Summary and Key Points

■ Assertive behavior helps individuals feel better about themselves by encouraging them to stand up for their own basic human rights.

■ Basic human rights have equal representation for all individuals.

■ Along with rights comes an equal number of responsibilities. Part of being assertive includes living up to these responsibilities.

■ Assertive behavior increases self-esteem and the ability to develop satisfying interpersonal relationships. This is accomplished through honesty, directness, appropriateness, and respecting one's own rights, and the rights of others.

■ Individuals develop patterns of responding in various ways, such as role modeling, by receiving positive or negative reinforcement, or by conscious choice.

■ Patterns of responding can take the form of nonassertiveness, assertiveness, aggressiveness, or passive-aggressiveness.

■ *Nonassertive* individuals seek to please others at the expense of denying their own basic human rights.

■ *Assertive* individuals stand up for their own rights while protecting the rights of others.

■ Those who respond *aggressively* defend their own rights by violating the basic rights of others.

■ Individuals who respond in a *passive-aggressive* manner defend their own rights by expressing resistance to social and occupational demands.

■ Some important behavioral considerations of assertive behavior include eye contact, body posture, distance/physical contact, gestures, facial expression, voice, fluency, timing, listening, thoughts, and content.

■ A discussion of techniques that have been developed to assist individuals in the process of becoming more assertive was presented.

■ Negative thinking can sometimes interfere with one's ability to respond assertively. Thought-stopping techniques help individuals remove negative, unwanted thoughts from awareness and promote the development of a more assertive attitude.

■ Nurses can assist individuals to learn and practice assertiveness techniques.

■ The nursing process is an effective vehicle for providing the information and support to clients as they strive to create positive change in their lives.

Davis*Plus* Additional info available @ davisplus.fadavis.com

Review Questions
Self-Examination/Learning Exercise

*Select the answer that is **most** appropriate for each of the following questions:*

1. Your husband says, "You're crazy to think about going to college! You're not smart enough to handle the studies and the housework, too." Which of the following is an example of a nonassertive response?
   a. "I will do what I can, and the best that I can."
   b. (Thinking to yourself): "We'll see how HE likes cooking dinner for a change."
   c. "You're probably right. Maybe I should reconsider."
   d. "I'm going to do what I want to do, when I want to do it, and you can't stop me!"

2. You are having company for dinner and they are due to arrive in 20 minutes. You are about to finish cooking and still have to shower and dress. The doorbell rings and it is a man selling a new product for cleaning windows. Which of the following is an example of an aggressive response?
   a. "I don't do windows!" and slam the door in his face.
   b. "I'll take a case," and write him a check.
   c. "Sure, I'll take three bottles." Then to yourself you think: "I'm calling this company tomorrow and complaining to the manager about their salespeople coming around at dinnertime!"
   d. "I'm very busy at the moment. I don't wish to purchase any of your product. Thank you."

3. You are in a movie theater that prohibits smoking. The person in the seat next to you just lit a cigarette and the smoke is very irritating. Which of the following is an example of an assertive response?
   a. You say nothing.
   b. "Please put your cigarette out. Smoking is prohibited."
   c. You say nothing, but begin to frantically fan the air in front of you and cough loudly and convulsively.
   d. "Put your cigarette out, you slob! Can't you read the 'no smoking' sign?"

4. You have been studying for a nursing exam all afternoon and lost track of time. Your husband expects dinner on the table when he gets home from work. You have not started cooking yet when he walks in the door and shouts, "Why the heck isn't dinner ready?" Which of the following is an example of a passive-aggressive response?
   a. "I'm sorry. I'll have it done in no time, honey." But then you move very slowly and take a long time to cook the meal.
   b. "I'm tired from studying all afternoon. Make your own dinner, you bum! I'm tired of being your slave!"
   c. "I haven't started dinner yet. I'd like some help from you."
   d. "I'm so sorry. I know you're tired and hungry. It's all my fault. I'm such a terrible wife!"

5. You and your best friend, Jill, have had plans for 6 months to go on vacation together to Hawaii. You have saved your money and have plane tickets to leave in 3 weeks. She has just called you and reported that she is not going. She has a new boyfriend, they are moving in together, and she does not want to leave him. You are very angry with Jill for changing your plans. Which of the following is an example of an assertive response?
   a. "I'm very disappointed and very angry. I'd like to talk to you about this later. I'll call you."
   b. "I'm very happy for you, Jill. I think it's wonderful that you and Jack are moving in together."
   c. You tell Jill that you are very happy for her, but then say to another friend, "Well, that's the end of my friendship with Jill!"
   d. "What? You can't do that to me! We've had plans! You're acting like a real slut!"

Continued

6. A typewritten report for your psychiatric nursing class is due tomorrow at 8:00 a.m. The assignment was made 4 weeks ago and, and yours is ready to turn in. Your roommate says, "I finally finished writing my report, but now I have to go to work, and I don't have time to type it. Please be a dear and type it for me, otherwise I'll fail!" You have a date with your boyfriend. Which of the following is an example of an aggressive response?
   a. "Okay, I'll call Ken and cancel our date."
   b. "I don't want to stay here and type your report. I'm going out with Ken."
   c. "You've got to be kidding! What kind of a fool do you take me for, anyway?"
   d. "Okay, I'll do it." However, when your roommate returns from work at midnight, you are asleep and the report has not been typed.

7. You are asked to serve on a committee on which you do not wish to serve. Which of the following is an example of a nonassertive response?
   a. "Thank you, but I don't wish to be a member of that committee."
   b. "I'll be happy to serve." But then you don't show up for any of the meetings.
   c. "I'd rather have my teeth pulled!"
   d. "Okay, if I'm really needed, I'll serve."

8. You're on your way to the laundry room when you encounter a fellow dorm tenant who often asks you to "throw a few of my things in with yours." You view this as an imposition. He asks you where you're going. Which of the following is an example of a passive-aggressive response?
   a. "I'm on my way to the Celtics game. Where do you think I'm going?"
   b. "I'm on my way to do some laundry. Do you have anything you want me to wash with mine?"
   c. "It's none of your damn business!"
   d. "I'm going to the laundry room. Please don't ask me to do some of yours. I resent being taken advantage of in that way."

9. At a hospital committee meeting, a fellow nurse who is the chairperson has interrupted you each time you have tried to make a statement. The next time it happens, you intend to respond assertively. Which of the following is an example of an assertive response?
   a. "You make a lousy leader! You won't even let me finish what I'm trying to say!"
   b. You say nothing.
   c. "Excuse me. I would like to finish my statement."
   d. You say nothing, but you fail to complete your assignment and do not show up for the next meeting.

10. A fellow worker often borrows small amounts of money from you with the promise that she will pay you back "tomorrow." She currently owes you $15.00, and has not yet paid back any of the money that she has borrowed. She asks if she can borrow a couple of dollars for lunch. Which of the following is an example of a nonassertive response?
    a. "I've decided not to loan you any more money until you pay me back what you already borrowed."
    b. "I'm so sorry. I only have enough to pay for my own lunch today."
    c. "Get a life, will you? I'm tired of you sponging off me all the time!"
    d. "Sure, here's two dollars." Then to the other workers in the office: "Be sure you never lend Cindy any money. She never pays her debts. I'd be sure never to go to lunch with her if I were you!"

References

Alberti, R. E., & Emmons, M. L. (2008). *Your perfect right* (9th ed.). Atascadero, CA: Impact Publishers.

American Psychiatric Association. (2000). *Diagnostic and statistical manual of mental disorders* (4th ed.). *Text revision.* Washington, DC: American Psychiatric Publishing.

Davis, M., McKay, M., & Eshelman, E. R. (2008). *The relaxation and stress reduction workbook* (6th ed). Oakland, CA: New Harbinger Publications.

Hopkins, L. (2010). Assertive communication: Six tips for effective use. *EzineArticles.* Retrieved August 5, 2010, from http://ezinearticles.com/?expert=Lee_Hopkins

Lloyd, S. R. (2002). *Developing positive assertiveness* (3rd ed.). Menlo Park, CA: Crisp Publications.

Powell, T. J., & Enright, S. J. (1990). *Anxiety and stress management.* London: Routledge.

Schuster, P. M. (2000). *Communication: The key to the therapeutic relationship.* Philadelphia: F.A. Davis.

Sobel, D. S., & Ornstein, R. (1996). *The healthy mind/healthy body handbook.* New York: Patient Education Media.

Wolpe, J. (1990). *The practice of behavior therapy* (4th ed.) Elmsford, NY: Pergamon Press.

Promoting Self-Esteem

CORE CONCEPTS

self-concept

self-esteem

CHAPTER OUTLINE

Objectives

Homework Assignment

Components of Self-Concept

Development of Self-Esteem

Manifestations of Low Self-Esteem

Boundaries

The Nursing Process

Summary and Key Points

Review Questions

KEY TERMS

body image

boundaries

contextual stimuli

enmeshed boundaries

flexible boundaries

focal stimuli

moral-ethical self

physical self

residual stimuli

rigid boundaries

self-consistency

self-expectancy

self-ideal

OBJECTIVES

After reading this chapter, the student will be able to:

1. Identify and define components of the self-concept.
2. Discuss influencing factors in the development of self-esteem and its progression through the life span.
3. Describe the verbal and nonverbal manifestations of low self-esteem.

4. Discuss the concept of boundaries and its relationship to self-esteem.
5. Apply the nursing process with clients who are experiencing disturbances in self-esteem.

HOMEWORK ASSIGNMENT

Please read the chapter and answer the following questions:

1. Children need unconditional love to promote positive self-esteem. How do parents demonstrate unconditional love?
2. Since her parents' divorce, 10-year-old Nancy and her mother have become inseparable. They spend all their spare time together, and Nancy has become her mother's confidant. This is an example of what type of boundary?

3. How does fulfillment of the developmental tasks described by Erikson promote a healthy self-esteem?
4. Name the three components of the self-concept and the meaning that individuals attach to each.

McKay and Fanning (2003) described self-esteem as an emotional *sine qua non,* a component that is essential for psychological survival. They stated, "Without some measure of self-worth, life can be enormously painful, with many basic needs going unmet" (p. 1).

The awareness of self (i.e., the ability to form an identity and then attach a value to it) is an important differentiating factor between humans and other animals. This capacity for judgment, then, becomes a contributing factor in disturbances of self-esteem.

The promotion of self-esteem is about stopping self-judgments. It is about helping individuals change how they perceive and feel about themselves. This chapter describes the developmental progression and the verbal and behavioral manifestations of self-esteem. The concept of **boundaries** and its relationship to self-esteem is explored. Nursing care of clients with disturbances in self-esteem is described in the context of the nursing process.

> ### CORE CONCEPT
> *Self-Concept*
> Self-concept is the cognitive or thinking component of the self, and generally refers to the totality of a complex, organized, and dynamic system of learned beliefs, attitudes and opinions that each person holds to be true about his or her personal existence (Huitt, 2009).

Components of Self-Concept

Physical Self or Body Image

An individual's **body image** is a subjective perception of one's physical appearance based on self-evaluation and on reactions and feedback from others. Gorman and Sultan (2008) stated:

> Body image is the mental picture a person has of his or her own body. It significantly influences the way a person thinks and feels about his or her body as a whole, about its functions, and about the internal and external sensations associated with it. It also includes perceptions of the way others see the person's body and is central to self-concept and self-esteem. (p. 9)

An individual's body image may not necessarily coincide with his or her actual appearance. For example, individuals who have been overweight for many years and then lose weight often have difficulty perceiving of themselves as thin. They may even continue to choose clothing in the size they were before they lost weight.

A disturbance in one's body image may occur with changes in structure or function. Examples of changes in bodily structure include amputations, mastectomy, and facial disfigurements. Functional alterations are conditions such as colostomy, paralysis, and impotence. Alterations in body image are often experienced as losses.

Personal Identity

This component of the self-concept is composed of the moral-ethical self, the self-consistency, and the self-ideal/self-expectancy.

The **moral-ethical self** is that aspect of the personal identity that evaluates who the individual says he or she is. This component of the personal self observes, compares, sets standards, and makes judgments that influence an individual's self-evaluation.

Self-consistency is the component of the personal identity that strives to maintain a stable self-image. Even if the self-image is negative, because of this need for stability and self-consistency, the individual resists letting go of the image from which he or she has achieved a measure of constancy.

Self-ideal/self-expectancy relates to an individual's perception of what he or she wants to be, to do, or to become. The concept of the ideal self arises out of the perception one has of the expectations of others. Disturbances in self-concept can occur when individuals are unable to achieve their ideals and expectancies.

> ### CORE CONCEPT
> *Self-Esteem*
> Self-esteem refers to the degree of regard or respect that individuals have for themselves and is a measure of worth that they place on their abilities and judgments.

Self-Esteem

Warren (1991) stated:

> Self-esteem breaks down into two components: (1) the ability to say that "I am important," "I matter," and (2) the ability to say "I am competent," "I have something to offer to others and the world." (p. 1)

Maslow (1970) postulated that individuals must achieve a positive self-esteem before they can achieve self-actualization (see Chapter 2). On a day-to-day basis, one's self-value is challenged by changes within the environment. With a positive self-worth, individuals are able to adapt successfully to the demands associated with situational and maturational crises that occur. The ability to adapt to these environmental changes is impaired when individuals hold themselves in low esteem.

Self-esteem is very closely related to the other components of the self-concept. Just as with body image and personal identity, the development of self-esteem is largely influenced by the perceptions of how one is viewed by significant others. It begins in early childhood and vacillates throughout the life span.

The Development of Self-Esteem

How self-esteem is established has been the topic of investigation for a number of theorists and clinicians. From a review of personality theories, Coopersmith (1981) identified the following antecedent conditions of positive self-esteem:

- **Power.** It is important for individuals to have a feeling of control over their own life situation and an ability to claim some measure of influence over the behaviors of others.

- **Significance.** Self-esteem is enhanced when individuals feel loved, respected, and cared for by significant others.

- **Virtue.** Individuals feel good about themselves when their actions reflect a set of personal, moral, and ethical values.

- **Competence.** Positive self-esteem develops out of one's ability to perform successfully or achieve self-expectations and the expectations of others.

- **Consistently set limits.** A structured lifestyle demonstrates acceptance and caring and provides a feeling of security.

Warren (1991) outlined the following focus areas to be emphasized by parents and others who work with children when encouraging the growth and development of positive self-esteem:

- **A Sense of Competence.** Everyone needs to feel skilled at something. Warren (1991) stated, "Children do not necessarily need to be THE best at a skill in order to have positive self-esteem; what they need to feel is that they have accomplished their PERSONAL best effort" (p. 1).

- **Unconditional Love.** Children need to know that they are loved and accepted by family and friends regardless of success or failure. This is demonstrated by expressive touch, realistic praise, and separation of criticism of the person from criticism of the behavior.

- **A Sense of Survival.** Everyone fails at something from time to time. Self-esteem is enhanced when individuals learn from failure and grow in the knowledge that they are stronger for having experienced it.

- **Realistic Goals.** Low self-esteem can be the result of not being able to achieve established goals. Individuals may "set themselves up" for failure by setting goals that are unattainable. Goals can be unrealistic when they are beyond a child's capability to achieve, require an inordinate amount of effort to accomplish, and are based on exaggerated fantasy.

- **A Sense of Responsibility.** Children gain positive self-worth when they are assigned areas of responsibility or are expected to complete tasks that they perceive are valued by others.

- **Reality Orientation.** Personal limitations abound within our world, and it is important for children to recognize and achieve a healthy balance between what they can possess and achieve, and what is beyond their capability or control.

Other factors that have been found to be influential in the development of self-esteem include:

- **The Responses of Others.** The development of self-esteem can be positively or negatively influenced by the responses of others, particularly significant others, and by how individuals perceive those responses.

- **Hereditary Factors.** Factors that are genetically determined, such as physical appearance, size, or inherited infirmity, can have an effect on the development of self-esteem.

- **Environmental Conditions.** The development of self-esteem can be influenced by demands from the environment. For example, intellectual prowess may be incorporated into the self-worth of an individual who is reared in an academic environment.

Developmental Progression of the Self-Esteem Through the Life Span

The development of self-esteem progresses throughout the life span. Erikson's (1963) theory of personality development provides a useful framework for illustration (see Chapter 3). Erikson describes eight transitional or maturational crises, the resolution of which can have a profound influence on self-esteem. If a crisis is successfully resolved at one stage, the individual develops healthy coping strategies that he or she can draw on to help fulfill tasks of subsequent stages. When an individual fails to achieve the tasks associated with a developmental stage, emotional growth is inhibited, and he or she is less able to cope with subsequent maturational or situational crises.

Trust Versus Mistrust (Birth to 18 Months)

The development of trust results in a feeling of confidence in the predictability of the environment. Achievement of trust results in positive self-esteem through the instillation of self-confidence, optimism, and faith in the gratification of needs.

Unsuccessful resolution results in the individual experiencing emotional dissatisfaction with the self and suspiciousness of others, thereby promoting negative self-esteem.

Autonomy Versus Shame and Doubt (18 Months to 3 Years)

With motor and mental development come greater movement and independence within the environment. The child begins active exploration and experimentation. Achievement of the task results in a sense of self-control and the ability to delay gratification, as well as a feeling of self-confidence in one's ability to perform.

This task remains unresolved when the child's independent behaviors are restricted or when the child fails because of unrealistic expectations. Negative self-esteem is promoted by a lack of self-confidence, a lack of pride in the ability to perform, and a sense of being controlled by others.

Initiative Versus Guilt (3 to 6 Years)

Positive self-esteem is gained through initiative when creativity is encouraged and performance is recognized and positively reinforced. In this stage, children strive to develop a sense of purpose and the ability to initiate and direct their own activities.

This is the stage during which the child begins to develop a conscience. He or she becomes vulnerable to the labeling of behaviors as "good" or "bad." Guidance and discipline that rely heavily on shaming the child create guilt and result in a decrease in self-esteem.

Industry Versus Inferiority (6 to 12 Years)

Self-confidence is gained at this stage through learning, competing, performing successfully, and receiving recognition from significant others, peers, and acquaintances.

Negative self-esteem is the result of nonachievement or unrealistic expectations, or when accomplishments are consistently met with negative feedback. The child develops a sense of personal inadequacy.

Identity Versus Role Confusion (12 to 20 Years)

During adolescence, the individual is striving to redefine the sense of self. Positive self-esteem occurs when individuals are allowed to experience independence by making decisions that influence their lives.

Failure to develop a new self-definition results in a sense of self-consciousness, doubt, and confusion about one's role in life. This can occur when adolescents are encouraged to remain in the dependent position; when discipline in the home has been overly harsh, inconsistent, or absent; and when parental support has been lacking. These conditions are influential in the development of low self-esteem.

Intimacy Versus Isolation (20 to 30 Years)

Intimacy is achieved when one is able to form a lasting relationship or a commitment to another person, a cause, an institution, or a creative effort (Murray, Zentner, & Yakimo, 2008). Positive self-esteem is promoted through this capacity for giving of oneself to another.

Failure to achieve intimacy results in behaviors such as withdrawal, social isolation, aloneness, and the inability to form lasting intimate relationships. Isolation occurs when love in the home has been deprived or distorted through the younger years, causing a severe impairment in self-esteem.

Generativity Versus Stagnation (30 to 65 Years)

Generativity promotes positive self-esteem through gratification from personal and professional achievements, and from meaningful contributions to others.

Failure to achieve generativity occurs when earlier developmental tasks are not fulfilled and the individual does not achieve the degree of maturity required to derive gratification out of a personal concern for the welfare of others. He or she lacks self-worth and becomes withdrawn and isolated.

Ego Integrity Versus Despair (65 Years to Death)

Ego integrity results in a sense of self-worth and self-acceptance as one reviews life goals, accepting that some were achieved and some were not. The individual has little desire to make major changes in how his or her life has progressed. Positive self-esteem is evident.

Individuals in despair possess a sense of self-contempt and disgust with how life has progressed. They feel worthless and helpless, and they would like to have a second chance at life. Earlier developmental tasks of self-confidence, self-identity, and concern for others remain unfulfilled. Negative self-esteem prevails.

The Manifestations of Low Self-Esteem

Individuals with low self-esteem perceive themselves to be incompetent, unlovable, insecure, and unworthy. The number of manifestations exhibited is influenced by the degree to which an individual experiences low self-esteem. Roy (1976) categorized behaviors according to the type of stimuli that give rise to these behaviors and affirmed the importance of including this type of information in the nursing assessment. Stimulus categories are identified as *focal,* *contextual,* and *residual.* A summary of these types of influencing factors is presented in Table 16-1.

Focal Stimuli

A **focal stimulus** is the immediate concern that is causing the threat to self-esteem and the stimulus that is engendering the current behavior. Examples of focal stimuli include termination of a significant relationship, loss of employment, and failure to pass the nursing state board examination.

Contextual Stimuli

Contextual stimuli are all of the other stimuli present in the person's environment that *contribute* to the behavior being caused by the focal stimulus. Examples of contextual stimuli related to the previously mentioned focal stimuli might be a child of the relationship becoming emotionally disabled in response to the divorce, advanced age interfering with obtaining employment, or a significant other who states, "I

TABLE 16-1 Factors That Influence Manifestations of Low Self-Esteem

FOCAL	CONTEXTUAL	RESIDUAL
1. Any experience or situation causing the individual to question or decrease his or her value of self; experiences of loss are particularly significant.	1. Body changes experienced because of growth or illness.	1. Age and coping mechanisms one has developed.
	2. Maturational crises associated with developmental stages.	2. Stressful situations previously experienced and how well one coped with them.
	3. Situational crises and the individual's ability to cope.	3. Previous feedback from significant others that contributed to self-worth.
	4. The individual's perceptions of feedback from significant others.	4. Coping strategies developed through experiences with previous developmental crises.
	5. Ability to meet expectations of self and others.	5. Previous experiences with powerlessness and hopelessness and how one coped with them.
	6. The feeling of control one has over life situation.	
	7. One's self-definition and the use of it to measure self-worth.	6. Coping with previous losses.
	8. How one copes with feelings of guilt, shame, and powerlessness.	7. Coping with previous failures.
	9. How one copes with the required changes in self-perception.	8. Previous experiences meeting expectations of self and others.
	10. Awareness of what affects self-concept and the manner with which these stimuli are dealt.	9. Previous experiences with control of self and the environment and quality of coping response.
	11. The number of failures experienced before judging self as worthless.	
	12. The degree of self-esteem one possesses.	10. Previous experience with decision making and subsequent consequences.
	13. How one copes with limits within the environment.	11. Previous experience with childhood limits, and whether or not those limits were clear, defined, and enforced.
	14. The type of support from significant others and how one responds to it.	
	15. One's awareness of and ability to express feelings.	
	16. One's current feeling of hope and comfort with the self.	

From Driever M. J. (1976). Problem of low self-esteem. In C. Roy (Ed.), Introduction to nursing: An adaptation model (pp. 232–242). Englewood Cliffs, NJ: Prentice-Hall, with permission.

knew you weren't smart enough to pass state boards."

Residual Stimuli

Residual stimuli are factors that may influence one's maladaptive behavior in response to focal and contextual stimuli. An individual conducting a self-esteem assessment might presume from previous knowledge that certain beliefs, attitudes, experiences, or traits have an effect on client behavior, even though it cannot be clearly substantiated. For example, being reared in an atmosphere of ridicule and deprecation may be affecting current adaptation to failure on the state board examination.

Symptoms of Low Self-Esteem

Driever (1976) identified a number of behaviors manifested by the individual with low self-esteem. These behaviors are presented in Box 16-1.

Boundaries

The word *boundary* is used to denote the personal space, both physical and psychological, that individuals identify as their own. Boundaries are sometimes referred to as limits: the limit or degree to which individuals feel comfortable in a relationship. Boundaries define and differentiate an individual's physical and psychological space from the physical and psychological space of others.

Boundaries help individuals define the self and are part of the individuation process. Individuals who are aware of their boundaries have a healthy self-esteem because they must know and accept their inner selves. The inner self includes beliefs, thoughts, feelings, decisions, choices, experiences, wants, needs, sensations, and intuitions.

Types of physical boundaries include physical closeness, touching, sexual behavior, eye contact, privacy (e.g., mail, diary, doors, nudity, bathroom, telephone), and pollution (e.g., noise and smoke), among others. Examples of invasions of physical boundaries are reading someone else's diary, smoking in a nonsmoking public area, and touching someone who does not wish to be touched.

Types of psychological boundaries include beliefs, feelings, choices, needs, time alone, interests, confidences, individual differences, and

---

BOX 16-1 Manifestations of Low Self-Esteem

1. Loss of appetite/weight loss
2. Overeating
3. Constipation or diarrhea
4. Sleep disturbances (insomnia or difficulty falling or staying asleep)
5. Hypersomnia
6. Complaints of fatigue
7. Poor posture
8. Withdrawal from activities
9. Difficulty initiating new activities
10. Decreased libido
11. Decrease in spontaneous behavior
12. Expression of sadness, anxiety, or discouragement
13. Expression of feeling of isolation, being unlovable, unable to express or defend oneself, and too weak to confront or overcome difficulties
14. Fearful of angering others
15. Avoidance of situations of self-disclosure or public exposure
16. Tendency to stay in background; be a listener rather than a participant
17. Sensitivity to criticism; self-conscious
18. Expression of feelings of helplessness
19. Various complaints of aches and pains
20. Expression of being unable to do anything "good" or productive; expression of feelings of worthlessness and inadequacy
21. Expressions of self-deprecation, self-dislike, and unhappiness with self
22. Denial of past successes/accomplishments and of possibility for success with current activities
23. Feeling that anything one does will fail or be meaningless
24. Rumination about problems
25. Seeking reinforcement from others; making efforts to gain favors, but failing to reciprocate such behavior
26. Seeing self as a burden to others
27. Alienation from others by clinging and self-preoccupation
28. Self-accusatory
29. Demanding reassurance but not accepting it
30. Hostile behavior
31. Angry at self and others but unable to express these feelings directly
32. Decreased ability to meet responsibilities
33. Decreased interest, motivation, concentration
34. Decrease in self-care, hygiene

From Driever M. J. (1976). Problem of low self-esteem. In C. Roy (Ed.), Introduction to nursing: An adaptation model (pp. 232–242). Englewood Cliffs, NJ: Prentice-Hall, with permission.

spirituality, among others. Examples of invasions of psychological boundaries are being criticized for doing something differently than others; having personal information shared in confidence told to others; and being told one "should" believe, feel, decide, choose, or think in a certain way.

Boundary Pliancy

Boundaries can be rigid, flexible, or enmeshed. The behavior of dogs and cats can be a good illustration of **rigid boundaries** and **flexible boundaries.** Most dogs want to be as close to people as possible. When "their people" walk into the room, the dog is likely to be all over them. They want to be where their people are and do what they are doing. Dogs have very flexible boundaries.

Cats, on the other hand, have very distinct boundaries. They do what they want, when they want. They decide how close they will be to their people, and when. Cats take notice when their people enter a room but may not even acknowledge their presence (until the cat decides the time is right). Their boundaries are less flexible than those of dogs.

Rigid Boundaries

Individuals who have rigid boundaries often have a hard time trusting others. They keep others at a distance and are difficult to communicate with. They reject new ideas or experiences, and often withdraw, both emotionally and physically.

EXAMPLE

Fred and Alice were seeing a marriage counselor because they were unable to agree on many aspects of raising their children and it was beginning to interfere with their relationship. Alice runs a day care service out of their home, and Fred is an accountant. Alice states, "He never once changed a diaper or got up at night with a child. Now that they are older, he refuses to discipline them in any way." Fred responds, "In my family, my Mom took care of the house and kids and my Dad kept us clothed and fed. That's the way it should be. It's Alice's job to raise the kids. It's my job to make the money." Fred's boundaries are considered rigid because he refuses to consider the ideas of others, or to experience alternative ways of doing things.

Flexible Boundaries

Healthy boundaries are flexible. That is, individuals must be able to let go of their boundaries and limits when appropriate. In order to have flexible boundaries, one must be aware of who is considered safe and when it is safe to let others invade our personal space.

EXAMPLE

Nancy always takes the hour from 4 to 5 p.m. for her own. She takes no phone calls and tells the children that she is not to be disturbed during that hour. She reads or takes a long leisurely bath and relaxes before it is time to start dinner. Today her private time was interrupted when her 15-year-old daughter came home from school crying because she had not made the cheerleading squad. Nancy used her private time to comfort her daughter who was experiencing a traumatic response to the failure.

Sometimes boundaries can be too flexible. Individuals with boundaries that are too loose are like chameleons. They take their "colors" from whomever they happen to be with at the time. That is, they allow others to make their choices and direct their behavior.

EXAMPLE

At a cocktail party, Diane agreed with one person that the winter had been so unbearable she had hardly been out of the house. Later at the same party, she agreed with another person that the winter had seemed milder than usual.

Enmeshed Boundaries

Enmeshed boundaries occur when two people's boundaries are so blended together that neither can be sure where one stops and the other begins, or one individual's boundaries may be blurred with another's. The individual with the enmeshed boundaries may be unable to differentiate his or her feelings, wants, and needs from the other person's.

EXAMPLE

1. Fran's parents are in town for a visit. They say to Fran, "Dear, we want to take you and Dave out to dinner tonight. What is your favorite restaurant?" Fran automatically responds, "Villa Roma," knowing that the Italian restaurant is Dave's favorite.

2. If a mother has difficulty allowing her daughter to individuate, the mother may perceive the daughter's experiences as happening to her. For example, Aileen got her hair cut without her mother's knowledge. It was styled with spikes across the top of her head. When her mother saw it, she said, "How dare you go around looking like that! What will people think of me?"

Establishing Boundaries

Boundaries are established in childhood. Unhealthy boundaries are the products of unhealthy, troubled, or dysfunctional families. The boundaries enclose painful feelings that have their origin in the dysfunctional family and that have not been dealt with. McKay and Fanning (2003) explained the correlation between unhealthy boundaries and self-esteem disturbances and how they can arise out of negative role models:

> Modeling self-esteem means valuing oneself enough to take care of one's own basic needs. When parents put themselves last, or chronically sacrifice for their kids, they teach them that a person is only worthy insofar as he or she is of service to others. When parents set consistent, supportive limits and protect themselves from overbearing demands, they send a message to their children that both are important and both have legitimate needs. (p. 312)

In addition to the lack of positive role models, unhealthy boundaries may also be the result of abuse or neglect. These circumstances can cause a delay in psychosocial development. The individual must then resume the grief process as an adult in order to continue the developmental progression.

They learn to recognize feelings, work through core issues, and learn to tolerate emotional pain as their own. They complete the individuation process, go on to develop healthy boundaries, and learn to appreciate their self-worth.

The Nursing Process

Assessment

Clients with self-esteem problems may manifest any of the symptoms presented in Box 16-1. Some clients with disturbances in self-esteem will make direct statements that reflect guilt, shame, or negative self-appraisal, but often it is necessary for the nurse to ask specific questions to obtain this type of information. In particular, clients who have experienced abuse or other severe trauma often have kept feelings and fears buried for years, and behavioral manifestations of low self-esteem may not be readily evident.

Various tools for measuring self-esteem exist. One is presented in Box 16-2. This particular tool can be used as a self-inventory by the client, or it can be adapted and used by the nurse to format questions for assessing level of self-esteem in the client.

BOX 16-2 Self-Esteem Inventory

Place a check mark in the column that most closely describes your answer to each statement. Each check is worth the number of points listed above each column.

	3 Often or A Great Deal	2 Sometimes	1 Seldom or Occasionally	0 Never or Not At All
1. I become angry or hurt when criticized.				
2. I am afraid to try new things.				
3. I feel stupid when I make a mistake.				
4. I have difficulty looking people in the eye.				
5. I have difficulty making small talk.				
6. I feel uncomfortable in the presence of strangers.				
7. I am embarrassed when people compliment me.				
8. I am dissatisfied with the way I look.				
9. I am afraid to express my opinions in a group.				
10. I prefer staying home alone than participating in group social situations.				
11. I have trouble accepting teasing.				
12. I feel guilty when I say "no" to people.				
13. I am afraid to make a commitment to a relationship for fear of rejection.				

Continued

BOX 16-2 Self-Esteem Inventory—cont'd

14. I believe that most people are more competent than I.
15. I feel resentment toward people who are attractive and successful.
16. I have trouble thinking of any positive aspects about my life.
17. I feel inadequate in the presence of authority figures.
18. I have trouble making decisions.
19. I fear the disapproval of others.
20. I feel tense, stressed out, or "uptight."

Problems with low self-esteem are indicated by items scored with a "3" or by a total score higher than 46.

Diagnosis/Outcome Identification

NANDA International has accepted, for use and testing, three nursing diagnoses that relate to self-esteem. These diagnoses are chronic low self-esteem, situational low self-esteem, and risk for situational low self-esteem (NANDA International, 2009). Each is described here with its definitions and defining characteristics.

Chronic Low Self-Esteem

Definition: Long-standing negative self-evaluating/feelings about self or self-capabilities.

Defining Characteristics

- Dependent on others' opinions
- Evaluation of self as unable to deal with events
- Exaggerates negative feedback about self
- Excessively seeks reassurance
- Expressions of guilt and shame
- Frequent lack of success in life events
- Hesitant to try new situations
- Hesitant to try new things
- Indecisive behavior
- Lack of eye contact
- Nonassertive behavior
- Overly conforming
- Passive
- Rejects positive feedback about self

Situational Low Self-Esteem

Definition: Development of a negative perception of self-worth in response to a current situation (specify)

Defining Characteristics

- Verbally reports current situational challenge to self-worth
- Self-negating verbalizations
- Indecisive, nonassertive behavior
- Evaluation of self as unable to deal with situations or events
- Expressions of helplessness and uselessness

Risk for Situational Low Self-Esteem

Definition: At risk for developing negative perception of self worth in response to a current situation (specify)

Risk Factors:

- Behavior inconsistent with values
- Decreased control over environment
- Developmental changes
- Disturbed body image
- Failures
- Functional impairment
- History of abandonment
- History of abuse
- History of learned helplessness
- History of neglect
- Lack of recognition
- Loss
- Physical illness
- Rejections
- Social role changes
- Unrealistic self-expectations

Outcome Criteria

Outcome criteria include short- and long-term goals. Timelines for achievement are individually determined. The following criteria may be used for measurement of outcomes in the care of the client with disturbances of self-esteem.

The client:

- Is able to express positive aspects about self and life situation.
- Is able to accept positive feedback from others.
- Is able to attempt new experiences.
- Is able to accept personal responsibility for own problems.
- Is able to accept constructive criticism without becoming defensive.
- Is able to make independent decisions about life situation.
- Uses good eye contact.
- Is able to develop positive interpersonal relationships.
- Is able to communicate needs and wants to others assertively.

Planning/Implementation

In Table 16-2, a plan of care using the three self-esteem diagnoses accepted by NANDA International is presented. Outcome criteria, appropriate nursing interventions, and rationales are included for each diagnosis.

> **CLINICAL PEARL** Ensure that client goals are realistic. Unrealistic goals set the client up for failure. Provide encouragement and positive reinforcement for attempts at change. Give recognition of accomplishments, however small.

Evaluation

Reassessment is conducted to determine if the nursing actions have been successful in achieving the objectives of care. Evaluation of the nursing actions for the client with self-esteem disturbances may be facilitated by gathering information using the following types of questions:

- Is the client able to discuss past accomplishments and other positive aspects about his or her life?
- Does the client accept praise and recognition from others in a gracious manner?
- Is the client able to try new experiences without extreme fear of failure?
- Can he or she accept constructive criticism now without becoming overly defensive and shifting the blame to others?

Table 16-2 CARE PLAN FOR THE CLIENT WITH PROBLEMS RELATED TO SELF-ESTEEM

NURSING DIAGNOSIS: CHRONIC LOW SELF-ESTEEM

RELATED TO: Lack of affection/approval; repeated failures; repeated negative reinforcement

EVIDENCED BY: Exaggerates negative feedback about self and expressions of shame and guilt

OUTCOME CRITERIA	NURSING INTERVENTIONS	RATIONALE
Client will verbalize positive aspects of self and abandon judgmental self-perceptions	1. Be supportive, accepting, and respectful without invading the client's personal space.	1. Individuals who have had long-standing feelings of low self-worth may be uncomfortable with personal attentiveness.
	2. Discuss inaccuracies in self-perception with client.	2. Client may not see positive aspects of self that others see, and bringing this to awareness may help change perception.
	3. Have client list success and strengths. Provide positive feedback.	3. Helps client to develop internal self-worth and new coping behaviors.
	4. Assess content of negative self-talk.	4. Self-blame, shame, and guilt promote feelings of low self-worth. Depending on chronicity and severity of the problem, this is likely to be the focus of long-term psychotherapy with this client.

Continued

Table 16-2 CARE PLAN FOR THE CLIENT WITH PROBLEMS RELATED TO SELF-ESTEEM—cont'd

NURSING DIAGNOSIS: SITUATIONAL LOW SELF-ESTEEM

RELATED TO: Failure (either real or perceived) in a situation of importance to the individual or loss (either real or perceived) of a concept of value to the individual

EVIDENCED BY: Indecisive behavior and expressions of helplessness and uselessness

OUTCOME CRITERIA	NURSING INTERVENTIONS	RATIONALE
Client will identify source of threat to self-esteem and work through the stages of the grief process to resolve the loss or failure.	1. Convey an accepting attitude; encourage client to express self openly.	1. An accepting attitude enhances trust and communicates to the client that you believe he or she is a worthwhile person, regardless of what is expressed.
	2. Encourage client to express anger. Do not become defensive if initial expression of anger is displaced on nurse/therapist. Assist client to explore angry feelings and direct them toward the intended object/person or other loss.	2. Verbalization of feelings in a nonthreatening environment may help client come to terms with unresolved issues related to the loss.
	3. Assist client to avoid ruminating about past failures. Withdraw attention if client persists.	3. Lack of attention to these undesirable behaviors may discourage their repetition.
	4. Client needs to focus on positive attributes if self-esteem is to be enhanced. Encourage discussion of past accomplishments and offer support in undertaking new tasks. Offer recognition of successful endeavors and positive reinforcement of attempts made.	4. Recognition and positive reinforcement enhance self-esteem and encourage repetition of desirable behaviors.

NURSING DIAGNOSIS: RISK FOR SITUATIONAL LOW SELF-ESTEEM

RISK FACTORS: Developmental changes; functional impairment; disturbed body image; loss; history of abuse or neglect; unrealistic self-expectations; physical illness; failures/rejections

OUTCOME CRITERIA	NURSING INTERVENTIONS	RATIONALE
Client's self-esteem will be preserved.	1. Provide an open environment and trusting relationship.	1. To facilitate client's ability to deal with current situation.
	2. Determine client's perception of the loss/failure and the meaning of it to him or her.	2. Assessment of the cause or contributing factor is necessary to provide assistance to the client.
	3. Identify response of family or significant others to client's current situation.	3. This provides additional background assessment data with which to plan client's care.
	4. Permit appropriate expressions of anger.	4. Anger is a stage in the normal grieving process and must be dealt with for progression to occur.
	5. Provide information about normalcy of individual grief reaction.	5. Individuals who are unaware of normal feelings associated with grief may feel guilty and try to deny certain feelings.
	6. Discuss and assist with planning for the future. Provide hope, but avoid giving false reassurance.	6. In a state of anxiety and grief, individuals need assistance with decision making and problem solving. They may find it difficult or impossible to envision any hope for the future.

- Does the client accept personal responsibility for problems, rather than attributing feelings and behaviors to others?

- Does the client participate in decisions that affect his or her life?

- Can the client make rational decisions independently?

- Has he or she become more assertive in interpersonal relations?

- Is improvement observed in the physical presentation of self-esteem, such as eye contact, posture, changes in eating and sleeping, fatigue, libido, elimination patterns, self-care, and complaints of aches and pains?

Summary and Key Points

- Emotional wellness requires that an individual have some degree of self-worth—a perception that he or she possesses a measure of value to self and others.

- Self-concept consists of body image, personal identity, and self-esteem.

- Body image encompasses one's appraisal of personal attributes, functioning, sexuality, wellness-illness state, and appearance.

- The personal identity component is composed of the moral-ethical self, the self-consistency, and the self-ideal.

- The moral-ethical self functions as observer, standard setter, dreamer, comparer, and most of all evaluator of who the individual says he or she is.

- Self-consistency is the component of the personal identity that strives to maintain a stable self-image.

- Self-ideal relates to an individual's perception of what he or she wants to be, do, or become.

- Self-esteem refers to the degree of regard or respect that individuals have for themselves and is a measure of worth that they place on their abilities and judgments. It is largely influenced by the perceptions of how one is viewed by significant others.

- Predisposing factors to the development of positive self-esteem include a sense of competence, unconditional love, a sense of survival, realistic goals, a sense of responsibility, and reality orientation. Genetics and environmental conditions may also be influencing factors.

- The development of self-esteem progresses throughout the life span. Erikson's theory of personality development was used in this chapter as a framework for illustration of this progression.

- The behaviors associated with low self-esteem are numerous.

- Stimuli that trigger these behaviors were presented according to focal, contextual, or residual types.

- Boundaries, or personal limits, help individuals define the self and are part of the individuation process.

- Boundaries are physical and psychological and may be rigid, flexible, or enmeshed.

- Unhealthy boundaries are often the result of dysfunctional family systems.

- The nursing process is the vehicle for delivery of care to clients needing assistance with self-esteem disturbances.

- The three nursing diagnoses relating to self-esteem that have been accepted by NANDA International are chronic low self-esteem, situational low self-esteem, and risk for situational low self-esteem.

DavisPlus   Additional info available @ davisplus.fadavis.com

Review Questions
Self-Examination/Learning Exercise

*Select the answer that is **most** appropriate for each of the following questions:*

1. Karen, age 23, graduated from nursing school with a 3.2/4.0 grade point average. She recently took the NCLEX exam and did not pass. Because of this, she had to give up her graduate nursing job until she can pass the exam. She has become very depressed and has sought counseling at the mental health clinic. Karen says to the psychiatric nurse, "I am a complete failure. I'm so dumb, I can't do anything right." What is the most appropriate nursing diagnosis for Karen?
   a. Chronic low self-esteem.
   b. Situational low self-esteem.
   c. Defensive coping.
   d. Risk for situational low self-esteem.

2. Which of the following outcome criteria would be most appropriate for the client described in question 1?
   a. Karen is able to express positive aspects about herself and her life situation.
   b. Karen is able to accept constructive criticism without becoming defensive.
   c. Karen is able to develop positive interpersonal relationships.
   d. Karen is able to accept positive feedback from others.

3. Nancy tried out for the cheerleading squad in junior high, but was rejected. At age 15, she had looked forward to trying out for the cheerleading squad in high school. She took cheerleading classes and practiced for many hours every day. However, when tryouts were held, she was not selected. She has become despondent, and her mother takes her to the mental health clinic for counseling. She tells the nurse, "What's the use of trying? I'm not good at anything!" Which of the following nursing interventions is best for Nancy's specific problem?
   a. Encourage Nancy to talk about her feeling of shame over the second failure.
   b. Assist Nancy to problem-solve her reasons for not making the team.
   c. Help Nancy understand the importance of good self-care and personal hygiene in the maintenance of self-esteem.
   d. Explore with Nancy her past successes and accomplishments.

4. The psychiatric nurse encourages Nancy (the client in question 3) to express her anger. Why is this an appropriate nursing intervention?
   a. Anger is the basis for self-esteem problems.
   b. The nurse suspects that Nancy was abused as a child.
   c. The nurse is attempting to guide Nancy through the grief process.
   d. The nurse recognizes that Nancy has long-standing repressed anger.

5. A nursing school graduate failing the NCLEX exam and a 15-year-old high school girl not being selected for the cheerleading squad are examples of which of the following?
   a. Focal stimuli.
   b. Contextual stimuli.
   c. Residual stimuli.
   d. Spatial stimuli.

6. The husband says to the wife, "What do you want to do tonight?" and the wife responds, "Whatever you want to do." This is an example of which of the following?
   a. Rigid boundary.
   b. A boundary violation.
   c. Too flexible boundary.
   d. Showing respect for the boundary of another.

Review Questions—cont'd
Self-Examination/Learning Exercise

7. Twins Jan and Jean still dress alike even though they are grown and married. This is an example of which of the following?
   a. Rigid boundary.
   b. Enmeshed boundary.
   c. A boundary violation.
   d. Boundary pliancy.

8. Karen's counselor asked her if she would like a hug. This is an example of which of the following?
   a. Rigid boundary.
   b. A boundary violation.
   c. Enmeshed boundary.
   d. Showing respect for the boundary of another.

9. Velma told Betty a secret that Mary had told her. This is an example of which of the following?
   a. Too flexible boundary.
   b. A boundary violation.
   c. Rigid boundary.
   d. Enmeshed boundary.

10. Tommy says to his friend, "I can't ever talk to my Daddy until after he has read his newspaper." This is an example of which of the following?
    a. Rigid boundary.
    b. A boundary violation.
    c. Enmeshed boundary.
    d. Too flexible boundary.

References

Gorman, L. M., & Sultan, D. F. (2008). *Psychosocial nursing for general patient care* (3rd ed.). Philadelphia: F.A. Davis.

Huitt, W. (2009). Self-concept and self-esteem. *Educational Psychology Interactive*. Valdosta, GA: Valdosta State University. Retrieved August 6, 2010, from http://www.edpsychinteractive.org/topics/regsys/self.html

McKay, M., & Fanning, P. (2003). *Self-esteem: A proven program of cognitive techniques for assessing, improving, and maintaining your self-esteem* (3rd ed.). New York: Fine Communications.

Murray, R. B., Zentner, J. P., & Yakimo, R. (2008). *Health promotion strategies through the life span* (8th ed.). Upper Saddle River, NJ: Prentice-Hall.

NANDA International. (2009). *Nursing diagnoses: Definitions and classification 2009–2011.* Hoboken, NJ: Wiley-Blackwell.

Warren, J. (1991). Your child and self-esteem. *The Prairie View, 30*(2):1.

Classical References

Coopersmith, S. (1981). *The antecedents of self-esteem* (2nd ed.). Palo Alto, CA: Consulting Psychologists Press.

Driever, M. J. (1976). Problem of low self-esteem. In C. Roy (Ed.), *Introduction to nursing: An adaptation model* (pp. 232–242). Englewood Cliffs, NJ: Prentice-Hall.

Erikson, E. H. (1963). *Childhood and society* (2nd ed.). New York: W.W. Norton.

Maslow, A. (1970). *Motivation and personality* (2nd ed.). New York: Harper & Row.

Roy, C. (1976). *Introduction to nursing: An adaptation model.* Englewood Cliffs, NJ: Prentice-Hall.

17 Anger/Aggression Management

CHAPTER OUTLINE

KEY TERMS

modeling
operant conditioning
prodromal syndrome

OBJECTIVES
After reading this chapter, the student will be able to:

1. Define and differentiate between *anger* and *aggression*.
2. Identify when the expression of anger becomes a problem.
3. Discuss predisposing factors to the maladaptive expression of anger.
4. Apply the nursing process to clients expressing anger or aggression.
   a. **Assessment:** Describe physical and psychological responses to anger.
   b. **Diagnosis/Outcome Identification:** Formulate nursing diagnoses and outcome criteria for clients expressing anger and aggression
   c. **Planning/Intervention:** Describe nursing interventions for clients demonstrating maladaptive expressions of anger.
   d. **Evaluation:** Evaluate achievement of the projected outcomes in the intervention with clients demonstrating maladaptive expression of anger.

HOMEWORK ASSIGNMENT
Please read the chapter and answer the following questions:

1. What symptoms often precede violent behavior?
2. What is the goal of anger management?
3. What psychiatric diagnoses are correlated with increased risk of violence?
4. Under what conditions might a nurse determine that a client should be placed in restraints?

Anger need not be a negative expression. It is a normal human emotion that, when handled appropriately and expressed assertively, can provide an individual with a positive force to solve problems and make decisions concerning life situations.

Anger becomes a problem when it is not expressed and when it is expressed aggressively. Violence occurs when individuals lose control of their anger. Violent acts are becoming commonplace in the United States. They are reported daily on the evening news, and health-care workers see the results on a regular basis in the emergency departments of general hospitals.

This chapter addresses the concepts of anger and aggression. Predisposing factors to the maladaptive expression of anger are discussed, and the nursing process as a vehicle for delivery of care to assist clients in the management of anger and aggression is described.

Anger and Aggression, Defined

CORE CONCEPT

Anger

Anger is an emotional state that varies in intensity from mild irritation to intense fury and rage. It is accompanied by physiological and biological changes, such as increases in heart rate, blood pressure, and levels of the hormones epinephrine and norepinephrine (American Psychological Association, 2010).

Anger is a normal, healthy emotion that serves as a warning signal and alerts us to potential threat or trauma. It triggers energy that sets us up for a good fight or quick flight, and can range from mild irritation to hot, fiery energy (Butterfield, 2000). Warren (1990) outlined some fundamental points about anger:

■ Anger is not a primary emotion, but it is typically experienced as an almost automatic inner response to hurt, frustration, or fear.

■ Anger is physiological arousal. It instills feelings of power and generates preparedness.

■ Anger and aggression are significantly different.

■ The expression of anger is learned.

■ The expression of anger can come under personal control.

Anger is a very powerful emotion. When it is denied or buried, it can precipitate a number of physical problems such as migraine headaches, ulcers, colitis, and even coronary heart disease. When turned inward on oneself, anger can result in depression and low self-esteem. When it is expressed inappropriately, it commonly interferes with relationships. When suppressed, anger may turn into resentment, which often manifests itself in negative, passive-aggressive behavior.

Anger creates a state of preparedness by arousing the sympathetic nervous system. The activation of this system results in increased heart rate and blood pressure, increased secretion of epinephrine (resulting in additional physiological arousal), and increased levels of serum glucose, among others. Anger prepares the body, physiologically, to fight. When anger goes unresolved, this physiological arousal can be the predisposing factor to a number of health problems. Even if the situation that created the anger is removed by miles or years, it can be replayed through the memory, reactivating the sympathetic arousal when this occurs.

Table 17-1 lists positive and negative functions of anger.

CORE CONCEPT

Aggression

Aggression is a behavior intended to threaten or injure the victim's security or self-esteem. It means "to go against," "to assault," or "to attack." It is a response that aims at inflicting pain or injury on objects or persons. Whether the damage is caused by words, fists, or weapons, the behavior is virtually always designed to punish. It is frequently accompanied by bitterness, meanness, and ridicule. An aggressive person is often vengeful (Warren, 1990, p. 81).

The term *anger* often takes on a negative connotation because of its link with aggression. Aggression is one way individuals express anger. It is sometimes used to try to force someone into compliance with the aggressor's wishes, but at other times the only objective seems to be the infliction of punishment and pain. In virtually all instances, aggression is a negative function or destructive use of anger.

Predisposing Factors to Anger and Aggression

A number of factors have been implicated in the way individuals express anger. Some theorists view aggression as purely biological, and some suggest that it results from individuals' interactions with their environments. It is likely a combination of both.

Modeling

Role **modeling** is one of the strongest forms of learning. Children model their behavior at a very early age after their primary caregivers, usually parents. How parents or significant others express anger becomes the child's method of anger expression.

TABLE 17-1 The Functions of Anger

POSITIVE FUNCTIONS OR CONSTRUCTIVE USES	NEGATIVE FUNCTIONS OR DESTRUCTIVE USES
Anger energizes and mobilizes the body for self-defense.	Without cognitive input, anger may result in impulsive behavior, disregarding possible negative consequences.
Communicated assertively, anger can promote conflict resolution.	Communicated passive-aggressively or aggressively, conflict escalates, and the problem that created the conflict goes unresolved.
Anger arousal is a personal signal of threat or injustice against the self. The signal elicits coping responses to deal with the distress.	Anger can lead to aggression when the coping response is displacement. Anger can be destructive if it is discharged against an object or person unrelated to the true target of the anger.
Anger is constructive when it provides a feeling of control over a situation and the individual is able to assertively take charge of a situation.	Anger can be destructive when the feeling of control is exaggerated and the individual uses the power to intimidate others.
Anger is constructive when it is expressed assertively, serves to increase self-esteem, and leads to mutual understanding and forgiveness.	Anger can be destructive when it masks honest feelings, weakens self-esteem, and leads to hostility and rage.

Adapted from Gorman and Sultan (2008) and Waughfield (2002).

Whether role modeling is positive or negative depends on the behavior of the models. Much has been written about the abused child becoming physically abusive as an adult.

Role models are not always in the home, however. Evidence supports the role of television violence as a predisposing factor to later aggressive behavior (American Psychological Association, 2004). The American Academy of Pediatrics (2001) suggested that monitoring what children view and regulation of violence in the media are necessary to prevent this type of violent modeling.

Operant Conditioning

Operant conditioning occurs when a specific behavior is reinforced. A positive reinforcement is a response to the specific behavior that is pleasurable or offers a reward. A negative reinforcement is a response to the specific behavior that prevents an undesirable result from occurring.

Anger responses can be learned through operant conditioning. For example, when a child wants something and has been told "no" by a parent, he or she might have a temper tantrum. If, when the temper tantrum begins, the parent lets the child have what is wanted, the anger has been positively reinforced (or rewarded).

An example of learning by negative reinforcement follows: A mother asks the child to pick up her toys and the child becomes angry and has a temper tantrum. If, when the temper tantrum

begins, the mother thinks, "Oh, it's not worth all this!" and picks up the toys herself, the anger has been negatively reinforced (child was rewarded by not having to pick up her toys).

Neurophysiological Disorders

Some research has implicated epilepsy of temporal and frontal lobe origin in episodic aggression and violent behavior (Sadock & Sadock, 2007). Clients with episodic dyscontrol often respond to anticonvulsant medication.

Tumors in the brain, particularly in the areas of the limbic system and the temporal lobes; trauma to the brain, resulting in cerebral changes; and diseases, such as encephalitis (or medications that may effect this syndrome), have all been implicated in the predisposition to aggression and violent behavior. A study by Lee and associates (1998) showed that destruction of the amygdaloid body in patients with intractable aggression resulted in a reduction in autonomic arousal levels and in the number of aggressive outbursts.

Biochemical Factors

Violent behavior may be associated with hormonal dysfunction caused by Cushing's disease or hyperthyroidism (Tardiff, 2003). Studies have not supported a correlation between violence and increased levels of androgens or alterations in hormone levels associated with hypoglycemia or premenstrual syndrome.

Some research indicates that various neurotransmitters (e.g., epinephrine, norepinephrine, dopamine, acetylcholine, and serotonin) may play a role in the facilitation and inhibition of aggressive impulses (Sadock & Sadock, 2007).

Socioeconomic Factors

High rates of violence exist within the subculture of poverty in the United States. This has been attributed to lack of resources, break-up of families, alienation, discrimination, and frustration (Tardiff, 2003). An ongoing controversy exists as to whether economic inequality or absolute poverty is most responsible for violent behavior within this subculture. That is, does violence occur because individuals perceive themselves as disadvantaged relative to other persons, or does violence occur because of the deprivation itself? These concepts are not easily understood and are still under investigation.

Environmental Factors

Physical crowding may be related to violence through increased contact and decreased defensible space (Tardiff, 2003). A relationship between heat and aggression also has been indicated (Anderson, 2001). Moderately uncomfortable temperature appears to be associated with an increase in aggression, while extremely hot temperatures seem to decrease aggression.

A number of epidemiological studies have found a strong link between use of alcohol and violent behavior. Other substances, including cocaine, amphetamines, hallucinogens, and anabolic steroids, have also been associated with violent behavior (Tardiff, 2003).

The Nursing Process

CORE CONCEPT

Anger Management
The use of various techniques and strategies to control responses to anger-provoking situations. The goal of anger management is to reduce both the emotional feelings and the physiological arousal that anger engenders.

Assessment

Nurses must be aware of the symptoms associated with anger and aggression in order to make an accurate assessment. The best intervention is prevention, so risk factors for assessing violence potential are also presented.

Anger

Anger can be associated with a number of typical behaviors, including (but not limited to) the following:

■ Frowning facial expression
■ Clenched fists
■ Low-pitched verbalizations forced through clenched teeth
■ Yelling and shouting
■ Intense eye contact or avoidance of eye contact
■ Easily offended
■ Defensive response to criticism
■ Passive-aggressive behaviors
■ Emotional overcontrol with flushing of the face
■ Intense discomfort; continuous state of tension

Anger has been identified as a stage in the grieving process. Individuals who become fixed in this stage may become depressed. In this instance, the anger is turned inward as a way for the individual to maintain control over the pent-up anger. Because of the negative connotation to the word *anger,* some clients will not acknowledge that what they are feeling is anger. These individuals need assistance to recognize their true feelings and to understand that anger is a perfectly acceptable emotion when it is expressed appropriately.

Aggression

Aggression can arise from a number of feeling states, including anger, anxiety, guilt, frustration, or suspiciousness. Aggressive behaviors can be classified as mild (e.g., sarcasm), moderate (e.g., slamming doors), severe (e.g., threats of physical violence against others), or extreme (e.g., physical acts of violence against others). Aggression may be associated with (but not limited to) the following defining characteristics:

■ Pacing, restlessness
■ Tense facial expression and body language
■ Verbal or physical threats
■ Loud voice, shouting, use of obscenities, argumentative
■ Threats of homicide or suicide
■ Increase in agitation, with overreaction to environmental stimuli
■ Panic anxiety, leading to misinterpretation of the environment
■ Disturbed thought processes; suspiciousness
■ Angry mood, often disproportionate to the situation

Kassinove and Tafrate (2002) stated, "In contrast to anger, aggression is almost always goal directed and has the aim of harm to a specific person or object. Aggression is one of the negative outcomes that may emerge from general arousal and anger" (pp. 40; 50).

Intent is a requisite in the definition of aggression. It refers to behavior that is *intended* to inflict harm or destruction. Accidents that lead to *unintentional* harm or destruction are not considered aggression.

Assessing Risk Factors

Prevention is the key issue in the management of aggressive or violent behavior. The individual who becomes violent usually feels an underlying helplessness. Three factors that have been identified as important considerations in assessing for potential violence include the following:

1. Past history of violence
2. Client diagnosis
3. Current behavior

Past history of violence is widely recognized as a major risk factor for violence in a treatment setting. Also highly correlated with assaultive behavior is diagnosis. Diagnoses that have a strong association with violent behavior are schizophrenia, major depression, bipolar disorder, and substance use disorders (Friedman, 2006). Substance abuse, in addition to mental illness, compounds the increased risk of violence. Dementia and antisocial, borderline, and intermittent explosive personality disorders have also been associated with a risk for violent behavior.

Novitsky, Julius, and Dubin (2009) stated:

> The successful management of violence is predicated on an understanding of the dynamics of violence. A patient's threatening behavior is commonly an overreaction to feelings of impotence, helplessness, and perceived or actual humiliation. Aggression rarely occurs suddenly and unexpectedly. (p. 50)

They described a "**prodromal syndrome**" that is characterized by anxiety and tension, verbal abuse and profanity, and increasing hyperactivity. These escalating behaviors usually do not occur in stages but most often overlap and sometimes occur simultaneously. Behaviors associated with this prodromal stage include rigid posture; clenched fists and jaws; grim, defiant affect; talking in a rapid, raised voice; arguing and demanding; using profanity and threatening verbalizations; agitation and pacing; and pounding and slamming.

Most assaultive behavior is preceded by a period of increasing hyperactivity. Behaviors associated with the prodromal syndrome should be considered emergent and demand immediate attention.

Keen observation skills and background knowledge for accurate assessment are critical factors in predicting potential for violent behavior. The Brøset Violence Checklist (BVC) is presented in Box 17-1. It is a quick, simple, and reliable checklist that can be used as a risk assessment for potential violence. Testing has shown a 63 percent accuracy for prediction of violence at a score of 2 and above (Almvik, Woods, & Rasmussen, 2000). De-escalation techniques are also included.

Diagnosis/Outcome Identification

NANDA International does not include a separate nursing diagnosis for anger. The nursing diagnosis

---

BOX 17-1 The Brøset Violence Checklist

Behaviors

Score (Score 1 point for each behavior observed. At a score of ≥ 2, begin de-escalation techniques.)

Confusion
Irritability
Boisterousness
Physical threats
Verbal threats
Attacks on objects
TOTAL SCORE

De-escalation techniques:

Calm voice	Walk outdoors or fresh air
Helpful attitude	Reduction in demands
Identify consequences	Group participation
Open hands and non-threatening posture	Relaxation techniques
Allow phone call	Express concern
Offer food or drink	Reduce stimulation and loud noise
Decrease waiting times and request refusals	Verbal redirection and limit setting
Distract with a more positive activity (e.g., soft music or a quiet room)	Time out–quiet time–open seclusion
	Offer prn medication

If de-escalation techniques fail:
1. Suggest prn medications
2. Time out or unlocked seclusion, which can progress to locked seclusion

From Almvik, R., Woods, P., & Rasmussen, K. (2000). The Brøset violence checklist: Sensitivity, specificity, and interrater reliability. Journal of Interpersonal Violence, 15(12), 1284–1296, with permission.
De-escalation techniques reprinted with permission from Barbara Barnes, Milwaukee County Behavioral Health Division.

of complicated grieving may be used when anger is expressed inappropriately and the etiology is related to a loss.

The following nursing diagnoses may be considered for clients demonstrating inappropriate expression of anger or aggression:

■ Ineffective coping related to negative role modeling and dysfunctional family system evidenced by yelling, name calling, hitting others, and temper tantrums as expressions of anger.

■ Risk for self-directed or other-directed violence related to having been nurtured in an atmosphere of violence; history of violence

Outcome Criteria

Outcome criteria include short- and long-term goals. Timelines are individually determined. The following criteria may be used for measurement of outcomes in the care of the client needing assistance with management of anger and aggression.

The client:

■ Is able to recognize when he or she is angry, and seeks out staff/support person to talk about his or her feelings.

■ Is able to take responsibility for own feelings of anger.

■ Demonstrates the ability to exert internal control over feelings of anger.

■ Is able to diffuse anger before losing control.

■ Uses the tension generated by the anger in a constructive manner.

■ Does not cause harm to self or others.

■ Is able to use steps of the problem-solving process rather than becoming violent as a means of seeking solutions.

Planning/Implementation

In Table 17-2, a plan of care is presented for the client who expresses anger inappropriately. Outcome criteria, appropriate nursing interventions, and rationales are included for each diagnosis.

Evaluation

Evaluation consists of reassessment to determine if the nursing interventions have been successful in achieving the objectives of care. The following type of information may be gathered to determine the success of working with a client exhibiting inappropriate expression of anger.

■ Is the client able to recognize when he or she is angry now?

■ Can the client take responsibility for these feelings and keep them in check without losing control?

■ Does the client seek out a staff/support person to talk about feelings of anger when they occur?

Table 17-2 CARE PLAN FOR THE INDIVIDUAL WHO EXPRESSES ANGER INAPPROPRIATELY

NURSING DIAGNOSIS: INEFFECTIVE COPING

RELATED TO: Negative role modeling and dysfunctional family system

EVIDENCED BY: Yelling, name calling, hitting others, and temper tantrums as expressions of anger.

OUTCOME CRITERIA	NURSING INTERVENTIONS	RATIONALE
Client will be able to recognize anger in self and take responsibility before losing control.	1. Remain calm when dealing with an angry client.	1. Anger expressed by the nurse will most likely incite increased anger in the client.
	2. Set verbal limits on behavior. Clearly delineate the consequences of inappropriate expression of anger and always follow through.	2. Consistency in enforcing the consequences is essential if positive outcomes are to be achieved. Inconsistency creates confusion and encourages testing of limits.
	3. Have the client keep a diary of angry feelings, what triggered them, and how they were handled.	3. This provides a more objective measure of the problem.
	4. Avoid touching the client when he or she becomes angry.	4. The client may view touch as threatening and could become violent.
	5. Help the client determine the true source of the anger.	5. Many times anger is being displaced onto a safer object or person. If resolution is to occur, the first step is to identify the source of the problem.

Continued

Table 17-2 CARE PLAN FOR THE INDIVIDUAL WHO EXPRESSES ANGER INAPPROPRIATELY—cont'd

OUTCOME CRITERIA	NURSING INTERVENTIONS	RATIONALE
	6. It may be constructive to ignore initial derogatory remarks by the client.	6. Lack of feedback often extinguishes an undesirable behavior.
	7. Help the client find alternate ways of releasing tension, such as physical outlets, and more appropriate ways of expressing anger, such as seeking out staff when feelings emerge.	7. Client will likely need assistance to problem-solve more appropriate ways of behaving.
	8. Role model appropriate ways of expressing anger assertively, such as, "I dislike being called names. I get angry when I hear you saying those things about me."	8. Role modeling is one of the strongest methods of learning.

NURSING DIAGNOSIS: RISK FOR SELF-DIRECTED OR OTHER-DIRECTED VIOLENCE

RISK FACTORS: Having been nurtured in an atmosphere of violence; history of violence

OUTCOME CRITERIA	NURSING INTERVENTIONS	RATIONALE
The client will not harm self or others. The client will verbalize anger rather than hit others.	1. Observe client for escalation of anger (called the prodromal syndrome): increased motor activity, pounding, slamming, tense posture, defiant affect, clenched teeth and fists, arguing, demanding, and challenging or threatening staff.	1. Violence may be prevented if risks are identified in time.
	2. When these behaviors are observed, first ensure that sufficient staff are available to help with a potentially violent situation. Attempt to defuse the anger beginning with the least restrictive means.	2. The initial consideration must be having enough help to diffuse a potentially violent situation. Client rights must be honored, while preventing harm to client and others.
	3. Techniques for dealing with aggression include:	3. Aggression control techniques promote safety and reduce risk of harm to client and others:
	💬 a. Talking down. Say, "John, you seem very angry. Let's go to your room and talk about it." (Ensure that client does not position self between door and nurse.)	a. Promotes a trusting relationship and may prevent the client's anxiety from escalating.
	💬 b. Physical outlets. "Maybe it would help if you punched your pillow or the punching bag for a while." "I'll stay here with you if you want."	b. Provides effective way for client to release tension associated with high levels of anger.
	c. Medication. If agitation continues to escalate, offer client choice of taking medication voluntarily. If he or she refuses, reassess the situation to determine if harm to self or others is imminent.	c. Tranquilizing medication may calm client and prevent violence from escalating.
	d. Call for assistance. Remove self and other clients from the immediate area. Call violence code, push "panic" button, call for assault team, or institute measures established by the institution. Sufficient staff to indicate a show of strength may be enough to de-escalate the situation, and client may agree to take the medication.	d. Client and staff safety are of primary concern.

Table 17-2 CARE PLAN FOR THE INDIVIDUAL WHO EXPRESSES ANGER INAPPROPRIATELY—cont'd

OUTCOME CRITERIA	NURSING INTERVENTIONS	RATIONALE
	e. Restraints. If client is not calmed by "talking down" or by medication, use of mechanical restraints and/or seclusion may be necessary. Be sure to have sufficient staff available to assist. Figures 17–1, 17–2, and 17–3 illustrate ways in which staff can safely and appropriately deal with an out-of-control client. Follow protocol for restraints/seclusion established by the institution. The Joint Commission (formerly the Joint Commission on Accreditation of Healthcare Organizations [JCAHO]) requires that an in-person evaluation by a physician or other licensed independent practitioner (LIP) be conducted within 1 hour of the initiation of the restraint or seclusion (The Joint Commission, 2010). The physician or LIP must reissue a new order for restraints every 4 hours for adults and every 1–2 hours for children and adolescents. Restraints should be used as a last resort, after all other interventions have been unsuccessful, and the client is clearly at risk of harm to self or others.	e. Clients who do not have internal control over their own behavior may require external controls, such as mechanical restraints, in order to prevent harm to self or others.

FIGURE 17–1   Walking a client to the seclusion room.

FIGURE 17–2   Staff restraint of a client in supine position. The client's head is controlled to prevent biting.

Continued

Table 17-2 CARE PLAN FOR THE INDIVIDUAL WHO EXPRESSES ANGER INAPPROPRIATELY—cont'd

OUTCOME CRITERIA	NURSING INTERVENTIONS	RATIONALE

FIGURE 17–3 Transporting a client to the seclusion room.

	NURSING INTERVENTIONS	RATIONALE
	f. Observation and documentation. The client in restraints should be observed on a one-to-one basis for the first hour. This in-person observation can progress to audio and visual monitoring after the first hour. Every 15 minutes the client should be monitored to ensure that circulation to extremities is not compromised (check temperature, color, pulses). Assist client with needs related to nutrition, hydration, and elimination. Position client so that comfort is facilitated and aspiration can be prevented. Document all observations.	f. Client well-being is a nursing priority.
	g. Ongoing assessment. As agitation decreases, assess client's readiness for restraint removal or reduction. With assistance from other staff members, remove one restraint at a time, while assessing client's response. This minimizes the risk of injury to client and staff.	g. Gradual removal of the restraints allows for testing of the client's self-control. Client and staff safety are of primary concern.
	h. Staff debriefing. It is important when a client loses control for staff to follow up with a discussion about the situation. Tardiff (2003) stated, "The violent episode should be discussed in terms of what happened, what would have prevented it, why seclusion or restraint was used (if it was), and how the patient or the staff felt in terms of using seclusion and restraint." It is also important to discuss the situation with other clients who witnessed the episode. It is important that they understand what happened. Some clients may fear that they could be secluded or restrained at some time for no apparent reason.	h. Debriefing helps to diminish the emotional impact of the intervention. Mutual feedback is shared, and staff has an opportunity to process and learn from the event.

■ Is the client able to transfer tension generated by the anger into constructive activities?

■ Has harm to the client and others been avoided?

■ Is the client able to solve problems adaptively without undue frustration and without becoming violent?

Summary and Key Points

■ Statistics show that violence is rampant in the United States.

■ The precursor to violence is anger, which is a normal human emotion, and need not necessarily be a negative response.

■ When used appropriately, anger can provide positive assistance with problem solving and decision making in everyday life situations.

■ Violence occurs when individuals lose control of their anger.

■ Anger is viewed as the emotional response to one's perception of a situation.

■ Anger is a very powerful emotion and, when denied or buried, can precipitate a number of psychophysiological disorders.

■ When anger is turned inward on the self, it can result in depression.

■ When expressed inappropriately, anger commonly interferes with interpersonal relationships.

■ When anger is suppressed, it often turns to resentment.

■ Anger generates a physiological arousal comparable to the stress response discussed in Chapter 1.

■ Aggression is one way in which individuals express anger.

■ Aggression is behavior intended to threaten or injure the victim's security or self-esteem.

■ Aggression can be physical or verbal, but it is virtually always designed to punish.

■ Aggression is a negative function or destructive use of anger.

■ Various predisposing factors to the way individuals express anger have been implicated. Some theorists suggest that the etiology is purely biological, whereas others believe it depends on psychological and environmental factors.

■ Some possible predisposing factors include role modeling, operant conditioning, neurophysiological disorders (e.g., brain tumors, trauma, or diseases), biochemical factors (e.g., increased levels of androgens or other alterations in hormone levels and neurotransmitter involvement), socioeconomic factors (e.g., living in poverty), and environmental factors (e.g., physical crowding, uncomfortable temperature, use of alcohol or drugs, and availability of firearms).

■ Nurses must be aware of the symptoms associated with anger and aggression in order to make an accurate assessment.

■ Prevention is the key issue in the management of aggressive or violent behavior.

■ Three elements have been identified as key risk factors in the potential for violence: (1) past history of violence, (2) client diagnosis, and (3) current behaviors.

 DavisPlus   Additional info available @ davisplus.fadavis.com

Review Questions
Self-Examination/Learning Exercise

Select the answer that is most appropriate for each of the following questions:

1. John, age 27, was brought to the emergency department by two police officers. He smelled strongly of alcohol and was combative. His blood alcohol level was measured at 293 mg/dl. His girlfriend reports that he drinks excessively every day and is verbally and physically abusive. The nurses give John the nursing diagnosis of Risk for Other-directed Violence. What would be appropriate outcome objectives for this diagnosis? (Select all that apply.)
   a. The client will not verbalize anger or hit anyone.
   b. The client will verbalize anger rather than hit others.
   c. The client will not harm self or others.
   d. The client will be restrained if he becomes verbally or physically abusive.

Continued

Review Questions—con'd
Self-Examination/Learning Exercise

2. John, who was hospitalized with alcohol intoxication and violent behavior, is sitting in the day-room watching TV with the other clients when the nurse approaches with his 5:00 p.m. dose of haloperidol. John says, "I feel in control now. I don't need any drugs." The nurse's best response is based on which of the following statements?
   a. John must have the medication, or he will become violent.
   b. John knows that if he will not take the medication orally, he will be restrained and given an intramuscular injection.
   c. John has the right to refuse the medication provided there is no immediate danger to self or others.
   d. John must take the medication at this time in order to maintain adequate blood levels.

3. The nurse hears John, a client with a history of violence, yelling in the dayroom. The nurse observes his increased agitation, clenched fists, and loud, demanding voice. He is challenging and threatening staff and the other clients. The nurse's *priority* intervention would be to:
   a. Call for assistance.
   b. Draw up a syringe of prn haloperidol.
   c. Ask John if he would like to talk about his anger.
   d. Tell John if he does not calm down he will have to be restrained.

4. John, a client with a history of violence, has been hospitalized on the psychiatric unit. He becomes agitated and begins to threaten the staff and other clients. When all other interventions fail, John is placed in restraints in the seclusion room for his and others' protection. Which of the following are interventions for the client in restraints? (Select all that apply.)
   a. Check temperature and pulse of extremities.
   b. Document all observations.
   c. Explain to the client that restraint is his punishment for violent behavior.
   d. Provide ongoing assessment and observation.
   e. Withhold food and fluid until client is calm and can be released from restraints.

5. When it has been assessed that a client is in control and no longer requires restraining, how does the nurse proceed?
   a. The nurse removes the restraints.
   b. The nurse calls for assistance to remove the restraints.
   c. With assistance, the nurse removes one restraint.
   d. The nurse tells the client he will have to wait until the doctor comes in.

6. Which of these procedures is important in following up an episode of violence on the unit? (Select all that apply.)
   a. Document all observations and occurrences.
   b. Conduct a debriefing with staff.
   c. Discuss what occurred with other clients who witnessed the incident.
   d. Warn the client that it could happen again if he becomes violent.

7. A client who has been in restraints is now calm. He apologizes to the nurse and says, "I hope I didn't hurt anyone." The nurse's best response is:
   a. "This is our job. We know how to handle violent clients."
   b. "We understand you were out of control and didn't really mean to hurt anyone."
   c. "It is fortunate that no one was hurt. You will not be placed in restraints as long as you can control your behavior."
   d. "It is an unpleasant situation to have to restrain someone, but we have to think of the other clients. We can't have you causing injury to others. I just hope it won't happen again."

Review Questions—con'd
Self-Examination/Learning Exercise

8. John and his girlfriend had an argument during her visit. Which behavior by John would indicate he is learning to adaptively problem-solve his frustrations?
   a. John says to the nurse, "Give me some of that medication before I end up in restraints!"
   b. When his girlfriend leaves, John goes to the exercise room and punches on the punching bag.
   c. John says to the nurse, "I guess I'm going to have to dump that broad!"
   d. John says to his girlfriend, "You'd better leave before I do something I'm sorry for."

9. Which of the following assessment data would the nurse consider as risk factors for possible violence in a client? (Select all that apply.)
   a. A diagnosis of somatization disorder.
   b. A diagnosis of bipolar disorder.
   c. Substance intoxication.
   d. Argumentative and demanding behavior.
   e. Past history of violence.

10. Which of the following is true about *aggression?* (Select all that apply.)
   a. It is goal directed.
   b. Its aim is to do harm to a person or object.
   c. It has a requisite of *intent.*
   d. It energizes and mobilizes the body for self-defense.

References

Almvik, R., Woods, P., & Rasmussen, K. (2000). The Brøset violence checklist: Sensitivity, specificity, and interrater reliability. *Journal of Interpersonal Violence, 15*(12), 1284–1296.

American Academy of Pediatrics. (2001). Media violence. *Pediatrics, 108,* 1222–1226.

American Psychological Association. (2004). *Violence in the media—Psychologists help protect children from harmful effects.* Retrieved August 8, 2010, from http://www.apa.org/research/action/protect.aspx

American Psychological Association. (2010). *Controlling anger before it controls you.* Retrieved August 8, 2010, from http://www.apa.org/topics/anger/control.aspx

Anderson, C.A. (2001). Heat and violence. *Current Directions in Psychological Science 10*(1), 33–38.

Butterfield, P. (2000). *Understanding and managing anger: Diagnosis, treatment, and prevention.* Sunnyvale, CA: CorText Mind Matters Educational Seminars.

Friedman, R. A. (2006). Violence and mental illness—How strong is the link? *New England Journal of Medicine, 355*(20), 2064–2066.

Gorman, L. M., & Sultan, D. F. (2008). *Psychosocial nursing for general patient care* (3rd ed.). Philadelphia: F.A. Davis.

Kassinove, H., & Tafrate, R. C. (2002). *Anger management.* Atascadero, CA: Impact Publishers.

Lee, G. P., Bechara, A., Adolphs, R., Arena, J., Meador, K. J., Loring, D. W., et al. (1998). Clinical and physiological effects of stereotaxic bilateral amygdalotomy for intractable aggression. *Journal of Neuropsychiatry and Clinical Neurosciences, 10,* 413–420.

Novitsky, M. A., Julius, R. J., & Dubin, W. R. (2009). Non-pharmacologic management of violence in psychiatric emergencies. *Primary Psychiatry, 16*(9), 49–53.

Sadock, B. J., & Sadock, V. A. (2007). *Synopsis of psychiatry: Behavioral sciences/clinical psychiatry* (10th ed.). Philadelphia: Lippincott Williams & Wilkins.

Tardiff, K. J. (2003). Violence. In R. E. Hales & S. C. Yudofsky (Eds.). *Textbook of clinical psychiatry* (4th ed., pp. 1485–1509). Washington, DC: American Psychiatric Publishing.

The Joint Commission. (2010). *The comprehensive accreditation manual for hospitals: The official handbook* (January, 2010). Oakbrook Terrace, IL: Joint Commission Resources.

Turgut, T., Lagace, D., Izmir, M., & Dursun, S. (2006). Assessment of violence and aggression in psychiatric settings: Descriptive approaches. *Bulletin of Clinical Psychopharmacology, 16*(3), 179–194.

Warren, N. C. (1990). *Make anger your ally* (3rd ed.). Colorado Springs, CO: Focus on the Family Publishing.

Waughfield, C. G. (2002). *Mental health concepts* (5th ed.). Albany, NY: Delmar.

CHAPTER 18 | The Suicidal Client

KEY TERMS

altruistic suicide

anomic suicide

egoistic suicide

OBJECTIVES
After reading this chapter, the student will be able to:

1. Discuss epidemiological statistics and risk factors related to suicide.
2. Describe predisposing factors implicated in the etiology of suicide.
3. Differentiate between facts and fables regarding suicide.
4. Apply the nursing process to individuals exhibiting suicidal behavior.

HOMEWORK ASSIGNMENT
Please read the chapter and answer the following questions:

1. How do age, race, and gender affect suicide risk?
2. Your neighbor tells you he is going to visit his sister-in-law in the hospital. The sister-in-law has been hospitalized after attempting suicide. Your neighbor asks, "What should I say when I go to visit Jane?" What suggestions might you give him?
3. John's father committed suicide when John was a teenager. John's wife, Mary, tells the mental health nurse that she is afraid John "inherited" that predisposition from his father. How should the nurse respond to Mary?
4. The nurse notes that the mood of a client being treated for depression and suicidal ideation suddenly brightens and the client states, "I feel fine now. I don't feel depressed anymore." Why would this statement alert the nurse of a potential problem?"

Suicide is not a diagnosis or a disorder; it is a behavior. The Judeo-Christian belief has been that life is a gift from God and that taking it is strictly forbidden (Carroll-Ghosh, Victor, & Bourgeois, 2003). A recent, and more secular, view has influenced how some individuals view suicide in our society. Growing support for an individual's right to choose death over pain has been evidenced.

Some individuals are striving to advance the cause of physician-assisted suicides for the terminally ill. Can suicide be a rational act? Most people in our society do not yet believe that it can.

Approximately 95 percent of all persons who commit or attempt suicide have a diagnosed mental disorder (Sadock & Sadock, 2007). This chapter explores suicide from an epidemiological and etiological perspective. Care of the suicidal client is presented in the context of the nursing process.

Historical Perspectives

In ancient Greece, suicide was an offense against the state and individuals who committed suicide were denied burial in community sites (Minois, 2001). In the culture of the imperial Roman army, individuals sometimes resorted to suicide to escape humiliation or abuse.

In the Middle Ages, suicide was viewed as a selfish or criminal act (Minois, 2001). Individuals who committed suicide were often denied cemetery burial and their property was confiscated and shared by the crown and the courts (MacDonald & Murphy, 1991). The issue of suicide changed during the period of the Renaissance. Although condemnation was still expected, the view became more philosophical, and intellectuals could discuss the issue more freely.

Most philosophers of the 17th and 18th centuries condemned suicide, but some writers recognized a connection between suicide and melancholy or other severe mental disturbances (Minois, 2001). Suicide was illegal in England until 1961, and only in 1993 was it decriminalized in Ireland.

Most religions consider suicide as a sin against God. Judaism, Christianity, Islam, Hinduism, and Buddhism all condemn suicide. In 1995, Pope John II restated Church opposition to suicide, euthanasia, and abortion as crimes against life, not unlike homicide and genocide (Tondo & Baldessarini, 2001).

Epidemiological Factors

More than 34,000 persons in the United States end their lives each year by suicide (Centers for Disease Control and Prevention [CDC], 2010). These statistics have established suicide as the third leading cause of death (behind accidents and homicide) among young Americans ages 15 to 24 years, the fourth leading cause of death for ages 25 to 44, and the eighth leading cause of death for individuals ages 45 to 64 (National Center for Health Statistics [NCHS], 2009). Many more people attempt suicide than succeed, and countless others seriously contemplate the act without carrying it out. Suicide has become a major health-care problem in the United States today.

Over the years confusion has existed over the reality of various notions regarding suicide. Some facts and fables relating to suicide are presented in Table 18-1.

TABLE 18-1 Facts and Fables About Suicide

FABLES	FACTS
People who talk about suicide do not commit suicide. Suicide happens without warning.	Eight out of 10 people who kill themselves have given definite clues and warnings about their suicidal intentions. Very subtle clues may be ignored or disregarded by others.
You cannot stop a suicidal person. He or she is fully intent on dying.	Most suicidal people are very ambivalent about their feelings regarding living or dying. Most are "gambling with death" and see it as a cry for someone to save them.
Once a person is suicidal, he or she is suicidal forever.	People who want to kill themselves are only suicidal for a limited time. If they are saved from feelings of self-destruction, they can go on to lead normal lives.
Improvement after severe depression means that the suicide risk is over.	Most suicides occur within about 3 months after the beginning of "improvement," when the individual has the energy to carry out suicidal intentions.
Suicide is inherited, or "runs in families."	Suicide is not inherited. It is an individual matter and can be prevented. However, suicide by a close family member increases an individual's risk factor for suicide.
All suicidal individuals are mentally ill, and suicide is the act of a psychotic person.	Although suicidal persons are extremely unhappy, they are not necessarily psychotic. They are merely unable at that point in time to see an alternative solution to what they consider an unbearable problem.

Continued

TABLE 18-1 Facts and Fables About Suicide—cont'd

FABLES	FACTS
Suicidal threats and gestures should be considered manipulative or attention-seeking behavior, and should not be taken seriously.	All suicidal behavior must be approached with the gravity of the potential act in mind. Attention should be given to the possibility that the individual is issuing a cry for help.
People usually commit suicide by taking an overdose of drugs.	Gunshot wounds are the leading cause of death among suicide victims.
If an individual has attempted suicide, he or she will not do it again.	Between 50% and 80% of all people who ultimately kill themselves have a history of a previous attempt.

SOURCES: Friends for Survival, Inc. (2010); National Alliance on Mental Illness (2010); and The Samaritans (2010).

Risk Factors

Marital Status

The suicide rate for single persons is twice that of married persons. Divorced, separated, or widowed persons have rates four to five times greater than those of the married (Jacobs et al., 2006).

Gender

Women attempt suicide more, but men succeed more often. Successful suicides number about 70 percent for men and 30 percent for women. This has to do with the lethality of the means. Women tend to overdose; men use more lethal means such as firearms. In the United States, from 1970 to 2006, annual suicide rates per 100,000 rose from 16.8 to 17.8 in men, but decreased from 6.6 to 4.6 in women (NCHS, 2009). These differences between men and women may also reflect a tendency for women to seek and accept help from friends or professionals, whereas men often view help-seeking as a sign of weakness.

Age

Suicide risk and age are positively correlated. This is particularly true with men. Although rates among women remain fairly constant throughout life, rates among men show a higher age correlation. The rate rises sharply during adolescence, peaks between 40 and 50, and levels off until age 65, when it rises again for the remaining years (NCHS, 2009).

The suicide rate among young people (ages 15 to 19) peaked in 1990 at 11.1 per 100,000 and declined to 7.3 per 100,000 in 2006 (NCHS, 2009). Several factors put adolescents at risk for suicide, including impulsive and high-risk behaviors, untreated mood disorders (e.g., major depression and bipolar disorder), access to lethal means (e.g., firearms), and substance abuse. Statistics from the Centers for Disease Control and Prevention indicate that the most common method of completed suicide for adolescent males is firearm; for adolescent females it is hanging/suffocation (CDC, 2007).

The suicide rate for the elderly peaked in 1990 at 20.5 per 100,000 and declined to 14.2 per 100,000 in 2006 (NCHS, 2009). While the elderly make up less than 13 percent of the population, they account for 16 percent of all suicides (American Association of Suicidology, 2009). White males over the age of 80 are at the greatest risk of all age/gender/race groups. Eighty-five percent of elderly suicides are male, which is 7.7 times greater than for females, and firearms are the most common means of committing suicide (American Association of Suicidology, 2009). The overall rate of suicide for females declines after age 65.

Religion

Historically, suicide rates among Roman Catholic populations have been lower than rates among Protestants and Jews (Sadock & Sadock, 2007). In a recent study published in the *Journal of Affective Disorders,* men and women who consider themselves affiliated with a religion are less likely to attempt suicide than their nonreligious counterparts (Rasic et al., 2009). The authors found that religious attendance is associated with decreased suicide attempts both in the general population and in those with a mental illness, independent of the availability of social support systems.

Socioeconomic Status

Individuals in the very highest and lowest social classes have higher suicide rates than those in the middle classes (Sadock & Sadock, 2007). With regard to occupation, suicide rates are higher among physicians, artists, dentists, law enforcement officers, lawyers, and insurance agents.

Ethnicity

With regard to ethnicity, statistics show that whites are at highest risk for suicide, followed by Native Americans, African Americans, Hispanic Americans, and Asian Americans (NCHS, 2009).

Other Risk Factors

More than 90 percent of people who kill themselves have a diagnosable mental disorder, most commonly a mood disorder or a substance abuse disorder (National Institute of Mental Health [NIMH], 2010). Suicide risk may increase early during treatment with antidepressants, as the return of energy brings about an increased ability to act out self-destructive wishes. Other psychiatric disorders that may account for suicidal behavior include schizophrenia, personality disorders, and anxiety disorders (Jacobs et al., 2006).

Severe insomnia is associated with increased suicide risk, even in the absence of depression. Use of alcohol, and particularly a combination of alcohol and barbiturates, increases the risk of suicide. Psychosis, especially with command hallucinations, poses a higher than normal risk. Affliction with a chronic painful or disabling illness also increases the risk of suicide.

Several studies have indicated a higher risk factor for suicide among gay men and lesbians (Cochran & Mays, 2000; Eisenberg & Resnick, 2006; King et al., 2008; Medscape Psychiatry, 2011). It is thought that this increased risk may be a function of the social stigma and discrimination associated with the gay and lesbian orientation. Additional personal stressors, including isolation, victimization, and stressful interpersonal relationships with family, peers, and community, are not uncommon. A report by the Suicide Prevention Resource Center (2008) stated:

> Research indicates that lesbian, gay, and bisexual (LGB) youth have significantly higher rates of suicide attempts and suicidal ideation than their heterosexual peers. Data limitations make it difficult to draw conclusions about higher rates of death by suicide among LGB youth; however, the higher number of suicide attempts, as well as the seriousness of attempts among LGB youth, make it probable that this group of youth has a higher rate of suicide deaths than their heterosexual counterparts. (p. 19)

Higher risk is also associated with a family history of suicide, especially in a same-sex parent. Persons who have made prior suicide attempts are at higher risk for suicide. About half of individuals who kill themselves have previously attempted suicide. Loss of a loved one through death or separation and lack of employment or increased financial burden also increase risk.

Predisposing Factors: Theories of Suicide

Psychological Theories

Anger Turned Inward

Freud (1957) believed that suicide was a response to the intense self-hatred that an individual possessed. The anger had originated toward a love object but was ultimately turned inward against the self. Freud believed that suicide occurred as a result of an earlier repressed desire to kill someone else. He interpreted suicide to be an aggressive act toward the self that often was really directed toward others.

Hopelessness

Carroll-Ghosh and associates (2003) identified hopelessness as a central underlying factor in the predisposition to suicide. Beck, Brown, and Berchick (1990) also found a high correlation between hopelessness and suicide.

Desperation and Guilt

Hendin (1991) identified desperation as another important factor in suicide. With desperation, an individual feels helpless to change, but he or she also feels that life is impossible without such change. Guilt and self-recrimination are other aspects of desperation. These affective components were found to be prominent in Vietnam veterans with posttraumatic stress disorder exhibiting suicidal behaviors (Carroll-Ghosh et al., 2003).

History of Aggression and Violence

Some studies have indicated that violent behavior often goes hand-in-hand with suicidal behavior (Carroll-Ghosh et al., 2003). These studies correlate the suicidal behavior in violent individuals to conscious rage, therefore citing rage as an important psychological factor underlying the suicidal behavior (Hendin, 1991).

Shame and Humiliation

Some individuals have viewed suicide as a "face-saving" mechanism—a way to prevent public humiliation following a social defeat such as a sudden loss of status or income. Often these individuals are too embarrassed to seek treatment or other support systems.

Developmental Stressors

Rich, Warsradt, and Nemiroff (1991) have associated developmental level with certain life stressors and their correlation to suicide. The stressors of conflict, separation, and rejection are associated with suicidal behavior in adolescence and early adulthood. The principal stressor associated with suicidal behavior in the 40- to 60-year-old group is economic problems. Medical illness plays an increasingly significant role after age 60 and becomes the leading predisposing factor to suicidal behavior in individuals older than age 80.

Sociological Theory

Durkheim (1951) studied the individual's interaction with the society in which he or she lived. He believed that the more cohesive the society, and the more that the individual felt an integrated part of the society, the less likely he or she was to commit suicide. Durkheim described three social categories of suicide:

Egoistic suicide is the response of the individual who feels separate and apart from the mainstream of society. Integration is lacking and the individual does not feel a part of any cohesive group (such as a family or a church).

Altruistic suicide is the opposite of egoistic suicide. The individual who is prone to altruistic suicide is excessively integrated into the group. The group is often governed by cultural, religious, or political ties, and allegiance is so strong that the individual will sacrifice his or her life for the group.

Anomic suicide occurs in response to changes that occur in an individual's life (e.g., divorce, loss of job) that disrupt feelings of relatedness to the group. An interruption in the customary norms of behavior instills feelings of "separateness," and fears of being without support from the formerly cohesive group.

Biological Theories

Genetics

Twin studies have shown a much higher concordance rate for monozygotic twins than for dizygotic twins. Some studies with suicide attempters have focused on the genotypic variations in the gene for tryptophan hydroxylase, with results indicating significant association to suicidality (Abbar et al.,

2001). These results suggest a possible existence of genetic predisposition toward suicidal behavior.

Neurochemical Factors

A number of studies have been conducted to determine if there is a correlation between neurochemical functioning in the central nervous system (CNS) and suicidal behavior. Some studies have revealed a deficiency of serotonin (measured as a decrease in the levels of 5-hydroxyindole acetic acid [5-HIAA] of the cerebrospinal fluid) in depressed clients who attempted suicide (Sadock & Sadock, 2007). Some changes in the noradrenergic system of suicide victims have also been reported.

Application of the Nursing Process With the Suicidal Client

Assessment

The following items should be considered when conducting a suicidal client assessment: demographics, presenting symptoms/medical-psychiatric diagnosis, suicidal ideas or acts, interpersonal support system, analysis of the suicidal crisis, psychiatric/medical/family history, and coping strategies. The Surgeon General, in his "Call to Action to Prevent Suicide," spoke of risk factors and protective factors (U.S. Public Health Service, 1999). Risk factors are associated with a greater potential for suicide and suicidal behavior, whereas protective factors are associated with reduced potential for suicide. These risk and protective factors are outlined in Box 18-1. Table 18-2 presents some additional guidelines for determining the degree of suicide potential.

Demographics

The following demographics are assessed:

■ **Age.** Suicide is highest in persons older than 50. Adolescents are also at high risk.

■ **Gender.** Males are at higher risk than females.

■ **Ethnicity.** Caucasians are at higher risk than are Native Americans, who are at higher risk than African Americans.

■ **Martial Status.** Single, divorced, and widowed are at higher risk than married.

■ **Socioeconomic Status.** Individuals in the highest and lowest socioeconomic classes are at higher risk than those in the middle classes.

■ **Occupation.** Professional health care personnel and business executives are at highest risk.

■ **Method.** Use of firearms presents a significantly higher risk than overdose of substances.

BOX 18-1 Suicide Risk Factors and Protective Factors

RISK FACTORS

- Previous suicide attempt
- Mental disorders—particularly mood disorders such as depression and bipolar disorder
- Co-occurring mental and alcohol and substance abuse disorders
- Family history of suicide
- Hopelessness
- Impulsive and/or aggressive tendencies
- Barriers to accessing mental health treatment
- Relational, social, work, or financial loss
- Physical illness
- Easy access to lethal methods, especially guns
- Unwillingness to seek help because of stigma attached to mental and substance abuse disorders and/or suicidal thoughts
- Influence of significant people—family members, celebrities, peers who have died by suicide—both through direct personal contact or inappropriate media representations
- Cultural and religious beliefs—for instance, the belief that suicide is a noble resolution of a personal dilemma
- Local epidemics of suicide that have a contagious influence
- Isolation, a feeling of being cut off from other people

PROTECTIVE FACTORS

- Effective and appropriate clinical care for mental, physical, and substance abuse disorders
- Easy access to a variety of clinical interventions and support for help seeking
- Restricted access to highly lethal methods of suicide
- Family and community support
- Support from ongoing medical and mental health care relationships
- Learned skills in problem solving, conflict resolution, and nonviolent handling of disputes
- Cultural and religious beliefs that discourage suicide and support self-preservation instincts

From U.S. Public Health Service. (1999). The Surgeon General's call to action to prevent suicide. Washington, DC: U.S. Government Printing Office.

TABLE 18-2 Assessing the Degree of Suicide Risk

BEHAVIOR	INTENSITY OF RISK		
	Low	Moderate	High
Anxiety	Mild	Moderate	High or panic
Depression	Mild	Moderate	Severe
Isolation; withdrawal	Some feelings of isolation; no withdrawal	Some feelings of helplessness, hopelessness, and withdrawal	Hopeless, helpless, withdrawn, and self-deprecating
Daily functioning	Fairly good in most activities	Moderately good in some activities	Not good in any activities
Resources	Several	Some	Few or none
Coping strategies being used	Generally constructive	Some that are constructive	Predominantly destructive
Significant others	Several who are available	Few or only one available	Only one or none available
Psychiatric help in past	None, or positive attitude toward	Yes, and moderately satisfied with results	Negative view of help received
Lifestyle	Stable	Moderately stable	Unstable
Alcohol or drug use	Infrequently to excess	Frequently to excess	Continual abuse

Continued

TABLE 18-2 Assessing the Degree of Suicide Risk—cont'd			
BEHAVIOR	**INTENSITY OF RISK**		
	Low	Moderate	High
Previous suicide attempts	None, or of low lethality	One or more of moderate lethality	Multiple attempts of high lethality
Disorientation; disorganization	None	Some	Marked
Hostility	Little or none	Some	Marked
Suicidal plan	Vague, fleeting thoughts but no plan	Frequent thoughts, occasional ideas about a plan	Frequent or constant thought with a specific plan

From Hatton, C. L., Valente, S. M., & Rink, A. (1984). Suicide: Assessment and intervention (2nd ed.). Norwalk, CT: Appleton & Lange, with permission.

■ **Religion.** Individuals who are not affiliated with any religious group are at higher risk than those who have this type of affiliation.

■ **Family History.** Higher risk if individual has family history of suicide.

Presenting Symptoms/Medical-Psychiatric Diagnosis

Assessment data must be gathered regarding any psychiatric or physical condition for which the client is being treated. Mood disorders (major depression and bipolar disorders) are the most common disorders that precede suicide. Individuals with substance use disorders are also at high risk. Other psychiatric disorders in which suicide may be a risk include anxiety disorders, schizophrenia, and borderline and antisocial personality disorders (Jacobs et al., 2006). Other chronic and terminal physical illnesses have also precipitated suicidal acts.

Suicidal Ideas or Acts

How serious is the intent? Does the person have a plan? If so, does he or she have the means? How lethal are the means? Has the individual ever attempted suicide before? These are all questions that must be answered by the person conducting the suicidal client assessment.

Individuals may leave both behavioral and verbal clues as to the intent of their act. Examples of behavioral clues include giving away prized possessions, getting financial affairs in order, writing suicide notes, or sudden lifts in mood (may indicate a decision to carry out the intent).

Verbal clues may be both direct and indirect. Examples of direct statements include "I want to die" or "I'm going to kill myself." Examples of indirect statements include "This is the last time you'll see me," "I won't be around much longer for the doctor to have to worry about," or "I don't have anything worth living for anymore."

Other assessments include determining whether the individual has a plan, and if so, whether he or she has the means to carry out that plan. If the person states the suicide will be carried out with a gun, does he or she have access to a gun? Bullets? If pills are planned, what kind of pills? Are they accessible?

Interpersonal Support System

Does the individual have support persons on whom he or she can rely during a crisis situation? Lack of a meaningful network of satisfactory relationships may implicate an individual as a high risk for suicide during an emotional crisis.

Analysis of the Suicidal Crisis

■ **The Precipitating Stressor:** Adverse life events in combination with other risk factors such as depression may lead to suicide. Life stresses accompanied by an increase in emotional disturbance include the loss of a loved person either by death or by divorce, problems in major relationships, changes in roles, or serious physical illness.

■ **Relevant History:** Has the individual experienced numerous failures or rejections that would increase his or her vulnerability for a dysfunctional response to the current situation?

■ **Life-Stage Issues:** The ability to tolerate losses and disappointments is often compromised if those losses and disappointments occur during various stages of life in which the individual struggles with developmental issues (e.g., adolescence, midlife).

Psychiatric/Medical/Family History

The individual should be assessed with regard to previous psychiatric treatment for depression or alcoholism, or for previous suicide attempts. Medical history should be obtained to determine presence of chronic, debilitating, or terminal illness. Is there a history of depressive disorder in the family, and has a close relative committed suicide in the past?

Coping Strategies

How has the individual handled previous crisis situations? How does this situation differ from previous ones?

Diagnosis/Outcome Identification

Nursing diagnoses for the suicidal client may include the following:

■ Risk for suicide related to feelings of hopelessness and desperation.

■ Hopelessness related to absence of support systems and perception of worthlessness.

Outcome Criteria

Outcome criteria include short- and long-term goals. Timelines are individually determined. The following criteria may be used for measurement of outcomes in the care of the suicidal client.

The client:

1. Has experienced no physical harm to self.

2. Sets realistic goals for self.

3. Expresses some optimism and hope for the future.

Planning/Implementation

Table 18-3 provides a plan of care for the hospitalized suicidal client. Nursing diagnoses are presented, along with outcome criteria, appropriate nursing interventions, and rationales for each.

Intervention With the Suicidal Client Following Discharge (or Outpatient Suicidal Client)

In some instances, it may be determined that suicidal intent is low and that hospitalization is not

---

Table 18-3 CARE PLAN FOR THE SUICIDAL CLIENT

NURSING DIAGNOSIS: RISK FOR SUICIDE
RELATED TO: Feelings of hopelessness and desperation

OUTCOME CRITERIA	NURSING INTERVENTIONS	RATIONALES
Client will not harm self.	1. Ask client directly: "Have you thought about harming yourself in any way? If so, what do you plan to do? Do you have the means to carry out this plan?"	1. The risk of suicide is greatly increased if the client has developed a plan and particularly if means exist for the client to execute the plan.
	2. Create a safe environment for the client. Remove all potentially harmful objects from client's access (sharp objects, straps, belts, ties, glass items, alcohol). Supervise closely during meals and medication administration. Perform room searches as deemed necessary.	2. Client safety is a nursing priority.
	3. Formulate a short-term verbal or written contract that the client will not harm self. When time is up, make another, and so forth. Secure a promise that the client will seek out staff when feeling suicidal.	3. A degree of the responsibility for his or her safety is given to the client. Increased feelings of self-worth may be experienced when client feels accepted unconditionally regardless of thoughts or behavior.
	4. Maintain close observation of client. Depending on level of suicide precaution, provide one-to-one contact, constant visual observation, or every-15-minute checks. Place in room close to nurse's station; do not assign to private room. Accompany to off-unit activities if attendance is indicated. May need to accompany to bathroom.	4. Close observation is necessary to ensure that client does not harm self in any way. Being alert for suicidal and escape attempts facilitates being able to prevent or interrupt harmful behavior.

Continued

Table 18-3 CARE PLAN FOR THE SUICIDAL CLIENT—cont'd

OUTCOME CRITERIA	NURSING INTERVENTIONS	RATIONALES
	5. Maintain special care in administration of medications.	5. Prevents saving up to overdose or discarding and not taking.
	6. Make rounds at frequent, *irregular* intervals (especially at night, toward early morning, at change of shift, or other predictably busy times for staff).	6. Prevents staff surveillance from becoming predictable. To be aware of client's location is important, especially when staff is busy and least available and observable.
	7. Encourage client to express honest feelings, including anger. Provide hostility release if needed.	7. Depression and suicidal behaviors may be viewed as anger turned inward on the self. If this anger can be verbalized in a non-threatening environment, the client may be able to eventually resolve these feelings.

NURSING DIAGNOSIS: HOPELESSNESS

RELATED TO: Absence of support systems and perception of worthlessness

EVIDENCED BY: Verbal cues (despondent content, "I can't"); decreased affect; lack of initiative; suicidal ideas or attempts

OUTCOME CRITERIA	NURSING INTERVENTIONS	RATIONALES
Client will verbalize a measure of hope and acceptance of life and situations over which he or she has no control.	1. Identify stressors in client's life that precipitated current crisis.	1. Important to identify causative or contributing factors in order to plan appropriate assistance.
	2. Determine coping behaviors previously used and client's perception of effectiveness then and now.	2. It is important to identify client's strengths and encourage their use in current crisis situation.
	3. Encourage client to explore and verbalize feelings and perceptions.	3. Identification of feelings underlying behaviors helps client to begin process of taking control of own life.
	4. 💬 Provide expressions of hope to client in positive, low-key manner (e.g., "I know you feel you cannot go on, but I believe that things can get better for you. What you are feeling is temporary. It is okay if you don't see it just now." "You are very important to the people who care about you.")	4. Even though the client feels hopeless, it is helpful to hear positive expressions from others. The client's current state of mind may prevent him or her from identifying anything positive in life. It is important to accept the client's feelings nonjudgmentally and to affirm the individual's personal worth and value.
	5. Help client identify areas of life situation that are under own control.	5. The client's emotional condition may interfere with ability to problem solve. Assistance may be required to perceive the benefits and consequences of available alternatives accurately.
	6. Identify sources that client may use after discharge when crises occur or feelings of hopelessness and possible suicidal ideation prevail.	6. Client should be made aware of local suicide hotlines or other local support services from which he or she may seek assistance following discharge from the hospital. A concrete plan provides hope in the face of a crisis situation.

required. Instead, the client with suicidal ideation may be treated in an outpatient setting. Guidelines for treatment of the suicidal client on an outpatient basis include the following:

■ The person should not be left alone. Arrangements must be made for the client to stay with family or friends. If this is not possible, hospitalization should be reconsidered.

■ Establish a no-suicide contract with the client. Formulate a written contract that the client will not harm himself or herself in a stated period of time. For example, the client writes, "I will not harm myself in any way between now and the time of our next counseling session," or "I will call the suicide hotline (or go to the emergency room) if I start to feel like harming myself." When the time period of this short-term contract has lapsed, a new contract is negotiated. (Some clinicians believe that suicide prevention contracting is not helpful [Knoll, 2011]. Obviously, the contract for safety comes with no guarantee, and it holds no legal credibility. It should never be used as a single intervention, but can be viewed as one among many that serve to ensure the client's safety.)

■ Enlist the help of family or friends to ensure that the home environment is safe from dangerous items, such as firearms or stockpiled drugs. Give support persons the telephone number of a counselor or an emergency contact person in the event that the counselor is not available.

■ Appointments may need to be scheduled daily or every other day at first until the immediate suicidal crisis has subsided.

■ Establish rapport and promote a trusting relationship. It is important for the suicide counselor to become a key person in the client's support system at this time.

■ Accept the client's feelings in a nonjudgmental manner.

> **CLINICAL PEARL** Be direct. Talk openly and matter-of-factly about suicide. Listen actively and encourage expression of feelings, including anger.

■ Discuss the current crisis situation in the client's life. Use the problem-solving approach (see Chapter 13). Offer alternatives to suicide. Macnab (1993) suggested the following statements:

 [It is my belief that] you are incorrect in your belief that suicide is the only and

the best solution to your problem. There are alternatives, and they are good. What is more, you will be alive to test them. (p. 265)

■ Help client identify areas of the life situation that are within his or her control and those that the client does not have the ability to control. Discuss feelings associated with these control issues. It is important for the client to feel some control over his or her life situation in order to perceive a measure of self-worth.

■ The physician may prescribe antidepressants for an individual who is experiencing suicidal depression. It is wise to prescribe no more than a 3-day supply of the medication with no refills. The prescription can then be renewed at the client's next counseling session.

NOTE: Sadock and Sadock (2007) stated:

As the depression lifts, patients become energized and are thus able to put their suicidal plans into action. Sometimes, depressed patients, with or without treatment, suddenly appear to be at peace with themselves because they have reached a secret decision to commit suicide. Clinicians should be especially suspicious of such a dramatic clinical change, which may portend a suicidal attempt. (p. 905)

■ Macnab (1993) suggested the following steps in crisis counseling with the suicidal client:
  • Focus on the current crisis and how it can be alleviated. Identify the client's appraisals of how things are, and how things will be. Note how these appraisals change in changing contexts.
  • Note the client's reactivity to the crisis and how this can be changed. Discuss strategies and procedures for the management of anxiety, anger, and frustration.
  • Work toward restoration of the client's self-worth, status, morale, and control. Introduce alternatives to suicide.
  • Rehearse cognitive reconstruction—more positive ways of thinking about the self, events, the past, the present, and the future.
  • Identify experiences and actions that affirm self-worth and self-efficacy.
  • Encourage movement toward the new reality, with the coping skills required to manage adaptively.
  • Be available for ongoing therapeutic support and growth.

Information for Family and Friends of the Suicidal Client

The following suggestions are made for family and friends of an individual who is suicidal:

■ Take any hint of suicide seriously. Anyone expressing suicidal feelings needs immediate attention.

■ Do not keep secrets. If a suicidal person says, "Promise you won't tell anyone," do not make that promise. Suicidal individuals are ambivalent about dying, and suicidal behavior is a cry for help. It is that ambivalence that leads the person to confide to you the suicidal thoughts. Get help for the person and for you. 1-800-SUICIDE is a national hotline that is available 24 hours a day.

■ Be a good listener. If people express suicidal thoughts or feel depressed, hopeless, or worthless, be supportive. Let them know you are there for them and are willing to help them seek professional help.

■ Many people find it awkward to put into words how another person's life is important for their own well-being, but it is important to stress that the person's life is important to you and to others. Emphasize in specific terms the ways in which the person's suicide would be devastating to you and to others.

■ Express concern for individuals who express thoughts about committing suicide. The individual may be withdrawn and reluctant to discuss what he or she is thinking. Acknowledge the person's pain and feelings of hopelessness, and encourage the individual to talk to someone else if he or she does not feel comfortable talking with you.

■ Familiarize yourself with suicide intervention sources, such as mental health centers and suicide hotlines.

■ Ensure that access to firearms or other means of self-harm is restricted.

■ The Mental Health Sanctuary (2010) offers the following tips:
  • Acknowledge and accept their feelings and be an active listener.
  • Try to give them hope and remind them that what they are feeling is temporary.
  • Stay with them. Do not leave them alone. Go to where they are, if necessary.
  • Show love and encouragement. Hold them, hug them, touch them. Allow them to cry and express anger.
  • Help them seek professional help.
  • Remove any items from the home with which the person may harm himself or herself.
  • If there are children present, try to remove them from the home. Perhaps another friend or relative can assist by taking them to their home. This type of situation can be extremely traumatic for children.
  • DO NOT: judge suicidal people, show anger toward them, provoke guilt in them, discount their feelings, or tell them to "snap out of it." This is a very real and serious situation to suicidal individuals. They are in real pain. They feel the situation is hopeless and that there is no other way to resolve it aside from taking their own life.

Intervention With Families and Friends of Suicide Victims

Cvinar (2005) stated:

> Suicide has a profound effect on the family, friends, and associates of the victim that transcends the immediate loss. As those close to the victim suffer through bereavement, a variety of reactions and coping mechanisms are engaged as each individual sorts through individual reactions to the difficult loss. Bereavement following suicide is complicated by the complex psychological impact of the act on those close to the victim. It is further complicated by the societal perception that the act of suicide is a failure by the victim and the family to deal with some emotional issue and ultimately society affixes blame for the loss on the survivors. This individual or societal stigma introduces a unique stress on the bereavement process that in some cases requires clinical intervention. (p. 14)

Suicide of a family member can induce a whole gamut of feelings in the survivors. Macnab (1993) identified the following symptoms, which may be evident following the suicide of a loved one.

■ A sense of guilt and responsibility.

■ Anger, resentment, and rage that can never find its "object."

■ A heightened sense of emotionality, helplessness, failure, and despair.

■ A recurring self-searching: "If only I had done something," "If only I had not done something," "If only . . . ."

■ A sense of confusion and search for an explanation: "Why did this happen?" "What does it mean?" "What could have stopped it?" "What will people think?"

■ A sense of inner injury. The family feels wounded. They do not know how they will ever get over it and get on with life.

■ A severe strain is placed on relationships. A sense of impatience, irritability, and anger exists between family members.

■ A heightened vulnerability to illness and disease exists with this added burden of emotional stress.

Strategies for assisting survivors of suicide victims include:

■ Encourage the clients to talk about the suicide, each responding to the others' viewpoints and reconstructing of events. Share memories.

■ Be aware of any blaming or scapegoating of specific family members. Discuss how each person fits into the family situation, both before and after the suicide.

■ Listen to feelings of guilt and self-persecution. Gently move the individuals toward the reality of the situation.

■ Encourage the family members to discuss individual relationships with the lost loved one. Focus on both positive and negative aspects of the relationships. Gradually, point out the irrationality of any idealized concepts of the deceased person. The family must be able to recognize both positive and negative aspects about the person before grief can be resolved.

■ No two people grieve in the same way. It may appear that some family members are "getting over" the grief faster than others. All family members must be made to understand that, if this occurs, it is not because they "care less," just that they "grieve differently." Variables that enter into this phenomenon include individual past experiences, personal relationship with the deceased person, and individual temperament and coping abilities.

■ Recognize how the suicide has caused disorganization in family coping. Reassess interpersonal relationships in the context of the event. Discuss coping strategies that have been successful in times of stress in the past, and work to reestablish these within the family. Identify new adaptive coping strategies that can be incorporated.

■ Identify resources that provide support: religious beliefs and spiritual counselors, close friends and relatives, support groups for survivors of suicide. One on-line connection that puts individuals in contact with survivors groups specific to each state is the American Foundation for Suicide Prevention at http://www.afsp.org. A list of resources that provide information and help for issues regarding suicide is presented in Box 18-2.

BOX 18-2 Sources for Information Related to Issues of Suicide

National Suicide Hotline
1-800-SUICIDE (24/7)

American Association of Suicidology
www.suicidology.org
1-202-237-2280

American Foundation for Suicide Prevention
www.afsp.org
1-888-333-AFSP

American Psychiatric Association
www.psych.org
1-703-907-7300

American Psychological Association
www.apa.org
1-800-374-2721

Boys Town
Cares for troubled boys and girls and families in crisis.
Staff is trained to handle calls related to violence and
  suicide.
www.boystown.org
1-800-448-3000 (24/7 National hotline)

National Suicide Prevention Lifeline
www.suicidepreventionlifeline.org
1-800-273-TALK (24/7)

Depression and Bipolar Support Alliance (DBSA)
http://www.dbsalliance.org/
1-800-826-3632

National Institute of Mental Health
www.nimh.nih.gov
1-866-615-6464

Mental Health America
www.nmha.org
1-703-684-7722
1-800-969-6642

Screening for Mental Health
Stop a Suicide Today!
www.stopasuicide.org
1-781-239-0071

Centre for Suicide Prevention
www.suicideinfo.ca
1-403-245-3900

Continued

BOX 18-2 Sources for Information Related to Issues of Suicide—cont'd

Centers for Disease Control and Prevention
National Center for Injury Prevention and Control
Division of Violence Prevention
www.cdc.gov/injury/index.html
1-800-CDC-INFO
The Center for Mental Health Services
http://www.mentalhealth.samhsa.gov/topics/explore/
   suicide/
1-800-789-2647

Suicide Prevention Advocacy Network
http://spanusa.org
1-202-449-3600
National Alliance on Mental Illness
www.nami.org
1-800-950-NAMI

Evaluation

Evaluation of the suicidal client is an ongoing process accomplished through continuous reassessment of the client, as well as determination of goal achievement. Once the immediate crisis has been resolved, extended psychotherapy may be indicated. The long-term goals of individual or group psychotherapy for the suicidal client would be for him or her to:

■ Develop and maintain a more positive self-concept.

■ Learn more effective ways to express feelings to others.

■ Achieve successful interpersonal relationships.

■ Feel accepted by others and achieve a sense of belonging.

A suicidal person feels worthless and hopeless. These goals serve to instill a sense of self-worth, while offering a measure of hope and a meaning for living.

Summary and Key Points

■ More than 90 percent of all persons who commit or attempt suicide have a diagnosed mental disorder.

■ Suicide is the third leading cause of death among young Americans ages 15 to 24 years, the fourth leading cause of death for ages 25 to 44, and the eighth leading cause of death for individuals ages 45 to 64.

■ Single people are at greater risk for suicide than married people.

■ Women attempt suicide more, but men succeed more often.

■ Suicide and age are positively correlated.

■ Depressed men and women who consider themselves affiliated with a religion are less likely to attempt suicide than their nonreligious counterparts.

■ Individuals in the very highest and lowest social classes have higher suicide rates than those in the middle classes.

■ Whites are at highest risk for suicide, followed by Native Americans, African Americans, Hispanic Americans, and Asian Americans.

■ Psychiatric disorders that predispose individuals to suicide include mood disorders, substance use disorders, schizophrenia, personality disorders, and anxiety disorders.

■ Predisposing factors include internalized anger, hopelessness, desperation and guilt, history of aggression and violence, shame and humiliation, developmental stressors, sociological influences, genetics, and neurochemical factors.

■ It is important for the nurse to determine the seriousness of the intent, the existence of a plan, and the availability and lethality of the method.

■ The suicidal person should not be left alone.

■ Once the crisis intervention is complete, the individual may require long-term psychotherapy, during which he or she works to:
  • Develop and maintain a more positive self-concept.
  • Learn more effective ways to express feelings.
  • Improve interpersonal relationships.
  • Achieve a sense of belonging and a measure of hope for living.

Additional info available @
davisplus.fadavis.com

Review Questions
Self-Examination/Learning Exercise

*Select the answer that is **most** appropriate for each of the following questions:*

1. Which of the following individuals is at highest risk for suicide?
   a. Nancy, age 33, Asian American, Catholic, middle socioeconomic group, alcoholic.
   b. John, age 72, white, Methodist, low socioeconomic group, diagnosis of metastatic cancer of the pancreas.
   c. Carol, age 15, African American, Baptist, high socioeconomic group, no physical or mental health problems.
   d. Mike, age 55, Jewish, middle socioeconomic group, suffered myocardial infarction a year ago.

2. Some biological factors may be associated with the predisposition to suicide. Which of the following biological factors have been implicated?
   a. Genetics and decreased levels of serotonin.
   b. Heredity and increased levels of norepinephrine.
   c. Temporal lobe atrophy and decreased levels of acetylcholine.
   d. Structural alterations of the brain and increased levels of dopamine.

3. Theresa, age 27, was admitted to the psychiatric unit from the medical intensive care unit, where she was treated for taking a deliberate overdose of her antidepressant medication, trazodone (Desyrel). She says to the nurse, "My boyfriend broke up with me. We had been together for 6 years. I love him so much. I know I'll never get over him." Which is the best response by the nurse?
   a. "You'll get over him in time, Theresa."
   b. "Forget him. There are other fish in the sea."
   c. "You must be feeling very sad about your loss."
   d. "Why do you think he broke up with you, Theresa?"

4. The nurse identifies the primary nursing diagnosis for Theresa as Risk for Suicide related to feelings of hopelessness from loss of relationship. Which is the outcome criterion that would most accurately measure achievement of this diagnosis?
   a. The client has experienced no physical harm to herself.
   b. The client sets realistic goals for herself.
   c. The client expresses some optimism and hope for the future.
   d. The client has reached a stage of acceptance in the loss of the relationship with her boyfriend.

5. Theresa is hospitalized following a suicide attempt after breaking up with her boyfriend. Freudian psychoanalytic theory would explain Theresa's suicide attempt in which of the following ways?
   a. She feels hopeless about her future without her boyfriend.
   b. Without her boyfriend, she feels like an outsider with her peers.
   c. She is feeling intense guilt because her boyfriend broke up with her.
   d. She is angry at her boyfriend for breaking up with her and has turned the anger inward on herself.

6. Theresa is hospitalized following a suicide attempt after breaking up with her boyfriend. Theresa says to the nurse, "When I get out of here, I'm going to try this again, and next time I'll choose a no-fail method." Which is the best response by the nurse?
   a. "You are safe here. We will make sure nothing happens to you."
   b. "You're just lucky your roommate came home when she did."
   c. "What exactly do you plan to do?"
   d. "I don't understand. You have so much to live for."

Continued

Review Questions—cont'd
Self-Examination/Learning Exercise

7. In determining degree of suicide risk with a suicidal client, the nurse assesses the following behavioral manifestations: severely depressed, withdrawn, statements of worthlessness, difficulty accomplishing activities of daily living, no close support systems. The nurse identifies the client's risk for suicide as:
   a. Low.
   b. Moderate.
   c. High.
   d. Unable to determine.

8. Theresa, who has been hospitalized following a suicide attempt, is placed on suicide precautions on the psychiatric unit. She admits that she is still feeling suicidal. Which of the following interventions is most appropriate in this instance?
   a. Obtain an order from the physician to place Theresa in restraints to prevent any attempts to harm herself.
   b. Check on Theresa every 15 minutes or assign a staff person to stay with her on a one-to-one basis.
   c. Obtain an order from the physician to give Theresa a sedative to calm her and reduce suicide ideas.
   d. Do not allow Theresa to participate in any unit activities while she is on suicide precautions.

9. Which of the following interventions are appropriate for a client on suicide precautions? (Select all that apply.)
   a. Remove all sharp objects, belts, and other potentially dangerous articles from the client's environment.
   b. Accompany the client to off-unit activities.
   c. Obtain a promise from the client that she will not do anything to harm herself for the next 12 hours.
   d. Put all of the client's possessions in storage and explain to her that she may have them back when she is off suicide precautions.

10. Success of long-term psychotherapy with Theresa (who attempted suicide following a break-up with her boyfriend) could be measured by which of the following behaviors?
    a. Theresa has a new boyfriend.
    b. Theresa has an increased sense of self-worth.
    c. Theresa does not take antidepressants anymore.
    d. Theresa told her old boyfriend how angry she was with him for breaking up with her.

References

Abbar, M., Courtet, P., Bellivier, F., Leboyer, M., Boulenger, J. P., Castelhau, D., et al. (2001). Suicide attempters and the tryptophan hydroxylase gene. *Molecular Psychiatry, 6,* 268–273.

American Association of Suicidology. (2009). *Elderly suicide fact sheet.* Retrieved August 9, 2010, from http://www.suicidology.org/

Beck, A. T., Brown, G., & Berchick, R. J. (1990). Relationship between hopelessness and ultimate suicide: A replication with psychiatric outpatients. *American Journal of Psychiatry, 147,* 190–195.

Carroll-Ghosh, T., Victor, B. S., & Bourgeois, J. A. (2003). Suicide. In R. E. Hales & S. C. Yudofsky (Eds.), *Textbook of clinical psychiatry* (4th ed., pp. 1457–1483). Washington, DC: American Psychiatric Publishing.

Centers for Disease Control and Prevention. (2007). *Morbidity and Mortality Weekly Report, 56*(35), 905–908.

Centers for Disease Control and Prevention. (2010). *Understanding suicide.* Retrieved August 9, 2010, from www.cdc.gov/violenceprevention

Cochran, S. D., & Mays, V. M. (2000). Lifetime prevalence of suicide symptoms and affective disorders among men reporting same-sex partners: Results from

NHANES III. *American Journal of Public Health, 90*(4), 573–578.

Cvinar, J. G. (2005). Do suicide survivors suffer social stigma: A review of the literature. *Perspectives in Psychiatric Care, 41*(1), 14–21.

Eisenberg, M. E., & Resnick, M. D. (2006). Suicidality among gay, lesbian and bisexual youth: The role of protective factors. *Journal of Adolescent Health, 39*(5), 662–668.

Friends for Survival, Inc. (2010). *Facts and fables.* Retrieved August 9, 2010, from http://www.friendsforsurvival.org/facts-and-fables

Hatton, C. L., Valente, S. M., & Rink, A. (1984). *Suicide: Assessment and intervention* (2nd ed.). Norwalk, CT: Appleton & Lange.

Hendin, H. (1991). Psychodynamics of suicide, with particular reference to the young. *American Journal of Psychiatry, 148,* 1150–1158.

Jacobs, D. G., Baldessarini, R. J., Conwell, Y., Fawcett, J. A., Horton, L., Meltzer, H., et al. (2006). Practice guideline for the assessment and treatment of patients with suicidal behaviors. *American Psychiatric Association practice guidelines for the treatment of psychiatric disorders, Compendium 2006.* Arlington, VA: American Psychiatric Association.

King, M., Semlyen, J., Tai, S. S., Killaspy, H., Osborn, D., Popelyuk, D., et al. (2008). A systematic review of mental disorder, suicide, and deliberate self harm in lesbian, gay, and bisexual people. *BMC Psychiatry, 8*(70). Available from http://www.biomedcentral.com/1471-244X/8/70

Knoll, J. (2011). The suicide prevention contract: Contracting for comfort. *Psychiatric Times.* Retrieved July 30, 2011 from http://www.psychiatrictimes.com/blog/couchincrisis/content/article/10168/1811702

MacDonald, M., & Murphy, T. R. (1991). *Sleepless souls: Suicide in early modern England.* New York: Oxford University Press.

Macnab, F. (1993). *Brief psychotherapy: An integrative approach in clinical practice.* West Sussex, England: John Wiley & Sons.

Medscape Psychiatry (2011). *Striking risk for suicidality, depression in gay teens.* Retrieved July 30, 2011 from http://www.medscape.com/viewarticle/740429

Mental Health Sanctuary. (2010). *How to help a suicidal person.* Retrieved August 10, 2010, from http://www.mhsanctuary.com/suicide/sui2.htm

Minois, G. (2001). *History of suicide: Voluntary death in Western culture.* Baltimore: Johns Hopkins University Press.

National Alliance on Mental Illness. (2010). *Suicide: Learn more, learn to help.* Retrieved August 9, 2010, from http://www.nami.org

National Center for Health Statistics. (2009). *Health, United States, 2009.* Library of Congress Catalog Number 76-641496. Washington, DC: U.S. Government Printing Office.

National Institute of Mental Health. (2010). *The numbers count: Mental disorders in America.* Retrieved August 9, 2010, from http://www.nimh.nih.gov/health/publications/the-numbers-count-mental-disorders-in-america/index.shtml

Rasic, D. T., Belik, S. L., Elias, B., Katz, L. Y., Enns, M., & Sareen, J. (2009). Spirituality, religion, and suicidal behavior in a nationally representative sample. *Journal of Affective Disorders, 114*(1), 32–40.

Rich, C. L., Warsradt, G. M., & Nemiroff, R. A. (1991). Suicide, stressors, and the life cycle. *American Journal of Psychiatry, 148,* 524–527.

Sadock, B. J., & Sadock, V. A. (2007). *Synopsis of psychiatry: Behavioral sciences/clinical psychiatry* (10th ed.). Philadelphia: Lippincott Williams & Wilkins.

Suicide Prevention Resource Center. (2008). *Suicide risk and prevention for lesbian, gay, bisexual, and transgender youth.* Newton, MA: Education Development Center.

The Samaritans. (2010). *Suicide myths and misconceptions.* Retrieved August 9, 2010, from http://www.samaritansnyc.org/myths.html

Tondo, L., & Baldessarini, R. J. (2001). *Suicide: Historical, descriptive, and epidemiological considerations.* Retrieved August 9, 2010, from http://www.medscape.com/viewarticle/413194

U.S. Public Health Service. (1999). *The Surgeon General's call to action to prevent suicide.* Washington, DC: U.S. Government Printing Office.

Classical References

Durkheim, E. (1951). *Suicide: A study of sociology.* Glencoe, IL: Free Press.

Freud, S. (1957). *Mourning and melancholia,* Vol. 14 (standard ed.) London: Hogarth Press. (Original work published 1917)

Behavior Therapy

19

CORE CONCEPTS
behavior therapy
stimulus

KEY TERMS

aversive stimulus
classical conditioning
conditioned response
conditioned stimulus
contingency contracting
covert sensitization
discriminative stimulus
extinction

flooding
modeling
negative reinforcement
operant conditioning
overt sensitization
positive reinforcement
Premack principle
reciprocal inhibition

shaping
stimulus generalization
systematic desensitization
time out
token economy
unconditioned response
unconditioned stimulus

OBJECTIVES
After reading this chapter, the student will be able to:

1. Discuss the principles of classical and operant conditioning as foundations for behavior therapy.
2. Identify various techniques used in the modification of client behavior.

3. Implement the principles of behavior therapy using the steps of the nursing process.

HOMEWORK ASSIGNMENT
Please read the chapter and answer the following questions:

1. A mother is teaching her young child how to dress himself. Each time he makes an attempt, she praises him profusely, even though he has made several mistakes. She does this until he is able to dress himself appropriately. What is this technique called?
2. Flooding (implosion therapy) is used to desensitize individuals to phobic stimuli. When is this technique contraindicated?

3. A nurse is working with parents of a toddler who they say falls to the ground, screams, and kicks his legs whenever he doesn't get his way. They usually just give in to his wishes to keep him from behaving this way. The nurse decides to teach the parents about the technique of extinction. What would this entail?

A behavior is considered to be maladaptive when it is age inappropriate, when it interferes with adaptive functioning, or when others misunderstand it in terms of cultural inappropriateness. The behavioral approach to therapy is that people have become what they are through learning processes or, more correctly, through the interaction of the environment with their genetic endowment. The basic assumption is that problematic behaviors occur when there has been inadequate learning and therefore can be corrected through the provision of appropriate learning experiences. The principles of behavior therapy as we know it today are based on the early studies of **classical conditioning** by Pavlov (1927) and **operant conditioning** by Skinner (1938). Although in this text the concepts are presented separately for reasons of clarification, behavioral change procedures are often combined with cognitive procedures, and many behavior therapies are referred to as *cognitive-behavioral* therapies. Concepts of cognitive therapy are presented in Chapter 20.

Classical Conditioning

Classical conditioning is a process of learning that was introduced by the Russian physiologist Pavlov. In his experiments with dogs, during which he hoped to learn more about the digestive process, he inadvertently discovered that organisms can learn to respond in specific ways if they are conditioned to do so.

In his trials he found that, as expected, the dogs salivated when they began to eat the food that was offered to them. This was a reflexive response that Pavlov called an **unconditioned response.** However, he also noticed that with time, the dogs began to salivate when the food came into their range of view, before it was even presented to them for consumption. Pavlov, concluding that this response was not reflexive but had been learned, called it a **conditioned response.** He carried the experiments even further by introducing an unrelated stimulus, one that had had no previous connection to the animal's food. He simultaneously presented the food with the sound of a bell. The animal responded with the expected reflexive salivation to the food. After a number of trials with the combined stimuli (food and bell), Pavlov found that the reflexive salivation began to occur when the dog was presented with the sound of the bell in the absence of food.

CORE CONCEPT

Stimulus
A stimulus is an environmental event that interacts with and influences an individual's behavior.

This was an important discovery in terms of how learning can occur. Pavlov found that unconditioned responses (salivation) occur in response

to unconditioned stimuli (eating food). He also found that, over time, an unrelated stimulus (sound of the bell) introduced with the **unconditioned stimulus** can elicit the same response alone—that is, the conditioned response. The unrelated stimulus is called the **conditioned stimulus.** A graphic of Pavlov's classical conditioning model is presented in Figure 19–1. An example of the application of Pavlov's classical conditioning model to humans is shown in Figure 19–2. The process by which the fear response is elicited from similar stimuli (all individuals in white uniforms) is called **stimulus generalization.**

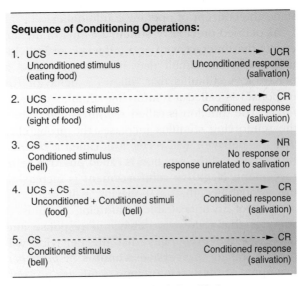

FIGURE 19–1   Pavlov's model of classical conditioning.

FIGURE 19–2   Example: Classical conditioning and stimulus generalization.

Operant Conditioning

The focus of operant conditioning differs from that of classical conditioning. With classical conditioning, the focus is on behavioral responses that are elicited by specific objects or events. With operant conditioning, additional attention is given to the consequences of the behavioral response.

Operant conditioning was introduced by Skinner (1953), an American psychologist whose work was largely influenced by Thorndike's (1911) law of effect—that is, that the connection between a stimulus and a response is strengthened or weakened by the consequences of the response. A number of terms must be defined in order to understand the concept of operant conditioning.

As defined previously, stimuli are environmental events that interact with and influence an individual's behavior. Stimuli may precede or follow a behavior. A stimulus that follows a behavior (or response) is called a reinforcing stimulus or *reinforcer.* The function is called *reinforcement.* When the reinforcing stimulus increases the probability that the behavior will recur, it is called a *positive reinforcer,* and the function is called **positive reinforcement. Negative reinforcement** is increasing the probability that a behavior will recur by removal of an undesirable reinforcing stimulus. A stimulus that follows a behavioral response and decreases the probability that the behavior will recur is called an **aversive stimulus** or *punisher.* Examples of these reinforcing stimuli are presented in Table 19-1.

Stimuli that precede a behavioral response and predict that a particular reinforcement will occur are called **discriminative stimuli.** Discriminative stimuli are under the control of the individual. The individual is said to be able to *discriminate* between stimuli and to *choose* according to the type of reinforcement he or she has come to associate with a specific stimulus. The following is an example of the concept of discrimination:

EXAMPLE

Mrs. M. was admitted to the hospital from a nursing home 2 weeks ago. She has no family, and no one visits her. She is very lonely. Nurse A and Nurse B have taken care of Mrs. M. on a regular basis during her hospital stay. When she is feeling particularly lonely, Mrs. M. calls Nurse A to her room, for she has learned that Nurse A will stay and talk to her for a while, but Nurse B only takes care of her physical needs and leaves. She no longer seeks out Nurse B for emotional support and comfort.

After several attempts, Mrs. M. is able to discriminate between stimuli. She can predict with assurance that calling Nurse A (and not Nurse B) will result in the reinforcement she desires.

CORE CONCEPT

Behavior Therapy

A form of psychotherapy, the goal of which is to modify maladaptive behavior patterns by reinforcing more adaptive behaviors.

Techniques for Modifying Client Behavior

Shaping

In **shaping** the behavior of another, reinforcements are given for increasingly closer approximations to the desired response. For example, in eliciting speech from an autistic child, the teacher may first reward the child for (a) watching the teacher's lips, then for (b) making any sound in imitation of the teacher, then for (c) forming sounds similar to the word uttered by the teacher. Shaping has been shown to be an effective way of modifying behavior for tasks that a child has not mastered on command or that are not in the child's repertoire (Souders, DePaul, Freeman, & Levy, 2002).

TABLE 19-1 Examples of Reinforcing Stimuli

TYPE	STIMULUS	BEHAVIORAL RESPONSE	REINFORCING STIMULUS
Positive	Messy room	Child cleans her messy room	Child gets allowance for cleaning room.
Negative	Messy room	Child cleans her messy room	Child does not receive scolding from the mother.
Aversive	Messy room	Child does not clean her messy room	Child receives scolding from the mother.

Modeling

Modeling refers to the learning of new behaviors by imitating the behavior in others. Role models are individuals who have qualities or skills that a person admires and wishes to imitate (Howard, 2000). Modeling occurs in various ways. Children imitate the behavior patterns of their parents, teachers, friends, and others. Adults and children alike model many of their behaviors after individuals observed on television and in movies. Unfortunately, modeling can result in maladaptive behaviors, as well as adaptive ones.

In the practice setting, clients may imitate the behaviors of practitioners who are charged with their care. This can occur naturally in the therapeutic community environment. It can also occur in a therapy session in which the client watches a model demonstrate appropriate behaviors in a role-play of the client's problem. The client is then instructed to imitate the model's behaviors in a similar role-play and is positively reinforced for appropriate imitation.

Premack Principle

This technique, named for its originator, states that a frequently occurring response (R_1) can serve as a positive reinforcement for a response (R_2) that occurs less frequently (Premack, 1959). This is accomplished by allowing R_1 to occur only after R_2 has been performed. For example, 13-year-old Jennie has been neglecting her homework for the past few weeks. She spends a lot of time on the telephone talking to her friends. Applying the **Premack principle,** being allowed to talk on the telephone to her friends could serve as a positive reinforcement for completing her homework. A schematic of the Premack principle for this situation is presented in Figure 19–3.

Extinction

Extinction is the gradual decrease in frequency or disappearance of a response when the positive reinforcement is withheld. A classic example of this technique is its use with children who have temper tantrums. The tantrum behaviors continue as long as the parent gives attention to them but decrease and often disappear when the parent simply leaves the child alone in the room.

Contingency Contracting

In **contingency contracting,** a contract is drawn up among all parties involved. The behavior change that is desired is stated explicitly in writing. The contract specifies the behavior change desired and the reinforcers to be given for performing the desired behaviors. The negative consequences or punishers that will be rendered for not fulfilling the terms of the contract are also delineated. The contract is specific about how reinforcers and punishment will be presented; however, flexibility is important so that renegotiations can occur if necessary.

Token Economy

Token economy is a type of contingency contracting (although there may or may not be a written and signed contract involved) in which the reinforcers for desired behaviors are presented in the form of *tokens*. Essential to this type of technique is the prior determination of items and situations of significance to the client that can be employed as reinforcements. With this therapy, tokens are awarded when desired behaviors are performed and may be exchanged for designated privileges. For example, a client may be able to "buy" a snack or cigarettes for 2 tokens, a trip to the coffee shop or library for 5 tokens, or even a trip outside the hospital (if that is a realistic possibility) for another designated number of tokens. The tokens themselves provide immediate positive feedback, and clients should be allowed to make the decision of whether to spend the token as soon as it is presented or to accumulate tokens that may be exchanged later for a more desirable reward.

Time Out

Time out is an aversive stimulus or punishment during which the client is removed from the environment where the unacceptable behavior is being exhibited. The client is usually isolated so that reinforcement from the attention of others is absent.

Reciprocal Inhibition

Also called counterconditioning, **reciprocal inhibition** decreases or eliminates a behavior by introducing a more adaptive behavior, but one

Discriminative stimulus (Homework assignment: to do or not to do) - - - - - → R_2 (Completion of homework assignment) - - - - - → R_1 (Talk to friends on telephone)

FIGURE 19–3   Example: Premack principle.

that is incompatible with the unacceptable behavior (Wolpe, 1958). An example is the introduction of relaxation exercises to an individual who is phobic. Relaxation is practiced in the presence of anxiety so that in time the individual is able to manage the anxiety in the presence of the phobic stimulus by engaging in relaxation exercises. Relaxation and anxiety are incompatible behaviors.

Overt Sensitization

Overt sensitization is a type of aversion therapy that produces unpleasant consequences for undesirable behavior. For example, disulfiram (Antabuse) is a drug that is given to individuals who wish to stop drinking alcohol. If an individual consumes alcohol while on Antabuse therapy, symptoms of severe nausea and vomiting, dyspnea, palpitations, and headache will occur. Instead of the euphoric feeling normally experienced from the alcohol (the positive reinforcement for drinking), the individual receives a severe punishment that is intended to extinguish the unacceptable behavior (drinking alcohol).

Covert Sensitization

Covert sensitization relies on the individual's imagination, rather than on medication, to produce unpleasant symptoms. The technique is under the client's control and can be used whenever and wherever it is required. The individual learns, through mental imagery, to visualize nauseating scenes and even to induce a mild feeling of nausea. This mental image is visualized when the individual is about to succumb to an attractive but undesirable behavior. It is most effective when paired with relaxation exercises that are performed instead of the undesirable behavior. The primary advantage of covert sensitization is that the individual does not have to perform the undesired behaviors but simply imagines them.

Systematic Desensitization

Systematic desensitization is a technique for assisting individuals to overcome their fear of a phobic stimulus. It is "systematic" in that there is a hierarchy of anxiety-producing events through which the individual progresses during therapy. An example of a hierarchy of events associated with a fear of elevators may be as follows:

1. Discuss riding an elevator with the therapist.
2. Look at a picture of an elevator.
3. Walk into the lobby of a building and see the elevators.
4. Push the button for the elevator.
5. Walk into an elevator with a trusted person; disembark before the doors close.
6. Walk into an elevator with a trusted person; allow doors to close; then open the doors and walk out.
7. Ride one floor with a trusted person, then walk back down the stairs.
8. Ride one floor with a trusted person and ride the elevator back down.
9. Ride the elevator alone.

As each of these steps is attempted, it is paired with relaxation exercises as an antagonistic behavior to anxiety. Generally, the desensitization procedures occur in the therapy setting by instructing the client to engage in relaxation exercises. When relaxation has been achieved, the client uses mental imagery to visualize the step in the hierarchy being described by the therapist. If the client becomes anxious, the therapist suggests relaxation exercises again, and presents a scene that is lower in the hierarchy. Therapy continues until the individual is able to progress through the entire hierarchy with manageable anxiety. The effects of relaxation in the presence of imagined anxiety-producing stimuli transfer to the real situation, once the client has achieved relaxation capable of suppressing or inhibiting anxiety responses (Ford-Martin, 2001). However, some clients are not successful in extinguishing phobic reactions through imagery. For these clients, *real-life desensitization* may be required. In these instances, the therapist may arrange for the client to be exposed to the hierarchy of steps in the desensitization process, but in real-life situations. Relaxation exercises may or may not be a part of real-life desensitization.

Flooding

This technique, sometimes called *implosion therapy,* is also used to desensitize individuals to phobic stimuli. It differs from systematic desensitization in that, instead of working up a hierarchy of anxiety-producing stimuli, the individual is "flooded" with a continuous presentation (through mental imagery) of the phobic stimulus until it no longer elicits anxiety. **Flooding** is believed to produce results faster than systematic desensitization; however, some therapists report more lasting behavioral changes with systematic desensitization.

Some questions have also been raised in terms of the psychological discomfort that this therapy produces for the client. Flooding is contraindicated with clients for whom intense anxiety would be hazardous (e.g., individuals with heart disease or fragile psychological adaptation) (Sadock & Sadock, 2007).

Role of the Nurse in Behavior Therapy

The nursing process is the vehicle for delivery of nursing care with the client requiring assistance with behavior modification. The steps of the nursing process are illustrated in the following example case study.

CASE STUDY

(This example focuses on inpatient care, but these interventions can be modified and are applicable to various health-care settings, including partial hospitalization, community outpatient clinic, home health, and private practice.)

ASSESSMENT

Sammy, age 8, has been admitted to the child psychiatric unit of a university medical center following evaluation by a child psychiatrist. His parents, Tom and Nancy, are at an impasse, and their marriage is suffering because of constant conflict over their son's behavior at home and at school. Tom complains bitterly that Nancy is overly permissive with their son. Tom reports that Sammy argues and has temper tantrums and insists on continuing games, books, and TV, whenever Nancy puts him to bed, so that an 8:30 p.m. bedtime regularly is delayed until 10:30 or later every night. Also, Nancy often cooks four or five different meals for her son's dinner if Sammy stubbornly insists that he will not eat what has been prepared. At school, several teachers have complained that the child is stubborn and argumentative, is often disruptive in the classroom, and refuses to follow established rules.

When asked by the psychiatric nurse about other maladaptive behaviors, such as destruction of property, stealing, lying, or setting fires, the parents denied that these had been a problem. During the interview, Sammy sat quietly without interrupting. He answered questions that were directed to him with brief responses and made light of the problems described by his parents and reported by his teachers.

During his first 3 days on the unit, the following assessments were made:

1. Sammy loses his temper when he cannot have his way. He screams, stomps his feet, and sometimes kicks the furniture.
2. Sammy refuses to follow directions given by staff. He merely responds, "No, I won't."
3. Sammy likes to engage in behaviors that annoy the staff and other children: belching loudly, scraping his fingernails across the blackboard, making loud noises when the other children are trying to watch television, opening his mouth when it is full of food.
4. Sammy blames others when he makes a mistake. He spilled his milk at lunchtime while racing to get to a specific seat he knew Tony wanted. He blamed the accident on Tony, saying, "He made me do it! He tripped me!"

Upon completion of the initial assessments, the psychiatrist diagnosed Sammy with oppositional defiant disorder.

DIAGNOSIS/OUTCOME IDENTIFICATION

Nursing diagnoses and outcome criteria for Sammy include:

Nursing Diagnoses	Outcome Criteria
Noncompliance with therapy	Sammy participates in and cooperates during therapeutic activities.
Defensive coping	Sammy accepts responsibility for own behaviors and interacts with others without becoming defensive.
Impaired social interaction	Sammy interacts with staff and peers using age-appropriate, acceptable behaviors.

PLANNING/IMPLEMENTATION

A contract for Sammy's care was drawn up by the admitting nurse and others on the treatment team. Sammy's contract was based on a system of token economies. He discussed with the nurse the kinds of privileges he would like to earn. They included:

■ Getting to wear his own clothes (5 tokens)
■ Having a can of pop for a snack (2 tokens)
■ Getting to watch 30 minutes of TV (5 tokens)
■ Getting to stay up later on Friday nights with the other clients (7 tokens)
■ Getting to play the video games (3 tokens)

Continued

CASE STUDY—cont'd

- Getting to walk with the nurse to the gift shop to spend some of his money (8 tokens)
- Getting to talk to his parents/grandparents on the phone (5 tokens)
- Getting to go on the outside therapeutic recreation activities such as movies, the zoo, and picnics (10 tokens)

    Tokens were awarded for appropriate behaviors:

- Gets out of bed when the nurse calls him (1 token)
- Gets dressed for breakfast (1 token)
- Presents himself for *all* meals in an appropriate manner, that is, no screaming, no belching, no opening his mouth when it is full of food, no throwing of food, staying in his chair during the meal, putting his tray away in the appropriate place when he is finished (2 tokens × 3 meals = 6 tokens)
- Completes hygiene activities (1 token)
- Accepts blame for own mistakes (1 token)
- Does not fight; uses no obscene language; does not "sass" staff (1 token)
- Remains quiet while others are watching TV (1 token)
- Participates and is not disruptive in unit meetings and group therapy sessions (2 tokens)
- Displays no temper tantrums (1 token)
- Follows unit rules (1 token)
- Goes to bed at designated hour without opposition (1 token)

    Tokens are awarded at bedtime for absence of inappropriate behaviors during the day. For example, if Sammy has no temper tantrums during the day, he is awarded 1 token. Likewise, if Sammy has a temper tantrum (or exhibits other inappropriate behavior), he must pay back the token amount designated for that behavior. No other attention is given to inappropriate behaviors other than withholding and payback of tokens.

    EXCEPTION: If Sammy is receiving reinforcement from peers for inappropriate behaviors, staff has the option of imposing time out or isolation until the behavior is extinguished.

The contract may be renegotiated at any time between Sammy and staff. Additional privileges or responsibilities may be added as they develop and are deemed appropriate.

All staff members are consistent with the terms of the contract and do not allow Sammy to manipulate. There are no exceptions without renegotiation of the contract.

NOTE: Parents meet regularly with the case manager from the treatment team. Effective parenting techniques are discussed, as are other problems identified within the marriage relationship. Parenting instruction coordinates with the pattern of behavior modification Sammy is receiving on the psychiatric unit. The importance of follow-through is emphasized, along with strong encouragement that the parents maintain a united front in disciplining Sammy. Oppositional behaviors are nurtured by divided management.

EVALUATION

Reassessment is conducted to determine if the nursing actions have been successful in achieving the objectives of Sammy's care. Evaluation can be facilitated by gathering information using the following questions:

- Does Sammy participate in and cooperate during therapeutic activities?
- Does he follow the rules of the unit (including mealtimes, hygiene, and bedtime) without opposition?
- Does Sammy accept responsibility for his own mistakes?
- Is he able to complete a task without becoming defensive?
- Does he refrain from interrupting when others are talking or making noise in situations where quiet is in order?
- Does he attempt to manipulate the staff?
- Is he able to express anger appropriately without tantrum behaviors?
- Does he demonstrate acceptable behavior in interactions with peers?

Summary and Key Points

- The basic assumption of behavior therapy is that problematic behaviors occur when there has been inadequate learning and, therefore, can be corrected through the provision of appropriate learning experiences.

- The antecedents of today's principles of behavior therapy are largely the products of laboratory efforts by Pavlov and Skinner.
- Pavlov introduced a process that came to be known as classical conditioning.
- Pavlov demonstrated in his trials with laboratory animals that a neutral stimulus could acquire

the ability to elicit a conditioned response through pairing with an unconditioned stimulus. He considered the conditioned response to be a new, learned response.

■ Skinner, in his model of operant conditioning, gave additional attention to the consequences of the response as an approach to learning new behaviors.

■ Skinner believed that the connection between a stimulus and a response is strengthened or weakened by the consequences of the response.

■ Various techniques for modifying client behavior include the following:
  • Shaping: a technique in which reinforcements are given for increasingly closer approximations to the desired response.
  • Modeling: refers to the learning of new behaviors by imitating the behavior of others.
  • Premack principle: this technique states that a frequently occurring response can serve as a positive reinforcement for a response that occurs less frequently.
  • Extinction: the gradual decrease in frequency or disappearance of a response when the positive reinforcement is withheld.
  • Contingency contracting: a contract is drawn up specifying a specific behavior change and the reinforcers to be given for performing the desired behaviors.
  • Token economy: a type of contingency contracting in which the reinforcers for desired behaviors are presented in the form of tokens.

  • Time out: an aversive stimulus or punishment during which the client is removed from the environment where the unacceptable behavior is being exhibited.
  • Reciprocal inhibition: a technique that decreases or eliminates a behavior by introducing a more adaptive behavior, but one that is incompatible with the unacceptable behavior.
  • Overt sensitization: a type of aversion therapy that produces unpleasant consequences for undesirable behavior.
  • Covert sensitization: relies on an individual's imagination to produce unpleasant consequences for undesirable behaviors.
  • Systematic desensitization: a technique for overcoming phobias in which there is a hierarchy of anxiety-producing events through which the individual progresses.
  • Flooding (also called implosion therapy): desensitizes individuals to phobic stimuli by "flooding" them with a continuous presentation (through mental imagery) of the phobic stimulus until it no longer elicits anxiety.

■ Nurses can implement behavior therapy techniques to help clients modify maladaptive behavior patterns.

■ The nursing process is a systematic method of directing care for clients who require this type of assistance.

 Additional info available @ davisplus.fadavis.com

Review Questions
Self-Examination/Learning Exercise

*Select the answer that is **most** appropriate for each of the following questions:*

1. A positive reinforcer:
   a. Increases the probability that a behavior will recur.
   b. Decreases the probability that a behavior will recur.
   c. Has nothing to do with modifying behavior.
   d. Always results in positive behavior.

2. A negative reinforcer:
   a. Increases the probability that a behavior will recur.
   b. Decreases the probability that a behavior will recur.
   c. Has nothing to do with modifying behavior.
   d. Always results in unacceptable behavior.

Continued

Review Questions—cont'd
Self-Examination/Learning Exercise

3. An aversive stimulus or punisher:
   a. Increases the probability that a behavior will recur.
   b. Decreases the probability that a behavior will recur.
   c. Has nothing to do with modifying behavior.
   d. Always results in unacceptable behavior.

Situation: B.J. has been out with his friends. He is late getting home. He knows his wife will be angry and will yell at him for being late. He stops at the florist's shop and buys a dozen red roses for her. Questions 4, 5, and 6 are related to this situation.

4. Which of the following behaviors represents positive reinforcement on the part of the wife?
   a. She meets him at the door, accepts the roses, and says nothing further about his being late.
   b. She meets him at the door, yelling that he is late, and makes him spend the night on the couch.
   c. She meets him at the door, expresses delight with the roses, and kisses him on the cheek.
   d. She meets him at the door and says, "How could you? You know I'm allergic to roses!"

5. Which of the following behaviors represents negative reinforcement on the part of the wife?
   a. She meets him at the door, accepts the roses, and says nothing further about his being late.
   b. She meets him at the door, yelling that he is late, and makes him spend the night on the couch.
   c. She meets him at the door, expresses delight with the roses, and kisses him on the cheek.
   d. She meets him at the door and says, "How could you? You know I'm allergic to roses!"

6. Which of the following behaviors represents an aversive stimulus on the part of the wife?
   a. She meets him at the door, accepts the roses, and says nothing further about his being late.
   b. She meets him at the door, yelling that he is late, and makes him spend the night on the couch.
   c. She meets him at the door, expresses delight with the roses, and kisses him on the cheek.
   d. She meets him at the door and says, "How could you? You know I'm allergic to roses!"

7. Fourteen-year-old Sally has been spending many hours after school watching TV. She has virtually stopped practicing her piano lessons. Sally's parents ask for advice about how to encourage Sally to practice more. The nurse believes the Premack principle may be helpful. Which of the following does she suggest to Sally's parents?
   a. She tells Sally's parents to reward Sally each time she practices the piano, even if it is only for 5 minutes.
   b. She tells Sally's parents to ignore this behavior and eventually she will start practicing on her own.
   c. She tells Sally's parents to draw up a contract with Sally stating what the consequences will be if she doesn't practice the piano.
   d. She tells Sally's parents to explain to Sally that she may watch TV only after she has practiced the piano for 1 hour.

8. Nancy has a fear of dogs. In helping her overcome this fear, the therapist is using systematic desensitization. List the following steps in the order in which the therapist would proceed. Having Nancy:
   a. Look at a real dog.
   b. Look at a stuffed toy dog.
   c. Pet a real dog.
   d. Pet the stuffed toy dog.
   e. Walk past a real dog.
   f. Look at a picture of a dog.

References

Ford-Martin, P. A. (2001). *Behavioral therapy.* Retrieved August 10, 2010, from http://www.findarticles.com/p/articles/mi_g2603/is_0001/ai_2603000194

Howard, D. (2000). *The effect of role modeling.* Retrieved August 10, 2010, from http://www.dianehoward.com/Effect_Role_Modeling.htm

Sadock, B. J., & Sadock, V. A. (2007). *Synopsis of psychiatry: Behavioral sciences/clinical psychiatry* (10th ed.). Philadelphia: Lippincott Williams & Wilkins.

Souders, M. C., DePaul, D., Freeman, K. G., & Levy, S. E. (2002). Caring for children and adolescents with autism who require challenging procedures. *Pediatric Nursing, 28*(6), 555–564.

Classical References

Pavlov, I. P. (1927). *Conditioned reflexes.* London: Oxford University Press.

Premack, D. (1959). Toward empirical behavior laws: I. Positive reinforcement. *Psychological Review, 66,* 219–233.

Skinner, B. F. (1938) *The behavior of organisms.* New York: Appleton-Century-Crofts.

Skinner, B. F. (1953). *Science and human behavior.* New York: Macmillan.

Thorndike, E. L. (1911). *Animal intelligence.* New York: Macmillan.

Wolpe, J. (1958). *Psychotherapy by reciprocal inhibition.* Stanford, CA: Stanford University Press.

Cognitive Therapy

KEY TERMS

arbitrary inference
automatic thoughts
catastrophic thinking
decatastrophizing
dichotomous thinking

distraction
magnification
minimization
overgeneralization
personalization

schemas
selective abstraction
Socratic questioning

OBJECTIVES

After reading this chapter, the student will be able to:

1. Discuss historical perspectives associated with cognitive therapy.
2. Identify various indications for cognitive therapy.
3. Describe goals, principles, and basic concepts of cognitive therapy.
4. Discuss a variety of cognitive therapy techniques.
5. Apply techniques of cognitive therapy within the context of the nursing process.

HOMEWORK ASSIGNMENT

Please read the chapter and answer the following questions:

1. Define *automatic thoughts.*
2. Why are automatic thoughts problematic for some people?
3. What are the three major components of cognitive therapy?
4. John submits his design of a house to some prospective clients. They ask for a few changes to be made. John thinks, "I'm a terrible architect!" What automatic thought does this statement represent?

Wright, Thase, and Beck (2008) stated, "The writing of Epictetus in the *Enchiridion, 'Men are disturbed not by things, but by the views which they take of them,'* captures the essence of the perspective that our ideas or thoughts are a controlling factor in our emotional lives." (p. 1212) This concept provides a foundation on which the cognitive model is established. In cognitive therapy, the therapist's objective is to use a variety of methods to create change in the client's thinking and belief system in an effort to bring about lasting emotional and behavioral change (Beck, 1995).

This chapter examines the historical development of the cognitive model, defines the goals of therapy, and describes various techniques of the cognitive approach. A discussion of the role of the nurse in the implementation of cognitive behavioral techniques with clients is presented.

NOTE: Although in this text the concepts are presented separately for reasons of clarification, cognitive therapy procedures are often combined with behavioral modification techniques and may be referred to as *cognitive-behavioral* therapy.

Historical Background

Cognitive therapy has its roots in the early 1960s research on depression conducted by Aaron Beck (1963, 1964). Beck had been trained in the Freudian psychoanalytic view of depression as "anger turned inward." In his clinical research, he began to observe a common theme of negative cognitive processing in the thoughts and dreams of his depressed clients (Beck & Weishaar, 2011).

A number of theorists have both taken from and expanded upon Beck's original concept. The common theme is the rejection of the passive listening of the psychoanalytic method in favor of active, direct dialogues with clients (Beck & Weishaar, 2011). The work of contemporary behavioral therapists has also influenced the evolution of cognitive therapy. Behavioral techniques such as expectancy of reinforcement and modeling are used within the cognitive domain.

Lazarus and Folkman (1984), upon whose premise of *personal appraisal* and *coping* the conceptual format of this book is founded, have also contributed a great deal to the cognitive approach to therapy. The model for cognitive therapy is based on an individual's cognition, or more specifically, an individual's personal cognitive appraisal of an event and the resulting emotions or behaviors. Personality—which undoubtedly influences our cognitive appraisal of an event—is viewed as having been shaped by the interaction between innate predisposition and environment (Beck, Freeman, & Davis, 2007). Whereas some therapies may be directed toward improvement in coping strategies or adaptiveness of behavioral response, cognitive therapy is aimed at modifying distorted cognitions about a situation.

Indications for Cognitive Therapy

Cognitive therapy was originally developed for use with depression. Today it is used for a broad range of emotional disorders. The proponents of cognitive therapy suggest that the emphasis of therapy must be varied and individualized for clients according to their specific diagnosis, symptoms, and level of functioning. In addition to depression, cognitive therapy may be used with the following clinical conditions: panic disorder, generalized anxiety disorder, social phobias, obsessive-compulsive disorder, post-traumatic stress disorder, eating disorders, substance abuse, personality disorders, schizophrenia, couples' problems, bipolar disorder, hypochondriasis, and somatoform disorder (Beck, 1995; Sadock & Sadock, 2007; Wright et al., 2008).

Goals and Principles of Cognitive Therapy

Beck and associates (1987) defined the goals of cognitive therapy in the following way:

The client will:

1. Monitor his or her negative, automatic thoughts.
2. Recognize the connections between cognition, affect, and behavior.
3. Examine the evidence for and against distorted automatic thoughts.
4. Substitute more realistic interpretations for these biased cognitions.
5. Learn to identify and alter the dysfunctional beliefs that predispose him or her to distort experiences.

Cognitive therapy is highly structured and short term, lasting from 12 to 16 weeks (Beck & Weishaar, 2011). Sadock and Sadock (2007) suggested that, if a client does not improve within 25 weeks of therapy, a reevaluation of the diagnosis should be made. Although therapy must be tailored to the individual, the following principles underlie cognitive therapy for all clients (Beck, 1995).

Principle 1. Cognitive therapy is based on an ever-evolving formulation of the client and his or her problems in cognitive terms. The therapist identifies the event that precipitated the distorted cognition. Current thinking patterns that serve to maintain the problematic behaviors are reviewed. The therapist then hypothesizes about certain developmental events and enduring patterns of cognitive appraisal that may have predisposed the client to specific emotional and behavioral responses.

Principle 2. Cognitive therapy requires a sound therapeutic alliance. A trusting relationship between therapist and client must exist for cognitive therapy to succeed. The therapist must convey warmth, empathy, caring, and genuine positive regard. Development of a working relationship between therapist and client is an individual process, and clients with various disorders will require varying degrees of effort to achieve this therapeutic alliance.

Principle 3. Cognitive therapy emphasizes collaboration and active participation. Teamwork between therapist and client is emphasized. They decide together what to work on during each session, how often they should meet, and what homework assignments should be completed between sessions.

Principle 4. Cognitive therapy is goal oriented and problem focused. At the beginning of therapy, the client is encouraged to identify what he or she perceives to be the problem or problems. With guidance from the therapist, goals are established as outcomes of therapy. Assistance in problem solving is provided as required as the client comes to recognize and correct distortions in thinking.

Principle 5. Cognitive therapy initially emphasizes the present. Resolution of distressing situations that are based in the present usually lead to symptom reduction. It is therefore of more benefit to begin with current problems and delay shifting attention to the past until (1) the client expresses a desire to do so, (2) the work on current problems produces little or no change, or (3) the therapist decides it is important to determine how dysfunctional ideas affecting the client's current thinking originated.

Principle 6. Cognitive therapy is educative, aims to teach the client to be his or her own therapist, and emphasizes relapse prevention. From the beginning of therapy, the client is taught about the nature and course of his or her disorder, about the cognitive model (i.e., how thoughts influence emotions and behavior), and about the process of cognitive therapy. The client is taught how to set goals, plan behavioral change, and intervene on his or her own behalf.

Principle 7. Cognitive therapy aims to be time limited. Clients often are seen weekly for a couple of months, followed by a number of biweekly sessions, then possibly a few monthly sessions. Some clients will want periodic "booster" sessions every few months.

Principle 8. Cognitive therapy sessions are structured. Each session has a set structure that includes (1) reviewing the client's week, (2) collaboratively setting the agenda for this session, (3) reviewing the previous week's session, (4) reviewing the previous week's homework, (5) discussing this week's agenda items, (6) establishing homework for next week, and (7) summarizing this week's session. This format focuses attention on what is important and maximizes the use of therapy time.

Principle 9. Cognitive therapy teaches clients to identify, evaluate, and respond to their dysfunctional thoughts and beliefs. Through gentle questioning and review of data, the therapist helps the client identify his or her dysfunctional thinking, evaluate the validity of the thoughts, and devise a plan of action. This is done by helping the client to examine evidence that supports or contradicts the accuracy of the thought, rather than directly challenging or confronting the belief.

Principle 10. Cognitive therapy uses a variety of techniques to change thinking, mood, and behavior. Techniques from various therapies may be used within the cognitive framework. Emphasis in treatment is guided by the client's particular disorder and directed toward modification of the client's dysfunctional cognitions that are contributing to the maladaptive behavior associated with their disorder. Examples of disorders and the dysfunctional thinking for which cognitive therapy may be of benefit are discussed later in this chapter.

Basic Concepts

Wright and associates (2008) stated, "The general thrust of cognitive therapy is that emotional responses are largely dependent upon cognitive appraisals of the significance of environmental cues" (p. 1213). Basic concepts include **automatic thoughts** and **schemas** or core beliefs.

Automatic Thoughts

Automatic thoughts are those that occur rapidly in response to a situation and without rational analysis.

These thoughts are often negative and based on erroneous logic. Beck and associates (1987) called these thoughts *cognitive errors*. Following are some examples of common cognitive errors:

Arbitrary Inference   In a type of thinking error known as **arbitrary inference,** the individual automatically comes to a conclusion about an incident without the facts to support it, or even sometimes despite contradictory evidence to support it.

EXAMPLE

Two months ago, Mrs. B. sent a wedding gift to the daughter of an old friend. She has not yet received acknowledgment of the gift. Mrs. B. thinks, "They obviously think I have poor taste."

Overgeneralization (Absolutistic Thinking)   Sweeping conclusions are **overgeneralizations** made based on one incident—a type of "all-or-nothing" thinking.

EXAMPLE

Frank submitted an article to a nursing journal and it was rejected. Frank thinks, "No journal will ever be interested in anything I write."

Dichotomous Thinking   An individual who is using **dichotomous thinking** views situations in terms of all-or-nothing, black-or-white, or good-or-bad.

EXAMPLE

Frank submits an article to a nursing journal and the editor returns it and asks Frank to rewrite parts of it. Frank thinks, "I'm a bad writer," instead of recognizing that revision is a common part of the publication process.

Selective Abstraction   A **selective abstraction** (sometimes referred to as a "mental filter") is a conclusion that is based on only a selected portion of the evidence. The selected portion is usually the negative evidence or what the individual views as a failure, rather than any successes that have occurred.

EXAMPLE

Jackie just graduated from high school with a 3.98/4.00 grade point average. She won a scholarship to the large state university near her home. She was active in sports and activities in high school and well liked by all her peers. However, she is very depressed and dwells on the fact that she did not earn a scholarship to a prestigious Ivy League college to which she had applied.

Magnification   Exaggerating the negative significance of an event is known as **magnification.**

EXAMPLE

Nancy hears that her colleague at work is having a cocktail party over the weekend and she is not invited. Nancy thinks, "She doesn't like me."

Minimization   Undervaluing the positive significance of an event is called **minimization.**

EXAMPLE

Mrs. M. is feeling lonely. She calls her granddaughter Amy, who lives in a nearby town, and invites her to visit. Amy apologizes that she must go out of town on business and would not be able to visit at that time. While Amy is out of town, she calls Mrs. M. twice, but Mrs. M. still feels unloved by her granddaughter.

Catastrophic Thinking   Always thinking that the worst will occur without considering the possibility of more likely positive outcomes is considered **catastrophic thinking.**

EXAMPLE

On Janet's first day in her secretarial job, her boss asked her to write a letter to another firm and put it on his desk for his signature. She did so and left for lunch. When she returned, the letter was on her desk with a typographical error circled in red and a note from her boss to redo the letter. Janet thinks, "This is it! I will surely be fired now!"

Personalization   With **personalization,** the person takes complete responsibility for situations without considering that other circumstances may have contributed to the outcome.

EXAMPLE

Jack, who sells vacuum cleaners door-to-door, has just given a 2-hour demonstration to Mrs. W. At the end of the demonstration, Mrs. W. tells Jack that she appreciates his demonstration, but she won't be purchasing a vacuum cleaner from him. Jack thinks, "I'm a lousy salesman," when in fact, Mrs. W.'s husband lost his job last week and they have no extra money to buy a new vacuum cleaner at this time.

Schemas (Core Beliefs)

Beck and Weishaar (2011) defined cognitive schemas as:

Structures that contain the individual's fundamental beliefs and assumptions. Schemas develop early in life from personal experience and identification with significant others.

These concepts are reinforced by further learning experiences and, in turn, influence the formation of beliefs, values, and attitudes. (p. 284)

These schemas, or core beliefs, may be adaptive or maladaptive. They may be general or specific, and they may be latent, becoming evident only when triggered by a specific stressful stimulus. Schemas differ from automatic thoughts in that they are deeper cognitive structures that serve to screen information from the environment. For this reason they are often more difficult to modify than automatic thoughts. However, the same techniques are used at the schema level as at the level of automatic thoughts. Schemas can be positive or negative, and generally fall into two broad categories: those associated with *helplessness* and those associated with *unlovability* (Beck, 1995). Some examples of types of schemas are presented in Table 20-1.

Techniques of Cognitive Therapy

The three major components of cognitive therapy are didactic or educational aspects, cognitive techniques, and behavioral interventions (Sadock & Sadock, 2007; Wright et al., 2008).

Didactic (Educational) Aspects

One of the basic principles of cognitive therapy is to prepare the client to eventually become his or her own cognitive therapist. The therapist provides information to the client about what cognitive therapy is, how it works, and the structure of the cognitive process. Explanation about expectations of both client and therapist is provided. Reading assignments are given in order to reinforce learning. Some therapists use audiotape or videotape sessions to teach clients about cognitive therapy. A full explanation about the relationship between depression (or anxiety, or whatever maladaptive response the client is experiencing) and distorted

thinking patterns is an essential part of cognitive therapy.

Cognitive Techniques

Strategies used in cognitive therapy include recognizing and modifying automatic thoughts (cognitive errors) and recognizing and modifying schemas (core beliefs). Wright and associates (2008) identified the following techniques commonly used in cognitive therapy.

Recognizing Automatic Thoughts and Schemas

Socratic Questioning

In **Socratic questioning** (also called *guided discovery*), the therapist questions the client about his or her situation. With Socratic questioning, the client is asked to describe feelings associated with specific situations. Questions are stated in a way that may stimulate in the client recognition of possible dysfunctional thinking and produce dissonance about the validity of the thoughts.

Imagery and Role Play

When Socratic questioning does not produce the desired results, the therapist may choose to guide the client through imagery exercises or role-play in an effort to elicit automatic thoughts. Through guided imagery, the client is asked to "relive" the stressful situation by imagining the setting in which it occurred. Where did it occur? Who was there? What happened just prior to the stressful situation? What feelings did the client experience in association with the situation?

Role-play is not used as commonly as imagery. It is a technique that should be used only when the relationship between client and therapist is exceptionally strong and there is little likelihood of maladaptive transference occurring. With role-play, the therapist assumes the role of an individual within a situation that produces a maladaptive response in the client. The situation is played out in an effort to elicit recognition of automatic thinking on the part of the client.

TABLE 20-1 Examples of Schemas (or Core Beliefs)		
SCHEMA CATEGORY	**MALADAPTIVE/NEGATIVE**	**ADAPTIVE/POSITIVE**
Helplessness	No matter what I do, I will fail.	If I try and work very hard, I will succeed.
	I must be perfect. If I make one mistake, I will lose everything.	I am not afraid of a challenge. If I make a mistake, I will try again.
Unlovability	I'm stupid. No one would love me.	I'm a loveable person.
	I'm nobody without a man.	People respect me for myself.

Thought Recording

This technique, one of the most frequently used methods of recognizing automatic thoughts, is taught to and discussed with the client in the therapy session. Thought recording is assigned as homework for the client outside of therapy. In thought recording, the client is asked to keep a written record of situations that occur and the automatic thoughts that are elicited by the situation. This is called a "two-column" thought recording. Some therapists ask their clients to keep a "three-column" recording, which includes a description of the emotional response also associated with the situation, as illustrated in Table 20-2.

Modifying Automatic Thoughts and Schemas

Generating Alternatives

To help the client see a broader range of possibilities than had originally been considered, the therapist guides the client in generating alternatives.

Examining the Evidence

With this technique, the client and therapist set forth the automatic thought as the hypothesis, and they study the evidence both for and against the hypothesis.

Decatastrophizing

With the technique of **decatastrophizing,** the therapist assists the client to examine the validity of a negative automatic thought. Even if some validity exists, the client is then encouraged to review ways to cope adaptively, moving beyond the current crisis situation.

Reattribution

It is believed that depressed clients attribute life events in a negatively distorted manner; that is, they have a tendency "to blame themselves for adverse life events, and to believe that these negative situations will last indefinitely" (Wright et al., 2008, p. 1216). Through Socratic questioning and testing of automatic thoughts, this technique is aimed at reversing the negative attribution of depressed clients from internal and enduring to the more external and transient manner of nondepressed individuals.

Daily Record of Dysfunctional Thoughts (DRDT)

The DRDT is a tool commonly used in cognitive therapy to help clients identify and modify automatic thoughts. Two more columns are added to the three-column thought record presented earlier. Clients are then asked to rate the intensity of the thoughts and emotions on a 0- to 100-percent scale. The fourth column of the DRDT asks the client to describe a more rational cognition than the automatic thought identified in the second column and rate the intensity of the belief in the rational thought. In the fifth column, the client records any changes that have occurred as a result of modifying the automatic thought and the new rate of intensity associated with it. With this tool, the client is able to modify automatic thoughts by identifying them and actually formulating a more rational alternative. Table 20-3 presents an example of a DRDT as an extension to the three-column thought recording presented in Table 20-2.

Cognitive Rehearsal

This technique uses mental imagery to uncover potential automatic thoughts in advance of their occurrence in a stressful situation. A discussion is held to identify ways to modify these dysfunctional cognitions. The client is then given "homework" assignments to try these newly learned methods in real situations.

Behavioral Interventions

It is believed that, in cognitive therapy, an interactive relationship exists between cognitions and behavior; that is, that cognitions affect behavior and behavior influences cognitions. With this concept in mind, a number of interventions are structured for the client to assist him or her to identify and modify maladaptive cognitions and behaviors.

The following procedures, which are behavior oriented, are directed toward helping clients learn more adaptive behavioral strategies that will in turn have a more positive effect on cognitions

TABLE 20-2 Three-Column Thought Recording		
SITUATION	**AUTOMATIC THOUGHTS**	**EMOTIONAL RESPONSE**
Girlfriend broke up with me.	I'm a stupid person. No one would ever want to marry me.	Sadness; depression
I was turned down for a promotion.	Stupid boss!! He doesn't know how to manage people. It's not fair!	Anger

TABLE 20-3 Daily Record of Dysfunctional Thoughts (DRDT)

SITUATION	AUTOMATIC THOUGHT	EMOTIONAL RESPONSE	RATIONAL RESPONSE	OUTCOME: EMOTIONAL RESPONSE
Girlfriend broke up with me.	I'm a stupid person. No one would ever want to marry me. (95%)	Sadness; depression (90%)	I'm not stupid. Lots of people like me. Just because one person doesn't want to date me doesn't mean that no one would want to. (75%)	Sadness; depression (50%)
I was turned down for a promotion.	Stupid boss!! He doesn't know how to manage people. It's not fair! (90%)	Anger (95%)	I guess I have to admit the other guy's education and experience fit the position better than mine. The boss was being fair because he filled the position based on qualifications. I'll try for the next promotion that fits my qualifications better. (70%)	Anger (20%) Disappointment (80%) Hope (80%)

(Basco, McDonald, Merlock, & Rush, 2004; Sadock & Sadock, 2007; Wright et al., 2008):

1. **Activity Scheduling.** With this intervention, clients are asked to keep a daily log of their activities on an hourly basis and rate each activity, for mastery and pleasure, on a 0-to-10 scale. The schedule is then shared with the therapist and used to identify important areas needing concentration during therapy.

2. **Graded Task Assignments.** This intervention is used with clients who are facing a situation that they perceive as overwhelming. The task is broken down into subtasks that clients can complete one step at a time. Each subtask will have a goal and a time interval attached to it. Successful completion of each subtask helps to increase self-esteem and decrease feelings of helplessness.

3. **Behavioral Rehearsal.** Somewhat akin to, and often used in conjunction with, cognitive rehearsal, this technique uses role-play to "rehearse" a modification of maladaptive behaviors that may be contributing to dysfunctional cognitions.

4. **Distraction.** When dysfunctional cognitions have been recognized, **distraction** can occur by engaging in activities that redirect the client's thinking and divert him or her from the intrusive thoughts or depressive ruminations that are contributing to the maladaptive responses.

5. **Miscellaneous Techniques.** Relaxation exercises, assertiveness training, role modeling, and social skills training are additional types of behavioral interventions that are used in cognitive therapy to assist clients to modify dysfunctional cognitions. Thought-stopping techniques (described in Chapter 15) may also be used to restructure dysfunctional thinking patterns.

Role of the Nurse in Cognitive Therapy

Many of the techniques used in cognitive therapy are well within the scope of nursing practice, from generalist through specialist levels. Cognitive therapy requires an understanding of educational principles and the ability to use problem-solving skills to guide clients' thinking through a reframing process. The scope of contemporary psychiatric nursing practice is expanding, and although psychiatric nurses have been using some of these techniques in various degrees within their practices for years, it is important that knowledge and skills related to this type of therapy be promoted further. The value of cognitive therapy as a useful and cost-effective tool has been observed in a number of inpatient and community outpatient mental health settings.

The following case study presents the role of the nurse in cognitive therapy in the context of the nursing process.

CASE STUDY

ASSESSMENT

Sam is a 45-year-old white male admitted to the psychiatric unit of a general medical center by his family physician, Dr. Jones, who reported that Sam had become increasingly despondent over the last month. His wife reported that he had made statements such as, "Life is not worth living," and "I think I could just take all those pills Dr. Jones prescribed at one time, then it would all be over." He was admitted at 6:40 p.m., via wheelchair from admissions, accompanied by his wife. He reports no known allergies. Vital signs upon admission were temperature, 97.9°F; pulse, 80; respirations, 16; and blood pressure, 132/77. He is 5 feet 11 inches tall and weighs 160 pounds. He was referred to the psychiatrist on call, Dr. Smith. Orders include suicide precautions, level I; regular diet; chemistry profile and routine urinalysis in a.m.; Desyrel, 200 mg tid; Dalmane, 30 mg hs prn for sleep.

Family Dynamics

Sam says he loves his wife and children and does not want to hurt them, but feels they no longer need him. He states, "They would probably be better off without me." His wife appears to be very concerned about his condition, although in his despondency, he seems oblivious to her feelings. His mother lives in a neighboring state, and he sees her infrequently. He admits that he is somewhat bitter toward her for allowing him and his siblings to "suffer from the physical and emotional brutality of their father." His siblings and their families live in distant states, and he sees them rarely, during holiday gatherings. He feels closest to the older of the two brothers.

Medical/Psychiatric History

Sam's father died 5 years ago at age 65 of a myocardial infarction. Sam and both his brothers have a history of high cholesterol and triglycerides from approximately age 30. During his regular physical examination 1 month ago, Sam's family doctor recognized symptoms of depression and prescribed fluoxetine. Sam's mother has a history of depressive episodes. She was hospitalized once about 7 years ago for depression, and she has taken various antidepressant medications over the years. Her family physician has also prescribed Valium for her on numerous occasions for her "nerves." No other family members have a history of psychiatric problems.

Past Experiences

Sam was the first child in a family of four. He is 2 years older than his sister and 4 years older than the third child, a brother. He was 6 years old when his youngest sibling, also a boy, was born. Sam's father was a career Army man, who moved his family many times during their childhood years. Sam attended 15 schools from the time he entered kindergarten until he graduated from high school.

Sam reports that his father was very autocratic and had many rules that he expected his children to obey without question. Infraction resulted in harsh discipline. Because Sam was the oldest child, his father believed he should assume responsibility for the behavior of his siblings. Sam describes the severe physical punishment he received from his father when he or his siblings allegedly violated one of the rules. It was particularly intense when Sam's father had been drinking, which he did most evenings and weekends.

Sam's mother was very passive. Sam believes she was afraid of his father, particularly when he was drinking, so she quietly conformed to his lifestyle and offered no resistance, even though she did not agree with his disciplining of the children. Sam reports that he observed his father physically abusing his mother on a number of occasions, most often when he had been drinking.

Sam states that he had very few friends when he was growing up. With all the family moves, he gave up trying to make new friends because it became too painful to give them up when it was time to leave. He took a paper route when he was 13 years old and then worked in fast-food restaurants from age 15 on. He was a hard worker and never seemed to have difficulty finding work in any of the places where the family relocated. He states that he appreciated the independence and the opportunity of being away from home as much as his job would allow. "I guess I can honestly say I hated my father, and working was my way of getting away from all the stress that was going on in that house. I guess my dad hated me, too, because he never was satisfied with anything I did. I never did well enough for him in school, on the job, or even at home. When I think of my dad now, the memories I have are of being criticized and beaten with a belt."

On graduation from high school, Sam joined the Navy, where he learned a skill that he used after discharge to obtain a job in a large aircraft plant. He also attended the local university at night, where he earned his accounting degree. When he completed his degree, he was reassigned to the administration department of the aircraft company, and he has been in the same position for 12 years without a promotion.

Precipitating Event

Over the last 12 years, Sam has watched while a number of his peers were promoted to management positions. Sam has been considered for several of these positions but has never been selected. Last month a management position became available for which Sam felt he was qualified. He applied for this position, believing he had a good chance of being promoted. However, when the announcement was made, the position had been given to a younger man who

Continued

CASE STUDY—cont'd

had been with the company only 5 years. Sam seemed to accept the decision, but over the last few weeks he has become more and more withdrawn. He speaks to very few people at the office and is becoming more and more behind in his work. At home, he eats very little, talks to family members only when they ask a direct question, withdraws to his bedroom very early in the evening, and does not come out until time to leave for work the next morning. Today, he refused to get out of bed or to go to work. His wife convinced him to talk to their family doctor, who admitted him to the hospital.

Client's Perception of the Stressor

Sam states that all his life he has "not been good enough at anything. I could never please my father. Now I can't seem to please my boss. What's the use of trying? I came to the hospital because my wife and my doctor are afraid I might try to kill myself. I must admit the thought has crossed my mind more than once. I seem to have very little motivation for living. I just don't care any more."

DIAGNOSES/OUTCOME IDENTIFICATION

The following nursing diagnoses were formulated for Sam:

1. Risk for suicide related to depressed mood and expressions of having nothing to live for.

2. Chronic low self-esteem related to lack of positive feedback and learned helplessness evidenced by a sense of worthlessness, lack of eye contact, social isolation, and negative/pessimistic outlook.

The following may be used as criteria for measurement of outcomes in the planning of care for Sam:

The client will:

1. Not harm self.

2. Acquire a feeling of hope for the future.

3. Demonstrate increased self-esteem and perception of self as a worthwhile person.

PLANNING/IMPLEMENTATION

Table 20-4 presents a nursing care plan for Sam employing some techniques associated with cognitive therapy that are within the scope of nursing practice. Rationales are presented for each intervention.

EVALUATION

Reassessment is conducted to determine if the nursing interventions have been successful in achieving the objectives of Sam's care. Evaluation can be facilitated by gathering information using the following questions:

1. Has self-harm to Sam been avoided?

2. Have Sam's suicidal ideations subsided?

3. Does Sam know where to seek help in a crisis situation?

4. Has Sam discussed the recent loss with staff and family?

5. Is Sam able to verbalize personal hope for the future?

6. Can Sam identify positive attributes about himself?

7. Does Sam demonstrate motivation to move on with his life without a fear of failure?

Table 20-4 CARE PLAN FOR "SAM" (AN EXAMPLE OF INTERVENTION WITH COGNITIVE THERAPY)

NURSING DIAGNOSIS: RISK FOR SUICIDE
RELATED TO: Depressed mood

OUTCOME CRITERIA	NURSING INTERVENTIONS*	RATIONALES*
Sam will not harm himself.	1. Acknowledge Sam's feelings of despair.	1. Cognitive therapists actively pursue the client's point of view.
	2. Convey warmth, accurate empathy, and genuineness.	2. Cognitive therapists use these skills to understand the client's personal view of the world and to establish rapport.
	3. Through Socratic questioning, challenge irrational pessimism. Ask Sam to discuss what problems suicide would solve. Then try to get him to think of reasons for *not* attempting suicide.	3. Cognitive therapists use problem-solving techniques to help the suicidal client think beyond the immediate future.
	4. Begin a serious discussion of alternatives.	4. Cognitive therapists use this strategy to decrease feelings of hopelessness in suicidal clients.

| Table 20-4 | CARE PLAN FOR "SAM" (AN EXAMPLE OF INTERVENTION WITH COGNITIVE THERAPY)—cont'd | |

NURSING DIAGNOSIS: CHRONIC LOW SELF-ESTEEM
RELATED TO: Lack of positive feedback and learned helplessness
EVIDENCED BY: A sense of worthlessness, lack of eye contact, social isolation, and negative/pessimistic outlook.

OUTCOME CRITERIA	NURSING INTERVENTIONS	RATIONALES
Sam will demonstrate increased self-esteem and perception of himself as a worthwhile person.	1. Ask Sam to keep a 3-column automatic thought recording.	1. Cognitive therapists use this tool to help clients identify automatic thoughts (cognitive errors).
	2. Help Sam to recognize that his worth as a person is not tied to his promotion at work. The world will go on and he can survive this loss.	2. Cognitive therapists use the technique of "decatastrophizing" to help clients get past a crisis situation.
	3. Help Sam to identify ways in which he could feel better about himself. For example, Sam states that he would like to update his computer skills, but he is afraid he is too old. Challenge his negative thinking about his age by using the cognitive therapy technique of "examining the evidence."	3. Cognitive therapists use the technique of "generating alternatives" to help clients recognize that a broader range of possibilities may exist than may be evident at the moment. "Examining the evidence" may help Sam understand that self-improvement is worthwhile at any age.
	4. Ask Sam to expand on his 3-column automatic thought recording and make a Daily Record of Dysfunctional Thoughts (DRDT).	4. Cognitive therapists use this tool to help clients identify their automatic thoughts and modify them by coming up with more rational responses.
	5. Discourage Sam's ruminating about his failures. May need to withdraw attention if he persists. Focus on past accomplishments and offer support in undertaking new tasks. Offer recognition of successful endeavors and positive reinforcement of attempts made.	5. Cognitive therapy employs some techniques of behavior therapy. Lack of attention to undesirable behavior may discourage its repetition. Recognition and positive reinforcement enhance self-esteem and encourage repetition of desirable behaviors.

Interventions and rationales for the diagnosis Risk for Suicide are adapted from Harvard Medical School (2003) and Beck and Weishaar (2011).

Summary and Key Points

■ Cognitive therapy is founded on the premise that how people think significantly influences their feelings and behavior.

■ The concept was initiated in the 1960s by Aaron Beck in his work with depressed clients. Since that time, it has been expanded for use with a number of emotional illnesses.

■ Cognitive therapy is short-term, highly structured, and goal-oriented therapy that consists of three major components: didactic, or educational, aspects; cognitive techniques; and behavioral interventions.

■ The therapist teaches the client about the relationship between his or her illness and the distorted thinking patterns. Explanation about cognitive therapy and how it works is provided.

■ The therapist helps the client to recognize his or her negative automatic thoughts (sometimes called *cognitive errors*).

■ Once these automatic thoughts have been identified, various cognitive and behavioral techniques are used to assist the client to modify the dysfunctional thinking patterns.

■ Independent homework assignments are an important part of the cognitive therapist's strategy.

■ Many of the cognitive therapy techniques are within the scope of nursing practice.

■ As the role of the psychiatric nurse continues to expand, the knowledge and skills associated with a variety of therapies will need to be broadened. Cognitive therapy is likely to be one in which nurses will become more involved.

 DavisPlus   Additional info available @ davisplus.fadavis.com

Review Questions
Self-Examination/Learning Exercise

*Select the answer that is **most** appropriate for each of the following questions:*

1. Janet failed her first test in nursing school. She thinks, "Well, that's it! I'll never be a nurse. What automatic thought does this statement represent?
   a. Overgeneralization.
   b. Magnification.
   c. Catastrophic thinking.
   d. Personalization.

2. When Jack is not accepted at the law school of his choice, he thinks, "I'm so stupid. No law school will ever accept me." What automatic thought does this statement represent?
   a. Overgeneralization.
   b. Magnification.
   c. Selective abstraction.
   d. Minimization.

3. Nancy's new in-laws came to dinner for the first time. When Nancy's mother-in-law left some food on her plate, Nancy thought, "I must be a lousy cook." What automatic thought does this statement represent?
   a. Dichotomous thinking.
   b. Overgeneralization.
   c. Minimization.
   d. Personalization.

4. Barbara burned the toast. She thinks, "I'm a totally incompetent person." What automatic thought does this statement represent?
   a. Selective abstraction.
   b. Magnification.
   c. Minimization.
   d. Personalization.

5. Opal is a 43-year-old woman who is suffering from depression and suicidal ideation. Opal says, "I'm such a worthless person. I don't deserve to live." The therapist responds, "I would like for you to think about what problems committing suicide would solve." The therapist is using which of the following cognitive therapy techniques?
   a. Imagery.
   b. Role-play.
   c. Problem solving.
   d. Thought recording.

6. The thought recording (2-column and 3-column) cognitive therapy techniques help clients:
   a. Identify automatic thoughts.
   b. Modify automatic thoughts.
   c. Identify rational alternatives.
   d. All of the above.

7. The purpose of the Daily Record of Dysfunctional Thoughts (DRDT) is used in cognitive therapy to help clients:
   a. Identify automatic thoughts.
   b. Modify automatic thoughts.
   c. Identify rational alternatives.
   d. All of the above.

Review Questions—cont'd
Self-Examination/Learning Exercise

8. A client tells the therapist, "I thought I would just die when my husband told me he was leaving me. If I had been a better wife, he wouldn't have fallen in love with another woman. It's all my fault." The therapist asks the client to think back to the day her husband told her he was leaving and to describe the situation and her feelings. What cognitive therapy technique is the therapist using?
   a. Imagery.
   b. Role-play.
   c. Problem solving.
   d. Thought recording.

9. A client tells the therapist, "I thought I would just die when my husband told me he was leaving me. If I had been a better wife, he wouldn't have fallen in love with another woman. It's all my fault." The therapist wants to use the technique of "examining the evidence." Which of the following statements reflects this technique:
   a. "How do you think you could have been a better wife?"
   b. "Okay, you say it's all your fault. Let's discuss why it might be your fault and then we will look at why it may not be."
   c. "Let's talk about what would make you a happier person."
   d. "Would you have wanted him to stay if he didn't really want to?"

10. The therapist teaches a client that, when the idea of herself as a worthless person starts to form in her mind, she should immediately start to whistle the tune of "Dixie." This is an example of the cognitive therapy technique of:
    a. Behavioral rehearsal.
    b. Social skills training.
    c. Distraction.
    d. Generating alternatives.

References

Basco, M. R., McDonald, N., Merlock, M., & Rush, A. J. (2004). A cognitive-behavioral approach to treatment of bipolar I disorder. In J. H. Wright (Ed.), *Cognitive-behavioral therapy* (pp. 25–53). Washington, DC: American Psychiatric Publishing.

Beck, A. T., Freeman, A., & Davis, D. D. (2007). *Cognitive therapy of personality disorders* (2nd ed.). New York: Guilford Publications.

Beck, A. T., Rush, A. H., Shaw, B. F., & Emery, G. (1987). *Cognitive therapy of depression.* New York: Guilford Press.

Beck, A. T., & Weishaar, M. E. (2011). Cognitive therapy. In R. J. Corsini & D. Wedding (Eds.), *Current psychotherapies* (9th ed., pp. 276–309). Belmont, CA: Brooks/Cole.

Beck, J. S. (1995). *Cognitive therapy: Basics and beyond.* New York: Guilford Press.

Harvard Medical School. (2003). Confronting suicide—part II. *Harvard Mental Health Letter, 19*(12), 1–5.

Sadock, B. J., & Sadock, V. A. (2007). *Synopsis of psychiatry: Behavioral sciences/clinical psychiatry* (10th ed.). Philadelphia: Lippincott Williams & Wilkins.

Wright, J. H., Thase, M. E., & Beck, A. T. (2008). Cognitive therapy. In R. E. Hales, S. C. Yudofsky, & G. O. Gabbard (Eds.), *Textbook of psychiatry* (5th ed., pp. 1211–1256). Washington, DC: American Psychiatric Publishing.

Classical References

Beck, A. T. (1963). Thinking and depression, I. Idiosyncratic content and cognitive distortions. *Archives of General Psychiatry, 9,* 324–333.

Beck, A. T. (1964). Thinking and depression, II. Theory and therapy. *Archives of General Psychiatry, 10,* 561–571.

Lazarus, R. S., & Folkman, S. (1984). *Stress, appraisal, and coping.* New York: Springer.

Electroconvulsive Therapy

21

CORE CONCEPT

electroconvulsive therapy

KEY TERMS

insulin coma therapy

pharmacoconvulsive therapy

OBJECTIVES

After reading this chapter, the student will be able to:

1. Define *electroconvulsive therapy.*
2. Discuss historical perspectives related to electroconvulsive therapy.
3. Discuss indications, contraindications, mechanism of action, and side effects of electroconvulsive therapy.
4. Identify risks associated with electroconvulsive therapy.
5. Describe the role of the nurse in the administration of electroconvulsive therapy.

HOMEWORK ASSIGNMENT

Please read the chapter and answer the following questions:

1. Mr. J. says to the nurse, "This consent form says there is a possibility of permanent memory loss with ECT. I don't want to lose my memory!" How should the nurse respond to Mr. J.?
2. What medication is commonly given before the ECT treatment to decrease secretions?
3. Why is the client given oxygen during the procedure?

Electroconvulsive therapy (ECT) has had very bad press. In the movie *One Flew Over the Cuckoo's Nest,* it is depicted as a physically and emotionally brutal procedure imposed on unwilling clients in order to calm them. Today, ECT remains one of the most controversial treatments for psychological disorders and continues to be the subject of impassioned debate among various factions of society, within both the professional and lay communities.

Despite its controversial image, ECT has been used continuously for more than 50 years, longer than any other physical treatment available for mental illness. It has achieved this longevity because, when administered properly, for the right illness, it can help as much as or more than any other treatment (Kellner, 2010).

This chapter explores the historical perspectives, indications and contraindications, mechanism of action, side effects, and risks associated with ECT. The role of the nurse in the care of the client receiving ECT is presented in the context of the nursing process.

Electroconvulsive Therapy, Defined

> ## CORE CONCEPT
> ### *Electroconvulsive therapy*
> The induction of a grand mal (generalized) seizure through the application of electrical current to the brain.

The stimulus is applied through electrodes that are placed either bilaterally in the frontotemporal region or unilaterally on the same side as the dominant hand (Marangell, Silver, Goff, & Yudofsky, 2003). Controversy exists over optimal placement of the electrodes in terms of possible greater efficacy with bilateral placement versus the potential in some clients for less confusion and acute amnesia with unilateral placement.

The amount of electrical stimulus applied is another point of controversy among clinicians. Dose of stimulation is based on the client's seizure threshold, which is highly variable among individuals. The duration of the seizure should be at least 15 to 25 seconds (Karasu, Gelenberg, Merriam, & Wang, 2006). Movements are very minimal because of the administration of a muscle relaxant before the treatment. The tonic phase of the seizure usually lasts 10 to 15 seconds and may be identified by a rigid plantar extension of the feet. The clonic phase follows and is usually characterized by rhythmic movements of the muscles that decrease in frequency and finally disappear. Because of the muscle relaxant, movements may be observed merely as a rhythmic twitching of the toes.

Most clients require an average of 6 to 12 treatments, but some may require up to 20 treatments (Sadock & Sadock, 2007). Treatments are usually administered every other day, three times per week. Treatments are performed on an inpatient basis for those who require close observation and care (e.g., clients who are suicidal, agitated, delusional, catatonic, or acutely manic). Those at less risk may have the option of receiving therapy at an outpatient treatment facility.

Historical Perspectives

The first electroconvulsive therapy treatment was performed in April 1938 by Italian psychiatrists Ugo Cerletti and Lucio Bini in Rome. Other somatic therapies had been tried before that time, in particular **insulin coma therapy** and **pharmacoconvulsive therapy.**

Insulin coma therapy was introduced by the German psychiatrist Manfred Sakel in 1933. His therapy was used for clients with schizophrenia. The insulin injection treatments would induce a hypoglycemic coma, which Sakel claimed was effective in alleviating schizophrenic symptoms. This therapy required vigorous medical and nursing intervention through the stages of induced coma. Some fatalities occurred when clients failed to respond to efforts directed at termination of the coma. The efficacy of insulin coma therapy has been questioned, and its use has been discontinued in the treatment of mental illness.

Pharmacoconvulsive therapy was introduced in Budapest in 1934 by Ladislas Meduna (Fink, 1999). He induced convulsions with intramuscular injections of camphor in oil in clients with schizophrenia. He based his treatment on clinical observation and on his theory that there was a biological antagonism between schizophrenia and epilepsy. Thus, by inducing seizures he hoped to reduce schizophrenic symptoms. Because he discovered that camphor was unreliable for inducing seizures, he began using pentylenetetrazol (Metrazol). Some successes were reported in terms of reduction of psychotic symptoms, and, until the advent of ECT in 1938, pentylenetetrazol was the most frequently used procedure for producing seizures in psychotic clients. There was a brief resurgence of pharmacoconvulsive therapy in the late 1950s, when flurothyl (Indoklon), a potent inhalant convulsant, was introduced as an alternative for individuals who were unwilling to consent to ECT for the treatment of depression and schizophrenia. Pharmacoconvulsive therapy is no longer used in psychiatry.

Periodic recognition of the important contribution of ECT in the treatment of mental illness has been evident in the United States. An initial acceptance was observed from 1940 to 1960, followed by a 20-year period in which ECT was considered objectionable by both the psychiatric profession and the lay public. A second wave of acceptance began around 1980 and has been increasing to the present. The period of nonacceptability coincided with the introduction of tricyclic and monoamine oxidase inhibitor antidepressant drugs and ended with the realization among many psychiatrists that the widely heralded replacement of ECT with these chemical agents had failed to materialize (Abrams, 2002). Some individuals showed improvement with ECT after failing to respond to other forms of therapy.

Currently, an estimated 100,000 people in the United States and about 2 million people worldwide receive ECT treatments each year (Dukakis &

Tye, 2006). The typical client is white, female, middle-aged and from a middle- to upper-income background, receiving treatment in a private or university hospital for major depression, usually after drug therapy has proved ineffective. Largely because of the expense involved, as well as the need for a team of highly skilled medical specialists, many public hospitals are not able to offer this service to their clients.

Indications

Major Depression

ECT has been shown to be effective in the treatment of severe depression. It appears to be particularly effective in depressed clients who are also experiencing psychotic symptoms and those with psychomotor retardation and neurovegetative changes, such as disturbances in sleep, appetite, and energy. These symptoms are associated with the diagnoses of major depressive disorder, major depressive disorder with psychotic or melancholic symptoms, and bipolar disorder depression (Sadock & Sadock, 2007). ECT is not often used as the treatment of choice for depressive disorders but is considered only after a trial of therapy with antidepressant medication has proved ineffective.

Mania

ECT is also indicated in the treatment of acute manic episodes of bipolar disorder (Black & Andreasen, 2011). At present it is rarely used for this purpose, having been superceded by the widespread use of antipsychotic drugs and/or lithium. However, it has been shown to be effective in the treatment of manic clients who do not tolerate or fail to respond to lithium or other drug treatment, or when life is threatened by dangerous behavior or exhaustion.

Schizophrenia

ECT can induce a remission in some clients who present with acute schizophrenia, particularly if it is accompanied by catatonic or affective (depression or mania) symptomatology (Black & Andreasen, 2011). It does not appear to be of value to individuals with chronic schizophrenic illness.

Other Conditions

ECT has also been tried with clients experiencing a variety of neuroses, obsessive-compulsive disorders, and personality disorders. Little evidence exists to support the efficacy of ECT in the treatment of these conditions.

Contraindications

The only absolute contraindication for ECT is increased intracranial pressure (from brain tumor, recent cardiovascular accident, or other cerebrovascular lesion). ECT is associated with a physiological rise in cerebrospinal fluid pressure during the treatment, resulting in increased intracranial pressure that could lead to brainstem herniation (Marangell et al., 2003).

Various other conditions, not considered absolute contraindications but rendering clients at high risk for the treatment, have been identified (Black & Andreasen, 2011; Eisendrath & Lichtmacher, 2009; Marangell et al., 2003). These conditions are largely cardiovascular in nature and include myocardial infarction or cerebrovascular accident within the preceding 3 to 6 months, aortic or cerebral aneurysm, severe underlying hypertension, and congestive heart failure. Clients with cardiovascular problems are placed at risk because of the response of the body to the seizure itself. The initial vagal response results in a sinus bradycardia and drop in blood pressure. This is followed immediately by tachycardia and a hypertensive response. These changes can be life threatening to an individual with an already compromised cardiovascular system. Other factors that place clients at risk from ECT include severe osteoporosis, acute and chronic pulmonary disorders, and high-risk or complicated pregnancy.

Mechanism of Action

The exact mechanism by which ECT effects a therapeutic response is unknown. Several theories exist, but the one to which the most credibility has been given is the biochemical theory. A number of researchers have demonstrated that electrical stimulation results in significant increases in the circulating levels of several neurotransmitters (Wahlund & von Rosen, 2003). These neurotransmitters include serotonin, norepinephrine, and dopamine, the same biogenic amines that are affected by antidepressant drugs. Additional evidence suggests that ECT may also result in increases in glutamate and gamma-aminobutyric acid (Grover, Mattoo, & Gupta, 2005). The results of studies relating to the mechanism underlying the effectiveness of ECT are still ongoing and continue to be controversial.

Side Effects

The most common side effects of ECT are temporary memory loss and confusion. Critics of the therapy argue that these changes represent irreversible brain damage. Proponents insist they are temporary and reversible. Black and Andreasen (2011) stated:

> Because ECT disrupts new memories that have not been incorporated into long-term memory stores, ECT can cause anterograde and retrograde amnesia that is most dense around the time of treatment. The anterograde component usually clears quickly, but the retrograde amnesia can extend back to months before treatment. It is unclear if the memory loss is due to the ECT or to ongoing depressive symptoms. (p. 550)

The controversy continues regarding the choice of unilateral versus bilateral ECT. Studies have shown that unilateral placement of the electrodes decreases the amount of memory disturbance. However, unilateral ECT often requires a higher stimulus dose or a greater number of treatments to match the efficacy of bilateral ECT in the relief of depression (Geddes, 2003).

Risks Associated With Electroconvulsive Therapy

Mortality

Studies indicate that the mortality rate from ECT is about 2 per 100,000 treatments (Marangell et al., 2003; Sadock & Sadock, 2007). Although the occurrence is rare, the major cause of death with ECT is from cardiovascular complications (e.g., acute myocardial infarction or cerebrovascular accident), usually in individuals with previously compromised cardiac status. Assessment and management of cardiovascular disease *prior to* treatment is vital in the reduction of morbidity and mortality rates associated with ECT.

Permanent Memory Loss

Most individuals report no problems with their memory, aside from the time immediately surrounding the ECT treatments. However, some clients have reported retrograde amnesia extending back to months before treatment. In rare instances, more extensive amnesia has occurred, resulting in memory gaps dating back years (Joska & Stein, 2008). Some clients have reported gaps in recollections of specific personal memories.

Sackeim and associates (2007) reported on the results of a longitudinal study of clinical and cognitive outcomes in patients with major depression treated with ECT at seven facilities in the New York City metropolitan area. Subjects were evaluated shortly following the ECT course and 6 months later. Data revealed that cognitive deficits at the 6-month interval were directly related to type of electrode placement and electrical waveform used. Bilateral electrode placement resulted in more severe and persisting (as evaluated at the 6-month follow-up) retrograde amnesia than unilateral placement. The extent of the amnesia was directly related to the number of ECT treatments received. The researchers also found that stimulation produced by sine wave (continuous) current resulted in greater short- and long-term deficits than that produced by short-pulse wave (intermittent) current.

Black and Andreasen (2011) suggested that all clients receiving ECT should be informed of the possibility for some degree of permanent memory loss. Although the potential for these effects appears to be minimal, the client must be made aware of the risks involved before consenting to treatment.

Brain Damage

Brain damage from ECT remains a concern for those who continue to believe in its usefulness and efficacy as a treatment for depression. Critics of the procedure remain adamant in their belief that ECT always results in some degree of immediate brain damage (Frank, 2002). However, evidence is based largely on animal studies in which the subjects received excessive electrical dosages, and the seizures were unmodified by muscle paralysis and oxygenation (Abrams, 2002). Although this is an area for continuing study, there is no evidence to substantiate that ECT produces any permanent changes in brain structure or functioning (McClintock & Husain, 2011).

The Role of the Nurse in Electroconvulsive Therapy

Nurses play an integral role in the teaching and preparation for and administration of ECT. They provide support before, during, and after the treatment to the client and family, and assist the medical professionals who are conducting the therapy. The nursing process provides a systematic approach to the provision of care for the client receiving ECT.

Assessment

A complete physical examination must be completed by the appropriate medical professional prior to the initiation of ECT. This evaluation should include a thorough assessment of cardiovascular and pulmonary status as well as laboratory blood and urine studies. A skeletal history and x-ray assessment should also be considered.

The nurse may be responsible for ensuring that informed consent has been obtained from the client. If the depression is severe and the client is clearly unable to consent to the procedure, permission may be obtained from family or another legally responsible individual. Consent is secured only after the client or responsible individual acknowledges understanding of the procedure, including possible side effects and potential risks involved. Client and family must also understand that ECT is voluntary, and that consent may be withdrawn at any time (American Psychiatric Association, 2001; Fetterman & Ying, 2011).

Nurses may also be required to assess:

■ The client's mood and level of interaction with others

■ Evidence of suicidal ideation, plan, and means

■ Level of anxiety and fears associated with receiving ECT

■ Thought and communication patterns

■ Baseline memory for short- and long-term events

■ Client and family knowledge of indications for, side effects of, and potential risks associated with ECT

■ Current and past use of medications

■ Baseline vital signs and history of allergies

■ The client's ability to carry out activities of daily living

Diagnosis/Outcome Identification

Selection of appropriate nursing diagnoses for the client undergoing ECT is based on continual assessment before, during, and after treatment. Selected potential nursing diagnoses with outcome criteria for evaluation are presented in Table 21-1.

Planning/Implementation

ECT treatments are usually performed in the morning. The client is given nothing by mouth (NPO) for 6 to 8 hours before the treatment. Some institutional policies require that the client be placed on NPO status at midnight prior to the treatment day. The treatment team routinely consists of the psychiatrist, anesthesiologist, and two or more nurses.

Nursing interventions before the treatment include:

■ Ensure that the physician has obtained informed consent and that a signed permission form is on the chart.

TABLE 21-1 Potential Nursing Diagnoses and Outcome Criteria for Client Receiving ECT

NURSING DIAGNOSES	OUTCOME CRITERIA
Anxiety (moderate to severe) related to impending therapy	Client verbalizes a decrease in anxiety following explanation of procedure and expression of fears.
Deficient knowledge related to necessity for and side effects or risks of ECT	Client verbalizes understanding of need for and side effects/risks of ECT following explanation.
Risk for injury related to risks associated with ECT	Client undergoes treatment without sustaining injury.
Risk for aspiration related to altered level of consciousness immediately following treatment	Client experiences no aspiration during ECT.
Decreased cardiac output related to vagal stimulation occurring during the ECT	Client demonstrates adequate tissue perfusion during and after treatment (absence of cyanosis or severe change in mental status).
Disturbed thought processes related to side effects of temporary memory loss and confusion	Client maintains reality orientation following ECT treatment.
Self-care deficit related to incapacitation during postictal stage	Client's self-care needs are fulfilled at all times.
Risk for activity intolerance related to post-ECT confusion and memory loss	Client gradually increases participation in therapeutic activities to the highest level of personal capability.

■ Ensure that the most recent laboratory reports (complete blood count, urinalysis) and results of electrocardiogram (ECG) and x-ray examination are available.

■ Approximately 1 hour before treatment is scheduled, take vital signs and record them. Have the client void and remove dentures, eyeglasses or contact lenses, jewelry, and hairpins. Following institutional requirements, the client should change into hospital gown or, if permitted, into own loose clothing or pajamas. Client should remain in bed with side rails up.

■ Approximately 30 minutes before treatment, administer the pretreatment medication as prescribed by the physician. The usual order is for atropine sulfate or glycopyrrolate (Robinul) given intramuscularly. Either of these medications may be ordered to decrease secretions (to prevent aspiration) and counteract the effects of vagal stimulation (bradycardia) induced by the ECT.

■ Stay with the client to help allay fears and anxiety. Maintain a positive attitude about the procedure, and encourage the client to verbalize feelings.

In the treatment room, the client is placed on the treatment table in a supine position. The anesthesiologist administers intravenously a short-acting anesthetic, such as etomidate (Amidate) or methohexital sodium (Brevital). A muscle relaxant, usually succinylcholine chloride (Anectine), is given intravenously to prevent severe muscle contractions during the seizure, thereby reducing the possibility of fractured or dislocated bones. Because succinylcholine paralyzes respiratory muscles as well, the client is oxygenated with pure oxygen during and after the treatment, except for the brief interval of electrical stimulation, until spontaneous respirations return (Sadock & Sadock, 2007). A blood pressure cuff may be placed on the lower leg and inflated above systolic pressure prior to the injection of the succinylcholine. This is to ensure that the seizure activity can be observed in this one limb that is unaffected by the muscle relaxant.

An airway/bite block is placed in the client's mouth and he or she is positioned to facilitate airway patency. Electrodes are placed (either bilaterally or unilaterally) on the temples to deliver the electrical stimulation.

Nursing interventions during the treatment include:

■ Ensure patency of airway. Provide suctioning if needed.

■ Assist anesthesiologist with oxygenation as required.

■ Observe readouts on machines monitoring vital signs and cardiac functioning.

■ Provide support to the client's arms and legs during the seizure.

■ Observe and record the type and amount of movement induced by the seizure.

After the treatment, the anesthesiologist continues to oxygenate the client with pure oxygen until spontaneous respirations return. Most clients awaken within 10 or 15 minutes of the treatment and are confused and disoriented; however, some clients will sleep for 1 to 2 hours following the treatment. All clients require close observation in this immediate post-treatment period.

Nursing interventions in the post-treatment period include:

■ Monitor pulse, respirations, and blood pressure every 15 minutes for the first hour, during which time the client should remain in bed.

■ Position the client on side to prevent aspiration.

■ Orient the client to time and place.

■ Describe what has occurred.

■ Provide reassurance that confusion and memory loss will subside, and memories should return following the course of ECT therapy.

■ Allow the client to verbalize fears and anxieties related to receiving ECT.

■ Stay with the client until he or she is fully awake, oriented, and able to perform self-care activities without assistance.

■ Provide the client with a highly structured schedule of routine activities in order to minimize confusion.

Evaluation

Evaluation of the effectiveness of nursing interventions is based on the achievement of the projected outcomes. Reassessment may be based on answers to the following questions:

■ Was the client's anxiety maintained at a manageable level?

■ Was the client/family teaching completed satisfactorily?

■ Did the client/family verbalize understanding of the procedure, its side effects, and risks involved?

■ Did the client undergo treatment without experiencing injury or aspiration?

■ Has the client maintained adequate tissue perfusion during and following treatment? Have vital signs remained stable?

■ With consideration to the individual client's condition and response to treatment, is the client reoriented to time, place, and situation?

■ Have all of the client's self-care needs been fulfilled?

■ Is the client participating in therapeutic activities to his or her maximum potential?

■ What is the client's level of social interaction?

Careful documentation is an important part of the evaluation process. Some routine observations may be evaluated on flow sheets specifically identified for ECT. However, progress notes with detailed descriptions of client behavioral changes are essential to evaluate improvement and help determine the number of treatments that will be administered. Continual reassessment, planning, and evaluation will ensure that the client receives adequate and appropriate nursing care throughout the course of therapy.

Summary and Key Points

■ Electroconvulsive therapy (ECT) is the induction of a grand mal seizure through the application of electrical current to the brain.

■ It is a safe and effective treatment alternative for individuals with depression, mania, or schizoaffective disorder who do not respond to other forms of therapy.

■ ECT is contraindicated for individuals with increased intracranial pressure.

■ Individuals with cardiovascular problems are at high risk for complications from ECT.

■ Other factors that place clients at risk include severe osteoporosis, acute and chronic pulmonary disorders, and high-risk or complicated pregnancy.

■ The exact mechanism of action of ECT is unknown, but it is thought that the electrical stimulation results in significant increases in the circulating levels of the neurotransmitters serotonin, norepinephrine, and dopamine.

■ The most common side effects with ECT are temporary memory loss and confusion.

■ Although it is rare, death must be considered a risk associated with ECT. When it does occur, the most common cause is cardiovascular complications.

■ There may be a risk for some degree of permanent long-term memory loss, and some opponents suggest that a risk for brain damage also exists (although there is little or no substantiating evidence).

■ The nurse assists with ECT using the steps of the nursing process before, during, and after treatment.

■ Important nursing interventions include ensuring client safety, managing client anxiety, and providing adequate client education.

■ Nursing input into the ongoing evaluation of client behavior is an important factor in determining the therapeutic effectiveness of ECT.

 Additional info available @ davisplus.fadavis.com

Review Questions
Self-Examination/Learning Exercise

*Select the answer that is **most appropriate** for each of the following questions:*

1. Electroconvulsive therapy is most commonly prescribed for:
   a. Bipolar disorder, manic.
   b. Paranoid schizophrenia.
   c. Major depression.
   d. Obsessive-compulsive disorder.

Review Questions—cont'd
Self-Examination/Learning Exercise

2. Which of the following best describes the average number of ECT treatments given and the timing of administration?
   a. One treatment per month for 6 months.
   b. One treatment every other day for a total of 6 to 12.
   c. One treatment three times per week for a total of 20 to 30.
   d. One treatment every day for a total of 10 to 15.

3. Which of the following conditions is considered to be the only absolute contraindication for ECT?
   a. Increased intracranial pressure.
   b. Recent myocardial infarction.
   c. Severe underlying hypertension.
   d. Congestive heart failure.

4. Electroconvulsive therapy is thought to effect a therapeutic response by:
   a. Stimulation of the CNS.
   b. Decreasing the levels of acetylcholine and monoamine oxidase.
   c. Increasing the levels of serotonin, norepinephrine, and dopamine.
   d. Altering sodium metabolism within nerve and muscle cells.

5. The most common side effects of ECT are:
   a. Permanent memory loss and brain damage.
   b. Fractured and dislocated bones.
   c. Myocardial infarction and cardiac arrest.
   d. Temporary memory loss and confusion.

6. Sam has a diagnosis of Major Depression. After an unsuccessful trial of antidepressant medication, Sam's physician has hospitalized Sam for a course of ECT treatments. Sam says to the nurse on admission, "I don't want to end up like McMurphy on *One Flew Over the Cuckoo's Nest!* I'm scared!" Sam's priority nursing diagnosis at this time would be:
   a. Anxiety related to deficient knowledge about ECT.
   b. Risk for injury related to risks associated with ECT.
   c. Deficient knowledge related to negative media presentation of ECT.
   d. Disturbed thought processes related to side effects of ECT.

7. Sam, who has been hospitalized for ECT treatments, says to the nurse on admission, "I don't want to end up like McMurphy on *One Flew Over the Cuckoo's Nest!* I'm scared!" Which of the following statements would be most appropriate by the nurse in response to Sam's expression of concern?
   a. "I guarantee you won't end up like McMurphy, Sam."
   b. "The doctor knows what he is doing. There's nothing to worry about."
   c. "I know you are scared, Sam, and we're going to talk about what you can expect from the therapy."
   d. "I'm going to stay with you as long as you are scared."

8. The priority nursing intervention before starting ECT therapy is to:
   a. Take vital signs and record.
   b. Have the patient void.
   c. Administer succinylcholine.
   d. Ensure that the consent form has been signed.

Continued

Review Questions—cont'd
Self-Examination/Learning Exercise

9. Atropine sulfate is administered to a client receiving ECT for what purpose?
   a. To alleviate anxiety.
   b. To decrease secretions.
   c. To relax muscles.
   d. As a short-acting anesthetic.

10. Succinylcholine is administered to a client receiving ECT for what purpose?
    a. To alleviate anxiety.
    b. To decrease secretions.
    c. To relax muscles.
    d. As a short-acting anesthetic.

References

Abrams, R. (2002). *Electroconvulsive therapy* (4th ed). New York: Oxford University Press.

American Psychiatric Association. (2001). *The practice of electroconvulsive therapy: Recommendations for treatment, training, and privileging* (2nd ed.). Washington, DC: American Psychiatric Publishing.

Black, D. W., & Andreasen, N. C. (2011). *Introductory textbook of psychiatry* (5th ed.). Washington, DC: American Psychiatric Publishing.

Dukakis, K., & Tye, L. (2006). *Shock: The healing power of electroconvulsive therapy.* New York: Penguin Group.

Eisendrath, S. J., & Lichtmacher, J. E. (2009). Psychiatric disorders. In S. J. McPhee & M. A. Papadakis (Eds.), *Current medical diagnosis & treatment* (48th ed., pp. 912–964). New York: McGraw-Hill.

Fetterman, T. C., & Ying, P. (2011). Informed consent and electroconvulsive therapy. *Journal of the American Psychiatric Nurses Association, 17*(3), 219–222.

Fink, M. (1999). Images in psychiatry: Ladislas J. Meduna. *American Journal of Psychiatry, 156,* 1807.

Frank, L. R. (2002). Electroshock: A crime against the spirit. *Ethical Human Sciences & Services, 4*(1), 63–71.

Geddes, J. R. (2003). Efficacy and safety of electroconvulsive therapy in depressive disorders: A systematic review and meta-analysis. *Lancet, 361,* 799–808.

Grover, S., Mattoo, S. K., & Gupta, N. (2005). Theories on mechanism of action of electroconvulsive therapy. *German Journal of Psychiatry, 8*(4), 70–84.

Joska, J. A., & Stein, D. J. (2008). Mood disorders. In R. E. Hales, S. C. Yudofsky, & G. O. Gabbard (Eds.), *Textbook of psychiatry* (5th ed., pp. 457–503). Washington, DC: American Psychiatric Publishing.

Karasu, T. B., Gelenberg, A., Merriam, A., & Wang, P. (2006). Practice guideline for the treatment of patients with major depressive disorder. *Practice guidelines for the treatment of psychiatric disorders, Compendium 2006.* Washington, DC: American Psychiatric Publishing.

Kellner, C. H. (2010, May 11). Speed of response to ECT. *Psychiatric Times, 27*(5). Retrieved August 21, 2010, from http://www.psychiatrictimes.com/display/article/10168/1567001

Marangell, L. B., Silver, J. M., Goff, D. C., & Yudofsky, S. C. (2003). Psychopharmacology and electroconvulsive therapy. In R. E. Hales & S. C. Yudofsky (Eds.), *Textbook of clinical psychiatry* (pp. 1047–1149). Washington, DC: American Psychiatric Publishing.

McClintock, S. M., & Husain, M. M. (2011). Electroconvulsive therapy does not damage the brain. *Journal of the American Psychiatric Nurses Association, 17*(3), 212–213.

Sackeim, H. A., Prudic, J., Fuller, R., Keilp, J., Lavori, P. W., & Olfson, M. (2007). The cognitive effects of electroconvulsive therapy in community settings. *Neuropsychopharmacology, 32,* 244-254.

Sadock, B. J., & Sadock, V. A. (2007). *Synopsis of psychiatry: Behavioral sciences/clinical psychiatry* (10th ed.). Philadelphia: Lippincott Williams & Wilkins.

Wahlund, B., & von Rosen, D. (2003). ECT of major depressed patients in relation to biological and clinical variables: A brief overview. *Neuropsychopharmacology, 28,* S21–S26.

Complementary Therapies

CORE CONCEPTS
alternative medicine
complementary
medicine

KEY TERMS

acupoints
acupressure
acupuncture
allopathic medicine
chiropractic medicine

meridians
qi
subluxation
yoga

OBJECTIVES
After reading this chapter, the student will be able to:

1. Compare and contrast various types of conventional and alternative therapies.
2. Describe the philosophies behind various complementary therapies, including herbal medicine, acupressure and acupuncture, diet and nutrition, chiropractic medicine,

therapeutic touch and massage, yoga, and pet therapy.
3. Discuss the historical background of various complementary therapies.
4. Describe the techniques used in various complementary therapies.

HOMEWORK ASSIGNMENT
Please read the chapter and answer the following questions:

1. How do alternative medicine and complementary medicine differ?
2. What is the Western medical philosophy regarding the efficacy of acupressure and acupuncture?
3. What herbal remedy has been used effectively for relief of migraine headaches?
4. What is the major difference in focus between conventional medicine and alternative/complementary medicine?

The History of Medicine

2000 BC—Here, eat this root.

1000 AD—That root is heathen. Here, say this prayer.

1850 AD—That prayer is superstition. Here, drink this potion.

1940 AD—That potion is snake oil. Here, swallow this pill.

1985 AD—That pill is ineffective. Here, take this antibiotic.

2000 AD—That antibiotic is ineffective and dangerous. Here, eat this root.

Anonymous

The connection between mind and body, and the influence of each on the other, is well recognized by all clinicians, and particularly by psychiatrists. Conventional medicine as it is currently practiced in the United States is based solely on scientific methodology. Conventional, science-based medicine, also known as **allopathic medicine**, is the type of medicine historically taught in U.S. medical schools. Many individuals today are choosing to move away from conventional medicine by trying a variety of alternative approaches to health care.

CORE CONCEPT

Alternative medicine

Interventions that differ from the traditional or conventional biomedical treatment of disease. "Alternative" refers to an intervention that is used *instead* of conventional treatment.

Some individuals do not completely abandon traditional medicine for alternative therapies. Instead, they may choose to *complement* the conventional methods with the addition of alternative strategies.

CORE CONCEPT

Complementary medicine

A complementary therapy is an intervention that is different from, but used *in conjunction with,* traditional or conventional medical treatment.

In the United States, approximately 38 percent of adults and 12 percent of children use some form of complementary or alternative therapy (National Institutes of Health [NIH], 2008). When prayer specifically for health reasons is included in the definition of complementary and alternative medicine, the numbers are even higher. More than $27 billion a year is spent on these types of therapies in the United States.

In 1991, an Office of Alternative Medicine (OAM) was established by the NIH to study nontraditional therapies and to evaluate their usefulness and their effectiveness. Since that time, the name has been changed to the National Center for Complementary and Alternative Medicine (NCCAM). According to the mission statement of NCCAM:

> NCCAM's mission is to explore complementary and alternative healing practices in the context of rigorous science, train CAM researchers, and disseminate authoritative information to the public and professionals. (NIH, 2008, p. 4)

Although there is no universal classification for complementary and alternative medicine (CAM), NCCAM has grouped CAM practices and modalities into five domains. Some types of practices may overlap; that is, they may fall within more than one domain (e.g., *qi gong* is considered both part of Chinese medicine and an energy therapy). Within the five major domains, the practices have been subdivided into three categories: (1) those that fall under CAM, (2) those that are found in conventional health care but are classified as behavioral medicine, and (3) those that overlap between the two (DeSantis, 2009). A list of the NCCAM classification of complementary and alternative medicine practices and examples of each is presented in Table 22-1. Figure 22–1 shows the 10 most common CAM therapies among adults.

Some health insurance companies and health maintenance organizations (HMOs) appear to be bowing to public pressure by including alternative providers in their networks of providers for

TABLE 22-1 Classification of Complementary and Alternative Medicine Practices		
CATEGORY	**EXAMPLES**	
I. Alternative Medical Systems	**a. Traditional Oriental Medicine[1]**	
	■ Acupuncture	■ Diet
	■ Herbal formulas	■ Tai Chi
	■ Massage & manipulation	■ Qi Gong
	b. Traditional Indigenous Systems[1]	
	■ Ayurvedic medicine	■ Unani-tibbi
	■ Native American	■ Kampo
	■ Traditional African	■ Curanderismo
	■ Traditional Aboriginal	■ SIDDHI
	■ Central and South American	

TABLE 22-1 Classification of Complementary and Alternative Medicine Practices—cont'd

CATEGORY	EXAMPLES

c. Unconventional Western Systems
- Homeopathy[1]
- Functional medicine[1]
- Orthomolecular medicine[1]
- Environmental medicine[1]
- Anthroposophically-extended medicine[2]

d. Naturopathy[1]
- Natural systems and therapies

II. Mind-Body Interventions

a. Mind-Body Methods

■ Yoga[1]	■ Hypnosis[2]	■ Humor[3]
■ Tai Chi[1]	■ Meditation[2]	■ Journaling[3]
■ Internal qi gong[1]	■ Biofeedback[2]	■ Art, music, & dance therapies[3]

b. Religion and Spirituality[1]

■ Confession	■ Soul retrieval
■ Nonlocality	■ "Special" healers
■ Nontemporality	■ Spiritual healing

c. Social and Contextual Areas
- Caring-based approaches (e.g., holistic nursing, pastoral care)[1]
- Intuitive diagnosis[1]
- Explanatory models[3]
- Placebo[3]
- Community-based approaches (e.g., Native American "sweat" rituals)[3]

III. Biologically-Based Therapies

a. Phytotherapy or Herbalism[1]

■ Aloe vera	■ Ginseng
■ Bee pollen	■ Green tea
■ Ginkgo biloba	■ Hawthorne
■ Feverfew	■ Kava kava
■ Cat's claw	■ Licorice root
■ Dong quai	■ Mistletoe
■ Echinacea	■ Peppermint oil
■ Evening primrose	■ Saw palmetto
■ Garlic	■ Witch hazel
■ Ginger	■ Valerian

b. Special Diet Therapies[1]

■ Atkins	■ Asian
■ Diamond	■ Fasting
■ Kelly-Gonzalez	■ High fiber
■ Gerson	■ Macrobiotic
■ Livingston-Wheeler	■ Mediterranean
■ McDougall	■ Natural hygiene
■ Ornish	■ Paleolithic
■ Pritikin	■ Vegetarian
■ Wigmore	

c. Orthomolecular Therapies[1]
Single nutrients (partial listing)

■ Ascorbic acid	■ Carotenes	■ Tocopherols
■ Folic acid	■ Niacin	■ Niacinamide

Continued

TABLE 22-1 Classification of Complementary and Alternative Medicine Practices—cont'd

CATEGORY	EXAMPLES

- Pantothenic acid
- Thiamine
- Vitamin K
- Calcium
- Potassium
- Tyrosine
- Manganese
- Coenzyme Q10
- Glutamine
- Lipoic acid
- Fatty acids

- Pyridoxine
- Vitamin A
- Biotin
- Magnesium
- Taurine
- Iodine
- Boron
- Carnitine
- Glucosamine
- Amino acids
- DHEA

- Riboflavin
- Vitamin D
- Choline
- Selenium
- Lycine
- Iron
- Silicon
- Probiotics
- Chondroitin
- Melatonin
- Medium-chain triglycerides

d. Pharmacological, Biological, and Instrumental Inverventions[1]

Products (partial listing)

- Coley's toxins
- Cartilage
- Cone therapy
- Cell therapy
- Antineoplastons

- Enderlin products
- Enzyme therapies
- Gallo immunotherapy
- H_2O_2
- Bee pollen

- Hyperbaric oxygen
- Ozone
- Revici system
- nduced remission therapy

Procedures/devices

- Apitherapy
- Bioresonance
- Chirography
- Electrodiagnostics

- Iridology
- MORA device
- Neural therapy

IV. Manipulative and Body-Based Methods

a. Chiropractic Medicine[1]

b. Massage and Bodywork[1]

- Osteopathic manipulative therapy
- Cranial-sacral OMT
- Swedish massage
- Applied kinesiology
- Reflexology
- Pilates method
- Polarity

- Trager bodywork
- Alexander technique
- Feldenkrais technique
- Chinese tui na massage
- Acupressure
- Rolfing
- Body psychotherapy

c. Unconventional Physical Therapies[1]

- Hydrotherapy
- Diathermy
- Light and color therapies

- Colonics
- Heat and electrotherapies
- Alternate nostril breathing

V. Energy Therapies

a. Biofield Therapies[1]

- External qi gong
- Healing science
- Healing touch
- Natural healing

- Huna
- Reiki
- Biorelax
- Therapeutic touch

b. Bioelectromagnetic-based Therapies[1]

- Unconventional use of electromagnetic fields for medical purposes

KEY: [1]*CAM therapies.*
[2]*Behavioral medicine therapies.*
[3]*Overlapping therapies (either CAM or behavioral medicine).*
SOURCES: *Ashar and Dobs (2006); DeSantis (2009); and National Center for Complementary and Alternative Medicine (2010).*

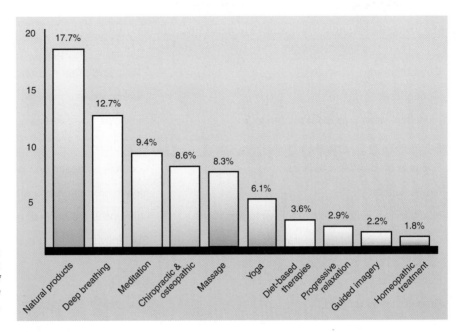

FIGURE 22–1 Ten most common CAM therapies among adults. (From National Institutes of Health. [2008]. *The use of complementary and alternative medicine in the United States.* NCCAM Publication No. D424. Bethesda, MD: Author.)

treatments such as acupuncture and massage therapy. Chiropractic care has been covered by some third-party payers for many years. Individuals who seek alternative therapy, however, are often reimbursed at lower rates than those who choose conventional practitioners.

Client education is an important part of complementary care. Positive lifestyle changes are encouraged, and practitioners serve as educators as well as treatment specialists. Complementary medicine is viewed as *holistic* health care, which deals not only with the physical perspective, but also the emotional and spiritual components of the individual. Interest in holistic health care is increasing worldwide. A large number of U.S. medical schools—among them Harvard, Yale, Johns Hopkins, and Georgetown Universities—now offer coursework in holistic methods (Neddermeyer, 2006). The American Medical Association (AMA, 2010), in its Policy #H-480-973, "encourages its members to become better informed regarding the practices and techniques of alternative or unconventional medicine."

This chapter examines various complementary therapies by describing the therapeutic approach and identifying the conditions for which the therapy is intended. Although most are not founded in scientific principle, they have been shown to be effective in the treatment of certain disorders, and merit further examination as a viable component of holistic health care.

Commonalities and Contrasts

A number of commonalities and contrasts exist between complementary medicine and conventional health care. DeSantis (2009) stated:

> Conventional medicine focuses on the physical or material part of the person, the body. It is concerned with the structure, function, and connections or communication between material elements that compose the body, such as bones, muscles, and nerves. Conventional medicine generally views all humans as being very similar biologically. Disease is seen as a deviation from what is generally considered to be a normal biological or somatic state.
>
> In contrast, the alternative approach views the person-body as consisting of multiple, integrated elements that incorporate both the materialistic and nonmaterialistic aspects of existence. These elements include the physical, spiritual, energetic, and social bodies. From this viewpoint, diagnostic measures and interventions cannot be based on only one aspect of the person's being, but must be tailored to the person-body of each individual. (pp. 510; 512)

A summary of these characteristics is presented in Table 22-2.

TABLE 22-2 Commonalities and Contrasts Between Conventional and Complementary or Alternative Therapies

CONVENTIONAL	COMPLEMENTARY/ALTERNATIVE
Chemotherapy	Plants and other natural products
Curing/treating	Healing/ministering care
Individual viewed as disease category	Individual is viewed as a unique being
End-stage	Hope/hopefulness
Focus is on disease and illness	Focus is on health and wellness
Illness treatment	Health promotion and illness prevention
Nutrition is adjunct and supportive to treatment	Nutrition is the basis of health, wellness, and treatment
Objectivism: Person is separate from his/her disease	Subjectivism: person is integral to the illness
Patient/Client	Person
Practitioner as authority	Practitioner as facilitator
Practitioner paternalism/patient dependency	Practitioner as partner/person empowerment
Positivism/materialism: data are physically measurable	Metaphysical: Entity is energy system or vital force
Reductionistic	Holistic
Specialist care	Self-care
Symptom relief	Alleviation of causative factors
Somatic (biological and physiological) model	Behavioral-psycho-social-spiritual model
Science is only source of knowledge and truth	Multiple sources of knowledge and truth
Technology/invasive	Natural/noninvasive

From DeSantis, L. (2009). Alternative and complementary healing practices. In J. T. Catalano (Ed.), Nursing now! Today's issues, tomorrow's trends (5th ed., p. 511). Philadelphia: F.A. Davis, with permission.

Types of Complementary Therapies

Herbal Medicine

The use of plants to heal is probably as old as humankind. Virtually every culture in the world has relied on herbs and plants to treat illness. Clay tablets from about 4000 B.C. reveal that the Sumerians had apothecaries for dispensing medicinal herbs. At the root of Chinese medicine is the *Pen Tsao,* a Chinese text written around 3000 B.C., which contained hundreds of herbal remedies. When the Pilgrims came to America in the 1600s, they brought with them a variety of herbs to be established and used for medicinal purposes. The new settlers soon discovered that the Native Americans also had their own varieties of plants that they used for healing.

Many people are seeking a return to herbal remedies, because they perceive them as being less potent than prescription drugs and as being free of adverse side effects. However, because the U.S. Food and Drug Administration (FDA) classifies herbal remedies as dietary supplements or food additives, their labels cannot indicate medicinal uses. They are not subject to FDA approval, and they lack uniform standards of quality control.

Several organizations have been established to attempt regulation and control of the herbal industry. They include the Council for Responsible Nutrition, the American Herbal Association, and the American Botanical Council. The Commission E of the German Federal Health Agency is the group responsible for researching and regulating the safety and efficacy of herbs and plant medicines in

Germany. All of the Commission E monographs of herbal medicines have been translated into English and compiled into one text (Blumenthal, 1998).

Until more extensive testing has been completed on humans and animals, the use of herbal medicines must be approached with caution and responsibility. *The notion that something being "natural" means it is therefore completely safe is a myth.* In fact, some of the plants from which prescription drugs are derived are highly toxic in their natural state. Also, because of lack of regulation and standardization, ingredients may be adulterated. Their method of manufacture also may alter potency. For example, dried herbs lose potency rapidly because of exposure to air. In addition, it is often safer to use preparations that contain only one herb. There is a greater likelihood of unwanted side effects with combined herbal preparations.

Table 22-3 lists information about common herbal remedies, with possible implications for psychiatric/mental health nursing. Botanical names, medicinal uses, and safety profiles are included.

TABLE 22-3 Herbal Remedies

COMMON NAME (BOTANICAL NAME)	MEDICINAL USES/POSSIBLE ACTION	SAFETY PROFILE
Black cohosh (*Cimicifuga racemosa*)	May provide relief of menstrual cramps; improved mood; calming effect. Extracts from the roots are thought to have action similar to estrogen.	Generally considered safe in low doses. Occasionally causes GI discomfort. Toxic in large doses, causing dizziness, nausea, headaches, stiffness, and trembling. Should not take with heart problems, concurrently with antihypertensives, or during pregnancy.
Cascara sagrada (*Rhamnus purshiana*)	Relief of constipation	Generally recognized as safe; sold as over-the-counter drug in the United States. Should not be used during pregnancy. Contraindicated in bowel obstruction or inflammation.
Chamomile (*Matricaria chamomilla*)	As a tea, is effective as a mild sedative in the relief of insomnia. May also aid digestion, relieve menstrual cramps, and settle upset stomach.	Generally recognized as safe when consumed in reasonable amounts.
Echinacea (*Echinacea angustifolia* and *Echinacea purpurea*)	Stimulates the immune system; may have value in fighting infections and easing the symptoms of colds and flu.	Considered safe in reasonable doses. Observe for side effects or allergic reaction.
Fennel (*Foeniculum vulgare* or *Foeniculum officinale*)	Used to ease stomachaches and to aid digestion. Taken in a tea or in extracts to stimulate the appetites of people with anorexia (1–2 tsp. seeds steeped in boiling water for making tea).	Generally recognized as safe when consumed in reasonable amounts.

Continued

TABLE 22-3 Herbal Remedies—cont'd

COMMON NAME (BOTANICAL NAME)	MEDICINAL USES/POSSIBLE ACTION	SAFETY PROFILE
Feverfew (Tanacetum parthenium)	Prophylaxis and treatment of migraine headaches. Effective in either the fresh leaf or freeze-dried forms (2–3 fresh leaves [or equivalent] per day).	A small percentage of individuals may experience the adverse effect of temporary mouth ulcers. Considered safe in reasonable doses.
Ginger (Zingiber officinale)	Ginger tea to ease stomachaches and to aid digestion. Two powdered gingerroot capsules have shown to be effective in preventing motion sickness.	Generally recognized as safe in designated therapeutic doses.
Ginkgo (Ginkgo biloba)	Used to treat senility, short-term memory loss, and peripheral insufficiency. Has been shown to dilate blood vessels. Usual dosage is 120–240 mg/day.	Safety has been established with recommended dosages. Possible side effects include headache, GI problems, and dizziness. Contraindicated in pregnancy and lactation and in patients with bleeding disorder. Possible compound effect with concomitant use of aspirin or anticoagulants.
Ginseng (Panax ginseng)	The ancient Chinese saw this herb as one that increased wisdom and longevity. Current studies support a possible positive effect on the cardiovascular system. Action not known.	Generally considered safe. Side effects may include headache, insomnia, anxiety, skin rashes, diarrhea. Avoid concomitant use with anticoagulants.
Hops (Humulus lupulus)	Used in cases of nervousness, mild anxiety, and insomnia. Also may relieve the cramping associated with diarrhea. May be taken as a tea, in extracts, or capsules.	Generally recognized as safe when consumed in recommended dosages.
Kava kava (Piper methysticum)	Used to reduce anxiety while promoting mental acuity. Dosage: 150–300 mg bid.	Scaly skin rash may occur when taken at high dosage for long periods. Motor reflexes and judgment when driving may be reduced while taking the herb. Concurrent use with CNS depressants may produce additive tranquilizing effects. Reports of potential for liver damage. Investigations continue. Should not be taken for longer than 3 months without a doctor's supervision.

TABLE 22-3 Herbal Remedies—cont'd

COMMON NAME (BOTANICAL NAME)	MEDICINAL USES/POSSIBLE ACTION	SAFETY PROFILE
Passion flower (*Passiflora incarnata*)	Used in tea, capsules, or extracts to treat nervousness and insomnia. Depresses the central nervous system to produce a mild sedative effect.	Generally recognized as safe in recommended doses.
Peppermint (*Mentha piperita*)	Used as a tea to relieve upset stomachs and headaches and as a mild sedative. Pour boiling water over 1 tbsp. dried leaves and steep to make a tea. Oil of peppermint is also used for inflammation of the mouth, pharynx, and bronchus.	Considered to be safe when consumed in designated therapeutic dosages.
Psyllium (*Plantago ovata*)	Psyllium seeds are a popular bulk laxative commonly used for chronic constipation. Also found to be useful in the treatment of hypercholesterolemia.	Approved as an over-the-counter drug in the United States.
Scullcap (*Scutellaria lateriflora*)	Used as a sedative for mild anxiety and nervousness.	Considered safe in reasonable amounts.
St. John's wort (*Hypericum perforatum*)	Used in the treatment of mild to moderate depression. May block reuptake of serotonin/norepinephrine and have a mild monoamine oxidase (MAO)-inhibiting effect. Effective dose: 900 mg/day. May also have antiviral, antibacterial, and anti-inflammatory properties.	Generally recognized as safe when taken at recommended dosages. Side effects include mild GI irritation that is lessened with food; photosensitivity when taken in high dosages over long periods. Should not be taken with other psychoactive medications.
Valerian (*Valeriana officinalis*)	Used to treat nervousness and insomnia. Produces restful sleep without morning "hangover." The root may be used to make a tea, or capsules are available in a variety of dosages. Mechanism of action is similar to benzodiazepines, but without addicting properties. Daily dosage range: 100–1,000 mg.	Generally recognized as safe when taken at recommended dosages. Side effects may include mild headache or upset stomach. Taking doses higher than recommended may result in severe headache, nausea, morning grogginess, blurry vision. Should not be taken concurrently with central nervous system depressants.

SOURCES: Adapted from Holt and Kouzi (2002); PDR for Herbal Medicines (2007); Pranthikanti (2007); Sadock and Sadock (2007); and Trivieri and Anderson (2002).

CLINICAL PEARL It is important to ask the client about any herbal preparations he or she may be taking. The client may not think to mention these when questioned about current medications being taken. Herbals may interact with other medications, resulting in adverse physiological reactions. Document and report the client's history and current use of any herbal and over-the-counter preparations.

Acupressure and Acupuncture

Acupressure and **acupuncture** are healing techniques based on the ancient philosophies of traditional Chinese medicine dating back to 3000 B.C. The main concept behind Chinese medicine is that healing energy (*qi*) flows through the body along specific pathways called **meridians**. It is believed that these meridians of *qi* connect various parts of the body in a way similar to the way in which lines on a road map link various locations. The pathways link a conglomerate of points, called **acupoints.** Therefore, it is possible to treat a part of the body distant to another because they are linked by a meridian. Trivieri and Anderson (2002) state, "The proper flow of *qi* along energy channels (meridians) within the body is crucial to a person's health and vitality" (p. 435).

In acupressure, the fingers, thumbs, palms, or elbows are used to apply pressure to the acupoints. This pressure is thought to dissolve any obstructions in the flow of healing energy and to restore the body to a healthier functioning. In acupuncture, hair-thin, sterile, disposable, stainless-steel needles are inserted into acupoints to dissolve the obstructions along the meridians. The needles may be left in place for a specified length of time, they may be rotated, or a mild electrical current may be applied. An occasional tingling or numbness is experienced, but little to no pain is associated with the treatment (NCCAM, 2009).

The Western medical philosophy regarding acupressure and acupuncture is that they stimulate the body's own painkilling chemicals—the morphine-like substances known as *endorphins.* These treatments have been found to be effective in the treatment of asthma, dysmenorrhea, cervical pain, insomnia, anxiety, depression, substance abuse, stroke rehabilitation, nausea of pregnancy, postoperative and chemotherapy-induced nausea and vomiting, tennis elbow, fibromyalgia, low back pain, carpal tunnel syndrome, and many other conditions (Council of Acupuncture and Oriental Medicine Associations [CAOMA], 2010a; NCCAM, 2009; Sadock & Sadock, 2007). Recent studies suggest that acupuncture may aid in the treatment of cocaine dependence and chronic daily headaches (Avants, Margolin, Holford, & Kosten, 2000; Coeytaux et al., 2005).

Acupuncture is gaining wide acceptance in the United States by both patients and physicians. This treatment can be administered at the same time other techniques are being used, such as conventional Western techniques, although it is essential that all health-care providers have knowledge of all treatments being received. Acupuncture should be administered by a physician or an acupuncturist who is licensed by the state in which the service is provided. Typical training for licensed acupuncturists, doctors of oriental medicine, and acupuncture physicians is a 3- or 4-year program of 2,500 to 3,500 hours. Medical doctors and chiropractors who practice acupuncture must undergo 50 to 200 hours of acupuncture training. The National Commission for the Certification of Acupuncture and Oriental Medicine (NCCAOM) is attempting to set minimal competency standards in the United States through certification by their organization. A number of states have adopted NCCAOM's examination as part of their licensing criteria. Others, such as California, have their own licensing examination and set higher standards than those established by NCCAOM (CAOMA, 2010b).

Diet and Nutrition

The value of nutrition in the healing process has long been underrated. Lutz and Przytulski (2011) stated:

> Good nutrition is essential for good health and important for physical growth and development, good body composition, and mental development. A person's nutritional state can protect him from or predispose him toward chronic disease. Only recently has it been discovered that nutrition influences our genetic code. Medical treatment for many diseases includes diet therapy. Nutrition is thus both a preventive and a therapeutic science. (p. 5)

Individuals select the foods they eat based on a number of factors, not the least of which is enjoyment. Eating must serve social and cultural, as well as nutritional, needs. The U.S. Departments of Agriculture (USDA) and Health and Human Services (USDHHS) have collaborated on a set of guidelines to help individuals understand what types of foods to eat and the healthy lifestyle they need to pursue in order to promote health and prevent disease. Following is a list of key recommendations from these guidelines (USDA/USDHHS, 2010).

Balancing Calories to Manage Weight

■ Prevent and/or reduce overweight and obesity through improved eating and physical activity behaviors.

■ Control total calorie intake to manage body weight. For people who are overweight or obese, this will mean consuming fewer calories from foods and beverages.

■ Increase physical activity and reduce time spent in sedentary behaviors.

■ Maintain appropriate calorie balance during each stage of life—childhood, adolescence, adulthood, pregnancy and breastfeeding, and older age.

Foods and Food Components to Reduce

■ Reduce daily sodium intake to less than 2,300 milligrams (mg) and further reduce intake to 1,500 mg among persons who are 51 and older and those of any age who are African American or have hypertension, diabetes, or chronic kidney disease. The 1,500 mg recommendation applies to about half of the U.S. population, including children, and the majority of adults.

■ Consume less than 10 percent of calories from saturated fatty acids by replacing them with monounsaturated and polyunsaturated fatty acids.

■ Consume less than 300 mg per day of dietary cholesterol.

■ Keep *trans*-fatty acid consumption as low as possible by limiting foods that contain synthetic sources of *trans*-fats, such as partially hydrogenated oils, and by limiting other solid fats.

■ Reduce the intake of calories from solid fats and added sugars.

■ Limit the consumption of foods that contain refined grains, especially refined grain foods that contain sold fats, added sugars, and sodium.

■ If alcohol is consumed, it should be consumed in moderation—up to one drink per day for women and two drinks per day for men—and only by adults of legal drinking age. One drink is defined as:

• 12 ounces of regular beer (150 calories)
• 5 ounces of wine (100 calories)
• 1.5 ounces of 80-proof distilled spirits (100 calories)

Alcohol should be avoided by individuals who are unable to restrict their intake; women who are pregnant, may become pregnant, or are breast-feeding; and individuals who are taking medications that may interact with alcohol or who have specific medical conditions.

Foods and Nutrients to Increase

Individuals should meet the following recommendations as part of a healthy eating pattern while staying within their calorie needs:

■ Increase vegetable and fruit intake.

■ Eat a variety of vegetables, especially dark-green and red and orange vegetables and beans and peas.

■ Consume at least half of all grains as whole grains. Increase whole-grain intake by replacing refined grains with whole grains.

■ Increase intake of fat-free or low-fat milk and milk products, such as milk, yogurt, cheese, or fortified soy beverages.

■ Choose a variety of protein foods, which include seafood, lean meat and poultry, eggs, beans and peas, soy products, and unsalted nuts and seeds.

■ Increase the amount and variety of seafood consumed by choosing seafood in place of some meat and poultry.

■ Replace protein foods that are higher in solid fats with choices that are lower in solid fats and calories and/or are sources of oils.

■ Use oils to replace solid fats where possible.

■ Choose foods that provide more potassium, dietary fiber, calcium, and vitamin D, which are nutrients of concern in American diets. These foods include vegetables, fruits, whole grains, and milk and milk products.

■ Meet recommended intakes within energy needs by adopting a balanced eating pattern, such as the USDA Food Guide (Table 22-4). Table 22-5 provides a summary of information about essential vitamins and minerals.

Building Healthy Eating Patterns

■ Select an eating pattern that meets nutrient needs over time at an appropriate calorie level.

■ Account for all foods and beverages consumed and assess how they fit within a total healthy eating pattern.

■ Follow food safety recommendations when preparing and eating foods to reduce the risk of food-borne illnesses.

TABLE 22-4 Sample USDA Food Guide at the 2,000-Calorie Level

FOOD GROUPS AND SUBGROUPS	USDA FOOD GUIDE DAILY AMOUNT	EXAMPLES/EQUIVALENT AMOUNTS
Fruit Group	2 cups (4 servings)	½ cup equivalent is: ■ ½ cup fresh, frozen, or canned fruit ■ 1 medium fruit ■ ¼ cup dried fruit ■ ½ cup fruit juice
Vegetable Group	2.5 cups (5 servings) ■ Dark green vegetables: 3 cups/week ■ Orange vegetables: 2 cups/week ■ Legumes (dry beans/peas): 3 cups/week ■ Starchy vegetables: 3 cups/week ■ Other vegetables: 6.5 cups/week	½ cup equivalent is: ■ ½ cup cut-up raw or cooked vegetable ■ 1 cup raw leafy vegetable ■ ½ cup vegetable juice
Grain Group	6 ounce-equivalents ■ Whole grains: 3 ounce-equivalents ■ Other grains: 3 ounce-equivalents	1 ounce-equivalent is: ■ 1 slice bread ■ 1 cup dry cereal ■ ½ cup cooked rice, pasta, cereal
Meat and Beans Group	5.5 ounce-equivalents	1 ounce-equivalent is: ■ 1 oz. cooked lean meat, poultry, or fish ■ 1 egg ■ ¼ cup cooked dry beans or tofu ■ 1 tbsp. peanut butter ■ ½ oz. nuts or seeds
Milk Group	3 cups	1 cup equivalent is: ■ 1 cup low-fat/fat-free milk ■ 1 cup low-fat/fat-free yogurt ■ 1½ oz. low-fat/fat-free natural cheese ■ 2 oz. low-fat/fat-free processed cheese

TABLE 22-4 Sample USDA Food Guide at the 2,000-Calorie Level—cont'd		
FOOD GROUPS AND SUBGROUPS	**USDA FOOD GUIDE DAILY AMOUNT**	**EXAMPLES/EQUIVALENT AMOUNTS**
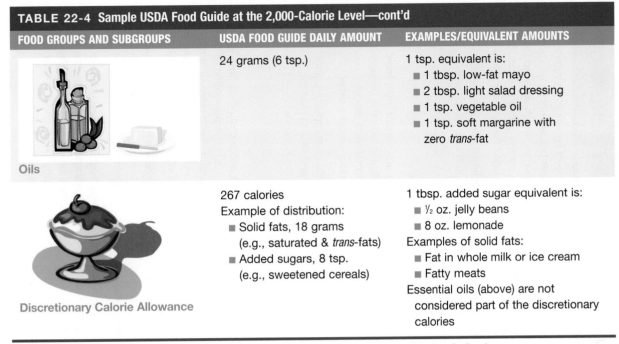 Oils	24 grams (6 tsp.)	1 tsp. equivalent is: ■ 1 tbsp. low-fat mayo ■ 2 tbsp. light salad dressing ■ 1 tsp. vegetable oil ■ 1 tsp. soft margarine with zero *trans*-fat
Discretionary Calorie Allowance	267 calories Example of distribution: ■ Solid fats, 18 grams (e.g., saturated & *trans*-fats) ■ Added sugars, 8 tsp. (e.g., sweetened cereals)	1 tbsp. added sugar equivalent is: ■ ½ oz. jelly beans ■ 8 oz. lemonade Examples of solid fats: ■ Fat in whole milk or ice cream ■ Fatty meats Essential oils (above) are not considered part of the discretionary calories

From U.S. Department of Agriculture & U.S. Department of Health and Human Services. (2010). Dietary Guidelines for Americans 2010. Washington, DC: U.S. Government Printing Office.

Chiropractic Medicine

Chiropractic medicine is one of the most widely used forms of alternative healing in the United States. It was developed in the late 1800s by a self-taught healer named David Palmer. It was later reorganized and expanded by his son Joshua, a trained practitioner. Palmer's objective was to find a cure for disease and illness that did not use drugs, but instead relied on more natural methods of healing (Trivieri & Anderson, 2002). Palmer's theory behind chiropractic medicine was that energy flows from the brain to all parts of the body through the spinal cord and spinal nerves. When vertebrae of the spinal column become displaced, they may press on a nerve and interfere with the normal nerve transmission. Palmer named the displacement of these vertebrae **subluxation,** and he alleged that the way to restore normal function was to manipulate the vertebrae back into their normal positions. These manipulations are called *adjustments.*

Adjustments are usually performed by hand, although some chiropractors have special treatment tables equipped to facilitate these manipulations (Figure 22–2). Other processes used to facilitate the outcome of the spinal adjustment by providing muscle relaxation include massage tables, application of heat or cold, and ultrasound treatments.

The chiropractor takes a medical history and performs a clinical examination, which usually includes x-ray films of the spine. Today's chiropractors may practice "straight" therapy, that is, the only therapy provided is that of subluxation adjustments. *Mixer* is a term applied to a chiropractor who combines adjustments with adjunct therapies, such as exercise, heat treatments, or massage.

Individuals seek treatment from chiropractors for many types of ailments and illnesses; the most common is back pain. In addition, chiropractors treat clients with headaches, neck injuries, scoliosis, carpal tunnel syndrome, respiratory and gastrointestinal disorders, menstrual difficulties, allergies, sinusitis, and certain sports injuries (Trivieri & Anderson, 2002). Some chiropractors are employed by professional sports teams as their team physicians.

Chiropractors are licensed to practice in all 50 states, and treatment costs are covered by government and most private insurance plans. They treat over 20 million people in the United States annually (Sadock & Sadock, 2007).

Therapeutic Touch and Massage

Therapeutic Touch

Therapeutic touch was developed in the 1970s by Dolores Krieger, a nurse associated with the New York University School of Nursing. It is based on

TABLE 22-5 Essential Vitamins and Minerals

VITAMIN/MINERAL	FUNCTION	DRI (UL)*	FOOD SOURCES	COMMENTS
Vitamin A	Prevention of night blindness; calcification of growing bones; resistance to infection	Men: 900 μg (3,000 μg) Women: 700 μg (3,000 μg)	Liver, butter, cheese, whole milk, egg yolk, fish, green leafy vegetables, carrots, pumpkin, sweet potatoes	May be of benefit in prevention of cancer because of its antioxidant properties, which are associated with control of free radicals that damage DNA and cell membranes.[1]
Vitamin D	Promotes absorption of calcium and phosphorus in the small intestine; prevention of rickets	Men and women: 5 μg (50 μg) (5 to 10 μg for ages 50–70 and 15 μg for >70)	Fortified milk and dairy products, egg yolk, fish liver oils, liver, oysters; formed in the skin by exposure to sunlight	Without vitamin D, very little dietary calcium can be absorbed.
Vitamin E	An antioxidant that prevents cell membrane destruction	Men and women: 15 mg (1,000 mg)	Vegetable oils, wheat germ, whole-grain or fortified cereals, green leafy vegetables, nuts	As an antioxidant, may have implications in the prevention of Alzheimer's disease, heart disease, breast cancer.[1]
Vitamin K	Synthesis of prothrombin and other clotting factors; normal blood coagulation	Men: 120 mg (ND)*** Women: 90 mg (ND)***	Green vegetables (collards, spinach, lettuce, kale, broccoli, brussel sprouts, cabbage), plant oils, and margarine	Individuals on anticoagulant therapy should monitor vitamin K intake.
Vitamin C	Formation of collagen in connective tissues; a powerful antioxidant; facilitates iron absorption; aids in the release of epinephrine from the adrenal glands during stress	Men: 90 mg (2,000 mg) Women: 75 mg (2,000 mg)	Citrus fruits, tomatoes, potatoes, green leafy vegetables, strawberries	As an antioxidant, may have implications in the prevention of cancer, cataracts, heart disease. It may stimulate the immune system to fight various types of infection.[1]
Vitamin B₁ (thiamine)	Essential for normal functioning of nervous tissue; coenzyme in carbohydrate metabolism	Men: 1.2 mg (ND)*** Women: 1.1 mg (ND)***	Whole grains, legumes, nuts, egg yolk, meat, green leafy vegetables	Large doses may improve mental performance in people with Alzheimer's disease
Vitamin B₂ (riboflavin)	Coenzyme in the metabolism of protein and carbohydrate for energy	Men: 1.3 mg (ND)*** Women: 1.1 mg (ND)***	Meat, dairy products, whole or enriched grains, legumes, nuts	May help in the prevention of cataracts; high-dose therapy may be effective in migraine prophylaxis (Schoenen, Jacquy, & Lenaerts, 1998).

	Function	Amount	Food Sources	Comments
Vitamin B₃ (niacin)	Coenzyme in the metabolism of protein and carbohydrates for energy	Men: 16 mg (35 mg) Women: 14 mg (35 mg)	Milk, eggs, meats, legumes, whole-grain and enriched cereals, nuts	High doses of niacin have been successful in decreasing levels of cholesterol in some individuals.
Vitamin B₆ (pyridoxine)	Coenzyme in the synthesis and catabolism of amino acids; essential for metabolism of tryptophan to niacin	Men and women: 1.3 mg (100 mg) After age 50: Men: 1.7 mg Women: 1.5 mg	Meat, fish, grains, legumes, bananas, nuts, white and sweet potatoes	May decrease depression in some individuals by increasing levels of serotonin; deficiencies may contribute to memory problems; also used in the treatment of migraines and premenstrual discomfort.
Vitamin B₁₂	Necessary in the formation of DNA and the production of red blood cells; associated with folic acid metabolism	Men and women: 2.4 µg (ND)***	Found in animal products (e.g., meats, eggs, dairy products)	Deficiency may contribute to memory problems. Vegetarians can get this vitamin from fortified foods. Intrinsic factor must be present in the stomach for absorption of vitamin B₁₂.
Folic acid (folate)	Necessary in the formation of DNA and the production of red blood cells	Men and women: 400 µg (1,000 µg) Pregnant women: 600 µg	Meat; green leafy vegetables; beans; peas; fortified cereals, breads, rice, and pasta	Important in women of childbearing age to prevent fetal neural tube defects; may contribute to prevention of heart disease and colon cancer
Calcium	Necessary in the formation of bones and teeth; neuron and muscle functioning; blood clotting	Men and women: 1,000 mg (2,500 mg) After age 50: Men and women: 1,200 mg	Dairy products, kale, broccoli, spinach, sardines, oysters, salmon	Calcium has been associated with preventing headaches, muscle cramps, osteoporosis, and premenstrual problems. Requires vitamin D for absorption.
Phosphorus	Necessary in the formation of bones and teeth; a component of DNA, RNA, ADP, and ATP; helps control acid-base balance in the blood	Men and women: 700 mg (4,000 mg)	Milk, cheese, fish, meat, yogurt, ice cream, peas, eggs	

Continued

TABLE 22-5 Essential Vitamins and Minerals—cont'd

VITAMIN/MINERAL	FUNCTION	DRI (UL)*	FOOD SOURCES	COMMENTS
Magnesium	Protein synthesis and carbohydrate metabolism; muscular relaxation following contraction; bone formation	Men: 420 mg (350 mg)** Women: 320 mg (350 mg)**	Green vegetables, legumes, seafood, milk, nuts, meat	May aid in prevention of asthmatic attacks and migraine headaches. Deficiencies may contribute to insomnia, premenstrual problems.
Iron	Synthesis of hemoglobin and myoglobin; cellular oxidation	Men: 8 mg (45 mg) Women: (45 mg) Childbearing age: 18 mg Over 50: 8 mg Pregnant: 27 mg Breastfeeding: 9 mg	Meat, fish, poultry, eggs, nuts, dark green leafy vegetables, dried fruit, enriched pasta and bread	Iron deficiencies can result in headaches and feeling chronically fatigued.
Iodine	Aids in the synthesis of T_3 and T_4	Men and women: 150 µg (1,100 µg)	Iodized salt, seafood	Exerts strong controlling influence on overall body metabolism.
Selenium	Works with vitamin E to protect cellular compounds from oxidation	Men and women: 55 µg (400 µg)	Seafood, low-fat meats, dairy products, liver	As an antioxidant combined with vitamin E, may have some anti-cancer effect. Deficiency has also been associated with depressed mood.[1]
Zinc	Involved in synthesis of DNA and RNA; energy metabolism and protein synthesis; wound healing; increased immune functioning; necessary for normal smell and taste sensation.	Men: 11 mg (40 mg) Women: 8 mg (40 mg)	Meat, seafood, fortified cereals, poultry, eggs, milk	An important source for the prevention of infection and improvement in wound healing.

[1]The health benefits of antioxidants continue to be investigated.
*Dietary Reference Intakes (UL), the most recent set of dietary recommendations for adults established by the Food and Nutrition Board of the Institute of Medicine, © 2004. UL is the upper limit of intake considered to be safe for use by adults (includes total intake from food, water, and supplements). In addition to the UL, DRIs are composed of the Recommended Dietary Allowance (RDA, the amount considered sufficient to meet the requirements of 97 to 98 percent of all healthy individuals) and the Adequate Intake (AI, the amount considered sufficient where no RDA has been established).
**UL for magnesium applies only to intakes from dietary supplements, excluding intakes from food and water.
***ND, not determined.
Adapted from National Academy of Sciences (2004). Dietary Reference Intakes (DRIs) Tables. Food and Nutrition Board, Institute of Medicine. Retrieved August 26, 2010, from http://fnic.nal.usda.gov/nal_display/index.php?info_center=4&tax_level=3&tax_subject=256&topic_id=1342&level3_id=5140

FIGURE 22–2 Chiropractic adjustments.

the philosophy that the human body projects a field of energy. When this field becomes blocked, pain or illness occurs. Practitioners of therapeutic touch use this method to correct the blockages, thereby relieving the discomfort and improving health.

Based on the premise that the energy field extends beyond the surface of the body, the practitioner need not actually touch the client's skin. The therapist's hands are passed over the client's body, remaining 2 to 4 inches from the skin. The goal is to re-pattern the energy field by performing slow, rhythmic, sweeping hand motions over the entire body. Heat should be felt where the energy is blocked. The therapist "massages" the energy field in that area, smoothing it out, and thus correcting the obstruction. Therapeutic touch is thought to reduce pain and anxiety and promote relaxation and health maintenance. It has proved to be useful in the treatment of chronic health conditions.

Massage

Massage is the technique of manipulating the muscles and soft tissues of the body. Chinese physicians prescribed massage for the treatment of disease more than 5,000 years ago. The Eastern style focuses on balancing the body's vital energy (*qi*) as it flows through pathways (meridians), as described earlier in the discussion of acupressure and acupuncture. The Western style of massage affects muscles, connective tissues, (e.g., tendons and ligaments), and the cardiovascular system. Swedish massage, which is probably the best-known Western style, uses a variety of gliding and kneading strokes along with deep circular movements and vibrations to relax the muscles, improve circulation, and increase mobility (Trivieri & Anderson, 2002).

Massage has been shown to be beneficial in the following conditions: anxiety, chronic back and neck pain, arthritis, sciatica, migraine headaches, muscle spasms, insomnia, pain of labor and delivery, stress-related disorders, and whiplash. Massage is contraindicated in certain conditions, such as high blood pressure, acute infection, osteoporosis, phlebitis, skin conditions, and varicose veins. It also should not be performed over the site of a recent injury, bruise, or burn.

Massage therapists require specialized training in a program accredited by the American Massage Therapy Association and must pass the National Certification Examination for Therapeutic Massage and Bodywork.

Yoga

Yoga is thought to have developed in India some 5,000 years ago and is attributed to an Indian physician and Sanskrit scholar named Patanjali. The objective of yoga is to integrate the physical, mental, and spiritual energies that enhance health and well-being (Trivieri & Anderson, 2002). Yoga has been found to be especially helpful in relieving stress and in improving overall physical and psychological wellness. Proper breathing is a major component of yoga. It is believed that yoga breathing—a deep, diaphramatic breathing—increases oxygen to brain and body tissues, thereby easing stress and fatigue, and boosting energy.

Another component of yoga is meditation. Individuals who practice the meditation and deep breathing associated with yoga find that they are able to achieve a profound feeling of relaxation (Figure 22–3).

The most familiar type of yoga practiced in Western countries is hatha yoga. Hatha yoga uses body postures, along with the meditation and breathing exercises, to achieve a balanced, disciplined workout that releases muscle tension, tones the internal organs, and energizes the mind, body, and spirit, to allow natural healing to occur. The complete routine of poses is designed to work all

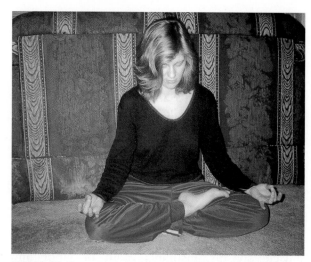

FIGURE 22–3 Achieving relaxation through the practice of yoga.

parts of the body—stretching and toning muscles, and keeping joints flexible. Studies have shown that yoga has provided beneficial effects to some individuals with back pain, stress, migraine, insomnia, high blood pressure, rapid heart rates, and limited mobility (Sadock & Sadock, 2007; Steinberg, 2002; Trivieri & Anderson, 2002).

Pet Therapy

The therapeutic value of pets is no longer just theory. Evidence has shown that animals can directly influence a person's mental and physical well-being. Many pet-therapy programs have been established across the country and the numbers are increasing regularly.

Several studies have provided information about the positive results of human interaction with pets. Some of these include:

1. Petting a dog or cat has been shown to lower blood pressure. In one study, volunteers experienced a 7.1-mm Hg drop in systolic and an 8.1-mm Hg decrease in diastolic blood pressure when they talked to and petted their dogs, as opposed to reading aloud or resting quietly (Whitaker, 2000).

2. Bringing a pet into a nursing home or other institution for the elderly has been shown to enhance a client's mood and social interaction (Godenne, 2001). Another study revealed that animal-assisted therapy with nursing home residents significantly reduced loneliness for those in the study group (Banks & Banks, 2002).

3. One study of 96 patients who had been admitted to a coronary care unit for heart attack or angina revealed that, in the year following hospitalization, the mortality rate among those who did not own pets was 22 percent higher than among pet owners (Whitaker, 2000).

4. Individuals with AIDS who have pets are less likely to suffer from depression than people with AIDS who don't own pets (Siegel, Angulo, Detels, Wesch, & Mullen, 1999).

Some researchers believe that animals actually may retard the aging process among those who live alone (Figure 22–4). Loneliness often results in premature death, and having a pet mitigates the effects of loneliness and isolation. Whitaker (2000) suggested:

> Though owning a pet doesn't make you immune to illness, pet owners are, on the whole, healthier than those who don't own pets. Study after study shows that people with pets have fewer minor health problems, require fewer visits to the doctor and less medication, and have fewer risk factors for heart disease, such as high blood pressure or cholesterol levels. (p. 7)

It may never be known precisely why animals affect humans they way they do, but for those who have pets to love, the therapeutic benefits come as no surprise. Pets provide unconditional, nonjudgmental

FIGURE 22–4 Healthy aging with a pet.

love and affection, which can be the perfect antidote for a depressed mood or a stressful situation. The role of animals in the human healing process still requires more research, but its validity is now widely accepted in both the medical and lay communities.

Summary and Key Points

■ *Alternative* medicine includes those practices that differ from the usual conventional ones in the treatment of disease.

■ *Complementary* therapies are those that work in partnership with conventional medical practice.

■ Complementary therapies help the practitioner view the client in a holistic manner.

■ Most complementary therapies consider the mind and body connection and strive to enhance the body's own natural healing powers.

■ The National Center for Complementary and Alternative Medicine of the National Institutes of Health has established a list of complementary and alternative therapies to be used in practice and for investigative purposes.

■ More than $27 billion a year is spent on alternative medical therapies in the United States.

■ Many people are seeking a return to herbal remedies. Because they do not require FDA approval, their use should be approached with caution and responsibility.

■ With acupressure and acupuncture, pressure is applied (or small needles are inserted) into points along specific pathways of the body called meridians. This is done in an effort to dissolve obstructions in the flow of healing energy and restore the body to a healthier functioning.

■ The value of nutrition in the healing process has long been underrated. Nutrition is, in part, a preventive science. The USDA and USDHHS have collaborated on a set of guidelines to help individuals understand what types of foods to eat and the healthy lifestyle they need to pursue in order to promote health and prevent disease.

■ The theory behind chiropractic medicine is that energy flows from the brain to all parts of the body through the spinal cord and spinal nerves. When vertebrae become displaced, there is interference with normal nerve transmission. Chiropractic adjustments manipulate the displacements back into position, thereby restoring normal functioning.

■ Therapeutic touch promotes relaxation and re-patterns the body's energy field by unblocking obstructions. Massage relaxes muscles, improves circulation, and increases mobility.

■ Yoga serves to integrate the physical, mental, and spiritual energies that enhance health and well-being. Body postures, breathing exercises, and meditation combine to achieve a balanced workout and allow natural healing to occur.

■ The therapeutic benefits of pet ownership are widely accepted. The role of animals in the human healing process still requires more research, but its validity is now widely accepted in both the medical and lay communities.

■ Nurses must be familiar with these therapies, as more and more clients seek out the healing properties of alternative and complementary care strategies.

 DavisPlus   Additional info available @ davisplus.fadavis.com

Review Questions
Self-Examination/Learning Exercise

*Select the answer that is **most** appropriate for the following questions:*

1. Which of the following herbs is thought to be helpful in cases of nervousness, anxiety, and/or insomnia? (Select all that apply.)
   a. Chamomile.
   b. Echinacea.
   c. Kava kava.
   d. Ginseng.
   e. Valerian.
   f. Hops.

Continued

Review Questions—cont'd
Self-Examination/Learning Exercise

2. Which of the following food groups do the USDA/USDHHS food guidelines recommend using in moderation? (Select all that apply.)
   a. Refined carbohydrates.
   b. Fats.
   c. Milk and milk products.
   d. Sodium chloride.
   e. Whole grains.

3. Which of the following herbs is thought to be helpful in relieving menstrual cramping? (Select all that apply.)
   a. Feverfew.
   b. Ginger.
   c. Chamomile.
   d. Black cohosh.

4. With which of the following conditions should massage not be performed? (Select all that apply.)
   a. High blood pressure.
   b. Neck pain.
   c. Arthritis.
   d. Phlebitis.
   e. Osteoporosis.

5. Which of the following applies to vitamin C?
   a. Coenzyme in protein metabolism; found in meat and dairy products.
   b. Necessary in formation of DNA; found in beans and other legumes.
   c. A powerful antioxidant; found in tomatoes and strawberries.
   d. Necessary for blood clotting; found in whole grains and bananas.

6. Which of the following applies to calcium?
   a. Coenzyme in carbohydrate metabolism; found in whole grains and citrus fruits.
   b. Facilitates iron absorption; found in vegetable oils and liver.
   c. Prevents night blindness; found in egg yolk and cantaloupe.
   d. Important for nerve and muscle functioning; found in dairy products and oysters.

7. *Subluxation* is a term used by chiropractic medicine to describe:
   a. Displacement of vertebrae in the spine.
   b. Adjustment of displaced vertebrae in the spine.
   c. Interference with the flow of energy from the brain.
   d. Pathways along which energy flows throughout the body.

8. Nancy has been diagnosed with Dysthymic Disorder. The physician has just prescribed fluoxetine 20 mg/day. Nancy tells the nurse that she has been taking St. John's wort, but still feels depressed. Which of the following is the appropriate response by the nurse?
   a. "St. John's wort is not effective for depression."
   b. "Do not take fluoxetine and St. John's wort together."
   c. "You probably just need to increase your dose of St. John's wort."
   d. "Go ahead and take the St. John's wort with the fluoxetine. Maybe both of them together will be more helpful."

Review Questions—cont'd
Self-Examination/Learning Exercise

9. Joann tells the nurse that she has painful menstrual periods and would like to try an alternative therapy to see if she can get some relief. Which of the following might the nurse suggest for Joann? (Select all that apply.)
   a. Chiropractic.
   b. Black cohosh.
   c. Accupuncture.
   d. Ginkgo biloba.

10. Large doses of which of the following vitamins has been shown to be effective in some people for migraine prophylaxis?
    a. Vitamin D.
    b. Vitamin K.
    c. Vitamin B_2 (riboflavin).
    d. Vitamin B_3 (niacin).

References

American Medical Association. (2010). *Unconventional medical care in the United States.* Policy #H-480-973. Advocacy Resource Center. Chicago: Author.

Ashar, B. H., & Dobs, A. S. (2006). Complementary and alternative medicine. In *The American College of Physicians ACP Medicine.* New York: WebMD Publishing.

Avants, S. K., Margolin, A., Holford, T. R., & Kosten, T. R. (2000). A randomized controlled trial of auricular acupuncture for cocaine dependence. *Archives of Internal Medicine, 160,* 2305–2312.

Banks, M. R., & Banks, W. A. (2002). The effects of animal-assisted therapy on loneliness in an elderly population in long-term care facilities. *Journals of Gerontology Series A: Biological Sciences and Medical Sciences, 57*(7), M428–M432.

Blumenthal, M. (Ed.). (1998). *The complete German Commission E monographs: Therapeutic guide to herbal medicines.* Austin, TX: American Botanical Council.

Coeytaux, R. R., Kaufman, J. S., Kaptchuk, T. J., Chen, W., Miller, W. M., Callahan, L. F., et al. (2005). A randomized, controlled trial of acupuncture for chronic daily headache. *Headache, 45,* 1113–1123.

Council of Acupuncture and Oriental Medicine Associations. (2010a). *Conditions treated by acupuncture and oriental medicine.* Retrieved August 26, 2010, from http://www.acucouncil.org/conditions_treated.htm

Council of Acupuncture and Oriental Medicine Associations. (2010b). *Standards for acupuncture and oriental medicine.* Retrieved August 26, 2010, from http://www.acucouncil.org/aom_standards.htm

DeSantis, L. (2009). Alternative and complementary healing practices. In J. T. Catalano (Ed.), *Nursing Now! Today's issues, tomorrow's trends* (5th ed., pp. 502–531). Philadelphia: F.A. Davis.

Godenne, G. (2001). The role of pets in nursing homes...and psychotherapy. *The Maryland Psychiatrist, 27*(3), 5–6.

Holt, G. A., & Kouzi, S. (2002). Herbs through the ages. In M. A. Bright (Ed.), *Holistic health and healing* (pp. 135–160). Philadelphia: F.A. Davis.

Lutz, C. A., & Przytulski, K. R. (2011). *Nutrition and diet therapy* (5th ed.). Philadelphia: F.A. Davis.

National Academy of Sciences. (2004). *Dietary Reference Intakes (DRIs) Tables.* Food and Nutrition Board, Institute of Medicine. Retrieved August 26, 2010, from http://fnic.nal.usda.gov/nal_display/index.php?info_center=4&tax_level=3&tax_subject=256&topic_id=1342&level3_id=5140

National Center for Complementary and Alternative Medicine. (2009). *Acupuncture: An introduction.* Retrieved August 26, 2010, from http://nccam.nih.gov/health/acupuncture/

National Center for Complementary and Alternative Medicine. (2010). *What is complementary and alternative medicine?* NCCAM Publication No. D347. Bethesda, MD: National Institutes of Health.

National Institutes of Health. (2008). *The use of complementary and alternative medicine in the United States.* NCCAM Publication No. D424. Bethesda, MD: Author.

Neddermeyer, D. M. (2006). Holistic health care increasing in popularity worldwide. *EzineArticles.* Retrieved August 26, 2010, from http://ezinearticles.com/?Holistic-Health-Care-Increasing-in-Popularity-Worldwide&id=373550

PDR for Herbal Medicines (4th ed.). (2007). Montvale, NJ: Thomson PDR.

Pranthikanti, S. (2007). Ayurvedic treatments. In J. H. Lake & D. Spiegel (Eds.), *Complementary and alternative treatments in mental health care* (pp. 225–272). Washington, DC: American Psychiatric Publishing.

Sadock, B. J., & Sadock, V. A. (2007). *Synopsis of psychiatry: Behavioral sciences/clinical psychiatry* (10th ed.). Philadelphia: Lippincott Williams & Wilkins.

Schoenen, J., Jacquy, J., & Lenaerts, M. (1998, February). Effectiveness of high-dose riboflavin in migraine prophylaxis: A randomized controlled trial. *Neurology, 50,* 466–469.

Siegel, J. M., Angulo, F. J., Detels, R., Wesch, J., & Mullen, A. (1999). AIDS diagnosis and depression in the Multicenter AIDS Cohort Study: the ameliorating impact of pet ownership. *AIDS Care, 11*(2), 157–170.

Steinberg, L. (2002). Yoga. In M. A. Bright (Ed.), *Holistic health and healing* (pp. 285–304). Philadelphia: F.A. Davis.

Trivieri, L., & Anderson, J. W. (2002). *Alternative medicine: The definitive guide.* Berkeley, CA: Celestial Arts.

U.S. Department of Agriculture & U.S. Department of Health and Human Services. (2010). *Dietary guidelines for Americans, 2010* (7th ed). Washington, DC: U.S. Government Printing Office.

Whitaker, J. (2000). Pet owners are a healthy breed. *Health & Healing 10*(10), 1–8.

Nursing Care of Clients With Alterations in Psychosocial Adaptation

23 Disorders Usually First Diagnosed in Infancy, Childhood, or Adolescence

CORE CONCEPTS

autism spectrum
  disorders

disruptive behavior
  disorders

hyperactivity

impulsiveness

temperament

CHAPTER OUTLINE

Objectives

Homework Assignment

Mental Retardation

Autistic Disorder

Attention-Deficit/Hyperactivity Disorder

Conduct Disorder

Oppositional Defiant Disorder

Tourette's Disorder

Separation Anxiety Disorder

General Therapeutic Approaches

Summary and Key Points

Review Questions

KEY TERMS

aggression

autistic disorder

clinging

echolalia

impulsivity

negativism

palilalia

OBJECTIVES
After reading this chapter, the student will be able to:

1. Identify psychiatric disorders usually first diagnosed in infancy, childhood, or adolescence.
2. Discuss predisposing factors implicated in the etiology of mental retardation, autistic disorder, attention-deficit/hyperactivity disorder, conduct disorder, oppositional defiant disorder, Tourette's disorder, and separation anxiety disorder.
3. Identify symptomatology and use the information in the assessment of clients with the aforementioned disorders.
4. Identify nursing diagnoses common to clients with these disorders and select appropriate nursing interventions for each.
5. Discuss relevant criteria for evaluating nursing care of clients with selected infant, childhood, and adolescent psychiatric disorders.
6. Describe treatment modalities relevant to selected disorders of infancy, childhood, and adolescence.

HOMEWORK ASSIGNMENT
Please read the chapter and answer the following questions:

1. What maternal prenatal activity has been associated with attention-deficit/hyperactivity disorder (ADHD) in children?
2. What antidepressant medication has been used with some success in treating ADHD?
3. Neuroimaging brain studies in children with Tourette's disorder have been consistent in finding dysfunction in what area of the brain?
4. What are some family behaviors that have been implicated as influential in the development of separation anxiety disorder?

This chapter examines various disorders in which the symptoms usually first become evident during infancy, childhood, or adolescence. That is not to say that some of the disorders discussed in this chapter do not appear later in life or that symptoms associated with other disorders, such as major depression or bipolar disorder, do not appear in childhood or adolescence. These disorders, with consideration of the variances in age and developmental level, are discussed in Chapters 27 and 28.

Developmental theories were discussed in Chapter 3. All nurses working with children or adolescents should be knowledgeable about "normal" stages of growth and development. At best, the developmental process is one that is fraught with frustrations and difficulties. Behavioral responses are individual and idiosyncratic. They are, indeed, *human* responses.

Whether or not a child's behavior indicates emotional problems is often difficult to determine. The *Diagnostic and Statistical Manual of Mental Disorders, Fourth Edition, Text Revision* (DSM-IV-TR) (American Psychiatric Association [APA], 2000) includes the following criteria among many of its diagnostic categories. An emotional problem exists if the behavioral manifestations:

- Are not age-appropriate.
- Deviate from cultural norms.
- Create deficits or impairments in adaptive functioning.

This chapter focuses on the nursing process in care of clients with mental retardation, autistic disorder, attention-deficit/hyperactivity disorder, conduct disorder, oppositional defiant disorder, Tourette's disorder, and separation anxiety disorder. Additional treatment modalities are included.

Mental Retardation

Mental retardation is defined by deficits in general intellectual functioning and adaptive functioning (APA, 2000). General intellectual functioning is measured by an individual's performance on intelligence quotient (IQ) tests. Adaptive functioning refers to the person's ability to adapt to the requirements of daily living and the expectations of his or her age and cultural group. The *DSM-IV-TR* diagnostic criteria for mental retardation are presented in Box 23-1.

Predisposing Factors

The *DSM-IV-TR* (APA, 2000) states that the etiology of mental retardation may be primarily biological

---

BOX 23-1 Diagnostic Criteria for Mental Retardation

A. Significantly subaverage general intellectual functioning: an IQ of approximately 70 or below on an individually administered IQ test (for infants, a clinical judgment of significantly subaverage intellectual functioning).
B. Concurrent deficits or impairments in adaptive functioning (i.e., the person's effectiveness in meeting the standards expected for his or her age by his or her cultural group) in at least two of the following areas: communication, self-care, home living, social/interpersonal skills, use of community resources, self-direction, functional academic skills, work, leisure, health, and safety.
C. The onset is before age 18 years.

From American Psychiatric Association. (2000). Diagnostic and statistical manual of mental disorders (4th ed.) Text revision. Washington, DC: American Psychiatric Publishing, with permission.

---

or primarily psychosocial, or some combination of both. In approximately 30 to 40 percent of individuals seen in clinical settings, the etiology cannot be determined. Five major predisposing factors have been identified.

Hereditary Factors

Hereditary factors are implicated as the cause in approximately 5 percent of the cases. These factors include inborn errors of metabolism, such as Tay-Sachs disease, phenylketonuria, and hyperglycinemia. Also included are chromosomal disorders, such as Down syndrome and Klinefelter syndrome, and single-gene abnormalities, such as tuberous sclerosis and neurofibromatosis.

Early Alterations in Embryonic Development

Prenatal factors that result in early alterations in embryonic development account for approximately 30 percent of mental retardation cases. Damages may occur in response to toxicity associated with maternal ingestion of alcohol or other drugs. Maternal illnesses and infections during embryonic development (e.g., rubella, cytomegalovirus) and complications of pregnancy (e.g., toxemia, uncontrolled diabetes) also can result in congenital mental retardation (Sadock & Sadock, 2007).

Pregnancy and Perinatal Factors

Approximately 10 percent of cases of mental retardation are the result of factors that occur during pregnancy (e.g., fetal malnutrition, viral and other infections, and prematurity) or during the birth process. Examples of the latter include trauma to the head incurred during the process of birth, placenta previa or premature separation of the placenta, and prolapse of the umbilical cord.

General Medical Conditions Acquired in Infancy or Childhood

General medical conditions acquired during infancy or childhood account for approximately 5 percent of cases of mental retardation. They include infections, such as meningitis and encephalitis; poisonings, such as from insecticides, medications, and lead; and physical trauma, such as head injuries, asphyxiation, and hyperpyrexia (Sadock & Sadock, 2007).

Environmental Influences and Other Mental Disorders

Between 15 and 20 percent of cases of mental retardation are attributed to deprivation of nurturance and social, linguistic, and other stimulation, and to severe mental disorders, such as autistic disorder (APA, 2000).

Recognition of the cause and period of inception provides information regarding what to expect in terms of behavior and potential. However, each child is different, and consideration must be given on an individual basis in every case.

Application of the Nursing Process to Mental Retardation

Background Assessment Data (Symptomatology)

The degree of severity of mental retardation is identified by the client's IQ level. Four levels have been delineated: mild, moderate, severe, and profound. The various behavioral manifestations and abilities associated with each of these levels of retardation are outlined in Table 23-1.

TABLE 23-1 Developmental Characteristics of Mental Retardation by Degree of Severity				
LEVEL (IQ)	**ABILITY TO PERFORM SELF-CARE ACTIVITIES**	**COGNITIVE/EDUCATIONAL CAPABILITIES**	**SOCIAL/COMMUNICATION CAPABILITIES**	**PSYCHOMOTOR CAPABILITIES**
Mild (50–70)	Capable of independent living, with assistance during times of stress.	Capable of academic skills to sixth-grade level. As adult, can achieve vocational skills for minimum self-support.	Capable of developing social skills. Functions well in a structured, sheltered setting.	Psychomotor skills usually not affected, although may have some slight problems with coordination.
Moderate (35–49)	Can perform some activities independently. Requires supervision.	Capable of academic skill to second-grade level. As adult, may be able to contribute to own support in sheltered workshop.	May experience some limitation in speech communication. Difficulty adhering to social convention may interfere with peer relationships.	Motor development is fair. Vocational capabilities may be limited to unskilled gross motor activities.
Severe (20–34)	May be trained in elementary hygiene skills. Requires complete supervision.	Unable to benefit from academic or vocational training. Profits from systematic habit training.	Minimal verbal skills. Wants and needs often communicated by acting-out behaviors.	Poor psychomotor development. Only able to perform simple tasks under close supervision.
Profound (below 20)	No capacity for independent functioning. Requires constant aid and supervision.	Unable to profit from academic or vocational training. May respond to minimal training in self-help if presented in the close context of a one-to-one relationship.	Little, if any, speech development. No capacity for socialization skills.	Lack of ability for both fine and gross motor movements. Requires constant supervision and care. May be associated with other physical disorders.

Adapted from American Psychiatric Association (2000); Black and Andreasen (2011); Sadock and Sadock (2007).

Nurses should assess and focus on each client's strengths and individual abilities. Knowledge regarding level of independence in the performance of self-care activities is essential to the development of an adequate plan for the provision of nursing care.

Diagnosis/Outcome Identification

Selection of appropriate nursing diagnoses for the client with mental retardation depends largely on the degree of severity of the condition and the client's capabilities. Possible nursing diagnoses include:

■ Risk for injury related to altered physical mobility or aggressive behavior

■ Self-care deficit related to altered physical mobility or lack of maturity

■ Impaired verbal communication related to developmental alteration

■ Impaired social interaction related to speech deficiencies or difficulty adhering to conventional social behavior

■ Delayed growth and development related to isolation from significant others; inadequate environmental stimulation; hereditary factors

■ Anxiety (moderate to severe) related to hospitalization and absence of familiar surroundings

■ Defensive coping related to feelings of powerlessness and threat to self-esteem

■ Ineffective coping related to inadequate coping skills secondary to developmental delay

Outcome Criteria

Outcome criteria include short- and long-term goals. Timelines are individually determined. The following criteria may be used for measurement of outcomes in the care of the client with mental retardation.

The client:

■ Has experienced no physical harm.

■ Has had self-care needs fulfilled.

■ Interacts with others in a socially appropriate manner.

■ Has maintained anxiety at a manageable level.

■ Is able to accept direction without becoming defensive.

■ Demonstrates adaptive coping skills in response to stressful situations.

Planning/Implementation

Table 23-2 provides a plan of care for the child with mental retardation using selected nursing

---

Table 23-2 CARE PLAN FOR THE CHILD WITH MENTAL RETARDATION

NURSING DIAGNOSIS: RISK FOR INJURY
RELATED TO: Altered physical mobility or aggressive behavior

OUTCOME CRITERIA	NURSING INTERVENTIONS	RATIONALE
Short- and Long-Term Goal • Client will not experience injury.	1. Create a safe environment for the client.	1–5. Client safety is a nursing priority.
	2. Ensure that small items are removed from area where client will be ambulating and that sharp items are out of reach.	
	3. Store items that client uses frequently within easy reach.	
	4. Pad side rails and headboard of client with history of seizures.	
	5. Prevent physical aggression and acting out behaviors by learning to recognize signs that client is becoming agitated.	

Continued

Table 23-2 CARE PLAN FOR THE CHILD WITH MENTAL RETARDATION—cont'd

NURSING DIAGNOSIS: SELF-CARE DEFICIT

RELATED TO: Altered physical mobility or lack of maturity

OUTCOME CRITERIA	NURSING INTERVENTIONS	RATIONALE
Short-Term Goal • Client will be able to participate in aspects of self-care. **Long-Term Goal** • Client will have all self-care needs met.	1. Identify aspects of self-care that may be within the client's capabilities. Work on one aspect of self-care at a time. Provide simple, concrete explanations. Offer positive feedback for efforts. 2. When one aspect of self-care has been mastered to the best of the client's ability, move on to another. Encourage independence but intervene when client is unable to perform.	1. Positive reinforcement enhances self-esteem and encourages repetition of desirable behaviors. 2. Client comfort and safety are nursing priorities.

NURSING DIAGNOSIS: IMPAIRED VERBAL COMMUNICATION

RELATED TO: Developmental alteration

OUTCOME CRITERIA	NURSING INTERVENTIONS	RATIONALE
Short-Term Goal • Client will establish trust with caregiver and a means of communication of needs. **Long-Term Goals** • Client's needs are being met through established means of communication. • If client cannot speak or communicate by other means, needs are met by caregiver's anticipation of client's needs.	1. Maintain consistency of staff assignments over time. 2. Anticipate and fulfill client's needs until satisfactory communication patterns are established. Learn (from family, if possible) special words client uses that are different from the norm. Identify nonverbal gestures or signals that client may use to convey needs if verbal communication is absent. Practice these communications skills repeatedly.	1. Consistency of staff assignments facilitates trust and the ability to understand client's actions and communications. 2. Some children with mental retardation, particularly at the severe level, can only learn by systematic habit training.

NURSING DIAGNOSIS: IMPAIRED SOCIAL INTERACTION

RELATED TO: Speech deficiencies or difficulty adhering to conventional social behavior

OUTCOME CRITERIA	NURSING INTERVENTIONS	RATIONALE
Short-Term Goal • Client will be able to interact with others using behaviors that are socially acceptable and appropriate to developmental level. **Long-Term Goal** • Client will be able to interact with others using behaviors that are socially acceptable and appropriate to developmental level.	1. Remain with client during initial interactions with others on the unit. 2. Explain to other clients the meaning behind some of the client's nonverbal gestures and signals. Use simple language to explain to client which behaviors are acceptable and which are not. Establish a procedure for behavior modification with rewards for appropriate behaviors and aversive reinforcement for inappropriate behaviors.	1. Presence of a trusted individual provides a feeling of security. 2. Positive, negative, and aversive reinforcements can contribute to desired changes in behavior. These privileges and penalties are individually determined as staff learns the likes and dislikes of the client.

diagnoses, outcome criteria, and appropriate nursing interventions and rationales.

Although this plan of care is directed toward the individual client, it is essential that family members or primary caregivers participate in the ongoing care of the client with mental retardation. They need to receive information regarding the scope of the condition, realistic expectations and client potentials, methods for modifying behavior as required, and community resources from which they may seek assistance and support.

Evaluation

Evaluation of care given to the client with mental retardation should reflect positive behavior changes. Evaluation is accomplished by determining if the goals of care have been met through implementation of the nursing actions selected. The nurse reassesses the plan and makes changes where required. Reassessment data may include information gathered by asking the following questions:

- Have nursing actions providing for the client's safety been sufficient to prevent injury?

- Have all of the client's self-care needs been fulfilled? Can he or she fulfill some of these needs independently?

- Has the client been able to communicate needs and desires so that he or she can be understood?

- Has the client learned to interact appropriately with others?

- When regressive behaviors surface, can the client accept constructive feedback and discontinue the inappropriate behavior?

- Has anxiety been maintained at a manageable level?

- Has the client learned new coping skills through behavior modification? Does the client demonstrate evidence of increased self-esteem because of the accomplishment of these new skills and adaptive behaviors?

- Have primary caregivers been taught realistic expectations of the client's behavior and methods for attempting to modify unacceptable behaviors?

- Have primary caregivers been given information regarding various resources from which they can seek assistance and support within the community?

> ## CORE CONCEPT
> ### Autism Spectrum Disorders
> A group of disorders that are characterized by impairment in several areas of development, including social interaction skills and interpersonal communication. Included in this category are autistic disorder, Rett's disorder, childhood disintegrative disorder, pervasive developmental disorder not otherwise specified, and Asperger's disorder (APA, 2000).

Autistic Disorder

Clinical Findings

Autistic disorder is characterized by a withdrawal of the child into the self and into a fantasy world of his or her own creation. The child has markedly abnormal or impaired development in social interaction and communication and a markedly restricted repertoire of activity and interests (APA, 2000). Activities and interests may be considered somewhat bizarre.

Epidemiology and Course

A study by the Autism and Developmental Disabilities Monitoring (ADDM) Network and funded by the Centers for Disease Control and Prevention (CDC) determined the prevalence of Autism Spectrum Disorders (ASDs) in the United States to be about 9 per 1,000 (CDC, 2009). Autistic disorder occurs about four times more often in boys than in girls. Onset of the disorder occurs before age 3, and in most cases it runs a chronic course, with symptoms persisting into adulthood.

Predisposing Factors
Neurological Implications

It is generally accepted that autistic disorder is caused by abnormalities in brain structures or functions (National Institute of Mental Health [NIMH], 2008). Imaging studies have implicated a number of major brain structures associated with the disorder. These include the cerebellum, cerebral cortex, limbic system, corpus callosum, basal ganglia, and brainstem (Black & Andreasen, 2011; NIMH, 2008). The role of neurotransmitters, such as serotonin, dopamine, and epinephrine, is currently under investigation.

Physiological Implications

Ursano, Kartheiser, and Barnhill (2008) identified a number of medical conditions that may be implicated in the predisposition to autistic disorder. These include tuberous sclerosis, fragile X syndrome, maternal rubella, congenital hypothyroidism, phenylketonuria, Down syndrome, neurofibromatosis, and Angelman's syndrome. Ursano and associates (2008) stated, "In the vast majority of cases (likely greater than 90 percent), there is no readily identifiable cause for autism" (p. 879).

Genetics

Research has revealed strong evidence that genetic factors play a significant role in the etiology of autistic disorder (Ursano et al., 2008). Studies have shown that parents who have one child with autistic disorder are at increased risk for having more than one child with the disorder. Other studies with both monozygotic and dizygotic twins also have provided evidence of a genetic involvement. Research into how genetic factors influence the development of autistic disorder is ongoing. A number of linkage studies have implicated areas on several chromosomes to the development of the disorder, most notably chromosomes 2, 7, 15, 16, and 17 (Brkanac, Raskind, & King, 2008; NIMH, 2010; Ursano et al., 2008). The results of a study by the Autism Genome Project Consortium, which was funded by the U.S. National Institutes of Health, have implicated a region on chromosome 11 and aberrations in a brain development gene called *neurexin 1* (Autism Genome Project Consortium, 2007). The researchers stress that these findings strongly suggest the need for further study in this area.

Perinatal Influences

In a study by researchers at Kaiser Permanente in Oakland, California, it was found that women who suffered from asthma and/or allergies around the time of pregnancy were at increased risk of having a child affected by autistic disorder (Croen, Grether, Yoskida, Odouli, & Van dewater, 2005). Women with asthma and allergies recorded during the second trimester had a greater than twofold elevated risk of having a child affected by autistic disorder. The researchers have postulated that this may be due to maternal immune response during pregnancy, or that asthma and allergy may share environmental risk factors with autism spectrum disorders.

Application of the Nursing Process to Autistic Disorder

Background Assessment Data (Symptomatology)

The symptomatology presented here is common among children with autistic disorder. This information, as well as knowledge about predisposing factors associated with the disorder, is important in creating an accurate plan of care for the client.

Impairment in Social Interaction

Children with autistic disorder do not form interpersonal relationships with others. They do not respond to or show interest in people. As infants, they may have an aversion to affection and physical contact. As toddlers, the attachment to a significant adult may be either absent or manifested as exaggerated adherence behaviors. In childhood, there is failure to develop cooperative play, imaginative play, and friendships. Those children with minimal handicaps may eventually progress to the point of recognizing other children as part of their environment, if only in a passive manner.

Impairment in Communication and Imaginative Activity

Both verbal and nonverbal skills are affected. Language may be totally absent, or characterized by immature structure or idiosyncratic utterances whose meaning is clear only to those who are familiar with the child's past experiences. Nonverbal communication, such as facial expression or gestures, is often absent or socially inappropriate. The pattern of imaginative play is often restricted and stereotypical.

Restricted Activities and Interests

Even minor changes in the environment are often met with resistance or sometimes with hysterical responses. Attachment to, or extreme fascination with, objects that move or spin (e.g., fans) is common. Routine may become an obsession, with minor alterations in routine leading to marked distress. Stereotyped body movements (hand clapping, rocking, whole-body swaying) and verbalizations (repetition of words or phrases) are typical. Diet abnormalities may include eating only a few specific foods or consuming an excessive amount of fluids. Behaviors that are self-injurious, such as head banging or biting the hands or arms, may be evident.

The *DSM-IV-TR* (APA, 2000) diagnostic criteria for autistic disorder are presented in Box 23-2.

Diagnosis/Outcome Identification

Based on data collected during the nursing assessment, possible nursing diagnoses for the client with autistic disorder include:

■ Risk for self-mutilation related to neurological alterations

■ Impaired social interaction related to inability to trust; neurological alterations

■ Impaired verbal communication related to withdrawal into the self; inadequate sensory stimulation; neurological alterations

BOX 23-2 Diagnostic Criteria for Autistic Disorder

A. A total of six (or more) items from (1), (2), and (3), with at least two from (1), and one each from (2) and (3):

　1. Qualitative impairment in social interaction, as manifested by at least two of the following:

　　(a) Marked impairment in the use of multiple nonverbal behaviors such as eye-to-eye gaze, facial expression, body postures, and gestures to regulate social interaction.

　　(b) Failure to develop peer relationships appropriate to developmental level.

　　(c) Lack of social or emotional reciprocity.

　2. Qualitative impairments in communication, as manifested by at least one of the following:

　　(a) Delay in, or total lack of, the development of spoken language (not accompanied by an attempt to compensate through alternative modes of communication such as gesture or mime).

　　(b) In individuals with adequate speech, marked impairment in the ability to initiate or sustain a conversation with others.

　　(c) Stereotyped and repetitive use of language or idiosyncratic language.

　　(d) Lack of varied, spontaneous make-believe play or social imitative play appropriate to developmental level.

　3. Restricted repetitive and stereotyped patterns of behavior, interests, and activities, as manifested by at least one of the following:

　　(a) Encompassing preoccupation with one or more stereotyped and restricted patterns of interest that is abnormal either in intensity or focus.

　　(b) Apparently inflexible adherence to specific, nonfunctional routines or rituals.

　　(c) Stereotyped and repetitive motor mannerisms (e.g., hand or finger flapping or twisting, or complex whole-body movements).

　　(d) Persistent preoccupation with parts of objects.

B. Delays or abnormal functioning in at least one of the following areas, with onset prior to age 3 years:

　(1) social interaction, (2) language as used in social communication, or (3) symbolic or imaginative play.

From American Psychiatric Association. (2000). Diagnostic and statistical manual of mental disorders (4th ed.) Text revision. Washington, DC: American Psychiatric Publishing, with permission.

■ Disturbed personal identity related to inadequate sensory stimulation; neurological alterations

Outcome Criteria

Outcome criteria include short- and long-term goals. Timelines are individually determined. The following criteria may be used for measurement of outcomes in the care of the client with autistic disorder.

The client:

■ Exhibits no evidence of self-harm.

■ Interacts appropriately with at least one staff member.

■ Demonstrates trust in at least one staff member.

■ Is able to communicate so that he or she can be understood by at least one staff member.

■ Demonstrates behaviors that indicate he or she has begun the separation/individuation process.

Planning/Implementation

Table 23-3 provides a plan of care for the child with autistic disorder, including selected nursing diagnoses, outcome criteria, and appropriate nursing interventions and rationales.

Evaluation

Evaluation of care for the child with autistic disorder reflects whether the nursing actions have been effective in achieving the established goals. The nursing process calls for reassessment of the plan. Questions for gathering reassessment data may include:

■ Has the child been able to establish trust with at least *one* caregiver?

■ Have the nursing actions directed toward preventing mutilative behaviors been effective in protecting the client from self-harm?

■ Has the child attempted to interact with others? Has he or she received positive reinforcement for these efforts?

■ Has eye contact improved?

■ Has the child established a means of communicating his or her needs and desires to others? Have all self-care needs been met?

■ Does the child demonstrate an awareness of self as separate from others? Can he or she

Table 23-3 CARE PLAN FOR THE CHILD WITH AUTISTIC DISORDER

NURSING DIAGNOSIS: RISK FOR SELF-MUTILATION

RELATED TO: Neurological alterations

OUTCOME CRITERIA	NURSING INTERVENTIONS	RATIONALE
Short-Term Goal • Client will demonstrate alternative behavior (e.g., initiating interaction between self and nurse) in response to anxiety within specified time. (Length of time required for this objective will depend on severity and chronicity of the disorder.) **Long-Term Goal** • Client will not harm self.	1. Work with the child on a one-to-one basis. 2. Try to determine if the self-mutilative behavior occurs in response to increasing anxiety, and if so, to what the anxiety may be attributed. 3. Try to intervene with diversion or replacement activities and offer self to the child as anxiety level starts to rise. 4. Protect the child when self-mutilative behaviors occur. Devices such as a helmet, padded hand mitts, or arm covers may provide protection when the risk for self-harm exists.	1. One-to-one interaction facilitates trust. 2. Mutilative behaviors may be averted if the cause can be determined and alleviated. 3. Diversion and replacement activities may provide needed feelings of security and substitute for self-mutilative behaviors. 4. Client safety is a priority nursing intervention.

NURSING DIAGNOSIS: IMPAIRED SOCIAL INTERACTION

RELATED TO: Inability to trust; neurological alterations

OUTCOME CRITERIA	NURSING INTERVENTIONS	RATIONALE
Short-Term Goal • Client will demonstrate trust in one caregiver (as evidenced by facial responsiveness and eye contract) within specified time (depending on severity and chronicity of disorder). **Long-Term Goal** • Client will initiate social interactions (physical, verbal, nonverbal) with caregiver by time of discharge from treatment.	1. Assign a limited number of caregivers to the child. Ensure that warmth, acceptance, and availability are conveyed. 2. Provide child with familiar objects, such as familiar toys or a blanket. Support child's attempts to interact with others. 3. Give positive reinforcement for eye contact with something acceptable to the child (e.g., food, familiar object). Gradually replace with social reinforcement (e.g., touch, smiling, hugging).	1. Warmth, acceptance, and availability, along with consistency of assignment, enhance the establishment and maintenance of a trusting relationship. 2. Familiar objects and presence of a trusted individual provide security during times of distress. 3. Being able to establish eye contact is essential to the child's ability to form satisfactory interpersonal relationships.

NURSING DIAGNOSIS: IMPAIRED VERBAL COMMUNICATION

RELATED TO: Withdrawal into the self; inadequate sensory stimulation; neurological alterations.

OUTCOME CRITERIA	NURSING INTERVENTIONS	RATIONALE
Short-Term Goal • Client will establish trust with one caregiver (as evidenced by facial responsiveness and eye contact) by specified time (depending on severity and chronicity of disorder).	1. Maintain consistency in assignment of caregivers. 2. Anticipate and fulfill the child's needs until communication can be established.	1. Consistency facilitates trust and enhances the caregiver's ability to understand the child's attempts to communicate. 2. Anticipating needs helps to minimize frustration while the child is learning communication skills.

Table 23-3 CARE PLAN FOR THE CHILD WITH AUTISTIC DISORDER—cont'd

OUTCOME CRITERIA	NURSING INTERVENTIONS	RATIONALE
Long-Term Goal • Client will establish a means of communicating needs and desires to others.	3. Seek clarification and validation. 4. Give positive reinforcement when eye contact is used to convey nonverbal expressions.	3. Validation ensures that the intended message has been conveyed. 4. Positive reinforcement increases self-esteem and encourages repetition.

NURSING DIAGNOSIS: DISTURBED PERSONAL IDENTITY

RELATED TO: Inadequate sensory stimulation; neurological alterations

OUTCOME CRITERIA	NURSING INTERVENTIONS	RATIONALE
Short-Term Goal • Client will name own body parts as separate and individual from those of others. **Long-Term Goal** • Client will develop ego identity (evidenced by ability to recognize physical and emotional self as separate from others) by time of discharge from treatment.	1. Assist child to recognize separateness during self-care activities, such as dressing and feeding. 2. Assist the child in learning to name own body parts. This can be facilitated by the use of mirrors, drawings, and pictures of the child. Encourage appropriate touching of, and being touched by, others.	1. Recognition of body parts during dressing and feeding increases the child's awareness of self as separate from others. 2. All of these activities may help increase the child's awareness of self as separate from others.

name own body parts and body parts of caregiver?

■ Can he or she accept touch from others? Does he or she willingly and appropriately touch others?

Psychopharmacological Intervention for Autistic Disorder

The U.S. Food and Drug Administration (FDA) has approved two medications for the treatment of irritability associated with autistic disorder: risperidone (Risperdal; in children and adolescents 5 to 16 years) and aripiprazole (Abilify; in children and adolescents 6 to 17 years). The behavior symptoms for which these medications are targeted include:

■ Aggression

■ Deliberate self-injury

■ Temper tantrums

■ Quickly changing moods

Dosage of risperidone for autistic disorder is based on weight of the child and the clinical response. In clinical trials, children weighing between 15 and 45 kg received 2.5 mg/day, and those weighing more than 45 kg received 3.5 mg/day. The most common

side effects were drowsiness, mild to moderate increase in appetite, nasal congestion, fatigue, constipation, drooling, dizziness, and weight gain. Although some reports of "abnormal movements" were described, no cases of tardive dyskinesia were reported in clinical studies (Research Units on Pediatric Psychopharmacology Autism Network, 2002, 2005). When administering risperidone, caution must be maintained concerning less common but more serious possible side effects, including neuroleptic malignant syndrome, tardive dyskinesia, hyperglycemia, and diabetes.

In clinical studies with aripiprazole, the most frequently reported adverse events included sedation, fatigue, weight gain, vomiting, somnolence, and tremor. The most common reasons for discontinuation of aripiprazole were sedation, drooling, tremor, vomiting, and extrapyramidal disorder.

Dosage with aripiprazole for irritability in autistic disorder is initiatied at 2 mg/day. Dosage may be increased by 5 mg/day at intervals of no less than 1 week, up to a maximum of 15 mg/day. The efficacy of maintenance therapy with aripiprazole has not been evaluated, and clients should be periodically reassessed to determine the need for continued treatment.

Attention-Deficit/Hyperactivity Disorder

Clinical Findings, Epidemiology, and Course

The essential feature of attention-deficit/hyperactivity disorder (ADHD) is a persistent pattern of inattention and/or hyperactivity-**impulsivity** that is more frequent and severe than is typically observed in individuals at a comparable level of development (APA, 2000). These children are highly distractible and unable to contain stimuli. Motor activity is excessive and movements are random and impulsive. Onset of the disorder is difficult to diagnose in children younger than age 4 years because their characteristic behavior is much more variable than that of older children. Frequently the disorder is not recognized until the child enters school. It is more common in boys than girls by a ratio of 2:1 to 4:1 and may occur in as many as 7 to 10 percent of school-age children (Ferguson-Noyes & Wilkinson, 2008). In about 60 to 70 percent of the cases, ADHD persists into young adulthood, and about 25 percent will subsequently meet the criteria for antisocial personality disorder as adults (Black & Andreasen, 2011).

The *DSM-IV-TR* further categorizes the disorder into the following subtypes:

- **Attention-Deficit/Hyperactivity Disorder, Combined Type.** This subtype is used if at least six symptoms of inattention and at least six symptoms of hyperactivity-impulsivity have persisted for at least 6 months. Most children and adolescents with the disorder have the combined type. It is not known whether the same is true of adults with the disorder.

- **Attention-Deficit/Hyperactivity Disorder, Predominantly Inattentive Type.** This subtype is used if at least six symptoms of inattention (but fewer than six symptoms of hyperactivity-impulsivity) have persisted for at least 6 months.

- **Attention-Deficit/Hyperactivity Disorder, Predominantly Hyperactive-Impulsive Type.** This subtype is used if at least six symptoms of hyperactivity-impulsivity (but fewer than six symptoms of inattention) have persisted for at least 6 months. In many cases, inattention still may be a significant clinical feature.

Predisposing Factors

Biological Influences

Genetics

A number of studies have revealed supportive evidence of genetic influences in the etiology of ADHD. Results have indicated that a large number of parents of hyperactive children showed signs of hyperactivity during their own childhood; that hyperactive children are more likely than normal children to have siblings who are also hyperactive; and that when one twin of an identical twin pair has the disorder, the other is likely to have it too (Kollins, 2008). Adoption studies reveal that biological parents of children with ADHD have more psychopathology than the adoptive parents.

One recent study of genetic evidence for ADHD found copy number variants on a specific region of chromosome 16 (Williams et al., 2010). The researchers also found that copy number variants overlap with chromosomal regions previously linked to autistic disorder and schizophrenia.

Biochemical Theory

Although it is believed that certain neurotransmitters—particularly dopamine, norepinephrine, and possibly serotonin—are involved in producing the symptoms associated with ADHD, their involvement is still under investigation. Abnormal levels of these neurotransmitters may be associated with the symptoms of inattention, hyperactivity, impulsivity, mood, and **aggression** often observed in individuals with the disorder (Faraone, 2006; Hunt, 2006) (see Figure 23–1).

Anatomical Influences

Recent studies have implicated alterations in specific areas of the brain in individuals with ADHD. These regions include the prefrontal lobes, basal ganglia, caudate nucleus, globus pallidus, and cerebellum (Ursano et al., 2008).

FIGURE 23–1 Neurobiology of ADHD.

Neurotransmitters

The major neurotransmitters implicated in the pathophysiology of ADHD are dopamine, norepinephrine, and possibly serotonin. Dopamine and norepinephrine appear to be depleted in ADHD. Serotonin in ADHD has been studied less extensively, but recent evidence suggests that it also is reduced in children with ADHD.

Neurotransmitter Functions

- Norepinephrine is thought to play a role in the ability to perform executive functions, such as analysis and reasoning, and in the cognitive alertness essential for processing stimuli and sustaining attention and thought (Hunt, 2006).
- Dopamine is thought to play a role in sensory filtering, memory, concentration, controlling emotions, locomotor activity, and reasoning.
- Deficits in norepinephrine and dopamine have both been implicated in the inattention, impulsiveness, and hyperactivity associated with ADHD.
- Serotonin appears to play a role in ADHD, although possibly less significant than norepinephrine and dopamine. It has been suggested that alterations in serotonin may be related to the disinhibition and impulsivity observed in children with ADHD. It may play a role in mood disorders, particularly depression, which is a common comorbid disorder associated with ADHD.

Functional Areas of the Brain Affected

- **Prefrontal cortex:** Associated with maintaining attention, organization, and executive function. Also serves to modulate behavior inhibition, with serotonin as the predominant central inhibiting neurotransmitter for this function.
- **Basal ganglia** (particularly the caudate nucleus and globus pallidus): Involved in the regulation of high-level movements. In association with its connecting circuits to the prefrontal cortex, may also be important in cognition. Interruptions in these circuits may result in inattention or impulsivity.
- **Hippocampus:** Plays an important role in learning and memory.
- **Limbic System** (composed of the amygdala, hippocampus, mammillary body, hypothalamus, thalamus, fornix, cingulate gyrus and septum pallucidum): Regulation of emotions. A neurotransmitter deficiency in this area may result in restlessness, inattention, or emotional volatility.
- **Reticular activating system** (composed of the reticular formation [located in the brain brainstem] and its connections): It is the major relay system among the many pathways that enter and leave the brain. It is thought to be the center of arousal and motivation and is crucial for maintaining a state of consciousness.

Continued

Medications for ADHD

CNS STIMULANTS

- Amphetamines (dextroamphetamine, lisdexamfetamine, methamphetamine, and mixtures): cause the release of norepinephrine from central noradrenergic neurons. At higher doses, dopamine may be released in the mesolimbic system.
- Methylphenidate and dexmethylphenidate: block the reuptake of norepinephrine and dopamine into the presynaptic neuron and increase the release of these monoamines into the extraneuronal space.
  Side effects of CNS stimulants include restlessness, insomnia, headache, palpitations, weight loss, suppression of growth in children (with long-term use), increased blood pressure, abdominal pain, anxiety, tolerance, and physical and psychological dependence.

OTHERS

- Atomoxatine: selectively inhibits the reuptake of norepinephrine by blocking the presynaptic transporter.
  Side effects include headache, upper abdominal pain, nausea and vomiting, anorexia, cough, dry mouth, constipation, increase in heart rate and blood pressure, and fatigue.
- Bupropion: inhibits the reuptake of norepinephrine and dopamine into presynaptic neurons.
  Side effects include headache, dizziness, insomnia or sedation, tachycardia, increased blood pressure, dry mouth, nausea and vomiting, weight gain or loss, and seizures (dose dependent).
- Alpha Agonists (clonidine, guanfacine): stimulate central alpha-adrenoreceptors in the brain, resulting in reduced sympathetic outflow from the CNS.
  Side effects include palpitations, bradycardia, constipation, dry mouth, and sedation.

Prenatal, Perinatal, and Postnatal Factors

Studies have linked maternal smoking during pregnancy and hyperkinetic-impulsive behavior in offspring (Linnet et al., 2005; Rizwan, Manning, & Brabin, 2007). Intrauterine exposure to toxic substances, including alcohol, can produce effects on behavior. Fetal alcohol syndrome includes hyperactivity, impulsivity, and inattention, as well as physical anomalies (see Chapter 25).

Perinatal influences that may contribute to ADHD are prematurity or low birth weight, signs of fetal distress, precipitated or prolonged labor, and perinatal asphyxia and low Apgar scores (Bhat, Grizenko, Ben-Amor, & Joober, 2005). Postnatal factors that have been implicated include cerebral palsy, seizures, and other central nervous system (CNS) abnormalities resulting from trauma, infections, or other neurological disorders (Ben-Amor et al., 2005; Popper, Gammon, West, & Bailey, 2003).

Environmental Influences

Environmental Lead

Studies continue to provide evidence of the adverse effects of elevated body levels of lead on cognitive and behavioral development in children. The government has placed tighter restrictions on the substance in recent years, making exposure to toxic levels less prevalent than it once was. Popper and associates (2003) stated:

Both prenatal and postnatal toxic lead exposure can precede ADHD and other cognitive deficits. Transient lead exposure during childhood produces neurocognitive and neurobehavioral abnormalities that may persist for ten or more years. Although its physical toxicity rises in a dose-dependent manner, there appears to be no minimal level below which lead ceases to have toxic effects on the development of cognition. (p. 840)

Diet Factors

The possible link between food dyes and additives, such as artificial flavorings and preservatives, was introduced in the mid-1970s. Studies on the effect of food and food-additive allergies remain controversial, largely because of the inconsistencies in the results. Striking improvement in behavior has been reported by some parents and teachers when hyperactive children are placed on a diet free of dyes and additives. Researchers in Great Britain recently reported on a study that revealed significant hyperactive behavior in 3-, 8-, and 9-year-old children who were given fruit drinks with food additives compared with children who received a placebo drink (McCann et al., 2007). Further study in this area is still required.

Another diet factor that has received much attention in its possible link to ADHD is sugar. A number of studies have been conducted in an effort to determine the effect of sugar on hyperactive behavior, and the results strongly suggest that sugar plays no role in hyperactivity.

Psychosocial Influences

Disorganized or chaotic environments or a disruption in family equilibrium may contribute to ADHD in some individuals. A high degree of psychosocial stress, maternal mental disorder, paternal criminality, low socioeconomic status, living in poverty, growing up in an institution, and unstable foster care have been shown to increase the risk of ADHD in predisposed individuals (Dopheide & Pliszka, 2009; Voeller, 2004).

Application of the Nursing Process to ADHD

Background Assessment Data (Symptomatology)

A major portion of the hyperactive child's problems relate to difficulties in performing age-appropriate tasks. Hyperactive children are highly distractible and have extremely limited attention spans. They often shift from one uncompleted activity to another. Impulsivity, or deficit in inhibitory control, is also common.

Hyperactive children have difficulty forming satisfactory interpersonal relationships. They demonstrate behaviors that inhibit acceptable social interaction. They are disruptive and intrusive in group endeavors. They have difficulty complying with social norms. Some children with ADHD are very aggressive or oppositional, whereas others exhibit more regressive and immature behaviors. Low frustration tolerance and outbursts of temper are common.

Children with ADHD have boundless energy, exhibiting excessive levels of activity, restlessness, and fidgeting. They have been described as "perpetual motion machines," continuously running, jumping, wiggling, or squirming. They experience a greater than average number of accidents, from minor mishaps to more serious incidents that may lead to physical injury or the destruction of property. The *DSM-IV-TR* diagnostic criteria for ADHD are presented in Box 23-3.

Comorbidity

The prevalence of comorbid psychiatric disorders with ADHD may be as high as 84 percent (Ferguson-Noyes & Wilkinson, 2008). Those commonly identified include oppositional defiant disorder, conduct disorder, anxiety, depression, bipolar disorder, and substance abuse. It is extremely

---

BOX 23-3 Diagnostic Criteria for Attention-Deficit/Hyperactivity Disorder

A. Either (1) or (2):

1. Six (or more) of the following symptoms of inattention have persisted for at least 6 months to a degree that is maladaptive and inconsistent with developmental level:

   Inattention

   (a) Often fails to give close attention to details or makes careless mistakes in school work, work, or other activities.

   (b) Often has difficulty sustaining attention in tasks or play activities.

   (c) Often does not seem to listen when spoken to directly.

   (d) Often does not follow through on instructions and fails to finish schoolwork, chores, or duties in the workplace (not because of oppositional behavior or failure to understand instructions).

   (e) Often has difficulty organizing tasks and activities.

   (f) Often avoids, dislikes, or is reluctant to engage in tasks that require sustained mental effort (such as schoolwork or homework).

   (g) Often loses things necessary for tasks or activities (e.g., toys, school assignments, pencils, books, or tools).

   (h) Is often easily distracted by extraneous stimuli.

   (i) Is often forgetful in daily activities.

2. Six (or more) of the following symptoms of hyperactivity-impulsivity have persisted for at least 6 months to a degree that is maladaptive and inconsistent with developmental level:

   Hyperactivity

   (a) Often fidgets with hands or feet or squirms in seat.

   (b) Often leaves seat in classroom or in other situations in which remaining seated is expected.

   (c) Often runs about or climbs excessively in situations in which it is inappropriate (in adolescents or adults, may be limited to subjective feelings of restlessness).

   (d) Often has difficulty playing or engaging in leisure activities quietly.

   (e) Is often "on the go" or often acts as if "driven by a motor."

   (f) Often talks excessively.

BOX 23-3 Diagnostic Criteria for Attention-Deficit/Hyperactivity Disorder—cont'd

Impulsivity

(g) Often blurts out answers before questions have been completed.

(h) Often has difficulty awaiting turn.

(i) Often interrupts or intrudes on others (e.g., butts into conversations or games).

B. Some hyperactive-impulsive or inattentive symptoms that caused impairment were present before age 7 years.

C. Some impairment from the symptoms is present in two or more settings (e.g., at school or work and at home).

D. There is clear evidence of clinically significant impairment in social, academic, or occupational functioning.

E. The symptoms do not occur exclusively during the course of a pervasive developmental disorder, schizophrenia, or other psychotic disorder and are not better accounted for by another mental disorder (e.g., mood disorder, anxiety disorder, dissociative disorder, or a personality disorder).

Subtypes:

1. **Attention-Deficit/Hyperactivity Disorder, Combined Type:** If both criteria A1 and A2 are met for the past 6 months.

2. **Attention-Deficit/Hyperactivity Disorder, Predominantly Inattentive Type:** If criterion A1 is met but criterion A2 is not met for the past 6 months.

3. **Attention-Deficit/Hyperactivity Disorder, Predominantly Hyperactive-Impulsive Type:** If criterion A2 is met but criterion A1 is not met for the past 6 months.

From American Psychiatric Association. (2000). Diagnostic and statistical manual of mental disorders (4th ed.) Text revision. Washington, DC: American Psychiatric Publishing, with permission.

important to identify and treat any comorbid psychiatric conditions in a child with ADHD. In some instances, as with anxiety and depression, the comorbid disorders may be treated concurrently with the symptoms of ADHD. Jenson (2005) suggested that comorbid depression and ADHD may respond to bupropion or atomoxetine as a single agent, and individuals with comorbid anxiety and ADHD may benefit from treatment with atomoxetine (Dopheide & Pliszka, 2009).

Other disorders may require separate treatment. Wilens and Upadhyaya (2007) stated, "In patients with coexisting substance use disorders and ADHD, the priority is to stabilize the addiction before treating the ADHD." Because stimulants can exacerbate mania, it is suggested that medication for ADHD be initiated only after bipolar symptoms have been controlled with a mood stabilizer (Dopheide & Pliszka, 2009). Types of conditions often seen with ADHD and their rate of comorbidity are presented in Table 23-4.

Diagnosis/Outcome Identification

Based on the data collected during the nursing assessment, possible nursing diagnoses for the child with ADHD include:

■ Risk for injury related to impulsive and accident-prone behavior and the inability to perceive self-harm

TABLE 23-4 Type and Frequency of Comorbidity with ADHD

COMORBIDITY	RATES
Oppositional defiant disorder	Up to 50%
Conduct disorder	~ 33%
Learning disorders	20% to 30%
Anxiety	25% to 35%
Depression	~ 26%
Bipolar disorder	11% to 20%
Substance use	13% to 26%

SOURCES: Dopheide and Pliszka (2009); Ferguson-Noyes and Wilkinson (2008); Jenson (2005); and Robb (2006).

■ Impaired social interaction related to intrusive and immature behavior

■ Low self-esteem related to dysfunctional family system and negative feedback

■ Noncompliance with task expectations related to low frustration tolerance and short attention span

Outcome Criteria

Outcome criteria include short- and long-term goals. Timelines are individually determined. The following criteria may be used for measurement of outcomes in the care of the child with ADHD.

The client:

■ Has experienced no physical harm.

■ Interacts with others appropriately.

■ Verbalizes positive aspects about self.

■ Demonstrates fewer demanding behaviors.

■ Cooperates with staff in an effort to complete assigned tasks.

Planning/Implementation

Table 23-5 provides a plan of care for the child with ADHD using nursing diagnoses common to the disorder, outcome criteria, and appropriate nursing interventions and rationales.

Table 23-5 CARE PLAN FOR THE CHILD WITH ATTENTION-DEFICIT/HYPERACTIVITY DISORDER

NURSING DIAGNOSIS: RISK FOR INJURY

RELATED TO: Impulsive and accident-prone behavior and the inability to perceive self-harm

OUTCOME CRITERIA	NURSING INTERVENTIONS	RATIONALE
Short- and Long-Term Goal • Client will be free of injury	1. Ensure that client has a safe environment. Remove from immediate area objects on which client could injure self as a result of random, hyperactive movements.	1. Objects that are appropriate to the normal living situation can be hazardous to the child whose motor activities are out of control.
	2. Identify deliberate behaviors that put the child at risk for injury. Institute consequences for repetition of this behavior.	2. Behavior can be modified with aversive reinforcement.
	3. If there is risk of injury associated with specific therapeutic activities, provide adequate supervision and assistance, or limit client's participation if adequate supervision is not possible.	3. Client safety is a nursing priority.

NURSING DIAGNOSIS: IMPAIRED SOCIAL INTERACTION

RELATED TO: Intrusive and immature behavior

OUTCOME CRITERIA	NURSING INTERVENTIONS	RATIONALE
Short-Term Goal • Client will interact in age-appropriate manner with nurse in one-to-one relationship within 1 week. **Long-Term Goal** • Client will observe limits set on intrusive behavior and will demonstrate ability to interact appropriately with others.	1. Develop a trusting relationship with the child. Convey acceptance of the child separate from the unacceptable behavior.	1. Unconditional acceptance increases feelings of self-worth.
	2. Discuss with client those behaviors that are and are not acceptable. Describe in a matter-of-fact manner the consequences of unacceptable behavior. Follow through.	2. Aversive reinforcement can alter undesirable behaviors.
	3. Provide group situations for client.	3. Appropriate social behavior is often learned from the positive and negative feedback of peers.

Continued

Table 23-5 CARE PLAN FOR THE CHILD WITH ATTENTION-DEFICIT/HYPERACTIVITY DISORDER—cont'd

NURSING DIAGNOSIS: LOW SELF-ESTEEM

RELATED TO: Dysfunctional family system and negative feedback

OUTCOME CRITERIA	NURSING INTERVENTIONS	RATIONALE
Short-Term Goal • Client will independently direct own care and activities of daily living within 1 week. **Long-Term Goal** • Client will demonstrate increased feelings of self-worth by verbalizing positive statements about self and exhibiting fewer demanding behaviors.	1. Ensure that goals are realistic. 2. Plan activities that provide opportunities for success. 3. Convey unconditional acceptance and positive regard. 4. Offer recognition of successful endeavors and positive reinforcement for attempts made. Give immediate positive feedback for acceptable behavior.	1. Unrealistic goals set client up for failure, which diminishes self-esteem. 2. Success enhances self-esteem. 3. Affirmation of client as worthwhile human being may increase self-esteem. 4. Positive reinforcement enhances self-esteem and may increase the desired behaviors.

NURSING DIAGNOSIS: NONCOMPLIANCE (WITH TASK EXPECTATIONS)

RELATED TO: Low frustration tolerance and short attention span

OUTCOME CRITERIA	NURSING INTERVENTIONS	RATIONALE
Short-Term Goal • Client will participate in and cooperate during therapeutic activities. **Long-Term Goal** • Client will be able to complete assigned tasks independently or with a minimum of assistance.	1. Provide an environment for task efforts that is as free of distractions as possible. 2. Provide assistance on a one-to-one basis, beginning with simple, concrete instructions. 3. Ask client to repeat instructions to you. 4. Establish goals that allow client to complete a part of the task, rewarding each step-completion with a break for physical activity. 5. Gradually decrease the amount of assistance given, while assuring the client that assistance is still available if deemed necessary.	1. Client is highly distractible and is unable to perform in the presence of even minimal stimulation. 2. Client lacks the ability to assimilate information that is complicated or has abstract meaning. 3. Repetition of the instructions helps to determine client's level of comprehension. 4. Short-term goals are not so overwhelming to one with such a short attention span. The positive reinforcement (physical activity) increases self-esteem and provides incentive for client to pursue the task to completion. 5. This encourages the client to perform independently while providing a feeling of security with the presence of a trusted individual.

The concept map care plan is an innovative approach to planning and organizing nursing care (see Chapter 9). It is a diagrammatic teaching and learning strategy that allows visualization of interrelationships between medical diagnoses, nursing diagnoses, assessment data, and treatments. An example of a concept map care plan for a client with ADHD is presented in Figure 23–2.

Clinical Vignette: Andy, age 9, has been admitted to the child and adolescent psychiatric unit with a diagnosis of Attention Deficit Hyperactivity Disorder (ADHD). He is unable to sit still, is constantly moving and running around the unit. In the short time since his admission, he has hit another patient, knocked over and broken a lamp, and yelled at the nurse, "I don't have to mind you! You're not the boss!" He became frustrated and left the occupational therapy group when he was having difficulty with the project. He denies any responsibility and blames others for his actions. He ridicules the other patients and calls them insulting names. The nurse develops the following concept map care plan for Andy.

S & Sx:
- Impulsivity
- Accident-prone behavior
- Inability to perceive self-harm

S & Sx:
- Intrusive and immature behavior

S & Sx:
- Denies responsibility
- Blames others
- Ridicules others

S & Sx:
- Low frustration tolerance
- Short attention span

Nsg Dx:
Risk for Injury

Nsg Dx:
Impaired Social Interaction

Nsg Dx:
Low Self-Esteem

Nsg Dx:
Noncompliance (with task expectations)

Nursing Actions:
- Ensure that environment is safe
- Identify and limit behaviors that put child at risk for injury
- Provide necessary supervision to prevent injury during therapeutic activities

Nursing Actions:
- Develop a trusting relationship
- Discuss with client which behaviors are and are not acceptable
- Employ consequences for unacceptable behavior
- Provide group situations for client

Nursing Actions:
- Ensure that goals are realistic
- Plan activities that provide opportunities for success
- Convey unconditional acceptance and positive regard
- Give positive reinforcement for achievements

Nursing Actions:
- Reduce environmental distraction
- Provide simple, concrete instructions
- Establish goals for completion of tasks in steps. Reward each step completion
- Encourage and reward independent achievement

Medical RX:
Ritalin 10 mg twice daily before breakfast and lunch

Outcomes:
- Has experienced no physical harm

Outcomes:
- Has developed trusting relationship with nurse
- Interacts with peers appropriately

Outcomes:
- Verbalizes positive statements about self
- Demonstrates fewer demanding behaviors

Outcomes:
- Completes tasks independently or with minimal assistance
- Cooperates with staff to complete assigned tasks

FIGURE 23–2   Concept map care plan for client with Attention-Deficit/Hyperactivity Disorder.

IMPLICATIONS OF RESEARCH FOR EVIDENCE-BASED PRACTICE

Frame, K., Kelly, L., & Bayley, E. (2003). Increasing perceptions of self-worth in preadolescents diagnosed with ADHD. *Journal of Nursing Scholarship, 35*(3), 225–229.

DESCRIPTION OF THE STUDY: The theoretical framework for this study was based on the Roy adaptation model. The sample in this study consisted of 65 preadolescents diagnosed with attention deficit disorder (ADD) or ADHD in an upper middle-class community in the United States. Participants were randomly assigned to either the control group or the experimental group, and all completed the Harter's Self-Perception Profile for Children instrument at the beginning of the study and 4 weeks later. This tool was designed to measure perceptions of scholastic competence, social acceptance, athletic competence, physical appearance, behavioral conduct, and global self-worth. Children in the experimental group participated in a school nurse–facilitated support group that met twice weekly for 4 weeks. In the group, the participants were assisted to learn strategies for effective interactions with their peers, teachers, and families. Interventions served to promote adaptive self-evaluations and to address the unfavorable self-perceptions of many children with ADHD.

RESULTS OF THE STUDY: On post-testing, participants in the support group scored significantly higher than controls on each of the six subscales, with significant increases on four of the subscales, including perceived social acceptance, perceived athletic competence, perceived physical appearance, and perceived global self-worth.

IMPLICATIONS FOR NURSING PRACTICE: This study has implications for nurses who work with children, and particularly those who work with children diagnosed with ADHD. Because preadolescence is a time when children compare themselves, either positively or negatively, with their peers, group interaction is an especially significant intervention. The authors stated, "The support group, with children helping children, enabled participants to engage in creative problem-solving and to develop solutions to their difficulties." This intervention was shown to promote positive perceptions and behaviors among children with ADD and ADHD. It is especially appropriate for the role of school nurse, but it is also consistent with the role of any nurse who interacts directly with children or adolescents who have similar problems.

Evaluation

Evaluation of the care of a client with ADHD involves examining client behaviors following implementation of the nursing actions to determine if the goals of therapy have been achieved. Collecting data by using the following types of questions may provide appropriate information for evaluation.

■ Have the nursing actions directed at client safety been effective in protecting the child from injury?

■ Has the child been able to establish a trusting relationship with the primary caregiver?

■ Is the client responding to limits set on unacceptable behaviors?

■ Is the client able to interact appropriately with others?

■ Is the client able to verbalize positive statements about self?

■ Is the client able to complete tasks independently or with a minimum of assistance? Can he or she follow through after listening to simple instructions?

■ Is the client able to apply self-control to decrease motor activity?

Psychopharmacological Intervention for ADHD

Indications

Examples of commonly used agents for ADHD are presented in Table 23-6. The medications discussed in this section are used for ADHD in children and adults. Amphetamines are also used in the treatment of narcolepsy and exogenous obesity. Bupropion is used in the treatment of major depression and for smoking cessation (Zyban only). Clonidine and guanfacine are used to treat hypertension.

Action

CNS stimulants increase levels of neurotransmitters (probably norepinephrine, dopamine, and serotonin) in the CNS. They produce CNS and respiratory stimulation, dilated pupils, increased motor activity and mental alertness, diminished sense of fatigue, and brighter spirits. The CNS stimulants discussed in this section include dextroamphetamine sulfate, methamphetamine, lisdexamphetamine, amphetamine mixtures, methylphenidate, and dexmethylphenidate. Action in the treatment of ADHD is unclear.

Atomoxetine inhibits the reuptake of norepinephrine, and bupropion blocks the neuronal

TABLE 23-6 Pharmaceutical Agents for Attention-Deficit/Hyperactivity Disorder

CHEMICAL CLASS	GENERIC (TRADE) NAME	DAILY DOSAGE RANGE (mg)	CONTROLLED CATEGORIES	PREGNANCY CATEGORIES/ HALF-LIFE (hr)
CNS Stimulants				
Amphetamines	Dextroamphetamine sulfate (Dexedrine; Dextrostat)	2.5–40	CII	C/ ~12
	Methamphetamine (Desoxyn)	5–25	CII	C/ 4–5
	Lisdexamphetamine (Vyvanse)	20–70	CII	C/ < 1
Amphetamine Mixtures	Dextroamphetamine/ amphetamine (Adderall; Adderall XR)	2.5–40	CII	C/ 9–13
Miscellaneous	Methylphenidate (Ritalin; Ritalin-SR; Ritalin LA; Methylin; Methylin ER; Metadate ER; Metadate CD; Concerta; Daytrana)	10–60	CII	C/ 2–4
	Dexmethylphenidate (Focalin)	5–20	CII	C/ 2.2
Alpha Agonists	Clonidine (Catapres)	0.05–0.3	—	C/ 12–16
	Guanfacine (Tenex; Intuniv)	1–4	—	B/ 10–30
Miscellaneous	Atomoxetine (Strattera)	>70 kg: 40–100; ≤ 70 kg: 0.5–1.4 mg/ kg (or 100 mg— whichever is less)	—	C/ 5.2 (metabolites 6–8)
	Bupropion (Wellbutrin; Wellbutrin SR; Wellbutrin XL)	3 mg/kg (ADHD); 100–300 (depression)	—	C/ 8–24

uptake of serotonin, norepinephrine, and dopamine. Clonidine and guanfacine stimulate central alpha-adrenoreceptors in the brain, resulting in reduced sympathetic outflow from the central nervous system. The exact mechanism by which these nonstimulant drugs produce the therapeutic effect in ADHD is unclear.

Contraindications/Precautions

CNS stimulants are contraindicated in individuals with hypersensitivity to sympathomimetic amines. They should not be used in advanced arteriosclerosis, cardiovascular disease, hypertension, hyperthyroidism, glaucoma, or agitated or hyperexcitability states; in clients with a history of drug abuse; during or within 14 days of receiving therapy with monoamine oxidase inhibitors (MAOIs); in children younger than 3 years of age; and in pregnancy and lactation. Atomoxetine and bupropion are contraindicated in clients with hypersensitivity to the drugs or their components, in lactation, and in concomitant use with, or within 2 weeks of using, MAOIs. Atomoxetine is contraindicted in clients with narrow-angle glaucoma. Bupropion is contraindicated in individuals with known or suspected seizure disorder, in the acute phase of myocardial infarction, and in clients with bulimia or anorexia nervosa. Alpha agonists are contraindicated in clients with known hypersensitivity to the drugs.

Caution is advised in using CNS stimulants in children with psychosis; in Tourette's disorder; in clients with anorexia or insomnia; in elderly, debilitated, or asthenic clients; and in clients with a history of suicidal or homicidal tendencies. Prolonged use may result in tolerance and physical or psychological dependence. Atomoxetine and bupropion should be used cautiously in clients with urinary retention; hypertension; hepatic, renal, or cardiovascular disease; suicidal clients; pregnancy; and elderly and debilitated clients. Alpha agonists should be used with caution in clients with coronary insufficiency, recent myocardial infarction, or cerebrovascular disease; in chronic renal or hepatic failure; in the elderly; and in pregnancy and lactation.

Interactions

CNS Stimulants (Amphetamines)

Effects of amphetamines are increased with furazolidone or urinary alkalinizers. Hypertensive crisis may occur with concomitant use of (and up to several weeks after discontinuing) MAOIs. Increased risk of serotonin syndrome occurs with coadministration of selective serotonin reuptake inhibitors (SSRIs). Decreased effects of amphetamines occur with urinary acidifiers, and decreased hypotensive effects of guanethidine occur with amphetamines.

Dexmethylphenidate and Methylphenidate

Effects of antihypertensive agents and pressor agents (e.g., dopamine, epinephrine, phenylephrine) are decreased with concomitant use of the methylphenidates. Effects of coumarin anticoagulants, anticonvulsants (e.g., phenobarbital, phenytoin, primidone), tricyclic antidepressants, and SSRIs are increased with the methylphenidates. Hypertensive crisis may occur with coadministration of MAOIs.

Atomoxatine

Effects of atomoxetine are increased with concomitant use of cytochrome P450 isozyme 2D6 (CYP2D6) inhibitors (e.g., paroxetine, fluoxetine, quinidine). Potentially fatal reactions may occur with concurrent use of (or within 2 weeks of discontinuation of) MAOIs. Risk of cardiovascular effects is increased with concomitant use of albuterol or vasopressors.

Bupropion

Effects of bupropion are increased with amantadine, levodopa, or ritonavir. Effects of bupropion are decreased with carbamazepine. There is increased risk of acute toxicity with MAOIs. Increased risk of hypertension may occur with nicotine replacement agents, and adverse neuropsychiatric events may occur with alcohol. Increased anticoagulant effects of warfarin occur with concomitant use, as well as increased effects of drugs metabolized by CYP2D6 (e.g., nortriptyline, imipramine, desipramine, paroxetine, fluoxetine, sertraline, haloperidol, risperidone, thioridazine, metoprolol, propafenone, and flecainide).

Alpha Agonists

Synergistic pharmacologic and toxic effects, possibly causing atrioventricular (AV) block, bradycardia, and severe hypotension, may occur with concomitant use of calcium channel blockers or beta blockers. Additive sedation occurs with CNS depressants, including alcohol, antihistamines, opioid analgesics, and sedative-hypnotics. Effects of clonidine may be decreased with concomitant use of tricyclic antidepressants and prozosin. Decreased effects of levodopa may occur with clonidine, and effects of guanfacine are decreased with barbiturates or phenytoin.

Side Effects

The plan of care should include monitoring for the following side effects from agents for ADHD. Nursing implications related to each side effect are designated by an asterisk (*).

■ Overstimulation, restlessness, insomnia (with CNS stimulants)
  *Assess mental status for changes in mood, level of activity, degree of stimulation, and aggressiveness.
  *Ensure that the client is protected from injury.
  *Keep stimuli low and environment as quiet as possible to discourage overstimulation.
  *To prevent insomnia, administer the last dose at least 6 hours before bedtime. Administer sustained-release forms in the morning.

■ Palpitations, tachycardia (with CNS stimulants; atomoxetine; bupropion; clonidine) or bradycardia (with clonidine; guanfacine)
  *Monitor and record vital signs at regular intervals (two or three times a day) throughout therapy. Report significant changes to the physician immediately.

NOTE: The FDA has issued warnings associated with CNS stimulants and atomoxetine of the risk for sudden death in patients who have cardiovascular disease. A careful personal and family history of heart disease, heart defects, or hypertension should be obtained before these medications are prescribed. Careful monitoring of cardiovascular function during administration must be ongoing.

■ Anorexia, weight loss (with CNS stimulants; atomoxetine; bupropion)
  *To reduce anorexia, the medication may be administered immediately after meals. The client should be weighed regularly (at least

weekly) when receiving therapy with CNS stimulants, atomoxetine, or bupropion because of the potential for anorexia and weight loss, and temporary interruption of growth and development.

■ Tolerance, physical and psychological dependence (with CNS stimulants)
*Tolerance develops rapidly.
*In children with ADHD, a drug "holiday" should be attempted periodically under direction of the physician to determine the effectiveness of the medication and the need for continuation.
*The drug should not be withdrawn abruptly. To do so could initiate the following syndrome of symptoms: nausea, vomiting, abdominal cramping, headache, fatigue, weakness, mental depression, suicidal ideation, increased dreaming, and psychotic behavior.

■ Nausea and vomiting (with atomoxetine and bupropion)
*May be taken with food to minimize GI upset.

■ Constipation (with atomoxetine; bupropion; clonidine; guanfacine)
*Increase fiber and fluid in diet, if not contraindicated.

■ Dry mouth (with clonidine and guanfacine)
*Offer the client sugarless candy, ice, frequent sips of water.
*Strict oral hygiene is very important.

■ Sedation (with clonidine and guanfacine)
*Warn client that this effect is increased by concomitant use of alcohol and other CNS drugs.
*Warn clients to refrain from driving or performing hazardous tasks until response has been established.

■ Potential for seizures (with bupropion)
*Protect client from injury if seizure should occur. Instruct family and significant others of clients on bupropion therapy how to protect client during a seizure if one should occur. Ensure that doses of the immediate-release medication are administered at l east 4 to 6 hours apart and doses of the sustained-release medication at least 8 hours apart.

■ Severe liver damage (with atomoxetine)
*Monitor for the following side effects and report to physician immediately: itching, dark urine, right upper quadrant pain, yellow skin or eyes, sore throat, fever, malaise.

■ New or worsened psychiatric symptoms (with CNS stimulants and atomoxetine)
*Monitor for psychotic symptoms (e.g., hearing voices, paranoid behaviors, delusions)
*Monitor for manic symptoms, including aggressive and hostile behaviors

■ Rebound syndrome (with clonidine and guanfacine)
*Client should be instructed not to discontinue therapy abruptly. To do so may result in symptoms of nervousness, agitation, headache, and tremor, and a rapid rise in blood pressure. Dosage should be tapered gradually under the supervision of the physician.

CORE CONCEPT

Disruptive Behavior Disorders

A disturbance of conduct severe enough to produce significant impairment in social, occupational, or academic functioning because of symptoms that range from oppositional defiant to moderate and severe conduct disturbances (Shahrokh & Hales, 2003).

Conduct Disorder

With conduct disorder, there is a repetitive and persistent pattern of behavior in which the basic rights of others or major age-appropriate societal norms or rules are violated (APA, 2000). Physical aggression is common. The *DSM-IV-TR* divides this disorder into two subtypes based on the age at onset:

1. **Childhood-Onset Type.** This subtype is defined by the onset of at least one criterion characteristic of conduct disorder prior to age 10. Individuals with this subtype are usually boys, frequently display physical aggression, and have disturbed peer relationships. They may have had oppositional defiant disorder during early childhood, usually meet the full criteria for conduct disorder by puberty, and are likely to develop antisocial personality disorder in adulthood.

2. **Adolescent-Onset Type.** This subtype is defined by the absence of any criteria characteristic of conduct disorder prior to age 10. These individuals are less likely to display aggressive behaviors and tend to have more normal peer relationships than those with

childhood-onset type. They are also less likely to have persistent conduct disorder or develop antisocial personality disorder than those with childhood-onset type. The ratio of boys to girls is lower in adolescent-onset type than in childhood-onset type.

CORE CONCEPT

Temperament
Personality characteristics that define an individual's mood and behavioral tendencies. The sum of physical, emotional, and intellectual components that affect or determine a person's actions and reactions.

Predisposing Factors
Biological Influences
Genetics
Studies with monozygotic and dizygotic twins as well as with non-twin siblings have revealed a significantly higher number of conduct disorders among those who have family members with the disorder (APA, 2000). Although genetic factors appear to be involved in the etiology of conduct disorders, little is yet known about the actual mechanisms involved in genetic transmission. One study found that regions on chromosomes 19 and 2 may contain genes conferring risk for conduct disorder (Dick et al., 2004). In this study, the same region on chromosome 2 was also linked to alcohol dependence. These researchers reported that childhood conduct disorder is known to be associated with the susceptibility for future alcohol problems. They have concluded that these findings suggest that some of the genes contributing to alcohol dependence in adulthood may also contribute to conduct disorder in childhood.

Temperament
The term *temperament* refers to personality traits that become evident very early in life and may be present at birth. Evidence suggests a genetic component in temperament and an association between temperament and behavioral problems later in life. Studies have shown that, without appropriate intervention, difficult temperament at age 3 has significant links to conduct disorder and movement into care or institutional life at age 17 (Bagley & Mallick, 2000).

Biochemical Factors
Researchers have investigated various chemicals as biological markers. Alterations in the neurotransmitters norepinephrine and serotonin have been suggested by some studies (Comings et al., 2000; Searight, Rottnek, & Abby, 2001). Some investigators have examined the possibility of testosterone association with violence. One study correlates higher levels of testosterone in pubertal boys with social dominance and association with deviant peers (Rowe, Maughan, Worthman, Costello, & Angold, 2004).

Psychosocial Influences
Peer Relationships
Social groups have a significant impact on a child's development. Peers play an essential role in the socialization of interpersonal competence, and skills acquired in this manner affect the child's long-term adjustment. Studies have shown that poor peer relations during childhood were consistently implicated in the etiology of later deviance (Ladd, 1999). Aggression was found to be the principal cause of peer rejection, thus contributing to a cycle of maladaptive behavior.

Family Influences
The following factors related to family dynamics have been implicated as contributors in the predisposition to this disorder (Foley et al., 2004; Sadock & Sadock, 2007; Ursano et al., 2008):

■ Parental rejection
■ Inconsistent management with harsh discipline
■ Early institutional living
■ Frequent shifting of parental figures
■ Large family size
■ Absent father
■ Parents with antisocial personality disorder and/or alcohol dependence
■ Marital conflict and divorce
■ Inadequate communication patterns
■ Parental permissiveness

Application of the Nursing Process to Conduct Disorder
Background Assessment Data (Symptomatology)
The classic characteristic of conduct disorder is the use of physical aggression in the violation of the rights of others. The behavior pattern manifests itself it virtually all areas of the child's life (home, school, with peers, and in the community). Stealing, lying, and truancy are common problems. The child lacks feelings of guilt or remorse.

IMPLICATIONS OF RESEARCH FOR EVIDENCE-BASED PRACTICE

Hall, L. A., Rayens, M. K., & Peden, A. R. (2008). **Maternal factors associated with child behavior.** *Journal of Nursing Scholarship, 40*(2), 124–130.

DESCRIPTION OF THE STUDY: The purpose of this study was to identify maternal predictors of children's internalizing behaviors (e.g., anxiety, depression, withdrawal, and somatic complaints) and externalizing behaviors (e.g., impulsivity, disruptiveness, and aggression). The sample included 205 low-income, single mothers with children between 2 and 6 years of age. Other criteria for inclusion in the study sample were not being in psychiatric care or counseling, not taking antidepressant medication, not being suicidal, not being pregnant, and having no children less than 1 year of age. Maternal variables were measured as follows: The Beck Depression Inventory was used to measure depressive symptoms; negative thinking was measured using the Crandell Cognitions Inventory; self-worth and self-acceptance were measured on the Rosenberg Self-esteem Scale; and chronic stress was measured on the Everyday Stressors Index, which assesses common problems faced daily by mothers with young children. Surveys were conducted using in-home interviews with the mothers.

RESULTS OF THE STUDY: Maternal stress exerted the largest total effects on children's internalizing and externalizing behaviors. Depressive symptoms had the second largest total effect, followed by negative thinking. Mothers' self-esteem displayed the weakest total effect on both child outcomes. Other studies have shown that maternal depression is associated with their children's poor school performance, slow cognitive and motor development, and elevated cortisol levels. Very young children with behavior problems are at risk for continuation of these problems into school age and adolescence.

IMPLICATIONS FOR NURSING PRACTICE: The authors suggested that the types of stressors faced by low-income women need to be identified, and attempts made at alleviation by intervention or referral to social services for support. Treatment of the mother's depression with antidepressant medication and cognitive-behavioral strategies to reduce negative thinking may also provide positive benefits for their children. The authors stated:

> The findings of this study indicate that a focus on decreasing mothers' negative thinking may provide a way to reduce their depressive symptoms and result in fewer behavior problems among their young children. Nurses working in primary care and community-based setting are in key positions to address this problem and improve the mental health of low-income mothers and positively affect the behavior of their children.

The use of tobacco, liquor, or nonprescribed drugs, as well as the participation in sexual activities, occurs earlier than at the expected age for the peer group. Projection is a common defense mechanism.

Low self-esteem is manifested by a "tough guy" image. Characteristics include poor frustration tolerance, irritability, and frequent temper outbursts. Symptoms of anxiety and depression are not uncommon.

Level of academic achievemenst may be low in relation to age and IQ. Manifestations associated with ADHD (e.g., attention difficulties, impulsiveness, and hyperactivity) are very common in children with conduct disorder.

The *DSM-IV-TR* diagnostic criteria for conduct disorder are presented in Box 23-4.

Diagnosis/Outcome Identification

Based on the data collected during the nursing assessment, possible nursing diagnoses for the client with conduct disorder include:

■ Risk for other-directed violence related to characteristics of temperament, peer rejection, negative parental role models, dysfunctional family dynamics

■ Impaired social interaction related to negative parental role models, impaired peer relations leading to inappropriate social behaviors

■ Defensive coping related to low self-esteem and dysfunctional family system

■ Low self-esteem related to lack of positive feedback and unsatisfactory parent/child relationship.

Outcome Criteria

Outcome criteria include short- and long-term goals. Timelines are individually determined. The following criteria may be used for measurement of outcomes in the care of the client with conduct disorder:

The client:

■ Has not harmed self or others.

■ Interacts with others in a socially appropriate manner.

■ Accepts direction without becoming defensive.

BOX 23-4 Diagnostic Criteria for Conduct Disorder

A. A repetitive and persistent pattern of behavior in which the basic rights of others or major age-appropriate societal norms or rules are violated, as manifested by the presence of three (or more) of the following criteria in the past 12 months, with at least one criterion present in the past 6 months:

  1. Aggression to people and animals

    a. Often bullies, threatens, or intimidates others.

    b. Often initiates physical fights.

    c. Has used a weapon that can cause serious physical harm to others (e.g., a bat, brick, broken bottle, knife, gun)

    d. Has been physically cruel to people.

    e. Has been physically cruel to animals.

    f. Has stolen while confronting a victim (e.g., mugging, purse snatching, extortion, armed robbery).

    g. Has forced someone into sexual activity.

  2. Destruction of property

    a. Has deliberately engaged in fire setting with the intention of causing serious damage.

    b. Has deliberately destroyed others' property (other than by fire setting).

  3. Deceitfulness or theft.

    a. Has broken into someone else's house, building, or car.

    b. Often lies to obtain goods or favors or to avoid obligations (i.e., "cons" others)

    c. Has stolen items of nontrivial value without confronting a victim (e.g., shoplifting, but without breaking and entering; forgery).

  4. Serious violations of rules

    a. Often stays out at night despite parental prohibitions, beginning before age 13 years.

    b. Has run away from home overnight at least twice while living in parental or parental surrogate home (or once without returning for a lengthy period).

    c. Is often truant from school, beginning before age 13 years.

B. The disturbance in behavior causes clinically significant impairment in social, academic, or occupational functioning.

C. If the individual is age 18 years or older, criteria are not met for antisocial personality disorder.

Subtypes:

  1. Childhood-Onset Type: Onset of at least one criterion characteristic of conduct disorder prior to age 10 years.

  2. Adolescent-Onset Type: Absence of any criteria characteristic of conduct disorder prior to age 10 years.

  3. Unspecified Onset: Age at onset is not known.

From American Psychiatric Association. (2000). Diagnostic and statistical manual of mental disorders (4th ed.) Text revision. Washington, DC: American Psychiatric Publishing, with permission.

■ Demonstrates evidence of increased self-esteem by discontinuing exploitative and demanding behaviors toward others.

Planning/Implementation

Table 23-7 provides a plan of care for the child with conduct disorder using nursing diagnoses common to the disorder, outcome criteria, and appropriate nursing interventions and rationales.

Evaluation

Following the planning and implementation of care, evaluation is made of the behavior changes in the child with conduct disorder. This is accomplished by determining if the goals of therapy have been achieved. Reassessment, the next step in the nursing process, may be initiated by gathering information using the following questions:

■ Have the nursing actions directed toward managing the client's aggressive behavior been effective?

■ Have interventions prevented harm to others or others' property?

■ Is the client able to express anger in an appropriate manner?

■ Has the client developed more adaptive coping strategies to deal with anger and feelings of aggression?

■ Does the client demonstrate the ability to trust others? Is he or she able to interact with staff and peers in an appropriate manner?

Table 23-7 CARE PLAN FOR THE CHILD/ADOLESCENT WITH CONDUCT DISORDER

NURSING DIAGNOSIS: RISK FOR OTHER-DIRECTED VIOLENCE

RELATED TO: Characteristics of temperament, peer rejection, negative parental role models, dysfunctional family dynamics

OUTCOME CRITERIA	NURSING INTERVENTIONS	RATIONALE
Short-Term Goal • Client will discuss feelings of anger with nurse or therapist. **Long-Term Goal** • Client will not harm others or others' property.	1. Observe client's behavior frequently through routine activities and interactions. Become aware of behaviors that indicate a rise in agitation. 2. Redirect violent behavior with physical outlets for suppressed anger and frustration. 3. Encourage client to express anger and act as a role model for appropriate expression of anger. 4. Ensure that a sufficient number of staff is available to indicate a show of strength if necessary. 5. Administer tranquilizing medication, if ordered, or use mechanical restraints or isolation room only if situation cannot be controlled with less restrictive means.	1. Recognition of behaviors that precede the onset of aggression may provide the opportunity to intervene before violence occurs. 2. Excess energy is released through physical activities, inducing a feeling of relaxation. 3. Discussion of situations that create anger may lead to more effective ways of dealing with them. 4. This conveys an evidence of control over the situation and provides physical security for staff. 5. It is the client's right to expect the use of techniques that ensure safety of the client and others by the least restrictive means.

NURSING DIAGNOSIS: IMPAIRED SOCIAL INTERACTION

RELATED TO: Negative parental role models; impaired peer relations leading to inappropriate social behavior

OUTCOME CRITERIA	NURSING INTERVENTIONS	RATIONALE
Short-Term Goal • Client will interact in age-appropriate manner with nurse in one-to-one relationship within 1 week. **Long-Term Goal** • Client will be able to interact with staff and peers using age-appropriate, acceptable behaviors.	1. Develop a trusting relationship with the client. Convey acceptance of the person separate from the unacceptable behavior. 2. Discuss with client which behaviors are and are not acceptable. Describe in matter-of-fact manner the consequence of unacceptable behavior. Follow through. 3. Provide group situations for client.	1. Unconditional acceptance increases feeling of self-worth. 2. Aversive reinforcement can alter or extinguish undesirable behaviors. 3. Appropriate social behavior is often learned from the positive and negative feedback of peers.

NURSING DIAGNOSIS: DEFENSIVE COPING

RELATED TO: Low self-esteem and dysfunctional family system

OUTCOME CRITERIA	NURSING INTERVENTIONS	RATIONALE
Short-Term Goal • Client will verbalize personal responsibility for difficulties experienced in interpersonal relationships within (time period reasonable for client).	1. Explain to client the correlation between feelings of inadequacy and the need for acceptance from others and how these feelings provoke defensive behaviors, such as blaming others for own behaviors.	1. Recognition of the problem is the first step in the change process toward resolution.

Continued

Table 23-7 CARE PLAN FOR THE CHILD/ADOLESCENT WITH CONDUCT DISORDER—cont'd

OUTCOME CRITERIA	NURSING INTERVENTIONS	RATIONALE
Long-Term Goal • Client will accept responsibility for own behaviors and interact with others without becoming defensive.	2. Provide immediate, matter-of-fact, nonthreatening feedback for unacceptable behaviors. 3. Help identify situations that provoke defensiveness and practice through role-play more appropriate responses. 4. Provide immediate positive feedback for acceptable behaviors.	2. Client may not realize how these behaviors are being perceived by others. 3. Role-playing provides confidence to deal with difficult situations when they actually occur. 4. Positive feedback encourages repetition, and immediacy is significant for these children who respond to immediate gratification.

NURSING DIAGNOSIS: LOW SELF-ESTEEM

RELATED TO: Lack of positive feedback and unsatisfactory parent/child relationship

OUTCOME CRITERIA	NURSING INTERVENTIONS	RATIONALE
Short-Term Goal • Client will participate in own self-care and discuss with nurse aspects of self about which he or she feels good. **Long-Term Goal** • Client will demonstrate increased feelings of self-worth by verbalizing positive statements about self and exhibiting fewer manipulative behaviors.	1. Ensure that goals are realistic. 2. Plan activities that provide opportunities for success. 3. Convey unconditional acceptance and positive regard. 4. Set limits on manipulative behavior. Take caution not to reinforce manipulative behaviors by providing desired attention. Identify the consequences of manipulation. Administer consequences matter-of-factly when manipulation occurs. 5. Help client understand that he or she uses this behavior in order to try to increase own self-esteem. Interventions should reflect other actions to accomplish this goal.	1. Unrealistic goals set client up for failure, which diminishes self-esteem. 2. Success enhances self-esteem. 3. Communicating that client is a worthwhile human being may increase self-esteem. 4. Aversive consequences may work to decrease unacceptable behaviors. 5. When the client feels better about self, the need to manipulate others will diminish.

■ Is the client able to accept responsibility for his or her own behavior? Is there less blaming of others?

■ Is the client able to accept feedback from others without becoming defensive?

■ Is the client able to verbalize positive statements about self?

■ Is the client able to interact with others without engaging in manipulation?

Oppositional Defiant Disorder

Clinical Findings, Epidemiology, and Course

Oppositional defiant disorder (ODD) is characterized by a pattern of negativistic, defiant, disobedient, and hostile behavior toward authority figures that occurs more frequently than is usually observed in individuals of comparable age and developmental level, and interferes with social, academic, or occupational functioning (APA, 2000). The disorder typically begins by 8 years of age, and usually not later than early adolescence. Prevalence estimates range from 2 to 12 percent, and common comorbid disorders include ADHD and anxiety and mood disorders (Ursano et al., 2008). It is more prevalent in boys than in girls before puberty, but the rates are more closely equal after puberty. In a significant proportion of cases, ODD is a developmental antecedent to conduct disorder (Tynan, 2008).

Predisposing Factors

Biological Influences

Because the behaviors associated with ODD are very similar to those of conduct disorder, with the exception of violation of the rights of others, it is reasonable to speculate that they may share at least *some* of the same biological influences. What role, if any, genetics, temperament, or biochemical alterations play in the etiology of ODD is still being investigated. The study by Comings and associates (2000) suggests the genes for metabolism of dopamine, serotonin, and norepinephrine may be contributing factors in the development of ODD.

Family Influences

Opposition during various developmental stages is both normal and healthy. Children first exhibit oppositional behaviors at around 10 or 11 months of age, again as toddlers between 18 and 36 months of age, and finally during adolescence. Pathology is considered only when the developmental phase is prolonged, or when there is overreaction in the child's environment to his or her behavior.

Some children exhibit these behaviors in a more intense form than others. Sadock and Sadock (2007) reported, "Epidemiological studies of negativistic traits in nonclinical populations found such behavior in 16 to 22 percent of school-age children" (p. 1218).

Some parents interpret average or increased level of developmental oppositional behavior as hostility and a deliberate effort on the part of the child to be in control. If power and control are issues for parents, or if they exercise authority for their own needs, a power struggle can be established between the parents and the child that sets the stage for the development of ODD.

Popper and associates (2003) suggested that the following familial influences may play an etiological role in the development of ODD:

■ Parental problems in disciplining, structuring, and limit setting

■ Identification by the child with an impulse-disordered parent who sets a role model for oppositional and defiant interactions with other people

■ Parental unavailability (e.g., separation, evening work hours)

Application of the Nursing Process to ODD

Background Assessment Data (Symptomatology)

ODD is characterized by passive-aggressive behaviors such as stubbornness, procrastination, disobedience, carelessness, **negativism,** testing of limits, resistance to directions, deliberately ignoring the communication of others, and unwillingness to compromise. Other symptoms that may be evident are running away, school avoidance, school underachievement, temper tantrums, fighting, and argumentativeness.

The oppositional attitude is directed toward adults, most particularly the parents. Symptoms of the disorder may or may not be evident in school or elsewhere in the community (APA, 2000).

Usually these children do not see themselves as being oppositional but view the problem as arising from others whom they believe are making unreasonable demands on them. Interpersonal relationships are fraught with difficulty, including those with peers. These children are often friendless, perceiving human relationships as negative and unsatisfactory. School performance is usually poor because of their refusal to participate and their resistance to external demands.

The *DSM-IV-TR* diagnostic criteria for ODD are presented in Box 23-5.

Diagnosis/Outcome Identification

Based on the data collected during the nursing assessment, possible nursing diagnoses for the client with ODD include:

■ Noncompliance with therapy related to negative temperament, denial of problems, underlying hostility

■ Defensive coping related to retarded ego development, low self-esteem, unsatisfactory parent/child relationship

■ Low self-esteem related to lack of positive feedback, retarded ego development

■ Impaired social interaction related to negative temperament, underlying hostility, manipulation of others

BOX 23-5 Diagnostic Criteria for Oppositional Defiant Disorder

A. A pattern of negativistic, hostile, and defiant behavior lasting at least 6 months, during which four (or more) of the following are present:
  1. Often loses temper.
  2. Often argues with adults
  3. Often actively defies or refuses to comply with adult requests or rules.
  4. Often deliberately annoys people.
  5. Often blames others for his or her mistakes or misbehavior.
  6. Is often touchy or easily annoyed by others.
  7. Is often angry and resentful.
  8. Is often spiteful or vindictive.
B. The disturbance in behavior causes clinically significant impairment in social, academic, or occupational functioning.
C. The behaviors do not occur exclusively during the course of a psychotic or mood disorder.
D. Criteria are not met for conduct disorder, and if the individual is age 18 years or older, criteria are not met for antisocial personality disorder.

From American Psychiatric Association. (2000). Diagnostic and statistical manual of mental disorders (4th ed.) Text revision. Washington, DC: American Psychiatric Publishing, with permission.

Outcome Criteria

Outcome criteria include short- and long-term goals. Timelines are individually determined. The following criteria may be used for measurement of outcomes in the care of the client with ODD.

The client:

■ Complies with treatment by participating in therapies without negativism.

■ Accepts responsibility for his or her part in the problem.

■ Takes direction from staff without becoming defensive.

■ Does not manipulate other people.

■ Verbalizes positive aspects about self.

■ Interacts with others in an appropriate manner.

Planning/Implementation

Table 23-8 provides a plan of care for the child with ODD using nursing diagnoses common to the disorder, outcome criteria, and appropriate nursing interventions and rationales.

Table 23-8 CARE PLAN FOR THE CHILD/ADOLESCENT WITH OPPOSITIONAL DEFIANT DISORDER

NURSING DIAGNOSIS: NONCOMPLIANCE WITH THERAPY

RELATED TO: Negative temperament; denial of problems; underlying hostility

OUTCOME CRITERIA	NURSING INTERVENTIONS	RATIONALE
Short-Term Goal • Client will participate in and cooperate during therapeutic activities. **Long-Term Goal** • Client will complete assigned tasks willingly and independently or with a minimum of assistance.	1. Set forth a structured plan of therapeutic activities. Start with minimum expectations and increase as client begins to manifest evidence of compliance.	1. Structure provides security, and one or two activities may not seem as overwhelming as the whole schedule of activities presented at one time.
	2. Establish a system of rewards for compliance with therapy and consequences for noncompliance. Ensure that the rewards and consequences are concepts of value to the client.	2. Positive, negative, and aversive reinforcements can contribute to desired changes in behavior.
	3. Convey acceptance of the client separate from the undesirable behaviors being exhibited. ("It is not *you*, but your *behavior*, that is unacceptable").	3. Unconditional acceptance enhances self-worth and may contribute to a decrease in the need for passive-aggressiveness toward others.

Table 23-8 CARE PLAN FOR THE CHILD/ADOLESCENT WITH OPPOSITIONAL DEFIANT DISORDER—cont'd

NURSING DIAGNOSIS: DEFENSIVE COPING

RELATED TO: Retarded ego development; low self-esteem; unsatisfactory parent/child relationship

OUTCOME CRITERIA	NURSING INTERVENTIONS	RATIONALE
Short-Term Goal • Client will verbalize personal responsibility for difficulties experienced in interpersonal relationships within (time period reasonable for client). **Long-Term Goal** • Client will accept responsibility for own behaviors and interact with others without becoming defensive.	1. Help client recognize that feelings of inadequacy provoke defensive behaviors, such as blaming others for problems, and the need to "get even." 2. Provide immediate, nonthreatening feedback for passive-aggressive behavior. 3. Help identify situations that provoke defensiveness and practice through role-play more appropriate responses. 4. Provide immediate positive feedback for acceptable behaviors.	1. Recognition of the problem is the first step toward initiating change. 2. Because client denies responsibility for problems, he or she is denying the inappropriateness of behavior. 3. Role-playing provides confidence to deal with difficult situations when they actually occur. 4. Positive feedback encourages repetition, and immediacy is significant for these children who respond to immediate gratification.

NURSING DIAGNOSIS: LOW SELF-ESTEEM

RELATED TO: Lack of positive feedback; retarded ego development

OUTCOME CRITERIA	NURSING INTERVENTIONS	RATIONALE
Short-Term Goal • Client will participate in own self-care and discuss with nurse aspects of self about which he or she feels good. **Long-Term Goal** • Client will demonstrate increased feelings of self-worth by verbalizing positive statements about self and exhibiting fewer manipulative behaviors.	1. Ensure that goals are realistic. 2. Plan activities that provide opportunities for success. 3. Convey unconditional acceptance and positive regard. 4. Set limits on manipulative behavior. Take caution not to reinforce manipulative behaviors by providing desired attention. Identify the consequences of manipulation. Administer consequences matter-of-factly when manipulation occurs. 5. Help client understand that he or she uses this behavior in order to try to increase own self-esteem. Interventions should reflect other actions to accomplish this goal.	1. Unrealistic goals set client up for failure, which diminishes self-esteem. 2. Success enhances self-esteem. 3. Affirmation of client as worthwhile human being may increase self-esteem. 4. Aversive reinforcement may work to decrease unacceptable behaviors. 5. When client feels better about self, the need to manipulate others will diminish.

NURSING DIAGNOSIS: IMPAIRED SOCIAL INTERACTION

RELATED TO: Negative temperament; underlying hostility; manipulation of others

OUTCOME CRITERIA	NURSING INTERVENTIONS	RATIONALE
Short-Term Goal • Client will interact in age-appropriate manner with nurse in one-to-one relationship within 1 week.	1. Develop a trusting relationship with the client. Convey acceptance of the person separate from the unacceptable behavior.	1. Unconditional acceptance increases feelings of self-worth and may serve to diminish feelings of rejection that have accumulated over a long period.

Continued

Table 23-8 CARE PLAN FOR THE CHILD/ADOLESCENT WITH OPPOSITIONAL DEFIANT DISORDER—cont'd

OUTCOME CRITERIA	NURSING INTERVENTIONS	RATIONALE
Long-Term Goal • Client will be able to interact with staff and peers using age-appropriate, acceptable behaviors.	2. Explain to the client about passive-aggressive behavior. Explain how these behaviors are perceived by others. Describe which behaviors are not acceptable and role-play more adaptive responses. Give positive feedback for acceptable behaviors. 3. Provide peer group situations for the client.	2. Role-playing is a way to practice behaviors that do not come readily to the client, making it easier when the situation actually occurs. Positive feedback enhances repetition of desirable behaviors. 3. Appropriate social behavior is often learned from the positive and negative feedback of peers. Groups also provide an atmosphere for using the behaviors rehearsed in role-play.

Evaluation

The evaluation step of the nursing process calls for reassessment of the plan of care to determine if the nursing actions have been effective in achieving the goals of therapy. The following questions can be used with the child or adolescent with ODD to gather information for the evaluation.

■ Is the client cooperating with the schedule of therapeutic activities? Is level of participation adequate?

■ Is the client's attitude toward therapy less negative?

■ Is the client accepting responsibility for problem behavior?

■ Is the client verbalizing the unacceptability of his or her passive-aggressive behavior?

■ Is he or she able to identify which behaviors are unacceptable and substitute more adaptive behaviors?

■ Is the client able to interact with staff and peers without defending behavior in an angry manner?

■ Is the client able to verbalize positive statements about self?

■ Is increased self-worth evident with fewer manifestations of manipulation?

■ Is the client able to make compromises with others when issues of control emerge?

■ Is anger and hostility expressed in an appropriate manner? Can the client verbalize ways of releasing anger adaptively?

■ Is he or she able to verbalize true feelings instead of allowing them to emerge through use of passive-aggressive behaviors?

Tourette's Disorder

Clinical Findings, Epidemiology, and Course

The essential feature of Tourette's disorder is the presence of multiple motor tics and one or more vocal tics (APA, 2000). They may appear simultaneously or at different periods during the illness. The disturbance causes marked distress or interferes with social, occupational, or other important areas of functioning. The age at onset of Tourette's disorder can be as early as 2 years, but the disorder occurs most commonly during childhood (around age 6 to 7 years). Prevalence of the disorder is related to age, affecting many more children (5 to 30 per 10,000) than adults (1 to 2 per 10,000) (APA, 2000). It is more common in boys than in girls. Although the disorder can be lifelong, the symptoms usually diminish during adolescence and adulthood, and in some cases, disappear altogether by early adulthood (Leckman, Bloch, Scahill, & King, 2006).

Predisposing Factors

Biological Factors

Genetics

Tics are noted in two thirds of relatives of Tourette's disorder clients (Popper et al., 2003).

Twin studies with both monozygotic and dizygotic twins suggest an inheritable component. Evidence suggests that Tourette's disorder may be transmitted in an autosomal pattern intermediate between dominant and recessive (Sadock & Sadock, 2007). Singer, Leffler, and Murray (2008) stated:

> The precise gene and mechanism of inheritance remain undetermined. A complex genetic mechanism is likely, perhaps one associated with multiple genes or an epigenetic effect, i.e., an environmental exposure influencing gene expression.

Biochemical Factors

Abnormalities in levels of dopamine, serotonin, dynorphin, gamma-aminobutyric acid (GABA), acetylcholine, and norepinephrine have been associated with Tourette's disorder (Popper et al., 2003). Neurotransmitter pathways through the basal ganglia, globus pallidus, and subthalamic regions appear to be involved.

Structural Factors

Neuroimaging brain studies have been consistent in finding dysfunction in the area of the basal ganglia. One recent study found a correlation between smaller size of the corpus callosum and Tourette's disorder in children (Plessen et al., 2007). Peterson and associates (2007) found larger volumes in subregions of the hippocampus and amygdala in children with Tourette's disorder.

Environmental Factors

Additional retrospective findings may be implicated in the etiology of Tourette's disorder. Complications of pregnancy (e.g., severe nausea and vomiting or excessive stress), low birthweight, head trauma, carbon monoxide poisoning, and encephalitis are thought to be associated with the onset of nongenetic Tourette's disorder. It is speculated that these environmental factors also may temper the genetic predisposition to the disorder. One study suggests that Tourette's disorder may arise as a result of a postinfection autoimmune phenomenon induced by childhood streptococcal infection (Mell, Davis, & Owens, 2005).

Application of the Nursing Process to Tourette's Disorder

Background Assessment Data (Symptomatology)

The motor tics of Tourette's disorder may involve the head, torso, and upper and lower limbs. Initial symptoms may begin with a single motor tic, most commonly eye blinking, or with multiple symptoms. The *DSM-IV-TR* identifies simple motor tics as eye blinking, neck jerking, shoulder shrugging, facial grimacing, and coughing. Common complex motor tics include touching, squatting, hopping, skipping, deep knee bends, retracing steps, and twirling when walking.

Vocal tics include various words or sounds such as clicks, grunts, yelps, barks, sniffs, snorts, coughs and, in about 10 percent of cases, a complex vocal tic involving the uttering of obscenities (APA, 2000). Vocal tics may include repeating certain words or phrases out of context, repeating one's own sounds or words (**palilalia**), or repeating what others say (**echolalia**).

The movements and vocalizations are experienced as compulsive and irresistible, but they can be suppressed for varying lengths of time. They are exacerbated by stress and attenuated during periods in which the individual becomes totally absorbed by an activity. In most cases, tics are diminished during sleep (Singer et al., 2008).

Comorbid disorders common with Tourette's disorder include ADHD, obsessive-compulsive disorder, depression, and anxiety. Episodic outbursts and school difficulties are also frequently observed. In severe cases, self-injurious behaviors may be exhibited (Singer et al., 2008).

The *DSM-IV-TR* diagnostic criteria for Tourette's disorder are presented in Box 23-6.

Diagnosis/Outcome Identification

Based on data collected during the nursing assessment, possible nursing diagnoses for the client with Tourette's disorder include:

- Risk for self-directed or other-directed violence related to low tolerance for frustration

- Impaired social interaction related to impulsiveness, oppositional and aggressive behavior

- Low self-esteem related to shame associated with tic behaviors

Outcome Criteria

Outcome criteria include short- and long-term goals. Timelines are individually determined. The following criteria may be used for measurement of outcomes in the care of the client with Tourette's disorder.

The client:

- Has not harmed self or others.

- Interacts with staff and peers in an appropriate manner.

- Demonstrates self-control by managing tic behavior.

- Follows rules of unit without becoming defensive.

- Verbalizes positive aspects about self.

BOX 23-6 Diagnostic Criteria for Tourette's Disorder

A. Both multiple motor and one or more vocal tics have been present at some time during the illness, although not necessarily concurrently. (A tic is a sudden, rapid, recurrent, non-rhythmic, stereotyped motor movement or vocalization.)

B. The tics occur many times a day (usually in bouts) nearly every day or intermittently throughout a period of more than 1 year, and during this period there was never a tic-free period of more than 3 consecutive months.

C. The disturbance causes marked distress or significant impairment in social, occupational, or other important areas of functioning.

D. The onset is before age 18 years.

E. The disturbance is not due to the direct physiological effects of a substance (e.g., stimulants) or a general medical condition (e.g., Huntington's disease or postviral encephalitis).

From American Psychiatric Association. (2000). Diagnostic and statistical manual of mental disorders (4th ed.) Text revision. Washington, DC: American Psychiatric Publishing, with permission.

Planning/Implementation

Table 23-9 provides a plan of care for the child or adolescent with Tourette's disorder using selected nursing diagnoses, outcome criteria, and appropriate nursing interventions and rationales.

Evaluation

Evaluation of care for the child with Tourette's disorder reflects whether or not the nursing actions have been effective in achieving the established goals. The nursing process calls for reassessment of the plan. Questions for gathering reassessment data may include:

■ Has the client refrained from causing harm to self or others during times of increased tension?

■ Has the client developed adaptive coping strategies for dealing with frustration to prevent resorting to self-destruction or aggression to others?

Table 23-9 CARE PLAN FOR THE CHILD/ADOLESCENT WITH TOURETTE'S DISORDER

NURSING DIAGNOSIS: RISK FOR SELF-DIRECTED OR OTHER-DIRECTED VIOLENCE
RELATED TO: Low tolerance for frustration

OUTCOME CRITERIA	NURSING INTERVENTIONS	RATIONALE
Short-Term Goal • Client will seek out staff or support person at any time if thoughts of harming self or others should occur. **Long-Term Goal** • Client will not harm self or others.	1. Observe client's behavior frequently through routine activities and interactions. Become aware of behaviors that indicate a rise in agitation.	1. Stress commonly increases tic behaviors. Recognition of behaviors that precede the onset of aggression may provide the opportunity to intervene before violence occurs.
	2. Monitor for self-destructive behavior and impulses. A staff member may need to stay with the client to prevent self-mutilation.	2. Client safety is a nursing priority.
	3. Provide hand coverings and other restraints that prevent the client from self-mutilative behaviors.	3. For the client's protection, provide immediate external controls against self-aggressive behaviors.
	4. Redirect violent behavior with physical outlets for frustration.	4. Excess energy is released through physical activities and a feeling of relaxation is induced.

Table 23-9 CARE PLAN FOR THE CHILD/ADOLESCENT WITH TOURETTE'S DISORDER—cont'd

NURSING DIAGNOSIS: IMPAIRED SOCIAL INTERACTION

RELATED TO: Impulsiveness; oppositional and aggressive behavior

OUTCOME CRITERIA	NURSING INTERVENTIONS	RATIONALE
Short-Term Goal • Client will develop a one-to-one relationship with a nurse or support person within 1 week. **Long-Term Goal** • Client will be able to interact with staff and peers using age-appropriate, acceptable behaviors.	1. Develop a trusting relationship with the client. Convey acceptance of the person separate from the unacceptable behavior. 2. Discuss with client which behaviors are and are not acceptable. Describe in matter-of-fact manner the consequences of unacceptable behavior. Follow through. 3. Provide group situations for client.	1. Unconditional acceptance increases feelings of self-worth. 2. Aversive reinforcement can alter undesirable behaviors. 3. Appropriate social behavior is often learned from the positive and negative feedback of peers.

NURSING DIAGNOSIS: LOW SELF-ESTEEM

RELATED TO: Shame associated with tic behaviors

OUTCOME CRITERIA	NURSING INTERVENTIONS	RATIONALE
Short-Term Goal • Client will verbalize positive aspects about self not associated with tic behaviors. **Long-Term Goal** • Client will exhibit increased feeling of self-worth as evidenced by verbal expression of positive aspects about self, past accomplishments, and future prospects.	1. Convey unconditional acceptance and positive regard. 2. Set limits on manipulative behavior. Take caution not to reinforce manipulative behaviors by providing desired attention. Identify the consequences of manipulation. Administer consequences matter-of-factly when manipulation occurs. 3. Help client understand that he or she uses manipulation to try to increase own self-esteem. Interventions should reflect other actions to accomplish this goal. 4. If client chooses to suppress tics in the presence of others, provide a specified "tic time," during which he or she "vents" tics, feelings, and behaviors (alone or with staff). 5. Ensure that client has regular one-to-one time with nursing staff.	1. Communicating a perception of the client as a worthwhile human being may increase self-esteem. 2. Aversive consequences may work to decrease unacceptable behaviors. 3. When client feels better about self, the need to manipulate others will diminish. 4. Allows for release of tics and assists in sense of control and management of symptoms. 5. One-to-one time gives the nurse the opportunity to provide the client with information about the illness and healthy ways to manage it. Exploring feelings about the illness helps the client incorporate the illness into a healthy sense of self.

- Is the client able to interact appropriately with staff and peers?
- Is the client able to suppress tic behaviors when he or she chooses to do so?
- Does the client set a time for "release" of the suppressed tic behaviors?
- Does the client verbalize positive aspects about self, particularly as they relate to his or her ability to manage the illness?
- Does the client comply with treatment in a nondefensive manner?

Psychopharmacological Intervention for Tourette's Disorder

Pharmacotherapy is often not recommended to treat Tourette's disorder unless it is causing significant functional impairment or physical discomfort, or is interfering with the individual's overall quality of life or psychological adjustment (Singer et al., 2008; Ursano et al., 2008). Pharmacotherapy is most effective when it is combined with psychosocial therapy, such as behavior therapy, individual counseling or psychotherapy, and/or family therapy. Medications that are used in the treatment of Tourette's disorder include antipsychotics and alpha agonists.

Antipsychotics

The conventional antipsychotics haloperidol (Haldol) and pimozide (Orap) have been approved by the FDA for control of tics and vocal utterances associated with Tourette's disorder. These drugs have been widely investigated, and have proved to be highly effective in alleviating these symptoms. They are often not the first-line choice of therapy, however, because of their propensity for severe adverse effects, such as extrapyramidal symptoms (EPS), neuroleptic malignant syndrome, tardive dyskinesia, and electrocardiographic changes. Haloperidol is not recommended for children younger than 3 years of age, and pimozide should not be administered to children younger than 12 years.

Although not presently approved by the FDA for use in Tourette's disorder, some clinicians prefer to prescribe the atypical antipsychotics, such as risperidone (Risperdal), olanzapine (Zyprexa), or ziprasidone (Geodon), because of their more favorable side-effect profiles. In clinical trials, these medications have been shown to be effective in treating the symptoms of Tourette's disorder. These drugs have a lower incidence of neurological side effects than the typical antipsychotics, although EPS has been observed with risperidone. Common side effects include weight gain and sedation. Ziprasidone has been associated with increased risk of QTc interval prolongation. Hyperglycemia has also been reported in some patients taking atypical antipsychotics.

Alpha Agonists

Clonidine (Catapres) and guanfacine (Tenex; Intuniv) are alpha-adrenergic agonists that are approved for use as antihypertensive agents. The extended-release forms have been approved by the FDA for the treatment of ADHD. These medications are often the first-line choice for treatment of Tourette's disorder because of their favorable side-effect profile, and because they are often effective for comorbid symptoms of ADHD, anxiety, and insomnia (Zinner, 2004). Common side effects include dry mouth, sedation, headaches, fatigue, and dizziness or postural hypotension. Guanfacine is longer lasting and less sedating than clonidine. Alpha agonists should not be prescribed for children and adolescents with preexisting cardiac or vascular disease. They should not be discontinued abruptly; to do so could result in symptoms of nervousness, agitation, tremor, and a rapid rise in blood pressure.

Separation Anxiety Disorder

Clinical Findings, Epidemiology, and Course

The essential feature of separation anxiety disorder is excessive anxiety concerning separation from the home or from those to whom the person is attached (APA, 2000). The anxiety is beyond that which would be expected for the individual's developmental level and interferes with social, academic, occupational, or others areas of functioning. Onset may occur anytime before age 18 years, but is most commonly diagnosed around age 5 or 6, when the child goes to school. Prevalence estimates for the disorder average about 4 percent in children and young adults, and it is more common in girls than in boys. Most children grow out of it, but in some instances the symptoms can persist into adulthood (Harvard Medical School, 2007).

Predisposing Factors

Biological Influences

Genetics

Studies have been conducted in which the children of adult clients diagnosed as having separation anxiety disorder were studied. A second method, studying parents and other relatives of children diagnosed as having separation anxiety disorder, has also been used. The results have shown that a greater number of children with relatives who manifest anxiety problems develop anxiety disorders themselves than do children with no such family patterns. The results are significant enough to speculate that there is a hereditary influence in the development of separation anxiety disorder, but the mode of genetic transmission has not been determined. Sadock and Sadock (2007) stated:

> Current consensus on the genetics of anxiety disorders suggests that what is inherited is a general predisposition toward anxiety, with resulting heightened levels of arousability, emotional reactivity, and increased negative affect, all of which increase the risk for the development of separation anxiety disorder [and other anxiety disorders]. (p. 1278)

Temperament

It is well established that children differ from birth, or shortly thereafter, on a number of temperamental characteristics. Shamir-Essakow, Ungerer, and Rapee (2005) stated:

> A temperament construct termed "behavioral inhibition to the unfamiliar" is characterized by the predisposition to be irritable as an infant, unusually shy and fearful as a toddler, and quiet, cautious, and withdrawn in the preschool and early school age years, with marked behavioral restraint and physiological arousal in unfamiliar situations. Integrated models propose that environmental factors, such as parent-child attachment, may combine with temperament to increase the risk for the development of childhood anxiety. (p. 131)

Individual differences in temperaments may be related to the acquisition of fear and anxiety disorders in childhood. This may be referred to as *anxiety proneness* or *vulnerability* and may denote an inherited "disposition" toward developing anxiety disorders.

Environmental Influences

Stressful Life Events

Studies have shown a relationship between life events and the development of anxiety disorders (Sadock & Sadock, 2007). It is thought that perhaps children who already are vulnerable or predisposed to developing anxiety disorders may be affected significantly by stressful life events. More research is needed before firm conclusions can be drawn.

Family Influences

Various theories expound on the idea that anxiety disorders in children are related to an overattachment to the mother. Attachment theorists attribute the major determinants of anxiety disorders to transactions relating to separation issues between mother (or mothering figure) and child (Shamir-Essakow et al., 2005). The *DSM-IV-TR* (APA, 2000) suggests that children with separation anxiety disorders come from close-knit families.

Some parents may instill anxiety in their children by overprotecting them from expectable dangers or by exaggerating the dangers of the present and the future (Sadock & Sadock, 2007). Some parents may also transfer their fears and anxieties to their children through role modeling. For example, a parent who becomes fearful in the presence of a small, harmless dog and retreats with dread and apprehension teaches the young child by example that this is an appropriate response.

Application of the Nursing Process to Separation Anxiety Disorder

Background Assessment Data (Symptomatology)

Age at onset of this disorder may be as early as preschool age; it rarely begins as late as adolescence. In most cases, the child has difficulty separating from the mother. Occasionally the separation reluctance is directed toward the father, siblings, or other significant individual to whom the child is attached. Anticipation of separation may result in tantrums, crying, screaming, complaints of physical problems, and **clinging** behaviors.

Reluctance or refusal to attend school is especially common in adolescence. Younger children may "shadow" or follow around the person from whom they are afraid to be separated. During middle childhood or adolescence, they may refuse to sleep away from home (e.g., at a friend's house or at camp). Interpersonal peer relationships are usually not a problem with these children. They are generally well liked by their peers and are reasonably socially skilled.

Worrying is common, and relates to the possibility of harm coming to self or to the attachment figure. Younger children may even have nightmares to this effect.

Specific phobias are not uncommon (e.g., fear of the dark, ghosts, animals). Depressed mood is frequently present and often precedes the onset of the anxiety symptoms, which commonly occur following a major stressor. The *DSM-IV-TR* diagnostic criteria for separation anxiety disorder are presented in Box 23-7.

Diagnosis/Outcome Identification

Based on the data collected during the nursing assessment, possible nursing diagnoses for the client with separation anxiety disorder include:

■ Anxiety (severe) related to family history, temperament, overattachment to parent, negative role modeling

■ Ineffective coping related to unresolved separation conflicts and inadequate coping skills evidenced by numerous somatic complaints

■ Impaired social interaction related to reluctance to be away from attachment figure

Outcome Criteria

Outcome criteria include short- and long-term goals. Timelines are individually determined. The following criteria may be used for measurement of outcomes in the care of the client with separation anxiety disorder.

The client:

■ Is able to maintain anxiety at manageable level.

■ Demonstrates adaptive coping strategies for dealing with anxiety when separation from attachment figure is anticipated.

■ Interacts appropriately with others and spends time away from attachment figure to do so.

Planning/Implementation

Table 23-10 provides a plan of care for the child or adolescent with separation anxiety, using nursing diagnoses common to this disorder, outcome criteria, and appropriate nursing interventions and rationales.

Evaluation

Evaluation of the child or adolescent with separation anxiety disorder requires reassessment of the behaviors for which the family sought treatment. Both the client and the family members will have to change their behavior. The following types of questions may provide assistance in gathering data required for evaluating whether the nursing interventions have been effective in achieving the goals of therapy:

■ Is the client able to maintain anxiety at a manageable level (i.e., without temper tantrums, screaming, or "clinging")?

■ Have complaints of physical symptoms diminished?

■ Has the client demonstrated the ability to cope in more adaptive ways in the face of escalating anxiety?

BOX 23-7 Diagnostic Criteria for Separation Anxiety Disorder

A. Developmentally inappropriate and excessive anxiety concerning separation from home or from those to whom the individual is attached, as evidenced by three (or more) of the following:
 1. Recurrent excessive distress when separation from home or major attachment figures occurs or is anticipated.
 2. Persistent and excessive worry about losing, or about possible harm befalling, major attachment figures.
 3. Persistent and excessive worry that an untoward event will lead to separation from a major attachment figure (e.g., getting lost or being kidnapped).
 4. Persistent reluctance or refusal to go to school or elsewhere because of fear of separation.
 5. Persistently and excessively fearful or reluctant to be alone or without major attachment figures at home or without significant adults in other setting.
 6. Persistent reluctance or refusal to go to sleep without being near a major attachment figure or to sleep away from home.
 7. Repeated nightmares involving the theme of separation.
 8. Repeated complaints of physical symptoms (such as headaches, stomachaches, nausea, or vomiting) when separation from major attachment figures occurs or is anticipated.
B. The duration of the disturbance is at least 4 weeks.
C. The onset is before age 18 years.
D. The disturbance causes clinically significant distress or impairment in social, academic (occupational), or other important areas of functioning.
E. The disturbance does not occur exclusively during the course of a pervasive developmental disorder, schizophrenia, or other psychotic disorder and, in adolescents and adults, is not better accounted for by panic disorder with agoraphobia.

From American Psychiatric Association. (2000). Diagnostic and statistical manual of mental disorders (4th ed.) Text revision. Washington, DC: American Psychiatric Publishing, with permission.

Table 23-10 CARE PLAN FOR THE CLIENT WITH SEPARATION ANXIETY DISORDER

NURSING DIAGNOSIS: ANXIETY (SEVERE)

RELATED TO: Family history; temperament; overattachment to parent; negative role modeling

OUTCOME CRITERIA	NURSING INTERVENTIONS	RATIONALE
Short-Term Goal • Client will discuss fears of separation with trusted individual. **Long-Term Goal** • Client will maintain anxiety at no higher than moderate level in the face of events that formerly have precipitated panic.	1. Establish an atmosphere of calmness, trust, and genuine positive regard. 2. Assure client of his or her safety and security. 3. Explore the child or adolescent's fears of separating from the parents. Explore with the parents possible fears they may have of separation from the child. 4. Help parents and child initiate realistic goals (e.g., child to stay with sitter for 2 hours with minimal anxiety; or, child to stay at friend's house without parents until 9 p.m. without experiencing panic anxiety). 5. Give, and encourage parents to give, positive reinforcement for desired behaviors.	1. Trust and unconditional acceptance are necessary for satisfactory nurse-client relationship. Calmness is important because anxiety is easily transmitted from one person to another. 2. Symptoms of panic anxiety are very frightening. 3. Some parents may have an underlying fear of separation from the child, of which they are unaware and which they are unconsciously transferring to the child. 4. Parents may be so frustrated with child's clinging and demanding behaviors that assistance with problem solving may be required. 5. Positive reinforcement encourages repetition of desirable behaviors.

NURSING DIAGNOSIS: INEFFECTIVE COPING

RELATED TO: Unresolved separation conflicts and inadequate coping skills

EVIDENCED BY: Numerous somatic complaints

OUTCOME CRITERIA	NURSING INTERVENTIONS	RATIONALE
Short-Term Goal • Client will verbalize correlation of somatic symptoms to fear of separation. **Long-Term Goal** • Client will demonstrate use of more adaptive coping strategies (than physical symptoms) in response to stressful situations.	1. Encourage child or adolescent to discuss specific situations in life that produce the most distress and describe his or her response to these situations. Include parents in the discussion. 2. Help the child or adolescent who is perfectionistic to recognize that self-expectations may be unrealistic. Connect times of unmet self-expectations to the exacerbation of physical symptoms. 3. Encourage parents and child to identify more adaptive coping strategies that the child could use in the face of anxiety that feels overwhelming. Practice through role-play.	1. Client and family may be unaware of the correlation between stressful situations and the exacerbation of physical symptoms. 2. Recognition of maladaptive patterns is the first step in the change process. 3. Practice facilitates the use of the desired behavior when the individual is actually faced with the stressful situation.

Continued

Table 23-10 CARE PLAN FOR THE CLIENT WITH SEPARATION ANXIETY DISORDER—cont'd

NURSING DIAGNOSIS: IMPAIRED SOCIAL INTERACTION

RELATED TO: Reluctance to be away from attachment figure

OUTCOME CRITERIA	NURSING INTERVENTIONS	RATIONALE
Short-Term Goal • Client will spend time with staff or other support person, without presence of attachment figure, without excessive anxiety. **Long-Term Goal** • Client will be able to spend time with others (without presence of attachment figure) without excessive anxiety.	1. Develop a trusting relationship with client. 2. Attend groups with the child and support efforts to interact with others. Give positive feedback. 3. Convey to the child the acceptability of his or her not participating in group in the beginning. Gradually encourage small contributions until client is able to participate more fully. 4. Help client set small personal goals (e.g., "Today I will speak to one person I don't know").	1. This is the first step in helping the client learn to interact with others. 2. Presence of a trusted individual provides security during times of distress. Positive feedback encourages repetition. 3. Small successes will gradually increase self-confidence and decrease self-consciousness, so that client will feel less anxious in the group situation. 4. Simple, realistic goals provide opportunities for success that increase self-confidence and may encourage the client to attempt more difficult objectives in the future.

■ Have the parents identified their role in the separation conflict? Are they able to discuss more adaptive coping strategies?

■ Does the client verbalize an intention to return to school?

■ Have nightmares and fears of the dark subsided?

■ Is the client able to interact with others away from the attachment figure?

■ Has the precipitating stressor been identified? Have strategies for coping more adaptively to similar stressors in the future been established?

Quality and Safety Education for Nurses (QSEN)

The Institute of Medicine (IOM), in its 2003 report, *Health Professions Education: A Bridge to Quality,* challenged faculties of medicine, nursing, and other health professions to ensure that their graduates have achieved a core set of competencies in order to meet the needs of the 21st-century health-care system. These competencies include *providing patient-centered care, working in interdisciplinary teams, employing evidence-based practice, applying quality improvement,* and *utilizing informatics.* A QSEN teaching strategy is included in Box 23-8. The use of this type of activity is intended to arm the instructor and the student with guidelines for attaining the knowledge,

skills, and attitudes necessary for achievement of quality and safety competencies in nursing.

General Therapeutic Approaches

Behavior Therapy

Behavior therapy is based on the concepts of classical conditioning and operant conditioning (see Chapter 19). Behavior therapy is a common and effective treatment with disruptive behavior disorders. With this approach, rewards are given for appropriate behaviors and withheld when behaviors are disruptive or otherwise inappropriate. The principle behind behavior therapy is that positive reinforcements encourage repetition of desirable behaviors and aversive reinforcements (punishments) discourage repetition of undesirable behaviors. Behavior modification techniques—the system of rewards and consequences—can be taught to parents to be used in the home environment. Consistency is an essential component.

In the treatment setting, individualized behavior modification programs are designed for each client. A case study example, based on a token economy, is presented in Chapter 19.

Family Therapy

Children cannot be separated from their family. Therapy for children and adolescents must involve

BOX 23-8 QSEN TEACHING STRATEGY

Assignment: Patient-Centered Care: Kleinman's Mini-Ethnography
Interviewing Families of Children with Psychiatric Disorders

Competency Domain: Patient-Centered Care
Learning Objectives: Student will:
- Demonstrate skills in hearing patients' and family members' stories of living with the disorder.
- Identify their own explanatory models of the disorder.
- Demonstrate attitudes that reflect a desire to cultivate cultural humility and cultural competence in nursing practice.

Strategy Overview:
1. Read the article, "Anthropology in the Clinic: The Problem of Cultural Competency and How to Fix it," by A. Kleinman and P. Benson. The article is available online at http://www.plosmedicine.org/article/info:doi/10.1371/journal.pmed.0030294
2. Based on the "mini-ethnography" described by Kleinman and Benson, interview a family member of a child with a psychiatric disorder and elicit a narrative of their experience in living with the disorder.
3. Drawing on notes from the interview, write one paper that is the narrative of the illness from the perspective of the interviewee and another paper that describes the student's own explanatory model.

Adapted from teaching strategy submitted by Lisa Day, Assistant Clinical Professor, UCSF, School of Nursing, San Francisco, CA. © 2009 QSEN; http://qsen.org. With permission.

the entire family if problems are to be resolved. Parents should be involved in designing and implementing the treatment plan for the child and should be involved in all aspects of the treatment process.

The genogram can be used to identify problem areas between family members (see Chapter 11). It provides an overall picture of the life of the family over several generations, including roles that various family members play and emotional distance between specific individuals. Areas for change can be easily identified.

The impact of family dynamics on disruptive behavior disorders has been identified. The impact of disruptive behavior on family dynamics cannot be ignored. Family coping can become severely compromised by the chronic stress of dealing with a child with a behavior disorder. It is therefore imperative that the treatment plan for the identified client be instituted within the context of family-centered care.

Group Therapy

Group therapy provides children and adolescents with the opportunity to interact within an association of their peers. This can be both gratifying and overwhelming, depending on the child.

Group therapy provides a number of benefits. Appropriate social behavior often is learned from the positive and negative feedback of peers. Opportunity is provided to learn to tolerate and accept differences in others, to learn that it is acceptable to disagree, to learn to offer and receive support from others, and to practice these new skills in a safe environment. It is a way to learn from the experiences of others.

Group therapy with children and adolescents can take several forms. Music therapy groups allow clients to express feelings through music, often when they are unable to express themselves in any other way. Art and activity/craft therapy groups allow individual expression through artistic means.

Group play therapy is the treatment of choice for many children between the ages of 3 and 9 years. Landreth and Bratton (2007) stated:

Play therapy is to children what counseling or psychotherapy is to adults. Play provides children with a means of expressing their inner world. The use of toys enables children to transfer anxieties, fears, fantasies, and guilt to objects rather than people. In the process, children are safe from their own feelings and reactions because play enables children to distance themselves from traumatic events and experiences. For children, play therapy changes what may be unmanageable in reality into manageable situations through symbolic representation. This provides children with opportunities for learning to cope.

Psychoeducational groups are very beneficial for adolescents. The only drawback to this type of group is that it works best when the group is closed-ended; that is, once the group has been formed, no one is allowed to join until the group has reached its preestablished closure. Members are allowed to propose topics for discussion. The leader serves as teacher much of the time and facilitates discussion of the proposed topic. Members may from time to time be presenters and serve as discussion leaders. Sometimes, psychoeducational groups evolve into traditional therapy discussion groups.

Psychopharmacology

Several of the disorders presented in this chapter are treated with medications. The appropriate pharmacology was presented following the section in which the disorder was discussed. Medication should never be the sole method of treatment. It is undeniable that medication can and does improve quality of life for families of children and adolescents with these disorders. However, research has indicated that medication alone is not as effective as a combination of medication and psychosocial therapy. It is important for families to understand that there is no way to "give him a pill and make him well." The importance of the psychosocial therapies cannot be overstressed. Some clinicians will not prescribe medications for a client unless he or she also participates in concomitant psychotherapy sessions. The beneficial effects of the medications promote improved coping ability, which in turn enhances the intent of the psychosocial therapy.

Summary and Key Points

■ Mental retardation is defined by deficits in general intellectual functioning and adaptive functioning.

■ Four levels of mental retardation—mild, moderate, severe, and profound—are associated with various behavioral manifestations and abilities.

■ Autistic disorder is characterized by a withdrawal of the child into the self and into a fantasy world of his or her own creation.

■ It is generally accepted that autistic disorder is caused by abnormalities in brain structures or

functions. Genetic factors are also thought to play a significant role.

■ Children with ADHD may exhibit symptoms of inattention or hyperactivity and impulsiveness or a combination of the two.

■ Genetics plays a role in the etiology of ADHD. Neurotransmitters that have been implicated include dopamine, norepinephrine, and serotonin. Maternal smoking during pregnancy has been linked to hyperactive behavior in offspring.

■ CNS stimulants, alpha agonists, atomoxetine, and bupropion are commonly used to treat ADHD.

■ With conduct disorder, there is a repetitive and persistent pattern of behavior in which the basic rights of others or major age-appropriate societal norms or rules are violated.

■ Oppositional defiant disorder is characterized by a pattern of negativitistic, defiant, disobedient, and hostile behavior toward authority figures that occurs more frequently than is usually observed in individuals of comparable age and developmental level.

■ The essential feature of Tourette's disorder is the presence of multiple motor tics and one or more vocal tics.

■ Common medications used with Tourette's disorder include haloperidol, pimozide, clonidine, guanfacine, and atypical antipsychotics such as, risperidone, olanzapine, and ziprasidone.

■ The essential feature of separation anxiety disorder is excessive anxiety concerning separation from the home or from those to whom the person is attached.

■ Children with separation anxiety disorder may have temperamental characteristics present at birth that predispose them to the disorder.

■ General therapeutic approaches for child and adolescent psychiatric disorders include behavior therapy, family therapy, group therapies (including music, art, crafts, play, and psychoeducation), and psychopharmacology.

Additional info available @ davisplus.fadavis.com

Review Questions
Self-Examination/Learning Exercise

*Select the answer that is **most** appropriate for each of the following questions:*

1. In an effort to help the child with mild to moderate mental retardation develop satisfying relationships with others, which of the following nursing interventions is most appropriate?
   a. Interpret the child's behavior for others.
   b. Set limits on behavior that is socially inappropriate.
   c. Allow the child to behave spontaneously, for he or she has no concept of right or wrong.
   d. This child is not capable of forming social relationships.

2. The child with autistic disorder has difficulty with trust. With this in mind, which of the following nursing actions would be most appropriate?
   a. Encourage all staff to hold the child as often as possible, conveying trust through touch.
   b. Assign a different staff member each day so the child will learn that everyone can be trusted.
   c. Assign the same staff person as often as possible to promote feelings of security and trust.
   d. Avoid eye contact, as it is extremely uncomfortable for the child, and may even discourage trust.

3. Which of the following nursing diagnoses would be considered the *priority* in planning care for the child with autistic disorder?
   a. Risk for self-mutilation evidenced by banging head against wall.
   b. Impaired social interaction evidenced by unresponsiveness to people.
   c. Impaired verbal communication evidenced by absence of verbal expression.
   d. Disturbed personal identity evidenced by inability to differentiate self from others.

4. Which of the following activities would be most appropriate for the child with ADHD?
   a. Monopoly.
   b. Volleyball.
   c. Pool.
   d. Checkers.

5. Which of the following groups are most commonly used for drug management of the child with ADHD?
   a. CNS depressants (e.g., diazepam [Valium]).
   b. CNS stimulants (e.g., methylphenidate [Ritalin]).
   c. Anticonvulsants (e.g., phenytoin [Dilantin]).
   d. Major tranquilizers (e.g., haloperidol [Haldol]).

6. The child with ADHD has a nursing diagnosis of impaired social interaction. Which of the following are appropriate nursing interventions for this child? (Select all that apply.)
   a. Socially isolate the child when interactions with others are inappropriate.
   b. Set limits with consequences on inappropriate behaviors.
   c. Provide rewards for appropriate behaviors.
   d. Provide group situations for the child.

7. The nursing history and assessment of an adolescent with a conduct disorder might reveal all of the following behaviors *except:*
   a. Manipulation of others for fulfillment of own desires.
   b. Chronic violation of rules.
   c. Feelings of guilt associated with the exploitation of others.
   d. Inability to form close peer relationships.

Continued

Review Questions—cont'd
Self-Examination/Learning Exercise

8. Certain family dynamics often predispose adolescents to the development of conduct disorder. Which of the following patterns is thought to be a contributing factor?
   a. Parents who are overprotective.
   b. Parents who have high expectations for their children.
   c. Parents who consistently set limits on their children's behavior.
   d. Parents who are alcohol dependent.

9. Which of the following is *least* likely to predispose a child to Tourette's disorder?
   a. Absence of parental bonding.
   b. Family history of the disorder.
   c. Abnormalities of brain neurotransmitters.
   d. Structural abnormalities of the brain.

10. Which of the following medications is used to treat Tourette's disorder?
   a. Methylphenidate (Ritalin).
   b. Haloperidol (Haldol).
   c. Imipramine (Tofranil).
   d. Phenytoin (Dilantin).

TEST YOUR CRITICAL THINKING SKILLS

Jimmy, age 9, has been admitted to the child psychiatric unit with a diagnosis of attention-deficit/hyperactivity disorder. He has been unmanageable at school and at home, and was recently suspended from school for continuous disruption of his class. He refuses to sit in his chair or do his work. He yells out in class, interrupts the teacher and the other students, and lately has become physically aggressive when he cannot have his way. He was suspended after hitting his teacher when she asked him to return to his seat.

Jimmy's mother describes him as a restless and demanding baby, who grew into a restless and demanding toddler. He has never gotten along well with his peers. Even as a small child, he would take his friends' toys away from them or bite them if they tried to hold their own with him. His 5-year-old sister is afraid of him and refuses to be alone with him.

During the nurse's intake assessment, Jimmy paced the room or rocked in his chair. He talked incessantly on a superficial level and jumped from topic to topic. He told the nurse that he did not know why he was there. He acknowledged that he had some problems at school but said that was only because the other kids picked on him and the teacher did not like him. He said he got into trouble at home sometimes but that was because his parents liked his little sister better than they liked him.

The physician has ordered methylphenidate 5 mg twice a day for Jimmy. His response to this order is, "I'm not going to take drugs. I'm not sick!"

Answer the following questions related to Jimmy:
1. What are the pertinent assessment data to be noted by the nurse?
2. What is the primary nursing diagnosis for Jimmy?
3. Aside from client safety, to what problems would the nurse want to direct intervention with Jimmy?

References

American Psychiatric Association. (2000). *Diagnostic and statistical manual of mental disorders* (4th ed.) *Text revision.* Washington, DC: American Psychiatric Publishing.

Autism Genome Project Consortium. (2007). Mapping autism risk loci using genetic linkage and chromosomal rearrangements. *Nature Genetics, 39,* 319–328.

Bagley, C., & Mallick, K. (2000). Spiraling up and spiraling down: Implications of a long-term study of temperament and conduct disorder for social work with children. *Child & Family Social Work, 5*(4), 291–301.

Ben-Amor, L., Grizenko, N., Schwartz, G., Lageix, P., Baron, C., Ter-Stepanian, M., et al. (2005). Perinatal complications in children with attention-deficit hyperactivity disorder and their unaffected siblings. *Journal of Psychiatry & Neuroscience, 30,* 120–126.

Bhat, M., Grizenko, N., Ben-Amor, L., & Joober, R. (2005). Obstetric complications in children with attention deficit/hyperactivity disorder and learning disability. *McGill Journal of Medicine, 8*(2), 109–113.

Black, D. W., & Andreasen, N. C. (2011). *Introductory textbook of psychiatry* (5th ed.). Washington, DC: American Psychiatric Publishing.

Brkanac, Z., Raskind, W. H., & King, B. H. (2008). Pharmacology and genetics of autism: Implications for diagnosis and treatment. *Personalized Medicine, 5*(6), 599–607.

Centers for Disease Control and Prevention. (2009, December 18). Prevalence of Autism Spectrum Disorders—Autism and Developmental Disabilities Monitoring Network, United States, 2006. *Morbidity and Mortality Weekly Report, 58*(SS-10), 1–20.

Comings, D. E., Gade-Andavolu, R., Gonzalez, N., Wu, S., Mahleman, D., Blake, H., et al. (2000). Comparison of the role of dopamine, serotonin, and noradrenaline genes in ADHD, ODD, and conduct disorder: Multivariate regression analysis of 20 genes. *Clinical Genetics, 57,* 178–196.

Croen, L. A., Grether, J. K., Yoshida, C. K., Odouli, R., & Van dewater, J. (2005). Maternal autoimmune diseases, asthma and allergies, and childhood autism spectrum disorders. *Archives of Pediatrics and Adolescent Medicine, 159,* 151–157.

Dick, D. M., Li, T.-K., Edenberg, H. J., Hesselbrock, V., Kramer, J., Kuperman, S., et al. (2004). A genome-wide screen for genes influencing conduct disorder. *Molecular Psychiatry, 9,* 81–86.

Dopheide, J. A., & Pliszka, S. R. (2009). Attention-deficit-hyperactivity disorder: An update. *Pharmacotherapy, 29,* 656–679.

Faraone, S. V. (2006). The genetics of attention-deficit/hyperactivity disorder: Current status and clinical implications. *Medscape Psychiatry & Mental Health, 11*(2). Retrieved August 24, 2010, from http://www.medscape.com/viewarticle/546469

Ferguson-Noyes, N., & Wilkinson, A. M. (2008). Caring for individuals with ADHD throughout the lifespan: An introduction to ADHD. *Psychiatric Nurse Counseling Points, 1*(1), 1–15.

Foley, D. L., Eaves, L. J., Wormley, B., Silberg, J. L., Maes, H. H., Kuh, J., et al. (2004). Childhood adversity, monoamine oxidase A genotype, and risk for conduct disorder. *Archives of General Psychiatry, 61*(7), 738–744.

Harvard Medical School. (2007). Separation anxiety. *Harvard Mental Health Letter, 23*(7), 1–3.

Hunt, R. D. (2006). The neurobiology of ADHD. *Medscape Psychiatry & Mental Health, 11*(2). Retrieved August 24, 2010, from http://www.medscape.com/viewarticle/541543

Institute of Medicine. (2003). *Health professions education: A bridge to quality.* Washington, DC: Author.

Jenson, J. (2005, Fall). Attention-deficit/hyperactivity disorder: Treatment update. *Pediatric Rounds: Newsletter of the Children's Specialty Group.* Milwaukee, WI: Medical College of Wisconsin.

Kollins, S. H. (2008). ADHD genetics, neurobiology, and neuropharmacology. *Medscape Psychiatry.* Retrieved August 23, 2010, from http://www.medscape.com/viewprogram/17290

Ladd, G. W. (1999). Peer relationships and social competence during early and middle childhood. *Annual Review of Psychology, 50,* 333–359.

Landreth, G., & Bratton, S. (2007). Play therapy. *ERIC Digests.* Retrieved August 25, 2010, from http://www.ericdigests.org/2000-1/play.html

Leckman, J. F., Bloch, M. H., Scahill, L., & King, R. A. (2006). Tourette syndrome: The self under siege. *Journal of Child Neurology, 21,* 642–649.

Linnet, K. M., Wisborg, K., Obel, C., Secher, N. J., Thomsen, P. H., Agerbo, E., et al. (2005). Smoking during pregnancy and the risk for hyperkinetic disorder in offspring. *Pediatrics, 116,* 462–467.

McCann, D., Barrett, A., Cooper, A., Crumpler, D., Dalen, L., Grimshaw, K., et al. (2007, November 3). Food additives and hyperactive behaviour in 3-year-old and 8/9-year-old children in the community: A randomized double-blinded, placebo-controlled trial. *Lancet, 370,* 1560–1567.

Mell, L. K., Davis, R. L., & Owens, D. (2005). Association between streptococcal infection and obsessive-compulsive disorder, Tourette's syndrome, and tic disorder. *Pediatrics, 116,* 56–60.

National Institute of Mental Health. (2008). *Autism Spectrum Disorders.* NIH Publication No. 08-5511. Retrieved August 23, 2010, from http://www.nimh.nih.gov/publicat/autism.cfm

National Institute of Mental Health. (2010). *Autism spectrum disorders research at NIMH—Part I.* NIH Publication No. 04-4508. Retrieved August 23, 2010, from http://counselingresource.com/distress/autistic/autism-research-1.html

Peterson, B. S., Choi, H. A., Hao, X., Amat, J. A., Zhu, H., Whiteman, R., et al. (2007). Morphologic features of the amygdala and hippocampus in children and adults with Tourette syndrome. *Archives of General Psychiatry, 65,* 1281–1291.

Plessen, K. J., Lundervold, A., Grunner, R., Hammar, A., Lundervold, A., Peterson, B. S., et al. (2007). Functional brain asymmetry, attentional modulation, and interhemispheric transfer in boys with Tourette syndrome. *Neuropsychologia, 45,* 767–774.

Popper, C. W., Gammon, G. D., West, S. A., & Bailey, C. E. (2003). Disorders usually first diagnosed in infancy, childhood, or adolescence. In R. E. Hales & S. C. Yudofsky (Eds.), *Textbook of clinical psychiatry* (4th ed., pp. 833–974). Washington, DC: American Psychiatric Publishing.

Research Units on Pediatric Psychopharmacology Autism Network. (2002). Risperidone in children with autism and serious behavioral problems. *New England Journal of Medicine, 347,* 314–321.

Research Units on Pediatric Psychopharmacology Autism Network. (2005). Risperidone treatment of autistic disorder: Longer-term benefits and blinded discontinuation after 6 months. *American Journal of Psychiatry, 162,* 1361–1369.

Rizwan, S., Manning, J. T., & Brabin, B. J. (2007). Maternal smoking during pregnancy and possible effects of in utero testosterone: Evidence from the 2D:4D finger length ratio. *Early Human Development, 83,* 87–90.

Robb, A. S. (2006). Managing ADHD in a patient with substance use disorder. *Medscape Psychiatry & Mental Health CME.* Retrieved August 24, 2010, from http://cme.medscape.com/viewarticle/549218

Rowe, R., Maughan, B., Worthman, C. M., Costello, E. J., & Angold, A. (2004). Testosterone, antisocial behavior, and social dominance in boys: pubertal development and biosocial interaction. *Biological Psychiatry, 55,* 546–552.

Sadock, B. J., & Sadock, V. A. (2007). *Synopsis of psychiatry: Behavioral sciences/clinical psychiatry* (10th ed.). Philadelphia: Lippincott Williams & Wilkins.

Searight, H. R., Rottnek, F., & Abby, S. L. (2001). Conduct disorder: Diagnosis and treatment in primary care. *American Family Physician, 63,* 1579–1588.

Shahrokh, N. C., & Hales, R. E. (2003). *American psychiatric glossary* (8th ed.). Washington, DC: American Psychiatric Publishing.

Shamir-Essakow, G., Ungerer, J. A., & Rapee, R. (2005). Attachment, behavioral inhibition, and anxiety in preschool children. *Journal of Abnormal Child Psychology, 33,* 131–143.

Singer, H. S., Leffler, J. B., & Murray, C. F. (2008). Tics and Tourette syndrome: A clinical review. *MedscapePsychiatry CME.* Retrieved August 25, 2010, from http://cme.medscape.com/viewarticle/574198

Tynan, W. D. (2008). Oppositional defiant disorder. Retrieved August 25, 2010, from http://www.emedicine.medscape.com/article/918095-overview

Ursano, A. M., Kartheiser, P. H., & Barnhill, L. J. (2008). Disorders usually first diagnosed in infancy, childhood, or adolescence. In R. E. Hales, S. C. Yudofsky, & G. O. Gabbard (Eds.), *Textbook of psychiatry* (5th ed., pp. 861–920). Washington, DC: American Psychiatric Publishing.

Voeller, K. K. S. (2004). Attention-deficit hyperactivity disorder (ADHD). *Journal of Child Neurology, 19,* 798–814.

Wilens, T. E., & Upadhyaya, H. P. (2007). ADHD and substance abuse: A frequent—and risky—combination. *Medscape Psychiatry & Mental Health CME.* Retrieved August 24, 2010, from http://www.medscape.com/viewprogram/6506

Williams, N. M., Zaharieva, I., Martin, A., Langley, K., Mantripragada, K., Fossdal, R., et al. (2010). Rare chromosomal deletions and duplications in attention-deficit hyperactivity disorder: A genome-wide analysis. *Lancet, 376,* 1401–1408.

Zinner, S. H. (2004). Tourette syndrome—much more than tics. *Contemporary Pediatrics, 21*(8), 38–49.

@ INTERNET REFERENCES

- Additional information about attention-deficit/hyperactivity disorder may be located at the following websites:
  - http://www.chadd.org
  - http://www.nimh.nih.gov/health/topics/attention-deficit-hyperactivity-disorder-adhd/index.shtml

- Additional information about autism may be located at the following websites:
  - http://www.autism-society.org
  - http://www.nimh.nih.gov/health/topics/autism-spectrum-disorders-pervasive-developmental-disorders/index.shtml

- Additional information about Tourette's disorder may be located at the following websites:
  - http://www.ninds.nih.gov/disorders/tourette/detail_tourette.htm
  - http://www.tsa-usa.org/

- Additional information about medications to treat ADHD and Tourette's disorder may be located at the following websites:
  - http://www.fadavis.com/townsend
  - http://www.drugs.com/
  - http://www.nimh.nih.gov/publicat/medicate.cfm

MOVIE CONNECTIONS

Bill (mental retardation) • *Bill, On His Own (mental retardation)* • *Sling Blade (mental retardation)* • *Forrest Gump (mental retardation)* • *Rain Man (autistic disorder)* • *Mercury Rising (autistic disorder)* • *Niagara, Niagara (Tourette's disorder)* • *Toughlove (conduct disorder)*

Delirium, Dementia, and Amnestic Disorders

CORE CONCEPTS

amnesia
delirium
dementia

KEY TERMS

aphasia
apraxia
ataxia
confabulation

primary dementia
pseudodementia
secondary dementia
sundowning

OBJECTIVES
After reading this chapter, the student will be able to:

1. Define and differentiate among *delirium, dementia,* and *amnestic disorder.*
2. Discuss predisposing factors implicated in the etiology of delirium, dementia, and amnestic disorders.
3. Describe clinical symptoms and use the information to assess clients with delirium, dementia, and amnestic disorders.
4. Identify nursing diagnoses common to clients with delirium, dementia, and

amnestic disorders, and select appropriate nursing interventions for each.
5. Identify topics for client and family teaching relevant to cognitive disorders.
6. Discuss criteria for evaluating nursing care of clients with delirium, dementia, and amnestic disorders.
7. Describe various treatment modalities relevant to care of clients with delirium, dementia, and amnestic disorders.

HOMEWORK ASSIGNMENT
Please read the chapter and answer the following questions:

1. An alteration in which neurotransmitter is most closely associated with the etiology of Alzheimer's disease?
2. How does vascular dementia differ from Alzheimer's disease?
3. What is pseudodementia?
4. What is the primary concern for nurses working with clients with cognitive disorders?

Cognitive disorders include those in which a clinically significant deficit in cognition or memory exists, representing a significant change from a previous level of functioning. The *Diagnostic and Statistical Manual of Mental Disorders, Fourth Edition, Text Revision* (DSM-IV-TR) (American Psychiatric Association [APA], 2000) describes the etiology of these disorders as a general medical condition, a substance, or a combination of these factors.

These disorders were previously identified as *organic mental syndromes and disorders*. With the publication of the *DSM-IV* in 1994, the name was changed to prevent the implication that *nonorganic* mental disorders do not have a biological basis.

This chapter presents predisposing factors, clinical symptoms, and nursing interventions for care of clients with delirium, dementia, and amnestic disorders. The objective is to provide these individuals with the dignity and quality of life they deserve, while offering guidance and support to their families or primary caregivers.

> ## CORE CONCEPT
>
> ### *Delirium*
> Delirium is a mental state characterized by a disturbance of cognition, which is manifested by confusion, excitement, disorientation, and a clouding of consciousness. Hallucinations and illusions are common.

Delirium

Clinical Findings and Course

A delirium is characterized by a disturbance of consciousness and a change in cognition that develop rapidly over a short period (APA, 2000). Symptoms of delirium include difficulty sustaining and shifting attention. The person is extremely distractible and must be repeatedly reminded to focus attention. Disorganized thinking prevails and is reflected by speech that is rambling, irrelevant, pressured, and incoherent, and that unpredictably switches from subject to subject. Reasoning ability and goal-directed behavior are impaired. Disorientation to time and place is common, and impairment of recent memory is invariably evident. Misperceptions of the environment, including illusions and hallucinations, prevail.

Level of consciousness is often affected, with a disturbance in the sleep-wakefulness cycle. The state of awareness may range from that of hypervigilance (heightened awareness to environmental stimuli) to stupor or semicoma. Sleep may fluctuate between hypersomnolence (excessive sleepiness) and insomnia. Vivid dreams and nightmares are common.

Psychomotor activity may fluctuate between agitated, purposeless movements (e.g., restlessness, hyperactivity, striking out at nonexistent objects) and a vegetative state resembling catatonic stupor. Various forms of tremor are frequently present.

Emotional instability may be manifested by fear, anxiety, depression, irritability, anger, euphoria, or apathy. These various emotions may be evidenced by crying, calls for help, cursing, muttering, moaning, acts of self-destruction, fearful attempts to flee, or attacks on others who are falsely viewed as threatening. Autonomic manifestations, such as tachycardia, sweating, flushed face, dilated pupils, and elevated blood pressure, are common.

The symptoms of delirium usually begin quite abruptly (e.g., following a head injury or seizure). At other times, they may be preceded by several hours or days of prodromal symptoms (e.g., restlessness, difficulty thinking clearly, insomnia or hypersomnolence, and nightmares). The slower onset is more common if the underlying cause is systemic illness or metabolic imbalance.

The duration of delirium is usually brief (e.g., 1 week; rarely more than 1 month) and, upon recovery from the underlying determinant, symptoms usually diminish over a 3- to 7-day period, but in some instances may take as long as 2 weeks (Sadock & Sadock, 2007). The age of the client and duration of the delirium influence rate of symptom resolution. Delirium may transition into a more permanent cognitive disorder (e.g., dementia) and also is associated with a high mortality rate (Bourgeois, Seaman, & Servis, 2008).

Predisposing Factors

The *DSM-IV-TR* (APA, 2000) differentiates between the disorders of delirium by their etiology, although they share a common symptom presentation. Categories of delirium include:

■ Delirium due to a general medical condition

■ Substance-induced delirium

■ Substance-intoxication delirium

■ Substance-withdrawal delirium

■ Delirium due to multiple etiologies

Delirium due to a General Medical Condition

In this type of delirium, evidence must exist (from history, physical examination, or laboratory findings) to show that the symptoms of delirium are a direct result of the physiological consequences of a general medical condition (APA, 2000). Such conditions include systemic infections, metabolic disorders (e.g., hypoxia, hypercarbia, hypoglycemia), fluid or electrolyte imbalances, hepatic or renal disease, thiamine deficiency, postoperative states, hypertensive encephalopathy, postictal states, sequelae of head trauma, and others (APA, 2000).

Substance-Induced Delirium

This disorder is characterized by the symptoms of delirium that are attributed to medication side effects or exposure to a toxin. The *DSM-IV-TR* (APA, 2000) lists the following examples of medications that have been reported to result in substance-induced delirium: anesthetics, analgesics, antiasthmatic agents, anticonvulsants, antihistamines, antihypertensive and cardiovascular medications, antimicrobials, antiparkinsonian drugs, corticosteroids, gastrointestinal medications, histamine H_2-receptor antagonists (e.g. cimetidine), immunosuppressive agents, lithium, muscle relaxants, and psychotropic medications with anticholinergic side effects. Toxins reported to cause delirium include organophosphate (anticholinesterase), insecticides, carbon monoxide, and volatile substances such as fuel or organic solvents.

Substance-Intoxication Delirium

With this disorder, the symptoms of delirium may arise within minutes to hours after taking relatively high doses of certain drugs such as cannabis, cocaine, and hallucinogens. It may take longer periods of sustained intoxication to produce delirium symptoms with alcohol, anxiolytics, or narcotics (APA, 2000).

Substance-Withdrawal Delirium

Withdrawal delirium symptoms develop after reduction or termination of sustained, usually high-dose use of certain substances, such as alcohol, sedatives, hypnotics, or anxiolytics (APA, 2000). The duration of the delirium is directly related to the half-life of the substance involved and may last from a few hours to 2 to 4 weeks.

Delirium due to Multiple Etiologies

This diagnosis is used when the symptoms of delirium are brought on by more than one cause. For example, the delirium may be related to more than one general medical condition or it may be a result of the combined effects of a general medical condition and substance use (APA, 2000).

CORE CONCEPT

Dementia
Dementia is defined by a loss of previous levels of cognitive, executive, and memory function in a state of full alertness (Bourgeois et al., 2008).

Dementia

Clinical Findings, Epidemiology, and Course

This disorder constitutes a large and growing public health problem. Scientists estimate that 5.3 million people in the United States currently have Alzheimer's disease (AD), the most common form of dementia, and the prevalence (the number of people with the disease at any one time) doubles for every 5-year age group beyond age 65 (National Institute on Aging [NIA], 2008). The NIA's Aging, Demographics, and Memory Study revealed that the disease affects 5 percent of people from ages 71 to 79, 24 percent of people ages 80 to 89, and 37 percent of those ages 90 and older (Plassman et al., 2007). Researchers estimate that by 2050, the number of individuals aged 65 and older with AD is projected to be between 11 million and 16 million, if current population trends continue and no preventive treatments become available (Alzheimer's Association, 2010a). After heart disease and cancer, AD is the third most costly disease to society, accounting for $100 billion in yearly costs (NIA, 2008). This proliferation is not the result of an "epidemic." It has occurred because more people now survive into the high-risk period for dementia, which is middle age and beyond.

Dementia can be classified as either primary or secondary. **Primary dementias** are those, such as AD, in which the dementia itself is the major sign of some organic brain disease not directly related to any other organic illness. **Secondary dementias** are caused by or related to another disease or condition, such as human immunodeficiency virus (HIV) disease or a cerebral trauma.

In dementia, impairment is evident in abstract thinking, judgment, and impulse control. The conventional rules of social conduct are often disregarded. Behavior may be uninhibited and inappropriate. Personal appearance and hygiene are often neglected.

Language may or may not be affected. Some individuals may have difficulty naming objects, or the language may seem vague and imprecise. In severe forms of dementia, the individual may not speak at all (**aphasia**). The client may know his or her needs, but may not know how to communicate those needs to a caregiver.

Personality change is common in dementia and may be manifested by either an alteration or accentuation of premorbid characteristics. For example, an individual who was previously very socially active may become apathetic and socially isolated. A previously neat person may become markedly untidy in his or her appearance. Conversely, an individual who may have had difficulty trusting others prior to the illness may exhibit extreme fear and paranoia as manifestations of the dementia.

The reversibility of a dementia is a function of the underlying pathology and of the availability and timely application of effective treatment (APA, 2000). Truly reversible dementia occurs in only a small percentage of cases and might be more appropriately termed *temporary* dementia. Reversible dementia can occur as a result of cerebral lesions, depression, side effects of certain medications, normal-pressure hydrocephalus, vitamin or nutritional deficiencies (especially B_{12} or folate), central nervous system infections, and metabolic disorders (Srikanth & Nagaraja, 2005). In most clients, dementia runs a progressive, irreversible course.

As the disease progresses, **apraxia,** which is the inability to carry out motor activities despite intact motor function, may develop. The individual may be irritable or moody, or exhibit sudden outbursts over trivial issues. The ability to work or care for personal needs independently will no longer be possible. These individuals can no longer be left alone because they do not comprehend their limitations and are therefore at serious risk for accidents. Wandering away from the home or care setting often becomes a problem.

Several causes have been described for the syndrome of dementia (see section on Predisposing Factors), but AD accounts for 50 to 60 percent of all cases (Black & Andreasen, 2011). The progressive nature of symptoms associated with AD has been described according to stages (Alzheimer's Association, 2010b; NIA, 2009; Stanley, Blair, & Beare, 2005).

Stage 1: No Apparent Symptoms In the first stage of the illness, there is no apparent decline in memory.

Stage 2: Forgetfulness The individual begins to lose things or forget names of people. Losses in short-term memory are common. The individual is aware of the intellectual decline and may feel ashamed, becoming anxious and depressed, which in turn may worsen the symptom. Maintaining organization with lists and a structured routine provides some compensation. These symptoms often are not observed by others.

Stage 3: Mild Cognitive Decline In this stage, there is interference with work performance, which becomes noticeable to coworkers. The individual may get lost when driving his or her car. Concentration may be interrupted. There is difficulty recalling names or words, which becomes noticeable to family and close associates. A decline occurs in the ability to plan or organize.

Stage 4: Mild-to-Moderate Cognitive Decline; Confusion At this stage, the individual may forget major events in personal history, such as his or her own child's birthday; experience declining ability to perform tasks, such as shopping and managing personal finances; or be unable to understand current news events. He or she may deny that a problem exists by covering up memory loss with **confabulation** (creating imaginary events to fill in memory gaps). Depression and social withdrawal are common.

Stage 5: Moderate Cognitive Decline; Early Dementia In the early stages of dementia, the individual loses the ability to perform some activities of daily living (ADLs) independently, such as hygiene, dressing, and grooming, and requires some assistance to manage these on an ongoing basis. They may forget addresses, phone numbers, and names of close relatives. They may become disoriented about place and time, but they maintain knowledge about themselves. Frustration, withdrawal, and self-absorption are common.

Stage 6: Moderate-to-Severe Cognitive Decline; Middle Dementia At this stage, the individual may be unable to recall recent major life events or even the name of his or her spouse. Disorientation to surroundings is common, and the person may be unable to recall the day, season, or year. The person is unable to manage ADLs without assistance. Urinary and fecal incontinence are common. Sleeping becomes a problem. Psychomotor symptoms include wandering, obsessiveness, agitation, and aggression. Symptoms seem to worsen in the late afternoon and evening—a phenomenon termed **sundowning.** Communication becomes more difficult, with increasing loss of language skills. Institutional care is usually required at this stage.

Stage 7: Severe Cognitive Decline; Late Dementia In the end stages of AD, the individual is unable to recognize family members. He or she most commonly is bedfast and aphasic. Problems of immobility, such as decubiti and contractures, may occur.

Stanley and associates (2005) described the late stages of dementia in the following manner:

> During late-stage dementia, the person becomes more chairbound or bedbound. Muscles are rigid, contractures may develop, and primitive reflexes may be present. The person may have very active hands and repetitive movements, grunting, or other vocalizations. There is depressed immune system function, and this impairment coupled with immobility may lead to the development of pneumonia, urinary tract infections, sepsis, and pressure ulcers. Appetite decreases and dysphagia is present; aspiration is common. Weight loss generally occurs. Speech and language are severely impaired, with greatly decreased verbal communication. The person may no longer recognize any family members. Bowel and bladder incontinence are present and caregivers need to complete most ADLs for the person. The sleep-wake cycle is greatly altered,

and the person spends a lot of time dozing and appears socially withdrawn and more unaware of the environment or surroundings. Death may be caused by infection, sepsis, or aspiration, although there are not many studies examining cause of death. (p. 358)

Predisposing Factors

The disorders of dementia are differentiated by their etiology, although they share a common symptom presentation. Categories of dementia include:

■ Dementia of the Alzheimer's type

■ Vascular dementia

■ Dementia due to HIV disease

■ Dementia due to head trauma

■ Dementia due to Lewy body disease

■ Dementia due to Parkinson's disease

■ Dementia due to Huntington's disease

■ Dementia due to Pick's disease

■ Dementia due to Creutzfeldt-Jakob disease

■ Dementia due to other general medical conditions

■ Substance-induced persisting dementia

■ Dementia due to multiple etiologies

Dementia of the Alzheimer's Type

Alzheimer's disease is characterized by the syndrome of symptoms identified as dementia in the *DSM-IV-TR* and in the seven stages described previously. The onset of symptoms is slow and insidious, and the course of the disorder is generally progressive and deteriorating. The *DSM-IV-TR* further categorizes this disorder as *early onset* (first symptoms occurring at age 65 or younger) or *late onset* (first symptoms occurring after age 65) and by the clinical presentation of behavioral disturbance (such as wandering or agitation) superimposed on the dementia.

Refinement of diagnostic criteria now enables clinicians to use specific clinical features to identify the disease with considerable accuracy. Examination by computed tomography (CT) scan or magnetic resonance imaging (MRI) reveals a degenerative pathology of the brain that includes atrophy, widened cortical sulci, and enlarged cerebral ventricles (Figures 24–1 and 24–2). Microscopic examinations reveal numerous neurofibrillary tangles and senile plaques in the brains of clients with AD. These changes apparently occur as a part of the normal aging process. However, in clients with AD, they are found in dramatically increased numbers and their

FIGURE 24–1   Changes in the Alzheimer's brain. *A.* Metabolic activity in a normal brain. *B.* Diminished metabolic activity in the Alzheimer's diseased brain. *C.* Late-stage Alzheimer's disease with generalized atrophy and enlargement of the ventricles and sulci. (Source: Alzheimer's Diease Education & Referral Center, A Service of the National Institute on Aging.)

profusion is concentrated in the hippocampus and certain parts of the cerebral cortex.

Etiology

The exact cause of AD is unknown. Several hypotheses have been supported by varying amounts and quality of data. These hypotheses include:

■ **Acetylcholine Alterations.** Research has indicated that, in the brains of Alzheimer's clients, the enzyme required to produce acetylcholine is dramatically reduced. The reduction seems to be greatest in the nucleus basalis of the inferior medial forebrain area (Cummings & Mega, 2003). This decrease in production of acetylcholine reduces the amount of the neurotransmitter that is released to cells in the cortex and hippocampus, resulting in a disruption of the cognitive processes. Other neurotransmitters implicated in the pathology and clinical symptoms of AD include norepinephrine, serotonin, dopamine, and the amino acid glutamate. It has been proposed that, in dementia, excess glutamate leads to overstimulation of the *N*-methyl-D-aspartate (NMDA) receptors, leading to increased intracellular calcium, and subsequent neuronal degeneration and cell death.

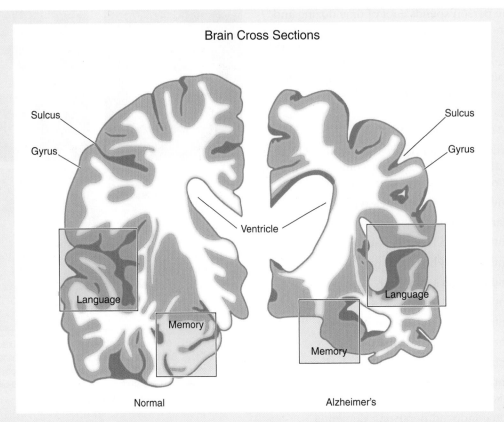

FIGURE 24–2 Neurobiology of Alzheimer's disease. (Source: American Health Assistance Foundation. (2010). http://www.ahaf.org/alzdis/about/BrainAlzheimer.htm, with permission.)

Neurotransmitters

A decrease in the neurotransmitter *acetylcholine* has been implicated in the etiology of Alzheimer's disease. Cholinergic sources arise from the brainstem and the basal forebrain to supply areas of the basal ganglia, thalamus, limbic structures, hippocampus, and cerebral cortex.

Cell bodies of origin for the *serotonin* pathways lie within the raphe nuclei located in the brainstem. Those for *norepinepherine* originate in the locus ceruleus. Projections for both neurotransmitters extend throughout the forebrain, prefrontal cortex, cerebellum, and limbic system. *Dopamine* pathways arise from areas in the midbrain and project to the frontal cortex, limbic system, basal ganglia, and thalamus. Dopamine neurons in the hypothalamus innervate the posterior pituitary.

Glutamate, an excitatory neurotransmitter, has largely descending pathways with highest concentrations in the cerebral cortex. It is also found in the hippocampus, thalamus, hypothalamus, cerebellum, and spinal cord.

Areas of the Brain Affected

Areas of the brain affected by Alzheimer's disease and associated symptoms include the following:

- Frontal lobe: Impaired reasoning ability; unable to solve problems and perform familiar tasks; poor judgment; inability to evaluate the appropriateness of behavior; aggressiveness.
- Parietal lobe: Impaired orientation ability; impaired visuospatial skills (unable to remain oriented within own environment).
- Occipital lobe: Impaired language interpretation; unable to recognize familiar objects.
- Temporal lobe: Inability to recall words; inability to use words correctly (language comprehension). In late stages, some clients experience delusions, and hallucinations.
- Hippocampus: Impaired memory. Short-term memory is affected initially. Later, the individual is unable to form new memories.
- Amygdala: Impaired emotions: depression, anxiety, fear, personality changes, apathy, paranoia.
- Neurotransmitters: Alterations in acetylcholine, dopamine, norepinephrine, serotonin and others may play a role in behaviors such as restlessness, sleep impairment, mood, and agitation.

Medications and Their Effects on the Brain

1. Cholinesterase inhibitors (e.g., tacrine, donepezil, rivastigmine, galantamine) act by inhibiting acetylcholinesterase, which slows the degradation of acetylcholine, thereby increasing concentrations of the neurotransmitter in the brain. Most common side effects include dizziness, gastrointestinal upset, fatigue, and headache.
2. NMDA receptor antagonists (e.g., memantine) act by blocking NMDA receptors from excessive glutamate, preventing continuous influx of calcium into the cells, and ultimately slowing down neuronal degradation. Possible side effects include dizziness, headache, and constipation.

■ **Plaques and Tangles.** As mentioned previously, an overabundance of structures called *plaques* and *tangles* appear in the brains of individuals with AD. The plaques are made of a protein called amyloid beta (Aβ), which is a fragment of a larger protein called amyloid precursor protein (APP) (NIA, 2008). Plaques are formed when these fragments clump together and mix with molecules and other cellular matter. Tangles are formed from a special kind of cellular protein called *tau protein,* whose function it is to provide stability to the neuron. In AD, the tau protein is chemically altered (NIA, 2008). Strands of the protein become tangled together, interfering with the neuronal transport system. It is not known whether the plaques and tangles cause AD or are a consequence of the AD process. It is thought that the plaques and tangles contribute to the destruction and death of neurons, leading to memory failure, personality changes, inability to carry out ADLs, and other features of the disease.

■ **Head Trauma.** The etiology of AD has been associated with serious head trauma (Tesco et al., 2007). Studies have shown that some individuals who had experienced head trauma had subsequently (after years) developed AD. This hypothesis is being investigated as a possible cause. Munoz and Feldman (2000) reported an increased risk for AD in individuals who are both genetically predisposed and experience traumatic head injury.

■ **Genetic Factors.** There is clearly a familial pattern with some forms of AD. Some families exhibit a pattern of inheritance that suggests possible autosomal dominant gene transmission (Sadock & Sadock, 2007). Some studies indicate that early-onset cases are more likely to be familial than late-onset cases, and that from one third to one half of all cases may be of the genetic form. Some research indicates that there is a link between AD and gene mutations found on chromosomes 21, 14, and 1 (Alzheimer's Disease Education & Referral [ADEAR], 2008). Mutations on chromosome 21 cause the formation of abnormal APP. Mutations on chromosome 14 cause abnormal presenilin 1 (*PS-1*) to be made, and mutations on chromosome 1 leads to the formation of abnormal presenilin 2 (*PS-2*). Each of these mutations results in an increased amount of the Aβ protein that is a major component of the plaques associated with AD. Individuals with Down syndrome (who carry an extra copy of chromosome 21) have been found to be unusually susceptible to AD (Blazer, 2008).

Two genetic variants have been identified as risk factors for late-onset AD. The apolipoprotein E epsilon 4 (*ApoE ∈4*) gene, found on chromosome 19, was identified in 1993. Its exact role in the development of AD is not yet clear (ADEAR, 2008). A second genetic variant, the *SORL1* gene, was identified in 2007 (Rogaeva et al., 2007). The researchers believe that the altered gene function results in increasing production of the toxic Aβ protein and subsequently the plaques associated with AD.

Vascular Dementia

In vascular dementia, the clinical syndrome of dementia is due to significant cerebrovascular disease. The blood vessels of the brain are affected, and progressive intellectual deterioration occurs. Vascular dementia is the second most common form of dementia, ranking after AD (Bourgeois et al., 2008).

Vascular dementia differs from AD in that it has a more abrupt onset and runs a highly variable course. Progression of the symptoms occurs in "steps" rather than as a gradual deterioration; that is, at times the dementia seems to clear up and the individual exhibits fairly lucid thinking. Memory may seem better, and the client may become optimistic that improvement is occurring, only to experience further decline of functioning in a fluctuating pattern of progression. This irregular pattern of decline appears to be an intense source of anxiety for the client with this disorder.

In vascular dementia, clients suffer the equivalent of small strokes that destroy many areas of the brain. The pattern of deficits is variable, depending on which regions of the brain have been affected (APA, 2000). Certain focal neurological signs are commonly seen with vascular dementia, including weaknesses of the limbs, small-stepped gait, and difficulty with speech.

The disorder is more common in men than in women (APA, 2000). Arvanitakis (2000) stated:

Prognosis for patients with vascular dementia is worse than that for Alzheimer's patients. The three-year mortality rate in cases over the age of 85 years old is quoted at 67 percent as compared to 42 percent in Alzheimer's disease, and 23 percent in non-demented individuals. However, outcome is ultimately dependent on the underlying risk factors and mechanism of disease, and further studies taking these distinctions into account are warranted.

The diagnosis can be subtyped when the dementia is superimposed with symptoms of delirium, delusions, or depressed mood.

Etiology

The cause of vascular dementia is directly related to an interruption of blood flow to the brain. Symptoms result from death of nerve cells in regions nourished by diseased vessels. Various diseases and conditions that interfere with blood circulation have been implicated.

High blood pressure is thought to be one of the most significant factors in the etiology of multiple small strokes or cerebral infarcts. Hypertension leads to damage to the lining of blood vessels. This can result in rupture of the blood vessel with subsequent hemorrhage or an accumulation of fibrin in the vessel with intravascular clotting and inhibited blood flow (DeMartinis, 2005). Dementia also can result from infarcts related to occlusion of blood vessels by particulate matter that travels

---

IMPLICATIONS OF RESEARCH FOR EVIDENCE-BASED PRACTICE

Heavy smoking in midlife and long-term risk of Alzheimer disease and vascular dementia. (2010). *Archives of Internal Medicine,* **online prepublication October 25, 2010, doi:10.1001/archinternmed. 2010.393**

DESCRIPTION OF THE STUDY: The purpose of this study was to investigate the correlation between midlife smoking and long-term risk of all-cause dementia 2 to 3 decades later. The study began with 33,108 individuals enrolled in a medical health plan in Northern California. They participated in a voluntary health examination called the Multiphasic Health Checkup (MHC) during 1978 through 1985, when they were 50 to 60 years old. The MHC collected large amounts of data on health habits (including smoking), health status, and medical and family history, and was given as part of routine care. The study participants consisted of 21,123 people who were still alive and members of the health plan in 1994. Diagnoses of dementia were ascertained from electronic medical records between January 1, 1994, and July 31, 2008, and results were adjusted for age, sex, education, race, marital status, hypertension, hyperlipidemia, body mass index (BMI), diabetes, heart disease, stroke, and alcohol use. The average age in 1994 at the onset of dementia follow-up was 71.6 years.

RESULTS OF THE STUDY: During a mean follow-up period of 23 years, about 25 percent of the group (5,367 people) were diagnosed as having dementia, with 1,136 identified as having Alzheimer disease and 416 as having vascular dementia. The study revealed the following data:

- Those diagnosed with dementia were older, had fewer years of education, and were more likely to be female.

- Compared to whites, African Americans were more likely to have dementia, whereas Asians were less likely.
- A higher percentage of those with a dementia diagnosis were divorced, widowed, or separated.
- A higher percentage of those with a dementia diagnosis were "never drinkers" of alcohol.
- Those with a dementia diagnosis had a higher mean BMI and all associated comorbidities.
- Former smoking or smoking less than 0.5 pack per day at midlife was not associated with dementia in later life.
- Compared to nonsmokers, smoking less than 2 packs per day at midlife was associated with an increased risk of dementia, but study statistics were not significant.
- Those who smoked more than 2 packs per day in midlife had a greater than 100 percent risk of developing dementia.

IMPLICATIONS FOR NURSING PRACTICE: This study provides yet another reason for nurses to be involved in helping individuals to stop smoking and, for those who do not smoke, to emphasize the importance of not starting. Educational programs aimed at individuals of all ages that emphasize the health hazards associated with smoking are well within the scope of nursing practice. The authors of this study stated, "The large detrimental impact that smoking already has on public health has the potential to become even greater as the population worldwide ages and dementia prevalence increases."

---

through the bloodstream to the brain. These emboli may be solid (e.g., clots, cellular debris, platelet aggregates), gaseous (e.g., air, nitrogen), or liquid (e.g., fat, following soft tissue trauma or fracture of long bones).

Cognitive impairment can occur with multiple small infarcts (sometimes called "silent strokes") over time or with a single cerebrovascular insult that occurs in a strategic area of the brain. An individual may have both vascular dementia and AD simultaneously. This is referred to as *mixed dementia,* the prevalence of which is likely to increase as the population ages (Langa, Foster, & Larson, 2004).

Dementia due to Human Immunodeficiency Virus

Infection with the human immunodeficiency virus type 1 (HIV-1) produces a dementing illness called *HIV-1–associated cognitive/motor complex.* A less severe form, known as HIV-1–associated minor cognitive/motor disorder, also occurs. The severity of symptoms is correlated to the extent of brain pathology. The immune dysfunction associated with HIV disease can lead to brain infections by other organisms, and the HIV-1 also appears to cause dementia directly. In the early stages, neuropsychiatric symptoms may be manifested by barely perceptible changes in a person's normal psychological presentation. Severe cognitive changes, particularly confusion, changes in behavior, and sometimes psychoses, are not uncommon in the later stages.

With the advent of highly active antiretroviral therapy (HAART), incidence rates of dementia associated with HIV disease have been on the decline. However, it is possible that the prolonged life span of HIV-infected patients taking medications may actually increase the numbers of individuals living with HIV-associated dementia.

Dementia due to Head Trauma

Serious head trauma can result in symptoms associated with the syndrome of dementia. Amnesia is the most common neurobehavioral symptom following head trauma, and a degree of permanent disturbance may persist (Bourgeois et al., 2008). Repeated head trauma, such as the type experienced by boxers, can result in *dementia pugilistica,* a syndrome characterized by emotional lability, dysarthria, ataxia, and impulsivity (Sadock & Sadock, 2007).

Dementia due to Lewy Body Disease

Clinically, Lewy body disease is fairly similar to AD; however, it tends to progress more rapidly, and there is an earlier appearance of visual hallucinations and parkinsonian features (Rabins et al., 2006). This disorder is distinctive by the presence of Lewy bodies— eosinophilic inclusion bodies—seen in the cerebral cortex and brainstem (Black & Andreasen, 2011). These patients are highly sensitive to extrapyramidal effects of antipsychotic medications. The disease is progressive and irreversible, and may account for as many as 25 percent of all dementia cases.

Dementia due to Parkinson's Disease

Dementia is observed in as many as 60 percent of clients with Parkinson's disease (Bourgeois et al.,

2008). In this disease, there is a loss of nerve cells located in the substantia nigra, and dopamine activity is diminished, resulting in involuntary muscle movements, slowness, and rigidity. Tremor in the upper extremities is characteristic. In some instances, the cerebral changes that occur in dementia of Parkinson's disease closely resemble those of AD.

Dementia due to Huntington's Disease

Huntington's disease is transmitted as a mendelian dominant gene. Damage is seen in the areas of the basal ganglia and the cerebral cortex. The onset of symptoms (i.e., involuntary twitching of the limbs or facial muscles, mild cognitive changes, depression, and apathy) usually occurs between ages 30 and 50 years. The client usually declines into a profound state of dementia and **ataxia.** The average duration of the disease is based on age at onset. One study concluded that juvenile-onset and late-onset clients have the shortest duration (Foroud, Gray, Ivashina, & Conneally, 1999). In this study, the median duration of the disease was 21.4 years.

Dementia due to Pick's Disease

The cause of Pick's disease is unknown, but a genetic factor appears to be involved. The clinical picture is strikingly similar to that of AD. One major difference is that the initial symptom in Pick's disease is usually personality change, whereas the initial symptom in AD is memory impairment. Studies reveal that pathology of Pick's disease results from atrophy in the frontal and temporal lobes of the brain, in contrast to AD, which is more widely distributed.

Dementia due to Creutzfeldt-Jakob Disease

Creutzfeldt-Jakob disease is an uncommon neurodegenerative disease caused by a transmissible agent known as a "slow virus" or prion (APA, 2000). Five to 15 percent of cases have a genetic component. The clinical presentation is typical of the syndrome of dementia, along with involuntary movements, muscle rigidity, and ataxia. Symptoms may develop at any age in adults, but typically occur between ages 40 and 60 years. The clinical course is extremely rapid, with the progression from diagnosis to death in less than 2 years (Rentz, 2008).

Dementia due to Other General Medical Conditions

A number of other general medical conditions can cause dementia. Some of these include endocrine conditions (e.g., hypoglycemia, hypothyroidism), pulmonary disease, hepatic or renal failure, cardiopulmonary insufficiency, fluid and electrolyte imbalances, nutritional deficiencies, frontal or temporal lobe lesions, central nervous system (CNS) or systemic infections, uncontrolled epilepsy, and other neurological conditions such as multiple sclerosis (APA, 2000).

Substance-Induced Persisting Dementia

The features associated with this type of dementia are those associated with dementias in general; however, evidence must exist from the history, physical examination, or laboratory findings to show that the deficits are etiologically related to the persisting effects of substance use or toxin exposure (APA, 2000). The term *persisting* is used to indicate that the dementia persists long after the effects of substance intoxication or substance withdrawal have subsided or toxin exposure has ended. The *DSM-IV-TR* identifies the following types of substances with which persisting dementia is associated:

1. Alcohol

2. Inhalants

3. Sedatives, hypnotics, and anxiolytics

4. Medications
   a. Anticonvulsants
   b. Intrathecal methotrexate

5. Toxins
   a. Lead
   b. Mercury
   c. Carbon monoxide
   d. Organophosphate insecticides
   e. Industrial solvents

The diagnosis is made according to the specific etiological substance involved. For example, if the substance known to cause the dementia is alcohol, the diagnosis is Alcohol-Induced Persisting Dementia. If the exact substance presumed to be causing the dementia is unknown, the diagnosis would be Unknown Substance-Induced Persisting Dementia.

Dementia due to Multiple Etiologies

This diagnosis is used when the symptoms of dementia are attributed to more than one cause. For example, the dementia may be related to more than one medical condition or to the combined effects of a general medical condition and the long-term use of a substance (APA, 2000).

The etiological factors associated with delirium and dementia are summarized in Box 24-1.

> ## CORE CONCEPT
> *Amnesia*
> The inability to retain or recall past experiences. The condition may be temporary or permanent, depending on etiology.

BOX 24-1 Etiological Factors Implicated in the Development of Delirium and/or Dementia

BIOLOGICAL FACTORS

- Hypoxia: any condition leading to a deficiency of oxygen to the brain
- Nutritional deficiencies: vitamins (particularly B and C); protein; fluid and electrolyte imbalances
- Metabolic disturbances: porphyria; encephalopathies related to hepatic, renal, pancreatic, or pulmonary insufficiencies; hypoglycemia
- Endocrine dysfunction: thyroid, parathyroid, adrenal, pancreas, pituitary
- Cardiovascular disease: stroke, cardiac insufficiency, atherosclerosis
- Primary brain disorders: epilepsy, Alzheimer's disease, Pick's disease, Huntington's chorea, multiple sclerosis, Parkinson's disease
- Infections: encephalitis, meningitis, pneumonia, septicemia, neurosyphilis (dementia paralytica), HIV disease, acute rheumatic fever, Creutzfeldt-Jakob disease
- Intracranial neoplasms
- Congenital defects: prenatal infections, such as first-trimester maternal rubella

EXOGENOUS FACTORS

- Birth trauma: prolonged labor, damage from use of forceps, other obstetric complications
- Cranial trauma: concussion, contusions, hemorrhage, hematomas
- Volatile inhalant compounds: gasoline, glue, paint, paint thinners, spray paints, cleaning fluids, typewriter correction fluid, varnishes, and lacquers
- Heavy metals: lead, mercury, manganese
- Other metallic elements: aluminum
- Organic phosphates: various insecticides
- Substance abuse/dependence: alcohol, amphetamines, caffeine, cannabis, cocaine, hallucinogens, inhalants, nicotine, opioids, phencyclidine, sedatives, hypnotics, anxiolytics
- Other medications: anticholinergics, antihistamines, antidepressants, antipsychotics, antiparkinsonians, antihypertensives, steroids, digitalis

Amnestic Disorders

Amnestic disorders are characterized by an inability to learn new information (short-term memory deficit) despite normal attention, and an inability to recall previously learned information (long-term memory deficit). Events from the remote past often are recalled more easily than recently occurring ones. The syndrome differs from dementia in that there is no impairment in abstract thinking or judgment, no other disturbances of higher cortical function, and no personality change.

Profound amnesia may result in disorientation to place and time, but rarely to self (APA, 2000). The individual may engage in confabulation—the creation of imaginary events to fill in memory gaps.

Some individuals will continue to deny that they have a problem despite evidence to the contrary. Others may acknowledge that a problem exists, but appear unconcerned. Apathy, lack of initiative, and emotional blandness are common. The person may appear friendly and agreeable, but the emotionality is superficial.

The onset of symptoms may be acute or insidious, depending on the pathological process causing the amnestic disorder. Duration and course of the illness may be quite variable and are also correlated with extent and severity of the cause.

Predisposing Factors

Amnestic disorders share a common symptom presentation of memory impairment but are differentiated in the *DSM-IV-TR* (APA, 2000) according to etiology:

■ Amnestic disorder due to a general medical condition

■ Substance-induced persisting amnestic disorder

Amnestic Disorder due to a General Medical Condition

In this type of amnestic disorder, evidence must exist from the history, physical examination, or laboratory findings to show that the memory impairment is the direct physiological consequence of a general medical condition (APA, 2000). The diagnosis is specified further by indicating whether the symptoms are *transient* (present for no more than 1 month) or *chronic* (present for more than 1 month).

General medical conditions that may be associated with amnestic disorder include head trauma, cerebrovascular disease, cerebral neoplastic disease, cerebral anoxia, herpes simplex encephalitis, poorly controlled insulin-dependent diabetes, and surgical intervention to the brain (APA, 2000; Black & Andreasen, 2011).

Transient amnestic syndromes can occur from cerebrovascular disease, cardiac arrhythmias, migraine, thyroid disorders, and epilepsy (Bourgeois et al., 2008).

Substance-Induced Persisting Amnestic Disorder

In this disorder, evidence must exist from the history, physical examination, or laboratory findings that the memory impairment is related to the persisting effects of substance use (e.g., a drug of abuse, a medication) or toxin exposure (APA, 2000). The term *persisting* is used to indicate that the symptoms exist long after the effects of substance intoxication or withdrawal have subsided or toxin exposure has ended. The *DSM-IV-TR* identifies the following substances with which amnestic disorder can be associated:

1. Alcohol

2. Sedatives, hypnotics, and anxiolytics

3. Medications
   a. Anticonvulsants
   b. Intrathecal methotrexate

4. Toxins
   a. Lead
   b. Mercury
   c. Carbon monoxide
   d. Organophosphate insecticides
   e. Industrial solvents

The diagnosis is made according to the specific etiological substance involved. For example, if the substance known to be the cause of the amnestic disorder is alcohol, the diagnosis would be Alcohol-Induced Persisting Amnestic Disorder.

Application of the Nursing Process

Assessment

Nursing assessment of the client with delirium, dementia, or persisting amnesia is based on knowledge of the symptomatology associated with the various disorders described in the beginning of this chapter. Subjective and objective data are gathered by various members of the health-care team. Clinicians report use of a variety of methods for obtaining assessment information.

Client History

Nurses play a significant role in acquiring the client history, including the specific mental and physical changes that have occurred and the age at which the changes began. If the client is unable to relate information adequately, the data should be obtained from family members or others who would be aware of the client's physical and psychosocial history.

From the client history, nurses should assess the following areas of concern: (1) type, frequency, and severity of mood swings, personality and behavioral changes, and catastrophic emotional reactions; (2) cognitive changes, such as problems with attention span, thinking process, problem solving, and memory (recent and remote); (3) language difficulties; (4) orientation to person, place, time, and situation; and (5) appropriateness of social behavior.

The nurse also should obtain information regarding current and past medication usage, history of other drug and alcohol use, and possible exposure to toxins. Knowledge regarding the history of related symptoms or specific illnesses (e.g., Huntington's disease, AD, Pick's disease, or Parkinson's disease) in other family members might be useful.

Physical Assessment

Assessment of physical systems by both the nurse and the physician has two main emphases: (1) signs of damage to the nervous system and (2) evidence of diseases of other organs that could affect mental function. Diseases of various organ systems can induce confusion, loss of memory, and behavioral changes. These causes must be considered in diagnosing cognitive disorders. In the neurological examination, the client is asked to perform maneuvers or answer questions that are designed to elicit information about the condition of specific parts of the brain or peripheral nerves. Testing will assess mental status and alertness, muscle strength, reflexes, sensory perception, language skills, and coordination. An example of a mental status examination for a client with dementia is presented in Box 24-2.

A battery of psychological tests may be ordered as part of the diagnostic examination. The results of these tests may be used to make a differential diagnosis between dementia and **pseudodementia** (depression). Depression is the most common mental illness in the elderly, but it

---

BOX 24-2 Mental Status Examination for Dementia

Patient Name _____ Date _____

Age _____ Sex _____ Diagnosis _____

	Maximum	Client's Score
1. VERBAL FLUENCY		
Ask client to name as many animals as he/she can. (Time: 60 seconds)	10 points	_____
(Score 1 point/2 animals)		
2. COMPREHENSION		
a. Point to the ceiling	1 point	_____
b. Point to your nose and the window	1 point	_____
c. Point to your foot, the door, and ceiling	1 point	_____
d. Point to the window, your leg, the door, and your thumb	1 point	_____
3. NAMING AND WORD FINDING		
Ask the client to name the following as you point to them:		
a. Watch stem (winder)	1 point	_____
b. Teeth	1 point	_____
c. Sole of shoe	1 point	_____
d. Buckle of belt	1 point	_____
e. Knuckles	1 point	_____
4. ORIENTATION		
a. Date	2 points	_____
b. Day of week	2 points	_____
c. Month	1 point	_____
d. Year	1 point	_____

5. NEW LEARNING ABILITY
Tell the client: "I'm going to tell you four words, which I want you to remember."
Have the client repeat the four words after they are initially presented, and then
say that you will ask him/her to remember the words later. Continue with the
examination, and at intervals of 5 and 10 minutes, ask the client to recall the
words. Three different sets of words are provided here.

		5 min.	10 min.
a. Brown (Fun) (Grape)	2 points each:	_____	_____
b. Honesty (Loyalty) (Happiness)	2 points each:	_____	_____
c. Tulip (Carrot) (Stocking)	2 points each:	_____	_____
d. Eyedropper (Ankle) (Toothbrush)	2 points each:	_____	_____

BOX 24-2 **Mental Status Examination for Dementia—cont'd**

6. VERBAL STORY FOR IMMEDIATE RECALL

Tell the client: "I'm going to read you a short story, which I want you to   13 points   _____
remember. Listen closely to what I read because I will ask you to tell me
the story when I finish." Read the story slowly and carefully, but without
pausing at the slash marks. After completing the paragraph, tell the client
to retell the story as accurately as possible. Record the number of correct
memories (information within the slashes) and describe confabulation if it
is present. (1 point = 1 remembered item [13 maximum points])
It was July / and the Rogers family, mom, dad, and four childern /
were packing up their station wagon / to go on vacation.
They were taking their yearly trip / to the beach at Gulf Shores.
This year they were making a special 1-day stop / at The Aquarium in New Orleans.
After a long day's drive they arrived at the motel / only to discover that in their excitement /
they had left the twins / and their suitcases / in the front yard.

7. VISUAL MEMORY (HIDDEN OBJECTS)

Tell the client that you are going to hide some objects around the
office (desk, bed) and that you want him/her to remember where
they are. Hide four or five common objects (e.g., keys, pen)
in various places in the client's sight. After a delay of several minutes,
ask the client to find the objects.   (1 point per item found)

a. Coin	1 point	_____
b. Pen	1 point	_____
c. Comb	1 point	_____
d. Keys	1 point	_____
e. Fork	1 point	_____

8. PAIRED ASSOCIATE LEARNING

Tell the client that you are going to read a list of words two at a time.
The client will be expected to remember the words that go together
(e.g., big—little). When he/she is clear on the directions, read the first
list of words at the rate of one pair per second. After reading the first
list, test for recall by presenting the first recall list. Give the first word
of a pair and ask for the word that was paired with it. Correct incorrect responses
and proceed to the next pair. After the first recall has been completed, allow
a 10-second delay and continue with the second presentation and
recall lists.

Presentation Lists

1	2
a. High—Low	a. Good—Bad
b. House—Income	b. Book—Page
c. Good—Bad	c. High—Low
d. Book—Page	d. House—Income

Recall Lists

1	2		
a. House _____	a. High _____	2 points	_____
b. Book _____	b. Good _____	2 points	_____
c. High _____	c. House _____	2 points	_____
d. Good _____	d. Book _____	2 points	_____

9. CONSTRUCTIONAL ABILITY

Ask client to reconstruct this drawing and to draw the other 2 items: 3 points   _____

Continued

BOX 24-2 **Mental Status Examination for Dementia—cont'd**

Draw a daisy in a flowerpot   3 points   _____

Draw a clock with all the numbers and set the clock at 2:30.   3 points   _____

10. WRITTEN COMPLEX CALCULATIONS

a. Addition 108 1 point   _____
$$+\,79$$

b. Subtraction 605 1 point   _____
$$-\,86$$

c. Multiplication 108 1 point   _____
$$\times\,36$$

d. Division $559 \div 43$ 1 point   _____

11. PROVERB INTERPRETATION

Tell the client to explain the following sayings. Record the answers.

a. Don't cry over spilled milk.   2 points   _____

b. Rome wasn't built in a day.   2 points   _____

c. A drowning man will clutch at a straw.   2 points   _____

d. A golden hammer can break down an iron door.   2 points   _____

e. The hot coal burns, the cold one blackens.   2 points   _____

12. SIMILARITIES

Ask the client to name the similarity or relationship between each of the two items.

a. Turnip...Cauliflower   2 points   _____
b. Car...Airplane   2 points   _____
c. Desk...Bookcase   2 points   _____
d. Poem..Novel   2 points   _____
e. Horse...Apple   2 points   _____

                         Maximum: 100 points   _____

Normal Individuals		Clients with Alzheimer's Disease	
Age Group	**Mean Score (standard deviation)**	**Stage**	**Mean Score (standard deviation)**
40–49	80.9 (9.7)	I	57.2 (9.1)
50–59	82.3 (8.6)	II	37.0 (7.8)
60–69	75.5 (10.5)	III	13.4 (8.1)
70–79	66.9 (9.1)		
80–89	67.9 (11.0)		

Adapted from Strub, R. L., & Black, F. W. (2000). *The mental status examination in neurology* (4th ed.). Philadelphia: F.A. Davis, with permission.

is often misdiagnosed and treated inadequately. Cognitive symptoms of depression may mimic dementia, and because of the prevalence of dementia in the elderly, diagnosticians are often too eager to make this diagnosis. A comparison of symptoms of dementia and pseudodementia (depression) is presented in Table 24-1. Nurses can assist in this assessment by carefully observing and documenting these sometimes subtle differences.

Diagnostic Laboratory Evaluations

The nurse also may be required to help the client fulfill the physician's orders for special diagnostic laboratory evaluations. Many of these tests are routinely included with the physical examination and may include evaluation of blood and urine samples to test for various infections; hepatic and renal dysfunction; diabetes or hypoglycemia; electrolyte imbalances; metabolic and endocrine disorders; nutritional deficiencies; and presence of toxic substances, including alcohol and other drugs.

Other diagnostic evaluations may be made by electroencephalogram (EEG), which measures and records the brain's electrical activity. With CT scanning, an image of the size and shape of the brain can be obtained. MRI is used to obtain a computerized image of soft tissue in the body. It provides a sharp detailed picture of the tissues

of the brain. A lumbar puncture may be performed to examine the cerebrospinal fluid for evidence of CNS infection or hemorrhage. Positron emission tomography (PET) is used to reveal the metabolic activity of the brain, an evaluation some researchers believe is important in the diagnosis of AD. Researchers at the University of California at Los Angeles used PET following injections of FDDNP (a molecule that binds to plaques and tangles in vitro) (Small et al., 2006). With this test, the researchers were able to distinguish between subjects with AD, those with mild cognitive impairment, and those with no cognitive impairment. With FDDNP-PET, researchers are able to accurately diagnose AD in its earlier stages and track disease progression noninvasively in a clinical setting. The researchers hope that this tool will help clinicians define therapeutic interventions before neuronal death occurs, thereby retarding the progression of the disease.

Nursing Diagnosis/Outcome Identification

Using information collected during the assessment, the nurse completes the client database, from which the selection of appropriate nursing diagnoses is determined. Table 24-2 presents a list of client behaviors and the NANDA nursing diagnoses that correspond to those behaviors, which

TABLE 24-1 A Comparison of Dementia and Pseudodementia (Depression)		
SYMPTOM ELEMENT	**DEMENTIA**	**PSEUDODEMENTIA (DEPRESSION)**
Progression of symptoms	Slow	Rapid
Memory	Progressive deficits; recent memory loss greater than remote; may confabulate for memory "gaps;" no complaints of loss	More like forgetfulness; no evidence of progressive deficit; recent and remote loss equal; complaints of deficits; no confabulation (will more likely answer "I don't know")
Orientation	Disoriented to time and place; may wander in search of the familiar	Oriented to time and place; no wandering
Task performance	Consistently poor performance, but struggles to perform	Performance is variable; little effort is put forth
Symptom severity	Worse as the day progresses	Better as the day progresses
Affective distress	Appears unconcerned	Communicates severe distress
Appetite	Unchanged	Diminished
Attention and concentration	Impaired	Intact

TABLE 24-2 Assigning Nursing Diagnoses to Behaviors Commonly Associated With Cognitive Disorders

BEHAVIORS	NURSING DIAGNOSES
Falls, wandering, poor coordination, confusion, misinterpretation of the environment (illusions, hallucinations), lack of under standing of environmental hazards, memory deficits	**Risk for trauma**
Disorientation, confusion, memory deficits, inaccurate interpretation of the environment, suspiciousness, paranoia	**Disturbed thought processes; Impaired memory**
Having hallucinations (ears voices, sees visions, feels crawling sensation on skin)	**Disturbed sensory perception**
Aggressiveness, assaultiveness (hitting, scratching, or kicking)	**Risk for other-directed violence**
Inability to name objects/people, loss of memory for words, difficulty finding the right word, confabulation, incoherent, screaming and demanding verbalizations	**Impaired verbal communication**
Inability to perform activities of daily living (ADLs): feeding, dressing, hygiene, toileting	**Self-care deficit (specify)**
Expressions of shame and self-degradation, progressive social isolation, apathy, decreased activity, withdrawal, depressed mood	**Situational low self-esteem; Grieving**

may be used in planning care for the client with a cognitive disorder.

Outcome Criteria

The following criteria may be used for measurement of outcomes in the care of the client with cognitive disorders.

The client:

■ Has not experienced physical injury.

■ Has not harmed self or others.

■ Has maintained reality orientation to the best of his or her capability.

■ Is able to communicate with consistent caregiver.

■ Fulfills activities of daily living with assistance (or for client who is unable: has needs met, as anticipated by caregiver).

■ Discusses positive aspects about self and life.

Planning/Implementation

Care for an individual with dementia must focus on immediate needs and keeping the individual safe from harm.

Risk for Trauma

Because the individual has impairments in cognitive and psychomotor functioning, it is important to ensure that the environment be made as safe as possible to prevent injury. NANDA defines *Risk for Trauma* as the "accentuated risk of accidental tissue injury (e.g., wound, burn, fracture)" (NANDA International [NANDA-I], 2009, p. 324). Table 24-3 presents this nursing diagnosis in care plan format.

Client Goals

Outcome criteria include short- and long-term goals. Timelines are individually determined.

Short-Term Goals

■ Client will call for assistance when ambulating or carrying out other activities (if it is within his or her cognitive ability).

■ Client will maintain a calm demeanor, with minimal agitated behavior.

■ Client will not experience physical injury.

Long-Term Goal

■ Client will not experience physical injury.

Interventions

Interventions for preventing injury in the cognitively impaired client include the following:

■ Arrange the furniture and other items in the room to accommodate the client's disabilities. Ensure that frequently used items are stored within easy access.

■ Keep the bed in its lowest position. If allowed by hospital regulation or accrediting body, limited use of bedrails may provide a measure of safety.

Table 24-3 CARE PLAN FOR THE CLIENT WITH A COGNITIVE DISORDER

NURSING DIAGNOSIS: RISK FOR TRAUMA

RELATED TO: Impairments in cognitive and psychomotor functioning

OUTCOME CRITERIA	NURSING INTERVENTIONS	RATIONALE
Short-Term Goals • Client will call for assistance when ambulating or carrying out other activities (if it is within his or her cognitive ability). • Client will maintain a calm demeanor, with minimal agitated behavior. • Client will not experience physical injury. **Long-Term Goal** • Client will not experience physical injury.	The following measures may be instituted: a. Arrange furniture and other items in the room to accommodate client's disabilities. b. Store frequently used items within easy access. c. Do not keep bed in an elevated position. Pad side rails and headboard if client has history of seizures. Keep bedrails up when client is in bed (if regulations permit). d. Assign room near nurses' station; observe frequently. e. Assist client with ambulation. f. Keep a dim light on at night. g. If client is a smoker, cigarettes and lighter or matches should be kept at the nurses' station and dispensed only when someone is available to stay with client while he or she is smoking. h. Frequently orient client to place, time, and situation. i. If client is prone to wander, provide an area within which wandering can be carried out safely. j. Soft restraints may be required if client is very disoriented and hyperactive.	To ensure client safety.

■ A room near the nurse's station may be helpful to ensure that the client has close observation. In some instances, one-to-one observation may be necessary, particularly for the delirious client.

■ If the client is a smoker, ensure that cigarettes and lighter are kept at the nurse's station and dispensed only when someone is available to stay with the client while he or she is smoking.

■ Assist the client with ambulation. Provide cane or walker for balance, and instruct client in their proper use. Transport client in wheelchair when longer excursions are necessary.

■ Teach client to hold on to hand railing, if one is available, or to call for assistance when ambulating, if he or she is cognitively able.

For the Agitated Client

■ Maintain as low a level of stimuli as possible in the environment of an individual with disruptions in cognitive processes. Irritability, hostility, aggression, and psychotic behaviors are troublesome problems that require management in individuals with cognitive disorders, particularly dementia. It is often these behaviors that make it difficult for family to care for their loved one, and this is a common cause for placement in an institution.

■ Antipsychotics have historically been used to help control behavioral problems in dementia patients. The conventional antipsychotics are problematic, however, because of their tendency to induce extrapyramidal side effects. The newer atypical antipsychotics have shown some effectiveness in controlling these behaviors. Although antipsychotic medications are still used for this purpose by some physicians, the FDA has issued black-box warnings against their use in elderly patients with dementia-related psychosis. They have been associated with increased mortality in this patient population.

■ Remain calm and undemanding, and avoid pressing the individual to perform activities that he or she is refusing. It may not be possible to reason with these clients; this may only increase the possibility for agitation. Practicing relaxation exercises and walking with the client may be of some help.

For the Client Who Wanders

A number of reasons have been proposed as to why individuals with dementia wander. Some clinicians associate wandering behavior with increased stress and anxiety or restless agitation. Others relate the behavior to stages of cognitive decline. When memory diminishes and fear sets in, individuals may wander in search of something that seems familiar to them. Increased walking at night corresponds with disruption of diurnal rhythm. In any event, wandering behavior in dementia can cause great problems for caregivers. Wandering is often a bigger problem in mid-stage dementia, and less so in later stages. Often patients new to a nursing home will wander in an attempt to become oriented to new surroundings. Wandering behavior can also be attributed to physical causes, such as hunger, thirst, and urinary or fecal urgency. When the wandering behavior begins after a long period of stability, it is likely that a new complication may be occurring—medical, psychiatric, or cognitive. Delirium may produce the abrupt onset of wandering behavior. The goals of wandering therapy are to keep the individual safe, to prevent intrusion into others' rooms, and to try to determine contributing factors to the behavior. When caring for a client who wanders, it is important to keep the following interventions in mind:

■ Keep the individual on a structured schedule of recreational activities and a strict feeding and toileting schedule.

■ Provide a safe, enclosed place for pacing and wandering.

■ Walk with the individual for a while and gently redirect him or her back to the care unit.

■ Ensure that outdoor exits are electronically controlled.

Disturbed Thought Processes and Sensory Perception

Disturbed thought processes and sensory perception are evidenced by disorientation, confusion, memory deficits, and inaccurate interpretation of the environment, including illusions, delusions, and hallucinations. NANDA defines *Disturbed Thought Processes* as a "disruption in cognitive operations and activities" (NANDA-I, 2009, p. 408). *Disturbed Sensory Perception* is defined as a "change in the amount or patterning of incoming stimuli accompanied by a diminished, exaggerated, distorted, or impaired response to such stimuli" (NANDA-I, 2009, p. 163).

Client Goals

Outcome criteria include short- and long-term goals. Timelines are individually determined.

Short-Term Goals

■ Client will utilize measures provided (e.g., clocks, calendars, room identification) to maintain reality orientation.

■ Client will experience fewer episodes of acute confusion.

Long-Term Goal

■ With assistance from caregiver, client will be able to interrupt non–reality-based thinking.

Interventions
For the Client Who Is Disoriented

■ Try to keep the client as oriented to reality as possible.

■ Use clocks and calendars with large numbers that are easy to read.

■ Place large colorful signs on the doors to identify clients' rooms, bathrooms, activity rooms, dining rooms, and chapel.

■ Allow the client to have as many of his or her personal items as possible. Even an old familiar chair in the room can provide a degree of comfort.

■ If at all possible, encourage family and close friends to be a part of the client's care, to promote feelings of security and orientation.

■ Provide the client with radio, television, and music if they are diversions the client enjoys; these may add a feeling of familiarity to the environment.

■ Ensure that noise level is controlled to prevent excess stimulation.

■ Allow the client to view old photograph albums and utilize reminiscence therapy. These are excellent ways to provide orientation to reality.

■ Maintain consistency of staff and caregivers to the best extent possible. Familiarity promotes comfort and feelings of security.

■ Continuously monitor for medication side effects. Physiological changes in the elderly can alter the body's response to certain medications. Toxic effects may intensify altered cognitive processes.

■ There has been some criticism in recent years about reality orientation of individuals with dementia (particularly those with moderate to severe disease process), suggesting that constant relearning of material contributes to problems with mood and self-esteem (Spector, Davies, Woods, & Orrell, 2000). (See Box 24-3, Validation Therapy.)

For the Client With Delusions and Hallucinations

■ Discourage rumination of delusional thinking. Do not disagree with made up stories. Instead, gently correct the client, and guide the conversation toward topics about real events and real people.

BOX 24-3 Validation Therapy

Some people believe it is not helpful (and sometimes even cruel) to try to insist that a person with moderate to severe dementia continually try to grasp what we know as the "real world." Allen (2000) stated,

> There is no successful alternative but to accept whatever the dementia person claims as their reality, no matter how untrue it is to us. There is no successful way to 'force' a person with dementia to join the 'real' world. The most frustrated caregivers are the ones who do not accept this simple fact: the world of dementia is defined by the dementia victim.

Validation therapy (VT) was originated by Naomi Feil, a gerontological social worker, who describes the process as "communicating with a disoriented elderly person by validating and respecting their feelings in whatever time or place is real to them at the time, even though this may not correspond with our 'here and now' reality" (Day, 2003). Feil suggests that the validation principle is truthful to the person with dementia because people live on several levels of awareness (Feil, 2007). She suggests that, if an individual asks to see his or her spouse, and the spouse has been dead for many years, that on some level of awareness, that person knows the truth. To keep reminding the person that the spouse is dead may only serve to cause repeated episodes of grief and distress, as he or she receives the information "anew" each time it is presented (Allen, 2000).

Validation therapy validates the feelings and emotions of a person with dementia. It often also integrates redirection techniques. Allen (2000) stated, "The key is to 'agree' with what they want but by conversation and 'steering' get them to do something else without them realizing they are actually being redirected. This is both validation and redirection therapy."

EXAMPLE:

Mrs. W. (agitated): "That old lady stole my watch! I know she did. She goes into people's rooms and takes our things. We call her 'sticky fingers!'"

Nurse: "That watch is very important to you. Have you looked around the room for it?"

Mrs. W.: "My husband gave it to me. He will be so upset that it is gone. I'm afraid to tell him."

Nurse: "I'm sure you miss your husband very much. Tell me what it was like when you were together. What kinds of things did you do for fun?"

Mrs. W.: "We did a lot of traveling. To Italy, and England, and France. We ate wonderful food."

Nurse: "Speaking of food, it is lunch time, and I will walk with you to the dining room."

Mrs. W.: "Yes, I'm getting really hungry."

In this situation, the nurse validated Mrs. W.'s feelings about not being able to find her watch. She did not deny that it had been stolen, nor did she remind Mrs. W. that her husband was deceased. (*Remember: a concept of VT is that, on some level, Mrs. W. knows that her husband is dead.*) The nurse validated the emotions Mrs. W. was feeling about missing her husband. She brought up special times that Mrs. W. and her husband

Continued

BOX 24-3 Validation Therapy—cont'd

had spent together, which served to elevate her mood and self-esteem. And lastly, she redirected Mrs. W. to the dining room to have her lunch. (The watch was eventually found in Mrs. W.'s medicine cabinet, where she had hidden it for safekeeping.)

Feil (2007) presented another example:

When a resident asks for his wife who is dead, caregivers reply, "She'll be here to see you later." The resident may not remember much, but he clings to that statement. He continues to ask for his wife on a daily basis, and the caregivers continue to lie. Eventually he loses trust in the caregivers, knowing that what they say is not true. With VT, the caregivers would encourage the resident to talk about his wife. They would validate his emotions, and encourage him to express his needs, accepting the fact that there is a reason behind his behavior. He has not simply "forgotten that his wife died;" he needs to grieve for her. This is unfinished business. When the emotion is expressed and someone listens with empathy, it is relieved. The old man no longer needs to search for his wife. He feels safe with the caregiver, whom he trusts. He always knew on a deep level of awareness that his wife had died. (pp. 3, 4)

■ Never argue a point with the client; to do so only serves to increase his or her anxiety and agitation.

■ Do not ignore reports of hallucinations when it is clear that the client is experiencing them. It is important for the nurse to hear an explanation of the hallucination from the client. These perceptions are very real and often very frightening to the client. Unless they are appropriately managed, hallucinations can escalate into disturbing and even hostile behaviors. Visual and auditory hallucinations are the most common type in dementia. Often the physician will treat these manifestations with antipsychotic medication.

■ Rule out the disturbed sensory perception as a possible side effect of certain physical conditions or medications.

■ Check to ensure that hearing aid is working properly and to ensure that faulty sounds are not being emitted.

■ Check eyeglasses to ensure that the individual is indeed wearing his or her own glasses.

■ Try to determine from where the visual hallucination is emanating. Clients often see faces in patterns on fabrics or in pictures on the wall. A mirror can also be the culprit of false perceptions. These may need to be moved or covered.

■ Provide reassurance that the client is safe. It may be necessary to stay with the client for a while until he or she is calm.

■ Never argue that the hallucination is not real. Try to let the client know that, although you are not sharing the experience, you understand how very distressing it is for him or her.

■ Distract the client. Hallucinations are less likely to occur when the person is occupied or involved in what is going on around them. Focus on real situations and real people.

■ Depending on the situation, it may be better to go along with the client rather than attempting to distract him or her (McShane, 2000). Not all hallucinations are upsetting.

EXAMPLE:

An elderly woman approaches the nurses station and says, "I'm so perturbed. The woman in my room refuses to turn down my bed so that I can go to sleep." The nurse may respond, "I'm sorry for the inconvenience, Mrs. G., but I will walk to your room with you and see that your bed is turned down." The nurse chats with Mrs. G. about something that occurred during the day, and by the time they arrive at her room, there is no further mention of a woman in her room.

Impaired Verbal Communication

When individuals who are cognitively impaired begin to lose their ability to process verbal communication, how words are expressed becomes as important as what is said. NANDA defines *Impaired Verbal Communication* as "decreased, delayed, or absent ability to receive, process, transmit, and/or use a system of symbols" (NANDA-I, 2009, p. 178).

Client Goals

Outcome criteria include short- and long-term goals. Timelines are individually determined.

IMPLICATIONS OF RESEARCH FOR EVIDENCE-BASED PRACTICE

Kovach, C. R., Noonan, P. E., Schlidt, A. M., & Wells, T. (2005). A model of consequences of need-driven, dementia-compromised behavior. *Journal of Nursing Scholarship, 37*(2), 134–140.

DESCRIPTION OF THE STUDY: Need-driven, dementia-compromised behavior (NDB) occurs because the caregiver is unable to comprehend needs, and the person with dementia cannot make needs known. The behaviors are viewed as an attempt on the part of the person with dementia to communicate a need and as a symptom that the need is not being met. The authors extended the primary need model to encompass secondary needs when primary needs go unresolved. From an extensive literature review, the authors proposed a framework for improving understanding of the person with dementia and the consequences of behavioral symptoms and unmet needs.

RESULTS OF THE STUDY: The experiences of people with dementia who have unmet needs are described as having "cascading effects." In people with dementia, basic needs (e.g., thirst/need for fluid) result in primary NDB (e.g., restlessness/ repetitive movements), which if left unmet may result in the negative outcome of constipation and abdominal discomfort. This need for relief may lead to the secondary NDB of aggression. The authors stated, "Secondary NDBs are iatrogenic outcomes of these cascading effects and the response of a vulnerable person to the recurrent and unpredictable stress of treatment targeted inappropriately or care providers who dismiss the NDB communication." Common problematic behaviors that may be associated with unmet needs include resistiveness to care, verbal complaining, restlessness, facial grimacing, aggression, crying, moaning, calling out, exiting behavior, tense body parts, and rubbing or holding a body part. Unmet needs may also influence affective status (e.g., depression or anxiety), physical status (e.g., immune suppression), and acceleration in functional status.

IMPLICATIONS FOR NURSING PRACTICE: The authors of this study stated, "The consequences of need-driven dementia-compromised behavior theory indicates that meeting needs of people with dementia will moderate the sequence of events that leads to negative outcomes." When caregivers cannot understand primary NDBs, they cannot provide anticipatory care. The anticipation and fulfillment of clients' needs is necessary to decrease the prevalence and severity of new unmet needs, thereby positively influencing comfort and quality of life for people with dementia.

Short-Term Goals

■ Client will be able to make needs known to primary caregiver.

■ Client is able to understand basic communications in interactions with primary caregiver.

Long-Term Goal

■ (In latter stages of the illness, when client is unable to communicate), needs are anticipated and fulfilled by primary caregiver.

Interventions

■ Keep interactions with the client calm and reassuring.

■ Use simple words, speak slowly and distinctly, and keep face-to-face contact with the client.

■ Always identify yourself to the client, and call the client by name at each meeting

■ Use nonverbal gestures to help the client understand what you want him or her to accomplish, if appropriate.

■ Ask only one question (or give only one direction) at a time, and give the client plenty of time to process the information and respond. The question may need to be rephrased if it is clear that the client has not understood the meaning of the direction.

■ Always try to approach the client from the front. An unexpected approach or touch from behind may startle and upset the client, and may even promote aggressive behavior.

■ Maintain consistency of staff and caregivers to the best extent possible. This facilitates comfort and security and promotes an effective communication process with the client.

■ Should the client become verbally aggressive, remain calm, and provide validation for his or her feelings. (e.g., "I know this is a hard time for you. You were always so busy and so active, and you took care of so many people. Maybe you could tell me about some of those people.")

■ When it is clearly appropriate, use touch and affection to communicate. Sometimes clients will respond to a hug or to a hand reaching for theirs when they will respond to nothing else.

Self-Care Deficit

It is important for clients to remain as independent as possible for as long as possible. They should be encouraged to accomplish ADLs to the best of their ability. NANDA defines *Self-Care Deficit* as "impaired ability to perform [activities of daily living] for self" (NANDA-I, 2009, pp. 153–156).

Client Goals

Outcome criteria include short- and long-term goals. Timelines are individually determined.

Short-Term Goal

■ Client will participate in ADLs with assistance from caregiver.

Long-Term Goals

■ Client will accomplish ADLs to the best of his or her ability.

■ Unfulfilled needs will be met by caregiver.

Interventions

■ Provide a simple, structured environment for the client, identify self-care deficits, and offer assistance as required.

■ Allow plenty of time for the client to complete tasks.

■ Provide guidance and support for independent actions by talking the client through the task one step at a time.

■ Provide a structured schedule of activities that does not change from day to day.

■ Ensure that ADLs follow the client's usual routine as closely as possible.

■ Minimize confusion by providing for consistency in assignment of daily caregivers.

■ Perform an ongoing assessment of the client's ability to fulfill his or her nutritional needs, ensure personal safety, follow the medication regimen, and communicate the need for assistance with activities that he or she cannot accomplish independently. Anticipate needs that are not verbally communicated.

■ If the client is to be discharged to family caregivers, assess those caregivers' ability to anticipate and fulfill client's unmet needs. Provide information to assist caregivers with this responsibility. Ensure that caregivers are aware of available community support systems from which they may seek assistance when required. Examples include adult day-care centers, housekeeping and homemaker services, respite care services, or the local chapter of a national support organization. Two of these include the following:

• For Alzheimer's disease information:

Alzheimer's Association

225 N. Michigan Ave., Fl. 17

Chicago, IL 60601-7633

1-800-272-3900

http://www.alz.org

• For Parkinson's disease information:

National Parkinson Foundation, Inc.

1501 N.W. 9th Ave.

Miami, FL 33136-1494

1-800-327-4545

http://www.parkinson.org

Concept Care Mapping

The concept map care plan is an innovative approach to planning and organizing nursing care (see Chapter 9). It is a diagrammatic teaching and learning strategy that allows visualization of interrelationships between medical diagnoses, nursing diagnoses, assessment data, and treatments. An example of a concept map care plan for a client with a cognitive disorder is presented in Figure 24–3.

Client/Family Education

The role of client teacher is important in the psychiatric area, as it is in all areas of nursing. A list of topics for client/family education relevant to cognitive disorders is presented in Box 24-4. Sample client teaching guides are presented in Appendix G.

Evaluation

In the final step of the nursing process, reassessment occurs to determine if the nursing interventions have been effective in achieving the intended goals of care. Evaluation of the client with a cognitive disorder is based on a series of short-term goals rather than on long-term goals. Resolution of identified problems is unrealistic for this client. Instead, outcomes must be measured in terms of slowing down the process rather than stopping or curing the problem. Evaluation questions may include the following:

■ Has the client experienced injury?

■ Does the client maintain orientation to time, person, place, and situation most of the time?

■ Is the client able to fulfill basic needs? Have those needs unmet by the client been fulfilled by caregivers?

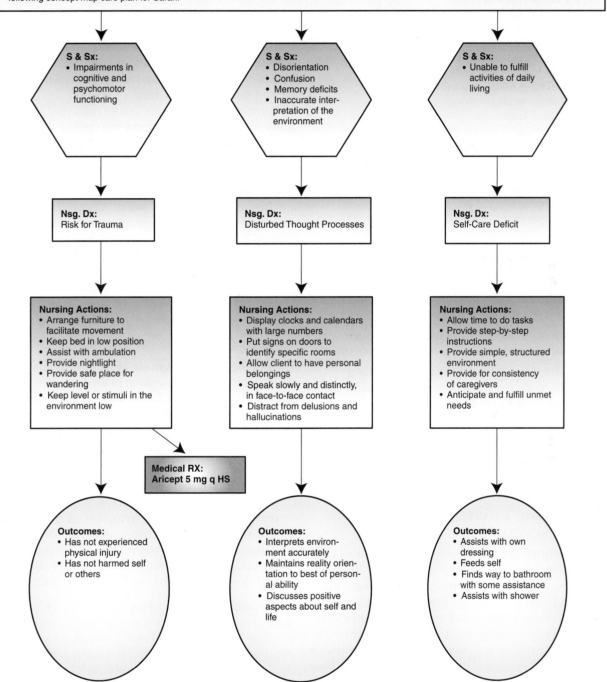

Clinical Vignette: Sarah, age 82, a widow of many years, has been admitted to a long-term care facility with a diagnosis of Alzheimer's disease. She is confused about her whereabouts and says to the nurse, "I think I've been here long enough now. It's time for me to go home. I'll just call my husband to come get me." She wanders around the unit and cannot find her room. She attempts to go out the locked door to the outside, and set off the alarm. With much reluctance, she allows the nurse to help her get ready for bed. The nurse discovers her awake in the middle of the night and wandering into other patients' rooms. She appears in the dining room the next morning barefoot and wearing her pajamas. The nurse develops the following concept map care plan for Sarah.

S & Sx:
- Impairments in cognitive and psychomotor functioning

S & Sx:
- Disorientation
- Confusion
- Memory deficits
- Inaccurate interpretation of the environment

S & Sx:
- Unable to fulfill activities of daily living

Nsg. Dx:
Risk for Trauma

Nsg. Dx:
Disturbed Thought Processes

Nsg. Dx:
Self-Care Deficit

Nursing Actions:
- Arrange furniture to facilitate movement
- Keep bed in low position
- Assist with ambulation
- Provide nightlight
- Provide safe place for wandering
- Keep level or stimuli in the environment low

Nursing Actions:
- Display clocks and calendars with large numbers
- Put signs on doors to identify specific rooms
- Allow client to have personal belongings
- Speak slowly and distinctly, in face-to-face contact
- Distract from delusions and hallucinations

Nursing Actions:
- Allow time to do tasks
- Provide step-by-step instructions
- Provide simple, structured environment
- Provide for consistency of caregivers
- Anticipate and fulfill unmet needs

Medical RX:
Aricept 5 mg q HS

Outcomes:
- Has not experienced physical injury
- Has not harmed self or others

Outcomes:
- Interprets environment accurately
- Maintains reality orientation to best of personal ability
- Discusses positive aspects about self and life

Outcomes:
- Assists with own dressing
- Feeds self
- Finds way to bathroom with some assistance
- Assists with shower

FIGURE 24–3   Concept map care plan for client with dementia.

■ Is confusion minimized by familiar objects and structured, routine schedule of activities?

■ Do the prospective caregivers have information regarding the progression of the client's illness?

■ Do caregivers have information regarding where to go for assistance and support in the care of their loved one?

■ Have the prospective caregivers received instruction in how to promote the client's safety, minimize confusion and disorientation, and cope with difficult client behaviors (e.g., hostility, anger, depression, agitation)?

Quality and Safety Education for Nurses (QSEN)

The Institute of Medicine (IOM), in its 2003 report, *Health Professions Education: A Bridge to Quality,* challenged faculties of medicine, nursing, and other health professions to ensure that their graduates have achieved a core set of competencies in order to meet the needs of the 21st-century health-care system. These competencies include *providing patient-centered care, working in interdisciplinary teams, employing evidence-based practice, applying quality improvement,* and *utilizing informatics.* A QSEN teaching strategy is included in Box 24-5. The use of this type of activity is intended to arm the instructor and the student with guidelines for attaining the knowledge, skills, and attitudes necessary for achievement of quality and safety competencies in nursing.

Medical Treatment Modalities

Delirium

The first step in the treatment of delirium should be the determination and correction of the underlying causes. Additional attention must be given to fluid and electrolyte status, hypoxia, anoxia, and diabetic problems. Staff members should remain with the client at all times to monitor behavior and provide reorientation and assurance. The room should maintain a low level of stimuli.

Some physicians prefer not to prescribe medications for the delirious client, reasoning that additional agents may only compound the syndrome of brain dysfunction. However, the agitation and aggression demonstrated by the delirious client may require chemical and/or mechanical restraint for his or her personal safety. Choice of specific therapy is made with consideration for the client's clinical condition and the underlying cause of the delirium. Low-dose neuroleptics are the pharmacological treatment of choice in most cases (Trzepacz et al., 2006). A benzodiazepine (e.g., lorazepam) is commonly used when the etiology is substance withdrawal (Eisendrath & Lichtmacher, 2009).

Dementia

Once a definitive diagnosis of dementia has been made, a primary consideration in the treatment of the disorder is the etiology. Focus must be directed to the identification and resolution of potentially reversible processes. Sadock and Sadock (2007) stated:

> Once dementia is diagnosed, patients must undergo a complete medical and neurological workup, because 10 to 15 percent of all patients with dementia have a potentially reversible condition if treatment is initiated before permanent brain damage occurs. [Causes of potentially-reversible dementia include] hypothyroidism, normal pressure hydrocephalus, and brain tumors. (p. 340)

The need for general supportive care, with provisions for security, stimulation, patience, and nutrition, has been recognized and accepted. A number of pharmaceutical agents have been tried, with varying degrees of success, in the treatment of clients with dementia. Some of these drugs are described in the following sections according to symptomatology for which they are indicated. A summary of medications for clients with dementia is provided in Table 24-4.

Cognitive Impairment

The cholinesterase inhibitor physostigmine (Antilirium) has been shown to enhance cognitive functioning in individuals with mild to moderate

BOX 24-5 QSEN TEACHING STRATEGY

Assignment: Linking Evidence-Based Practice With a Nursing Procedure
Reality Orientation of Clients With Dementia

Competency Domain: Evidence-Based Practice
Learning Objectives: Student will:
- Locate an evidence-based practice article on a hospital protocol, and compare and contrast this information with the facility's protocol.
- Identify whether evidence-based practice is utilized with this protocol, and identify barriers or challenges with implementing evidence-based practice in the clinical setting.

Strategy Overview:
1. Research the nursing intervention of reality orientation of clients with dementia. Identify the pros and cons and ethical issues associated with this intervention (particularly with clients who have advanced dementia).
2. Find an evidence-based practice journal article about the intervention.
3. Locate the facility's protocol for reality orientation of clients with dementia.
4. Compare and contrast the facility's protocol with how unit staff carry out this intervention. If there are deviations from the written protocol, what are they and why do the nurses deviate from the written protocol?
5. Compare and contrast the hospital's protocol with the information found in the evidence-based practice article.
6. At postconference, summarize the article on evidence-based practice to the clinical group, and report information gathered throughout the clinical day. Discuss any ethical dilemmas associated with the intervention.
7. Write a paper discussing personal reflections and feelings about this intervention.

Adapted from teaching strategy submitted by Chris Tesch, Instructor, University of South Dakota, Sioux Falls, SD. © 2009 QSEN; http://qsen.org. With permission.

TABLE 24-4 Selected Medications Used in the Treatment of Clients With Dementia

MEDICATION	CLASSIFICATION	DAILY DOSAGE RANGE (mg)	SIDE EFFECTS
For Treatment of Cognitive Impairment			
Tacrine (Cognex)	Cholinesterase inhibitor	40–160	Dizziness, headache, GI upset, elevated transaminase
Donepezil (Aricept)	Cholinesterase inhibitor	5–10	Insomnia, dizziness, GI upset, headache
Rivastigmine (Exelon)	Cholinesterase inhibitor	6–12	Dizziness, headache, GI upset, fatigue
Galantamine (Razadyne)	Cholinesterase inhibitor	8–24	Dizziness, headache, GI upset
Memantine (Namenda)	NMDA receptor antagonist	5–20	Dizziness, headache, constipation
For Treatment of Agitation, Aggression, Hallucinations, Thought Disturbances, Wandering			
Risperidone* (Risperdal)	Antipsychotic	1–4 (Increase dosage cautiously)	Agitation, insomnia, headache, extrapyramidal symptoms
Olanzapine* (Zyprexa)	Antipsychotic	5 (Increase dosage cautiously)	Hypotension, dizziness, sedation, constipation, weight gain, dry mouth

Continued

TABLE 24-4 Selected Medications Used in the Treatment of Clients With Dementia—cont'd

MEDICATION	CLASSIFICATION	DAILY DOSAGE RANGE (mg)	SIDE EFFECTS
Quetiapine* (Seroquel)	Antipsychotic	Initial dose 25 (Titrate slowly)	Hypotension, tachycardia, dizziness, drowsiness, headache, constipation, dry mouth
Haloperidol* (Haldol)	Antipsychotic	1–4 (Increase dosage cautiously)	Dry mouth, blurred vision, orthostatic hypotension, extrapyramidal symptoms, sedation
For Treatment of Depression			
Sertraline (Zoloft)	Antidepressant (SSRI)	50–100	Fatigue, insomnia, sedation, GI upset, headache, dizziness
Paroxetine (Paxil)	Antidepressant (SSRI)	10–40	Dizziness, headache, insomnia, somnolence, GI upset
Nortriptyline (Pamelor)	Antidepressant (tricyclic)	30–50	Anticholinergic, orthostatic hypotension, sedation, arrhythmia
For Treatment of Anxiety			
Lorazepam (Ativan)	Antianxiety (benzodiazepine)	1–2	Drowsiness, dizziness, GI upset, hypotension, tolerance, dependence
Oxazepam (Serax)	Antianxiety (benzodiazepine)	10–30	Drowsiness, dizziness, GI upset, hypotension, tolerance, dependence
For Treatment of Insomnia			
Temazepam (Restoril)	Sedative-Hypnotic (benzodiazepine)	15	Drowsiness, dizziness, GI upset, hypotension, tolerance, dependence
Zolpidem (Ambien)	Sedative-Hypnotic (nonbenzodiazepine)	5	Headache, drowsiness, dizziness, GI upset
Zaleplon (Sonata)	Sedative-Hypnotic (nonbenzodiazepine)	5	Headache, drowsiness, dizziness, GI upset
Eszopiclone (Lunesta)	Sedative-Hypnotic (nonbenzodiazepine)	1–2	Headache, drowsiness, dizziness, GI upset, unpleasant taste
For Treatment of Depression and Insomnia			
Trazodone (Desyrel)	Antidepressant (heterocyclic)	50	Dizziness, drowsiness, dry mouth, blurred vision, GI upset
Mirtazapine (Remeron)	Antidepressant (tetracyclic)	7.5–15	Somnolence, dry mouth, constipation, increased appetite

*Although clinicians may still prescribe these drugs in low-risk patients, no antipsychotics have been approved by the FDA for the treatment of patients with dementia-related psychosis. All antipsychotics include black-box warnings about increased risk of death in elderly dementia patients.

AD, although its short half-life makes it less desirable than the newer medications (Coelho Filho & Birks, 2001).

Other cholinesterase inhibitors are also being used for treatment of mild to moderate cognitive impairment in AD. Some of the clinical manifestations of AD are thought to be the result of a deficiency of the neurotransmitter acetylcholine. In the brain, acetylcholine is inactivated by the enzyme acetylcholinesterase. Tacrine (Cognex), donepezil (Aricept), rivastigmine (Exelon), and galantamine (Razadyne) act by inhibiting acetylcholinesterase, which slows the degradation of acetylcholine, thereby increasing concentrations of the neurotransmitter in the cerebral cortex. Because their action relies on functionally intact cholinergic neurons, the effects of these medications may lessen as the disease process advances, and there is no evidence that these medications alter the course of the underlying dementing process.

Another medication, an *N*-methyl-D-aspartate (NMDA) receptor antagonist, was approved by the U.S. Food and Drug Administration (FDA) in 2003. The medication, memantine (Namenda), was approved for the treatment of moderate to severe AD. High levels of glutamate in the brains of AD patients are thought to contribute to the symptomatology and decline in functionality. These high levels are caused by a dysfunction in glutamate transmission. In normal neurotransmission, glutamate plays an essential role in learning and memory by triggering NMDA receptors to allow a controlled amount of calcium to flow into a nerve cell (Alzheimer's Association, 2007b). This creates the appropriate environment for information processing. In AD, there is a sustained release of glutamate, which results in a continuous influx of calcium into the nerve cells. This increased intracellular calcium concentration ultimately leads to disruption and death of the neurons. Memantine may protect cells against excess glutamate by partially blocking NMDA receptors. Memantine has shown in clinical trials to be effective in improving cognitive function and the ability to perform ADLs in clients with moderate to severe AD. Although it does not stop or reverse the effects of the disease, it has been shown to slow down the progression of the decline in cognition and function (Salloway & Correia, 2009). Because memantine's action differs from that of the cholinesterase inhibitors, consideration is being given to possible coadministration of these medications. Ongoing research is revealing a greater improvement in cognitive function, ADLs, behavior, and clinical global status in clients who are administered a combination of memantine and a cholinesterase inhibitor than those administered either drug alone (Diamond, 2008).

Agitation, Aggression, Hallucinations, Thought Disturbances, and Wandering

Historically, physicians have prescribed antipsychotic medications to control agitation, aggression, hallucinations, thought disturbances, and wandering in clients with dementia. The newer antipsychotic medications such as risperidone, olanzapine, quetiapine, and ziprasidone are often favored because of their lessened propensity to cause anticholinergic and extrapyramidal side effects. In 2005, however, following review of a number of studies, the FDA ordered black-box warnings on drug labels of all the atypical antipsychotics noting that the drugs are associated with

an increased risk of death in elderly patients with psychotic behaviors associated with dementia. Most of the deaths appeared to be cardiovascular related. In July 2008, based on the results of several studies, the FDA extended this warning to include all first-generation antipsychotics as well, such as haloperidol and perphenazine (Yan, 2008). This poses a clinical dilemma for physicians who have found these medications to be helpful to their clients, and some have chosen to continue to use them in clients without significant cerebrovascular disease, in whom previous behavioral programs have failed, and with consent from relatives or guardians who are clearly aware of the risks and benefits.

Anticholinergic Effects Many antipsychotic, antidepressant, and antihistaminic medications produce anticholinergic side effects, which include confusion, blurred vision, constipation, dry mouth, dizziness, and difficulty urinating. Older people, and especially those with dementia, are particularly sensitive to these effects. Beers and Jones (2004) explained this phenomenon as follows:

> Older people are more likely to experience anticholinergic effects because as people age, the body produces less acetylcholine. Also, cells in many part of the body (such as the digestive tract) have fewer sites where acetylcholine can attach to them. Thus, the acetylcholine produced is less likely to have an effect, and the effect of anticholinergic drugs is greater. (p. 48)

Depression

It is estimated that up to 40 percent of people with AD also suffer from major depression (Alzheimer's Association, 2007a). Recognizing the symptoms of depression in these individuals is often a challenge. Depression—which affects thinking, memory, sleep, and appetite and interferes with daily life—is sometimes difficult to distinguish from dementia. Clearly, the existence of depression in the client with dementia complicates and worsens the individual's functioning.

Antidepressant medication is sometimes used in treatment of depression in dementia. The selective serotonin reuptake inhibitors (SSRIs) are considered by many to be the first-line drug treatment for depression in the elderly because of their favorable side-effect profile. Although still used by some physicians, tricyclic antidepressants are often avoided because of cardiac and anticholinergic side effects. Trazodone may be a good choice, used at bedtime, for depression and insomnia.

Dopaminergic agents (e.g., methylphenidate, amantadine, bromocriptine, and bupropion) may be helpful in the treatment of severe apathy (Rabins et al., 2006).

Not only is depression common in AD, but research has recently suggested that it may be a risk factor for the disease (Geerlings, den Heijer, Koudstaal, Hofman, & Breteler, 2008). This study found that individuals with a history of depression, particularly those with onset before age 60, had a 2.5 times greater risk of developing AD than people who had not suffered from depression. The authors suggested that further studies are required to understand the relationship between depression and AD. It is not completely understood whether depression contributes to the development of AD or whether another unknown factor is involved in the etiology of both depression and dementia.

Anxiety

The progressive loss of mental functioning is a significant source of anxiety in the early stages of dementia. It is important that clients be encouraged to verbalize their feelings and fears associated with this loss. These interventions may be useful in reducing the anxiety of clients with dementia.

Antianxiety medications may be helpful but should not be used routinely or for prolonged periods. The least toxic and most effective of the antianxiety medications are the benzodiazepines. Examples include diazepam (Valium), chlordiazepoxide (Librium), alprazolam (Xanax), lorazepam (Ativan), and oxazepam (Serax). The drugs with shorter half-lives (e.g., lorazepam and oxazepam) are preferred to the longer-acting medications (e.g., diazepam), which promote a higher risk of oversedation and falls. Barbiturates are not appropriate as antianxiety agents because they frequently induce confusion and paradoxical excitement in elderly individuals.

Sleep Disturbances

Sleep problems are common in clients with dementia and often intensify as the disease progresses. Wakefulness and nighttime wandering create much distress and anguish in family members who are charged with protection of their loved one. Indeed, sleep disturbances are among the problems that most frequently initiate the need for placement of the client in a long-term care facility.

Some physicians treat sleep problems with sedative-hypnotic medications. The benzodiazepines may be useful for some clients but are indicated for relatively brief periods only. Examples include flurazepam (Dalmane), temazepam (Restoril), and triazolam (Halcion). Daytime sedation and cognitive impairment, in addition to paradoxical agitation in elderly clients, are of particular concern with these medications (Beers & Jones, 2004). The nonbenzodiazepine sedative-hypnotics zolpidem (Ambien), zaleplon (Sonata), eszopiclone (Lunesta), and ramelteon (Rozerem), and the antidepressants trazodone (Desyrel) and mirtazapine (Remeron), are also prescribed. Daytime sedation may also be a problem with these medications. As previously stated, barbiturates should not be used in elderly clients. Sleep problems are usually ongoing, and most clinicians prefer to use medications only to help an individual through a short-term stressful situation. Rising at the same time each morning; minimizing daytime sleep; participating in regular physical exercise (but no later than 4 hours before bedtime); getting proper nutrition; avoiding alcohol, caffeine, and nicotine; and retiring at the same time each night are behavioral approaches to sleep problems that may eliminate the need for sleep aids, particularly in the early stages of dementia. Because of the tremendous potential for adverse drug reactions in the elderly, many of whom are already taking multiple medications, pharmacological treatment of insomnia should be considered only after attempts at nonpharmacological strategies have failed.

CASE STUDY AND SAMPLE CARE PLAN

NURSING HISTORY AND ASSESSMENT

Carmen is an 81-year-old widow who lives in the same small town, in the same house that she shared with her husband until his death 16 years ago. She and her husband raised two daughters, Joan and Nancy, who have been living with their husbands in a large city about 2 hours away from Carmen. They have always visited Carmen every 1 or 2 months. She has four grown grandchildren who live in distant states, and who see their grandmother on holidays.

About a year ago, Carmen's daughters began to receive reports from friends and other family members about incidents in which Carmen was becoming forgetful (e.g., forgetting to go to a cousin's birthday party, taking a wrong turn and getting lost on the way to a niece's house [where she had driven many times], returning to church to search for something she thought she "had forgotten," [although she could not explain what it was], sending birthday gifts to people when it was not their birthday). During routine visits,

CASE STUDY AND SAMPLE CARE PLAN — cont'd

the elder daughter, Joan, found bills left unpaid, sometimes months overdue. Housekeepers and yard workers reported to Joan that Carmen would forget she had paid them, and try to pay them again...and sometimes a third time. She became very confused when she would attempt to fill her weekly pillboxes, a task she had completed in the past without difficulty. Hundreds of dollars would disappear from her wallet, and she could not tell Joan what happened to it.

Joan and her husband subsequently moved to the small town where Carmen lived. They bought a home, and Joan visited her mother every day, took care of finances, and ensured that Carmen took her daily medications, although Joan worked in a job that required occasional out-of-town travel. As the months progressed, Carmen's cognitive abilities deteriorated. She burned food on the stove, left the house with the broiler-oven on, forgot to take her medication, got lost in her car, missed appointments, and forgot the names of her neighbors whom she had known for many years. She began to lose weight because she began forgetting to eat her meals.

Carmen was evaluated by a neurologist, who diagnosed her with Dementia of the Alzheimer's Type, Late Onset. Because they believed that Carmen needed 24-hour care, Joan and Nancy made the painful decision to place Carmen in long-term care. In the nursing home, her condition has continued to deteriorate. Carmen wanders up and down the halls (day and night), and she has fallen twice, once while attempting to get out of bed. She requires assistance to shower and dress, and has become incontinent of urine. The nurses found her attempting to leave the building, saying, "I'm going across the street to visit my daughter." One morning at breakfast she appeared in her pajamas in the communal dining room, not realizing that she had not dressed. She is unable to form new memories, and sometimes uses confabulation to fill in the blanks. She asks the same questions repeatedly, sometimes struggling for the right word. She can no longer provide the correct names of items in her environment. She has no concept of time.

Joan visits Carmen daily, and Nancy visits weekly, each offering support to the other in person and by phone. Carmen always seems pleased to see them, but can no longer call either of them by name. They are unsure if she knows who they are.

NURSING DIAGNOSES/OUTCOME IDENTIFICATION

From the assessment data, the nurse develops the following nursing diagnoses for Carmen:

1. **Risk for trauma** related to impairments in cognitive and psychomotor functioning; wandering; falls
   a. **Outcome Criteria:** Carmen will remain injury free during her nursing home stay.

   b. **Short-term goals:**
      ■ Carmen will not fall while wandering the halls.
      ■ Carmen will not fall out of bed.

2. **Disturbed thought processes** related to cerebral degeneration evidenced by disorientation, confusion, and memory deficits
   a. **Outcome Criteria:** Carmen will maintain reality orientation to the best of her cognitive ability.
   b. **Short-term goals:**
      ■ Carmen will be able to find her room.
      ■ Carman will be able to communicate her needs to staff.

3. **Self-care deficit** related to cognitive impairments, disorientation, confusion, and memory deficits
   a. **Outcome Criteria:** Carmen will accomplish ADLs to the best of her ability.
   b. **Short-term goals:**
      ■ Carmen will assist with dressing herself.
      ■ Carmen will cooperate with trips to the bathroom.
      ■ Carmen will wash herself in the shower, with help from the nurse.

PLANNING/IMPLEMENTATION

Risk for Trauma

The following nursing interventions may be implemented ***in an effort to ensure client safety:***

1. Arrange the furniture in Carmen's room so that it will accommodate her moving around freely.

2. Store frequently used items within her easy reach.

3. Provide a "low bed," or possibly move her mattress from the bed to the floor, to prevent falls from bed.

4. Attach a bed alarm to alert the nurse's station when Carmen has alighted from her bed.

5. Keep a dim light on in her room at night.

6. During the day and evening, provide a well-lighted area where Carmen can safely wander.

7. Ensure that all outside doors are electronically controlled.

8. Play soft music and maintain a low level of stimuli in the environment.

Disturbed Thought Processes

The following nursing interventions may be implemented ***to help maintain orientation and aid in memory and recognition:***

1. Use clocks and calendars with large numbers that are easy to read.

2. Put a sign on Carmen's door with her name on it, and hang a personal item of hers on the door.

Continued

CASE STUDY AND SAMPLE CARE PLAN — cont'd

3. Ask Joan to bring some of Carmen's personal items for her room, even a favorite comfy chair, if possible. Ask also for some old photograph albums if they are available.

4. Keep staff and caregivers to a minimum to promote familiarity.

5. Speak slowly and clearly while looking into Carmen's face.

6. Use reminiscence therapy with Carmen. Ask her to share happy times from her life with you. This technique helps decrease depression and boost self-esteem.

7. Mention the date and time in casual conversation. Refer to "spring rain," "summer flowers," "fall leaves." Emphasize holidays.

8. Correct misperceptions gently and matter-of-factly, and focus on real events and real people if false ideas should occur. Validate her feelings associated with current and past life situations.

9. Monitor for medication side effects, because toxic effects from certain medications can intensify altered thought processes.

Self-Care Deficit

The following nursing interventions may be implemented **to ensure that all Carmen's needs are fulfilled.**

1. Assess what Carmen can do independently and with what she needs assistance.

2. Allow plenty of time for her to accomplish tasks that are within her ability. Clothing with easy removal or replacement, such as Velcro, facilitates independence.

3. Provide guidance and support for independent actions by talking her through tasks one step at a time.

4. Provide a structured schedule of activities that does not change from day to day.

5. Ensure that Carmen has snacks between meals.

6. Take Carmen to the bathroom regularly (according to her usual pattern, e.g., after meals, before bedtime, on arising)

7. To minimize nighttime wetness, offer fluid every 2 hours during the day and restrict fluid after 6:00 p.m.

8. To promote more restful nighttime sleep (and less wandering at night), reduce naps during late afternoon and encourage sitting exercises, walking, and ball toss. Carbohydrate snacks at bedtime may also be helpful.

EVALUATION

The outcome criteria identified for Carmen have been met. She has experienced no injury. She has not fallen out of bed. She continues to wander in a safe area. She can find her room by herself, but occasionally requires some assistance when she is anxious and more confused. She has some difficulty communicating her needs to the staff, but those who work with her on a consistent basis are able to anticipate her needs. All ADLs are being fulfilled, and Carmen assists with dressing and grooming, accomplishing about half on her own. Nighttime wandering has been minimized. Soft bedtime music helps to relax her.

Summary and Key Points

■ Cognitive disorders constitute a large and growing public health concern.

■ Cognitive disorders include delirium, dementia, and amnestic disorders.

■ A delirium is a disturbance of consciousness and a change in cognition that develop rapidly over a short period. Level of consciousness is often affected and psychomotor activity may fluctuate between agitated purposeless movements and a vegetative state resembling catatonic stupor.

■ The symptoms of delirium usually begin quite abruptly and often are reversible and brief.

■ Delirium may be caused by a general medical condition, substance intoxication or withdrawal, or ingestion of a medication or exposure to a toxin.

■ Dementia is a syndrome of acquired, persistent intellectual impairment with compromised function in multiple spheres of mental activity, such as memory, language, visuospatial skills, emotion or personality, and cognition.

■ Symptoms of dementia are insidious and develop slowly over time. In most clients, dementia runs a progressive, irreversible course.

■ Dementia may be caused by genetics, cardiovascular disease, infections, neurophysiological disorders, and other general medical conditions.

■ Amnestic disorders are characterized by an inability to learn new information despite normal attention and an inability to recall previously learned information. Remote past events are often more easily recalled than recent ones.

■ The onset of amnestic symptoms may be acute or insidious, depending on the pathological process causing the disorder. Duration and course of the illness may be quite variable and are also correlated with extent and severity of the cause.

■ Nursing care of the client with a cognitive disorder is presented around the six steps of the nursing process.

■ Objectives of care for the client experiencing an acute syndrome are aimed at eliminating the etiology, promoting client safety, and a return to the highest possible level of functioning.

■ Objectives of care for the client experiencing a chronic, progressive disorder are aimed at preserving the dignity of the individual, promoting deceleration of the symptoms, and maximizing functional capabilities.

■ Nursing interventions are also directed toward helping the client's family or primary caregivers learn about a chronic, progressive cognitive disorder.

■ Education is provided about the disease process, expectations of client behavioral changes, methods for facilitating care, and sources of assistance and support as they struggle, both physically and emotionally, with the demands brought on by a disease process that is slowly taking their loved one away from them.

DavisPlus   Additional info available @ davisplus.fadavis.com

Review Questions
Self-Examination/Learning Exercise

*Select the answer that is **most** appropriate for each of the following questions:*

1. An example of a treatable (reversible) form of dementia is one that is caused by which of the following? (Select all that apply.)
   a. Multiple sclerosis.
   b. Multiple small brain infarcts.
   c. Electrolyte imbalances.
   d. HIV disease.
   e. Folate deficiency.

2. Mrs. G. has been diagnosed with dementia of the Alzheimer's type. The cause of this disorder is which of the following?
   a. Multiple small brain infarcts.
   b. Chronic alcohol abuse.
   c. Cerebral abscess.
   d. Unknown.

3. Mrs. G. has been diagnosed with dementia of the Alzheimer's type. The *primary* nursing intervention in working with Mrs. G. is which of the following?
   a. Ensuring that she receives food she likes, to prevent hunger.
   b. Ensuring that the environment is safe, to prevent injury.
   c. Ensuring that she meets the other patients, to prevent social isolation.
   d. Ensuring that she takes care of her own ADLs, to prevent dependence.

4. Which of the following medications have been indicated for improvement in cognitive functioning in mild to moderate Alzheimer's disease? (Select all that apply.)
   a. Donepezil (Aricept).
   b. Rivastigmine (Exelon).
   c. Risperidone (Risperdal).
   d. Sertraline (Zoloft).
   e. Tacrine (Cognex).

Continued

Review Questions—cont'd
Self-Examination/Learning Exercise

5. Mrs. G., who has Alzheimer's disease, says to the nurse, "I have a date tonight. I always have a date on Christmas." Which of the following is the most appropriate response?
   a. "Don't be silly. It's not Christmas, Mrs. G."
   b. "Today is Tuesday, October 21, Mrs. G. We will have supper soon, and then your daughter will come to visit."
   c. "Who is your date with, Mrs. G.?"
   d. "I think you need some more medication, Mrs. G. I'll bring it to you now."

6. In addition to disturbances in cognition and orientation, individuals with Alzheimer's disease may also show changes in which of the following? (Select all that apply.)
   a. Personality.
   b. Vision.
   c. Speech.
   d. Hearing.
   e. Mobility.

7. Mrs. G., who has Alzheimer's disease, has trouble sleeping and wanders around at night. Which of the following nursing actions would be *best* to promote sleep in Mrs. G.?
   a. Ask the doctor to prescribe flurazepam (Dalmane).
   b. Ensure that Mrs. G. gets an afternoon nap so she will not be overtired at bedtime.
   c. Make Mrs. G. a cup of tea with honey before bedtime.
   d. Ensure that Mrs. G. gets regular physical exercise during the day.

8. The night nurse finds Mrs. G., a client with Alzheimer's disease, wandering the hallway at 4 a.m. and trying to open the door to the side yard. Which statement by the nurse probably reflects the most accurate assessment of the situation?
   a. "That door leads out to the patio, Mrs. G. It's nighttime. You don't want to go outside now."
   b. "You look confused, Mrs. G. What is bothering you?"
   c. "This is the patio door, Mrs. G. Are you looking for the bathroom?"
   d. "Are you lonely? Perhaps you'd like to go back to your room and talk for a while."

9. A client says to the nurse: "I read an article about Alzheimer's and it said the disease is hereditary. My mother has Alzheimer's disease. Does that mean I'll get it when I'm old?" The nurse bases her response on the knowledge that which of the following factors is *not* associated with increased incidence of dementia of the Alzheimer's type?
   a. Multiple small strokes.
   b. Family history of Alzheimer's disease.
   c. Head trauma.
   d. Advanced age.

10. Mr. Stone is a client in the hospital with a diagnosis of Vascular Dementia. In explaining this disorder to Mr. Stone's family, which of the following statements by the nurse is correct?
    a. "He will probably live longer than if his dementia was of the Alzheimer's type."
    b. "Vascular dementia shows stepwise progression. This is why he sometimes seems okay."
    c. "Vascular dementia is caused by plaques and tangles that form in the brain."
    d. "The cause of vascular dementia is unknown."

Review Questions—cont'd
Self-Examination/Learning Exercise

11. Which of the following interventions is most appropriate in helping a client with Alzheimer's disease with her ADLs? (Select all that apply.)
    a. Perform ADLs for her while she is in the hospital.
    b. Provide her with a written list of activities she is expected to perform.
    c. Assist her with step-by-step instructions.
    d. Tell her that, if her morning care is not completed by 9:00 a.m., it will be performed for her by the nurse's aide so that she can attend group therapy.
    e. Encourage her and give her plenty of time to perform as many of her ADLs as possible independently.

TEST YOUR CRITICAL THINKING SKILLS

Joe, a 62-year-old accountant, began having difficulty remembering details necessary to perform his job. He was also having trouble at home, failing to keep his finances straight, and forgetting to pay bills. It became increasingly difficult for him to function properly at work, and eventually he was forced to retire. Cognitive deterioration continued, and behavioral problems soon began. He became stubborn, verbally and physically abusive, and suspicious of most everyone in his environment. His wife and son convinced him to see a physician, who recommended hospitalization for testing.

At Joe's initial evaluation, he was fully alert and cooperative but obviously anxious and fidgety. He thought he was at his accounting office and he could not state what year it was. He could not say the names of his parents or siblings, nor did he know who was currently the president of the United States. He could not perform simple arithmetic calculations, write a proper sentence, or copy a drawing. He interpreted proverbs concretely and had difficulty stating similarities between related objects.

Laboratory serum studies revealed no abnormalities, but a CT scan showed marked cortical atrophy. The physician's diagnosis was Dementia of the Alzheimer's Type, Early Onset. *Answer the following questions related to Joe:*

1. Identify the pertinent assessment data from which nursing care will be devised.
2. What is the primary nursing diagnosis for Joe?
3. How would outcomes be identified?

References

Allen, J. (2000). Using validation therapy to manage difficult behaviors. *Prism Innovations. ElderCare Online.* Retrieved August 28, 2010, from http://www.ec-online.net/community/Activists/difficultbehaviors.htm

Alzheimer's Association (2007a). *Depression and Alzheimer's.* Retrieved August 28, 2010, from http://www.alz.org/living_with_alzheimers_depression.asp

Alzheimer's Association (2007b). *FDA-approved treatments for Alzheimer's.* Retrieved August 28, 2010, from http://www.alz.org/national/documents/topicsheet_treatments.pdf

Alzheimer's Association. (2010a). *2010 Alzheimer's disease facts and figures.* Chicago, IL: Alzheimer's Association.

Alzheimer's Association. (2010b). *Stages of Alzheimer's disease.* Retrieved August 28, 2010, from http://www.alz.org/alzheimers_disease_stages_of_alzheimers.asp

Alzheimer's Disease Education & Referral. (2008). *Alzheimer's disease genetics.* NIH Publication No. 08-6424. Washington, DC: National Institutes of Health.

American Psychiatric Association. (2000). *Diagnostic and statistical manual of mental disorders* (4th ed.) *Text revision.* Washington, DC: American Psychiatric Publishing.

Arvanitakis, Z. (2000). *Dementia and vascular disease.* Duval County Medical Society. Retrieved August 28, 2010, from http://www.dcmsonline.org/jax-medicine/2000journals/February2000/vascdement.htm

Beers, M. H., & Jones, T. V. (Eds.). (2004). Drugs and aging. In *The Merck manual of health and aging.* Whitehouse Station, NJ: Merck Research Laboratories.

Black, D. W., & Andreasen, N. C. (2011). *Introductory textbook of psychiatry* (5th ed.). Washington, DC: American Psychiatric Publishing.

Blazer, D. G. (2008). Treatment of seniors. In R. E. Hales, S. C. Yudofsky, & G. O. Gabbard (Eds.), *Textbook of psychiatry* (5th ed., pp. 1449–1469). Washington, DC: American Psychiatric Publishing.

Bourgeois, J. A., Seaman, J. S., & Servis, M. E. (2008). Delirium, dementia, and amnestic disorders. In R. E. Hales, S. C. Yudofsky, & G. O. Gabbard (Eds.), *Textbook of clinical psychiatry* (5th ed., pp. 259–308). Washington, DC: American Psychiatric Publishing.

Coelho Filho, J. M., & Birks, J. (2001). Physostigmine for dementia due to Alzheimer's disease (Cochrane Review). *The Cochrane Database of Systematic Reviews,* Issue 2, Art. No. CD001499.

Cummings, J. L., & Mega, M. S. (2003). *Neuropsychiatry and behavioral neuroscience.* New York: Oxford University Press.

Day, C. R. (2003). Validation therapy: A review of the literature. *The Validation Training Institute, Inc.* Retrieved August 28, 2010, from http://www.vfvalidation.org/web.php?request=article1

DeMartinis, J. E. (2005). Management of clients with hypertensive disorders. In J. M. Black & J. H. Hawks (Eds.), *Medical surgical nursing: Clinical management for positive outcomes* (7th ed., pp. 1489–1508). St. Louis: Elsevier Saunders.

Diamond, J. (2008). *A report on Alzheimer's disease and current research.* Alzheimer Society of Canada. Retrieved

August 28, 2010, from http://www.alzheimer.ca/english/research/current-chol.htm

Eisendrath, S. J., & Lichtmacher, J. E. (2009). Psychiatric disorders. In L. M. Tierney, S. J. McPhee, & M. A. Papadakis (Eds.), *Current medical diagnosis and treatment 2009* (pp. 912–964). New York: McGraw-Hill.

Feil, N. (2007). It is never good to lie to a person who has dementia. *The Validation Training Institute, Inc.* Retrieved August 28, 2010, from http://www.vfvalidation.org//web.php?request=article5

Foroud, T., Gray, J., Ivashina, J., & Conneally, P. M. (1999). Differences in duration of Huntington's disease based on age at onset. *Journal of Neurology, Neurosurgery and Psychiatry, 66,* 52–56.

Geerlings, M. I., den Heijer, T., Koudstaal, P. J., Hofman, A., & Breteler, M. M. B. (2008). History of depression, depressive symptoms, and medial temporal lobe atrophy and the risk of Alzheimer disease. *Neurology, 70,* 1258–1264.

Institute of Medicine. (2003). *Health professions education: A bridge to quality.* Washington, DC: Author.

Langa, K. M., Foster, N. L., & Larson, E. B. (2004). Mixed dementia: Emerging concepts and therapeutic implications. *Journal of the American Medical Association, 292,* 2901–2908.

McShane, R. (2000). *Hallucinations and delusions.* London: The Alzheimer's Society.

Munoz, D. G., & Feldman, H. (2000). Causes of Alzheimer's disease. *Canadian Medical Association Journal, 162,* 65–72.

NANDA International. (2009). *Nursing diagnoses: Definitions & classification 2009–2011.* Hoboken, NJ: Wiley-Blackwell.

National Institute on Aging. (2008). *Alzheimer's disease: Unraveling the mystery.* NIH Publication No. 08-3782. Washington, DC: National Institutes of Health, U.S. Department of Health and Human Services.

National Institute on Aging. (2009). *Understanding stages and symptoms of Alzheimer's disease.* Retrieved August 28, 2010, from http://www.nia.nih.gov/Alzheimers/Publications/stages.htm

Plassman, B. L., Langa, K. M., Fisher, G. G., Heeringa, S. G., Weir, D. R., Ofstedal, M. B., et al. (2007). Prevalence of dementia in the United States: The Aging, Demographics, and Memory Study. *Neuroepidemiology, 29*(1-2), 125–132.

Rabins, P., Bland, W., Bright-Long, L., Cohen, E., Katz, I., Rovner, B., et al. (2006). Practice guideline for the treatment of patients with Alzheimer's disease and other dementias of late life. *American Psychiatric Association Practice Guidelines for the Treatment of Psychiatric Disorders, Compendium 2006.* Washington, DC: American Psychiatric Publishing.

Rentz, C. (2008). Nursing care of the person with sporadic Creutzfeldt-Jakob disease. *Journal of Hospice and Palliative Nursing, 10*(5), 272–282.

Rogaeva, E., Meng, Y., Lee, J. H., Gu, Y., Kawarai, T., Zou, F., et al. (2007). The neuronal sortilin-related receptor SOR1 is genetically associated with Alzheimer disease. *Nature Genetics, 39,* 168–177.

Sadock, B. J., & Sadock, V. A. (2007). *Synopsis of psychiatry: behavioral sciences/clinical psychiatry* (10th ed.). Philadelphia: Lippincott Williams & Wilkins.

Salloway, S., & Correia, S. (2009). Alzheimer disease: Time to improve its diagnosis and treatment. *Cleveland Clinic Journal of Medicine 76*(1), 49–58.

Small, G. W., Kepe, V., Ercoli, L. M., Siddarth, P., Bookheimer, S. Y., Miller, K. J., et al. (2006). PET of brain amyloid and tau in mild cognitive impairment. *New England Journal of Medicine, 355,* 2652–2663.

Spector, A., Davies, S., Woods, B., & Orrell, M. (2000). Reality orientation for dementia: A systematic review of the evidence of effectiveness from randomized controlled trials. *Gerontologist, 40,* 206–212.

Srikanth, S., & Nagaraja, A. V. (2005). A prospective study of reversible dementias: Frequency, causes, clinical profile and results of treatment. *Neurology India, 53,* 291–294.

Stanley, M., Blair, K. A., & Beare, P. G. (2005). *Gerontological nursing: Promoting successful aging with older adults* (3rd ed.). Philadelphia: F.A. Davis.

Tesco, G., Koh, Y. H., Kang, E. L., Cameron, A. N., Das, S., Sena-Esteves, M., et al. (2007). Depletion of GGA3 stabilizes BACE and enhances β-secretase activity. *Neuron, 54,* 721–737.

Trzepacz, P., Breitbart, W., Franklin, J., Levenson, J., Martini, D. R., & Wang, P. (2006). Practice guideline for the treatment of patients with delirium. *American Psychiatric Association Practice Guidelines for the Treatment of Psychiatric Disorders, Compendium 2006.* Washington, DC: American Psychiatric Publishing.

Yan, J. (2008). FDA extends black-box warning to all antipsychotics. *Psychiatric News, 43*(14), 1–4. American Psychiatric Association. Retrieved August 28, 2010, from http://pn.psychiatryonline.org/content/43/14/1.1.full

@ INTERNET REFERENCES

- Additional information about Alzheimer's disease may be located at the following websites:
  - http://www.alz.org
  - http://www.nia.nih.gov/alzheimers
  - http://www.ninds.nih.gov/disorders/alzheimersdisease/alzheimersdisease.htm
- Information on caregiving can be located at the following website:
  - http://www.aarp.org
- Additional information about medications to treat Alzheimer's disease may be located at the following websites:
  - http://www.fadavis.com/townsend
  - http://www.nlm.nih.gov/medlineplus/druginformation.html
  - http://www.nimh.nih.gov/publicat/medicate.cfm

MOVIE CONNECTIONS

The Notebook (Alzheimer's disease) • *Away From Her* (Alzheimer's disease) • *Iris* (Alzheimer's disease)

Substance-Related Disorders

KEY TERMS

Alcoholics Anonymous

amphetamines

ascites

cannabis

codependency

detoxification

disulfiram

dual diagnosis

esophageal varices

hepatic encephalopathy

Korsakoff's psychosis

opioids

peer assistance programs

phencyclidine

substitution therapy

Wernicke's encephalopathy

OBJECTIVES

After reading this chapter, the student will be able to:

1. Define *abuse, dependence, intoxication,* and *withdrawal.*
2. Discuss predisposing factors implicated in the etiology of substance-related disorders.
3. Identify symptomatology and use the information in assessment of clients with various substance-use disorders and substance-induced disorders.
4. Identify nursing diagnoses common to clients with substance-use disorders and substance-induced disorders, and select appropriate nursing interventions for each.
5. Identify topics for client and family teaching relevant to substance-use disorders and substance-induced disorders.
6. Describe relevant outcome criteria for evaluating nursing care of clients with substance-use disorders and substance-induced disorders.
7. Discuss the issue of substance-related disorders within the profession of nursing.
8. Define codependency and identify behavioral characteristics associated with the disorder.
9. Discuss treatment of codependency.
10. Describe various modalities relevant to treatment of individuals with substance-use disorders and substance-induced disorders.

HOMEWORK ASSIGNMENT

Please read the chapter and answer the following questions:

1. What are the physical consequences of thiamine deficiency in chronic alcohol abuse?
2. Define *tolerance* as it relates to physical dependence on a substance.
3. Describe two types of toxic reactions that can occur with the use of hallucinogens.
4. What is substitution therapy?

Substance-related disorders are composed of two groups: the substance-use disorders (dependence and abuse) and the substance-induced disorders (intoxication, withdrawal, delirium, dementia, amnesia, psychosis, mood disorder, anxiety disorder, sexual dysfunction, and sleep disorders). This chapter discusses dependence, abuse, intoxication, and withdrawal. The remainder of the substance-induced disorders are included in the chapters with which they share symptomatology (e.g., substance-induced anxiety disorders are included in Chapter 29).

Drugs are a pervasive part of our society. Certain mood-altering substances are quite socially acceptable and are used moderately by many adult Americans. They include alcohol, caffeine, and nicotine. Society has even developed a relative indifference to an occasional abuse of these substances, despite documentation of their negative impact on health.

A wide variety of substances are produced for medicinal purposes. These include central nervous system (CNS) stimulants (e.g., **amphetamines**) and CNS depressants (e.g., sedatives, tranquilizers), as well as numerous over-the-counter preparations designed to relieve nearly every kind of human ailment, real or imagined.

Some illegal substances have achieved a degree of social acceptance by various subcultural groups within our society. These drugs, such as marijuana and hashish, are by no means harmless, and the long-term effects are still being studied. On the other hand, the dangerous effects of other illegal substances (e.g., lysergic acid diethylamide [LSD], **phencyclidine,** cocaine, and heroin) have been well documented.

This chapter discusses the physical and behavioral manifestations and personal and social consequences related to the abuse of or dependence on alcohol, other CNS depressants, CNS stimulants, **opioids,** hallucinogens, and cannabinols. Wide cultural variations in attitudes exist regarding substance consumption and patterns of use. Substance abuse is especially prevalent among individuals between the ages of 18 and 24. Substance-related disorders are diagnosed more commonly in men than in women, but the gender ratios vary with the class of the substance (American Psychiatric Association [APA], 2000).

Codependency is described in this chapter, as are aspects of treatment for the disorder. The issue of substance impairment within the profession of nursing is also explored. Nursing care for substance abuse, dependence, intoxication, and withdrawal is presented in the context of the six steps of the nursing process. Various medical and other treatment modalities are also discussed.

Substance-Use Disorders

CORE CONCEPT

Abuse

To use wrongfully or in a harmful way. Improper treatment or conduct that may result in injury.

Substance Abuse

The *Diagnostic and Statistical Manual of Mental Disorders, Fourth Edition, Text Revision (DSM-IV-TR)* (APA, 2000) identifies substance abuse as a maladaptive pattern of substance use manifested by recurrent and significant adverse consequences related to repeated use of the substance. Substance abuse has also been referred to as any use of substances that poses significant hazards to health.

DSM-IV-TR Criteria for Substance Abuse

Substance abuse is described as a maladaptive pattern of substance use leading to clinically significant impairment or distress, as manifested by one (or more) of the following, occurring within a 12-month period:

1. Recurrent substance use resulting in a failure to fulfill major role obligations at work, school, or home (e.g., repeated absences or poor work performance related to substance use; substance-related absences, suspensions, or expulsions from school; neglect of children or household).

2. Recurrent substance use in situations in which it is physically hazardous (e.g., driving an automobile or operating a machine when impaired by substance use).

3. Recurrent substance-related legal problems (e.g., arrests for substance-related disorderly conduct).

4. Continued substance use despite having persistent or recurrent social or interpersonal problems caused or exacerbated by the effects of the substance (e.g., arguments with spouse about consequences of intoxication, physical fights).

CORE CONCEPT

Dependence

A compulsive or chronic requirement. The need is so strong as to generate distress (either physical or psychological) if left unfulfilled.

Substance Dependence

Physical Dependence

Physical dependence on a substance is evidenced by a cluster of cognitive, behavioral, and physiological symptoms indicating that the individual continues use of the substance despite significant substance-related problems (APA, 2000). As this condition develops, the repeated administration of the substance necessitates its continued use to prevent the appearance of unpleasant effects characteristic of the withdrawal syndrome associated with that particular drug. The development of physical dependence is promoted by the phenomenon of *tolerance*. Tolerance is defined as the need for increasingly larger or more frequent doses of a substance in order to obtain the desired effects originally produced by a lower dose.

Psychological Dependence

An individual is considered to be psychologically dependent on a substance when there is an overwhelming desire to repeat the use of a particular drug in order to produce pleasure or avoid discomfort. This desire can be extremely powerful, producing intense craving for a substance as well as its compulsive use.

DSM-IV-TR Criteria for Substance Dependence

At least three of the following characteristics must be present for a diagnosis of substance dependence:

1. Evidence of tolerance, as defined by either of the following:
   a. A need for markedly increased amounts of the substance to achieve intoxication or desired effects.
   b. Markedly diminished effect with continued use of the same amount of the substance.
2. Evidence of withdrawal symptoms, as manifested by either of the following:
   a. The characteristic withdrawal syndrome for the substance.
   b. The same (or a closely related) substance is taken to relieve or avoid withdrawal symptoms.
3. The substance is often taken in larger amounts or over a longer period than was intended.
4. There is a persistent desire or unsuccessful efforts to cut down or control substance use.
5. A great deal of time is spent in activities necessary to obtain the substance (e.g., visiting multiple doctors or driving long distances), use the substance (e.g., chain smoking), or recover from its effects.
6. Important social, occupational, or recreational activities are given up or reduced because of substance use.
7. The substance use is continued despite knowledge of having a persistent or recurrent physical or psychological problem that is likely to have been caused or exacerbated by the substance (e.g., current cocaine use despite recognition of cocaine-induced depression, or continued drinking despite recognition that an ulcer was made worse by alcohol consumption).

Substance-Induced Disorders

CORE CONCEPT

Intoxication

A physical and mental state of exhilaration and emotional frenzy or lethargy and stupor.

Substance Intoxication

Substance intoxication is defined as the development of a reversible substance-specific syndrome caused by the recent ingestion of (or exposure to) a substance (APA, 2000). The behavior changes can be attributed to the physiological effects of the substance on the CNS and develop during or shortly after use of the substance. This category does not apply to nicotine.

DSM-IV-TR Criteria for Substance Intoxication

1. The development of a reversible substance-specific syndrome caused by recent ingestion of (or exposure to) a substance.

   NOTE: Different substances may produce similar or identical syndromes.

2. Clinically significant maladaptive behavior or psychological changes that are due to the effect of the substance on the CNS (e.g., belligerence, mood lability, cognitive impairment, impaired judgment, impaired social or

occupational functioning) and develop during or shortly after use of the substance.

3. The symptoms are not due to a general medical condition and are not better accounted for by another mental disorder.

CORE CONCEPT

Withdrawal
The physiological and mental readjustment that accompanies the discontinuation of an addictive substance.

Substance Withdrawal

Substance withdrawal is the development of a substance-specific maladaptive behavior change, with physiological and cognitive concomitants, that is due to the cessation of, or reduction in, heavy and prolonged substance use (APA, 2000). Withdrawal is usually, but not always, associated with substance dependence.

DSM-IV-TR Criteria for Substance Withdrawal

1. The development of a substance-specific syndrome caused by the cessation of (or reduction in) heavy and prolonged substance use.

2. The substance-specific syndrome causes clinically significant distress or impairment in social, occupational, or other important areas of functioning.

3. The symptoms are not due to a general medical condition and are not better accounted for by another mental disorder.

Classes of Psychoactive Substances

The following 11 classes of psychoactive substances are associated with substance-use and substance-induced disorders:

1. Alcohol
2. Amphetamines and related substances
3. Caffeine
4. Cannabis
5. Cocaine
6. Hallucinogens
7. Inhalants
8. Nicotine
9. Opioids
10. Phencyclidine (PCP) and related substances
11. Sedatives, hypnotics, or anxiolytics

Predisposing Factors

A number of factors have been implicated in the predisposition to abuse of substances. At present, there is no single theory that can adequately explain the etiology of this problem. No doubt the interaction between various elements forms a complex collection of determinants that influence a person's susceptibility to abuse substances.

Biological Factors

Genetics

An apparent hereditary factor is involved in the development of substance-use disorders. This is especially evident with alcoholism, but less so with other substances. Children of alcoholics are three times more likely than other children to become alcoholics (Harvard Medical School, 2001). Studies with monozygotic and dizygotic twins have also supported the genetic hypothesis. Monozygotic (one egg, genetically identical) twins have a higher rate for concordance of alcoholism than dizygotic (two eggs, genetically nonidentical) twins (Black & Andreasen, 2011). Other studies have shown that biological offspring of alcoholic parents have a significantly greater incidence of alcoholism than offspring of nonalcoholic parents. This is true whether the child was reared by the biological parents or by nonalcoholic adoptive parents (Choudary & Knowles, 2008).

Biochemical

A second biological hypothesis relates to the possibility that alcohol may produce morphine-like substances in the brain that are responsible for alcohol addiction. These substances are formed by the reaction of biologically active amines (e.g., dopamine, serotonin) with products of alcohol metabolism, such as acetaldehyde (Jamal et al., 2003). Examples of these morphine-like substances include tetrahydropapaveroline and salsolinol. Some tests with animals have shown that injection of these compounds into the brain in small amounts results in patterns of alcohol addiction in animals who had previously avoided even the most dilute alcohol solutions (McCoy, Strawbridge, McMurtrey, Kane, & Ward, 2003).

Psychological Factors

Developmental Influences

The psychodynamic approach to the etiology of substance abuse focuses on a punitive superego and fixation at the oral stage of psychosexual development (Sadock & Sadock, 2007). Individuals with punitive superegos turn to alcohol to diminish unconscious anxiety and increase feelings of power and self-worth. Sadock and Sadock (2007) stated, "As a form of self-medication, alcohol may be used to control panic, opioids to diminish anger, and amphetamines to alleviate depression" (p. 386).

Personality Factors

Certain personality traits have been associated with an increased tendency toward addictive behavior. Some clinicians believe a low self-esteem, frequent depression, passivity, the inability to relax or to defer gratification, and the inability to communicate effectively are common in individuals who abuse substances. These personality characteristics cannot be called *predictive* of addictive behavior, yet for reasons not completely understood, they have been found to accompany addiction in many instances.

Substance abuse has also been associated with antisocial personality and depressive response styles. This may be explained by the inability of the individual with antisocial personality to anticipate the aversive consequences of his or her behavior. It is likely an effort on the part of the depressed person to treat the symptoms of discomfort associated with dysphoria. Achievement of relief then provides the positive reinforcement to continue abusing the substance.

Sociocultural Factors

Social Learning

The effects of modeling, imitation, and identification on behavior can be observed from early childhood onward. In relation to drug consumption, the family appears to be an important influence. Various studies have shown that children and adolescents are more likely to use substances if they have parents who provide a model for substance use. Peers often exert a great deal of influence in the life of the child or adolescent who is being encouraged to use substances for the first time. Modeling may continue to be a factor in the use of substances once the individual enters the work force, particularly if the work setting provides plenty of leisure time with coworkers and drinking is valued as a way to express group cohesiveness.

Conditioning

Another important learning factor is the effect of the substance itself. Many substances create a pleasurable experience that encourages the user to repeat it. Thus, it is the intrinsically reinforcing properties of addictive drugs that "condition" the individual to seek out their use again and again. The environment in which the substance is taken also contributes to the reinforcement. If the environment is pleasurable, substance use is usually increased. Aversive stimuli within an environment are thought to be associated with a decrease in substance use within that environment.

Cultural and Ethnic Influences

Factors within an individual's culture help to establish patterns of substance use by molding attitudes, influencing patterns of consumption based on cultural acceptance, and determining the availability of the substance. For centuries, the French and Italians have considered wine an essential part of the family meal, even for the children. The incidence of alcohol dependence is low, and acute intoxication from alcohol is not common. However, the possibility of chronic physiological effects associated with lifelong alcohol consumption cannot be ignored.

Historically, a high incidence of alcohol dependence has existed within the Native American culture. Alcohol-attributable deaths among Native Americans are approximately twice that of the U.S. general population (Centers for Disease Control and Prevention [CDC], 2008). Veterans Administration records show that 45 percent of the Native American veterans are alcohol dependent, or twice the rate for non–Native American veterans. A number of reasons have been postulated for alcohol abuse among Native Americans: a possible physical cause (difficulty metabolizing alcohol), children modeling their parents' drinking habits, unemployment and poverty, and loss of the traditional Native American religion that some believe has led to the increased use of alcohol to fill the spiritual gap.

The incidence of alcohol dependence is higher among northern Europeans than southern Europeans. The Finns and the Irish use excessive alcohol consumption for the release of aggression, and the English and Irish "pubs" are known for their attraction as social meeting places (Ehrlander, 2007; Wilson, 2008).

Incidence of alcohol dependence among Asians is relatively low. This may be a result of a possible genetic intolerance of the substance. Some Asians develop unpleasant symptoms, such as flushing, headaches, nausea, and palpitations, when they drink alcohol. Research indicates that this is because of an isoenzyme variant that quickly converts alcohol to acetaldehyde, as well as the absence of an isoenzyme that is needed to oxidize acetaldehyde. This results in a rapid accumulation of acetaldehyde, which produces the unpleasant symptoms (Hanley, 2008).

The Dynamics of Substance-Related Disorders

Alcohol Abuse and Dependence

A Profile of the Substance

Alcohol is a natural substance formed by the reaction of fermenting sugar with yeast spores. Although there are many alcohols, the kind in alcoholic beverages is known scientifically as ethyl alcohol and chemically as C_2H_5OH. Its abbreviation, ETOH, is sometimes seen in medical records and in various other documents and publications.

By strict definition, alcohol is classified as a food because it contains calories; however, it has no nutritional value. Different alcoholic beverages are produced by using different sources of sugar for the fermentation process. For example, beer is made from malted barley, wine from grapes or berries, whiskey from malted grains, and rum from molasses. Distilled beverages (e.g., whiskey, scotch, gin, vodka, and other "hard" liquors) derive their name from further concentration of the alcohol through a process called distillation.

The alcohol content varies by type of beverage. For example, most American beers contain 3 to 6 percent alcohol, wines average 10 to 20 percent, and distilled beverages range from 40 to 50 percent alcohol. The average-sized drink, regardless of beverage, contains a similar amount of alcohol. That is, 12 ounces of beer, 3 to 5 ounces of wine, and a cocktail with 1 ounce of whiskey all contain approximately 0.5 ounce of alcohol. If consumed at the same rate, they all would have an equal effect on the body.

Alcohol exerts a depressant effect on the CNS, resulting in behavioral and mood changes. The effects of alcohol on the CNS are proportional to the alcoholic concentration in the blood. Most states consider that an individual is legally intoxicated with a blood alcohol level of 0.08 to 0.10 percent.

The body burns alcohol at the rate of about 0.5 ounce per hour, so behavioral changes would not be expected to occur in an individual who slowly consumed only one averaged-sized drink per hour. Other factors do influence these effects, however, such as individual size and whether or not the stomach contains food at the time the alcohol is consumed. Alcohol is thought to have a more profound effect when an individual is emotionally stressed or fatigued (National Institute on Alcohol Abuse and Alcoholism [NIAAA], 2000).

Historical Aspects

The use of alcohol can be traced back to the Neolithic age. Beer and wine are known to have been used around 6400 B.C. With the introduction of distillation by the Arabs in the Middle Ages, alchemists believed that alcohol was the answer to all of their ailments. The word *whiskey,* meaning "water of life," became widely known.

In America, Native Americans had been drinking beer and wine prior to the arrival of the first white immigrants. Refinement of the distillation process made beverages with high alcohol content readily available. By the early 1800s, one renowned physician of the time, Benjamin Rush, had begun to identify the widespread excessive, chronic alcohol consumption as a disease and an addiction. The strong religious mores on which this country was founded soon led to a driving force aimed at prohibiting the sale of alcoholic beverages. By the middle of the 19th century, 13 states had passed prohibition laws. The most notable prohibition of major proportions was that in effect in the United States from 1920 to 1933. The mandatory restrictions on national social habits resulted in the creation of profitable underground markets that led to flourishing criminal enterprises. Furthermore, millions of dollars in federal, state, and local revenues from taxes and import duties on alcohol were lost. It is difficult to measure the value of this dollar loss against the human devastation and social costs that occur as a result of alcohol abuse in the United States today.

Patterns of Use/Abuse

About half of Americans ages 12 years and older report being current drinkers of alcohol (Substance Abuse and Mental Health Services Administration [SAMHSA], 2009). Of these about one fifth are binge drinkers or engage in heavy alcohol use.

IMPLICATIONS OF RESEARCH FOR EVIDENCE-BASED PRACTICE

Stevenson, J. S., & Masters, J. A. (2005). Predictors of alcohol misuse and abuse in older women. *Journal of Nursing Scholarship, 37,* **329–335.**

DESCRIPTION OF THE STUDY: The purpose of this study was to determine the predictive ability of self-report questions, physical measures, and biomarkers to detect alcohol misuse and abuse among older women. Older women are not routinely screened in health-care settings for alcohol use. Because they often have many other health concerns, health-care providers often fail to assess these older patients for an underlying alcohol problem. The sample included 135 healthy women ages 60 and older divided into two groups: drinkers (those who consumed 12 or more standard drinks [SD] in the past year) and nondrinkers (those who consumed no alcohol during the past year). A standard drink is identified by the National Institute on Alcohol Abuse and Alcoholism as 1.5 oz. of distilled liquor, 12 oz. of regular beer, or 5 oz. of wine. Data were gathered from an alcohol-enhanced assessment interview (the T-ACE), a physical examination, and biomarker-enhanced standard intake blood work. Biomarkers collected in this study were gamma-glutamyltransferase (GGT), mean corpuscular volume (MCV), total cholesterol (TC), high-density lipoprotein (HDL), low-density lipoprotein (LDL), and the ratio of HDL to TC. Other physical data collected were systolic and diastolic blood pressures, body mass index (BMI), exercise habits, past experiences of trauma, hemoglobin (Hgb), and hematocrit (Hct).

RESULTS OF THE STUDY: The T-ACE questionnaire discriminated strongly between the two groups. This test is similar to the CAGE questionnaire, with one exception. The question related to "guilt" is replaced with a question related to "tolerance." ("How many drinks does it take to make you feel high?"). Analyses of the biomarkers showed significant differences in MCV, HDL, Hgb, Hct, and GGT, with drinkers showing higher levels. Drinkers also were found to consume more coffee and over-the-counter (OTC) drugs, and were more likely to be (or have been) smokers and to use alcohol to fall asleep. Nutrition, trauma, and blood pressure showed no significant differences between the groups.

IMPLICATIONS FOR NURSING PRACTICE: This study suggests a way in which to identify older women who may be at risk for problems related to alcohol abuse. Results reveal promising predictors of alcohol use and abuse that can be part of clinical data collection during intake assessments in primary care and acute care. Indications suggest that the best predictors of high-risk drinkers include the T-ACE tool (a score of 1 or higher), elevated MCV and Hgb levels, smoking or having been a smoker, drinking large amounts of coffee, using alcohol to sleep at night, and self-medicating with two or more OTC drugs on a routine basis. The authors suggested that biological markers are significant predictors because alcohol is documented to have a powerful physiological effect on women.

Why do people drink? Drinking patterns in the United States show that people use alcoholic beverages to enhance the flavor of food with meals; at social gatherings to encourage relaxation and conviviality among the guests; and to promote a feeling of celebration at special occasions such as weddings, birthdays, and anniversaries. An alcoholic beverage (wine) is also used as part of the sacred ritual in some religious ceremonies. Therapeutically, alcohol is the major ingredient in many over-the-counter and prescription medicines that are prepared in concentrated form. Therefore, alcohol can be harmless and enjoyable—sometimes even beneficial—if it is used responsibly and in moderation. Like any other mind-altering drug, however, alcohol has the potential for abuse. Indeed, it is the most widely abused drug in the United States today. The National Council on Alcoholism and Drug Dependence (2010) reported:

Alcoholism is the third leading cause of preventable death in the U.S. As the nation's number one health problem, addiction strains the health care system, the economy, harms family life and threatens public safety. One-quarter of all emergency room admissions, one-third of all suicides, and more than half of all homicides and incidents of domestic violence are alcohol-related. Heavy drinking contributes to illness in each of the top three causes of death: heart disease, cancer, and stroke. Almost half of all traffic fatalities are alcohol-related. Fetal alcohol syndrome is the leading known cause of mental retardation.

Jellinek (1952) outlined four phases through which the alcoholic's pattern of drinking progresses. Some variability among individuals is to be expected within this model of progression.

Phase I: The Prealcoholic Phase

This phase is characterized by the use of alcohol to relieve the everyday stress and tensions of life. As a child, the individual may have observed parents or other adults drinking alcohol and enjoying the effects. The child learns that use of alcohol is an acceptable method of coping with stress. Tolerance develops, and the amount required to achieve the desired effect increases steadily.

Phase II: The Early Alcoholic Phase

This phase begins with blackouts—brief periods of amnesia that occur during or immediately following a period of drinking. Now the alcohol is no longer a source of pleasure or relief for the individual but rather a drug that is *required* by the individual. Common behaviors include sneaking drinks or secret drinking, preoccupation with drinking and maintaining the supply of alcohol, rapid gulping of drinks, and further blackouts. The individual feels enormous guilt and becomes very defensive about his or her drinking. Excessive use of denial and rationalization is evident.

Phase III: The Crucial Phase

In this phase, the individual has lost control, and physiological dependence is clearly evident. This loss of control has been described as the inability to choose whether or not to drink. Binge drinking, lasting from a few hours to several weeks, is common. These episodes are characterized by sickness, loss of consciousness, squalor, and degradation. In this phase, the individual is extremely ill. Anger and aggression are common manifestations. Drinking is the total focus, and he or she is willing to risk losing everything that was once important, in an effort to maintain the addiction. By this phase of the illness, it is not uncommon for the individual to have experienced the loss of job, marriage, family, friends, and most especially, self-respect.

Phase IV: The Chronic Phase

This phase is characterized by emotional and physical disintegration. The individual is usually intoxicated more than he or she is sober. Emotional disintegration is evidenced by profound helplessness and self-pity. Impairment in reality testing may result in psychosis. Life-threatening physical manifestations may be evident in virtually every system of the body. Abstention from alcohol results in a terrifying syndrome of symptoms that include hallucinations, tremors, convulsions, severe agitation, and panic. Depression and ideas of suicide are not uncommon.

Effects on the Body

Alcohol can induce a general, nonselective, reversible depression of the CNS. About 20 percent of a single dose of alcohol is absorbed directly and immediately into the bloodstream through the stomach wall. Unlike other "foods," it does not

have to be digested. The blood carries it directly to the brain, where the alcohol acts on the brain's central control areas, slowing down or depressing brain activity. The other 80 percent of the alcohol in one drink is processed only slightly slower through the upper intestinal tract and into the bloodstream. Only moments after alcohol is consumed, it can be found in all tissues, organs, and secretions of the body. Rapidity of absorption is influenced by various factors. For example, absorption is delayed when the drink is sipped, rather than gulped; when the stomach contains food, rather than being empty; and when the drink is wine or beer, rather than distilled beverages.

At low doses, alcohol produces relaxation, loss of inhibitions, lack of concentration, drowsiness, slurred speech, and sleep. Chronic abuse results in multisystem physiological impairments. These complications include (but are not limited to) those outlined in the following sections.

Peripheral Neuropathy

Peripheral neuropathy, characterized by peripheral nerve damage, results in pain, burning, tingling, or prickly sensations of the extremities. Researchers believe it is the direct result of deficiencies in the B vitamins, particularly thiamine. Nutritional deficiencies are common in chronic alcoholics because of insufficient intake of nutrients as well as the toxic effect of alcohol that results in malabsorption of nutrients. The process is reversible with abstinence from alcohol and restoration of nutritional deficiencies. Otherwise, permanent muscle wasting and paralysis can occur.

Alcoholic Myopathy

Alcoholic myopathy may occur as an acute or chronic condition. In the acute condition, the individual experiences a sudden onset of muscle pain, swelling, and weakness; a reddish tinge in the urine caused by myoglobin, a breakdown product of muscle excreted in the urine; and a rapid rise in muscle enzymes in the blood (Klopstock, Haller, & DiMauro, 2010). Muscle symptoms are usually generalized, but pain and swelling may selectively involve the calves or other muscle groups. Laboratory studies show elevations of the enzymes creatine phosphokinase (CPK), lactate dehydrogenase (LDH), aldolase, and aspartate aminotransferase (AST). The symptoms of chronic alcoholic myopathy include a gradual wasting and weakness in skeletal muscles. Neither the pain and tenderness nor the elevated muscle enzymes seen in acute myopathy are evident in the chronic condition.

Alcoholic myopathy is thought to be a result of the same B vitamin deficiency that contributes to peripheral neuropathy. Improvement is observed with abstinence from alcohol and the return to a nutritious diet with vitamin supplements.

Wernicke's Encephalopathy

Wernicke's encephalopathy represents the most serious form of thiamine deficiency in alcoholics. Symptoms include paralysis of the ocular muscles, diplopia, ataxia, somnolence, and stupor. If thiamine replacement therapy is not undertaken quickly, death will ensue.

Korsakoff's Psychosis

Korsakoff's psychosis is identified by a syndrome of confusion, loss of recent memory, and confabulation in alcoholics. It is frequently encountered in clients recovering from Wernicke's encephalopathy. In the United States, the two disorders are usually considered together and are called *Wernicke-Korsakoff syndrome.* Treatment is with parenteral or oral thiamine replacement.

Alcoholic Cardiomyopathy

The effect of alcohol on the heart is an accumulation of lipids in the myocardial cells, resulting in enlargement and a weakened condition. The clinical findings of alcoholic cardiomyopathy generally relate to congestive heart failure or arrhythmia. Symptoms include decreased exercise tolerance, tachycardia, dyspnea, edema, palpitations, and nonproductive cough. Laboratory studies may show elevation of the enzymes CPK, AST, alanine aminotransferase (ALT), and LDH. Changes may be observed by electrocardiogram, and congestive heart failure may be evident on chest x-ray films (Bashore, Granger, Hranitzky, & Patel, 2009).

The treatment is total permanent abstinence from alcohol. Treatment of the congestive heart failure may include rest, oxygen, digitalization, sodium restriction, and diuretics. Prognosis is encouraging if treated in the early stages. The death rate is high for individuals with advanced symptomatology.

Esophagitis

Esophagitis—inflammation and pain in the esophagus—occurs because of the toxic effects of alcohol on the esophageal mucosa. It also occurs because of frequent vomiting associated with alcohol abuse.

Gastritis

The effects of alcohol on the stomach include inflammation of the stomach lining characterized by epigastric distress, nausea, vomiting, and distention. Alcohol breaks down the stomach's protective mucosal barrier, allowing hydrochloric acid to erode the stomach wall. Damage to blood vessels may result in hemorrhage.

Pancreatitis

Pancreatitis may be categorized as *acute* or *chronic.* Acute pancreatitis usually occurs 1 or 2 days after a binge of excessive alcohol consumption. Symptoms include constant, severe epigastric pain, nausea and vomiting, and abdominal distention. The chronic condition leads to pancreatic insufficiency resulting in steatorrhea, malnutrition, weight loss, and diabetes mellitus.

Alcoholic Hepatitis

Alcoholic hepatitis is inflammation of the liver caused by long-term heavy alcohol use. Clinical manifestations include an enlarged and tender liver, nausea and vomiting, lethargy, anorexia, elevated white blood cell count, fever, and jaundice. **Ascites** and weight loss may be evident in more severe cases. With treatment—which includes strict abstinence from alcohol, proper nutrition, and rest—the individual can experience complete recovery. Severe cases can lead to cirrhosis or **hepatic encephalopathy.**

Cirrhosis of the Liver

Cirrhosis of the liver may be caused by anything that results in chronic injury to the liver. It is the end stage of alcoholic liver disease and results from long-term chronic alcohol abuse. There is widespread destruction of liver cells, which are replaced by fibrous (scar) tissue. Clinical manifestations include nausea and vomiting, anorexia, weight loss, abdominal pain, jaundice, edema, anemia, and blood coagulation abnormalities. Treatment includes abstention from alcohol, correction of malnutrition, and supportive care to prevent complications of the disease. Complications of cirrhosis include the following:

■ **Portal Hypertension.** Elevation of blood pressure through the portal circulation results from defective blood flow through the cirrhotic liver.

■ **Ascites.** Ascites, a condition in which an excessive amount of serous fluid accumulates in the abdominal cavity, occurs in response to portal hypertension. The increased pressure results in the seepage of fluid from the surface of the liver into the abdominal cavity.

■ **Esophageal Varices. Esophageal varices** are veins in the esophagus that become distended because of excessive pressure from defective blood flow through the cirrhotic liver. As this pressure increases, these varicosities can rupture, resulting in hemorrhage and sometimes death.

■ **Hepatic Encephalopathy.** This serious complication occurs in response to the inability of the diseased liver to convert ammonia to urea for excretion. The continued rise in serum ammonia results in progressively impaired mental functioning, apathy, euphoria or depression, sleep disturbance, increasing confusion, and progression to coma and eventual death. Treatment requires complete abstention from alcohol, temporary elimination of protein from the diet, and reduction of intestinal ammonia using neomycin or lactulose (National Library of Medicine, 2010).

Leukopenia

The production, function, and movement of the white blood cells are impaired in chronic alcoholics. This condition, called leukopenia, places the individual at high risk for contracting infectious diseases as well as for complicated recovery.

Thrombocytopenia

Platelet production and survival are impaired as a result of the toxic effects of alcohol. This places the alcoholic at risk for hemorrhage. Abstinence from alcohol rapidly reverses this deficiency.

Sexual Dysfunction

Alcohol interferes with the normal production and maintenance of female and male hormones (Sadock & Sadock, 2007). For women, this can mean changes in the menstrual cycles and a decreased or loss of ability to become pregnant. For men, the decreased hormone levels result in a diminished libido, decreased sexual performance, and impaired fertility (Schuckit, 2006).

Use During Pregnancy

Fetal Alcohol Syndrome

Prenatal exposure to alcohol can result in a broad range of disorders to the fetus, known as fetal alcohol spectrum disorders (FASDs), the most common of which is fetal alcohol syndrome (FAS). Fetal alcohol syndrome includes physical, mental, behavioral, and/or learning disabilities with lifelong implications. There may be problems with learning, memory, attention span, communication, vision, hearing, or a combination of these (CDC, 2005). Other FASDs include alcohol-related neurodevelopmental disorder (ARND) and alcohol-related birth defects (ARBDs).

No amount of alcohol during pregnancy is considered safe, and alcohol can damage a fetus at any stage of pregnancy (Carmona, 2005). Therefore, drinking alcohol should be avoided by women who are pregnant or by women who could become pregnant. Estimates of the prevalence of FAS range from 0.2 to 1.5 per 1,000 live births (CDC, 2005). The rate is higher among African Americans and Native Americans (possibly as high as 9 per 1,000

in the latter group) (Dannaway & Mulvihill, 2009). Maier and West (2001) stated:

> The number of women who engage in heavy alcohol consumption during pregnancy surpasses the total number of children diagnosed with either FAS or ARND, meaning that not every child whose mother drank alcohol during pregnancy develops FAS or ARND. Moreover, the degree to which people with FAS or ARND are impaired differs from person to person. Several factors may contribute to this variation in the consequences of maternal drinking. These factors include, but are not limited to, the following:

- Maternal drinking pattern
- Differences in maternal metabolism
- Differences in genetic susceptibility
- Timing of the alcohol consumption during pregnancy
- Variation in the vulnerability of different brain regions (p. 168)

Children with FAS may have the following characteristics or exhibit the following behaviors (CDC, 2005):

- Small size for gestational age or small stature in relation to peers
- Facial abnormalities (Fig. 25–1)
- Poor coordination or delays in psychomotor development
- Hyperactive behavior
- Learning disabilities (e.g., speech and language delays)
- Mental retardation or low IQ
- Problems with daily living
- Vision or hearing problems
- Poor reasoning and judgment skills
- Sleep and sucking disturbances in infancy
- Heart and kidney defects

Neuroimaging of children with FAS shows abnormalities in the size and shape of their brains. The frontal lobes and cerebellum are often smaller than normal, and the corpus callosum and basal ganglia are commonly affected (Dannaway & Mulvihill, 2009). Studies show that children with FAS are often at risk for psychiatric disorders, commonly attention-deficit/hyperactivity disorder, mood disorders, anxiety disorders, eating disorders, and drug and alcohol dependence (Harvard Medical School, 2004; Hoffman, 2006).

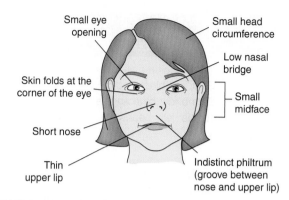

Small eye opening

Small head circumference

Low nasal bridge

Skin folds at the corner of the eye

Small midface

Short nose

Thin upper lip

Indistinct philtrum (groove between nose and upper lip)

FIGURE 25–1 Facial features of FAS. (From the National Institute on Alcohol Abuse and Alcoholism of the National Institutes of Health, Washington, DC.)

Children with FAS require lifelong care and treatment. There is no cure for FAS, but FAS can be prevented. The Surgeon General's Advisory on Alcohol Use in Pregnancy states:

> Health professionals should inquire routinely about alcohol consumption by women of childbearing age, inform them of the risks of alcohol consumption during pregnancy, and advise them not to drink alcoholic beverages during pregnancy. (Carmona, 2005, p. 1)

Alcohol Intoxication

Symptoms of alcohol intoxication include disinhibition of sexual or aggressive impulses, mood lability, impaired judgment, impaired social or occupational functioning, slurred speech, incoordination, unsteady gait, nystagmus, and flushed face. Intoxication usually occurs at blood alcohol levels between 100 and 200 mg/dL. Death has been reported at levels ranging from 400 to 700 mg/dL.

Alcohol Withdrawal

Within 4 to 12 hours of cessation of or reduction in heavy and prolonged (several days or longer) alcohol use, the following symptoms may appear: coarse tremor of hands, tongue, or eyelids; nausea or vomiting; malaise or weakness; tachycardia; sweating; elevated blood pressure; anxiety; depressed mood or irritability; transient hallucinations or illusions; headache; and insomnia. A complicated withdrawal syndrome may progress to *alcohol withdrawal delirium.* Onset of delirium is usually on the second or third day following cessation of or reduction in prolonged, heavy alcohol use. Symptoms include those described under the syndrome of delirium (see Chapter 24).

Sedative, Hypnotic, or Anxiolytic Abuse and Dependence

A Profile of the Substance

The sedative-hypnotic compounds are drugs of diverse chemical structures that are all capable of inducing varying degrees of CNS depression, from tranquilizing relief of anxiety to anesthesia, coma, and even death. They are generally categorized as (1) barbiturates, (2) nonbarbiturate hypnotics, and (3) antianxiety agents. Effects produced by these substances depend on size of dose and potency of drug administered.

Table 25-1 presents a selected list of drugs included in these categories. Generic names are followed in parentheses by the trade names. Common street names for each category are also included.

Several principles have been identified that apply fairly uniformly to all CNS depressants:

1. **The effects of CNS depressants are additive with one another and with the behavioral state of the user.** For example, when these drugs are used in combination with each other or in combination with alcohol, the depressive effects are compounded. These intense depressive effects are often unpredictable and can even be fatal. Similarly, a person who is mentally depressed or physically fatigued may have an exaggerated response to a dose of the drug that would only slightly affect a person in a normal or excited state.

2. **CNS depressants are capable of producing physiological dependence.** If large doses of CNS depressants are repeatedly administered over a prolonged duration, a period of CNS hyperexcitability occurs on withdrawal of the drug. The response can be quite severe, even leading to convulsions and death.

3. **CNS depressants are capable of producing psychological dependence.** CNS depressants have the potential to generate within the individual a psychic drive for periodic or continuous administration of the drug to achieve a maximum level of functioning or feeling of well-being.

4. **Cross-tolerance and cross-dependence may exist between various CNS depressants.** Cross-tolerance is exhibited when one drug results in a lessened response to another drug. Cross-dependence is a condition in which one drug can prevent withdrawal symptoms associated with physical dependence on a different drug (Julien, 2008).

TABLE 25-1 Sedative, Hypnotic, and Anxiolytic Drugs

CATEGORIES	GENERIC (TRADE) NAMES	COMMON STREET NAMES
Barbiturates	Pentobarbital (Nembutal) Secobarbital (Seconal) Amobarbital (Amytal) Secobarbital/amobarbital (Tuinal) Phenobarbital Butabarbital	Yellow jackets; yellow birds GBs; red birds; red devils Blue birds; blue angels Tooies; jelly beans
Nonbarbiturate hypnotics	Chloral hydrate (Noctec) Triazolam (Halcion) Flurazepam (Dalmane) Temazepam (Restoril) Quazepam (Doral)	Peter, Mickey Sleepers
Antianxiety agents	Diazepam (Valium) Chlordiazepoxide (Librium) Meprobamate (Miltown) Oxazepam (Serax) Alprazolam (Xanax) Lorazepam (Ativan) Clorazepate (Tranxene)	Vs (color designates strength) Green and whites; roaches Dolls; dollies Candy, downers (the benzodiazepines)
Club drugs	Flunitrazepam (Rohypnol) Gamma-hydroxybutyric acid (gamma-hydroxybutyrate; GHB)	Date rape drug; roofies, R-2, rope G, liquid X, grievous bodily harm, easy lay

Historical Aspects

Anxiety and insomnia, two of the most common human afflictions, were treated during the 19th century with opiates, bromide salts, chloral hydrate, paraldehyde, and alcohol (Julien, 2008; Sateia, 2009). Because the opiates were known to produce physical dependence, the bromides carried the risk of chronic bromide poisoning, and chloral hydrate and paraldehyde had an objectionable taste and smell, alcohol became the prescribed depressant drug of choice. However, some people refused to use alcohol either because they did not like the taste or for moral reasons, and others tended to take more than was prescribed. Therefore, a search for a better sedative drug continued.

Although barbituric acid was first synthesized in 1864, it was not until 1912 that phenobarbital was introduced into medicine as a sedative drug, the first of the structurally classified group of drugs called barbiturates (Julien, 2008). Since that time, more than 2,500 barbiturate derivatives have been synthesized, but currently, fewer than a dozen remain in medical use. Illicit use of the drugs for recreational purposes grew throughout the 1930s and 1940s.

Efforts to create depressant medications that were not barbiturate derivatives accelerated. By the mid-1950s, the market for depressants had been expanded by the appearance of the nonbarbiturates glutethimide, ethchlorvynol, methyprylon, and meprobamate. Introduction of the benzodiazepines occurred around 1960 with the marketing of chlordiazepoxide (Librium), followed shortly by its derivative diazepam (Valium). The use of these drugs, and others within their group, grew very rapidly, and they are prescribed widely in medical practice. Their margin of safety is greater than that of barbiturates and the other nonbarbiturates. However, prolonged use of even moderate doses is likely to result in physical and psychological dependence, with a characteristic syndrome of withdrawal that can be severe.

Patterns of Use/Abuse

Sadock and Sadock (2007) reported that about 15 percent of all persons in the United States have had a benzodiazepine prescribed by a physician. Of all the drugs used in clinical practice, the sedative-hypnotic/antianxiety drugs are among the most widely prescribed. The *DSM-IV-TR* states:

In the United States, up to 90 percent of individuals hospitalized for medical care or surgery receive orders for sedative, hypnotic, or anxiolytic medications during their hospital stay, and more than 15 percent of American adults use these medications (usually by prescription) during any one year. (p. 291)

Two patterns of development of dependence and abuse are described. The first pattern is one of an individual whose physician originally prescribed the CNS depressant as treatment for anxiety or insomnia. Independently, the individual has increased the dosage or frequency from that which was prescribed. Use of the medication is justified on the basis of treating symptoms, but as tolerance grows, more and more of the medication is required to produce the desired effect. Substance-seeking behavior is evident as the individual seeks prescriptions from several physicians in order to maintain sufficient supplies.

The second pattern, which the *DSM-IV-TR* reports is more frequent than the first, involves young people in their teens or early 20s who, in the company of their peers, use substances that were obtained illegally. The initial objective is to achieve a feeling of euphoria. The drug is usually used intermittently during recreational gatherings. This pattern of intermittent use leads to regular use and extreme levels of tolerance. Combining use with other substances is not uncommon. Physical and psychological dependence leads to intense substance-seeking behaviors, most often through illegal channels.

Effects on the Body

The sedative-hypnotic compounds induce a general depressant effect; that is, they depress the activity of the brain, nerves, muscles, and heart tissue. They reduce the rate of metabolism in a variety of tissues throughout the body, and in general, they depress any system that uses energy (Julien, 2008). Large doses are required to produce these effects. In lower doses these drugs appear to be more selective in their depressant actions. Specifically, in lower doses these drugs appear to exert their action on the centers within the brain that are concerned with arousal (e.g., the ascending reticular activating system, in the reticular formation, and the diffuse thalamic projection system).

As stated previously, the sedative-hypnotics are capable of producing all levels of CNS depression—from mild sedation to death. The level is determined by dosage and potency of the drug used. In Figure 25–2, a continuum of the CNS depressant effects is presented to demonstrate how increasing doses of sedative-hypnotic drugs affect behavioral depression.

The primary action of sedative-hypnotics is on nervous tissue. However, large doses may have an effect on other organ systems. Following is a discussion of the physiological effects of sedative-hypnotic/anxiolytic agents.

Effects on Sleep and Dreaming

Barbiturate use decreases the amount of sleep time spent in dreaming. During drug withdrawal, dreaming becomes vivid and excessive. Rebound insomnia and increased dreaming (termed *REM rebound*) are not uncommon with abrupt withdrawal from long-term use of these drugs as sleeping aids (Julien, 2008).

Respiratory Depression

Barbiturates are capable of inhibiting the reticular activating system, resulting in respiratory depression (Sadock & Sadock, 2007). Additive effects can occur with the concurrent use of other CNS depressants, effecting a life-threatening situation.

Cardiovascular Effects

Hypotension may be a problem with large doses. Only a slight decrease in blood pressure is noted with normal oral dosage. High dosages of barbiturates may result in decreased cardiac output, decreased cerebral blood flow, and direct impairment of myocardial contractility (Lafferty & Abdel-Kariem, 2010).

Renal Function

In doses high enough to produce anesthesia, barbiturates may suppress renal function. At the usual sedative-hypnotic dosage, however, there is

Normal - - → Relief From Anxiety - - → Disinhibition - - → Sedation - - → Hypnosis (sleep) - - → General Anesthesia - - → Coma - - → Death

- - - - - - - - - - → - - - - → Increasing Dosage of the Drug - - - - - - - - - → - - - - →

FIGURE 25–2 Continuum of behavioral depression with increasing doses of sedative-hypnotic drugs.

no evidence that they have any direct action on the kidneys.

Hepatic Effects

The barbiturates may produce jaundice with doses large enough to produce acute intoxication. Barbiturates stimulate the production of liver enzymes, resulting in a decrease in the plasma levels of both the barbiturates and other drugs metabolized in the liver. Preexisting liver disease may predispose an individual to additional liver damage with excessive barbiturate use.

Body Temperature

High doses of barbiturates can greatly decrease body temperature. It is not significantly altered with normal dosage levels.

Sexual Functioning

CNS depressants have a tendency to produce a biphasic response. There is an initial increase in libido, presumably from the primary disinhibitory effects of the drug. This initial response is then followed by a decrease in the ability to maintain an erection.

Sedative, Hypnotic, or Anxiolytic Intoxication

The *DSM-IV-TR* (APA, 2000) describes sedative, hypnotic, or anxiolytic intoxication as the presence of clinically significant maladaptive behavior or psychological changes that develop during, or shortly after, use of one of these substances. These maladaptive changes may include inappropriate sexual or aggressive behavior, mood lability, impaired judgment, or impaired social or occupational functioning. Other symptoms that may develop with excessive use of sedatives, hypnotics, or anxiolytics include slurred speech, incoordination, unsteady gait, nystagmus, impairment in attention or memory, and stupor or coma.

"Club drugs" in this category include gamma-hydroxybutyric acid (GHB) and flunitrazepam (Rohypnol). Like all of the depressants, they can produce a state of disinhibition, excitement, drunkenness, and amnesia (Julien, 2008). They have been widely implicated as "date rape" drugs, their presence being easily disguised in drinks. They produce anterograde amnesia, rendering the inability to remember events experienced while under their influence (*Street Drugs*, 2009).

Sedative, Hypnotic, or Anxiolytic Withdrawal

Withdrawal from sedatives, hypnotics, or anxiolytics produces a characteristic syndrome of symptoms that develops after a marked decrease in or cessation of intake after several weeks or more of regular use (APA, 2000). Onset of the symptoms depends on the drug from which the individual is withdrawing. A short-acting anxiolytic (e.g., lorazepam or oxazepam) may produce symptoms within 6 to 8 hours of decreasing blood levels, whereas withdrawal symptoms from substances with longer half-lives (e.g., diazepam) may not develop for more than a week, peak in intensity during the second week, and decrease markedly during the third or fourth week (APA, 2000).

Severe withdrawal is most likely to occur when a substance has been used at high dosages for prolonged periods. However, withdrawal symptoms also have been reported with moderate dosages taken over a relatively short duration. Withdrawal symptoms associated with sedatives, hypnotics or anxiolytics include autonomic hyperactivity (e.g., sweating or pulse rate greater than 100), increased hand tremor, insomnia, nausea or vomiting, hallucinations, illusions, psychomotor agitation, anxiety, or grand mal seizures.

CNS Stimulant Abuse and Dependence

A Profile of the Substance

The CNS stimulants are identified by the behavioral stimulation and psychomotor agitation that they induce. They differ widely in their molecular structures and in their mechanisms of action. The amount of CNS stimulation caused by a certain drug depends on both the area in the brain or spinal cord that is affected by the drug and the cellular mechanism fundamental to the increased excitability.

Groups within this category are classified according to similarities in mechanism of action. The *psychomotor stimulants* induce stimulation by augmentation or potentiation of the neurotransmitters norepinephrine, epinephrine, or dopamine. The *general cellular stimulants* (caffeine and nicotine) exert their action directly on cellular activity. Caffeine inhibits the enzyme phosphodiesterase, allowing increased levels of 3', 5'-cyclic adenosine monophosphate (cAMP), a chemical substance that promotes increased rates of cellular metabolism. Nicotine stimulates ganglionic synapses. This results in increased acetylcholine, which stimulates nerve impulse transmission to the entire autonomic nervous system. A selected list of drugs included in these categories is presented in Table 25-2.

The two most prevalent and widely used stimulants are caffeine and nicotine. Caffeine is readily available in every supermarket and grocery store as a common ingredient in coffee, tea, colas, and

TABLE 25-2 CNS Stimulants

CATEGORIES	GENERIC (TRADE) NAMES	COMMON STREET NAMES
Amphetamines	Dextroamphetamine (Dexedrine) Methamphetamine (Desoxyn) 3,4-methylenedioxyamphetamine (MDMA)* Amphetamine + dextroamphetamine (Adderall)	Dexies, uppers, truck drivers Meth, speed, crystal, ice Adam, Ecstasy, Eve, XTC
Nonamphetamine stimulants	Phendimetrazine (Bontril) Benzphetamine (Didrex) Diethylpropion (Tenuate) Phentermine (Adipex-P) Sibutramine (Meridia)† Methylphenidate (Ritalin) Dexmethylphenidate (Focalin) Modafinil (Provigil)	Diet pills Speed, uppers
Cocaine	Cocaine hydrochloride	Coke, blow, toot, snow, lady, flake, crack
Caffeine	Coffee, tea, colas, chocolate	Java, mud, brew, cocoa
Nicotine	Cigarettes, cigars, pipe tobacco, snuff	Weeds, fags, butts, chaw, cancer sticks

*Cross-listed with the hallucinogens.
†No longer marketed in the U.S.

chocolate. Nicotine is the primary psychoactive substance found in tobacco products. When used in moderation, these stimulants tend to relieve fatigue and increase alertness. They are a generally accepted part of our culture; however, with increased social awareness regarding the health risks associated with nicotine, its use has become stigmatized in some circles.

The more potent stimulants, because of their potential for physiological dependence, are under regulation by the Controlled Substances Act. These controlled stimulants are available for therapeutic purposes by prescription only; however, they are also clandestinely manufactured and widely distributed on the illicit market.

Historical Aspects

Cocaine is the most potent stimulant derived from nature. It is extracted from the leaves of the coca plant, which has been cultivated in the Andean highlands of South America since prehistoric times. Natives of the region chew the leaves of the plant for refreshment and relief from fatigue.

The coca leaves must be mixed with lime to release the cocaine alkaloid. The chemical formula for the pure form of the drug was developed in 1960. Physicians began using the drug as an anesthetic in eye, nose, and throat surgeries. It has also been used therapeutically in the United States in a morphine-cocaine elixir designed to relieve the suffering associated with terminal illness. These therapeutic uses are now obsolete.

Cocaine has achieved a degree of acceptability within some social circles. It is illicitly distributed as a white crystalline powder, often mixed with other ingredients to increase its volume and, therefore, create more profits. The drug is most commonly "snorted," and chronic users may manifest symptoms that resemble the congested nose of a common cold. The intensely pleasurable effects of the drug create the potential for extraordinary psychological dependence.

Another form of cocaine commonly used in the United States, called "crack," is a cocaine alkaloid that is extracted from its powdered hydrochloride salt by mixing it with sodium bicarbonate and allowing it to dry into small "rocks" (APA, 2000). Because this type of cocaine can be easily vaporized and inhaled, its effects have an extremely rapid onset.

Amphetamine was first prepared in 1887. Various derivatives of the drug soon followed, and clinical use of the drug began in 1927. Amphetamines were used quite extensively for medical purposes through the 1960s, but recognition of their abuse potential has sharply decreased clinical use. Today, they are prescribed only to treat narcolepsy (a rare disorder resulting in an uncontrollable desire for sleep), to treat hyperactivity disorders in children, and in certain cases of obesity.

Clandestine production of amphetamines for distribution on the illicit market has become a thriving business. U.S. government estimates, based on data from 2005, report the economic cost to society of methamphetamine use at between $16.2 billion and $48.3 billion (Office of National Drug Control Policy [ONDCP], 2010). Most of these expenses are related to the costs "that addiction places on dependent users and their premature mortality and from crime and criminal justice costs" (ONDCP, p. 1). Methamphetamine can be smoked, snorted, injected, or taken orally. The effects range from an intense rush from smoking or intravenous injection to a slower onset of euphoria as a result of snorting or oral ingestion. Another form of the drug, crystal methamphetamine, is produced by slowly recrystallizing powder methamphetamine from a solvent such as methanol, ethanol, isopropanol, or acetone (*Street Drugs,* 2009). It is a colorless, odorless, large-crystal form of *d*-methamphetamine, and is commonly called glass or ice because of its appearance. Crystal meth is usually smoked in a glass pipe like crack cocaine.

The earliest history of caffeine is unknown and is shrouded by legend and myth. Caffeine was first discovered in coffee in 1820 and in tea 7 years later. Both beverages have been widely accepted and enjoyed as a "pick-me-up" by many cultures.

Tobacco was used by the aborigines from remote times. Introduced in Europe in the mid-16th century, its use grew rapidly and soon became prevalent in the Orient. Tobacco came to America with the settlement of the earliest colonies. Today, it is grown in many countries of the world, and although smoking is decreasing in most industrialized nations, it is increasing in the developing areas (APA, 2000).

Patterns of Use/Abuse

Because of their pleasurable effects, CNS stimulants have a high abuse potential. In 2008, about 2 million Americans were current cocaine users (SAMHSA, 2009). Use was highest among Americans ages 18 to 25.

Many individuals who abuse or are dependent on a CNS stimulant began using the substance for the appetite-suppressant effect in an attempt at weight control (APA, 2000). Higher and higher doses are consumed in an effort to maintain the pleasurable effects. With continued use, the pleasurable effects diminish, and there is a corresponding increase in dysphoric effects. There is a persistent craving for the substance, however, even in the face of unpleasant adverse effects from the continued drug taking.

CNS stimulant abuse and dependence are usually characterized by either episodic or chronic daily, or almost daily, use. Individuals who use the substances on an episodic basis often "binge" on the drug with very high dosages followed by a day or two of recuperation. This recuperation period is characterized by extremely intense and unpleasant symptoms (called a "crash").

The daily user may take large or small doses and may use the drug several times a day or only at a specific time during the day. The amount consumed usually increases over time as tolerance occurs. Chronic users tend to rely on CNS stimulants to feel more powerful, more confident, and more decisive. They often fall into a pattern of taking "uppers" in the morning and "downers," such as alcohol or sleeping pills, at night.

The average American consumes two cups of coffee (about 200 mg of caffeine) per day. Caffeine is consumed in various amounts by 90 percent of the population. At a level of 500 to 600 mg of daily caffeine consumption, symptoms of anxiety, insomnia, and depression are not uncommon. It is also at this level that caffeine dependence and withdrawal can occur. Caffeine consumption is prevalent among children as well as adults. Table 25-3 lists some common sources of caffeine.

Next to caffeine, nicotine, an active ingredient in tobacco, is the most widely used psychoactive substance in U.S. society. Of the U.S. population ages 12 years or older, 28.4 percent reported current use of a tobacco product in 2008 (SAMHSA, 2009). Since 1964, when the results of the first public health report on smoking were issued, the percentage of total smokers has been on the decline. However, the percentage of women and teenage smokers has declined more slowly than that of adult men. Approximately 400,000 people die annually because of tobacco use, and an estimated 60 percent of the direct health-care costs in the United States go to treat tobacco-related illnesses (Sadock & Sadock, 2007).

Effects on the Body

The CNS stimulants are a group of pharmacological agents that are capable of exciting the entire nervous system. This is accomplished by increasing the activity or augmenting the capability of the neurotransmitter agents known to be directly involved in bodily activation and behavioral stimulation. Physiological responses vary markedly according to the potency and dosage of the drug.

Central Nervous System Effects

Stimulation of the CNS results in tremor, restlessness, anorexia, insomnia, agitation, and increased motor activity. Amphetamines, nonamphetamine

TABLE 25-3 Common Sources of Caffeine

SOURCE	CAFFEINE CONTENT (mg)
Food and Beverages	
5-6 oz. brewed coffee	90-125
5-6 oz. instant coffee	60-90
5-6 oz. decaffeinated coffee	3
5-6 oz. brewed tea	70
5-6 oz. instant tea	45
8 oz. green tea	15-30
8- to 12-oz. cola drinks	60
12 oz. Red Bull energy drink	115
5-6 oz. cocoa	20
8 oz. chocolate milk	2-7
1-oz. chocolate bar	22
Prescription Medications	
APCs (aspirin, phenacetin, caffeine)	32
Cafergot	100
Fiorinal	40
Migralam	100
Over-the-Counter Analgesics	
Anacin, Empirin, Midol, Vanquish	32
Excedrin Migraine (aspirin, acetaminophen, caffeine)	65
Over-the-Counter Stimulants	
No Doz Tablets	100
Vivarin	200
Caffedrine	250

stimulants, and cocaine produce increased alertness, decrease in fatigue, elation and euphoria, and subjective feelings of greater mental agility and muscular power. Chronic use of these drugs may result in compulsive behavior, paranoia, hallucinations, and aggressive behavior (*Street Drugs,* 2009).

Cardiovascular/Pulmonary Effects

Amphetamines can induce increased systolic and diastolic blood pressure, increased heart rate, and cardiac arrhythmias (*Street Drugs,* 2009). These drugs also relax bronchial smooth muscle.

Cocaine intoxication typically produces a rise in myocardial demand for oxygen and an increase in heart rate. Severe vasoconstriction may occur and can result in myocardial infarction, ventricular fibrillation, and sudden death. Inhaled cocaine can cause pulmonary hemorrhage, chronic bronchiolitis, and pneumonia. Nasal rhinitis is a result of chronic cocaine snorting.

Caffeine ingestion can result in increased heart rate, palpitations, extrasystoles, and cardiac arrhythmias. Caffeine induces dilation of pulmonary and general systemic blood vessels and constriction of cerebral blood vessels.

Nicotine stimulates the sympathetic nervous system, resulting in an increase in heart rate, blood pressure, and cardiac contractility, thereby increasing myocardial oxygen consumption and demand for blood flow (Royal College of Physicians, 2000). Contractions of gastric smooth muscle associated with hunger are inhibited, thereby producing a mild anorectic effect.

Gastrointestinal and Renal Effects

Gastrointestinal (GI) effects of amphetamines are somewhat unpredictable; however, a decrease in GI tract motility commonly results in constipation. Contraction of the bladder sphincter makes urination difficult. Caffeine exerts a diuretic effect on the kidneys. Nicotine stimulates the hypothalamus to release antidiuretic hormone, reducing the excretion of urine. Because nicotine increases the tone and activity of the bowel, it may occasionally cause diarrhea.

IMPLICATIONS OF RESEARCH FOR EVIDENCE-BASED PRACTICE

Gaffney, K. F. (2001). Infant exposure to environmental tobacco smoke. *Journal of Nursing Scholarship, 33,* 343–347.

DESCRIPTION OF THE STUDY: A review of 10 studies with a range of 100 to more than 1,000 participants was conducted. The studies took place in a variety of health-care settings in the United States, Australia, and Europe. The studies measured infant exposure to environmental tobacco smoke (ETS). Parents of the infants completed the self-reports that inquired about number of people in the household who smoked and the proximity of the infant to the smoking. The studies focused on children in the first year of life.

IMPLICATIONS OF RESEARCH FOR EVIDENCE-BASED PRACTICE—cont'd

RESULTS OF THE STUDY: In one of the studies, questionnaire information was supported by hair analysis of the subjects. Median level of hair nicotine was over 1.5 times higher among infants in homes reported by means of questionnaires to have smokers than among those in homes reported to have no smokers. Eight of the 10 studies demonstrated increased risk for poor infant health outcomes associated with ETS exposure. Positive associations were found between infant ETS exposure and gastroesophageal reflux, colic, sudden infant death syndrome, lower respiratory tract infections, ear infections, and altered thyroid function.

IMPLICATIONS FOR NURSING PRACTICE: The author suggested that nurses may use these results to document the need for identifying mothers who smoke as an important target group for clinical intervention. She stated, "This review shows the importance of identifying and assisting mothers who smoke so that this critical proximity with their infants may provide optimal health promotion. Nurses who care for infants as part of the regular health maintenance visits conducted during the first year of life are particularly well-prepared and logically situated to advise and assist these mothers as they initiate the long-term process of smoking cessation." (pp. 346–347)

Most CNS stimulants induce a small rise in metabolic rate and various degrees of anorexia. Amphetamines and cocaine can cause a rise in body temperature.

Sexual Functioning

CNS stimulants apparently promote the coital urge in both men and women. Women, more than men, report that stimulants make them feel sexier and have more orgasms. In fact, some men may experience sexual dysfunction with the use of stimulants. For the majority of individuals, however, these drugs exert a powerful aphrodisiac effect.

CNS Stimulant Intoxication

CNS stimulant intoxication produces maladaptive behavior and psychological changes that develop during, or shortly after, use of these drugs. Amphetamine and cocaine intoxication typically produces euphoria or affective blunting; changes in sociability; hypervigilance; interpersonal sensitivity; anxiety, tension, or anger; stereotyped behaviors; or impaired judgment. Physical effects include tachycardia or bradycardia, pupillary dilation, elevated or lowered blood pressure, perspiration or chills, nausea or vomiting, weight loss, psychomotor agitation or retardation, muscular weakness, respiratory depression, chest pain, cardiac arrhythmias, confusion, seizures, dyskinesias, dystonias, or coma (APA, 2000).

Intoxication from caffeine usually occurs following consumption in excess of 250 mg. Symptoms include restlessness, nervousness, excitement, insomnia, flushed face, diuresis, GI disturbance, muscle twitching, rambling flow of thought and speech, tachycardia or cardiac arrhythmia, periods of inexhaustibility, and psychomotor agitation (APA, 2000).

CNS Stimulant Withdrawal

CNS stimulant withdrawal is the presence of a characteristic withdrawal syndrome that develops within a few hours to several days after cessation of, or reduction in, heavy and prolonged use (APA, 2000). Withdrawal from amphetamines and cocaine causes dysphoria, fatigue, vivid unpleasant dreams, insomnia or hypersomnia, increased appetite, and psychomotor retardation or agitation (APA, 2000). The *DSM-IV-TR* states:

Marked withdrawal symptoms ("crashing") often follow an episode of intense, high-dose use (a "speed run"). This "crash" is characterized by intense and unpleasant feelings of lassitude and depression, generally requiring several days of rest and recuperation. Weight loss commonly occurs during heavy stimulant use, whereas a marked increase in appetite with rapid weight gain is often observed during withdrawal. Depressive symptoms may last several days to weeks and may be accompanied by suicidal ideation. (p. 227)

The *DSM-IV-TR* does not include a diagnosis of caffeine withdrawal. However, Sadock and Sadock (2007) stated that a number of well-controlled research studies indicate that caffeine withdrawal exists. They cite the following symptoms as typical: headache, fatigue, anxiety, irritability, depression, impaired psychomotor performance, nausea, vomiting, craving for caffeine, and muscle pain and stiffness.

Withdrawal from nicotine results in dysphoric or depressed mood; insomnia; irritability, frustration, or anger; anxiety; difficulty concentrating; restlessness; decreased heart rate; and increased appetite or weight gain (APA, 2000). A mild syndrome of nicotine withdrawal can appear when a smoker switches from regular cigarettes to low-nicotine cigarettes (Sadock & Sadock, 2007).

Inhalant Abuse and Dependence

A Profile of the Substance

Inhalant disorders are induced by inhaling the aliphatic and aromatic hydrocarbons found in substances such as fuels, solvents, adhesives, aerosol propellants, and paint thinners. Specific examples of these substances include gasoline, varnish remover, lighter fluid, airplane glue, rubber cement, cleaning fluid, spray paint, shoe conditioner, and typewriter correction fluid.

Patterns of Use/Abuse

Inhalant substances are readily available, legal, and inexpensive. These three factors make inhalants the drug of choice among poor people and among children and young adults. Use may begin by ages 9 to 12 and peak in the adolescent years; it is less common after age 35 (APA, 2000). A national government survey of drug use indicated that 8.9 percent of people in the United States ages 12 years or older acknowledged having used inhalants (SAMHSA, 2009). The highest use was seen in the 12- to 17-year-old age group.

Methods of use include "huffing"—a procedure in which a rag soaked with the substance is applied to the mouth and nose and the vapors breathed in. Another common method is called "bagging," in which the substance is placed in a paper or plastic bag and inhaled from the bag by the user. The substance may also be inhaled directly from the container or sprayed in the mouth or nose.

Sadock and Sadock (2007) reported that:

> Inhalant use among adolescents may be most common in those whose parents or older siblings use illegal substances. Inhalant use among adolescents is also associated with an increased likelihood of conduct disorder or antisocial personality disorder. (p. 435)

Tolerance to inhalants has been reported with heavy use. A mild withdrawal syndrome has been documented but does not appear to be clinically significant (APA, 2000).

Children with inhalant disorder may use inhalants several times a week, often on weekends and after school (APA, 2000). Adults with inhalant dependence may use the substance at varying times during each day, or they may binge on the substance during a period of several days.

Effects on the Body

Inhalants are absorbed through the lungs and reach the CNS very rapidly. Inhalants generally act as a CNS depressant (Sadock & Sadock, 2007). The effects are relatively brief, lasting from several minutes to a few hours, depending on the specific substance and amount consumed.

Central Nervous System

Inhalants can cause both central and peripheral nervous system damage, which may be permanent (APA, 2000). Neurological deficits, such as generalized weakness and peripheral neuropathies, may be evident. Other CNS effects that have been reported with heavy inhalant use include cerebral atrophy, cerebellar degeneration, and white matter lesions resulting in cranial nerve or pyramidal tract signs.

Respiratory Effects

The *DSM-IV-TR* reports the following respiratory effects with inhalant use: upper- or lower-airway irritation, including increased airway resistance; pulmonary hypertension; acute respiratory distress; coughing; sinus discharge; dyspnea; rales; or rhonchi. Rarely, cyanosis may result from pneumonitis or asphyxia. Death may occur from respiratory or cardiovascular depression.

Gastrointestinal Effects

Abdominal pain, nausea, and vomiting may occur. A rash may be present around the individual's nose and mouth. Unusual breath odors are common.

Renal System Effects

Chronic renal failure, hepatorenal syndrome, and proximal renal tubular acidosis have been reported (APA, 2000).

Inhalant Intoxication

The *DSM-IV-TR* defines inhalant intoxication as "clinically significant maladaptive behavior or psychological changes (e.g., confusion, belligerence, assaultiveness, apathy, impaired judgment, impaired social or occupational functioning) that developed during or shortly after, use of or exposure to volatile inhalants" (APA, p. 259). Two or more of the following signs are present:

- Dizziness
- Nystagmus
- Incoordination
- Slurred speech
- Unsteady gait
- Lethargy
- Depressed reflexes

■ Psychomotor retardation

■ Tremor

■ Generalized muscle weakness

■ Blurred vision or diplopia

■ Stupor or coma

■ Euphoria

The symptoms are not due to a general medical condition and are not better accounted for by another mental disorder.

Opioid Abuse and Dependence

A Profile of the Substance

The term *opioid* refers to a group of compounds that includes opium, opium derivatives, and synthetic substitutes. Opioids exert both a sedative and an analgesic effect, and their major medical uses are for the relief of pain, the treatment of diarrhea, and the relief of coughing. These drugs have addictive qualities; that is, they are capable of inducing tolerance and physiological and psychological dependence.

Opioids are popular drugs of abuse in that they desensitize an individual to both psychological and physiological pain and induce a sense of euphoria. Lethargy and indifference to the environment are common manifestations.

Opioid abusers usually spend much of their time nourishing their habit. Individuals who are opioid dependent are seldom able to hold a steady job that will support their need. They must therefore secure funds from friends, relatives, or whomever they have not yet alienated with their dependence-related behavior. It is not uncommon for individuals who are opioid dependent to resort to illegal means of obtaining funds, such as burglary, robbery, prostitution, or selling drugs.

Methods of administration of opioid drugs include oral, snorting, or smoking, and by subcutaneous, intramuscular, and intravenous injection. A selected list of opioid substances is presented in Table 25-4.

Under close supervision, opioids are indispensable in the practice of medicine. They are the most effective agents known for the relief of intense pain. However, they also induce a pleasurable effect on the CNS that promotes their abuse. The physiological and psychological dependence that occurs with opioids, as well as the development of profound tolerance, contribute to the addict's ongoing quest for more of the substance, regardless of the means.

Historical Aspects

In its crude form, opium is a brownish-black, gummy substance obtained from the ripened pods of the opium poppy. References to the use of opiates have been found in the Egyptian, Greek, and Arabian cultures as early as 3000 B.C. The drug became widely used both medicinally and recreationally throughout Europe during the 16th and 17th centuries. Most of the opium supply came from China, where the drug was introduced by

TABLE 25-4 Opioids and Related Substances		
CATEGORIES	**GENERIC (TRADE) NAMES**	**COMMON STREET NAMES**
Opioids of natural origin	Opium (ingredient in various antidiarrheal agents)	Black stuff, poppy, tar, big O
	Morphine (Astramorph)	M, white stuff, Miss Emma
	Codeine (ingredient in various analgesics and cough suppressants)	Terp, schoolboy, syrup, cody
Opioid derivatives	Heroin	H, horse, junk, brown sugar, smack, skag, TNT, Harry
	Hydromorphone (Dilaudid)	DLs, 4s, lords, little D
	Oxycodone (Percodan; OxyContin)	Perks, perkies, Oxy, O.C.
	Hydrocodone (Vicodin)	Vike
Synthetic opiate-like drugs	Meperidine (Demerol)	Doctors
	Methadone (Dolophine)	Dollies, done
	Pentazocine (Talwin)	Ts
	Fentanyl (Fentora)	Apache, China girl, China town, dance fever, goodfella, jackpot

Arabic traders in the late 17th century. Morphine, the primary active ingredient of opium, was isolated in 1803 by the European chemist Frederich Serturner. Since that time, morphine, rather than crude opium, has been used throughout the world for the medical treatment of pain and diarrhea. This process was facilitated in 1853 by the development of the hypodermic syringe, which made it possible to deliver the undiluted morphine quickly into the body for rapid relief from pain.

This development also created a new variety of opiate user in the United States: one who was able to self-administer the drug by injection. During this time, there was also a large influx of Chinese immigrants into the United States, who introduced opium smoking to this country. By the early part of the 20th century, opium addiction was widespread.

In response to the concerns over widespread addiction, in 1914 the U.S. government passed the Harrison Narcotic Act, which created strict controls on the accessibility of opiates. Until that time, these substances had been freely available to the public without a prescription. The Harrison Act banned the use of opiates for other than medicinal purposes and drove the use of heroin underground. To this day, the beneficial uses of these substances are widely acclaimed within the medical profession, but the illicit trafficking of the drugs for recreational purposes continues to resist most efforts aimed at control.

Patterns of Use/Abuse

The development of opioid abuse and dependence may follow one of two typical behavior patterns. The first occurs in the individual who has obtained the drug by prescription from a physician for the relief of a medical problem. Abuse and dependence occur when the individual increases the amount and frequency of use, justifying the behavior as symptom treatment. He or she becomes obsessed with obtaining more and more of the substance, seeking out several physicians in order to replenish and maintain supplies.

The second pattern of behavior associated with abuse of and dependence on opioids occurs among individuals who use the drugs for recreational purposes and obtain them from illegal sources. Opioids may be used alone to induce the euphoric effects or in combination with stimulants or other drugs to enhance the euphoria or to counteract the depressant effects of the opioid. Tolerance develops and dependence occurs, leading the individual to procure the substance by whatever means is required to support the habit.

A recent government survey reported that there were 213,000 current heroin users ages 12 years and older in the United States in 2008 (SAMHSA, 2009). The same survey revealed an estimated 4.7 million current users of narcotic pain relievers.

Effects on the Body

Opiates are sometimes classified as *narcotic analgesics*. They exert their major effects primarily on the CNS, the eyes, and the GI tract. Chronic morphine use or acute morphine toxicity is manifested by a syndrome of sedation, chronic constipation, decreased respiratory rate, and pinpoint pupils. Intensity of symptoms is largely dose dependent. The following physiological effects are common with opioid use.

Central Nervous System

All opioids, opioid derivatives, and synthetic opioid-like drugs affect the CNS. Common manifestations include euphoria, mood changes, and mental clouding. Other common CNS effects include drowsiness and pain reduction. Pupillary constriction occurs in response to stimulation of the oculomotor nerve. CNS depression of the respiratory centers within the medulla results in respiratory depression. The antitussive response is due to suppression of the cough center within the medulla. The nausea and vomiting commonly associated with opiate ingestion are related to the stimulation of the centers within the medulla that trigger this response.

Gastrointestinal Effects

These drugs exert a profound effect on the GI tract. Both stomach and intestinal tone are increased, whereas peristaltic activity of the intestines is diminished. These effects lead to a marked decrease in the movement of food through the GI tract. This is a notable therapeutic effect in the treatment of severe diarrhea. In fact, no drugs have yet been developed that are more effective than the opioids for this purpose. However, constipation, and even fecal impaction, may be a serious problem for the chronic opioid user.

Cardiovascular Effects

In therapeutic doses, opioids have minimal effect on the action of the heart. Morphine is used extensively to relieve pulmonary edema and the pain of myocardial infarction in cardiac clients. At high doses, opioids induce hypotension, which may be caused by direct action on the heart or by opioid-induced histamine release.

Sexual Functioning

With opioid use, there is decreased sexual function and diminished libido (National Cancer Institute, 2010). Retarded ejaculation, impotence, and orgasm failure (in both men and women) may occur. Sexual side effects from opioids appear to be largely influenced by dosage.

Opioid Intoxication

Opioid intoxication constitutes clinically significant maladaptive behavior or psychological changes that develop during, or shortly after, opioid use (APA, 2000). Symptoms include initial euphoria followed by apathy, dysphoria, psychomotor agitation or retardation, and impaired judgment. Physical symptoms include pupillary constriction (or dilation due to anoxia from severe overdose), drowsiness, slurred speech, and impairment in attention or memory (APA, 2000). Symptoms are consistent with the half-life of most opioid drugs, and usually last for several hours. Severe opioid intoxication can lead to respiratory depression, coma, and death.

Opioid Withdrawal

Opioid withdrawal produces a syndrome of symptoms that develops after cessation of, or reduction in, heavy and prolonged use of an opiate or related substance. Symptoms include dysphoric mood, nausea or vomiting, muscle aches, lacrimation or rhinorrhea, pupillary dilation, piloerection, sweating, abdominal cramping, diarrhea, yawning, fever, and insomnia. With short-acting drugs such as heroin, withdrawal symptoms occur within 6 to 12 hours after the last dose, peak within 1 to 3 days, and gradually subside over a period of 5 to 7 days (APA, 2000). With longer-acting drugs such as methadone, withdrawal symptoms begin within 1 to 3 days after the last dose, peak between days 4 and 6, and are complete in 14 to 21 days (Leamon, Wright, & Myrick, 2008). Withdrawal from the ultra-short-acting meperidine begins quickly, reaches a peak in 8 to 12 hours, and is complete in 4 to 5 days (Sadock & Sadock, 2007).

Hallucinogen Abuse and Dependence

A Profile of the Substance

Hallucinogenic substances are capable of distorting an individual's perception of reality. They have the ability to alter sensory perception and induce hallucinations. For this reason they have sometimes been referred to as "mind expanding." Some of the manifestations have been likened to a psychotic break. The hallucinations experienced by an individual with schizophrenia, however, are most often auditory, whereas substance-induced hallucinations are usually visual (Mack, Franklin, & Frances, 2003). Perceptual distortions have been reported by some users as spiritual, as giving a

sense of depersonalization (observing oneself having the experience), or as being at peace with self and the universe. Others, who describe their experiences as "bad trips," report feelings of panic and a fear of dying or going insane. A common danger reported with hallucinogenic drugs is that of "flashbacks," or a spontaneous reoccurrence of the hallucinogenic state without ingestion of the drug. These can occur months after the drug was last taken.

Recurrent use can produce tolerance, encouraging users to resort to higher and higher dosages. No evidence of physical dependence is detectable when the drug is withdrawn; however, recurrent use appears to induce a psychological dependence to the insight-inducing experiences that a user may associate with episodes of hallucinogen use (Sadock & Sadock, 2007). This psychological dependence varies according to the drug, the dose, and the individual user. Hallucinogens are highly unpredictable in the effects they may induce each time they are used.

Many of the hallucinogenic substances have structural similarities. Some are produced synthetically; others are natural products of plants and fungi. A selected list of hallucinogens is presented in Table 25-5.

Historical Aspects

Archeological data obtained with carbon-14 dating suggest that hallucinogens have been used as part of religious ceremonies and at social gatherings by Native Americans for as long as 7,000 years (Goldstein, 2002). Use of the peyote cactus as part of religious ceremonies in the southwestern part of the United States still occurs today, although this ritual use has greatly diminished.

LSD was first synthesized in 1943 by Dr. Albert Hoffman (Goldstein, 2002). It was used as a clinical research tool to investigate the biochemical etiology of schizophrenia. It soon reached the illicit market, however, and its abuse began to overshadow the research effort.

The abuse of hallucinogens reached a peak in the late 1960s, waned during the 1970s, and returned to favor in the 1980s with the so-called designer drugs (e.g., 3,4-methylene-dioxymethamphetamine [MDMA] and methoxy-amphetamine [MDA]). One of the most commonly abused hallucinogens today is PCP, even though many of its effects are perceived as undesirable. A number of deaths have been directly attributed to the use of PCP, and numerous accidental deaths have occurred as a result of overdose and of the behavioral changes the drug precipitates. A derivative of PCP, ketamine, which is a preoperative anesthetic,

TABLE 25-5 HALLUCINOGENS		
CATEGORIES	**GENERIC (TRADE) NAMES**	**COMMON STREET NAMES**
Naturally occurring hallucinogens	Mescaline (the primary active ingredient of the peyote cactus)	Cactus, mesc, mescal, half moon, big chief, bad seed, peyote
	Psilocybin and psilocin (active ingredients of *Psilocybe* mushrooms)	Magic mushroom, God's flesh, shrooms
	Ololiuqui (morning glory seeds)	Heavenly blue, pearly gates, flying saucers
Synthetic compounds	Lysergic acid diethylamide (LSD)—synthetically produced from a fungal substance found on rye or a chemical substance found in morning glory seeds	Acid, cube, big D, California sunshine, microdots, blue dots, sugar, orange wedges, peace tablets, purple haze, cupcakes
	Dimethyltryptamine (DMT) and diethyltryptamine (DET)—chemical analogues of tryptamine	Businessman's trip
	2,5-Dimethoxy-4-methylamphetamine (STP, DOM)	STP (serenity, tranquility, peace)
	Phencyclidine (PCP)	Angel dust, hog, peace pill, rocket fuel
	Ketamine (Ketalar)	Special K, vitamin K, kit kat
	3,4-Methylene-dioxyamphetamine (MDMA)*	XTC, ecstasy, Adam, Eve
	Methoxy-amphetamine (MDA)	Love drug

Cross-listed with the CNS stimulants.

also is abused for its psychedelic properties. It produces effects similar to, but somewhat less intense than, those of PCP.

Several therapeutic uses of LSD have been proposed, including the treatment of chronic alcoholism and the reduction of intractable pain such as occurs in malignant disease. A great deal more research is required regarding the therapeutic uses of LSD. At this time, there is no real evidence of the safety and efficacy of the drug in humans.

Patterns of Use/Abuse

Use of hallucinogens is usually episodic. Because cognitive and perceptual abilities are so markedly affected by these substances, the user must set aside time from normal daily activities for indulging in the consequences. According to the SAMHSA (2009) report, hallucinogens were used in the previous 30-day period before the survey in 2008 by more than 1 million persons (0.4 percent) ages 12 or older. This number included 555,000 (0.2 percent) who had used Ecstasy.

The use of LSD does not lead to the development of physical dependence or withdrawal symptoms (Sadock & Sadock, 2007). However, tolerance does develop quickly and to a high degree. In fact, an individual who uses LSD repeatedly for a period of 3 to 4 days may develop complete tolerance to the drug. Recovery from the tolerance also occurs very rapidly (in 4 to 7 days), so that the individual is able to achieve the desired effect from the drug repeatedly and often.

PCP is usually taken episodically, in binges that can last for several days. However, some chronic users take the substance daily. Physical dependence does not occur with PCP; however, psychological dependence characterized by craving for the drug has been reported in chronic users, as has the development of tolerance. Tolerance apparently develops quickly with frequent use.

Psilocybin is an ingredient of the *Psilocybe* mushroom indigenous to the United States and Mexico. Ingestion of these mushrooms produces an effect similar to that of LSD but of a shorter duration. This hallucinogenic chemical can now be produced synthetically.

Mescaline is the only hallucinogenic compound used legally for religious purposes today by members of the Native American Church of the United States. It is the primary active ingredient of the peyote cactus. Neither physical nor psychological dependence occurs with the use of mescaline, although, as with other hallucinogens, tolerance can develop quickly with frequent use.

Among the very potent hallucinogens of the current drug culture are those that are categorized as derivatives of amphetamines. These include 2,5-dimethoxy-4-methylamphetamine (DOM, STP), MDMA, and MDA. At lower doses, these drugs produce the "high" associated with CNS stimulants. At higher doses, hallucinogenic effects occur. These drugs have existed for many years but were *rediscovered* in the mid-1980s. Because of the rapid increase in recreational use, the Drug Enforcement Agency (DEA) imposed an emergency classification of MDMA as a schedule I drug in 1985. MDMA, or Ecstasy, is a synthetic drug with both stimulant and hallucinogenic qualities. It has a chemical structure similar to methamphetamine and mescaline, and it has become widely available throughout the world. Because of its growing popularity, the demand for this drug has led to tablets and capsules being sold as "Ecstasy," but that are not pure MDMA. Many contain drugs such as methamphetamine, PCP, amphetamine, ketamine, and *p*-methoxyamphetamine (PMA, a stimulant with hallucinogenic properties; more toxic than MDMA). This practice has increased the dangers associated with MDMA use (*Street Drugs,* 2009).

Effects on the Body

The effects produced by the various hallucinogenics are highly unpredictable. The variety of effects may be related to dosage, the mental state of the individual, and the environment in which the substance is used. Some common effects have been reported (APA, 2000; Julien, 2008; Sadock & Sadock, 2007):

Physiological Effects

- Nausea and vomiting
- Chills
- Pupil dilation
- Increased pulse, blood pressure, and temperature
- Mild dizziness
- Trembling
- Loss of appetite
- Insomnia
- Sweating
- A slowing of respirations
- Elevation in blood sugar

Psychological Effects

- Heightened response to color, texture, and sounds
- Heightened body awareness
- Distortion of vision

- Sense of slowing of time
- All feelings magnified: love, lust, hate, joy, anger, pain, terror, despair
- Fear of losing control
- Paranoia, panic
- Euphoria, bliss
- Projection of self into dreamlike images
- Serenity, peace
- Depersonalization
- Derealization
- Increased libido

The effects of hallucinogens are not always pleasurable for the user. Two types of toxic reactions are known to occur. The first is the *panic reaction,* or "bad trip." Symptoms include an intense level of anxiety, fear, and stimulation. The individual hallucinates and fears going insane. Paranoia and acute psychosis may be evident.

The second type of toxic reaction to hallucinogens is the *flashback.* This phenomenon refers to the transient, spontaneous repetition of a previous LSD-induced experience that occurs in the absence of the substance. Various studies have reported that 15 to 80 percent of hallucinogen users report having experienced flashbacks (Sadock & Sadock, 2007).

Hallucinogen Intoxication

Symptoms of hallucinogen intoxication develop during, or shortly after (within minutes to a few hours), hallucinogen use (APA, 2000). Maladaptive behavior or psychological changes include marked anxiety or depression, ideas of reference (a type of delusional thinking that all activity within one's environment is "referred to" [about] one's self), fear of losing one's mind, paranoid ideation, and impaired judgment. Perceptual changes occur in a state of full wakefulness and alertness and include intensification of perceptions, depersonalization, derealization, illusions, hallucinations, and synesthesias (APA, 2000). Physical symptoms include pupillary dilation, tachycardia, sweating, palpitations, blurring of vision, tremors, and incoordination (APA, 2000).

Symptoms of PCP intoxication develop within an hour of use (or less when it is smoked, snorted, or taken intravenously) (APA, 2000). Specific symptoms are dose related and include belligerence, assaultiveness, impulsiveness, unpredictability, psychomotor agitation, and impaired judgment. Physical symptoms include vertical or horizontal nystagmus, hypertension or tachycardia, numbness or diminished responsiveness to pain, ataxia, dysarthria, muscle rigidity, seizures or coma, and hyperacusis.

General effects of MDMA (Ecstasy) include increased heart rate, blood pressure, and body temperature; dehydration; confusion; insomnia; and paranoia. Overdose can result in panic attacks, hallucinations, blurred vision, rhabdomyolysis, and death from kidney or cardiovascular failure (*Street Drugs,* 2009).

Cannabis Abuse and Dependence

A Profile of the Substance

Cannabis is second only to alcohol as the most widely abused drug in the United States. The major psychoactive ingredient of this class of substances is delta-9-tetrahydrocannabinol (THC). It occurs naturally in the plant *Cannabis sativa,* which grows readily in warm climates. Marijuana, the most prevalent type of cannabis preparation, is composed of the dried leaves, stems, and flowers of the plant. Hashish is a more potent concentrate of the resin derived from the flowering tops of the plant. Hash oil is a very concentrated form of THC made by boiling hashish in a solvent and filtering out the solid matter (*Street Drugs,* 2009). Cannabis products are usually smoked in the form of loosely rolled cigarettes. Cannabis can also be taken orally when it is prepared in food, but about two to three times the amount of cannabis must be ingested orally to equal the potency of that obtained by the inhalation of its smoke (Sadock & Sadock, 2007).

At moderate dosages, cannabis drugs produce effects resembling alcohol and other CNS depressants. By depressing higher brain centers, they release lower centers from inhibitory influences. There has been some controversy in the past over the classification of these substances. They are not narcotics, although they are legally classified as controlled substances. They are not hallucinogens, although in very high dosages they can induce hallucinations. They are not sedative-hypnotics, although they most closely resemble these substances. Like sedative-hypnotics, their action occurs in the ascending reticular activating system.

Psychological dependence has been shown to occur with cannabis, and tolerance can occur. Controversy exists about whether physiological dependence occurs with cannabis. Sadock and Sadock (2007) stated:

> Withdrawal symptoms in humans are limited to modest increases in irritability, restlessness, insomnia, and anorexia and mild nausea; all these symptoms appear only when a person abruptly stops taking high doses of cannabis. (p. 418)

Common cannabis preparations are presented in Table 25-6.

Historical Aspects

Products of *Cannabis sativa* have been used therapeutically for nearly 5,000 years (Julien, 2008). Cannabis was first employed in China and India as an antiseptic and an analgesic. Its use later spread to the Middle East, Africa, and Eastern Europe.

In the United States, medical interest in the use of cannabis arose during the early part of the 19th century. Many articles were published espousing its use for many and varied reasons. The drug was almost as commonly used for medicinal purposes as aspirin is today and could be purchased without a prescription in any drug store. It was purported to have antibacterial and anticonvulsant capabilities, to decrease intraocular pressure, decrease pain, help in the treatment of asthma, increase appetite, and generally raise one's morale.

The drug went out of favor primarily because of the huge variation in potency within batches of medication caused by the variations in the THC content of different plants. Other medications were favored for their greater degree of solubility and faster onset of action than cannabis products. A federal law put an end to its legal use in 1937, after an association between marijuana and criminal activity became evident. In the 1960s, marijuana became the symbol of the "antiestablishment" generation, at which time it reached its peak as a drug of abuse.

Research continues in regard to the possible therapeutic uses of cannabis. It has been shown to be an effective agent for relieving the nausea and vomiting associated with cancer chemotherapy, when other antinausea medications fail. It has also been used in the treatment of chronic pain, glaucoma, multiple sclerosis, and acquired immunodeficiency syndrome (Sadock & Sadock, 2007).

Advocates who praise the therapeutic usefulness and support the legalization of the cannabinoids persist within the United States today. Such groups

TABLE 25-6 Cannabinoids		
CATEGORY	COMMON PREPARATIONS	STREET NAMES
Cannabis	Marijuana	Joint, weed, pot, grass, Mary Jane, Texas tea, locoweed, MJ, hay, stick
	Hashish	Hash, bhang, ganja, charas

as the Alliance for Cannabis Therapeutics (ACT) and the National Organization for the Reform of Marijuana Laws (NORML) have lobbied extensively to allow disease sufferers easier access to the drug. The medical use of marijuana has been legalized by a number of states. The DEA (2006) stated:

> DEA has approved and will continue to approve research into whether THC has any medicinal use. The Center for Medicinal Cannabis Research (CMCR) conducts studies to ascertain the general medical safety and efficacy of cannabis and cannabis products and examine alternative forms of cannabis administration. The CMCR currently has [a number of] ongoing studies involving marijuana and the efficacy of cannabis and cannabis compounds as they relate to medical conditions such as HIV, cancer pain, MS, and nausea. At present, however, the clear weight of the evidence is that smoked marijuana is harmful. No matter what medical condition has been studied, other drugs already approved by the FDA, such as Marinol—a pill form of synthetic THC—have been proven to be safer and more effective than smoked marijuana.

A great deal more research is required to determine the long-term effects of the drug. Until results indicate otherwise, it is safe to assume that the harmful effects of the drug outweigh the benefits.

Patterns of Use/Abuse

In its 2008 National Survey on Drug Use and Health, SAMHSA (2009) reported that an estimated 20 million Americans ages 12 years or older were current illicit drug users, meaning they had used an illicit drug during the month before the survey interview. This estimate represents 8 percent of the population ages 12 years old or older. Marijuana is the most commonly used illicit drug. In 2008, it was used by 75.7 percent of current illicit drug users. This constitutes about 15.2 million users of marijuana in the United States in the year 2008.

Many people incorrectly regard cannabis as a substance of low abuse potential. This lack of knowledge has promoted use of the substance by some individuals who believe it is harmless. Tolerance, although it tends to decline rapidly, does occur with chronic use. As tolerance develops, physical dependence also occurs, resulting in a mild withdrawal syndrome (as previously described) upon cessation of drug use.

One controversy that exists regarding marijuana is whether its use leads to the use of other illicit drugs. Leamon, Wright, and Myrick (2008) stated, "A relationship has consistently been shown between early, regular cannabis use and subsequent abuse of other drugs" (p. 381).

Effects on the Body

Following is a summary of some of the effects that have been attributed to marijuana in recent years. Undoubtedly, as research continues, evidence of additional physiological and psychological effects will be made available.

Cardiovascular Effects

Cannabis ingestion induces tachycardia and orthostatic hypotension (National Institutes of Health [NIH], 2008). With the decrease in blood pressure, myocardial oxygen supply is decreased. Tachycardia in turn increases oxygen demand.

Respiratory Effects

Marijuana produces a greater amount of "tar" than its equivalent weight in tobacco. Because of the method by which marijuana is smoked—that is, the smoke is held in the lungs for as long as possible to achieve the desired effect—larger amounts of tar are deposited in the lungs, promoting deleterious effects to the lungs.

Although the initial reaction to the marijuana is bronchodilation, thereby facilitating respiratory function, chronic use results in obstructive airway disorders (NIH, 2008). Frequent marijuana users often have laryngitis, bronchitis, cough, and hoarseness. Cannabis smoke contains more carcinogens than tobacco smoke; therefore, lung damage and cancer are real risks for heavy users (NIH, 2008).

Reproductive Effects

Some studies have shown that, with heavy marijuana use, men may have a decrease in sperm count, motility, and structure. In women, heavy marijuana use may result in a suppression of ovulation, disruption in menstrual cycles, and alteration of hormone levels.

Central Nervous System Effects

Acute CNS effects of marijuana are dose related. Many people report a feeling of being "high"—the equivalent of being "drunk" on alcohol. Symptoms include feelings of euphoria, relaxed inhibitions, disorientation, depersonalization, and relaxation. At higher doses, sensory alterations may occur, including impairment in judgment of time and distance, recent memory, and learning ability. Physiological symptoms may include tremors, muscle rigidity, and conjunctival redness. Toxic effects are generally characterized by panic reactions. Very heavy usage has been shown to precipitate an acute psychosis that is self-limited and short lived once the drug is removed from the body (Julien, 2008).

Heavy long-term cannabis use is also associated with a syndrome called *amotivational syndrome.* When this syndrome occurs, the individual is totally preoccupied with using the substance. Symptoms include lethargy, apathy, social and personal deterioration, and lack of motivation. This syndrome appears to be more common in countries in which the most potent preparations are used and where the substance is more freely available than it is in the United States.

Sexual Functioning

Marijuana is reported to enhance the sexual experience in both men and women. The intensified sensory awareness and the subjective slowness of time perception are thought to increase sexual satisfaction. Marijuana also enhances sexual functioning by releasing inhibitions for certain activities that would normally be restrained.

Cannabis Intoxication

Cannabis intoxication is evidenced by the presence of clinically significant maladaptive behavior or psychological changes that develop during, or shortly after, cannabis use (APA, 2000). Symptoms include impaired motor coordination, euphoria, anxiety, a sensation of slowed time, and impaired judgment. Physical symptoms include conjunctival injection, increased appetite, dry mouth, and tachycardia. The impairment of motor skills lasts for 8 to 12 hours and interferes with the operation of motor vehicles. These effects are additive to those of alcohol, which is commonly used in combination with cannabis (Sadock & Sadock, 2007).

Tables 25-7 and 25-8 include summaries of the psychoactive substances, including symptoms of intoxication, withdrawal, use, overdose, possible therapeutic uses, and trade and common names by which they may be referred. The dynamics of substance-use disorders using the Transactional Model of Stress/Adaptation are presented in Figure 25–3.

Application of the Nursing Process

Assessment

In the pre-introductory phase of relationship development, the nurse must examine his or her feelings about working with a client who abuses substances. If these behaviors are viewed as morally wrong and the nurse has internalized these attitudes from very early in life, it may be very difficult to suppress judgmental feelings. The role that alcohol or other substances has played (or plays) in the life of the nurse most certainly will affect the way in which he or she approaches interaction with the substance-abusing client.

How are attitudes examined? Some individuals may have sufficient ability for introspection to be able to recognize on their own whether they have unresolved issues related to substance abuse. For others, it may be more helpful to discuss these issues in a group situation, where insight may be gained from feedback regarding the perceptions of others.

Whether alone or in a group, the nurse may gain a greater understanding about attitudes and feelings related to substance abuse by responding to the following types of questions. As written here, the questions are specific to alcohol, but they could be adapted for any substance.

- What are my drinking patterns?
- If I drink, why do I drink? When, where, and how much?
- If I don't drink, why do I abstain?
- Am I comfortable with my drinking patterns?
- If I decided not to drink any more, would that be a problem for me?
- What did I learn from my parents about drinking?
- Have my attitudes changed as an adult?
- What are my feelings about people who become intoxicated?
- Does it seem more acceptable for some individuals than for others?
- Do I ever use terms like "sot," "drunk," or "boozer," to describe some individuals who overindulge, yet overlook it in others?
- Do I ever overindulge myself?
- Has the use of alcohol (by me or others) affected my life in any way?
- Do I see alcohol/drug abuse as a sign of weakness? A moral problem? An illness?

Unless nurses fully understand and accept their own attitudes and feelings, they cannot be empathetic toward clients' problems. Clients in recovery need to know they are accepted for themselves, regardless of past behaviors. Nurses must be able to separate the client from the behavior and to

TABLE 25-7 Psychoactive Substances: A Profile Summary

CLASS OF DRUGS	SYMPTOMS OF USE	THERAPEUTIC USES	SYMPTOMS OF OVERDOSE	TRADE NAMES	COMMON NAMES
CNS Depressants					
Alcohol	Relaxation, loss of inhibitions, lack of concentration, drowsiness, slurred speech, sleep	Antidote for methanol consumption; ingredient in many pharmacological concentrates	Nausea, vomiting; shallow respirations; cold, clammy skin; weak, rapid pulse; coma; possible death	Ethyl alcohol, beer, gin, rum, vodka, bourbon, whiskey, liqueurs, wine, brandy, sherry, champagne	Booze, alcohol, liquor, drinks, cocktails, highballs, nightcaps, moonshine, white lightening, firewater
Other (barbiturates and nonbarbiturates)	Same as alcohol	Relief from anxiety and insomnia; as anticonvulsants and anesthetics	Anxiety, fever, agitation, hallucinations, disorientation, tremors, delirium, convulsions, possible death	Seconal, Amytal, Nembutal Valium Librium Noctec Miltown	Red birds, yellow birds, blue birds Blues/yellows Green & whites Mickies Downers
CNS Stimulants					
Amphetamines and related drugs	Hyperactivity, agitation, euphoria, insomnia, loss of appetite	Management of narcolepsy, hyperkinesia, and weight control	Cardiac arrhythmias, headache, convulsions, hypertension, rapid heart rate, coma, possible death	Dexedrine, Didrex, Tenuate, Bontril, Ritalin, Focalin, Provigil	Uppers, pep pills, wakeups, bennies, eye-openers, speed, black beauties, sweet As
Cocaine	Euphoria, hyperactivity, restlessness, talkativeness, increased pulse, dilated pupils, rhinitis		Hallucinations, convulsions, pulmonary edema, respiratory failure, coma, cardiac arrest, possible death	Cocaine hydrochloride	Coke, flake, snow, dust, happy dust, gold dust, girl, cecil, C, toot, blow, crack
Opioids	Euphoria, lethargy, drowsiness, lack of motivation, constricted pupils	As analgesics; antidiarrheals, and antitussives; methadone in substitution therapy; heroin has no therapeutic use	Shallow breathing, slowed pulse, clammy skin, pulmonary edema, respiratory arrest, convulsions, coma, possible death	Heroin Morphine Codeine Dilaudid Demerol Dolophine Percodan Talwin Opium	Snow, stuff, H, harry, horse M, morph, Miss Emma Schoolboy Lords Doctors Dollies Perkies Ts Big O, black stuff

	Symptoms	Therapeutic Uses	Symptoms of Overdose	Agents	Common/Street Names
Hallucinogens	Visual hallucinations, disorientation, confusion, paranoid delusions, euphoria, anxiety, panic, increased pulse	LSD has been proposed in the treatment of chronic alcoholism, and in the reduction of intractable pain	Agitation, extreme hyperactivity, violence, hallucinations, psychosis, convulsions, possible death	LSD PCP Mescaline DMT STP, DOM MDMA Ketamine	Acid, cube, big D Angel dust, hog, peace pill Mesc Businessman's trip Serenity and peace Ecstasy, XTC Special K, vitamin K, kit kat
Cannabinols	Relaxation, talkativeness, lowered inhibitions, euphoria, mood swings	Marijuana has been used for relief of nausea and vomiting associated with antineoplastic chemotherapy and to reduce eye pressure in glaucoma	Fatigue, paranoia, delusions, hallucinations, possible psychosis	Cannabis Hashish	Marijuana, pot, grass, joint, Mary Jane, MJ Hash, rope, Sweet Lucy

Table 25-8 Summary of Symptoms Associated With the Syndromes of Intoxication and Withdrawal

CLASS OF DRUGS	INTOXICATION	WITHDRAWAL	COMMENTS
Alcohol	Aggressiveness, impaired judgment, impaired attention, irritability, euphoria, depression, emotional lability, slurred speech, incoordination, unsteady gait, nystagmus, flushed face	Tremors, nausea/vomiting, malaise, weakness, tachycardia, sweating, elevated blood pressure, anxiety, depressed mood, irritability, hallucinations, headache, insomnia, seizures	Alcohol withdrawal begins within 4-6 hours after last drink. May progress to delirium tremens on 2nd or 3rd day. Use of Librium or Serax is common for substitution therapy.
Amphetamines and related substances	Fighting, grandiosity, hypervigilance, psychomotor agitation, impaired judgment, tachycardia, pupillary dilation, elevated blood pressure, perspiration or chills, nausea and vomiting.	Anxiety, depressed mood, irritability, craving for the substance, fatigue, insomnia or hypersomnia, psychomotor agitation, paranoid and suicidal ideation.	Withdrawal symptoms usually peak within 2-4 days, although depression and irritability may persist for months. Antidepressants may be used.
Caffeine	Restlessness, nervousness, excitement, insomnia, flushed face, diuresis, gastrointestinal complaints, muscle twitching, rambling flow of thought and speech, cardiac arrhythmia, periods of inexhaustibility, psychomotor agitation	Headache	Caffeine is contained in coffee, tea, colas, cocoa, chocolate, some over-the-counter analgesics, "cold" preparations, and stimulants.
Cannabis	Euphoria, anxiety, suspiciousness, sensation of slowed time, impaired judgment, social withdrawal, tachycardia, conjunctival redness, increased appetite, hallucinations	Restlessness, irritability, insomnia, loss of appetite	Intoxication occurs immediately and lasts about 3 hours. Oral ingestion is more slowly absorbed and has longer lasting effects.
Cocaine	Euphoria, fighting, grandiosity, hypervigilance, psychomotor agitation, impaired judgment, tachycardia, elevated blood pressure, pupillary dilation, perspiration or chills, nausea/vomiting, hallucinations, delirium	Depression, anxiety, irritability, fatigue, insomnia or hypersomnia, psychomotor agitation, paranoid or suicidal ideation, apathy, social withdrawal	Large doses of the drug can result in convulsions or death from cardiac arrhythmias or respiratory paralysis.
Inhalants	Belligerence, assaultiveness, apathy, impaired judgment, dizziness, nystagmus, slurred speech, unsteady gait, lethargy, depressed reflexes, tremor, blurred vision, stupor or coma, euphoria, irritation around eyes, throat, and nose		Intoxication occurs within 5 minutes of inhalation. Symptoms last 60-90 minutes. Large doses can result in death from CNS depression or cardiac arrhythmia.

Table 25-8 Summary of Symptoms Associated With the Syndromes of Intoxication and Withdrawal—cont'd

CLASS OF DRUGS	INTOXICATION	WITHDRAWAL	COMMENTS
Nicotine		Craving for the drug, irritability, anger, frustration, anxiety, difficulty concentrating, restlessness, decreased heart rate, increased appetite, weight gain, tremor, headaches, insomnia	Symptoms of withdrawal begin within 24 hours of last drug use and decrease in intensity over days, weeks, or sometimes longer.
Opioids	Euphoria, lethargy, somnolence, apathy, dysphoria, impaired judgment, pupillary constriction, drowsiness, slurred speech, constipation, nausea, decreased respiratory rate and blood pressure	Craving for the drug, nausea/vomiting, muscle aches, lacrimation or rhinorrhea, pupillary dilation, piloerection or sweating, diarrhea, yawning, fever, insomnia	Withdrawal symptoms appear within 6–8 hours after last dose, reach a peak in the 2nd or 3rd day, and disappear in 7–10 days. Times are shorter with meperidine and longer with methadone.
Phencyclidine and related substances	Belligerence, assaultiveness, impulsiveness, psychomotor agitation, impaired judgment, nystagmus, increased heart rate and blood pressure, diminished pain response, ataxia, dysarthria, muscle rigidity, seizures, hyperacusis, delirium		Delirium can occur within 24 hours after use of phencyclidine, or may occur up to a week following recovery from an overdose of the drug.
Sedatives, hypnotics, and anxiolytics	Disinhibition of sexual or aggressive impulses, mood lability, impaired judgment, slurred speech, incoordination, unsteady gait, impairment in attention or memory disorientation, confusion	Nausea/vomiting, malaise, weakness, tachycardia, sweating, anxiety, irritability, orthostatic hypotension, tremor, insomnia, seizures	Withdrawal may progress to delirium, usually within 1 week of last use. Long-acting barbiturates or benzodiazepines may be used in withdrawal substitution therapy.

accept that individual with unconditional positive regard.

Assessment Tools

Nurses are often the individuals who perform the admission interview. A variety of assessment tools are appropriate for use in chemical dependency units. A nursing history and assessment tool was presented in Chapter 9 of this text. With some adaptation, it is an appropriate instrument for creating a database on clients who abuse substances. Box 25-1 presents a drug history and

assessment that could be used in conjunction with the general biopsychosocial assessment.

The Clinical Institute Withdrawal Assessment for Alcohol Scale, Revised (CIWA-Ar) is an excellent tool that is used by many hospitals to assess risk and severity of withdrawal from alcohol. It may be used for initial assessment as well as ongoing monitoring of alcohol withdrawal symptoms. A copy of the CIWA-Ar is presented in Box 25-2.

Other screening tools exist for determining whether an individual has a problem with substances. Two such tools developed by the American

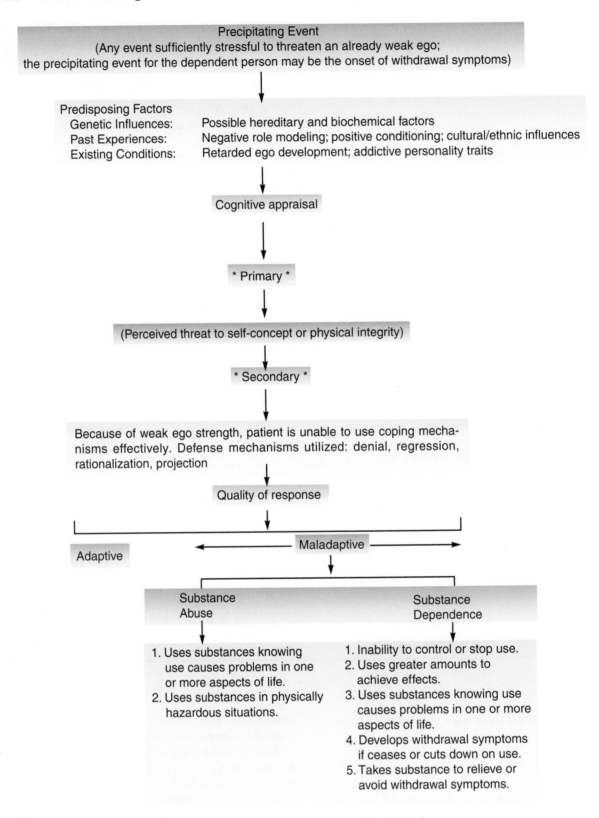

FIGURE 25–3 The dynamics of substance-use disorders using the Transactional Model of Stress/Adaptation.

BOX 25-1 **Drug History and Assessment***

1. When you were growing up, did anyone in your family drink alcohol or take other kinds of drugs?
2. If so, how did the substance use affect the family situation?
3. When did you have your first drink/drugs?
4. How long have you been drinking/taking drugs on a regular basis?
5. What is your pattern of substance use?
   a. When do you use substances?
   b. What do you use?
   c. How much do you use?
   d. Where are you and with whom when you use substances?
6. When did you have your last drink/drug? What was it and how much did you consume?
7. Does using the substance(s) cause problems for you? Describe. Include family, friends, job, school, other.
8. Have you ever experienced injury as a result of substance use?
9. Have you ever been arrested or incarcerated for drinking/using drugs?
10. Have you ever tried to stop drinking/using drugs? If so, what was the result? Did you experience any physical symptoms, such as tremors, headache, insomnia, sweating, or seizures?
11. Have you ever experienced loss of memory for times when you have been drinking/using drugs?
12. Describe a typical day in your life.
13. Are there any changes you would like to make in your life? If so, what?
14. What plans or ideas do you have for seeing that these changes occur?

*To be used in conjunction with a general biopsychosocial nursing history and assessment tool (Chapter 9).

BOX 25-2 **Clinical Institute Withdrawal Assessment for Alcohol Scale, Revised (CIWA-Ar)**

Patient: **Date:**   **Time:**

Pulse or heart rate, taken for one minute: **Blood pressure:**

Nausea and Vomiting—Ask "Do you feel sick to your stomach? Have you vomited?" Observation.

Tactile Disturbances—Ask "Have you any itching, pins and needles sensations, any burning, any numbness, or do you feel bugs crawling on or under your skin?" Observation.

0 no nausea and no vomiting
1 mild nausea with no vomiting
2
3
4 intermittent nausea with dry heaves
5
6
7 constant nausea, frequent dry heaves and vomiting

0 none
1 very mild itching, pins and needles, burning or numbness
2 mild itching, pins and needles, burning or numbness
3 moderate itching, pins and needles, burning or numbness
4 moderately severe hallucinations
5 severe hallucinations
6 extremely severe hallucinations
7 continuous hallucinations

Tremor—Arms extended and fingers spread apart. Observation.

Auditory Disturbances—Ask "Are you more aware of sounds around you? Are they harsh? Do they frighten you? Are you hearing anything that is disturbing to you? Are you hearing things you know are not there?" Observation.

0 no tremor
1 not visible, but can be felt fingertip to fingertip
2
3
4 moderate, with patient's arms extended
5
6
7 severe, even with arms not extended

0 not present
1 very mild harshness or ability to frighten
2 mild harshness or ability to frighten
3 moderate harshness or ability to frighten
4 moderately severe hallucinations
5 severe hallucinations
6 extremely severe hallucinations
7 continuous hallucinations

Continued

BOX 25-2 Clinical Institute Withdrawal Assessment for Alcohol Scale, Revised (CIWA-Ar)—cont'd

Paroxysmal Sweats—Observation.

0 no sweat visible
1 barely perceptible sweating, palms moist
2
3
4 beads of sweat obvious on forehead
5
6
7 drenching sweats

Anxiety—Ask "Do you feel nervous?" Observation.

0 no anxiety, at ease
1 mildly anxious
2
3
4 moderately anxious, or guarded, so anxiety is inferred
5
6
7 equivalent to acute panic states as seen in severe delirium or acute schizophrenic reactions

Agitation—Observation.

0 normal activity
1 somewhat more than normal activity
2
3
4 moderately fidgety and restless
5
6
7 paces back and forth during most of the interview, or constantly thrashes about

The CIWA-Ar is not copyrighted and may be reproduced freely. This assessment for monitoring withdrawal symptoms requires approximately 5 minutes to administer. The maximum score is 67 (see instrument). Patients scoring less than 10 do not usually need additional medication for withdrawal. _____

Visual Disturbances—Ask "Does the light appear to be too bright? Is its color different? Does it hurt your eyes? Are you seeing anything that is disturbing to you? Are you seeing things you know are not there?" Observation.
0 not present
1 very mild sensitivity
2 mild sensitivity
3 moderate sensitivity
4 moderately severe hallucinations
5 severe hallucinations
6 extremely severe hallucinations
7 continuous hallucinations

Headache, Fullness In Head—Ask "Does your head feel different? Does it feel like there is a band around your head?" Do not rate for dizziness or lightheadedness. Otherwise, rate severity.
0 not present
1 very mild
2 mild
3 moderate
4 moderately severe
5 severe
6 very severe
7 extremely severe

Orientation and Clouding of Sensorium—Ask "What day is this? Where are you? Who am I?"
0 oriented and can do serial additions
1 cannot do serial additions or is uncertain about date
2 disoriented for date by no more than 2 calendar days
3 disoriented for date by more than 2 calendar days
4 disoriented for place and/or person

Total CIWA-Ar Score _____
Rater's Initials _____

From Sullivan, J. T., Sykora, K., Schneiderman, J., Naranjo, C. A., & Sellers, E. M. (1989). Assessment of alcohol withdrawal: The revised Clinical Institute Withdrawal Assessment for Alcohol scale (CIWA-Ar). British Journal of Addiction, 84, 1353–1357.

Psychiatric Association for the diagnosis of alcoholism include the Michigan Alcoholism Screening Test and the CAGE Questionnaire (Boxes 25-3 and 25-4). Some psychiatric units administer these surveys to all clients who are admitted to help determine if there is a secondary alcoholism problem in addition to the psychiatric problem for which the client is being admitted (sometimes called **dual diagnosis**). It would be possible to adapt these tools to use in diagnosing problems with other drugs as well.

BOX 25-3 Michigan Alcoholism Screening Test (MAST)

Answer the following questions by placing an X under yes or no.*	Yes	No
1. Do you enjoy a drink now and then?	0	0
2. Do you feel you are a normal drinker? (By normal we mean you drink less than or as much as most people.)		2
3. Have you ever awakened the morning after some drinking the night before and found that you could not remember a part of the evening?	2	
4. Does your wife, husband, parent, or other near relative ever worry or complain about your drinking?	1	
5. Can you stop drinking without a struggle after one or two drinks?		2
6. Do you ever feel guilty about your drinking?	1	
7. Do friends or relatives think you are a normal drinker?		2
8. Are you able to stop drinking when you want to?		2
9. Have you ever attended a meeting of Alcoholics Anonymous (AA)?	5	
10. Have you gotten into physical fights when drinking?	1	
11. Has your drinking ever created problems between you and your wife, husband, a parent, or other relative?	2	
12. Has your wife, husband, or another family member ever gone to anyone for help about your drinking?	2	
13. Have you ever lost friends because of your drinking?	2	
14. Have you ever gotten into trouble at work or school because of drinking?	2	
15. Have you ever lost a job because of drinking?	2	
16. Have you ever neglected your obligations, your family, or your work for 2 or more days in a row because you were drinking?	2	
17. Do you drink before noon fairly often?	1	
18. Have you ever been told you have liver trouble? Cirrhosis?	2	
19. After heavy drinking have you ever had delirium tremens (DTs) or severe shaking or heard voices or seen things that really were not there?	5	
20. Have you ever gone to anyone for help about your drinking?	5	
21. Have you ever been in a hospital because of drinking?	5	
22. Have you ever been a patient in a psychiatric hospital or on a psychiatric ward of a general hospital where drinking was part of the problem that resulted in hospitalization?	2	
23. Have you ever been seen at a psychiatric or mental health clinic or gone to any doctor, social worker, or clergyman for help with any emotional problem, where drinking was part of the problem?	2	
24. Have you ever been arrested for drunk driving, driving while intoxicated, or driving under the influence of alcoholic beverages? (If yes, how many times? _____)	2 ea	
25. Have you ever been arrested, or taken into custody, even for a few hours, because of other drunk behavior? (If yes, how many times? _____)	2 ea	

*Items are scored under the response that would indicate a problem with alcohol.

Method of scoring: 0–3 points = no problem with alcohol

4 points = possible problem with alcohol

5 or more = indicates problem with alcohol

From Selzer, M. L. (1971). The Michigan alcohol screening test: The quest for a new diagnostic instrument. American Journal of Psychiatry, 127, 1653–1658, with permission.

BOX 25-4 The CAGE Questionnaire

1. Have you ever felt you should **C**ut down on your drinking?
2. Have people **A**nnoyed you by criticizing your drinking?
3. Have you ever felt bad or **G**uilty about your drinking?
4. Have you ever had a drink first thing in the morning to steady your nerves or get rid of a hangover (**E**ye-opener)?

Scoring: 2 or 3 "yes" answers strongly suggest a problem with alochol.

From Mayfield, D., McLeod, G., & Hall, P. (1974). The CAGE questionnaire: Validation of a new alcoholism screening instrument. American Journal of Psychiatry, 131, 1121–1123, with permission.

Dual Diagnosis

If it is determined that the client has a coexisting substance disorder and mental illness, he or she may be assigned to a special program that targets both problems. Counseling for the mentally ill person who abuses substances takes a different approach than that which is directed at individuals who abuse substances but are not mentally ill. In the latter, many counselors use direct confrontation of the substance-use behaviors. This approach is thought to be detrimental to the treatment of a person with mental illness (Mack et al., 2003). Most dual diagnosis programs take a more supportive and less confrontational approach.

Peer support groups are an important part of the treatment program. Group members offer encouragement and practical advice to each other. Psychodynamic therapy can be useful for some individuals with dual diagnosis by delving into the personal history of how psychiatric disorders and substance abuse have reinforced one another and how the cycle can be broken (Harvard Medical School, 2003). Cognitive and behavior therapies are helpful in training clients to monitor moods and thought patterns that lead to substance abuse. With these therapies, clients also learn to avoid substance use and to cope with cravings and the temptation to relapse (Harvard Medical School, 2003).

Individuals with dual diagnoses should be encouraged to attend 12-step recovery programs (e.g., Alcoholics Anonymous or Narcotics Anonymous). Dual diagnosis clients are sometimes resistant to attending 12-step programs, and they often do better in groups specifically designed for people with psychiatric disorders.

Substance-abuse groups are usually integrated into regular programming for the psychiatric client with a dual diagnosis. An individual in a psychiatric facility or day treatment program will attend a substance-abuse group periodically in lieu of another scheduled activity therapy. Topics are directed toward areas that are unique to clients with a mental illness, such as mixing medications with other substances, as well as topics that are common to primary substances abusers. Individuals are encouraged to discuss their personal problems.

Mack and associates (2003) stated:

> The dual diagnosis patient often falls through the cracks of the treatment system. Severe psychiatric disorders often preclude full treatment in substance abuse clinics or self-help groups. The addition of other Axis I, II, and III disorders to a substance use disorder greatly complicates diagnosis and makes treatment more difficult. (p. 359)

Continued attendance at 12-step group meetings is encouraged on discharge from treatment. Family involvement is enlisted, and preventive strategies are outlined. Individual case management is common, and success is often promoted by this close supervision.

Diagnosis/Outcome Identification

The next step in the nursing process is to identify appropriate nursing diagnoses by analyzing the data collected during the assessment phase. The individual who abuses or is dependent on substances undoubtedly has many unmet physical and emotional needs. Table 25-9 presents a list of client behaviors and the NANDA nursing diagnoses that correspond to those behaviors, which may be used in planning care for the client with a substance-use disorder.

Outcome Criteria

The following criteria may be used for measurement of outcomes in the care of the client with substance-related disorders.

The client:

■ Has not experienced physical injury.

■ Has not caused harm to self or others.

■ Accepts responsibility for own behavior.

■ Acknowledges association between personal problems and use of substance(s).

■ Demonstrates more adaptive coping mechanisms that can be used in stressful situations (instead of taking substances).

■ Shows no signs or symptoms of infection or malnutrition.

■ Exhibits evidence of increased self-worth by attempting new projects without fear of failure and by demonstrating less defensive behavior toward others.

■ Verbalizes importance of abstaining from use of substances in order to maintain optimal wellness.

Planning/Implementation

Implementation with clients who abuse substances is a long-term process, often beginning with **detoxification** and progressing to total abstinence. The following section presents a group of selected nursing diagnoses, with short- and long-term goals and nursing interventions for each.

Table 25-9 Assigning Nursing Diagnoses to Behaviors Commonly Associated with Substance-Related Disorders

BEHAVIORS	NURSING DIAGNOSES
Makes statements such as, "I don't have a problem with (substance). I can quit any time I want to." Delays seeking assistance; does not perceive problems related to use of substances; minimizes use of substances; unable to admit impact of disease on life pattern	**Ineffective denial**
Abuse of chemical agents; destructive behavior toward others and self; inability to meet basic needs; inability to meet role expectations; risk taking	**Ineffective coping**
Loss of weight, pale conjunctiva and mucous membranes, decreased skin turgor, electrolyte imbalance, anemia, drinks alcohol instead of eating	**Imbalanced nutrition: Less than body requirements/Deficient fluid volume**
Risk factors: Malnutrition, altered immune condition, failing to avoid exposure to pathogens	**Risk for infection**
Criticizes self and others, self-destructive behavior (abuse of substances as a coping mechanism), dysfunctional family background	**Chronic low self-esteem**
Denies that substance is harmful; continues to use substance in light of obvious consequences	**Deficient knowledge**
For the Client Withdrawing From CNS Depressants: Risk factors: CNS agitation (tremors, elevated blood pressure, nausea and vomiting, hallucinations, illusions, tachycardia, anxiety, seizures)	**Risk for injury**
For the Client Withdrawing From CNS Stimulants: Risk factors: Intense feelings of lassitude and depression; "crashing," suicidal ideation	**Risk for suicide**

Risk for Injury

Risk for injury is defined as "at risk for injury as a result of [internal or external] environmental conditions interacting with the individual's adaptive and defensive resources" (NANDA International [NANDA-I], 2009, p. 314).

Client Goals

Outcome criteria include short- and long-term goals. Timelines are individually determined.

Short-Term Goal

■ Client's condition will stabilize within 72 hours.

Long-Term Goal

■ Client will not experience physical injury.

Interventions

For the Client in Substance Withdrawal

■ Assess the client's level of disorientation to determine specific requirements for safety.

■ Obtain a drug history, if possible. It is important to determine the type of substance(s) used, the time and amount of last use, the length and frequency of use, and the amount used on a daily basis.

■ Because subjective history is often not accurate, obtain a urine sample for laboratory analysis of substance content.

■ It is important to keep the client is as quiet an environment as possible. Excessive stimuli may increase client agitation. A private room is ideal.

■ Observe the client's behaviors frequently. If seriousness of the condition warrants, it may be necessary to assign a staff person on a one-to-one basis.

■ Accompany and assist the client when ambulating, and use a wheelchair for transporting the client long distances.

■ Pad the headboard and side rails of the bed with thick towels to protect the client in case of a seizure.

■ Suicide precautions may need to be instituted for the client withdrawing from CNS stimulants.

■ Ensure that smoking materials and other potentially harmful objects are stored away from the client's access.

■ Frequently orient the client to reality and the surroundings.

■ Monitor the client's vital signs every 15 minutes initially and less frequently as acute symptoms subside.

■ Follow the medication regimen, as ordered by the physician. Common psychopharmacological intervention for substance intoxication and withdrawal is presented later in this chapter under the section entitled, Treatment Modalities for Substance-Related Disorders."

Ineffective Denial

Ineffective denial is defined as a "conscious or unconscious attempt to disavow the knowledge or meaning of an event to reduce anxiety/fear, but leading to the detriment of health" (NANDA-I, 2009, p. 259). Table 25-10 presents this nursing diagnosis in care plan format.

Client Goals

Outcome criteria include short- and long-term goals. Timelines are individually determined.

Short-Term Goal

■ Client will divert attention away from external issues and focus on behavioral outcomes associated with substance use.

Long-Term Goal

■ Client will verbalize acceptance of responsibility for own behavior and acknowledge association between substance use and personal problems.

Interventions

■ Begin by working to develop a trusting nurse-client relationship. Be honest and keep all promises.

Table 25-10 CARE PLAN FOR THE CLIENT WITH A SUBSTANCE-RELATED DISORDER

NURSING DIAGNOSIS: INEFFECTIVE DENIAL

RELATED TO: Weak, underdeveloped ego

EVIDENCED BY: Statements indicating no problem with substance use

OUTCOME CRITERIA	NURSING INTERVENTIONS	RATIONALE
Short-Term Goal • Client will divert attention away from external issues and focus on behavioral outcomes associated with substance use. **Long-Term Goal** • Client will verbalize acceptance of responsibility for own behavior and acknowledge association between substance use and personal problems.	1. Begin by working to develop a trusting nurse-client relationship. Be honest. Keep all promises. 2. Convey an attitude of acceptance to the client. Ensure that he or she understands "It is not *you* but your *behavior* that is unacceptable." 3. Provide information to correct misconceptions about substance abuse. Client may rationalize his or her behavior with statements such as, "I'm not an alcoholic. I can stop drinking any time I want. Besides, I only drink beer." Or "I only smoke pot to relax before class. So what? I know lots of people who do. Besides, you can't get hooked on pot." 4. Identify recent maladaptive behaviors or situations that have occurred in the client's life, and discuss how use of substances may have been a contributing factor.	1. Trust is the basis of a therapeutic relationship. 2. An attitude of acceptance promotes feelings of dignity and self-worth. 3. Many myths abound regarding use of specific substances. Factual information presented in a matter-of-fact, nonjudgmental way explaining what behaviors constitute substance-related disorders may help the client focus on his or her own behaviors as an illness that requires help. 4. The first step in decreasing use of denial is for client to see the relationship between substance use and personal problems.

Table 25-10 CARE PLAN FOR THE CLIENT WITH A SUBSTANCE-RELATED DISORDER—cont'd

NURSING DIAGNOSIS: INEFFECTIVE DENIAL
RELATED TO: Weak, underdeveloped ego
EVIDENCED BY: Statements indicating no problem with substance use

OUTCOME CRITERIA	NURSING INTERVENTIONS	RATIONALE
	5. Use confrontation with caring. Do not allow client to fantasize about his or her lifestyle (for example: "It is my understanding that the last time you drank alcohol, you . . ." or "The lab report shows that you were under the influence of alcohol when you had the accident that injured three people").	5. Confrontation interferes with client's ability to use denial; a caring attitude preserves self-esteem and avoids putting the client on the defensive.
	6. Do not accept rationalization or projection as client attempts to make excuses for or blame his or her behavior on other people or situations.	6. Rationalization and projection prolong denial that problems exist in the client's life because of substance use.
	7. Encourage participation in group activities.	7. Peer feedback is often more accepted than feedback from authority figures. Peer pressure can be a strong factor, as can association with individuals who are experiencing or who have experienced similar problems.
	8. Offer immediate positive recognition of client's expressions of insight gained regarding illness and acceptance of responsibility for own behavior.	8. Positive reinforcement enhances self-esteem and encourages repetition of desirable behaviors.

■ Convey an attitude of acceptance to the client. Ensure that he or she understands "It is not *you* but your *behavior* that is unacceptable." An attitude of acceptance helps to promote the client's feelings of dignity and self-worth.

■ Provide information to correct misconceptions about substance abuse. The client may rationalize his or her behavior with statements such as, "I'm not an alcoholic. I can stop drinking any time I want. Besides, I only drink beer." or "I only smoke pot to relax before class. So what? I know lots of people who do. Besides, you can't get hooked on pot." Many myths abound regarding use of specific substances. Factual information presented in a matter-of-fact, non-judgmental way explaining what behaviors constitute substance-related disorders may help the client focus on his or her own behaviors as an illness that requires help.

■ Identify recent maladaptive behaviors or situations that have occurred in the client's life, and discuss how use of substances may have been a contributing factor. The first step in decreasing use of denial is for the client to see the relationship between substance use and personal problems.

■ Use confrontation with caring. Do not allow the client to fantasize about his or her lifestyle. Confrontation interferes with the client's ability to use denial; a caring attitude preserves self-esteem and avoids putting the client on the defensive.

CLINICAL PEARL

It is important to speak objectively and nonjudgmentally to a person in denial. Examples: "It is my understanding that the last time you drank alcohol, you . . ." or "The lab report shows that your blood alcohol level was 250 when you were involved in that automobile accident."

■ Do not accept the use of rationalization or projection as the client attempts to make excuses for or blame his or her behavior on other people or situations. Rationalization and projection prolong the stage of denial that problems exist in the client's life because of substance use.

■ Encourage participation in group activities. Peer feedback is often more accepted than feedback from authority figures. Peer pressure can be a strong factor, as can the association with individuals who are experiencing or who have experienced similar problems.

■ Offer immediate positive recognition of the client's expressions of insight gained regarding illness and acceptance of responsibility for own behavior. Positive reinforcement enhances self-esteem and encourages repetition of desirable behaviors.

Ineffective Coping

Ineffective coping is defined as the "inability to form a valid appraisal of the stressors, inadequate choices of practiced responses, and/or inability to use available resources" (NANDA-I, 2009, p. 254).

Client Goals

Outcome criteria include short- and long-term goals. Timelines are individually determined.

Short-Term Goal

■ Client will express true feelings about using substances as a method of coping with stress.

Long-Term Goal

■ Client will be able to verbalize use of adaptive coping mechanisms, instead of substance abuse, in response to stress.

Interventions

■ Spend time with the client and establish a trusting relationship.

■ Set limits on manipulative behavior. Be sure that the client knows what is acceptable, what is not, and the consequences for violating the limits set. Ensure that all staff maintain consistency with this intervention. The client is unable to establish his or her own limits, so limits must be set for the client. Unless administration of consequences for violation of limits is consistent, manipulative behavior will not be eliminated.

■ Encourage the client to verbalize feelings, fears, and anxieties. Answer any questions he or she may have regarding the disorder. Verbalization of feelings in a nonthreatening environment may help the client come to terms with long-unresolved issues.

■ Explain the effects of substance abuse on the body. Emphasize that the prognosis is closely related to abstinence. Many clients lack knowledge regarding the deleterious effects of substance abuse on the body.

■ Explore with the client the options available to assist with stressful situations rather than resorting to substance abuse (e.g., contacting various members of Alcoholics Anonymous or Narcotics Anonymous; physical exercise; relaxation techniques; meditation). The client may have persistently resorted to chemical abuse and thus may possess little or no knowledge of adaptive responses to stress.

■ Provide positive reinforcement for evidence of gratification delayed appropriately. Encourage the client to be as independent as possible in performing his or her self-care. Provide positive feedback for independent decision making and effective use of problem-solving skills.

Dysfunctional Family Processes

Dysfunctional family processes is defined as "psychosocial, spiritual, and physiological functions of the family unit are chronically disorganized, which leads to conflict, denial of problems, resistance to change, ineffective problem solving, and a series of self-perpetuating crises" (NANDA-I, 2009, p. 211).

Client Goals

Outcome criteria include short- and long-term goals. Timelines are individually determined.

Short-Term Goals

■ Family members will participate in individual family programs and support groups.

■ Family members will identify ineffective coping behaviors and consequences.

■ Family will initiate and plan for necessary lifestyle changes.

Long-Term Goal

■ Family members will take action to change self-destructive behaviors and alter behaviors that contribute to client's addiction.

Interventions

■ Review family history; explore roles of family members, circumstances involving alcohol use, strengths, and areas of growth. Explore how family members have coped with the client's addiction (e.g., denial, repression, rationalization, hurt, loneliness, projection). Persons who enable also suffer from the same feelings as the client and use ineffective methods for dealing with the situation, necessitating help in learning new and effective coping skills.

■ Determine the family's understanding of the current situation and previous methods of coping with life's problems. Assess family members' current level of functioning.

■ Determine the extent of enabling behaviors being evidenced by family members; explore with each individual and client. Enabling is doing for the client what he or she needs to do for self (rescuing). People want to be helpful and do not want to feel powerless to help their loved one to stop substance use and change the behavior that is so destructive. However, the substance abuser often relies on others to cover up for his or her inability to cope with daily responsibilities.

■ Provide information about enabling behavior and addictive disease characteristics for both the user and nonuser. Achieving awareness and knowledge of behaviors (e.g., avoiding and shielding, taking over responsibilities, rationalizing, and subserving) provides an opportunity for individuals to begin the process of change.

■ Identify and discuss the possibility of sabotage behaviors by family members. Even though family member(s) may verbalize a desire for the individual to become substance free, the reality of interactive dynamics is that they may unconsciously not want the individual to recover, as this would affect the family members' own role in the relationship. Additionally, they may receive sympathy or attention from others (secondary gain).

■ Assist the client's partner to understand that the client's abstinence and drug use are not the partner's responsibility, and that the client's use of substances may or may not change despite involvement in treatment. Partners must come to realize and accept that the only behavior they can control is their own.

■ Involve the family in plans for discharge from treatment. Alcohol abuse is a family illness. Because the family has been so involved in dealing with the substance-abuse behavior,

family members need help adjusting to the new behavior of sobriety/abstinence. Encourage involvement with self-help associations, such as Alcoholics Anonymous, Al-Anon, Alateen, and professional family therapy. This puts client and family in direct contact with support systems necessary for continued sobriety and assists with problem resolution.

Concept Care Mapping

The concept map care plan is an innovative approach to planning and organizing nursing care (see Chapter 9). It is a diagrammatic teaching and learning strategy that allows visualization of interrelationships between medical diagnoses, nursing diagnoses, assessment data, and treatments. An example of a concept map care plan for a client with a substance-related disorder is presented in Figure 25–4.

Client/Family Education

The role of client teacher is important in the psychiatric area, as it is in all areas of nursing. A list of topics for client/family education relevant to substance-related disorders is presented in Box 25-5. Sample client teaching guides are presented in Appendix G.

Evaluation

The final step of the nursing process involves reassessment to determine if the nursing interventions have been effective in achieving the intended goals of care. Evaluation of the client with a substance-related disorder may be accomplished by using information gathered from the following reassessment questions:

■ Has detoxification occurred without complications?

■ Is the client still in denial?

■ Does the client accept responsibility for his or her own behavior? Has he or she acknowledged a personal problem with substances?

■ Has a correlation been made between personal problems and the use of substances?

■ Does the client still make excuses or blame others for use of substances?

■ Has the client remained substance-free during hospitalization?

■ Does the client cooperate with treatment?

■ Does the client refrain from manipulative behavior and violation of limits?

Clinical Vignette: John, age 56, was arrested for driving while under the influence of alcohol. He ran a red light and caused an accident in which another person was injured. He was taken to the hospital and admitted to the alcohol and drug detoxification unit. Following an unremarkable detoxifaction, he was transferred to the rehab unit. He says to the nurse, "I don't have a problem with alcohol. I can quit any time I want to. Besides... what does is hurt?" He tells the nurse that he has a very stressful job and drinking helps him relax. His is pale and underweight for his height. He admits that sometimes he doesn't eat regular meals, but rather just drinks until he goes to sleep. His skin is dry and flaky. Laboratory results indicate evidence of malnutrition and dehydration. The nurse develops the following concept map care plan for John.

S & Sx:
- "I don't have a problem with alcohol. I can quit any time I want to."

S & Sx:
- Use of alcohol as a coping mechanism

S & Sx:
- Dry skin
- Pale
- Underweight
- Lab reports positive for malnutrition

S & Sx:
- Unable to verbalize physiological effects of alcohol abuse
- "What does it hurt?"

Nsg Dx:
Ineffective Denial

Nsg Dx:
Ineffective Coping

Nsg Dx:
Imbalanced Nutrition: Less than body requirements

Nsg Dx:
Deficient Knowledge

Nursing Actions:
- Accept client unconditionally
- Identify ways in which use of alcohol has contributed to maladaptive behaviors
- Do not allow client to blame others for behaviors associated with alcohol abuse

Nursing Actions:
- Set limits on manipulative behavior
- Practice alternative, more adaptive coping strategies
- Give positive feedback for delaying gratification and using adaptive coping strategies

Nursing Actions:
- Consult dietitian
- I&O and daily weights
- Monitor protein intake of client with impaired liver function
- Restrict sodium intake to minimize fluid retention
- Provide small frequent feedings of nonirritating foods

Nursing Actions:
- Assess client's level of knowledge and readiness to learn
- Include significant others in teaching
- Provide information about physical effects of alcohol on body
- Teach about disulfiram

Outcomes:
- Verbalizes correlation between use of alcohol and personal problems
- Accepts responsibility for own behaviors

Outcomes:
- Verbalizes and demonstrates adaptive coping strategies as alternatives to alcohol use in response to stress

Outcomes:
- Vital signs, blood pressure and lab values are within normal limits
- Verbalizes importance of adequate nutrition

Outcomes:
- Verbalizes effects of alcohol on body
- Verbalizes knowledge about use of medication to assist with abstinence

FIGURE 25–4 Concept map care plan for client with alcoholism.

BOX 25-5 Topics for Client/Family Education Related to Substance-Use Disorders

NATURE OF THE ILLNESS

1. Effects of (substance) on the body
   a. Alcohol
   b. Other CNS depressants
   c. CNS stimulants
   d. Hallucinogens
   e. Inhalants
   f. Opioids
   g. Cannabinols
2. Ways in which use of (substance) affects life.

MANAGEMENT OF THE ILLNESS

1. Activities to substitute for (substance) in times of stress
2. Relaxation techniques
   a. Progressive relaxation
   b. Tense and relax
   c. Deep breathing
   d. Autogenics
3. Problem-solving skills
4. The essentials of good nutrition

SUPPORT SERVICES

1. Financial assistance
2. Legal assistance
3. Alcoholics Anonymous (or other support group specific to another substance)
4. One-to-one support person

■ Is the client able to verbalize alternative adaptive coping strategies to substitute for substance use? Has the use of these strategies been demonstrated? Does positive reinforcement encourage repetition of these adaptive behaviors?

■ Has nutritional status been restored? Does the client consume diet adequate for his or her size and level of activity? Is the client able to discuss the importance of adequate nutrition?

■ Has the client remained free of infection during hospitalization?

■ Is the client able to verbalize the effects of substance abuse on the body?

■ Does the client verbalize that he or she wants to recover and lead a life free of substances?

The Chemically-Impaired Nurse

Substance abuse and dependence is a problem that has the potential for impairment in an individual's social, occupational, psychological, and physical functioning. This becomes an especially serious problem when the impaired person is responsible for the lives of others on a daily basis. Approximately 10 percent of the general population suffers from the disease of chemical dependency. It is estimated that 10 to 15 percent of nurses suffer from this disease (Raia, 2004a). Alcohol is the most widely abused drug, followed closely by narcotics.

For years, the impaired nurse was protected, promoted, transferred, ignored, or fired. These types of responses promoted the growth of the problem. Programs are needed that involve early reporting and treatment of chemical dependency as a disease, with a focus on public safety and rehabilitation of the nurse.

How does one identify the impaired nurse? It is still easiest to overlook what *might* be a problem. Denial, on the part of the impaired nurse as well as nurse colleagues, is still the strongest defense for dealing with substance abuse problems. Some states have mandatory reporting laws that require observers to report substance-abusing nurses to the state board of nursing. They are difficult laws to enforce, and hospitals are not always compliant with mandatory reporting. Some hospitals may choose not to report to the state board of nursing if the impaired nurse is actively seeking treatment and is not placing clients in danger.

A number of clues for recognizing substance impairment in nurses have been identified (Ellis & Hartley, 2008; Raia, 2004b). They are not easy to detect and will vary according to the substance being used. There may be high absenteeism if the person's source is outside the work area, or the individual may rarely miss work if the substance source is at work. There may be an increase in "wasting" of drugs, higher incidences of incorrect narcotic counts, and a higher record of signing out drugs than for other nurses.

Poor concentration, difficulty meeting deadlines, inappropriate responses, and poor memory or recall are usually late in the disease process. The person may also have problems with relationships. Some other possible signs are irritability, mood swings, tendency to isolate, elaborate excuses for behavior, unkempt appearance, impaired motor coordination, slurred speech, flushed face, inconsistent job performance, and frequent use of the restroom. He or she may frequently medicate other nurses' patients, and there may be patient complaints of inadequate pain control. Discrepancies in documentation may occur.

If suspicious behavior occurs, it is important to keep careful, objective records. Confrontation with the impaired nurse will undoubtedly result in hostility and denial. Confrontation should occur in the presence of a supervisor or other nurse and should include the offer of assistance in seeking treatment. If a report is made to the state board of nursing, it should be a factual documentation of specific events and actions, not a diagnostic statement of impairment.

What will the state board do? Each case is generally decided on an individual basis. A state board may deny, suspend, or revoke a license based on a report of chemical abuse by a nurse. Several state boards of nursing have passed diversionary laws that allow impaired nurses to avoid disciplinary action by agreeing to seek treatment. Some of these state boards administer the treatment programs themselves, and others refer the nurse to community resources or state nurses' association assistance programs. This may require successful completion of inpatient, outpatient, group, or individual counseling treatment program(s); evidence of regular attendance at nurse support groups or 12-step program; random negative drug screens; and employment or volunteer activities during the suspension period. When a nurse is deemed safe to return to practice, he or she may be closely monitored for several years and required to undergo random drug screenings. The nurse also may be required to practice under specifically circumscribed conditions for a designated period of time.

In 1982, the American Nurses Association (ANA) House of Delegates adopted a national resolution to provide assistance to impaired nurses. Since that time, the majority of state nurses' associations have developed (or are developing) programs for nurses who are impaired by substances or psychiatric illness. The individuals who administer these efforts are nurse members of the state associations, as well as nurses who are in recovery themselves. For this reason, they are called **peer assistance programs.**

The peer assistance programs strive to intervene early, to reduce hazards to clients, and increase prospects for the nurse's recovery. Most states provide either a hot-line number that the impaired nurse or intervening colleague may call or phone numbers of peer assistance committee members, which are made available for the same purpose. Typically, a contract is drawn up detailing the method of treatment, which may be obtained from various sources, such as employee assistance programs, Alcoholics Anonymous, Narcotics Anonymous, private counseling, or outpatient clinics. Guidelines for monitoring the course of treatment are established. Peer support is provided through regular contact with the impaired nurse, usually for a period of 2 years. Peer assistance programs serve to assist impaired nurses to recognize their impairment, to obtain necessary treatment, and to regain accountability within their profession.

Codependency

The concept of **codependency** arose out of a need to define the dysfunctional behaviors that are evident among members of the family of a chemically dependent person. The term has been expanded to include all individuals from families that harbor secrets of physical or emotional abuse, other cruelties, or pathological conditions. Living under these conditions results in unmet needs for autonomy and self-esteem and a profound sense of powerlessness. The codependent person is able to achieve a sense of control only through fulfilling the needs of others. Personal identity is relinquished and boundaries with the other person become blurred. The codependent person disowns his or her own needs and wants in order to respond to external demands and the demands of others. Burney (1996) referred to codependency as a dysfunctional relationship with oneself.

The traits associated with a codependent personality are varied. The *DSM-IV-TR* (APA, 2000) states that personality traits only become disorders when they are "inflexible and maladaptive and cause significant functional impairment or subjective distress." To date, no diagnostic criteria exist for the diagnosis of codependent personality disorder.

A codependent individual is confused about his or her own identity. In a relationship, the codependent person derives self-worth from that of the partner, whose feelings and behaviors determine how the codependent should feel and behave. In order for the codependent to feel good, his or her partner must be happy and behave in appropriate ways. If the partner is not happy, the codependent feels responsible for *making* him or her happy. The codependent's home life is fraught with stress. Ego boundaries are weak and behaviors are often enmeshed with those of the pathological partner. Denial that problems exist is common. Feelings are kept in control, and anxiety may be released in the form of stress-related illnesses or compulsive behaviors such as eating, spending, working, or use of substances.

Wesson (2010) described the following behaviors characteristic of codependency. She stated that codependents:

■ Have a long history of focusing thoughts and behavior on other people.

■ Are "people pleasers" and will do almost anything to get the approval of others.

■ Outwardly appear very competent, but actually feel quite needy, helpless, or perhaps nothing at all.

■ Have experienced abuse or emotional neglect as a child.

■ Are outwardly focused toward others, and know very little about how to direct their own lives from their own sense of self.

The Codependent Nurse

Certain characteristics of codependency have been associated with the profession of nursing. A shortage of nurses combined with the increasing ranks of seriously ill clients may result in nurses providing care and fulfilling everyone's needs but their own. Many health-care workers who are reared in homes with a chemically dependent person or otherwise dysfunctional family are at risk for having any unresolved codependent tendencies activated. Nurses, who as children assumed the "fixer" role in their dysfunctional families of origin, may attempt to resume that role in their caregiving professions. They are attracted to a profession in which they are needed, but they nurture feelings of resentment for receiving so little in return. Their emotional needs go unmet; however, they continue to deny that these needs exist. Instead, these unmet emotional needs may be manifested through use of compulsive behaviors, such as working or spending excessively, or addictions, such as to food or substances.

Codependent nurses have a need to be in control. They often strive for an unrealistic level of achievement. Their self-worth comes from the feeling of being needed by others and of maintaining control over their environment. They nurture the dependence of others and accept the responsibility for the happiness and contentment of others. They rarely express their true feelings, and do what is necessary to preserve harmony and maintain control. They are at high risk for physical and emotional burnout.

Treating Codependency

Cermak (1986) identified four stages in the recovery process for individuals with codependent personality:

Stage I: The Survival Stage In this first stage, codependent persons must begin to let go of the denial that problems exist or that their personal capabilities are unlimited. This initiation of abstinence from blanket denial may be a very emotional and painful period.

Stage II: The Reidentification Stage Reidentification occurs when the individuals are able to glimpse their true selves through a break in the denial system. They accept the label of codependent and take responsibility for their own dysfunctional behavior. Codependents tend to enter reidentification only after being convinced that it is more painful not to. They accept their limitations and are ready to face the issues of codependency.

Stage III: The Core Issues Stage In this stage, the recovering codependent must face the fact that relationships cannot be managed by force of will. Each partner must be independent and autonomous. The goal of this stage is to detach from the struggles of life that exist because of prideful and willful efforts to control those things that are beyond the individual's power to control.

Stage IV: The Reintegration Stage This is a stage of self-acceptance and willingness to change when codependents relinquish the power *over others* that was not rightfully theirs but reclaim the *personal* power that they do possess. Integrity is achieved out of awareness, honesty, and being in touch with one's spiritual consciousness. Control is achieved through self-discipline and self-confidence.

Self-help groups have been found to be helpful in the treatment of codependency. Groups developed for families of chemically dependent people, such as Al-Anon, may be of assistance. Groups specific to the problem of codependency also exist. Two of these groups include:

Co-Dependents Anonymous (CoDA)

P.O. Box 33577

Phoenix, AZ 85067-3577

888-444-2359

www.coda.org

Co-Dependents Anonymous for Helping
Professionals (CODAHP)

P.O. Box 42253

Mesa, AZ 85274-2253

602-644-8605

Both of these groups apply the Twelve Steps and Twelve Traditions developed by Alcoholics Anonymous to codependency (see section on Alcoholics Anonymous below).

Treatment Modalities for Substance-Related Disorders

Alcoholics Anonymous

Alcoholics Anonymous (AA) is a major self-help organization for the treatment of alcoholism. It was founded in 1935 by two alcoholics—a stockbroker, Bill Wilson, and a physician, Dr. Bob Smith—who discovered that they could remain sober through mutual support. This they accomplished not as professionals, but as peers who were able to share their common experiences. Soon they were working with other alcoholics, who in turn worked with others. The movement grew, and remarkably, individuals who had been treated unsuccessfully by professionals were able to maintain sobriety through helping one another.

Today AA chapters exist in virtually every community in the United States. The self-help groups are based on the concept of peer support—acceptance and understanding from others who have experienced the same problems in their lives. The only requirement for membership is a desire on the part of the alcoholic person to stop drinking. Each new member is assigned a support person from whom he or she may seek assistance when the temptation to drink occurs.

A survey by the General Service Office of Alcoholics Anonymous in 2007 (Alcoholics Anonymous [AA], 2008) revealed the following statistics: members ages 30 and younger comprised 13.6 percent of the membership and the average age of an AA member was 47; women comprised 33 percent; 85.1 percent were white, 5.7 percent were African American, 4.8 percent were Hispanic, 1.6 percent were Native American, and 2.8 percent were Asian American and other minorities. By occupation, the highest percentages included the following: 16 percent were retired; 11 percent were self-employed; 10 percent were managers or administrators; and 10 percent were in professional or technical fields.

The sole purpose of AA is to help members stay sober. When sobriety has been achieved, they in turn are expected to help other alcoholic persons. The Twelve Steps that embody the philosophy of AA provide specific guidelines on how to attain and maintain sobriety (Box 25-6).

AA accepts alcoholism as an illness and promotes total abstinence as the only cure, emphasizing that the alcoholic person can never safely

---

BOX 25-6 Alcoholics Anonymous

THE TWELVE STEPS

1. We admitted we were powerless over alcohol—that our lives have become unmanageable.
2. Came to believe that a Power greater than ourselves could restore us to sanity.

3. Made a decision to turn our will and our lives over to the care of God as we understood Him.
4. Made a searching and fearless moral inventory of ourselves.
5. Admitted to God, to ourselves, and to another human being the exact nature of our wrongs.
6. Were entirely ready to have God remove all these defects of character.

7. Humbly asked Him to remove our shortcomings.

THE TWELVE TRADITIONS

1. Our common welfare should come first; personal recovery depends upon AA unity.
2. For our group purpose there is but one ultimate authority—a loving God as He may express Himself in our group conscience. Our leaders are but trusted servants; they do not govern.
3. The one requirement for AA membership is a desire to stop drinking.
4. Each group should be autonomous except in matters affecting other groups or AA as a whole.
5. Each group has but one primary purpose—to carry its message to the alcoholic who still suffers.
6. An AA group ought never endorse, finance, or lend the AA name to any related facility or outside enterprise, lest problems of money, property, and prestige divert us from our primary purpose.
7. Every AA group ought to be fully self-supporting, declining outside contributions.

BOX 25-6 Alcoholics Anonymous—cont'd

8. Made a list of all persons we had harmed and became willing to make amends to them all.

9. Made direct amends to such people wherever possible except when to do so would injure them or others.

10. Continued to take personal inventory and when we were wrong promptly admitted it.

11. Sought through prayer and meditation to improve our conscious contact with God as we understood Him, praying only for knowledge of His will for us and the power to carry that out.

12. Having had a spiritual awakening as the result of these steps, we tried to carry this message to alcoholics and to practice these principles in all our affairs.

8. Alcoholics Anonymous should remain forever non-professional, but our service centers may employ special workers.

9. Alcoholics Anonymous, as such, ought never be organized; but we may create service boards of committees directly responsible to those they serve.

10. Alcoholics Anonymous has no opinion on outside issues; hence, the Alcoholics Anonymous name ought never be drawn into public controversy.

11. Our public relations policy is based on attraction rather than promotion; we need always maintain personal anonymity at the level of press, radio, and films.

12. Anonymity is the spiritual foundation of all our traditions, ever reminding us to place principles before personalities.

The Twelve Steps and Twelve Traditions are reprinted with permission of Alcoholics Anonymous World Services, Inc. (AAWS). Permission to reprint the Twelve Steps and Twelve Traditions does not mean that AAWS has reviewed or approved the contents of this publication, or that AA necessarily agrees with the views expressed herein. AA is a program of recovery from alcoholism only. Use of the Twelve Steps and Twelve Traditions in connection with programs and activities which are patterned after AA, but which address other problems, or in any other non-AA context, does not imply otherwise.

return to social drinking. They encourage the members to seek sobriety, taking one day at a time. The Twelve Traditions are the statements of principles that govern the organization (see Box 25-6).

AA has been the model for various other self-help groups associated with abuse or dependence problems. Some of these groups and the memberships for which they are organized are listed in Table 25-11. Nurses need to be fully and accurately informed about available self-help groups and their importance as a treatment resource on the healthcare continuum so that they can use them as a referral source for clients with substance-related disorders.

Pharmacotherapy

Disulfiram (Antabuse)

Disulfiram (Antabuse) is a drug that can be administered as a deterrent to drinking to individuals who abuse alcohol. Ingestion of alcohol while disulfiram is in the body results in a syndrome of symptoms that can produce a good deal of discomfort for the individual. It can even result in death if the blood alcohol level is high. The reaction varies according to the sensitivity of the individual and how much alcohol was ingested.

Disulfiram works by inhibiting the enzyme aldehyde dehydrogenase, thereby blocking the oxidation of alcohol at the stage when acetaldehyde is converted to acetate. This results in an accumulation of acetaldehyde in the blood, which is thought to produce the symptoms associated with the disulfiram-alcohol reaction. These symptoms persist as long as alcohol is being metabolized. The rate of alcohol elimination does not appear to be affected.

Symptoms of disulfiram-alcohol reaction can occur within 5 to 10 minutes of ingestion of alcohol. Mild reactions can occur at blood alcohol levels as low as 5 to 10 mg/dL. Symptoms are fully developed at approximately 50 mg/dL, and may include flushed skin, throbbing in the head and neck, respiratory difficulty, dizziness, nausea and vomiting, sweating, hyperventilation, tachycardia, hypotension, weakness, blurred vision, and confusion. With a blood alcohol level of approximately 125 to 150 mg/dL, severe reactions can occur, including respiratory depression, cardiovascular collapse, arrhythmias, myocardial infarction, acute congestive heart failure, unconsciousness, convulsions, and death.

Disulfiram should not be administered until it has been ascertained that the client has abstained from alcohol for at least 12 hours. If disulfiram is

TABLE 25-11 Addiction Self-Help Groups

GROUP	MEMBERSHIP
Adult Children of Alcoholics (ACOA)	Adults who grew up with an alcoholic in the home
Al-Anon	Families of alcoholics
Alateen	Adolescent children of alcoholics
Children Are People	School-age children with an alcoholic family member
Cocaine Anonymous	Cocaine addicts
Families Anonymous	Parents of children who abuse substances
Fresh Start	Nicotine addicts
Narcotics Anonymous	Narcotics addicts
Nar-Anon	Families of narcotics addicts
Overeaters Anonymous	Food addicts
Pills Anonymous	Polysubstance addicts
Pot Smokers Anonymous	Marijuana smokers
Smokers Anonymous	Nicotine addicts
Women for Sobriety	Female alcoholics

discontinued, it is important for the client to understand that the sensitivity to alcohol may last for as long as 2 weeks. Consuming alcohol or alcohol-containing substances during this 2-week period could result in the disulfiram-alcohol reaction.

The client receiving disulfiram therapy should be aware of the large number of alcohol-containing substances. These products, such as liquid cough and cold preparations, vanilla extract, aftershave lotions, colognes, mouthwash, nail polish removers, and isopropyl alcohol, if ingested or even rubbed on the skin, are capable of producing the symptoms described. The individual must read labels carefully and must inform any doctor, dentist, or other healthcare professional from whom assistance is sought that he or she is taking disulfiram. In addition, it is important that the client carry a card explaining participation in disulfiram therapy, possible consequences of the therapy, and symptoms that may indicate an emergency situation.

The client must be assessed carefully before beginning disulfiram therapy. A thorough medical screening is performed before starting therapy, and written informed consent is usually required. The drug is contraindicated for clients who are at high risk for alcohol ingestion. It is also contraindicated for psychotic clients and clients with severe cardiac, renal, or hepatic disease.

Disulfiram therapy is not a cure for alcoholism. It provides a measure of control for the individual who desires to avoid impulse drinking. Clients receiving disulfiram therapy are encouraged to seek other assistance with their problem, such as AA or other support group, to aid in the recovery process.

Other Medications for Treatment of Alcoholism

The narcotic antagonist naltrexone (ReVia) was approved by the Food and Drug Administration (FDA) in 1994 for the treatment of alcohol dependence. Naltrexone, which was approved in 1984 for the treatment of heroin abuse, works on the same receptors in the brain that produce the feelings of pleasure when heroin or other opiates bind to them, but it does not produce the "narcotic high" and is not habit forming. Although alcohol does not bind to these same brain receptors, studies have shown that naltrexone works equally well against it (O'Malley et al., 1992; Volpicelli, Alterman, Hayashida, & O'Brien, 1992). In comparison to the placebo-treated clients, subjects on naltrexone therapy showed significantly lower overall relapse rates and fewer drinks per drinking day among those clients who did resume drinking. A study with an oral form of nalmefene (Revex) produced similar results (Mason et al., 1994).

The efficacy of selective serotonin reuptake inhibitors (SSRIs) in the decrease of alcohol craving among alcohol-dependent individuals has yielded mixed results (NIAAA, 2000). A greater degree of success was observed with moderate drinkers than with heavy drinkers.

In August, 2004, the FDA approved acamprosate (Campral), which is indicated for the maintenance of abstinence from alcohol in patients with alcohol dependence who are abstinent at treatment initiation. The mechanism of action of acamprosate in maintenance of alcohol abstinence is not completely understood. It is hypothesized to restore the normal balance between neuronal excitation and inhibition by interacting with glutamate and gamma-aminobutyric acid (GABA) neurotransmitter systems. Acamprosate is ineffective in clients who have not undergone detoxification and not achieved alcohol abstinence prior to beginning treatment. It is recommend for concomitant use with psychosocial therapy.

Counseling

Counseling on a one-to-one basis is often used to help the client who abuses substances. The relationship is goal directed, and the length of the counseling may vary from weeks to years. The focus is on current reality, development of a working treatment relationship, and strengthening ego assets. The counselor must be warm, kind, and nonjudgmental, yet able to set limits firmly. The primary characteristic of counselors that influences treatment outcome appears to be interpersonal functioning, including therapists' empathy, genuineness, and respect for patients (Najavits & Weiss, 1994).

Counseling of the client who abuses substances passes through various phases, each of which is of indeterminate length. In the first phase, an assessment is conducted. Factual data are collected to determine whether the client does indeed have a problem with substances; that is, that substances are regularly impairing effective functioning in a significant life area.

Following the assessment, in the working phase of the relationship, the counselor assists the individual to work on acceptance of the fact that the use of substances causes problems in significant life areas and that he or she is not able to prevent it from occurring. The client states a desire to make changes. The strength of the denial system is determined by the duration and extent of substance-related adverse effects in the person's life. Thus, those individuals with rather minor substance-related problems of recent origin have less difficulty with this stage than those with long-term extensive impairment. The individual also works to gain self-control and abstain from substances.

Once the problem has been identified and sobriety is achieved, the client must have a concrete and workable plan for getting through the early weeks of abstinence. Anticipatory guidance through role-play helps the individual practice how he or she will respond when substances are readily obtainable and the impulse to partake is strong.

Counseling often includes the family or specific family members. In family counseling, the therapist tries to help each member see how he or she has affected, and been affected by, the substance-abuse behavior. Family strengths are mobilized, and family members are encouraged to move in a positive direction. Referrals are often made to self-help groups such as Al-Anon, Nar-Anon, Alateen, Families Anonymous, and Adult Children of Alcoholics.

Group Therapy

Group therapy with substance abusers has long been regarded as a powerful agent of change. In groups, individuals are able to share their experiences with others who are going through similar problems. They are able to "see themselves in others," and confront their defenses about giving up the substance. They may confront similar attitudes and defenses in others. Groups also give individuals the capacity for communicating needs and feelings directly.

Some groups may be task-oriented education groups in which the leader is charged with presenting material associated with substance abuse and its various effects on the person's life. Other educational groups that may be helpful with individuals who abuse substances include those that provide instruction in assertiveness techniques and methods of relaxation. Teaching groups differ from psychotherapy groups, whose focus is more on helping individuals understand and manage difficult feelings and situations, particularly as they relate to use of substances.

Therapy groups and self-help groups such as AA are complementary to each other. Whereas the self-help group focus is on achieving and maintaining sobriety, in the therapy group the individual may learn more adaptive ways of coping, how to deal with problems that may have arisen or were exacerbated by the former substance use, and ways to improve quality of life and to function more effectively without substances.

Psychopharmacology for Substance Intoxication and Substance Withdrawal

Various medications have been used to decrease the intensity of symptoms in an individual who is withdrawing from, or who is experiencing the effects of excessive use of, alcohol and other drugs. **Substitution therapy** may be required to reduce the life-threatening effects of intoxication or withdrawal from some substances. The severity of the withdrawal syndrome depends on the particular drug used, how long it has been used, the dose used, and the rate at which the drug is eliminated from the body.

Alcohol

Benzodiazepines are the most widely used group of drugs for substitution therapy in alcohol withdrawal. Chlordiazepoxide (Librium), oxazepam (Serax), lorazepam (Ativan), and diazepam (Valium) are the most commonly used agents. The approach to treatment with benzodiazepines for alcohol withdrawal is to start with relatively high doses and reduce the dosage by 20 to 25 percent each day until withdrawal is complete. Additional doses may be given for breakthrough signs or symptoms (Black & Andreasen, 2011). In clients with liver disease, accumulation of the longer-acting agents (chlordiazepoxide and diazepam) may be problematic, and use of the shorter-acting benzodiazepines (lorazepam or oxazepam) is more appropriate.

Some physicians may order anticonvulsant medication (e.g., carbamazepine, valproic acid, or gabapentin) for management of withdrawal seizures. These drugs are particularly useful in individuals who undergo repeated episodes of alcohol withdrawal. Repeated episodes of withdrawal appear to "kindle" even more serious withdrawal episodes, including the production of withdrawal seizures that can result in brain damage (Julien, 2008). These anticonvulsants have been used successfully in both acute withdrawal and longer-term craving situations.

Multivitamin therapy, in combination with daily injections or oral administration of thiamine, is common protocol. Thiamine is commonly deficient in chronic alcoholics. Replacement therapy is required to prevent neuropathy, confusion, and encephalopathy.

Opioids

Examples of opioids are heroin, morphine, opium, meperidine, codeine, and methadone. With short-acting drugs such as heroin, withdrawal symptoms occur within 6 to 12 hours after the last dose, peak within 1 to 3 days, and gradually subside over a period of 5 to 7 days (APA, 2000). With longer-acting drugs such as methadone, withdrawal symptoms begin within 1 to 3 days after the last dose, peak between days 4 and 6, and are complete in 14 to 21 days (Leamon, Wright, & Myrick, 2008). Withdrawal from the ultra-short-acting meperidine begins quickly, reaches a peak in 8 to 12 hours, and is complete in 4 to 5 days (Sadock & Sadock, 2007).

Opioid intoxication is treated with narcotic antagonists such as naloxone (Narcan), naltrexone (ReVia), or nalmefene (Revex). Withdrawal therapy includes rest, adequate nutritional support, and methadone substitution. Methadone is given on the first day in a dose sufficient to suppress withdrawal symptoms. The dose is then gradually tapered over a specified time. As the dose of methadone diminishes, renewed abstinence symptoms may be ameliorated by the addition of clonidine.

In October 2002, the FDA approved two forms of the drug buprenorphine for treating opiate dependence. Buprenorphine is less powerful than methadone but is considered to be somewhat safer and causes fewer side effects, making it especially attractive for clients who are mildly or moderately addicted. Individuals will be able to access treatment with buprenorphine in office-based settings, providing an alternative to methadone clinics. Physicians are deemed qualified to prescribe buprenorphine if they hold an addiction certification from the American Society of Addiction Medicine, the American Academy of Addiction Psychiatry, the American Psychiatric Association, or other associations deemed appropriate. The number of patients to whom individual physicians may provide outpatient buprenorphine treatment is limited to 100 (Daly, 2007).

Clonidine (Catapres) also has been used to suppress opiate withdrawal symptoms. As monotherapy, it is not as effective as substitution with methadone, but it is nonaddicting and serves effectively as a bridge to enable the client to stay opiate free long enough to facilitate termination of methadone maintenance.

Depressants

Substitution therapy for CNS depressant withdrawal (particularly barbiturates) is most commonly with the long-acting barbiturate phenobarbital (Luminal). The dosage required to suppress withdrawal symptoms is administered. When stabilization has been achieved, the dose is gradually decreased by 30 mg/day until withdrawal is complete. Long-acting benzodiazepines are commonly used for substitution therapy when the abused substance is a nonbarbiturate CNS depressant (Ashton, 2002).

Stimulants

Treatment of stimulant intoxication usually begins with minor tranquilizers such as chlordiazepoxide and progresses to major tranquilizers such as haloperidol (Haldol). Antipsychotics should be administered with caution because of their propensity to lower seizure threshold (Mack et al., 2003). Repeated seizures are treated with intravenous diazepam.

Withdrawal from CNS stimulants is not the medical emergency observed with CNS depressants. Treatment is usually aimed at reducing drug craving and managing severe depression. The client is placed in a quiet atmosphere and allowed to sleep and eat as much as is needed or desired. Suicide precautions may need to be instituted. Antidepressant therapy may be helpful in treating symptoms of depression. Desipramine has been especially successful with symptoms of cocaine withdrawal and abstinence (Mack et al., 2003).

Hallucinogens and Cannabinols

Substitution therapy is not required with these drugs. When adverse reactions, such as anxiety or panic, occur, benzodiazepines (e.g., diazepam or chlordiazepoxide) may be prescribed to prevent harm to the client or others. Psychotic reactions may be treated with antipsychotic medications.

CASE STUDY AND SAMPLE CARE PLAN

NURSING HISTORY AND ASSESSMENT

The police bring Dan to the emergency department of the local hospital around 9:00 p.m. His wife, Carol, called 911 when Dan became violent and she began to fear for her safety. Dan was fired from his job as a foreman in a manufacturing plant for refusing to follow his supervisor's directions on a project. When cleaning up after his move, several partially used bottles of liquor were found in his work area.

Carol reports that Dan has been drinking since he came home shortly after noon today. He bloodied her nose and punched her in the stomach when she poured the contents of a bottle from which he was drinking down the kitchen sink. The police responded to her call and brought Dan to the hospital in handcuffs. By the time they arrive at the hospital, Dan has calmed down, and appears drugged and drowsy. His blood alcohol level measures 247 mg/dL. He is admitted to the detoxification unit of the hospital with a diagnosis of Alcohol Intoxication.

Carol tells the admitting nurse that she and Dan have been married for 12 years. He was a social drinker before they were married, but his drinking has increased over the years. He has been under a lot of stress at work; hates his job, his boss, and his coworkers; and is depressed a lot of the time. He never had a loving relationship with his parents, who are now deceased. For the past few years, his pattern has been to come home, start drinking immediately, and drink until he passes out for the night. She states that she has tried to get him to go for help with his drinking, but he refuses, and says that he doesn't have a problem.

Carol begins to cry and says to the nurse, "We can't go on like this. I don't know what to do!"

NURSING DIAGNOSES/OUTCOME IDENTIFICATION

From the assessment data, the nurse develops the following nursing diagnoses for Dan:

1. **Risk for injury** related to CNS agitation from alcohol withdrawal.
   a. **Short-Term Goal:** Dan's condition will stabilize within 72 hours.
   b. **Long-Term Goal:** Dan will not experience physical injury.

2. **Ineffective denial** related to low self-esteem, weak ego development, and underlying fears and anxieties.
   a. **Short-Term Goal:** Dan will focus immediate attention on behavioral changes required to achieve sobriety.
   b. **Long-Term Goal:** Dan will accept responsibility for his drinking behaviors, and acknowledge the association between his drinking and personal problems.

PLANNING/IMPLEMENTATION

Risk for Injury

The following nursing interventions may be implemented *in an effort to ensure client safety:*

1. Assess his level of disorientation; frequently orient him to reality and his surroundings.

2. Obtain a drug history.

3. Obtain a urine sample for analysis.

4. Place Dan in a quiet room (private, if possible).

5. Ensure that smoking materials and other potentially harmful objects are stored away.

6. Observe Dan frequently. Take vital signs every 15 to 30 minutes.

Continued

CASE STUDY AND SAMPLE CARE PLAN — Cont'd

7. Monitor for signs of withdrawal within a few hours after admission. Watch for signs of:

   ▪ Increased heart rate
   ▪ Tremors
   ▪ Headache
   ▪ Diaphoresis
   ▪ Agitation; restlessness
   ▪ Nausea
   ▪ Fever
   ▪ Convulsions

8. Follow medication regimen, as ordered by physician (commonly a benzodiazepine, thiamine, multivitamin).

Ineffective Denial

The following nursing interventions may be implemented *in an effort to help Dan accept responsibility for the behavioral consequences associated with his drinking:*

1. Develop Dan's trust by spending time with him, being honest, and keeping all promises.

2. Ensure that Dan understands that it is not *him,* but his *behavior,* that is unacceptable.

3. Provide Dan with accurate information about the effects of alcohol. Do this in a matter-of-fact, nonjudgmental way.

4. Point out recent negative events that have occurred in Dan's life, and associate the use of alcohol with these events. Help him to see the association.

5. Use confrontation with caring: "Yes, your wife called the police. You were physically abusive. She was afraid. And your blood alcohol level was 247 when you were brought in. You were obviously not in control of your behavior at the time."

6. Don't accept excuses for his drinking. Point out rationalization and projection behaviors. These behaviors prolong denial that he has a problem. He must directly accept responsibility for his drinking (not make excuses and blame it on the behavior of others). He must come to understand that only HE has control of his behavior.

7. Encourage Dan to attend group therapy during treatment, and Alcoholics Anonymous following treatment. Peer feedback is a strong factor in helping individuals to recognize their problems and to ultimately remain sober.

8. Encourage Carol to attend Al-Anon meetings. She can benefit from the experiences of others who have experienced and are experiencing the same types of problems as she.

9. Help Dan to identify ways that he can cope besides using alcohol (e.g., exercise, sports, relaxation). He should choose what is most appropriate for him, and should be given positive feedback for efforts made toward change.

EVALUATION

The outcome criteria identified for Dan have been met. He experienced an uncomplicated withdrawal from alcohol and exhibits no evidence of physical injury. He verbalizes understanding of the relationship between his personal problems and his drinking, and accepts responsibility for his own behavior. He verbalizes understanding that alcohol dependence is an illness that requires ongoing support and treatment, and regularly attends AA meetings. Carol regularly attends Al-Anon meetings.

Summary and Key Points

▪ An individual is considered to be dependent on a substance when he or she is unable to control its use, even knowing that it interferes with normal functioning; when more and more of the substance is required to produce the desired effects; and when characteristic withdrawal symptoms develop upon cessation or drastic decrease in use of the substance.

▪ Abuse is considered when there is continued use of the substance despite having a persistent or recurrent problem that is caused or exacerbated by its use or when the substance is used in physically hazardous situations.

▪ Substance intoxication is defined as the development of a reversible syndrome of maladaptive behavior or psychological changes that are due to the direct physiological effects of a substance on the CNS and develop during or shortly after ingestion of (or exposure to) a substance.

▪ Substance withdrawal is the development of a substance-specific maladaptive behavior change, with physiological and cognitive concomitants, that is due to the cessation of, or reduction in, heavy and prolonged substance use.

■ The etiology of substance-use disorders is unknown. Various contributing factors have been implicated, such as genetics, biochemical changes, developmental influences, personality factors, social learning, conditioning, and cultural and ethnic influences.

■ Seven classes of substances are presented in this chapter in terms of a profile of the substance, historical aspects, patterns of use and abuse, and effects on the body. These are: alcohol, other CNS depressants, CNS stimulants, opioids, hallucinogens, inhalants, and cannabinols.

■ The nurse uses the nursing process as the vehicle for delivery of care of the client with a substance-related disorder.

■ The nurse must first examine his or her own feelings regarding personal substance use and the substance use by others. Only the nurse who can be accepting and nonjudgmental of substance-abuse behaviors will be effective in working with these clients.

■ Special care is given to clients with dual diagnoses of mental illness and substance-use disorders.

■ Substance abuse is a problem for many members of the nursing profession. Most state boards of nursing and state nurses' associations have established avenues for peer assistance to provide help to impaired members of the profession.

■ Individuals who are reared in families with chemically dependent persons learn patterns of dysfunctional behavior that carry over into adult life. These dysfunctional behavior patterns have been termed *codependency*. Codependent persons sacrifice their own needs for the fulfillment of others' in order to achieve a sense of control. Many nurses also have codependent traits.

■ Treatment modalities for substance-related disorders include self-help groups, deterrent therapy, individual counseling, and group therapy. Substitution pharmacotherapy is frequently implemented with clients experiencing substance intoxication or substance withdrawal. Treatment modalities are implemented on an inpatient basis or in outpatient settings, depending on the severity of the impairment.

 DavisPlus   Additional info available @ davisplus.fadavis.com

Review Questions
Self-Examination/Learning Exercise

*Select the answer that is **most** appropriate for each of the following questions:*

1. Mr. White is admitted to the hospital after an extended period of binge alcohol drinking. His wife reports that he has been a heavy drinker for a number of years. Laboratory reports reveal he has a blood alcohol level of 250 mg/dL. He is placed on the chemical dependency unit for detoxification. When would the first signs of alcohol withdrawal symptoms be expected to occur?
   a. Several hours after the last drink.
   b. 2 to 3 days after the last drink.
   c. 4 to 5 days after the last drink.
   d. 6 to 7 days after the last drink.

2. Symptoms of alcohol withdrawal include:
   a. Euphoria, hyperactivity, and insomnia.
   b. Depression, suicidal ideation, and hypersomnia.
   c. Diaphoresis, nausea and vomiting, and tremors.
   d. Unsteady gait, nystagmus, and profound disorientation.

3. Which of the following medications is the physician most likely to order for a client experiencing alcohol withdrawal syndrome?
   a. Haloperidol (Haldol).
   b. Chlordiazepoxide (Librium).
   c. Methadone (Dolophine).
   d. Phenytoin (Dilantin).

Review Questions—cont'd
Self-Examination/Learning Exercise

4. Dan, who has been admitted to the alcohol rehabilitation unit after being fired for drinking on the job, states to the nurse, "I don't have a problem with alcohol. I can handle my booze better than anyone I know. My boss is a jerk! I haven't missed any more days than my coworkers." The nurse's best response is:
   a. "Maybe your boss is mistaken, Dan."
   b. "You are here because your drinking was interfering with your work, Dan."
   c. "Get real, Dan! You're a boozer and you know it!"
   d. "Why do you think your boss sent you here, Dan?"

5. Dan, who has been admitted to the alcohol rehabilitation unit after being fired for drinking on the job, states to the nurse, "I don't have a problem with alcohol. I can handle my booze better than anyone I know. My boss is a jerk! I haven't missed any more days than my coworkers." The defense mechanism that Dan is using is:
   a. Denial.
   b. Projection.
   c. Displacement.
   d. Rationalization.

6. Dan has been admitted to the alcohol rehabilitation unit after being fired for drinking on the job. Dan's drinking buddies come for a visit, and when they leave, the nurse smells alcohol on Dan's breath. Which of the following would be the best intervention with Dan at this time?
   a. Search his room for evidence.
   b. Ask, "Have you been drinking alcohol, Dan?"
   c. Send a urine specimen from Dan to the lab for drug screening.
   d. Tell Dan, "These guys cannot come to the unit to visit you again."

7. Dan begins attendance at AA meetings. Which of the statements by Dan reflects the purpose of this organization?
   a. "They claim they will help me stay sober."
   b. "I'll dry out in AA, then I can have a social drink now and then."
   c. "AA is only for people who have reached the bottom."
   d. "If I lose my job, AA will help me find another."

8. From which of the following symptoms might the nurse identify a chronic cocaine user?
   a. Clear, constricted pupils.
   b. Red, irritated nostrils.
   c. Muscle aches.
   d. Conjunctival redness.

9. An individual who is addicted to heroin is likely to experience which of the following symptoms of withdrawal?
   a. Increased heart rate and blood pressure.
   b. Tremors, insomnia, and seizures.
   c. Incoordination and unsteady gait.
   d. Nausea and vomiting, diarrhea, and diaphoresis.

10. A polysubstance abuser makes the statement, "The green and whites do me good after speed." How might the nurse interpret the statement?
    a. The client abuses amphetamines and anxiolytics.
    b. The client abuses alcohol and cocaine.
    c. The client is psychotic.
    d. The client abuses narcotics and marijuana.

TEST YOUR CRITICAL THINKING SKILLS

Kelly, age 23, is a first-year law student. She is engaged to a surgical resident at the local university hospital. She has been struggling to do well in law school because she wants to make her parents, two prominent local attorneys, proud of her. She had never aspired to do anything but go into law, and that is also what her parents expected her to do.

Kelly's midterm grades were not as high as she had hoped, so she increased the number of hours of study time, staying awake all night several nights a week to study. She started drinking large amounts of coffee to stay awake, but still found herself falling asleep as she tried to study at the library and in her apartment. As final exams approached, she began to panic that she would not be able to continue the pace of studying she felt she needed in order to make the grades she hoped for.

One of Kelly's classmates told her that she needed some "speed" to give her that extra energy to study. Her classmate said, "All the kids do it. Hardly anyone I know gets through law school without it." She gave Kelly the name of a source.

Kelly contacted the source, who supplied her with enough amphetamines to see her through final exams. Kelly was excited, because she had so much energy, did not require sleep, and was able to study the additional hours she thought she needed for the exams. However, when the results were posted, Kelly had failed two courses and would have to repeat them in summer school if she was to continue with her class in the fall. She continued to replenish her supply of amphetamines from her "contact" until he told her he could not get her anymore. She became frantic and stole a prescription blank from her fiancé and forged his name for more pills.

She started taking more and more of the medication in order to achieve the "high" she wanted to feel. Her behavior became erratic. Yesterday, her fiancé received a call from a pharmacy to clarify an order for amphetamines that Kelly had written. He insisted that she admit herself to the chemical dependency unit for detoxification.

On the unit, she appears tired and depressed, moves very slowly, and wants to sleep all the time. She keeps saying to the nurse, "I'm a real failure. I'll never be an attorney like my parents. I'm too dumb. I just wish I could die."

Answer the following questions related to Kelly:

1. What is the primary nursing diagnosis for Kelly?
2. Describe important nursing interventions to be implemented with Kelly.
3. In addition to physical safety, what would be the primary short-term goal the nurses would strive to achieve with Kelly?

References

Alcoholics Anonymous. (2008). *Alcoholics Anonymous 2007 membership survey.* Retrieved September 2, 2010, from http://www.aa.org/

American Psychiatric Association. (2000). *Diagnostic and statistical manual of mental disorders* (4th ed.) *Text revision.* Washington, DC: American Psychiatric Publishing.

Ashton, C. H. (2002). *Benzodiazepines: How they work and how to withdraw.* Newcastle upon Tyne, UK: University of Newcastle.

Bashore, T. M., Granger, C. B., Hranitzky, P., & Patel, M. R. (2009). Heart disease. In S. J. McPhee & M. A. Papadakis (Eds.), *2009 Current medical diagnosis & treatment* (pp. 287–375). New York: McGraw Hill Medical.

Black, D. W., & Andreasen, N. C. (2011). *Introductory textbook of psychiatry* (5th ed.). Washington, DC: American Psychiatric Publishing.

Burney, R. (1996). *Codependence—the dance of wounded souls.* Cambria, CA: Joy to You & Me Enterprises.

Carmona, R. H. (2005). *Surgeon General's advisory on alcohol use in pregnancy.* Washington, DC: U.S. Department of Health and Human Services.

Centers for Disease Control and Prevention. (2005). Guidelines for identifying and referring persons with fetal alcohol syndrome. *MMWR Recommendations and Reports, 54*(RR-11).

Centers for Disease Control and Prevention. (2008, August 29). Alcohol-attributable deaths and years of potential life lost among American Indians and Alaska Natives—United States, 2001–2005. *MMWR Morbidity and Mortality Weekly Report, 57*(34), 938–941.

Choudary, P. V., & Knowles, J. A. (2008). Genetics. In R. E. Hales, S. C. Yudofsky, & G. O. Gabbard (Eds.), *Textbook of psychiatry* (5th ed., pp. 191–243). Washington, DC: American Psychiatric Publishing.

Daly, R. (2007). Congress lets MDs treat more buprenorphine patients. *Psychiatric News, 42*(1), 4.

Dannaway, D. C., & Mulvihill, J. J. (2009). Fetal alcohol spectrum disorder. *NeoReviews 10*(5), e230–e238.

Ehrlander, M. (2007). Alcohol cultures in Finland and Alaska: Explosive drinking patterns and their consequences. *Northern Review.* Number 27 (Fall 2007). Retrieved August 31, 2010, from http://www.yukoncollege.yk.ca/research/pages/the_northern_review

Ellis, J. R., & Hartley, C. L. (2008). *Nursing in today's world: Trends, issues, and mangement.* Philadelphia: Lippincott Williams & Wilkins.

Goldstein, A. (2002). *Addiction: From biology to drug policy* (2nd ed.). New York: Oxford University Press.

Hanley, C. E. (2008). Navajos. In J. N. Giger & R. E. Davidhizar (Eds.), *Transcultural nursing* (5th ed., pp. 276–299). St. Louis: Mosby Elsevier.

Harvard Medical School. (2001). *Alcohol use and abuse.* Boston: Harvard Health Publications.

Harvard Medical School. (2003, September). Dual diagnosis: Part II. *Harvard Mental Health Letter, 20*(3), 1–5.

Harvard Medical School. (2004, September). Alcohol before birth. *Harvard Mental Health Letter, 21*(3), 1–8.

Hoffman, M. T. (2006). ADHD related to fetal alcohol syndrome. *Medscape Psychiatry & Mental Health.* Retrieved September 1, 2010, from http://www.medscape.com/viewarticle/546475

Jamal, M., Ameno, K., Kubota, T., Ameno, S., Zhang, X., Kumihashi, M., et al. (2003). In vivo formation of salsolinol induced by high acetaladehyde concentration in rat striatum employing microdialysis. *Alcohol and Alcoholism, 38,* 197–201.

Julien, R. M. (2008). *A primer of drug action: A comprehensive guide to actions, uses and side effects of psychoactive drugs* (11th ed.). New York: Worth Publishers.

Klopstock, T., Haller, R. G., & DiMauro, S. (2010). Alcoholic myopathy. *MedlinkNeurology.* Retrieved August 31, 2010, from http://www.medlink.com/medlinkcontent.asp

Lafferty, K. A., & Abdel-Kariem, R. (2010). *Toxicity, barbiturate*. Retrieved September 1, 2010, from http://emedicine.medscape.com/article/813155-overview

Leamon, M. H., Wright, T. M., & Myrick, H. (2008). Substance-related disorders. In R. E. Hales, S. C. Yudofsky, & G. O. Gabbard (Eds.), *Textbook of psychiatry* (5th ed., pp. 365–406). Washington, DC: American Psychiatric Publishing.

Mack, A. H., Franklin, J. E., & Frances, R. J. (2003). Substance use disorders. In R. E. Hales & S. C. Yudofsky (Eds.), *Textbook of clinical psychiatry* (4th ed., pp. 309–377). Washington, DC: American Psychiatric Publishing.

Maier, S. E., & West, J. R. (2001). Drinking patterns and alcohol-related birth defects. *Alcohol Research & Health, 25,* 168–174.

Mason, G. J., Ritvo, E. C., Morgan, R. O., Salvanto, F. R., Goldberg, G., Welch, B., et al. (1994). Double-blind, placebo-controlled pilot study to evaluate the efficacy and safety of oral nalmefene HCl for alcohol dependence. *Alcoholism, Clinical and Experimental Research 18,* 1162–1167.

McCoy, J. G., Strawbridge, C., McMurtrey, K. D., Kane, V. B., & Ward, C. P. (2003). A re-evaluation of the role of tetrahydropapaveroline in ethanol consumption in rats. *Brain Research Bulletin, 60*(1-2), 59–65.

Najavits, L. M., & Weiss, R. D. (1994). Variations in therapist effectiveness in the treatment of patients with substance use disorders: An empirical review. *Addiction 89,* 679–688.

NANDA International. (2009). *Nursing diagnoses: Definitions & classification 2009-2011.* Hoboken, NJ: Wiley-Blackwell.

National Cancer Institute. (2010). Pharmacological effects of supportive care medications on sexual function. Retrieved September 1, 2010, from http://www.cancer.gov/cancertopics/pdq/supportivecare/sexuality/HealthProfessional/page4

National Council on Alcoholism and Drug Dependence. (2010). *Alcohol and drug dependence are America's number one health problem.* Retrieved August 31, 2010, from http://www.ncadd.org/facts/numberoneprob.html

National Institute on Alcohol Abuse and Alcoholism. (2000). *Tenth special report to the U.S. Congress on alcohol and health.* Bethesda, MD: Author.

National Institutes of Health. (2008). What are the acute effects of marijuana abuse? *Research Report Series—Marijuana Abuse.* Retrieved September 1, 2010, from http://www.drugabuse.gov/ResearchReports/marijuana/marijuana3.html

National Library of Medicine. (2010). *Hepatic encephalopathy.* Retrieved August 31, 2010, from http://www.nlm.nih.gov/medlineplus/ency/article/000302.htm

Office of National Drug Control Policy. (2010, May). *Methamphetamine trends in the United States.* Retrieved September 1, 2010, from http://www.whitehousedrugpolicy.gov/publications/pdf/Pseudoephedrine.pdf

O'Malley, S. S., Jaffe, A. J., Chang, G., Schottenfeld, R. S., Meyer, R. E., & Rounsaville, B. (1992). Naltrexone and coping skills therapy for alcohol dependence: A controlled study. *Archives of General Psychiatry, 49,* 881–887.

Raia, S. (2004a). The problem of impaired practice. *New Jersey Nurse, 34*(6), 8.

Raia, S. (2004b). Understanding chemical dependency. *New Jersey Nurse, 34*(7), 8.

Royal College of Physicians. (2000). *Nicotine addiction in Britain.* London: Author.

Sadock, B. J., & Sadock, V. A. (2007). *Synopsis of psychiatry: Behavioral sciences/clinical psychiatry* (10th ed.). Philadelphia: Lippincott Williams & Wilkins.

Sateia, M. J. (2009). Description of insomnia. In C. A. Kushida (Ed.), *Handbook of sleep disorders* (2nd ed., pp. 3–13). New York: Informa Healthcare.

Schuckit, M. A. (2006). *Drug and alcohol abuse.* New York: Springer.

Street Drugs. (2009). Plymouth, MN: The Publishers Group.

Substance Abuse and Mental Health Services Administration. (2009). *Results from the 2008 National Survey on Drug Use and Health: National findings.* Office of Applied Studies, NSDUH Series H-36, HHS Publication No. SMA 09-4434. Rockville, MD: Author.

Sullivan, J. T., Sykora, K., Schneiderman, J., Naranjo, C. A., & Sellers, E. M. (1989). Assessment of alcohol withdrawal: The revised Clinical Institute Withdrawal Assessment for Alcohol scale (CIWA-Ar). *British Journal of Addiction, 84,* 1353–1357.

U.S. Drug Enforcement Agency. (2006). *The DEA Position on Marijuana.* Retrieved September 1, 2010, from http://www.justice.gov/dea/marijuana_position.html

Volpicelli, J. R., Alterman, A. I., Hayashida, M., & O'Brien, C. P. (1992). Naltrexone in the treatment of alcohol dependence. *Archives of General Psychiatry, 49,* 876-880.

Wesson, N. (2010). *Codependence: What is it? How do I know if I am codependent?* Retrieved September 2, 2010, from http://www.wespsych.com/codepend.html

Wilson, S. A. (2008). People of Irish heritage. In L. D. Purnell & B. J. Paulanka (Eds.), *Transcultural health care* (3rd ed.). Philadelphia: F.A. Davis. Retrieved from http://davisplus.fadavis.com

Classical References

Cermak, T. L. (1986). *Diagnosing and treating co-dependence.* Center City, MN: Hazelton Publishing.

Jellinek, E. M. (1952). Phases of alcohol addiction. *Quarterly Journal of Studies on Alcohol, 13,* 673–684.

Mayfield, D., McLeod, G., & Hall, P. (1974). The CAGE questionnaire: Validation of a new alcoholism screening instrument. *American Journal of Psychiatry, 131,* 1121–1123.

Seltzer, M. L. (1971). The Michigan Alcoholism Screening Test: The quest for a new diagnostic instrument. *American Journal of Psychiatry, 127,* 1653–1658.

@ INTERNET REFERENCES

- Additional information on addictions may be located at the following websites:
  - http://www.samhsa.gov/index.aspx
  - http://www.ccsa.ca/
  - http://www.well.com/user/woa/
  - http://www.addictions.org/

- Additional information on self-help organizations may be located at the following websites:
  - http://www.ca.org (Cocaine Anonymous)
  - http://www.aa.org (Alcoholics Anonymous)
  - http://www.na.org (Narcotics Anonymous)
  - http://www.al-anon.org

- Additional information about medications for treatment of alcohol and drug dependence may be located at the following websites:
  - http://www.fadavis.com/Townsend
  - http://www.nlm.nih.gov/medlineplus/
  - http://www.drugs.com/condition/alcoholism.html

MOVIE CONNECTIONS

Affliction (alcoholism) • *Days of Wine and Roses* (alcoholism) • *I'll Cry Tomorrow* (alcoholism) • *When a Man Loves a Woman* (alcoholism) • *Clean and Sober* (addiction—cocaine) • *28 Days (alcoholism)* • *Lady Sings the Blues (addiction—heroin)* • *I'm Dancing as Fast as I Can* (addiction—sedatives) • *The Rose* (polysubstance addiction)

Schizophrenia and Other Psychotic Disorders

KEY TERMS

agranulocytosis

akathisia

akinesia

amenorrhea

anhedonia

associative looseness

autism

catatonic

circumstantiality

clang association

delusions

dystonia

echolalia

echopraxia

extrapyramidal symptoms

gynecomastia

hallucinations

illusion

magical thinking

neologism

neuroleptic malignant
    syndrome

neuroleptics

oculogyric crisis

paranoia

perseveration

pseudoparkinsonism

religiosity

retrograde ejaculation

social skills training

tangentiality

tardive dyskinesia

waxy flexibility

word salad

OBJECTIVES
After reading this chapter, the student will be able to:

1. Discuss the concepts of schizophrenia and related psychotic disorders.
2. Identify predisposing factors in the development of these disorders.
3. Describe various types of schizophrenia and related psychotic disorders.
4. Identify symptomatology associated with these disorders and use this information in client assessment.
5. Formulate nursing diagnoses and outcomes of care for clients with schizophrenia and other psychotic disorders.

6. Identify topics for client and family teaching relevant to schizophrenia and other psychotic disorders.
7. Describe appropriate nursing interventions for behaviors associated with these disorders.
8. Describe relevant criteria for evaluating nursing care of clients with schizophrenia and related psychotic disorders.
9. Discuss various modalities relevant to treatment of schizophrenia and related psychotic disorders.

1. An alteration in which of the neurotransmitters is most closely associated with the symptoms of schizophrenia?
2. What is schizoaffective disorder?
3. How do delusions differ from hallucinations?
4. What was the first atypical antipsychotic to be developed? Why is it not considered a first-line treatment for schizophrenia?

The term *schizophrenia* was coined in 1908 by the Swiss psychiatrist Eugen Bleuler. The word was derived from the Greek "skhizo" (split) and "phren" (mind).

Over the years, much debate has surrounded the concept of schizophrenia. Various definitions of the disorder have evolved, and numerous treatment strategies have been proposed, but none has proven to be uniformly effective or sufficient.

Although the controversy lingers, two general factors appear to be gaining acceptance among clinicians. The first is that schizophrenia is probably not a homogeneous disease entity with a single cause but results from a variable combination of genetic predisposition, biochemical dysfunction, physiological factors, and psychosocial stress. The second factor is that there is not now and probably never will be a single treatment that cures the disorder. Instead, effective treatment requires a comprehensive, multidisciplinary effort, including pharmacotherapy and various forms of psychosocial care, such as living skills and **social skills training,** rehabilitation, and family therapy.

Of all the mental illnesses that cause suffering in society, schizophrenia probably is responsible for lengthier hospitalizations, greater chaos in family life, more exorbitant costs to individuals and governments, and more fears than any other. Because it is such an enormous threat to life and happiness and because its causes are an unsolved puzzle, it has probably been studied more than any other mental disorder.

Potential for suicide is a major concern among patients with schizophrenia. Radomsky and associates (1999) reported that suicide is the primary cause of premature death among individuals with the disorder. They estimated that approximately 10 percent of patients with schizophrenia die by suicide. Other studies estimate evidence of suicidal ideation in individuals with schizophrenia to be in the range of 40 to 55 percent and attempted suicide to be in the range of 20 to 50 percent (Addington, 2006).

Black and Andreasen (2011) stated:

[Schizophrenia] is probably the most devastating illness that psychiatrists treat. [It]

strikes people just when they are preparing to enter the phase of their lives in which they can achieve their highest growth and productivity—typically in the teens or early 20s—leaving most of them unable to return to normal young adult lives: to go to school, to find a job, or to marry and have children. According to *The Global Burden of Disease,* a World Health Organization-sponsored study of the cost of medical illnesses worldwide, schizophrenia is among the 10 leading causes of disability in the world among people in the 15–44 age range. (p. 107)

This chapter explores various theories of predisposing factors that have been implicated in the development of schizophrenia. Symptomatology associated with different diagnostic categories of the disorder is discussed. Nursing care is presented in the context of the six steps of the nursing process. Various dimensions of medical treatment are explored.

Nature of the Disorder

CORE CONCEPT

Psychosis

A severe mental condition in which there is disorganization of the personality, deterioration in social functioning, and loss of contact with, or distortion of, reality. There may be evidence of hallucinations and delusional thinking. Psychosis can occur with or without the presence of organic impairment.

Perhaps no psychological disorder is more crippling than schizophrenia. Characteristically, disturbances in thought processes, perception, and affect invariably result in a severe deterioration of social and occupational functioning.

In the United States, the lifetime prevalence of schizophrenia is about 1 percent (Minzenberg, Yoon, & Carter, 2008). Symptoms generally appear in late adolescence or early adulthood, although they may occur in middle or late adult life. Some studies have indicated that symptoms occur earlier in men than in women. The pattern of development of schizophrenia can be viewed in four phases: the premorbid phase, the prodromal phase, the active psychotic phase (schizophrenia), and the residual phase.

Phase I: The Premorbid Phase

The premorbid personality often indicates social maladjustment, social withdrawal, irritability, and antagonistic thoughts and behavior (Minzenberg et al., 2008). Premorbid personality and behavioral measurements that have been noted include being very shy and withdrawn, having poor peer relationships, doing poorly in school, and demonstrating antisocial behavior. Sadock and Sadock (2007) stated:

> In the typical, but not invariable, premorbid history of schizophrenia, patients had schizoid or schizotypal personalities characterized as quiet, passive, and introverted; as children, they had few friends. Preschizophrenic adolescents may have no close friends and no dates and may avoid team sports. They may enjoy [solitary activities] to the exclusion of social activities. (p. 481)

Phase II: The Prodromal Phase

The prodrome of an illness refers to certain signs and symptoms that precede the characteristic manifestations of the acute, fully developed illness. The prodromal phase of schizophrenia begins with a change from premorbid functioning and extends until the onset of frank psychotic symptoms. This phase can be as brief as a few weeks or months, but most studies indicate that the average length of the prodromal phase is between 2 and 5 years. Lehman and associates (2006) stated:

> During the prodromal phase the person experiences substantial functional impairment and nonspecific symptoms such as a sleep disturbance, anxiety, irritability, depressed mood, poor concentration, fatigue, and behavioral deficits such as deterioration in role functioning and social withdrawal. Positive symptoms such as perceptual abnormalities, ideas of reference, and suspiciousness develop late in the prodromal phase and herald the imminent onset of psychosis. (pp. 625–626)

Recognition of the behaviors associated with the prodromal phase provides an opportunity for early intervention with a possibility for improvement in long-term outcomes. Current treatment guidelines suggest therapeutic interventions that offer support with identified problems, cognitive therapies to minimize functional impairment, family interventions to improve coping, and involvement with the schools to reduce the possibility of failure. Some controversy exists as to the benefit of using pharmaceutical therapy during the prodromal phase. Can providing interventions, including pharmacologic treatments, delay (or even prevent) the onset of psychosis? Minzenberg and associates (2008) stated, "The use of [antipsychotic] medications to treat symptoms that are below the threshold of psychosis has to date been poorly studied" (p. 423).

Phase III: Schizophrenia

In the active phase of the disorder, psychotic symptoms are prominent. Following are the diagnostic criteria for schizophrenia from the *Diagnostic and Statistical Manual of Mental Disorders, Fourth Edition, Text Revision* (DSM-IV-TR) (American Psychiatric Association [APA], 2000):

1. **Characteristic Symptoms:** Two (or more) of the following, each present for a significant portion of time during a 1-month period (or less if successfully treated):
   a. **Delusions**
   b. **Hallucinations**
   c. Disorganized speech (e.g., frequent derailment or incoherence)
   d. Grossly disorganized or **catatonic** behavior
   e. Negative symptoms (i.e., affective flattening, alogia, or avolition)

2. **Social/Occupational Dysfunction:** For a significant portion of the time since the onset of the disturbance, one or more major areas of functioning, such as work, interpersonal relations, or self-care, are markedly below the level achieved before the onset (or, when the onset is in childhood or adolescence, failure to achieve expected level of interpersonal, academic, or occupational achievement).

3. **Duration:** Continuous signs of the disturbance persist for at least 6 months. This 6-month period must include at least 1 month of symptoms (or less if successfully treated) that meet criterion 1 (i.e., active-phase symptoms) and may include periods of prodromal or residual symptoms. During these prodromal or residual periods, the signs of the disturbance may be manifested by only negative symptoms or two or more symptoms listed in criterion 1 present

in an attenuated form (e.g., odd beliefs, unusual perceptual experiences).

4. **Schizoaffective and Mood Disorder Exclusion:** Schizoaffective disorder and mood disorder with psychotic features have been ruled out because (a) no major depressive, manic, or mixed episodes have occurred concurrently with the active-phase symptoms; or (b) if mood episodes have occurred during active-phase symptoms, their total duration has been brief relative to the duration of the active and residual periods.

5. **Substance/General Medical Condition Exclusion:** The disturbance is not due to the direct physiological effects of a substance (e.g., a drug of abuse, a medication) or a general medical condition.

6. **Relationship to a Pervasive Developmental Disorder:** If there is a history of autistic disorder or another pervasive developmental disorder, the additional diagnosis of schizophrenia is made only if prominent delusions or hallucinations are also present for at least 1 month (or less if successfully treated).

Phase IV: Residual Phase

Schizophrenia is characterized by periods of remission and exacerbation. A residual phase usually follows an active phase of the illness. During the residual phase, symptoms of the acute stage are either absent or no longer prominent. Negative symptoms may remain, and flat affect and impairment in role functioning are common. Residual impairment often increases between episodes of active psychosis.

Prognosis

A return to full premorbid functioning is not common (APA, 2000). However, several factors have been associated with a more positive prognosis, including good premorbid adjustment, later age at onset, female gender, abrupt onset of symptoms precipitated by a stressful event (as opposed to gradual insidious onset of symptoms), associated mood disturbance, brief duration of active-phase symptoms, good interepisode functioning, minimal residual symptoms, absence of structural brain abnormalities, normal neurological functioning, a family history of mood disorder, and no family history of schizophrenia (APA, 2000; Black & Andreasen, 2011).

Predisposing Factors

The cause of schizophrenia is still uncertain. Most likely no single factor can be implicated in the etiology; rather, the disease probably results from a combination of influences including biological, psychological, and environmental factors.

Biological Influences

Refer to Chapter 4 for a more thorough review of the biological implications of psychiatric illness.

Genetics

The body of evidence for genetic vulnerability to schizophrenia is growing. Studies show that relatives of individuals with schizophrenia have a much higher probability of developing the disease than does the general population. Whereas the lifetime risk for developing schizophrenia is about 1 percent in most population studies, the siblings or offspring of an identified client have a 10 percent risk of developing schizophrenia, and offspring with one parent who has schizophrenia have a 5 to 6 percent chance of developing the disorder (Black & Andreasen, 2011).

How schizophrenia is inherited is uncertain. No definitive biological marker has as yet been found. Studies are ongoing to determine which genes are important in the vulnerability to schizophrenia, and whether one or many genes are implicated. Some individuals have a strong genetic link to the illness, whereas others may have only a weak genetic basis. This theory gives further credence to the notion of multiple causations.

Twin Studies

The rate of schizophrenia among monozygotic (identical) twins is four times that of dizygotic (fraternal) twins and approximately 50 times that of the general population (Sadock & Sadock, 2007). Identical twins reared apart have the same rate of development of the illness as do those reared together. Because in about half of the cases only one of a pair of monozygotic twins develops schizophrenia, some investigators believe environmental factors interact with genetic ones.

Adoption Studies

In studies conducted by both American and Danish investigators, adopted children born of schizophrenic mothers were compared with adopted children whose mothers had no psychiatric disorder. Children who were born to mothers with schizophrenia were more likely to develop the illness than the comparison control groups (Minzenberg et al., 2008). Studies also indicate that children born to nonschizophrenic parents, but reared by parents afflicted with the illness, do not seem to suffer more often from schizophrenia than general controls. These findings provide additional evidence for the genetic basis of schizophrenia.

Biochemical Influences

The oldest and most thoroughly explored biological theory in the explanation of schizophrenia attributes a pathogenic role to abnormal brain biochemistry. Notions of a "chemical disturbance" as an explanation for insanity were suggested by some theorists as early as the mid-19th century.

The Dopamine Hypothesis

This theory suggests that schizophrenia (or schizophrenia-like symptoms) may be caused by an excess of dopamine-dependent neuronal activity in the brain (Fig. 26–1). This excess activity may be related to increased production or release of the substance at nerve terminals, increased receptor sensitivity, too many dopamine receptors, or a combination of these mechanisms (Sadock & Sadock, 2007).

Pharmacological support for this hypothesis exists. Amphetamines, which increase levels of dopamine, induce psychotomimetic symptoms. The **neuroleptics** (e.g., chlorpromazine or haloperidol) lower brain levels of dopamine by blocking dopamine receptors, thus reducing the schizophrenic symptoms, including those induced by amphetamines.

Postmortem studies of brains of schizophrenic individuals have reported a significant increase in the average number of dopamine receptors in approximately two thirds of the brains studied. This suggests that an increased dopamine response may not be important in *all* schizophrenic clients. Clients with acute manifestations (e.g., delusions and hallucinations) respond with greater efficacy to neuroleptic drugs than do clients with chronic manifestations (e.g., apathy, poverty of ideas, and loss of drive). The current position, in terms of the dopamine hypothesis, is that manifestations of acute schizophrenia may be related to increased numbers of dopamine receptors in the brain and respond to neuroleptic drugs that block these receptors. Manifestations of chronic schizophrenia are probably unrelated to numbers of dopamine receptors, and neuroleptic drugs are unlikely to be as effective in treating these chronic symptoms.

Other Biochemical Hypotheses

Various other biochemicals have been implicated in the predisposition to schizophrenia. Abnormalities in the neurotransmitters norepinephrine, serotonin, acetylcholine, and gamma-aminobutyric acid and in the neuroregulators, such as prostaglandins and endorphins, have been suggested.

Physiological Influences

A number of physical factors of possible etiological significance have been identified in the medical literature. However, their specific mechanisms in the implication of schizophrenia are unclear.

Viral Infection

Sadock and Sadock (2007) reported that epidemiological data indicate a high incidence of schizophrenia after prenatal exposure to influenza. They stated:

> Other data supporting a viral hypothesis are an increased number of physical anomalies at birth, an increased rate of pregnancy and birth complications, seasonality of birth consistent with viral infection, geographical clusters of adult cases, and seasonality of hospitalizations. (p. 469)

Another study found an association between viral infections of the central nervous system during childhood and adult-onset schizophrenia (Rantakallio, Jones, Moring, & VonWendt, 1997).

Anatomical Abnormalities

With the use of neuroimaging technologies, structural brain abnormalities have been observed in individuals with schizophrenia. Ventricular enlargement is the most consistent finding; however, sulci enlargement and cerebellar atrophy are also reported. Black and Andreasen (2011) suggested that "ventricular enlargement is associated with poor premorbid functioning, negative symptoms, poor response to treatment, and cognitive impairment" (p. 122).

Magnetic resonance imaging (MRI) provides a greater ability to image in multiple planes. Studies with MRI have revealed a possible decrease in cerebral and intracranial size in clients with schizophrenia. Studies have also revealed a decrease in frontal lobe size, but this has been less consistently replicated. MRI has been used to explore possible abnormalities in specific subregions such as the amygdala, hippocampus, temporal lobes, and basal ganglia in the brains of people with schizophrenia.

Histological Changes

Cerebral changes in schizophrenia have also been studied at the microscopic level. A "disordering" or disarray of the pyramidal cells in the area of the hippocampus has been suggested (Jonsson, Luts, Guldberg-Kjaer, & Brun, 1997). This disarray of cells has been compared to the normal alignment of the cells in the brains of clients without the disorder. Some researchers have hypothesized that this alteration in hippocampal cells occurs during the second trimester of pregnancy and may be related to an influenza virus encountered by the mother during this period. Further research is required to determine the possible link between this birth defect and the development of schizophrenia.

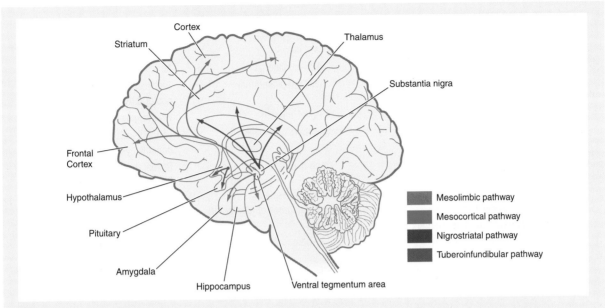

FIGURE 26–1 Neurobiology of schizophrenia.

Neurotransmitters

A number of neurotransmitters have been implicated in the etiology of schizophrenia. These include dopamine, norepinephrine, serotonin, glutamate, and gamma-aminobutyric acid (GABA). The dopaminergic system has been most widely studied and closely linked to the symptoms associated with the disease.

Areas of the Brain Affected

Four major dopaminergic pathways have been identified:
- *Mesolimbic pathway:* originates in the ventral tegmentum area and projects to areas of the limbic system, including the nucleus accumbens, amygdala, and hippocampus. The mesolimbic pathway is associated with functions of memory, emotion, arousal, and pleasure. Excess activity in the mesolimbic tract has been implicated in the positive symptoms of schizophrenia (e.g., hallucinations, delusions).
- *Mesocortical pathway:* originates in the ventral tegmentum area and has projections into the cortex. The mesocortical pathway is concerned with cognition, social behavior, planning, problem solving, motivation, and reinforcement in learning. Negative symptoms of schizophrenia (e.g., flat affect, apathy, lack of motivation, and anhedonia) have been associated with diminished activity in the mesocortical tract.
- *Nigrostriatal pathway:* originates in the substantia nigra and terminates in the striatum of the basal ganglia. This pathway is associated with the function of motor control. Degeneration in this pathway is associated with Parkinson's disease and involuntary psychomotor symptoms of schizophrenia.
- *Tuberoinfundibular pathway:* originates in the hypothalamus and projects to the pituitary gland. It is associated with endocrine function, digestion, metabolism, hunger, thirst, temperature control, and sexual arousal. Implicated in certain endocrine abnormalities associated with schizophrenia.

Two major groups of dopamine receptors and their highest tissue locations include:
- The D_1 Family:

  D_1 receptors: basal ganglia, nucleus accumbens, and cerebral cortex

  D_5 receptors: hippocampus and hypothalamus, with lower concentrations in the cerebral cortex and basal ganglia

- The D_2 Family:

  D_2 receptors: basal ganglia, anterior pituitary, cerebral cortex, limbic structures

  D_3 receptors: limbic regions, with lower concentrations in basal ganglia

  D_4 receptors: frontal cortex, hippocampus, amygdala

ANTIPSYCHOTIC MEDICATIONS

Type	Receptor Affinity	Associated Side Effects
Conventional (typical) antipsychotics: Phenothiazines, haloperidol Provide relief of psychosis, improvement	Strong D_2 (dopamine)	Extrapyramidal symptoms (EPS), hyperprolactinemia, neuroleptic malignant syndrome

Continued

ANTIPSYCHOTIC MEDICATIONS—cont'd

Type	Receptor Affinity	Associated Side Effects
in positive symptoms, worsening of negative symptoms.	Varying degrees of affinity for:	
	ACh (cholinergic)	Anticholinergic effects
	α_1 (norepinephrine)	Tachycardia, tremors, insomnia, postural hypotension
	H_1 (histamine)	Weight gain, sedation
	Weak 5-HT (serotonin)	Low potential for ejaculatory difficulty
Novel (atypical) antipsychotics: Clozapine, olanzapine, quetiapine, aripiprazole, risperidone, iloperidone, ziprasidone, paliperidone, asenapine, lurasidone	Strong 5-HT	Sexual dysfunction, GI disturbance, headache
	Low to moderate D_2	Low potential for EPS
	Varying degrees of affinity for:	
Provide relief of psychosis, improvement in positive symptoms, improvement in negative symptoms.	ACh	Anticholinergic effects
	α-adrenergic	Tachycardia, tremors, insomnia, postural hypotension
	H_1	Weight gain, sedation

Physical Conditions

Some studies have reported a link between schizophrenia and epilepsy (particularly temporal lobe), Huntington's disease, birth trauma, head injury in adulthood, alcohol abuse, cerebral tumor (particularly in the limbic system), cerebrovascular accidents, systemic lupus erythematosus, myxedema, parkinsonism, and Wilson's disease.

Psychological Influences

Early conceptualizations of schizophrenia focused on family relationship factors as major influences in the development of the illness, probably in light of the conspicuous absence of information related to a biological connection. These early theories implicated poor parent-child relationships and dysfunctional family systems as the cause of schizophrenia, but they no longer hold any credibility. Researchers now focus their studies in terms of schizophrenia as a brain disorder. Nevertheless, Sadock and Sadock (2007) stated:

> Clinicians should consider both the psychosocial and biological factors affecting schizophrenia. The disorder affects individual patients, each of whom has a unique psychological makeup. Although many psychodynamic theories about the pathogenesis of schizophrenia seem outdated, perceptive clinical observations can help contemporary clinicians understand how the disease may affect a patient's psyche. (p. 474)

Environmental Influences

Sociocultural Factors

Many studies have been conducted that have attempted to link schizophrenia to social class.

Indeed, epidemiological statistics have shown that greater numbers of individuals from the lower socioeconomic classes experience symptoms associated with schizophrenia than do those from the higher socioeconomic groups (Ho, Black, & Andreasen, 2003). Explanations for this occurrence include the conditions associated with living in poverty, such as congested housing accommodations, inadequate nutrition, absence of prenatal care, few resources for dealing with stressful situations, and feelings of hopelessness for changing one's lifestyle of poverty.

An alternative view is that of the *downward drift hypothesis,* which suggests that, because of the characteristic symptoms of the disorder, individuals with schizophrenia have difficulty maintaining gainful employment and "drift down" to a lower socioeconomic level (or fail to rise out of a lower socioeconomic group). Proponents of this view consider poor social conditions to be a consequence rather than a cause of schizophrenia.

Stressful Life Events

Studies have been conducted in an effort to determine whether psychotic episodes may be precipitated by stressful life events. There is no scientific evidence to indicate that stress causes schizophrenia. It is very probable, however, that stress may contribute to the severity and course of the illness. It is known that extreme stress can precipitate psychotic episodes. Stress may indeed precipitate symptoms in an individual who possesses a genetic vulnerability to schizophrenia.

Stressful life events also may be associated with exacerbation of schizophrenic symptoms and increased rates of relapse.

The Transactional Model

The etiology of schizophrenia remains unclear. No single theory or hypothesis has been postulated that substantiates a clear-cut explanation for the disease. Indeed, it seems the more research that is conducted, the more evidence is compiled to support the concept of multiple causation in the development of schizophrenia. The most current theory seems to be that schizophrenia is a biologically based disease, the onset of which is influenced by factors within the environment (either internal or external). The dynamics of schizophrenia using the Transactional Model of Stress/Adaptation are presented in Figure 26–2.

Types of Schizophrenia and Other Psychotic Disorders

The *DSM-IV-TR* (APA, 2000) identifies various types of schizophrenia and other psychotic disorders. Differential diagnosis is made according to the total symptomatic clinical picture presented.

Disorganized Schizophrenia

This type previously was called *hebephrenic schizophrenia*. Onset of symptoms is usually before age 25, and the course is commonly chronic. Behavior is markedly regressive and primitive. Contact with reality is extremely poor. Affect is flat or grossly inappropriate, often with periods of silliness and incongruous giggling. Facial grimaces and bizarre mannerisms are common, and communication is consistently incoherent. Personal appearance is generally neglected, and social impairment is extreme.

Catatonic Schizophrenia

Catatonic schizophrenia is characterized by marked abnormalities in motor behavior and may be manifested in the form of *stupor* or *excitement*.

Catatonic stupor is characterized by extreme psychomotor retardation. The individual exhibits a pronounced decrease in spontaneous movements and activity. Mutism (i.e., absence of speech) is common, and negativism (i.e., an apparently motiveless resistance to all instructions or attempts to be moved) may be evident. **Waxy flexibility** may be exhibited. This term describes a type of "posturing," or voluntary assumption of bizarre positions, in which the individual may remain for long periods. Efforts to move the individual may be met with rigid bodily resistance.

Catatonic excitement is manifested by a state of extreme psychomotor agitation. The movements are frenzied and purposeless, and are usually accompanied by continuous incoherent verbalizations and shouting. Clients in catatonic excitement urgently require physical and medical control because they are often destructive and violent toward others, and their excitement may cause them to injure themselves or to collapse from complete exhaustion.

This type of schizophrenia, which was relatively common in the past, has become quite rare since the advent of antipsychotic medications for use in psychiatry.

Paranoid Schizophrenia

Paranoid schizophrenia is characterized mainly by the presence of delusions of persecution or grandeur and auditory hallucinations related to a single theme. The individual is often tense, suspicious, and guarded, and may be argumentative, hostile, and aggressive. Onset of symptoms is usually later (perhaps in the late 20s or 30s), and less regression of mental faculties, emotional response, and behavior is seen than in the other subtypes of schizophrenia. Social impairment may be minimal, and there is some evidence that prognosis, particularly with regard to occupational functioning and capacity for independent living, is promising (APA, 2000).

Undifferentiated Schizophrenia

Sometimes clients with schizophrenic symptoms do not meet the criteria for any of the subtypes, or they may meet the criteria for more than one subtype. These individuals may be given the diagnosis of undifferentiated schizophrenia. The behavior is clearly psychotic; that is, there is evidence of delusions, hallucinations, incoherence, and bizarre behavior. However, the symptoms cannot be easily classified into any of the previously listed diagnostic categories.

Residual Schizophrenia

This diagnostic category is used when the individual has a history of at least one previous episode of schizophrenia with prominent psychotic symptoms. Residual schizophrenia occurs in an individual who has a chronic form of the disease and is the stage that follows an acute episode (prominent delusions, hallucinations, incoherence, bizarre behavior, and violence). In the residual stage, there is continuing evidence of the illness, although there are no prominent psychotic symptoms. Residual symptoms may include social isolation, eccentric behavior, impairment in personal hygiene and grooming, blunted or inappropriate affect,

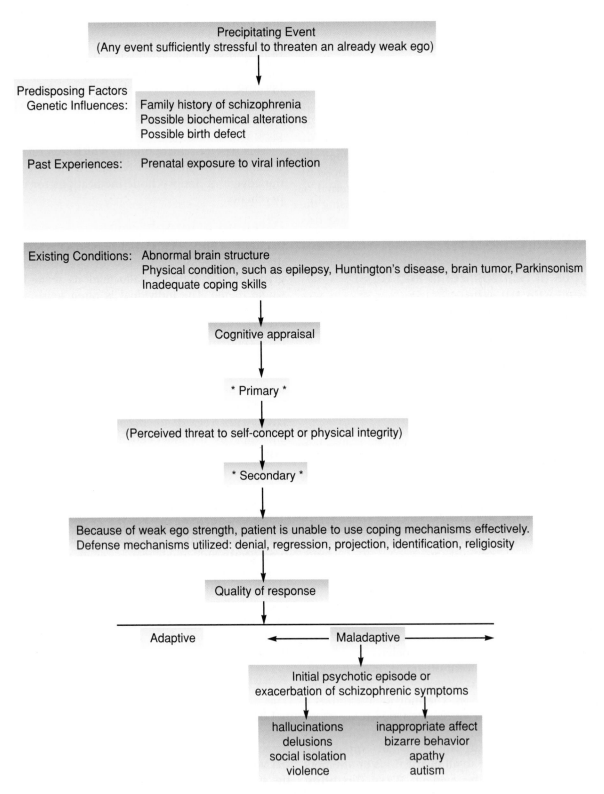

FIGURE 26–2 The dynamics of schizophrenia using the Transactional Model of Stress/Adaptation.

poverty of or overly elaborate speech, illogical thinking, and apathy.

Schizoaffective Disorder

This disorder is manifested by schizophrenic behaviors, with a strong element of symptomatology associated with the mood disorders (depression or mania). The client may appear depressed, with psychomotor retardation and suicidal ideation, or symptoms may include euphoria, grandiosity, and hyperactivity. However, the decisive factor in the diagnosis of schizoaffective disorder is the presence of characteristic schizophrenic symptoms. For example, in addition to the dysfunctional mood, the individual exhibits bizarre delusions, prominent hallucinations, incoherent speech, catatonic behavior, or blunted or inappropriate affect. The prognosis for schizoaffective disorder is generally better than that for other schizophrenic disorders but worse than that for mood disorders alone (Black & Andreasen, 2011).

Brief Psychotic Disorder

The essential feature of this disorder is the sudden onset of psychotic symptoms that may or may not be preceded by a severe psychosocial stressor. These symptoms last at least 1 day but less than 1 month, and there is an eventual full return to the premorbid level of functioning (APA, 2000). The individual experiences emotional turmoil or overwhelming perplexity or confusion. Evidence of impaired reality testing may include incoherent speech, delusions, hallucinations, bizarre behavior, and disorientation. Individuals with preexisting personality disorders (most commonly, histrionic, narcissistic, paranoid, schizotypal, and borderline personality disorders) appear to be susceptible to this disorder (Sadock & Sadock, 2007).

Schizophreniform Disorder

The essential features of this disorder are identical to those of schizophrenia, with the exception that the duration, including prodromal, active, and residual phases, is at least 1 month but less than 6 months (APA, 2000). If the diagnosis is made while the individual is still symptomatic but has been so for less than 6 months, it is qualified as "provisional." The diagnosis is changed to schizophrenia if the clinical picture persists beyond 6 months. Schizophreniform disorder is thought to have a good prognosis if the individual's affect is not blunted or flat, if there is a rapid onset of psychotic symptoms from the time the unusual behavior is noticed, or if the premorbid social and occupational functioning was satisfactory.

Delusional Disorder

The essential feature of this disorder is the presence of one or more nonbizarre delusions that persist for at least 1 month (APA, 2000). If present at all, hallucinations are not prominent, and apart from the delusions, behavior is not bizarre. The subtype of delusional disorder is based on the predominant delusional theme.

Erotomanic Type

With this type of delusion, the individual believes that someone, usually of a higher status, is in love with him or her. Famous persons are often the subjects of erotomanic delusions. Sometimes the delusion is kept secret, but some individuals may follow, contact, or otherwise try to pursue the object of their delusion.

Grandiose Type

Individuals with grandiose delusions have irrational ideas regarding their own worth, talent, knowledge, or power. They may believe that they have a special relationship with a famous person, or even assume the identity of a famous person (believing that the actual person is an imposter). Grandiose delusions of a religious nature may lead to assumption of the identity of a deity or religious leader.

Jealous Type

The content of jealous delusions centers on the idea that the person's sexual partner is unfaithful. The idea is irrational and without cause, but the individual with the delusion searches for evidence to justify the belief. The sexual partner is confronted (and sometimes physically attacked) regarding the imagined infidelity. The imagined "lover" of the sexual partner may also be the object of the attack. Attempts to restrict the autonomy of the sexual partner in an effort to stop the imagined infidelity are common.

Persecutory Type

In persecutory delusions, which are the most common type, individuals believe they are being malevolently treated in some way. Frequent themes include being conspired against, cheated, spied on, followed, poisoned or drugged, maliciously maligned, harassed, or obstructed in the pursuit of long-term goals (APA, 2000). The individual may obsess about and exaggerate a slight rebuff (either real or imagined) until it becomes the focus of a delusional system. Repeated complaints may be directed at legal authorities, lack of satisfaction from which may result in violence toward the object of the delusion.

Somatic Type

Individuals with somatic delusions believe they have some physical defect, disorder, or disease. The *DSM-IV-TR* (APA, 2000) identifies the most common types of somatic delusions as those in which the individual believes that he or she:

■ Emits a foul odor from the skin, mouth, rectum, or vagina

■ Has an infestation of insects in or on the skin

■ Has an internal parasite

■ Has misshapen and ugly body parts

■ Has dysfunctional body parts

Shared Psychotic Disorder

The essential feature of this disorder, also called *folie à deux,* is a delusional system that develops in a second person as a result of a close relationship with another person who already has a psychotic disorder with prominent delusions (APA, 2000). The person with the primary delusional disorder is usually the dominant person in the relationship, and the delusional thinking is gradually imposed on the more passive partner. This occurs within the context of a long-term close relationship, particularly when the couple has been socially isolated from other people. The course is usually chronic, and is more common in women than in men.

Psychotic Disorder Due to a General Medical Condition

The essential features of this disorder are prominent hallucinations and delusions that can be directly attributed to a general medical condition (APA, 2000). The diagnosis is not made if the symptoms occur during the course of a delirium or chronic, progressing dementia. A number of medical conditions can cause psychotic symptoms. Common ones identified by the *DSM-IV-TR* (APA, 2000) are presented in Table 26-1.

Substance-Induced Psychotic Disorder

The essential features of this disorder are the presence of prominent hallucinations and delusions that are judged to be directly attributable to the physiological effects of a substance (i.e., a drug of abuse, a medication, or toxin exposure) (APA, 2000). The diagnosis is made in the absence of reality testing and when history, physical examination, or laboratory findings indicate use of substances. When reality testing has been retained in the presence of substance-induced psychotic symptoms, the diagnosis would be substance-related disorder (Sadock & Sadock, 2007). Substances

TABLE 26-1 General Medical Conditions That May Cause Psychotic Symptoms	
Neurological conditions	Neoplasms
	Cerebrovascular disease
	Huntington's disease
	Epilepsy
	Auditory nerve injury
	Deafness
	Migraine headache
	CNS infections
Endocrine conditions	Hyperthyroidism
	Hypothyroidism
	Hyperparathyroidism
	Hypoparathyroidism
	Hypoadrenocorticism
Metabolic conditions	Hypoxia
	Hypercarbia
	Hypoglycemia
Autoimmune disorders	Systemic lupus erythematosus
Others	Fluid or electrolyte imbalances
	Hepatic or renal diseases

identified by the *DSM-IV-TR* (APA, 2000) that are believed to induce psychotic disorders are presented in Table 26-2.

Application of the Nursing Process

Background Assessment Data

In the first step of the nursing process, the nurse gathers a database from which nursing diagnoses are derived and a plan of care is formulated. This first step of the nursing process is extremely important because without an accurate assessment, problem identification, objectives of care, and outcome criteria cannot be accurately determined.

Assessment of the client with schizophrenia may be a complex process, based on information gathered from a number of sources. Clients in an acute episode of their illness are seldom able to make a significant contribution to their history. Data may be obtained from family members, if possible; from old records, if available; or from other individuals who have been in a position to report on the progression of the client's behavior.

The nurse must be familiar with behaviors common to the disorder to be able to obtain an

TABLE 26-2	Substances That May Cause Psychotic Disorders
Drugs of abuse	Alcohol
	Amphetamines and related substances
	Cannabis
	Cocaine
	Hallucinogens
	Inhalants
	Opioids
	Phencyclidine and related substances
	Sedatives, hypnotics, and anxiolytics
Medications	Anesthetics and analgesics
	Anticholinergic agents
	Anticonvulsants
	Antidepressant medication
	Antihistamines
	Antihypertensive agents
	Antimicrobial medications
	Antiparkinsonian agents
	Cardiovascular medications
	Chemotherapeutic agents
	Corticosteroids
	Disulfiram
	Gastrointestinal medications
	Muscle relaxants
	Nonsteroidal anti-inflammatory agents
Toxins	Anticholinesterase
	Carbon monoxide
	Carbon dioxide
	Nerve gases
	Organophosphate insecticides
	Volatile substances (e.g., fuel or paint)

adequate assessment of the client with schizophrenia. Symptoms of schizophrenia are commonly described as positive or negative. Positive symptoms tend to reflect an excess or distortion of normal functions, whereas negative symptoms reflect a diminution or loss of normal functions (APA, 2000). Most clients exhibit a mixture of both types of symptoms.

Positive symptoms are associated with normal brain structures on computed tomography (CT) scan and relatively good responses to treatment. Regarding negative symptoms, Ho and associated (2003) stated, "Not only are [they] difficult to treat and respond less well to neuroleptics than positive symptoms, but they are also the most destructive because they render the patient inert and unmotivated" (p. 386).

Behavioral disturbances are categorized as positive or negative and considered in eight areas of functioning: content of thought, form of thought, perception, affect, sense of self, volition, impaired interpersonal functioning and relationship to the external world, and psychomotor behavior. A summary of positive and negative symptoms is presented in Box 26-1. Additional impairments outside the limits of these eight areas are also presented.

Positive Symptoms

Content of Thought

Delusions Delusions are false personal beliefs that are inconsistent with the person's intelligence or cultural background. The individual continues to have the belief in spite of obvious proof that it is false or irrational. Delusions are subdivided according to their content. Some of the more common ones are listed here.

■ **Delusion of Persecution.** The individual feels threatened and believes that others intend harm or persecution toward him or her in some way (e.g., "The FBI has 'bugged' my room and intends to kill me." "I can't take a shower in this bathroom; the nurses have put a camera in there so that they can watch everything I do.").

■ **Delusion of Grandeur.** The individual has an exaggerated feeling of importance, power, knowledge, or identity (e.g., "I am Jesus Christ").

■ **Delusion of Reference.** All events within the environment are referred by the psychotic person to him- or herself (e.g., "Someone is trying to get a message to me through the articles in this magazine [or newspaper or TV program]; I must break the code so that I can receive the message."). *Ideas* of reference are less rigid than delusions of reference. An example of an idea of reference is irrationally thinking that one is being talked about or laughed at by other people.

■ **Delusion of Control or Influence.** The individual believes certain objects or persons have control over his or her behavior (e.g., "The

BOX 26-1 Positive and Negative Symptoms of Schizophrenia

POSITIVE SYMPTOMS

Content of Thought

Delusions
Religiosity
Paranoia
Magical thinking

Form of Thought

Associative looseness
Neologisms
Concrete thinking
Clang associations
Word salad
Circumstantiality
Tangentiality
Mutism
Perseveration

Perception

Hallucinations
Illusions

Sense of Self

Echolalia
Echopraxia
Identification and imitation
Depersonalization

NEGATIVE SYMPTOMS

Affect

Inappropriate affect
Bland or flat affect
Apathy

Volition

Inability to initiate goal-directed activity
Emotional ambivalence

Impaired Interpersonal Functioning and Relationship to the External World

Autism
Deteriorated appearance

Psychomotor Behavior

Anergia
Waxy flexibility
Posturing
Pacing and rocking

Associated Features

Anhedonia
Regression

---

dentist put a filling in my tooth; I now receive transmissions through the filling that control what I think and do.").

- **Somatic Delusion.** The individual has a false idea about the functioning of his or her body (e.g., "I'm 70 years old and I will be the oldest person ever to give birth. The doctor says I'm not pregnant, but I know I am.").

- **Nihilistic Delusion.** The individual has a false idea that the self, a part of the self, others, or the world is nonexistent (e.g., "The world no longer exists." "I have no heart.").

Religiosity **Religiosity** is an excessive demonstration of or obsession with religious ideas and behavior. Because individuals vary greatly in their religious beliefs and level of spiritual commitment, religiosity is often difficult to assess. The individual with schizophrenia may use religious ideas in an attempt to provide rational meaning and structure to his or her behavior. Religious preoccupation in this vein may therefore be considered a manifestation of

the illness. However, clients who derive comfort from their religious beliefs should not be discouraged from employing this means of support. An example of religiosity is the individual who believes the voice he or she hears is God and incessantly searches the Bible for interpretation.

Paranoia Individuals with **paranoia** have extreme suspiciousness of others and of their actions or perceived intentions (e.g., "I won't eat this food. I know it has been poisoned.").

Magical Thinking With **magical thinking**, the person believes that his or her thoughts or behaviors have control over specific situations or people (e.g., the mother who believed that, if she scolded her son in any way, he would be taken away from her). Magical thinking is common in children (e.g., "It's raining; the sky is sad." "It snowed last night because I wished very, very hard that it would.").

Form of Thought

Associative Looseness Thinking is characterized by speech in which ideas shift from one unrelated subject to another. With **associative looseness,** the individual is unaware that the topics are unconnected. When the condition is severe, speech may be incoherent (e.g., "We wanted to take the bus, but the airport took all the traffic. Driving is the ticket when you want to get somewhere. No one needs a ticket to heaven. We have it all in our pockets.")

Neologisms The psychotic person invents new words, or **neologisms,** that are meaningless to others but have symbolic meaning to the psychotic person (e.g., "She wanted to give me a ride in her new *uniphorum*.").

Concrete Thinking Concreteness, or literal interpretations of the environment, represents a regression to an earlier level of cognitive development. Abstract thinking is very difficult. For example, the client with schizophrenia would have great difficulty describing the abstract meaning of sayings such as "I'm climbing the walls," or "It's raining cats and dogs."

Clang Associations Choice of words is governed by sounds. **Clang associations** often take the form of rhyming, for instance "It is very cold. I am cold and bold. The gold has been sold."

Word Salad A **word salad** is a group of words that are put together randomly, without any logical connection (e.g., "Most forward action grows life double plays circle uniform.").

Circumstantiality With **circumstantiality,** the individual delays in reaching the point of a communication because of unnecessary and tedious details. The point or goal is usually met but only with numerous interruptions by the interviewer to keep the person on track of the topic being discussed.

Tangentiality **Tangentiality** differs from circumstantiality in that the person never really gets to the point of the communication. Unrelated topics are introduced, and the focus of the original discussion is lost.

Mutism Mutism is an individual's inability or refusal to speak.

Perseveration The individual who exhibits **perseveration** persistently repeats the same word or idea in response to different questions.

Perception

Hallucinations Hallucinations, or false sensory perceptions not associated with real external stimuli, may involve any of the five senses. Types of hallucinations include the following:

- **Auditory.** Auditory hallucinations are false perceptions of sound. Most commonly they are of voices, but the individual may report clicks, rushing noises, music, and other noises. Command hallucinations may place the individual or others in a potentially dangerous situation. "Voices" that issue commands for violence to self or others may or may not be heeded by the psychotic person. Auditory hallucinations are the most common type in psychiatric disorders.

- **Visual.** These are false visual perceptions. They may consist of formed images, such as of people, or of unformed images, such as flashes of light.

- **Tactile.** Tactile hallucinations are false perceptions of the sense of touch, often of something on or under the skin. One specific tactile hallucination is formication, the sensation that something is crawling on or under the skin.

- **Gustatory.** This type is a false perception of taste. Most commonly, gustatory hallucinations are described as unpleasant tastes.

- **Olfactory.** Olfactory hallucinations are false perceptions of the sense of smell.

IMPLICATIONS OF RESEARCH FOR EVIDENCE-BASED PRACTICE

Trygstad, L., Buccheri, R., Dowling, G., Zin, R., White, K., Griffin, J. J., et al. (2002). Behavioral management of persistent auditory hallucinations in schizophrenia: Outcomes from a 10-week course. *Journal of the American Psychiatric Nurses Association, 8*(3), 84–91.

DESCRIPTION OF THE STUDY: The purpose of this study was to examine the effects of a 10-week course in which behavior management strategies were taught to participants with schizophrenia who experienced persistent auditory hallucinations. The primary aim was to examine the effects of the intervention on seven specific characteristics of auditory hallucinations: frequency, loudness, self-control, clarity, tone, distractibility, and distress. The secondary aim was to examine level of anxiety and depression. The sample consisted of 62 subjects who had been diagnosed with schizophrenia by a board-certified psychiatrist using *DSM-IV* diagnostic criteria. They all reported having persistent auditory hallucinations for at least 10 minutes a day for the past 3 months; reported a desire to learn new strategies to manage their auditory hallucinations; were taking stable doses of antipsychotic medication for at least 4 weeks

Continued

IMPLICATIONS OF RESEARCH FOR EVIDENCE-BASED PRACTICE—cont'd

before entry into the study; were able to read and write in English; and did not have a severe cognitive deficit. The 10-week course was taught in nine different outpatient settings by nurses who had experience caring for patients with schizophrenia and were knowledgeable in group facilitation skills. In each class, participants were taught and practiced one behavior strategy. The following strategies were taught in the course: self-monitoring, talking with someone, listening to music with or without earphones, watching television, saying "stop"/ignoring what the voices say to do, using ear plugs, learning relaxation techniques, keeping busy with an enjoyable activity and/or helping others, and practicing communication related to taking medication and not using drugs and alcohol. Measurement of the outcomes was based on subjects' scores on the Characteristics of Auditory Hallucinations Questionnaire (CAHQ), the Profile of Mood States (POMS) scale, and the Beck Depression Inventory, second edition (BDI-II).

RESULTS OF THE STUDY: The outcome of this study strongly supported the expectation that subjects who attended the behavior-management strategy classes for auditory hallucinations would experience improvement in the characteristics of their auditory hallucinations and have less anxiety and depression. Postintervention scores on the POMS and BDI-II were significantly lower than preintervention scores, indicating an overall decrease in anxiety and depression.

Postintervention mean scores on the CAHQ were significantly lower than preintervention mean scores on all hallucination characteristics, with the exception of loudness, which did not change significantly. In a 5-point self-report rating helpfulness of the course, 25% of the participants reported that the course was *extremely helpful,* 42% reported that it was *helpful,* 23% *moderately helpful,* 8% *minimally helpful,* and 2% *not helpful.*

IMPLICATIONS FOR NURSING PRACTICE: This study shows that individuals can manage their auditory hallucinations by learning and using specific behavioral strategies. The group setting also proved to be beneficial, as clients were able to have their own experiences validated, to see that others had similar experiences, and to learn how others managed them. They gained encouragement and hope from learning that certain strategies were effective for others in the group. The authors stated, "This low cost, low-tech intervention could be incorporated into the practice of psychiatric nurses or other mental health professionals who have group training and experience facilitating groups with people who have schizophrenia. Teaching behavior management of persistent auditory hallucinations to clients who wish to learn has minimal risks and could be easily incorporated into existing outpatient programs." (p. 90)

Illusions **Illusions** are misperceptions or misinterpretations of real external stimuli.

Sense of Self

Sense of self describes the uniqueness and individuality a person feels. Because of extremely weak ego boundaries, the individual with schizophrenia lacks this feeling of uniqueness and experiences a great deal of confusion regarding his or her identity.

Echolalia The client with schizophrenia may repeat words that he or she hears, which is called **echolalia.** This is an attempt to identify with the person speaking. (For instance, the nurse says, "John, it's time for lunch." The client may respond, "It's time for lunch, it's time for lunch." or sometimes, "Lunch, lunch, lunch, lunch.").

Echopraxia The client who exhibits **echopraxia** may purposelessly imitate movements made by others.

Identification and Imitation Identification, which occurs on an unconscious level, and imitation, which occurs on a conscious level, are ego defense mechanisms used by individuals with schizophrenia

and reflect their confusion regarding self-identity. Because they have difficulty knowing where their ego boundaries end and another person's begin, their behavior often takes on the form of that which they see in the other person.

Depersonalization The unstable self-identity of an individual with schizophrenia may lead to feelings of unreality (e.g., feeling that one's extremities have changed in size; or a sense of seeing oneself from a distance).

Negative Symptoms

Affect

Affect describes the behavior associated with an individual's feeling state or emotional tone.

Inappropriate Affect Affect is inappropriate when the individual's emotional tone is incongruent with the circumstances (e.g., a young woman who laughs when told of the death of her mother).

Bland or Flat Affect Affect is described as bland when the emotional tone is very weak. The individual with flat affect appears to be void of emotional tone (or overt expression of feelings).

Apathy The client with schizophrenia often demonstrates an indifference to or disinterest in the environment. The bland or flat affect is a manifestation of the emotional apathy.

Volition

Impaired volition has to do with the inability to initiate goal-directed activity. In the individual with schizophrenia, this may take the form of inadequate interest, motivation, or ability to choose a logical course of action in a given situation.

Emotional Ambivalence Ambivalence in the client with schizophrenia refers to the coexistence of opposite emotions toward the same object, person, or situation. These opposing emotions may interfere with the person's ability to make even a very simple decision (e.g., whether to have coffee or tea with lunch). Underlying the ambivalence is the difficulty the client with schizophrenia has in fulfilling a satisfying human relationship. This difficulty is based on the *need-fear dilemma*—the simultaneous need for and fear of intimacy.

Impaired Interpersonal Functioning and Relationship to the External World

Some clients with acute schizophrenia cling to others and intrude on the personal space of others, exhibiting behaviors that are not socially and culturally acceptable. Impairment in social functioning may also be reflected in social isolation, emotional detachment, and lack of regard for social convention.

Autism **Autism** describes the condition created by the person with schizophrenia who focuses inward on a fantasy world, while distorting or excluding the external environment.

Deteriorated Appearance Personal grooming and self-care activities may be neglected. The client with schizophrenia may appear disheveled and untidy and may need to be reminded of the need for personal hygiene.

Psychomotor Behavior

Anergia Anergia is a deficiency of energy. The individual with schizophrenia may lack sufficient energy to carry out activities of daily living or to interact with others.

Waxy Flexibility Waxy flexibility describes a condition in which the client with schizophrenia allows body parts to be placed in bizarre or uncomfortable positions. Once placed in position, the arm, leg, or head remains in that position for long periods, regardless of how uncomfortable it is for the client. For example, the nurse may position the client's arm in an outward position to take a blood pressure measurement. When the cuff is removed, the client may maintain the arm in the position in which it was placed to take the reading.

Posturing This symptom is manifested by the voluntary assumption of inappropriate or bizarre postures.

Pacing and Rocking Pacing back and forth and body rocking (a slow, rhythmic, backward-and-forward swaying of the trunk from the hips, usually while sitting) are common psychomotor behaviors of the client with schizophrenia.

Associated Features

Anhedonia **Anhedonia** is the inability to experience pleasure. This is a particularly distressing symptom that compels some clients to attempt suicide.

Regression Regression is the retreat to an earlier level of development. Regression, a primary defense mechanism of schizophrenia, is a dysfunctional attempt to reduce anxiety. It provides the basis for many of the behaviors associated with schizophrenia.

Diagnosis/Outcome Identification

Using information collected during the assessment, the nurse completes the client database, from which the selection of appropriate nursing diagnoses is determined. Table 26-3 presents a list of client behaviors and the NANDA nursing diagnoses that correspond to those behaviors, which may be used in planning care for clients with psychotic disorders.

Outcome Criteria

The following criteria may be used for measurement of outcomes in the care of the client with schizophrenia.

The client:

■ Demonstrates an ability to relate satisfactorily with others.

■ Recognizes distortions of reality.

■ Has not harmed self or others.

■ Perceives self realistically.

■ Demonstrates the ability to perceive the environment correctly.

■ Maintains anxiety at a manageable level.

■ Relinquishes the need for delusions and hallucinations.

TABLE 26-3 Assigning Nursing Diagnoses to Behaviors Commonly Associated with Psychotic Disorders

BEHAVIORS	NURSING DIAGNOSES
Impaired communication (inappropriate responses), disordered thought sequencing, rapid mood swings, poor concentration, disorientation, stops talking in midsentence, tilts head to side as if listening	**Disturbed sensory perception**
Delusional thinking; inability to concentrate; impaired volition; inability to problem-solve, abstract, or conceptualize; extreme suspiciousness of others; inaccurate interpretation of the environment	**Disturbed thought processes**
Withdrawal, sad dull affect, need-fear dilemma, preoccupation with own thoughts, expression of feelings of rejection or of aloneness imposed by others, uncommunicative, seeks to be alone	**Social isolation**
Risk factors: Aggressive body language (e.g., clenching fists and jaw, pacing, threatening stance), verbal aggression, catatonic excitement, command hallucinations, rage reactions, history of violence, overt and aggressive acts, goal-directed destruction of objects in the environment, self-destructive behavior, or active aggressive suicidal acts	**Risk for violence: Self-directed or other-directed**
Loose association of ideas, neologisms, word salad, clang associations, echolalia, verbalizations that reflect concrete thinking, poor eye contact, difficulty expressing thoughts verbally, inappropriate verbalization	**Impaired verbal communication**
Difficulty carrying out tasks associated with hygiene, dressing, grooming, eating, and toileting	**Self-care deficit**
Neglectful care of client in regard to basic human needs or illness treatment, extreme denial or prolonged overconcern regarding client's illness, depression, hostility and aggression	**Disabled family coping**
Inability to take responsibility for meeting basic health practices, history of lack of health-seeking behavior, lack of expressed interest in improving health behaviors, demonstrated lack of knowledge regarding basic health practices	**Ineffective health maintenance**
Unsafe, unclean, disorderly home environment; household members express difficulty in maintaining their home in a safe and comfortable condition	**Impaired home maintenance**

■ Demonstrates the ability to trust others.

■ Uses appropriate verbal communication in interactions with others.

■ Performs self-care activities independently.

Planning/Implementation

The following section presents a group of selected nursing diagnoses, with short- and long-term goals and nursing interventions for each.

Some institutions are using a case management model to coordinate care (see Chapter 9 for more detailed explanation). In case management models, the plan of care may take the form of a critical pathway.

Disturbed Thought Processes

Disturbed thought processes is defined as "disruption in cognitive operations and activities" (NANDA International [NANDA-I], 2009, p. 408).

Client Goals

Outcome criteria include short- and long-term goals. Timelines are individually determined.

Short-Term Goal

■ By the end of 2 weeks, client will recognize and verbalize that false ideas occur at times of increased anxiety.

Long-Term Goal

Depending on chronicity of the disease process, choose the most realistic long-term goal for the client:

■ By time of discharge from treatment, client's verbalizations will reflect reality-based thinking with no evidence of delusional ideation.

■ By time of discharge from treatment, the client will be able to differentiate between delusional thinking and reality.

Interventions

■ Convey acceptance of the client's need for the false belief, but indicate that you do not share the belief. The client must understand that you do not view the idea as real.

■ Do not argue or deny the belief. Arguing with the client or denying the belief serves no useful purpose, because delusional ideas are not eliminated by this approach, and the development of a trusting relationship may be impeded.

CLINICAL PEARL 💬

Use *reasonable doubt* as a therapeutic technique: "I understand that you believe this is true, but I personally find it hard to accept."

■ Reinforce and focus on reality. Discourage long ruminations about the irrational thinking. Talk about real events and real people. Discussions that focus on the false ideas are purposeless and useless, and may even aggravate the psychosis.

■ If the client is highly suspicious, the following interventions may be helpful:
- To promote the development of trust, use the same staff as much as possible; be honest and keep all promises.
- Avoid physical contact. Warn the client before touching to perform a procedure, such as taking a blood pressure. Suspicious clients often perceive touch as threatening and may respond in an aggressive or defensive manner.
- Avoid laughing, whispering, or talking quietly where the client can see but cannot hear what is being said.

- Suspicious clients may believe they are being poisoned and refuse to eat food from an individually prepared tray. It may be necessary to provide canned food with a can opener or serve food family style.
- They may believe they are being poisoned with their medication and attempt to discard the tablets or capsules. Mouth checks may be necessary following medication administration to verify whether the client is actually swallowing the pills.
- Competitive activities are very threatening to suspicious clients. Activities that encourage a one-to-one relationship with the nurse or therapist are best.
- Maintain an assertive, matter-of-fact, yet genuine approach with suspicious clients. They do not have the capacity to relate to, and therefore often feel threatened by, a friendly or overly cheerful attitude.

Disturbed Sensory Perception: Auditory/Visual

Disturbed sensory perception is defined as "change in the amount or patterning of incoming stimuli accompanied by a diminished, exaggerated, distorted, or impaired response to such stimuli" (NANDA-I, 2009, p. 163). Table 26-4 presents this nursing diagnosis in care plan format.

Client Goals

Outcome criteria include short- and long-term goals. Timelines are individually determined.

Short-Term Goal

■ Client will discuss content of hallucinations with nurse or therapist within 1 week.

Long-Term Goal

■ Client will be able to define and test reality, reducing or eliminating the occurrence of hallucinations.

This goal may not be realistic for the individual with severe and persistent illness who has experienced auditory hallucinations for many years. A more realistic goal may be:

■ Client will verbalize understanding that the voices are a result of his or her illness and demonstrate ways to interrupt the hallucination.

Interventions

■ Observe the client for signs of hallucinations (listening pose, laughing or talking to self, stopping in mid-sentence). Ask, "Are you hearing the voices again?" Early intervention

Table 26-4 CARE PLAN FOR A CLIENT EXPERIENCING HALLUCINATIONS

NURSING DIAGNOSIS: DISTURBED SENSORY PERCEPTION: AUDITORY/VISUAL
RELATED TO: Panic anxiety, extreme loneliness and withdrawal into the self
EVIDENCED BY: Inappropriate responses, disordered thought sequencing, rapid mood swings, poor concentration, disorientation

OUTCOME CRITERIA	NURSING INTERVENTIONS	RATIONALE
Short-Term Goal • Client will discuss content of hallucinations with nurse or therapist within 1 week. **Long-Term Goal** • Client will be able to define and test reality, reducing or eliminating the occurrence of hallucinations. This goal may not be realistic for the individual with severe and persistent illness who has experienced auditory hallucinations for many years. A more realistic goal may be: • Client will verbalize understanding that the voices are a result of his or her illness and demonstrate ways to interrupt the hallucination.	1. Observe the client for signs of hallucinations (listening pose, laughing or talking to self, stopping in mid-sentence). 2. Avoid touching the client without warning him or her that you are about to do so. 3. An attitude of acceptance will encourage the client to share the content of the hallucination with you. Ask, "What do you hear the voices saying to you?" 4. 💬 Do not reinforce the hallucination. Use "the voices" instead of words such as "they" that imply validation. Let the client know that you do not share the perception. Say, "Even though I realize the voices are real to you, I do not hear any voices speaking." 5. Help the client understand the connection between increased anxiety and the presence of hallucinations. 6. Try to distract the client from the hallucination. 7. For some clients, auditory hallucinations persist after the acute psychotic episode has subsided. Listening to the radio or watching television helps distract some clients from attention to the voices. Others have benefited from an intervention called *voice dismissal*. With this technique, the client is taught to say loudly, "Go away!" or "Leave me alone!" in a conscious effort to dismiss the auditory perception.	1. Early intervention may prevent aggressive response to command hallucinations. 2. The client may perceive touch as threatening and may respond in an aggressive manner. 3. This is important to prevent possible injury to the client or others from command hallucinations. 4. It is important for the nurse to be honest, and the client must accept the perception as unreal before hallucinations can be eliminated. 5. If the client can learn to interrupt escalating anxiety, hallucinations may be prevented. 6. Involvement in interpersonal activities and explanation of the actual situation will help bring the client back to reality. 7. These activities assist the client to exert some conscious control over the hallucination.

may prevent aggressive responses to command hallucinations.

■ Avoid touching the client before warning him or her that you are about to do so. The client may perceive touch as threatening and respond in an aggressive or defensive manner.

■ An attitude of acceptance will encourage the client to share the content of the hallucination with you. Ask, "What do you hear the voices saying to you?" This is important in order to prevent possible injury to the client or others from command hallucinations.

CLINICAL PEARL

Do not reinforce the hallucination. Use "the voices" instead of words like "they" that imply validation. Let the client know that you do not share the perception. Say, "Even though I realize that the voices are real to you, I do not hear any voices speaking." It is important for the nurse to be honest, and the client must accept the perception as unreal before hallucinations can be eliminated.

■ Help the client to understand the connection between increased anxiety and the presence of hallucinations. If the client can learn to interrupt escalating anxiety, hallucinations may be prevented.

■ Try to distract the client from the hallucination. Involvement in interpersonal activities and explanation of the actual situation will help bring the client back to reality.

■ For some clients, auditory hallucinations persist after the acute psychotic episode has subsided. Listening to the radio or watching television helps distract some clients from attention to the voices. Others have benefited from an intervention called *voice dismissal*. With this technique, the client is taught to say loudly, "Go away!" or "Leave me alone!", thereby exerting some conscious control over the behavior.

Risk for Violence: Self-Directed or Other-Directed

Risk for self- or other-directed violence is defined as "at risk for behaviors in which an individual demonstrates that he or she can be physically, emotionally, and/or sexually harmful either to self or to others" (NANDA-I, 2009, pp. 332–333).

NOTE: Please refer to Chapter 17 for additional concepts related to anger and aggression management.

Client Goals

Outcome criteria include short- and long-term goals. Timelines are individually determined.

Short-Term Goals

■ Within [a specified time], client will be able to recognize signs of increasing anxiety and agitation and report to staff (or other care provider) for assistance with intervention.

■ Client will not harm self or others.

Long-Term Goal

■ Client will not harm self or others.

Interventions

■ Maintain a low level of stimuli in the client's environment (low lighting, few people, simple decor, low noise level). Anxiety level rises in a stimulating environment. A suspicious, agitated client may perceive individuals as threatening.

■ Observe the client's behavior frequently. Do this while carrying out routine activities so as to avoid creating suspiciousness in the individual. Close observation is necessary so that intervention can occur if required to ensure the client's (and others') safety.

■ Remove all dangerous objects from the client's environment so that, in his or her agitated, confused state, the client may not use them to harm self or others.

CLINICAL PEARL

Intervene at the first sign of increased anxiety, agitation, or verbal or behavioral aggression. Offer empathetic response to the client's feelings: "You seem anxious (or frustrated, or angry) about this situation. How can I help?" Validation of the client's feelings conveys a caring attitude and offering assistance reinforces trust.

■ It is important to maintain a calm attitude toward the client. As the client's anxiety increases, offer some alternatives: participating in a physical activity (e.g., punching bag, physical exercise), talking about the situation, taking some antianxiety medication. Offering alternatives to the client gives him or her a feeling of some control over the situation.

■ Have sufficient staff available to indicate a show of strength to the client if it becomes necessary. This shows the client evidence of control over the situation and provides some physical security for staff.

■ If the client is not calmed by "talking down" or by medication, use of mechanical restraints may be necessary. The avenue of the "least restrictive alternative" must be selected when planning interventions for a violent client. Restraints should be used only as a last resort, after all other interventions have been unsuccessful, and the client is clearly at risk of harm to self or others.

■ If restraint is deemed necessary, ensure that sufficient staff is available to assist. Follow protocol established by the institution. The Joint Commission (formerly the Joint Commission on Accreditation of Healthcare Organizations [JCAHO]) requires that an in-person evaluation by a physician or other licensed independent practitioner (LIP) be conducted within 1 hour of the initiation of the restraint or seclusion (The Joint Commission, 2010). The physician or

LIP must reissue a new order for restraints every 4 hours for adults and every 1 to 2 hours for children and adolescents.

■ The Joint Commission requires that the client in restraints be observed at least every 15 minutes to ensure that circulation to extremities is not compromised (check temperature, color, pulses); to assist the client with needs related to nutrition, hydration, and elimination; and to position the client so that comfort is facilitated and aspiration is prevented. Some institutions may require continuous one-to-one monitoring of restrained clients, particularly those who are highly agitated, and for whom there is a high risk of self- or accidental injury.

■ As agitation decreases, assess the client's readiness for restraint removal or reduction. Remove one restraint at a time while assessing the client's response. This minimizes the risk of injury to client and staff.

Impaired Verbal Communication

Impaired verbal communication is defined as "decreased, delayed, or absent ability to receive, process, transmit, and/or use a system of symbols" (NANDA-I, 2009, p. 178).

Client Goals

Outcome criteria include short- and long-term goals. Timelines are individually determined.

Short-Term Goal

■ Client will demonstrate ability to remain on one topic, using appropriate, intermittent eye contact, for 5 minutes with the nurse or therapist.

Long-Term Goal

■ By time of discharge from treatment, client will demonstrate ability to carry on a verbal communication in a socially acceptable manner with health-care providers and peers.

Interventions

■ Facilitate trust and understanding by maintaining staff assignments as consistently as possible. In a nonthreatening manner, explain to the client how his or her behavior and verbalizations are viewed by and may alienate others.

CLINICAL PEARL

Attempt to decode incomprehensible communication patterns. Seek validation and clarification by stating, "Is it that you mean ...?" or "I don't understand what you mean by that. Would you please explain it to me?" These techniques reveal to the client how he or she is being perceived by others, and the responsibility for not understanding is accepted by the nurse.

■ Anticipate and fulfill the client's needs until functional communication has been established.

■ Orient the client to reality as required. Call the client by name. Validate those aspects of communication that help differentiate between what is real and not real. These techniques may facilitate restoration of functional communication patterns in the client.

CLINICAL PEARL

If the client is unable or unwilling to speak (mutism), using the technique of verbalizing the implied is therapeutic. (Example: "That must have been very difficult for you when your mother left. You must have felt very alone.") This approach conveys empathy, facilitates trust, and eventually may encourage the client to discuss painful issues.

■ Because concrete thinking prevails, abstract phrases and clichés must be avoided, as they are likely to be misinterpreted. Explanations must be provided at the client's level of comprehension.

CLINICAL PEARL

Speak plainly and clearly in words that cannot be misinterpreted. Example: "Pick up the spoon, scoop some mashed potatoes into it, and put it in your mouth."

Concept Care Mapping

The concept map care plan is an innovative approach to planning and organizing nursing care (see Chapter 9). It is a diagrammatic teaching and learning strategy that allows visualization of interrelationships between medical diagnoses, nursing diagnoses, assessment data, and treatments. An example of a concept map care plan for a client with schizophrenia is presented in Figure 26–3.

Client/Family Education

The role of client teacher is important in the psychiatric area, as it is in all areas of nursing. A list of topics for client/family education relevant to schizophrenia is presented in Box 26-2. Sample client teaching guides are presented in Appendix G.

Evaluation

In the final step of the nursing process, a reassessment is conducted to determine if the nursing actions have been successful in achieving the objectives of care. Evaluation of the nursing actions for the client with exacerbation of schizophrenic

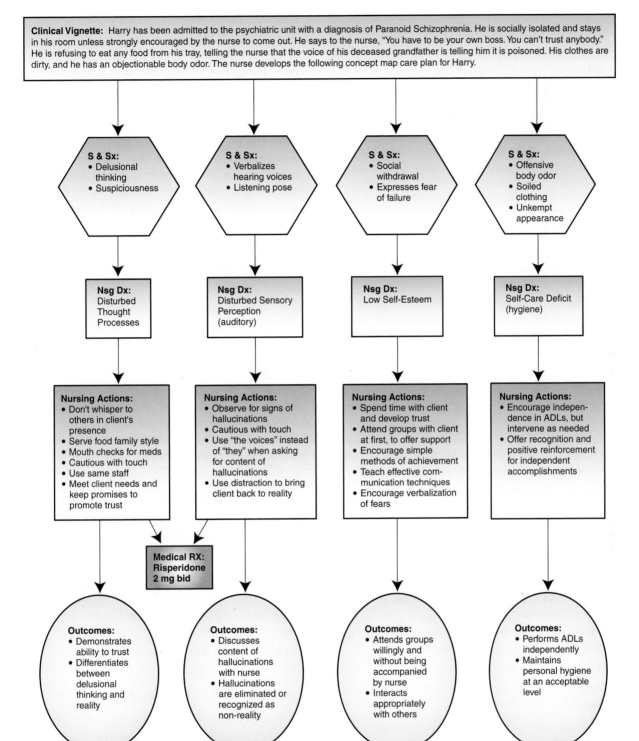

Clinical Vignette: Harry has been admitted to the psychiatric unit with a diagnosis of Paranoid Schizophrenia. He is socially isolated and stays in his room unless strongly encouraged by the nurse to come out. He says to the nurse, "You have to be your own boss. You can't trust anybody." He is refusing to eat any food from his tray, telling the nurse that the voice of his deceased grandfather is telling him it is poisoned. His clothes are dirty, and he has an objectionable body odor. The nurse develops the following concept map care plan for Harry.

S & Sx:
- Delusional thinking
- Suspiciousness

S & Sx:
- Verbalizes hearing voices
- Listening pose

S & Sx:
- Social withdrawal
- Expresses fear of failure

S & Sx:
- Offensive body odor
- Soiled clothing
- Unkempt appearance

Nsg Dx:
Disturbed Thought Processes

Nsg Dx:
Disturbed Sensory Perception (auditory)

Nsg Dx:
Low Self-Esteem

Nsg Dx:
Self-Care Deficit (hygiene)

Nursing Actions:
- Don't whisper to others in client's presence
- Serve food family style
- Mouth checks for meds
- Cautious with touch
- Use same staff
- Meet client needs and keep promises to promote trust

Nursing Actions:
- Observe for signs of hallucinations
- Cautious with touch
- Use "the voices" instead of "they" when asking for content of hallucinations
- Use distraction to bring client back to reality

Nursing Actions:
- Spend time with client and develop trust
- Attend groups with client at first, to offer support
- Encourage simple methods of achievement
- Teach effective communication techniques
- Encourage verbalization of fears

Nursing Actions:
- Encourage independence in ADLs, but intervene as needed
- Offer recognition and positive reinforcement for independent accomplishments

Medical RX:
Risperidone 2 mg bid

Outcomes:
- Demonstrates ability to trust
- Differentiates between delusional thinking and reality

Outcomes:
- Discusses content of hallucinations with nurse
- Hallucinations are eliminated or recognized as non-reality

Outcomes:
- Attends groups willingly and without being accompanied by nurse
- Interacts appropriately with others

Outcomes:
- Performs ADLs independently
- Maintains personal hygiene at an acceptable level

FIGURE 26–3   Concept map care plan for client with schizophrenia.

BOX 26-2 Topics for Client/Family Education Related to Schizophrenia

NATURE OF THE ILLNESS
1. What to expect as the illness progresses.
2. Symptoms associated with the illness.
3. Ways for family to respond to behaviors associated with the illness.

MANAGEMENT OF THE ILLNESS
1. Connection of exacerbation of symptoms to times of stress.
2. Appropriate medication management.
3. Side effects of medications.
4. Importance of not stopping medications.
5. When to contact health-care provider.
6. Relaxation techniques.
7. Social skills training.
8. Daily living skills training.

SUPPORT SERVICES
1. Financial assistance
2. Legal assistance
3. Caregiver support groups
4. Respite care
5. Home health care

---

psychosis may be facilitated by gathering information utilizing the following types of questions:

■ Has the client established trust with at least one staff member?

■ Is the anxiety level maintained at a manageable level?

■ Is delusional thinking still prevalent?

■ Is hallucinogenic activity evident? Does the client share content of hallucinations, particularly if commands are heard?

■ Is the client able to interrupt escalating anxiety with adaptive coping mechanisms?

■ Is the client easily agitated?

■ Is the client able to interact with others appropriately?

■ Does the client voluntarily attend therapy activities?

■ Is verbal communication comprehensible?

■ Is the client compliant with medication? Does the client verbalize the importance of taking medication regularly and on a long-term basis? Does he or she verbalize understanding of possible side effects, and when to seek assistance from the physician?

■ Does the client spend time with others rather than isolating self?

■ Is the client able to carry out all activities of daily living independently?

■ Is the client able to verbalize resources from which he or she may seek assistance outside the hospital?

■ Does the family have information regarding support groups in which they may participate, and from which they may seek assistance in dealing with their family member who is ill?

■ If the client lives alone, does he or she have a source for assistance with home maintenance and health management?

Quality and Safety Education for Nurses (QSEN)

The Institute of Medicine (IOM), in its 2003 report, *Health Professions Education: A Bridge to Quality*, challenged faculties of medicine, nursing, and other health professions to ensure that their graduates have achieved a core set of competencies in order to meet the needs of the 21st century health-care system. These competencies include *providing patient-centered care, working in interdisciplinary teams, employing evidence-based practice, applying quality improvement*, and *utilizing informatics*. A QSEN teaching strategy is included in Box 26-3. The use of this type of activity is intended to arm the instructor and the student with guidelines for attaining the knowledge, skills, and attitudes necessary for achievement of quality and safety competencies in nursing.

Treatment Modalities for Schizophrenia and Other Psychotic Disorders

Psychological Treatments

Individual Psychotherapy

Ho and associates (2003) stated:

Although intensive psychodynamic- and insight-oriented psychotherapy is generally not recommended, the form of individual psychotherapy that psychiatrists employ when providing pharmacological treatment typically involves a synthesis of various psychotherapeutic strategies and interventions. These include problem solving, reality testing, psychoeducation, and supportive and cognitive-behavioral techniques anchored on

BOX 26-3 QSEN TEACHING STRATEGY

Assignment: Using Evidence to Address Clinical Problems
Intervention with a Combative Client

Competency Domain: Evidence-Based Practice

Learning Objectives: Student will:
• Differentiate clinical opinion from research and evidence summaries.
• Explain the role of evidence in determining the best clinical practice for intervening with combative clients.
• Identify gaps between what is observed in the treatment setting and what has been identified as best practice.
• Discriminate between valid and invalid reasons for modifying evidence-based clinical practice based on clinical expertise or other reasons.
• Participate effectively in appropriate data collection and other research activities.
• Acknowledge own limitations in knowledge and clinical expertise before determining when to deviate from evidence-based best practices.

Strategy Overview:

1. Investigate the research related to intervening with a combative client.

2. Identify best practices described in the literature. How were these best practices determined?

3. Compare and contrast staff intervention with best practices described in the literature.

4. Investigate staff perceptions related to intervening with a combative client. How have they developed these perceptions?

5. Do staff members view any problems associated with their practice versus best practice described in the literature? If so, how would they like to see the problem addressed?

6. Describe ethical issues associated with intervening with a combative client.

7. What is your personal perception regarding the best evidence available to date related to intervening with a combative client? Are there situations that you can think of when you might deviate from the best practice model?

8. What questions do you have about intervening with a combative client that are not being addressed by current researchers?

Adapted from teaching strategy submitted by Pamela M. Ironside, Associate Professor, Indiana University School of Nursing, Indianapolis, IN. © 2010 QSEN; http://qsen.org, with permission.

an empathetic therapeutic alliance with the patient. The goals of such individual psychotherapy are to improve medication compliance, enhance social and occupational functioning, and prevent relapse. (p. 419)

Reality-oriented individual therapy is the most suitable approach to individual psychotherapy for schizophrenia. The primary focus in all cases must reflect efforts to decrease anxiety and increase trust.

Establishing a relationship is often particularly difficult because the individual with schizophrenia is desperately lonely yet defends against closeness and trust. He or she is likely to respond to attempts at closeness with suspiciousness, anxiety, aggression, or regression. Successful intervention may be achieved with honesty, simple directness, and a manner that respects the client's privacy and

human dignity. Exaggerated warmth and professions of friendship are likely to be met with confusion and suspicion.

Once a therapeutic interpersonal relationship has been established, reality orientation is maintained through exploration of the client's behavior within relationships. Education is provided to help the client identify sources of real or perceived danger and ways of reacting appropriately. Methods for improving interpersonal communication, emotional expression, and frustration tolerance are attempted.

Individual psychotherapy for clients with schizophrenia is seen as a long-term endeavor that requires patience on the part of the health-care provider, as well as the ability to accept that a great deal of change may not occur. Some cases report treatment durations of many years before clients regain some degree of independent functioning.

Group Therapy

Group therapy for individuals with schizophrenia has been shown to be effective, particularly with outpatients and when combined with drug treatment. Sadock and Sadock (2007) stated:

> Group therapy for persons with schizophrenia generally focuses on real-life plans, problems, and relationships. Some investigators doubt that dynamic interpretation and insight therapy are valuable for typical patients with schizophrenia. But group therapy is effective in reducing social isolation, increasing the sense of cohesiveness, and improving reality testing for patients with schizophrenia. (p. 492)

Group therapy in inpatient settings is less productive. Inpatient treatment usually occurs when symptomatology and social disorganization are at their most intense. At this time, the least amount of stimuli possible is most beneficial for the client. Because group therapy can be intensive and highly stimulating, it may be counterproductive early in treatment.

Group therapy for schizophrenia has been most useful over the long-term course of the illness. The social interaction, sense of cohesiveness, identification, and reality testing achieved within the group setting have proven to be highly therapeutic processes for these clients. Groups that offer a supportive environment appear to be more helpful to clients with schizophrenia than those that follow a more confrontational approach.

Behavior Therapy

Behavior modification has a history of qualified success in reducing the frequency of bizarre, disturbing, and deviant behaviors and increasing appropriate behaviors. Features that have led to the most positive results include:

- Clearly defining goals and how they will be measured.
- Attaching positive, negative, and aversive reinforcements to adaptive and maladaptive behavior.
- Using simple, concrete instructions and prompts to elicit the desired behavior.

Behavior therapy can be a powerful treatment tool for helping clients change undesirable behaviors. In the treatment setting, the health-care provider can use praise and other positive reinforcements to help the client with schizophrenia reduce the frequency of maladaptive or deviant behaviors. A limitation of this type of therapy is the inability of some individuals with schizophrenia to generalize what they have learned from the treatment setting to the community setting.

Social Skills Training

Social skills training has become one of the most widely used psychosocial interventions in the treatment of schizophrenia. Mueser, Bond, and Drake (2002) stated:

> The basic premise of social skills training is that complex interpersonal skills involve the smooth integration of a combination of simpler behaviors, including *nonverbal behaviors* (e.g., facial expression, eye contact); *paralinguistic features* (e.g., voice loudness and affect); *verbal content* (i.e., the appropriateness of what is said); and *interactive balance* (e.g., response latency, amount of time talking). These specific skills can be systematically taught, and, through the process of *shaping* (i.e., rewarding successive approximations toward the target behavior), complex behavioral repertoires can be acquired.

Social dysfunction is a hallmark of schizophrenia. Indeed, impairment in social functioning is included as one of the defining diagnostic criteria for schizophrenia in the *DSM-IV-TR* (APA, 2000). Considerable attention is now being given to enhancement of social skills in these clients.

The educational procedure in social skills training focuses on role-play. A series of brief scenarios are selected. These should be typical of situations clients experience in their daily lives and be graduated in terms of level of difficulty. The health-care provider may serve as a role model for some behaviors. For example, "See how I sort of nod my head up and down and look at your face while you talk." This demonstration is followed by the client's role-playing. Immediate feedback is provided regarding the client's presentation. Only by countless repetitions does the response gradually become smooth and effortless.

Progress is geared toward the client's needs and limitations. The focus is on small units of behavior, and the training proceeds very gradually. Highly threatening issues are avoided, and emphasis is placed on functional skills that are relevant to activities of daily living.

Social Treatment

Milieu Therapy

Some clinicians believe that milieu therapy can be an appropriate treatment for the client with schizophrenia. Research suggests that psychotropic medication is more effective at all levels of care when used along with milieu therapy and that milieu therapy is more successful if used in conjunction with these medications.

Sadock and Sadock (2007) stated:

> Most milieu therapy programs emphasize group and social interaction; rules and expectations are mediated by peer pressure for normalization of adaptation. When patients are viewed as responsible human beings, the patient role becomes blurred. Milieu therapy stresses a patient's rights to goals and to have freedom of movement and informal relationship with staff; it also emphasizes interdisciplinary participation and goal-oriented, clear communication. (p. 970)

Individuals with schizophrenia who are treated with milieu therapy alone require longer hospital stays than do those treated with drugs and psychosocial therapy. Other economic considerations, such as the need for a high staff-to-client ratio, in addition to the longer admission, limit the use of milieu therapy in the treatment of schizophrenia. The milieu environment can be successfully employed in outpatient settings, however, such as day and partial hospitalization programs.

Family Therapy

Some health-care providers treat schizophrenia as an illness not of the client alone, but of the entire family. Even when families appear to cope well, there is a notable impact on the mental health status of relatives when a family member has the illness. Safier (1997) stated:

> When a family member has a serious mental illness, the family must deal with a major upheaval in their lives, a terrible event that causes great pain and grief for the loss of a once-promising child or relationship. (p. 5)

The importance of the expanded role of family in the aftercare of relatives with schizophrenia has been recognized, thereby stimulating interest in family intervention programs designed to support the family system, prevent or delay relapse, and help to maintain the client in the community. These psychoeducational programs treat the family as a resource rather than a stressor, with the focus on concrete problem solving and specific helping behaviors for coping with stress. These programs recognize the biological basis for schizophrenia and the impact that stress has on the client's ability to function. By providing the family with information about the illness and suggestions for effective coping, psychoeducational programs reduce the likelihood of the client's relapse and the possible emergence of mental illness in previously nonaffected relatives.

Mueser and associates (2002) stated that, although models of family intervention with schizophrenia differ in their characteristics and methods, effective treatment programs share a number of common features:

- All programs are long term (usually 9 months to 2 years or more).
- They all provide client and family with information about the illness and its management.
- They focus on improving adherence to prescribed medications.
- They strive to decrease stress in the family, and improve family functioning.

Asen (2002) suggested the following interventions with families of individuals with schizophrenia:

- Forming a close alliance with the caregivers
- Lowering the emotional intrafamily climate by reducing stress and burden on relatives
- Increasing the capacity of relatives to anticipate and solve problems
- Reducing the expressions of anger and guilt by family members
- Maintaining reasonable expectations for how the ill family member should perform
- Encouraging relatives to set appropriate limits while maintaining some degree of separateness
- Promoting desirable changes in the relatives' behaviors and belief systems

Family therapy typically consists of a brief program of family education about schizophrenia, and a more extended program of family contact designed to reduce overt manifestations of conflict and to improve patterns of family communication and problem solving. The response to this type of therapy has been very dramatic. Studies have clearly revealed that a more positive outcome in the treatment of the client with schizophrenia can be achieved by including the family system in the program of care.

Program of Assertive Community Treatment (PACT)

The Program of Assertive Community Treatment (PACT) is case management that takes a team approach in providing comprehensive, community-based psychiatric treatment, rehabilitation, and support to persons with serious and persistent mental illness such as schizophrenia. (The National Alliance for the Mentally Ill [NAMI] uses the terms PACT and Assertive Community Treatment [ACT] interchangeably. Some states use other terms for this type of treatment, such as Mobile Treatment Teams [MTTs] and Community Support Programs [CSPs].) Aggressive programs of treatment are individually tailored for each client and include the teaching of basic living skills, helping clients work with community agencies, and assisting clients in developing a social support network (Ho et al., 2003). There is emphasis on vocational expectations, and supported work settings (i.e., sheltered workshops) are an important part of the treatment program. Other services include substance abuse treatment, psychoeducational programs, family support and education, mobile crisis intervention, and attention to health-care needs.

Responsibilities are shared by multiple team members, including psychiatrists, nurses, social workers, vocational rehabilitation therapists, and substance abuse counselors. Services are provided in the person's home; within the neighborhood; in local restaurants, parks, and stores; or wherever assistance by the client is required. These services are available to the client 24 hours a day, 365 days a year. NAMI (2010) listed the primary goals of PACT as follows:

■ To meet basic needs and enhance quality of life

■ To improve functioning in adult social and employment roles

■ To enhance an individual's ability to live independently in his or her own community

■ To lessen the family's burden of providing care

■ To lessen or eliminate the debilitating symptoms of mental illness

■ To minimize or prevent recurrent acute episodes of the illness

Individuals best served by PACT are identified by the Assertive Community Treatment Association (ACTA) (2010) as follows:

Clients served by ACT are individuals with serious and persistent mental illness or personality disorders, with severe functional impairments, who have avoided or not responded well to traditional outpatient mental health care and psychiatric rehabilitation services. Persons served by ACT often have co-existing problems such as homelessness, substance abuse problems, or involvement with the judicial system.

PACT has been shown to reduce the number of hospitalizations and decrease costs of care for these clients. Although it has been called "paternalistic" and "coercive" by its critics, PACT has provided a much-needed service and increased quality of life for many clients who are unable to manage in a less-structured environment.

The Recovery Model

The concept of recovery is not new. It originally began in the addictions field, referring to a person recovering from a substance-related disorder. The term has recently been adopted by mental health professionals who believe that recovery from mental illness is also possible.

A number of definitions of recovery as it applies to mental illness have been proposed. The Substance Abuse and Mental Health Services Administration (SAMHSA) suggested the following:

Mental health recovery is a journey of healing and transformation enabling a person with a mental health problem to live a meaningful life in a community of his or her choice while striving to achieve his or her full potential. (SAMHSA, 2010)

William A. Anthony, Executive Director of the Center for Psychiatric Rehabilitation at Boston University, offered this definition:

Recovery is described as a deeply personal, unique process of changing one's attitudes, values, feelings, goals, skills, and/or roles. It is a way of living a satisfying, hopeful, and contributing life even with limitations caused by illness. Recovery involves the development of new meaning and purpose in one's life as one grows beyond the catastrophic effects of mental illness. (Anthony, 1993, p. 13)

The President's New Freedom Commission on Mental Health (2003) has proposed to transform the mental health system by shifting the paradigm of care of persons with serious mental illness from traditional medical psychiatric treatment toward the concept of recovery, and the APA has endorsed a recovery model from a psychiatric services perspective (Sharfstein, 2005).

The basic concept of a recovery model is empowerment of the consumer. The recovery model is designed to allow consumers primary control over decisions about their own care. The National Association of Social Workers (NASW, 2010) suggested that this means, "Consumers need to be as fully informed as possible about the potential benefits and consequences of each decision. They also need to know the possible results if they become a danger to themselves or others."

SAMSHA (2010) outlined the following 10 fundamental components of the recovery model:

1. **Self-direction.** Consumers lead, control, exercise choice over, and determine their own path of recovery by optimizing autonomy, independence, and control of resources to achieve a self-determined life.

2. **Individualized and person centered.** Multiple pathways to recovery exist and are based on an individual's unique strengths, needs, preferences, experiences, and cultural background. Recovery is identified as an ongoing journey and an end result as well as an overall paradigm for achieving wellness and optimal mental health.

3. **Empowerment.** Through empowerment, individuals gain control of their own destiny and influence the organizational and societal structures in their lives. They have the authority to choose from a range of options and to participate in all decisions—including the allocation of resources—that will affect their lives, and are educated and supported in doing so.

4. **Holistic.** Recovery encompasses an individual's whole life, including mind, body, spirit, and community. Recovery embraces all aspects of life, including housing, employment, education, mental health and health-care treatment and services, complementary and naturalistic services, addictions treatment, spirituality, creativity, social networks, community participation, and family supports as determined by the person.

5. **Nonlinear.** Recovery is not a step-by-step process, but one based on continual growth, occasional setbacks, and learning from experience. It begins with an initial stage of awareness in which a person recognizes that positive change is possible, and progresses to full engagement in the work of recovery.

6. **Strengths based.** Recovery builds on the multiple capacities, resiliencies, talents, coping abilities, and inherent worth of the individual, encouraging consumers to leave stymied life roles behind and engage in new life roles (e.g., partner, caregiver, friend, student, employee). The process of recovery moves forward through interaction with others in supportive, trust-based relationships.

7. **Peer support.** Mutual support—including the sharing of experiential knowledge and skills and social learning—plays an invaluable role in recovery. Individuals provide each other with a sense of belonging, supportive relationships, valued roles, and community.

8. **Respect.** Community, systems, and societal acceptance and appreciation of consumers—including protecting their rights and eliminating discrimination and stigma—are crucial in achieving recovery. Self-acceptance and regaining belief in one's self are particularly vital. Respect ensures the inclusion and full participation of consumers in all aspects of their lives.

9. **Responsibility.** Consumers have a personal responsibility for their own self-care and journeys of recovery. They must strive to understand and give meaning to their experiences and identify coping strategies and healing processes to promote their own wellness.

10. **Hope.** Recovery provides the essential and motivating message of a better future—that people can and do overcome the barriers and obstacles that confront them. Hope is internalized, but can be fostered by peers, families, friends, providers, and others. Hope is the catalyst of the recovery process.

The recovery model integrates services provided by professionals (e.g., medication, therapy, case management), services provided by consumers (e.g., advocacy, peer support programs, hotlines, mentoring), and services provided in collaboration (e.g., recovery education, crisis planning, community integration, consumer rights education) (Jacobson & Greenley, 2001). Jacobson and Greenley (2001) stated,

> Although many of these services may sound similar to services currently being offered in many mental health systems, it is important to recognize that no service is recovery-oriented unless it incorporates the attitude that recovery is possible and has the goal of promoting hope, healing, empowerment, and connection. (p. 485)

Organic Treatment

Psychopharmacology

Chlorpromazine (Thorazine) was first introduced in the United States in 1952. At that time, it was used in conjunction with barbiturates in surgical anesthesia. With increased use, the drug's psychic properties were recognized, and by 1954 it was marketed as an antipsychotic medication in the United States. The manufacture and sale of other antipsychotic drugs followed in rapid succession.

Antipsychotic medications are also called *neuroleptics* or major tranquilizers. They are effective in the treatment of acute and chronic manifestations of schizophrenia and in maintenance therapy to prevent exacerbation of schizophrenic symptoms. Without drug treatment, an estimated 72 percent of individuals who have experienced a psychotic episode relapse within a year. This relapse rate can be reduced to about 23 percent with continuous medication administration (Dixon, Lehman, & Levine, 2009).

The prognosis of schizophrenia is often reported in the paradigm of thirds. One third of the people achieve significant and lasting improvement. They may never experience another episode of psychosis following the initial occurrence. One third may achieve some improvement with intermittent relapses and residual disability. Their occupational level may have decreased because of their illness, or they may be socially isolated. Finally, one third experience severe and permanent incapacity. They often do not respond to medication and remain chronically ill for much of their lives. Men have poorer outcomes than women do; women respond better to treatment with antipsychotic medications.

As mentioned earlier, the efficacy of antipsychotic medications is enhanced by adjunct psychosocial therapy. Because the psychotic manifestations of the illness subside with use of the drugs, clients are generally more cooperative with the psychosocial therapies. However, it takes several weeks for the antipsychotics to effectively treat positive symptoms, a fact that often leads to discontinuation of the medication. Clients and families need to be educated about the importance of waiting, often for several weeks, to determine if the drug will be effective.

IMPLICATIONS OF RESEARCH FOR EVIDENCE-BASED PRACTICE

Beebe, L. H., Smith, K., Crye, C., Addonizio, C., Strunk, D. J., Martin, W., et al. (2008). Telenursing intervention increases psychiatric medication adherence in schizophrenia outpatients. *Journal of the American Psychiatric Nurses Association, 14*(3), 217–224.

DESCRIPTION OF THE STUDY: The purpose of this study was to evaluate the impact of telephone intervention problem solving (TIPS), a problem-based telenursing intervention, on both psychiatric and nonpsychiatric medication adherence in outpatients with schizophrenia. The study sample included 25 outpatients (age range 25 to 69) receiving care at a Community Mental Health Center (CMHC) in the southeastern United States; 60% were male and 44% were African American. The majority lived alone and were unemployed. All had chart diagnoses of schizophrenia (any subtype) according to the criteria in the *DMS-IV-TR*. Thirteen study participants and 12 control subjects completed the research study. The intervention included weekly telephone calls throughout the 3-month study by registered nurses with graduate degrees who had received TIPS training from one of the authors. The calls were designed "to foster problem solving, offer coping alternatives, provide reminders so clients remember to use alternatives, and assess the effectiveness of coping efforts. Effective use of problem solving may assist patients to cope with common medication adherence barriers such as forgetfulness or lack of knowledge about prescribed medications. Nurses guide the participant through the problem-solving process for any difficulties identified, generating solutions, choosing a solution, and following up on the effectiveness of the solution at the next call" (p. 220). Medication adherence was measured by pill counts performed monthly in the participants' homes. Both psychiatric and nonpsychiatric medications were counted.

RESULTS OF THE STUDY: As had been expected, there was a statistically significant improvement in adherence to psychiatric medications in the experimental group compared to the control group. However, nonpsychiatric medication adherence was not significantly affected by the TIPS intervention. The authors suggest that this may have occurred "because participants were recruited at a CMHC, they associated TIPS providers with the CMHC and tended to generalize adherence suggestions to psychiatric medications for this reason" (p. 223).

IMPLICATIONS FOR NURSING PRACTICE: The telenursing intervention described in this study may provide nurses with a tool for assisting clients with schizophrenia to maintain greater medication adherence. Prior work by the primary author demonstrated fewer rehospitalizations in persons receiving TIPS, indicating that there is a strong association between lack of psychiatric medication adherence and symptom relapse and psychiatric readmission. TIPS may be considered as part of an outpatient or partial hospitalization program for clients with schizophrenia.

These medications are classified as either "typical" (first-generation, conventional antipsychotics) or "atypical" (the newer, novel antipsychotics). Examples of commonly used antipsychotic agents are presented in Table 26-5. A detailed description of these medications follows.

Indications

Antipsychotics medications are used in the treatment of schizophrenia and other psychotic disorders. Selected agents are used in the treatment of bipolar mania (olanzapine, aripiprazole, chlorpromazine, quetiapine, risperidone, asenapine, ziprasidone). Others are used as antiemetics (chlorpromazine, perphenazine, prochlorperazine), in the treatment of intractable hiccoughs (chlorpromazine), and for the control of tics and vocal utterances in Tourette's disorder (haloperidol, pimozide).

Action

Typical antipsychotics work by blocking postsynaptic dopamine receptors in the basal ganglia, hypothalamus, limbic system, brainstem, and medulla. They also demonstrate varying affinity for cholinergic, alpha$_1$-adrenergic, and histaminic receptors. Antipsychotic effects may also be related to inhibition of dopamine-mediated transmission of neural impulses at the synapses.

Atypical antipsychotics are weaker dopamine receptor antagonists than the conventional antipsychotics, but are more potent antagonists of the serotonin (5-hydroxytryptamine) type 2A (5HT$_{2A}$) receptors. They also exhibit antagonism for cholinergic, histaminic, and adrenergic receptors.

Contraindications/Precautions

Typical antipsychotics are contraindicated in clients with known hypersensitivity (cross-sensitivity may exist among phenothiazines). They should not be used in comatose states or when central nervous system (CNS) depression is evident; when blood dyscrasias exist; in clients with Parkinson's disease or narrow-angle glaucoma; in those with

TABLE 26-5 Antipsychotic Agents

CHEMICAL CLASS	GENERIC (TRADE) NAME	PREGNANCY CATEGORIES/ HALF-LIFE (hr)	DAILY DOSAGE RANGE (mg)
Typical Antipsychotic Agents (first generation; conventional)	Chlorpromazine	C/ 24	40–400
	Fluphenazine	C/ HCl: 18 hr Decanoate: 6.8–9.6 days	2.5–10
	Haloperidol (Haldol)	C/ ~18 (oral); ~3 wk (IM decanoate)	1–100
	Loxapine	C/ 8	20–250
	Perphenazine	C/ 9–12	12–64
	Pimozide (Orap)	C/ ~55	1–10
	Prochlorperazine	C/ 3–5 (oral) 6.9 (IV)	15–150
	Thioridazine	C/ 24	150–800
	Thiothixene (Navane)	C/ 34	6–30
	Trifluoperazine	C/ 18	4–40
Atypical Antipsychotic Agents (second generation; novel)	Aripiprazole (Abilify)	C/ 75–146	10–30
	Asenapine (Saphris)	C/ 24	10–20
	Clozapine (Clozaril)	B/ 8 (single dose); 12 (at steady state)	300–900
	Iloperidone (Fanapt)	C/ 18–33	12–24
	Lurasidone (Latuda)	B/ 18	40–80
	Olanzapine (Zyprexa)	C/ 21–54	5–20
	Paliperidone (Invega)	C/ 23	6–12
	Quetiapine (Seroquel)	C/ ~6	300–400
	Risperidone (Risperdal)	C/ 3–20	4–8
	Ziprasidone (Geodon)	C/ ~7 (oral); 2–5 (IM)	40–160

liver, renal, or cardiac insufficiency; in individuals with poorly controlled seizure disorders; or in elderly clients with dementia-related psychosis. Thioridazine, pimozide, and haloperidol have been shown to prolong the QT interval, and are contraindicated if the client is taking other drugs that also produce this side effect.

Caution should be taken in administering these drugs to clients who are elderly, severely ill, or debilitated, and to diabetic clients or clients with respiratory insufficiency, prostatic hypertrophy, or intestinal obstruction. Antipsychotics may lower seizure threshold. Individuals should avoid exposure to extremes in temperature while taking antipsychotic medication. Safety in pregnancy and lactation has not been established.

Atypical antipsychotics are contraindicated in hypersensitivity, comatose or severely depressed patients, elderly patients with dementia-related psychosis, and lactation. Ziprasidone, risperidone, paliperidone, asenapine, and iloperidone are contraindicated in patients with a history of QT prolongation or cardiac arrhythmias, recent myocardial infarction (MI), uncompensated heart failure, and concurrent use with other drugs that prolong the QT interval. Clozapine is contraindicated in patients with myeloproliferative disorders, with a history of clozapine-induced agranulocytosis or severe granulocytopenia, and with uncontrolled epilepsy. Lurasidone is contraindicated in concomitant use with strong inhibitors of cytochrome P450 isozyme 3A4 (CYP3A4) (e.g., ketoconazole) and strong CYP3A4 inducers (e.g., rifampin).

Caution should be taken in administering these drugs to elderly or debilitated patients; to patients with cardiac, hepatic, or renal insufficiency; to those with a history of seizures; to patients with diabetes or risk factors for diabetes; to clients exposed to temperature extremes; under conditions that cause hypotension (dehydration, hypovolemia, treatment with antihypertensive medication); and to pregnant clients or children (safety not established).

Interactions

Typical antipsychotics have additive hypotensive effects with antihypertensive agents, additive CNS effects when taken with CNS depressants, and additive anticholinergic effects when taken with drugs that have anticholinergic properties. Phenothiazines may reduce effectiveness of oral anticoagulants. Concurrent use of phenothiazines or haloperidol with epinephrine or dopamine may result in severe hypotension. Additive effects of QT prolongation occur when haloperidol, thioridazine, or pimozide are taken concurrently with other drugs that prolong the QT interval. Pimozide is contraindicated

with CYP3A inhibitors, and thioridazine is contraindicated with cytochrome P450 isozyme 2D6 (CYP2D6) inhibitors. Concurrent use of haloperidol and carbamazepine results in decreased therapeutic effects of haloperidol and increased effects of carbamazepine.

Atypical antipsychotics have additive hypotensive effects when taken with antihypertensive agents and additive CNS effects with CNS depressants. There are additive anticholinergic effects when resperidone or paliperidone are taken with other drugs that have anticholinergic properties. There are additive effects of QT prolongation with ziprasidone, risperidone, paliperidone, asenapine, and iloperidone and other drugs that prolong the QT interval. Decreased effects of levodopa and dopamine agonists occur with concurrent use of ziprasidone, olanzapine, quetiapine, resperidone, or paliperidone. Increased effects of ziprasidone, clozapine, quetiapine, aripiprazole, lurasidone, and iloperidone occur with CYP3A4 inhibitors. Decreased effects of lurasidone occur with CYP3A4 inducers. Increased effects of iloperidone occur with CYP2D6 inhibitors. Decreased effects of ziprasidone, clozapine, olanzapine, risperidone, paliperidone, asenapine, and aripiprazole occur with cytochrome P450 isozyme 1A2 (CYP1A2) inducers, and increased effects occur with CYP1A2 inhibitors. Concurrent use of asenapine and paroxetine results in decreased therapeutic effects of asenapine and increased effects of paroxetine. Additive orthostatic hypotension occurs with risperidone, paliperidone, or iloperidone and other drugs that also cause this adverse reaction.

Side Effects

The effects of these medications are related to blockage of a number of receptors for which they exhibit various degrees of affinity. Blockage of the dopamine receptors is thought to be responsible for controlling positive symptoms of schizophrenia. Dopamine blockage also results in **extrapyramidal symptoms** (EPS) and prolactin elevation (galactorrhea; gynecomastia). Cholinergic blockade causes anticholinergic side effects (dry mouth, blurred vision, constipation, urinary retention, tachycardia). Blockage of the alpha$_1$-adrenergic receptors produces dizziness, orthostatic hypotension, tremors, and reflex tachycardia. Histamine blockade is associated with weight gain and sedation.

The plan of care should include monitoring for the following side effects from antipsychotic medications. Nursing implications related to each side effect are designated by an asterisk (*). A profile of side effects comparing various antipsychotic medications is presented in Table 26-6.

TABLE 26-6 Comparison of Side Effects Among Antipsychotic Agents

CLASS	GENERIC (TRADE) NAME‡	EPS†	SEDATION	ANTICHOLINERGIC	ORTHOSTATIC HYPOTENSION	WEIGHT GAIN
Typical Antipsychotic Agents	Chlorpromazine	3	4	3	4	*
	Fluphenazine	5	2	2	2	
	Haloperidol (Haldol)	5	2	2	2	
	Loxapine	3	2	2	2	*
	Perphenazine	4	2	2	2	*
	Pimozide (Orap)	4	2	3	2	*
	Prochlorperazine	3	2	2	2	*
	Thioridazine	2	4	4	4	*
	Thiothixene (Navane)	4	2	2	2	*
	Trifluoperazine	4	2	2	2	*
Atypical Antipsychotic Agents	Aripiprazole (Abilify)	1	2	1	3	2
	Asenapine (Saphris)	1	3	1	3	4
	Clozapine (Clozaril)	1	5	5	4	5
	Iloperidone (Fanapt)	1	3	2	3	3
	Lurasidone (Latuda)	1	3	1	3	3
	Olanzapine (Zyprexa)	1	3	2	2	5
	Paliperidone (Invega)	1	2	1	3	2
	Quetiapine (Seroquel)	1	3	1	3	4
	Risperidone (Risperdal)	1	2	1	3	4
	Ziprasidone (Geodon)	1	3	1	2	2

Key: 1 = Very low; 2 = Low; 3 = Moderate; 4 = High; 5 = Very high.
*Weight gain occurs, but incidence is unknown.
†EPS = extrapyramidal symptoms.
‡Drugs without trade names are available in generic form only.
Adapted from Black and Andreasen (2011); Drug Facts and Comparisons (2011); and Schatzberg, Cole, and DeBattista (2010).

■ Anticholinergic effects (see Table 26-6 for differences between typical and atypical antipsychotics)
- Dry mouth
  *Provide client with sugarless candy or gum, ice, and frequent sips of water.
  *Ensure that client practices strict oral hygiene.
- Blurred vision
  *Explain that this symptom will most likely subside after a few weeks.
  *Advise client not to drive a car until vision clears.
  *Clear small items from pathway to prevent falls.
- Constipation
  *Order foods high in fiber; encourage increase in physical activity and fluid intake if not contraindicated.
- Urinary retention
  *Instruct client to report any difficulty urinating; monitor intake and output.

■ Nausea; gastrointestinal (GI) upset (may occur with all classifications)
  *Tablets or capsules may be administered with food to minimize GI upset.
  *Concentrates may be diluted and administered with fruit juice or other liquid; they should be mixed immediately before administration.

■ Skin rash (may occur with all classifications)
  *Report appearance of any rash on skin to physician.
  *Avoid spilling any of the liquid concentrate on skin; contact dermatitis can occur with some medications.

■ Sedation (see Table 26-6 for differences between typical and atypical antipsychotics)
  *Discuss with physician the possibility of administering the drug at bedtime.
  *Discuss with physician a possible decrease in dosage or an order for a less-sedating drug.

*Instruct client not to drive or operate dangerous equipment while experiencing sedation.

■ Orthostatic hypotension (see Table 26-6 for differences between typical and atypical antipsychotics)
*Instruct client to rise slowly from a lying or sitting position
*Monitor blood pressure (lying and standing) each shift; document and report significant changes.

■ Photosensitivity (may occur with all classifications)
*Ensure that client wears a sunblock lotion, protective clothing, and sunglasses while spending time outdoors.

■ Hormonal effects (may occur with all classifications, but more common with typical antipsychotics)
• Decreased libido, **retrograde ejaculation**, **gynecomastia** (men)
*Provide explanation of the effects and reassurance of reversibility. If necessary, discuss with physician possibility of ordering alternate medication.
• Amenorrhea (women)
*Offer reassurance of reversibility; instruct client to continue use of contraception, because **amenorrhea** does not indicate cessation of ovulation.
• Weight gain (may occur with all classifications; has been problematic with the atypical antipsychotics)
*Weigh client every other day; order calorie-controlled diet; provide opportunity for physical exercise; provide diet and exercise instruction.

■ Electrocardiogram (ECG) changes. ECG changes, including prolongation of the QT interval, are possible with most of the antipsychotics. This is particularly true with ziprasidone, thioridazine, pimozide, haloperidol, paliperidone, iloperidone, asenapine, and clozapine. Caution is advised in prescribing these medications to individuals with history of arrhythmias. Conditions that produce hypokalemia and/or hypomagnesemia, such as diuretic therapy or diarrhea, should be taken into consideration when prescribing. Routine ECG should be taken before initiation of therapy and periodically during therapy. Clozapine has also been associated with other cardiac events, such as ischemic changes, arrhythmias, congestive heart failure, myocarditis, and cardiomyopathy.
*Monitor vital signs every shift.

*Observe for symptoms of dizziness, palpitations, syncope, weakness, dyspnea, and peripheral edema.

■ Reduction of seizure threshold (more common with the typical than the atypical antipsychotics, with the exception of clozapine)
*Closely observe clients with history of seizures.
***NOTE:** This is particularly important with clients taking clozapine (Clozaril), with which seizures have been frequently associated. Dose appears to be an important predictor, with a greater likelihood of seizures occurring at higher doses. Extreme caution is advised in prescribing clozapine for clients with history of seizures.

■ **Agranulocytosis** (more common with the typical than the atypical antipsychotics, with the exception of clozapine)
*Agranulocytosis usually occurs within the first 3 months of treatment. Observe for symptoms of sore throat, fever, malaise. A complete blood count should be monitored if these symptoms appear.

EXCEPTION: There is a significant risk of agranulocytosis with clozapine (Clozaril). Agranulocytosis is a potentially fatal blood disorder in which the client's white blood cell (WBC) count can drop to extremely low levels. A baseline WBC count and absolute neutrophil count (ANC) must be taken before initiation of treatment with clozapine and weekly for the first 6 months of treatment. Only a 1-week supply of medication is dispensed at a time. If the counts remain within the acceptable levels (i.e., WBC at least $3,500/mm^3$ and the ANC at least $2,000/mm^3$) during the 6-month period, blood counts may be monitored biweekly, and a 2-week supply of medication may then be dispensed. If the counts remain within the acceptable level for the biweekly period, counts may then be monitored every 4 weeks thereafter. When the medication is discontinued, weekly WBC counts are continued for an additional 4 weeks.

■ Hypersalivation (most common with clozapine)
*A significant number of clients receiving clozapine (Clozaril) therapy experience extreme salivation. Offer support to the client because this may be an embarrassing situation. It may even be a safety issue (e.g., risk of aspiration) if the problem is severe. Management has included the use of sugar-free gum to increase the

swallowing rate, as well as the prescription of medications such as an anticholinergic (e.g., scopolamine patch) or alpha$_2$-adrenoceptor agonist (e.g., clonidine).

■ Extrapyramidal symptoms (see Table 26-6 for differences between typical and atypical antipsychotics)

*Observe for symptoms and report; administer antiparkinsonian drugs, as ordered (see Table 26-7).

• **Pseudoparkinsonism** (tremor, shuffling gait, drooling, rigidity)

*Symptoms may appear 1 to 5 days following initiation of antipsychotic medication; occurs most often in women, the elderly, and dehydrated clients.

• **Akinesia** (muscular weakness)

*Same as for pseudoparkinsonism.

• **Akathisia** (continuous restlessness and fidgeting)

*This occurs most frequently in women; symptoms may occur 50 to 60 days following initiation of therapy.

• **Dystonia** (involuntary muscular movements [spasms] of face, arms, legs, and neck)

*This occurs most often in men and in people younger than 25 years of age.

• **Oculogyric crisis** (uncontrolled rolling back of the eyes)

*This may appear as part of the syndrome described as dystonia. It may be mistaken for seizure activity. Dystonia and oculogyric crisis should be treated as an emergency situation. The physician should be contacted, and intravenous benztropine mesylate (Cogentin) is commonly administered. Stay with the client and offer reassurance and support during this frightening time.

■ **Tardive dyskinesia** (bizarre facial and tongue movements, stiff neck, and difficulty swallowing; may occur with all classifications, but more common with typical antipsychotics)

*All clients receiving long-term (months or years) antipsychotic therapy are at risk.

*The symptoms are potentially irreversible.

*The drug should be withdrawn at the first sign, which is usually vermiform movements of the tongue; prompt action may prevent irreversibility.

TABLE 26-7 Antiparkinsonian Agents Used to Treat Extrapyramidal Side Effects of Antipsychotic Drugs

Indication	Used to treat parkinsonism of various causes and drug-induced extrapyramidal reactions.
Action	Restores the natural balance of acetylcholine and dopamine in the CNS. The imbalance is a deficiency in dopamine that results in excessive cholinergic activity.
Contraindications/ Precautions	Antiparkinsonian agents are contraindicated in individuals with hypersensitivity. Anticholinergics should be avoided by individuals with angle-closure glaucoma; pyloric, duodenal, or bladder neck obstructions; prostatic hypertrophy; or myasthenia gravis. Caution should be used in administering these drugs to clients with hepatic, renal, or cardiac insufficiency; elderly and debilitated clients; those with a tendency toward urinary retention; or those exposed to high environmental temperatures.
Common side effects	Anticholinergic effects (dry mouth, blurred vision, constipation, paralytic ileus, urinary retention, tachycardia, elevated temperature, decreased sweating), nausea/GI upset, sedation, dizziness, orthostatic hypotension, exacerbation of psychoses.

CHEMICAL CLASS	GENERIC (TRADE) NAME	PREGNANCY CATEGORIES/ HALF-LIFE (hr)	DAILY DOSAGE RANGE (mg)
Anticholinergics	Benztropine (Cogentin)	C/ UKN	1–8
	Biperiden (Akineton)	C/ 18.4–24.3	2–6
	Trihexyphenidyl (Artane)	C/ 5.6–10.2	1–15
Antihistamines	Diphenhydramine (Benadryl)	C/ 4–15	25–200
Dopaminergic Agonists	Amantadine (Symmetrel)	C/ 10–25	200–300

UKN = unknown.

*The Abnormal Involuntary Movement Scale (AIMS) is a rating scale that was developed in the 1970s by the National Institute of Mental Health to measure involuntary movements associated with tardive dyskinesia. The AIMS aids in early detection of movement disorders and provides a means for ongoing surveillance. The AIMS assessment tool, examination procedure, and interpretation of scoring are presented in Box 26-4.

■ **Neuroleptic malignant syndrome** (NMS) (more common with the typical than the atypical antipsychotics)
*This is a relatively rare, but potentially fatal, complication of treatment with neuroleptic drugs. Routine assessments should include

---

BOX 26-4 Abnormal Involuntary Movement Scale (AIMS)

NAME _____ RATER NAME _____ DATE _____

INSTRUCTIONS: Complete the examination procedure before making ratings. For movement ratings, circle the highest severity observed. Rate movements that occur upon activation one *less* than those observed spontaneously. Circle movement as well as code number that applies.

Code: 0 = None
      1 = Minimal, may be normal
      2 = Mild
      3 = Moderate
      4 = Severe

	1. Muscles of Facial Expression (e.g., movements of forehead, eyebrows, periorbital area, cheeks, including frowning, blinking, smiling, grimacing)	0 1 2 3 4
Facial and Oral Movements	**2. Lips and Perioral Area** (e.g., puckering, pouting, smacking)	0 1 2 3 4
	3. Jaw (e.g., biting, clenching, chewing, mouth opening, lateral movement)	0 1 2 3 4
	4. Tongue (Rate only increases in movement both in and out of mouth. NOT inability to sustain movement. Darting in and out of mouth.)	0 1 2 3 4
Extremity Movements	**5. Upper (arms, wrists, hands, fingers)** (Include choreic movements [i.e., rapid, objectively purposeless, irregular, spontaneous] and athetoid movements [i.e., slow, irregular, complex serpentine]. *Do not include tremor* [i.e., repetitive, regular, rhythmic])	0 1 2 3 4
	6. Lower (legs, knees, ankles, toes) (e.g., lateral knee movement, foot tapping, heel dropping, foot squirming, inversion and eversion of foot)	0 1 2 3 4
Trunk Movements	**7. Neck, shoulders, hips** (e.g., rocking, twisting, squirming, pelvic gyrations)	0 1 2 3 4
	8. Severity of abnormal movements overall	0 1 2 3 4
	9. Incapacitation due to abnormal movements	0 1 2 3 4
Global Judgments	**10. Patient's awareness of abnormal movements** (Rate only the client's report)	
	No awareness	0
	Aware, no distress	1
	Aware, mild distress	2
	Aware, moderate distress	3
	Aware, severe distress	4
Dental Status	**11. Current problems with teeth and/or dentures?**	No Yes
	12. Are dentures usually worn?	No Yes
	13. Edentia?	No Yes
	14. Do movements disappear in sleep?	No Yes

BOX 26-4 **Abnormal Involuntary Movement Scale (AIMS)—cont'd**

AIMS EXAMINATION PROCEDURE

Either before or after completing the Examination Procedure, observe the client unobtrusively, at rest (e.g. in waiting room). The chair to be used in this examination should be a hard, firm one without arms.

1. Ask client to remove shoes and socks.
2. Ask client whether there is anything in his/her mouth (i.e., gum, candy, etc.), and if there is, to remove it.
3. Ask client about the current condition of his/her teeth. Ask client if he/she wears dentures. Do teeth or dentures bother client now?
4. Ask client whether he/she notices any movements in mouth, face, hands, or feet. If yes, ask to describe and to what extent they currently bother client or interfere with his/her activities.
5. Have client sit in chair with both hands on knees, legs slightly apart, and feet flat on floor. (Look at entire body for movements while in this position.)
6. Ask client to sit with hands hanging unsupported. If male, between legs, if female and wearing a dress, hanging over knees. (Observe hands and other body areas.)
7. Ask client to open mouth. (Observe tongue at rest within mouth.) Do this twice.
8. Ask client to protrude tongue. (Observe abnormalities of tongue movement.) Do this twice.
9. Ask client to tap thumb with each finger as rapidly as possible for 10 to 15 seconds; separately with right hand, then with left hand. (Observe facial and leg movements.)
10. Flex and extend client's left and right arms (one at a time). (Note any rigidity.)
11. Ask client to stand up. (Observe in profile. Observe all body areas again, hips included.)
12. Ask client to extend both arms outstretched in front with palms down. (Observe trunk, legs, and mouth.)
13. Have client walk a few paces, turn, and walk back to chair. (Observe hands and gait.) Do this twice.

INTERPRETATION OF AIMS SCORE

Add client scores and note areas of difficulty.
Score of:

- 0 to 1 = low risk
- 2 in only ONE of the areas assessed = borderline/observe closely
- 2 in TWO or more of the areas assessed **or** 3 to 4 in ONLY ONE area = indicative of TD

From U.S. Department of Health and Human Services. Available for use in the public domain.

---

temperature and observation for parkinsonian symptoms.

*Onset can occur within hours or as long as years after drug initiation, and progression is rapid over the following 24 to 72 hours.

*Symptoms include severe parkinsonian muscle rigidity, very high fever, tachycardia, tachypnea, fluctuations in blood pressure, diaphoresis, and rapid deterioration of mental status to stupor and coma.

*Discontinue neuroleptic medication immediately.

*Monitor vital signs, degree of muscle rigidity, intake and output, level of consciousness.

*The physician may order bromocriptine (Parlodel) or dantrolene (Dantrium) to counteract the effects of NMS.

■ Hyperglycemia and diabetes (more common with atypical antipsychotics). Studies have suggested an increased risk of treatment-emergent hyperglycemia-related adverse events in clients using atypical antipsychotics (e.g., risperidone, clozapine, olanzapine, quetiapine, ziprasidone, paliperidone, iloperidone, asenapine, lurasidone, and aripiprazole). The U.S. Food and Drug Administration (FDA) recommends that clients with diabetes starting on atypical antipsychotic drugs be monitored regularly for worsening of glucose control. Clients with risk factors for diabetes should undergo fasting blood glucose testing at the beginning of treatment and periodically thereafter. All clients taking these medications should be monitored for symptoms of hyperglycemia (polydipsia, polyuria, polyphagia, and weakness). If these symptoms appear during treatment, the client should undergo fasting blood glucose testing.

■ Increased risk of mortality in elderly patients with dementia-related psychosis. Recent studies have indicated that elderly patients with dementia-related psychosis who are treated with antipsychotic drugs are at increased risk of death compared with those taking a placebo. Causes of death are most commonly related to infections or cardiovascular problems. All antipsychotic drugs now carry black-box warnings to this effect. They are not approved for treatment of elderly patients with dementia-related psychosis.

Client/Family Education Related to Antipsychotics

The client should:

■ Use caution when driving or operating dangerous machinery. Drowsiness and dizziness can occur.

■ Not stop taking the drug abruptly after long-term use. To do so might produce withdrawal symptoms, such as nausea, vomiting, dizziness, gastritis, headache, tachycardia, insomnia, and tremulousness.

■ Use sunblock lotion and wear protective clothing when spending time outdoors. Skin is more susceptible to sunburn, which can occur in as little as 30 minutes.

■ Report weekly (if receiving clozapine therapy) to have blood levels drawn and to obtain a weekly supply of the drug.

■ Report the occurrence of any of the following symptoms to the physician immediately: sore throat, fever, malaise, unusual bleeding, easy bruising, persistent nausea and vomiting, severe headache, rapid heart rate, fainting, difficulty urinating, muscle twitching, tremors, darkly colored urine, excessive urination, excessive thirst, excessive hunger, weakness, pale stools, yellow skin or eyes, muscular incoordination, or skin rash.

■ Rise slowly from a sitting or lying position to prevent a sudden drop in blood pressure.

■ Take frequent sips of water, chew sugarless gum, or suck on hard candy if dry mouth is a problem. Good oral care (frequent brushing, flossing) is very important.

■ Consult the physician regarding smoking while on neuroleptic therapy. Smoking increases the metabolism of neuroleptics, requiring an adjustment in dosage to achieve a therapeutic effect.

■ Dress warmly in cold weather and avoid extended exposure to very high or low temperatures. Body temperature is harder to maintain with this medication.

■ Avoid drinking alcohol while on neuroleptic therapy. These drugs potentiate each other's effects.

■ Not consume other medications (including over-the-counter products) without the physician's approval. Many medications contain substances that interact with neuroleptics in a way that may be harmful.

■ Be aware of possible risks of taking neuroleptics during pregnancy. Safe use during pregnancy has not been established. Neuroleptics are thought to readily cross the placental barrier; if so, a fetus could experience adverse effects of the drug. Inform the physician immediately if pregnancy occurs, is suspected, or is planned.

■ Be aware of side effects of neuroleptic drugs. Refer to written materials furnished by health-care providers for safe self-administration.

■ Continue to take the medication, even if feeling well and as though it is not needed. Symptoms may return if medication is discontinued.

■ Carry a card or other identification at all times describing medications being taken.

CASE STUDY AND SAMPLE CARE PLAN

NURSING HISTORY AND ASSESSMENT

Frank is 22 years old. He joined the Marines just out of high school at age 18 for a 3-year enlistment. His final year was spent in Iraq. When his 3-year enlistment was up, he returned to his hometown and married a young woman with whom he had been a high school classmate. Frank has always been quiet, somewhat withdrawn, and had very few friends. He was the only child of a single mom who never married, and he does not know his father. His mother was killed in an automobile accident the spring before he enlisted in the Marines.

During the past year, he has become more and more isolated and withdrawn. He is without regular employment, but finds work as a day laborer when he can. His wife, Suzanne, works as a secretary and is the primary wage earner. Lately he has become very suspicious of her, and sometimes follows her to work. He also drops in on her at work and accuses her of having affairs with some of the men in the office.

Last evening when Suzanne got home from work, Frank was hiding in the closet. She didn't know he was home. When she started to undress, he jumped out of the closet holding a large kitchen knife and threatened to kill her "for being unfaithful." Suzanne managed to flee their home and ran to the neighbor's house and called the police.

Frank told the police that he received a message over the radio from his Marine commanding officer telling him that he couldn't allow his wife to continue to commit adultery, and the only way he could stop it was to kill her. The police took Frank to the emergency department of the VA Hospital, where he was admitted to the psychiatric unit. Suzanne is helping with the admission history.

Suzanne tells the nurse that she has never been unfaithful to Frank and she doesn't know why he believes that she has. Frank tells the nurse that he has been "taking orders from my commanding officer through my car radio ever since I got back from Iraq." He survived a helicopter crash in Iraq in which all were killed except Frank and one other man. Frank says, "I have to follow my CO's orders. God saved me to annihilate the impure."

Following an evaluation, the psychiatrist diagnoses Frank with paranoid schizophrenia. He orders olanzapine 10 mg PO to be given daily and olanzapine 10 mg IM q6h prn for agitation.

NURSING DIAGNOSES/OUTCOME IDENTIFICATION

From the assessment data, the nurse develops the following nursing diagnoses for Frank:

1. **Risk for self-directed or other-directed violence** related to unresolved grief over loss of mother; survivor's guilt associated with helicopter crash; command hallucinations; and history of violence.
   a. **Short-Term Goals:**
      - Frank will seek out staff when anxiety and agitation start to increase.
      - Frank will not harm self or others.
   b. **Long-Term Goal:** Frank will not harm self or others.
2. **Disturbed sensory perception: Auditory** related to increased anxiety and agitation, withdrawal into self, and stress of sufficient intensity to threaten an already weak ego
   a. **Short-Term Goals:**
      - Frank will discuss the content of the hallucinations with the nurse.
      - Frank will maintain anxiety at a manageable level.
   b. **Long-Term Goal:** Frank will be able to define and test reality, reducing or eliminating the occurrence of hallucinations.

PLANNING/IMPLEMENTATION

Risk for Self-Directed or Other-Directed Violence

1. Keep the stimuli as low as possible in Frank's environment.
2. Monitor Frank's behavior frequently, but in a manner of carrying out routine activities so as not to create suspiciousness on his part.

3. Watch for the following signs (considered the prodrome to aggressive behavior): increased motor activity, pounding, slamming, tense posture, defiant affect, clenched teeth and fists, arguing, demanding, and challenging or threatening staff.
4. If Frank should become aggressive, maintain a calm attitude. Try talking. Offer medication. Provide physical activities.
5. If these interventions fail, indicate a show of strength with a team of staff members.
6. Utilize restraints only as a last resort and if Frank is clearly at risk of harm to self or others.
7. Help Frank recognize unresolved grief and fixation in denial or anger stage of grief process.
8. Encourage him to talk about the loss of his mother and fellow Marines in Iraq.
9. Encourage him to talk about guilt feelings associated with survival when others died.
10. Make a short-term contract with Frank that he will seek out staff if considering harming self or others. When this contract expires, make another, etc.

Disturbed Sensory Perception: Auditory

1. Monitor Frank's behavior for signs that he is hearing voices: listening pose, talking and laughing to self, stopping in mid-sentence.
2. If these behaviors are observed, ask Frank, "Are you hearing the voices again?"
3. Encourage Frank to share the content of the hallucinations. Ask, "What do you hear the voices saying to you?" This is important for early intervention in case the content contains commands to harm self or others.
4. Say to Frank, "I understand that the voice is real to you, but I do not hear any voices speaking." It is important for him to learn the difference between what is real and what is not real.
5. Try to help Frank recognize that the voices often appear at times when he becomes anxious about something and his agitation increases.
6. Help him to recognize this increasing anxiety, and teach him methods to keep it from escalating.
7. Use distracting activities to bring him back to reality. Involvement with real people and real situations will help to distract him from the hallucination.
8. Teach him to use **voice dismissal.** When he hears the CO's (or others') voice, he should shout, "Go

Continued

CASE STUDY AND SAMPLE CARE PLAN— cont'd

away!" or "Leave me alone!" These commands may help to diminish the sounds and give him a feeling of control over the situation.

EVALUATION

The outcome criteria identified for Frank have been met. When feeling especially anxious or becoming agitated, he seeks out staff for comfort and for assistance in maintaining his anxiety at a manageable level. He establishes short-term contracts with staff not to harm himself. He is experiencing fewer auditory hallucinations, and has learned to use voice dismissal to interrupt the behavior. He is beginning to recognize his position in the grief process, and working toward resolution at his own pace.

Summary and Key Points

- Of all mental illness, schizophrenia undoubtedly results in the greatest amount of personal, emotional, and social costs. It presents an enormous threat to life and happiness, yet it remains an enigma to the medical community.

- For many years there was little agreement as to a definition of the concept of schizophrenia. The *DSM-IV-TR* (APA, 2000) identifies specific criteria for diagnosis of the disorder.

- The initial symptoms of schizophrenia most often occur in early adulthood. Development of the disorder can be viewed in four phases: (1) the premorbid phase, (2) the prodromal phase, (3) the active psychotic phase (schizophrenia), and (4) the residual phase.

- The cause of schizophrenia remains unclear. Research continues, and most contemporary psychiatrists view schizophrenia as a brain disorder with little if any emphasis on psychosocial influences.

- The disease most likely results from a combination of influences including genetics, biochemical dysfunction, and physiological and environmental factors.

- Various types of schizophrenic and related psychotic disorders have been identified and are differentiated by their total picture of clinical symptomatology. They include disorganized schizophrenia, catatonic schizophrenia, paranoid schizophrenia, undifferentiated schizophrenia, residual schizophrenia, schizoaffective disorder, brief psychotic disorder, schizophreniform disorder, delusional disorder, shared psychotic disorder, psychotic disorder caused by a general medical condition, and substance-induced psychotic disorder.

- Nursing care of the client with schizophrenia is accomplished using the six steps of the nursing process.

- Nursing assessment is based on knowledge of symptomatology related to thought content and form, perception, affect, sense of self, volition, impaired interpersonal functioning and relationship to the external world, and psychomotor behavior.

- These behaviors are categorized as *positive* (an excess or distortion of normal functions) or *negative* (a diminution or loss of normal functions).

- Antipsychotic medications remain the mainstay of treatment for psychotic disorders. Atypical antipsychotics have become the first line of therapy, and treat both positive and negative symptoms of schizophrenia. They have a more favorable side-effect profile than the conventional (typical) antipsychotics.

- Individuals with schizophrenia require long-term integrated treatment with pharmacological and other interventions. Some of these include individual psychotherapy, group therapy, behavior therapy, social skills training, milieu therapy, family therapy, and assertive community treatment. For the majority of clients, the most effective treatment appears to be a combination of psychotropic medication and psychosocial therapy.

- Some clinicians are choosing a course of therapy based on a model of recovery, somewhat like that which has been used for many years with problems of addiction. The basic premise of a recovery model is empowerment of the consumer. The recovery model is designed to allow consumers primary control over decisions about their own care, and to enable a person with a mental health problem to live a meaningful life in a community of his or her choice while striving to achieve his or her full potential.

■ Families generally require support and education about psychotic illnesses. The focus is on coping with the diagnosis, understanding the illness and its course, teaching about medication, and learning ways to manage symptoms.

DavisPlus.

Additional info available @ davisplus.fadavis.com

Review Questions
Self-Examination/Learning Exercise

*Select the answer that is **most** appropriate for each of the following questions:*

1. Tony, age 21, has been diagnosed with paranoid schizophrenia. He has been socially isolated and hearing voices telling him to kill his parents. He has been admitted to the psychiatric unit from the emergency department. The *initial* nursing intervention for Tony is to:
   a. Give him an injection of Thorazine.
   b. Ensure a safe environment for him and others.
   c. Place him in restraints.
   d. Order him a nutritious diet.

2. The primary goal in working with an actively psychotic, suspicious client would be to:
   a. Promote interaction with others.
   b. Decrease his anxiety and increase trust.
   c. Improve his relationship with his parents.
   d. Encourage participation in therapy activities.

3. The nurse is caring for a client with paranoid schizophrenia. Orders from the physician include 100 mg chlorpromazine STAT and then 50 mg bid; 2 mg benztropine (Cogentin) bid prn. Why is chlorpromazine ordered?
   a. To reduce extrapyramidal symptoms.
   b. To prevent neuroleptic malignant syndrome.
   c. To decrease psychotic symptoms.
   d. To induce sleep.

4. The nurse is caring for a client with paranoid schizophrenia. Orders from the physician include 100 mg chlorpromazine STAT and then 50 mg bid; 2 mg benztropine (Cogentin) bid prn. Because benztropine was ordered on a prn basis, which of the following assessments by the nurse would convey a need for this medication?
   a. The client's level of agitation increases.
   b. The client complains of a sore throat.
   c. The client's skin has a yellowish cast.
   d. The client develops tremors and a shuffling gait.

5. Clint, a client on the psychiatric unit, has been diagnosed with paranoid schizophrenia. He begins to tell the nurse about how the CIA is looking for him and will kill him if they find him. The most appropriate response by the nurse is:
   a. "That's ridiculous, Clint. No one is going to hurt you."
   b. "The CIA isn't interested in people like you, Clint."
   c. "Why do you think the CIA wants to kill you?"
   d. "I know you believe that, Clint, but it's really hard for me to believe."

Continued

Review Questions—cont'd
Self-Examination/Learning Exercise

6. Clint, a client on the psychiatric unit, has been diagnosed with paranoid schizophrenia. He begins to tell the nurse about how the CIA is looking for him and will kill him if they find him. Clint's belief is an example of a:
   a. Delusion of persecution.
   b. Delusion of reference.
   c. Delusion of control or influence.
   d. Delusion of grandeur.

7. The nurse is interviewing a client on the psychiatric unit. The client tilts his head to the side, stops talking in mid-sentence, and listens intently. The nurse recognizes from these signs that the client is likely experiencing:
   a. Somatic delusions.
   b. Catatonic stupor.
   c. Auditory hallucinations.
   d. Pseudoparkinsonism.

8. The nurse is interviewing a client on the psychiatric unit. The client tilts his head to the side, stops talking in mid-sentence, and listens intently. The nurse recognizes these behaviors as a symptom of the client's illness. The most appropriate nursing intervention for this symptom is to:
   a. Ask the client to describe his physical symptoms.
   b. Ask the client to describe what he is hearing.
   c. Administer a dose of benztropine.
   d. Call the physician for additional orders.

9. When a client suddenly becomes aggressive and violent on the unit, which of the following approaches would be best for the nurse to use *first*?
   a. Provide gross motor activities to relieve the client's pent-up tension.
   b. Administer a dose of prn chlorpromazine to keep the client calm.
   c. Call for sufficient help to control the situation safely.
   d. Convey to the client that his behavior is unacceptable and will not be permitted.

10. The primary focus of family therapy for clients with schizophrenia and their families is:
    a. To discuss concrete problem solving and adaptive behaviors for coping with stress.
    b. To introduce the family to others with the same problem.
    c. To keep the client and family in touch with the health-care system.
    d. To promote family interaction and increase understanding of the illness.

TEST YOUR CRITICAL THINKING SKILLS

Sara, a 23-year-old single woman, has just been admitted to the psychiatric unit by her parents. They explain that over the past few months she has become more and more withdrawn. She stays in her room alone, but lately has been heard talking and laughing to herself.

Sara left home for the first time at age 18 to attend college. She performed well during her first semester, but when she returned after Christmas, she began to accuse her roommate of stealing her possessions. She started writing to her parents that her roommate wanted to kill her and that her roommate was turning everyone against her. She said she feared for her life. She started missing classes and stayed in her bed most of the time. Sometimes she locked herself in her closet. Her parents took her home, and she was hospitalized and diagnosed with paranoid schizophrenia. She has since been maintained on antipsychotic medication while taking a few classes at the local community college.

Sara tells the admitting nurse that she quit taking her medication 4 weeks ago because the pharmacist who fills the prescriptions is plotting to have her killed. She believes he is trying to poison her. She says she got this information from a television message. As Sara speaks, the nurse notices that she sometimes stops in mid-sentence and listens; sometimes she cocks her head to the side and moves her lips as though she is talking.

Answer the following questions related to Sara:

1. From the assessment data, what would be the most immediate nursing concern in working with Sara?

2. What is the nursing diagnosis related to this concern?

3. What interventions must be accomplished before the nurse can be successful in working with Sara?

References

Addington, D. E. (2006). Reducing suicide risk in patients with schizophrenia. *Medscape Psychiatry & Mental Health*. Retrieved September 10, 2010, from http://www.medscape.com/viewprogram/5616

American Psychiatric Association. (2000). *Diagnostic and statistical manual of mental disorders* (4th ed.). *Text revision*. Washington, DC: American Psychiatric Publishing.

Anthony, W. A. (1993). Recovery from mental illness: The guiding vision of the mental health service system in the 1990s. *Psychosocial Rehabilitation Journal, 16*(4), 11–23.

Asen, E. (2002). Outcome research in family therapy: Family intervention for psychosis. *Advances in Psychiatric Treatment, 8,* 230–238.

Assertive Community Treatment Association. (2010). *ACT Model*. Retrieved September 8, 2010, from http://www.actassociation.org/actModel

Black, D. W., & Andreasen, N. C. (2011). *Introductory textbook of psychiatry* (5th ed.). Washington, DC: American Psychiatric Publishing.

Dixon, L. B., Lehman, A. F., & Levine, J. (2009). *Conventional antipsychotic medications for schizophrenia*. Retrieved September 10, 2010, from http://www.mental-health-matters.com

Drug facts and comparisons. (2011). St. Louis: Wolters Kluwer.

Ho, B. C., Black, D. W., & Andreasen, N. C. (2003). Schizophrenia and other psychotic disorders. In R. E. Hales & S. C. Yudofsky (Eds.), *Textbook of clinical psychiatry* (4th ed.,

pp. 379–438). Washington, DC: American Psychiatric Publishing.

Institute of Medicine. (2003). *Health professions education: A bridge to quality*. Washington, DC: Author.

Jacobson, N., & Greenley, D. (2001). What is recovery? A conceptual model and explication. *Psychiatric Services, 52*(4), 482–485.

Jonsson, S. A., Luts, A., Guldberg-Kjaer, N., & Brun, A. (1997). Hippocampal pyramidal cell disarray correlates negatively to cell number: Implications for the pathogenesis of schizophrenia. *European Archives of Psychiatry and Clinical Neuroscience, 247,* 120–127.

Lehman, A. F., Lieberman, J. A., Dixon, L. B., McGlashan, T. H., Miller, A. L., Perkins, D. O., et al. (2006). Practice guideline for the treatment of patients with schizophrenia (2nd ed.). *American Psychiatric Association practice guidelines for the treatment of psychiatric disorders, Compendium 2006*. Washington, DC: American Psychiatric Publishing.

Minzenberg, M. J., Yoon, J. H., & Carter, C. S. (2008). Schizophrenia. In R. E. Hales, S. C. Yudofsky, & G. O. Gabbard (Eds.), *Textbook of psychiatry* (5th ed., pp. 407–456). Washington, DC: American Psychiatric Publishing.

Mueser, K. T., Bond, G. R., & Drake, R. E. (2002). Community-based treatment of schizophrenia and other severe mental disorders: Treatment outcomes. *Medscape Psychiatry & Mental Health eJournal 6*(1). Retrieved September 8, 2010, from http://www.medscape.com/viewarticle/430529

NANDA International. (2009). *Nursing diagnoses: Definitions & classification 2009–2011*. Hoboken, NJ: Wiley-Blackwell.

National Alliance for the Mentally Ill. (2010). *Program of Assertive Community Treatment (PACT)*. Retrieved September 8, 2010, from http://www.nami.org/

National Association of Social Workers. (2010). *NASW practice snapshot: The mental health recovery model*. Retrieved September 8, 2010, from http://www.socialworkers.org/practice/behavioral_health/0206snapshot.asp?

President's New Freedom Commission on Mental Health. (2003). *Achieving the promise: Transforming mental health care in America*. Retrieved September 8, 2010, from http://www.mentalhealthcommission.gov/

Radomsky, E. D., Haas, G. L., Mann, J. J., & Sweeney, J. A. (1999). Suicidal behavior in patients with schizophrenia and other psychotic disorders. *American Journal of Psychiatry, 156,* 1590–1595.

Rantakallio, P., Jones, P., Moring, J., & VonWendt, L. (1997). Association between central nervous system infections during childhood and adult onset schizophrenia and other psychoses: A 28-year follow-up. *International Journal of Epidemiology, 26,* 837–843.

Sadock, B. J., & Sadock, V. A. (2007). *Synopsis of psychiatry: Behavioral sciences/clinical psychiatry* (10th ed.). Philadelphia: Lippincott Williams & Wilkins.

Safier, E. (1997). Our families, the context of our lives. *Menninger Perspective, 28*(1), 4–9.

Schatzberg, A. F., Cole, J. O., & DeBattista, C. (2010). *Manual of clinical psychopharmacology* (7th ed.). Washington, DC: American Psychiatric Publishing.

Sharfstein, S. (2005). Recovery model will strengthen psychiatrist-patient relationship. *Psychiatric News, 40*(20), 3.

Substance Abuse and Mental Health Services Administration, Center for Mental Health Services. (2010). *National consensus statement on mental health recovery*. Retrieved September 8, 2010, from http://www.samhsa.gov

The Joint Commission. (2010, January). *The comprehensive accreditation manual for hospitals: The official handbook*. Oakbrook Terrace, IL: Joint Commission Resources.

@ INTERNET REFERENCES

- Additional information about schizophrenia may be located at the following websites:
  - http://www.nimh.nih.gov
  - http://www.nami.org
  - http://mentalhealth.com
  - http://www.narsad.org/

- Additional information about medications to treat schizophrenia may be located at the following websites:
  - http://www.medicinenet.com/medications/article.htm
  - http://www.fadavis.com/townsend
  - http://www.nlm.nih.gov/medlineplus
  - http://www.drugs.com/

MOVIE CONNECTIONS

I Never Promised You a Rose Garden (schizophrenia) • *A Beautiful Mind* (schizophrenia) • *The Fisher King* (schizophrenia) • *Bennie & Joon* (schizophrenia) • *Out of Darkness* (schizophrenia) • *Conspiracy Theory* (paranoia) • *The Fan* (delusional disorder)

Mood Disorders—Depression

CORE CONCEPTS
depression
mood

KEY TERMS

cognitive therapy
dysthymic disorder
melancholia

postpartum depression
premenstrual dysphoric
  disorder

psychomotor retardation
tyramine

OBJECTIVES
After reading this chapter, the student will be able to:

1. Recount historical perspectives of depression.
2. Discuss epidemiological statistics related to depression.
3. Describe various types of depressive disorders.
4. Identify predisposing factors in the development of depression.
5. Discuss implications of depression related to developmental stage.
6. Identify symptomatology associated with depression and use this information in client assessment.
7. Formulate nursing diagnoses and goals of care for clients with depression.
8. Identify topics for client and family teaching relevant to depression.
9. Describe appropriate nursing interventions for behaviors associated with depression.
10. Describe relevant criteria for evaluating nursing care of clients with depression.
11. Discuss various modalities relevant to treatment of depression.

HOMEWORK ASSIGNMENT
Please read the chapter and answer the following questions:

1. Alterations in which of the neurotransmitters are most closely associated with depression?
2. Depression in adolescence is very hard to differentiate from the normal stormy behavior associated with adolescence. What is the best clue for determining a problem with depression in adolescence?
3. Behaviors of depression often change with the diurnal variation in the level of neurotransmitters. Describe the difference in this phenomenon between moderate and severe depression.
4. All antidepressants carry a black-box warning. What is it?

Depression is likely the oldest and still one of the most frequently diagnosed psychiatric illnesses. Symptoms of depression have been described almost as far back as there is evidence of written documentation.

An occasional bout with the "blues," a feeling of sadness or downheartedness, is common among healthy people and considered to be a normal response to everyday disappointments in life. These episodes are short-lived as the individual adapts to the loss, change, or failure (real or perceived) that has been experienced. Pathological depression occurs when adaptation is ineffective.

CORE CONCEPT

Mood

Also called *affect*. Mood is a pervasive and sustained emotion that may have a major influence on a person's perception of the world. Examples of mood include depression, joy, elation, anger, and anxiety. *Affect* is described as the emotional reaction associated with an experience.

This chapter focuses on the consequences of complicated grieving as it is manifested by depression. A historical perspective and epidemiological statistics related to depression are presented. Predisposing factors that have been implicated in the etiology of depression provide a framework for studying the dynamics of the disorder.

The implications of depression relevant to individuals of various developmental stages are discussed. An explanation of the symptomatology is presented as background knowledge for assessing the client with depression. Nursing care is described in the context of the six steps of the nursing process. Various medical treatment modalities are explored.

CORE CONCEPT

Depression

An alteration in mood that is expressed by feelings of sadness, despair, and pessimism. There is a loss of interest in usual activities, and somatic symptoms may be evident. Changes in appetite and sleep patterns are common.

Historical Perspective

Many ancient cultures (e.g., Babylonian, Egyptian, Hebrew) have believed in the supernatural or divine origin of mood disorders. The Old Testament states in the Book of Samuel that King Saul's depression was inflicted by an "evil spirit" sent from God to "torment" him.

A clearly nondivine point of view regarding depression was held by the Greek medical community from the fifth century B.C. through the third century A.D. This represented the thinking of Hippocrates, Celsus, and Galen, among others. They strongly rejected the idea of divine origin and considered the brain as the seat of all emotional states. Hippocrates believed that **melancholia** was caused by an excess of black bile, a heavily toxic substance produced in the spleen or intestine, which affected the brain. Melancholia is a severe form of depressive disorder in which symptoms are exaggerated and interest or pleasure in virtually all activities is lost.

During the Renaissance, several new theories evolved. Depression was viewed by some as being the result of obstruction of vital air circulation, excessive brooding, or helpless situations beyond the client's control. Depression was reflected in major literary works of the time, including Shakespeare's *King Lear, Macbeth,* and *Hamlet.*

Contemporary thinking has been shaped a great deal by the works of Sigmund Freud, Emil Kraepelin, and Adolf Meyer. Having evolved from these early 20th-century models, current thinking about mood disorders generally encompasses the intrapsychic, behavioral, and biological perspectives. These various perspectives support the notion of multiple causation in the development of mood disorders.

Epidemiology

Major depression is one of the leading causes of disability in the United States. In 2008, 6.4 percent of persons ages 18 or older (14.3 million persons) had at least one major depressive episode in the past year. Over 1 in 25 adults (4.2 percent, or 9.5 million persons) reported that they had had a major depressive episode with severe impairment in the previous year (Substance Abuse and Mental Health Services Administration [SAMHSA], 2009). During their lifetime, about 21 percent of women and 13 percent of men will become clinically depressed. This preponderance has led to the consideration of depression by some researchers as "the common cold of psychiatric disorders" and this generation as an "age of melancholia."

Age and Gender

Research indicates that the incidence of depressive disorder is higher in women than it is in men by almost 2 to 1. Women experience more depression than men beginning at about age 10 and continuing through midlife (Kornstein, 2006). The gender difference is less pronounced between ages 44 and 65, but after the age of 65, women are again more likely to be depressed than men. This occurrence may be related to gender differences in social roles and economic and social opportunities and the shifts that occur with age. The construction of gender stereotypes, or *gender socialization,* promotes typical female characteristics, such as helplessness, passivity, and emotionality, that are associated with depression. In contrast, some studies have suggested that "masculine" characteristics are associated with higher self-esteem and less depression.

Social Class

Results of studies have indicated an inverse relationship between social class and report of depressive symptoms. However, there has yet to be a definitive causal structure in the socioeconomic status–mental illness relationship. Hudson (2005) stated:

> Do poor socioeconomic conditions predispose people to mental disability? Or do preexisting, biologically based mental illnesses result in the drift of individuals into poor socioeconomic circumstances? (p. 3)

Hudson (2005) reported that both depression and personality disorders have most commonly been found to be outcomes of low socioeconomic status.

IMPLICATIONS OF RESEARCH FOR EVIDENCE-BASED PRACTICE

Peden, A. R., Rayens, M. K., Hall, L. A., & Grant, E. (2004). Negative thinking and the mental health of low-income single mothers. *Journal of Nursing Scholarship, (36)*4, 337–344.

DESCRIPTION OF THE STUDY: The aims of this study were to: (1) examine the prevalence of a high level of depressive symptoms in low-income, single mothers with children 2 to 6 years of age; (2) evaluate the relationships of personal sociodemographic characteristics with self-esteem, chronic stressors, negative thinking, and depressive symptoms; and (3) determine whether negative thinking mediates the effects of self-esteem and chronic stressors on depressive symptoms. Single mothers are a particularly high-risk group for clinical depression because of life circumstances such as poverty, low self-esteem, and few social resources. The average age of the mothers in the study was 27 years. The ethnicity of the sample was approximately half Caucasian and half African American. The majority had never been married; most were employed, but had annual incomes at or below $15,000. The Beck Depression Inventory was used to measure symptoms of depression, the Crandell Cognitions Inventory was used to measure negative thoughts, and the Rosenberg Self-Esteem Scale was used to measure self-worth and self-acceptance.

RESULTS OF THE STUDY: More than 75 percent of the mothers scored somewhere in the mild to high range for depression. Negative thinking mediated the effect of self-esteem on depressive symptoms and partially mediated the effect of chronic stressors. Those subjects who were employed measured higher self-esteem, less negative thinking, fewer chronic stressors, and less depression. No differences in predictors of depression were found between Caucasian and African American mothers in this study.

IMPLICATIONS FOR NURSING PRACTICE: The results of this study suggest the importance of intervening to address negative thinking among low-income single mothers to help them lessen their stress and decrease their risk of depression. The authors stated, "Depression may interfere with parenting and participation in educational and employment opportunities, significantly undermining the quality of life in these families. [A number of studies] have indicated that mothers' depression may also negatively influence their children's behavior." (p. 342) Psychiatric nurses may employ cognitive-behavioral strategies to help women minimize negative thinking. Strategies such as writing affirmations and use of positive self-talk have been supported in nursing research. Targeting the symptom of negative thinking, which can be modified, may serve to break the links of chronic stressors and low self-esteem to depressive symptoms, resulting in improved mental health for the mother and the subsequent well-being of her children.

Race and Culture

Studies have shown no consistent relationship between race and affective disorder. One problem encountered in reviewing racial comparisons has to do with the socioeconomic class of the race being investigated. Sample populations of nonwhite clients are many times predominantly lower class and are often compared with white populations from middle and upper social classes.

Other studies suggest a second problematic factor in the study of racial comparisons. Clinicians tend to underdiagnose mood disorders and to overdiagnose schizophrenia in clients who have racial or cultural backgrounds different from their own (Sadock & Sadock, 2007). This misdiagnosis may result from language barriers between clients and physicians who are unfamiliar with cultural aspects of nonwhite clients' language and behavior.

Recent findings from the National Study of American Life, a survey of mental health among blacks in the United States, reveal that depression is more prevalent in whites than it is in blacks, but that depression tends to be more severe, persistent, and disabling in blacks, and they are less likely to be treated (Williams et al., 2007). Even among blacks whose symptoms were rated severe or very severe, only 48.5 percent of African Americans and 21.9 percent of Caribbean blacks received any treatment at all. The authors concluded that these findings highlight the importance of identifying high-risk subgroups in racial populations and the need for targeting cost-effective interventions to them.

Marital Status

A number of studies have suggested that marriage has a positive effect on the psychological well-being of an individual (as compared to those who are single or do not have a close relationship with another person). LaPierre (2004) suggested that marital status alone may lack validity, and that the effect of marital status on depression may be contingent on age. She found in her study that being single was a significant predictor of depression in the 37- to 49-year-old age group, but was not a significant predictor of depression in any of the other age groups (18 to 25; 26 to 36; 50+). She explained her finding in the following way:

> The realization that the normative ideal of marriage (and accompanying children) is becoming a remote possibility is likely to occur in the 37-49 year old age group, causing a decrease in mental health and corresponding increase in depressive symptomatology. This is particularly true for women who reach the end of their childbearing years in this age category, and feel they may have to forfeit the normative role of motherhood if they do not find a partner to have a child with. The subsequent decline in depressive symptomatology (observed in the 50+ age group) could occur because with time the never-married/childless individual comes to accept their non-normative behavior and find ways to adjust.

Other studies also have indicated that age may moderate the effect of marital status on depression. George (1992) found that marriage (versus separated/divorced) had a protective effect against major depression only in the oldest age category (65+). Her results also showed that being never married (versus separated/divorced) was associated with increased risk of major depression in the 40- to 64-year-old age group and the 65+ age group.

Seasonality

A number of studies have examined seasonal patterns associated with mood disorders. These studies have revealed two prevalent periods of seasonal involvement: one in the spring (March, April, and May) and one in the fall (September, October, and November). This pattern tends to parallel the seasonal pattern for suicide, which shows a large peak in the spring and a smaller one in October (Davidson, 2005). A number of etiologies associated with this trend have been postulated (Hakko, 2000). Some of these include the following:

- A meteorological factor, associating drastic temperature and barometric pressure changes to human mental instability
- Sociodemographic variables, such as the seasonal increase in social intercourse (e.g., increased social activity with the commencement of an academic year)
- Biochemical variables due to possible seasonal variations in peripheral and central aspects of serotonergic function involved in depression and suicide

Types of Depressive Disorders

Major Depressive Disorder

Major depressive disorder (MDD) is characterized by depressed mood or loss of interest or pleasure in usual activities. Evidence will show impaired social and occupational functioning that has existed for at least 2 weeks, no history of manic behavior, and symptoms that cannot be attributed to use of substances or a general medical condition. Additionally, the diagnosis of MDD is specified according to whether it is a *single episode* (the individual's first encounter) or *recurrent episode* (the individual has a history of previous episodes). The diagnosis will also identify the degree of severity of symptoms (mild, moderate, or severe), whether there is evidence of psychotic or catatonic features, and if a seasonal pattern can be detected. It is noted as *postpartum onset* if the symptoms appear within 4 weeks of childbirth. The *Diagnostic and Statistical Manual of Mental Disorders, Fourth Edition, Text*

Revision (DSM-IV-TR) (American Psychiatric Association [APA], 2000) diagnostic criteria for major depressive disorder are presented in Box 27-1.

Dysthymic Disorder

Characteristics of **dysthymic disorder** are similar to, if somewhat milder than, those ascribed to MDD. Individuals with this mood disturbance describe their mood as sad or "down in the dumps" (APA, 2000). There is no evidence of psychotic symptoms. The essential feature is a chronically depressed mood (or possibly an irritable mood in children or adolescents) for most of the day, more days than not, for at least 2 years (1 year for children and adolescents). The diagnosis is identified as *early onset* (occurring before age 21 years) or *late onset* (occurring at age 21 years or older). The *DSM-IV-TR* diagnostic criteria for dysthymic disorder are presented in Box 27-2.

Premenstrual Dysphoric Disorder

The *DSM-IV-TR* (APA, 2000) does not include **premenstrual dysphoric disorder** as an official diagnostic category, but provides a set of research criteria to promote further study of the disorder. The essential features include markedly depressed mood, excessive anxiety, mood swings, and decreased interest in activities during the week prior to menses and subsiding shortly after the onset of menstruation (APA, 2000). The *DSM-IV-TR* research criteria for premenstrual dysphoric disorder are presented in Box 27-3.

Other Depressive Disorders

Mood Disorder (Depression) due to a General Medical Condition

This disorder is characterized by prominent and persistent depression that is judged to be the result of direct physiological effects of a general medical condition (APA, 2000). The depression causes clinically significant distress or impairment in social, occupational, or other important areas of functioning. Types of physiological influences are included in the discussion of etiological implications for depression.

BOX 27-1 Diagnostic Criteria for Major Depressive Disorder

A. Five (or more) of the following symptoms have been present during the same 2-week period and represent a change from previous functioning; at least one of the symptoms is either (1) depressed mood, or (2) loss of interest or pleasure.
   1. Depressed mood most of the day, nearly every day, as indicated by either subjective report (e.g., feels sad or empty) or observation made by others (e.g., appears tearful). In children and adolescents, symptom can be irritable mood.
   2. Markedly diminished interest or pleasure in all, or almost all, activities most of the day, nearly every day (as indicated either by subjective account or observation made by others).
   3. Significant weight loss when not dieting or weight gain (e.g., a change of more than 5% of body weight in a month), or a decrease or increase in appetite nearly every day. In children, consider failure to make expected weight gains.
   4. Insomnia or hypersomnia nearly every day.
   5. Psychomotor agitation or retardation nearly every day (observable by others, not merely subjective feelings of restlessness or being slowed down).
   6. Fatigue or loss of energy nearly every day.
   7. Feelings of worthlessness or excessive or inappropriate guilt (which may be delusional) nearly every

day (not merely self-reproach or guilt about being sick).
   8. Diminished ability to think or concentrate, or indecisiveness, nearly every day (either by subjective account or as observed by others).
   9. Recurrent thoughts of death (not just fear of dying), recurrent suicidal ideation without a specific plan, or a suicide attempt or a specific plan for committing suicide.

B. There has never been a manic episode, a mixed episode, or a hypomanic episode that was not substance or treatment induced or due to the direct physiological effects of a general medical condition.

C. The symptoms cause clinically significant distress or impairment in social, occupational, or other important areas of functioning.

D. The symptoms are not due to the direct physiological effects of a substance (e.g., a drug of abuse, a medication) or a general medical condition (e.g., hypothyroidism).

E. The symptoms are not better accounted for by bereavement (i.e., after the loss of a loved one), the symptoms persist for longer than 2 months or are characterized by marked functional impairment, morbid preoccupation with worthlessness, suicidal ideation, psychotic symptoms, or psychomotor retardation.

From American Psychiatric Association. (2000). *Diagnostic and statistical manual of mental disorders (4th ed.). Text Revision.* Washington, DC: American Psychiatric Publishing, with permission.

BOX 27-2 Diagnostic Criteria for Dysthymic Disorder

A. Depressed mood for most of the day, more days than not, as indicated either by subjective account or observation by others, for at least 2 years. In children and adolescents, mood can be irritable and duration must be at least 1 year.

B. Presence, while depressed, of two (or more) of the following:
1. Poor appetite or overeating.
2. Insomnia or hypersomnia.
3. Low energy or fatigue.
4. Low self-esteem.
5. Poor concentration or difficulty making decisions.
6. Feelings of hopelessness.

C. During the 2-year period (1 year for children or adolescents) of the disturbance, the person has never been without the symptoms in A or B for more than 2 months at a time.

D. No major depressive disorder has been present during the first 2 years of the disturbance (1 year for children and adolescents)

E. There has never been a manic, mixed or hypomanic episode, and criteria have never been met for cyclothymic disorder.

F. The disturbance does not occur exclusively during the course of a chronic psychotic disorder, such as schizophrenia or delusional disorder.

G. The symptoms are not due to the direct physiological effects of a substance (e.g., a drug of abuse, a medication) or a general medical condition (e.g., hypothyroidism).

H. The symptoms cause clinically significant distress or impairment in social, occupational, or other important areas of functioning.

Specify if:

Early onset: Before age 21 years.

Late onset: Age 21 years or older.

From American Psychiatric Association. (2000). Diagnostic and statistical manual of mental disorders (4th ed.). Text Revision. Washington, DC: American Psychiatric Publishing, with permission.

BOX 27-3 Research Criteria for Premenstrual Dysphoric Disorder

A. In most menstrual cycles during the past year, five (or more) of the following symptoms were present for most of the time during the last week of the luteal phase, began to remit within a few days after the onset of the follicular phase, and were absent in the week postmenses, with at least one of the symptoms being 1, 2, 3, or 4:
1. Markedly depressed mood, feelings of hopelessness, or self-deprecating thoughts.
2. Marked anxiety, tension, feelings of being "keyed up," or "on edge."
3. Marked affective lability (e.g., feeling suddenly sad or tearful or increased sensitivity to rejection).
4. Persistent and marked anger or irritability or increased interpersonal conflicts.
5. Decreased interest in usual activities (e.g., work, school, friends, hobbies).
6. Subjective sense of difficulty in concentrating.
7. Lethargy, easy fatigability, or marked lack of energy.

8. Marked change in appetite, overeating, or specific food cravings.
9. Hypersomnia or insomnia.
10. A subjective sense of being overwhelmed or out of control.
11. Other physical symptoms, such as breast tenderness or swelling, headaches, joint or muscle pain, a sensation of "bloating," weight gain.

B. The disturbance markedly interferes with work or school or with usual social activities and relationships with others (e.g., avoidance of social activities, decreased productivity and efficiency at work or school).

C. The disturbance is not merely an exacerbation of the symptoms of another disorder, such as major depressive disorder, panic disorder, dysthymic disorder, or a personality disorder (although it may be superimposed on any of these disorders).

D. Criteria A, B, and C must be confirmed by prospective daily ratings during at least two consecutive symptomatic cycles.

From American Psychiatric Association. (2000). Diagnostic and statistical manual of mental disorders (4th ed.). Text Revision. Washington, DC: American Psychiatric Publishing, with permission.

Substance-Induced Mood Disorder (Depression)

The depressed mood associated with a substance-induced mood disorder is considered to be the direct result of physiological effects of a substance (e.g., a drug of abuse, a medication, or toxin exposure), and causes clinically significant distress or impairment in social, occupational, or other important areas of functioning.

Mood disturbances are associated with *intoxication* from substances such as alcohol, amphetamines, cocaine, hallucinogens, inhalants, opioids, phencyclidine, sedatives, hypnotics, and anxiolytics. Symptoms can occur with *withdrawal* from substances such as alcohol, amphetamines, cocaine, sedatives, hypnotics, and anxiolytics. Heavy metals and toxins, such as gasoline, paint, organophosphate insecticides, nerve gases, carbon monoxide, and carbon dioxide, may also cause mood symptoms (APA, 2000).

A number of medications have been known to evoke mood symptoms. Classifications include anesthetics, analgesics, anticholinergics, anticonvulsants, antihypertensives, antiparkinsonian agents, antiulcer agents, cardiac medications, oral contraceptives, psychotropic medications, muscle relaxants, steroids, and sulfonamides. Some specific examples are included in the discussion of predisposing factors to mood disorders.

Predisposing Factors

The etiology of depression is unclear. No single theory or hypothesis has been postulated that substantiates a clear-cut explanation for the disease. Evidence continues to mount in support of multiple causations, recognizing the combined effects of genetic, biochemical, and psychosocial influences on an individual's susceptibility to depression. A number of theoretical postulates are presented here.

Biological Theories

Genetics

Affective illness has been the subject of considerable research on the relevance of hereditary factors. A genetic link has been suggested in numerous studies; however, a definitive mode of genetic transmission has yet to be demonstrated.

Twin Studies

Twin studies suggest a strong genetic factor in the etiology of affective illness. Joska and Stein (2008) reported that studies of monozygotic twins indicate that heritability of recurrent major depression is approximately 37 percent. They stated:

> In individuals who share all or almost all of their genetic material, genes account for about 37 percent of the risk of developing major depression. The effect of the individual environment and the interaction between genes and the said environment probably account for a large portion of the remaining risk. (p. 474)

Family Studies

Most family studies have shown that major depression is 1.5 to 3 times more common among first-degree biological relatives of people with the disorder than among the general population (APA, 2000). Indeed, the evidence to support an increased risk of depressive disorder in individuals with positive family history is quite compelling. It is unlikely that random environmental factors could cause the concentration of illness that is seen within families.

Adoption Studies

Further support for heritability as an etiological influence in depression comes from studies of the adopted offspring of affectively ill biological parents. These studies have indicated that biological children of parents with mood disorders are at increased risk of developing a mood disorder, even when they are reared by adoptive parents who do not have the disorder (Dubovsky, Davies, & Dubovsky, 2003).

Biochemical Influences

Biogenic Amines

It has been hypothesized that depressive illness may be related to a deficiency of the neurotransmitters norepinepherine, serotonin, and dopamine at functionally important receptor sites in the brain. Historically, the biogenic amine hypothesis of mood disorders grew out of the observation that reserpine, which depletes the brain of amines, was associated with the development of a depressive syndrome (Slattery, Hudson, & Nutt, 2004). The catecholamine norepinephrine has been identified as a key component in the mobilization of the body to deal with stressful situations. Neurons that contain serotonin are critically involved in the regulation of many psychobiological functions, such as mood, anxiety, arousal, vigilance, irritability, thinking, cognition, appetite, aggression, and circadian rhythm (Dubovsky et al., 2003). Tryptophan, the amino acid precursor of serotonin, has been shown to enhance the efficacy of antidepressant medications and, on occasion, to be effective as an antidepressant itself. The level of dopamine in the mesolimbic system of the brain is thought to exert a strong influence over human mood and behavior. A diminished supply of these biogenic amines inhibits the transmission of impulses from one neuronal fiber to another, causing a failure of the cells to fire or become charged (see Figure 27–1).

More recently, the biogenic amine hypothesis has been expanded to include another neurotransmitter, acetylcholine. Because cholinergic agents do have profound effects on mood, electroencephalograms, sleep, and neuroendocrine function, it has been suggested that the problem in depression and mania may be an imbalance between the biogenic amines and acetylcholine.

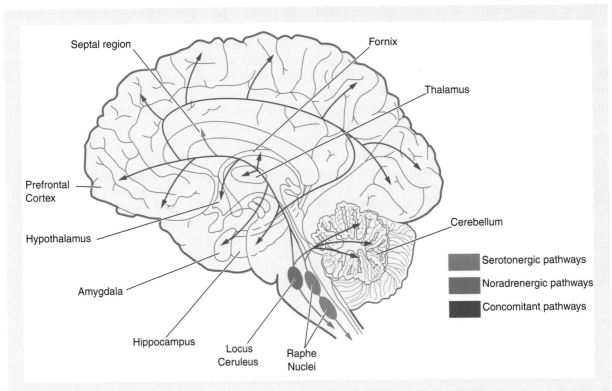

FIGURE 27–1 Neurobiology of depression.

Neurotransmitters

Although other neurotransmitters have also been implicated in the pathophysiology of depression, disturbances in serotonin and norepinephrine have been the most extensively scrutinized.

Cell bodies of origin for the serotonin pathways lie within the raphe nuclei located in the brainstem. Those for norepinepherine originate in the locus ceruleus. Projections for both neurotransmitters extend throughout the forebrain, prefrontal cortex, cerebellum, and limbic system.

Areas of the Brain Affected

Areas of the brain affected by depression and the symptoms that they mediate include the following:
- Hippocampus: Memory impairments, feelings of worthlessness, hopelessness, and guilt
- Amygdala: Anhedonia, anxiety, reduced motivation
- Hypothalamus: Increased or decreased sleep and appetite; decreased energy and libido
- Other limbic structures: Emotional alterations
- Frontal cortex: Depressed mood; problems concentrating
- Cerebellum: Psychomotor retardation/agitation

Medications and their Effects on the Brain

All medications that increase serotonin, norepinephrine, or both can improve the emotional and vegetative symptoms of depression. Medications that produce these effects include those that block the presynaptic reuptake of the neurotransmitters or block receptors at nerve endings (tricyclics; SSRIs; SNRIs) and those that inhibit monoamine oxidase, an enzyme that is involved in the metabolism of the monoamines serotonin, norepinephrine, and dopamine (MAOIs).

Side effects of these medications relate to their specific neurotransmitter receptor-blocking action. Tricyclic and tetracyclic drugs (e.g., imipramine, amitriptyline, mirtazapine) block reuptake and/or receptors for serotonin, norepinephrine, acetylcholine, and histamine. SSRIs are selective serotonin reuptake inhibitors. Others, such as bupropion, venlafaxine, and duloxetine, block serotonin and norepinephrine reuptake, and also are weak inhibitors of dopamine.

Blockade of norepinephrine reuptake results in side effects of tremors, cardiac arrhythmias, sexual dysfunction, and hypertension. Blockade of serotonin reuptake results in side effects of GI disturbances, increased agitation, and sexual dysfunction. Blockade of dopamine reuptake results in side effects of psychomotor activation. Blockade of acetylcholine reuptake results in dry mouth, blurred vision, constipation, and urinary retention. Blockade of histamine reuptake results in sedation, weight gain, and hypotension.

Cholinergic transmission is thought to be excessive in depression and inadequate in mania (Dubovsky et al., 2003).

The precise role that any of the neurotransmitters plays in the etiology of depression is unknown. As the body of research grows, there is no doubt that increased knowledge regarding the biogenic amines will contribute to a greater capacity for understanding and treating affective illness.

Neuroendocrine Disturbances

Neuroendocrine disturbances may play a role in the pathogenesis or persistence of depressive illness. This notion has arisen in view of the marked disturbances in mood observed with the administration of certain hormones or in the presence of spontaneously occurring endocrine disease.

Hypothalamic-Pituitary-Adrenocortical Axis

In clients who are depressed, the normal system of hormonal inhibition fails, resulting in a hypersecretion of cortisol. This elevated serum cortisol is the basis for the dexamethasone suppression test that is sometimes used to determine if an individual has somatically treatable depression.

Hypothalamic-Pituitary-Thyroid Axis

Thyrotropin-releasing factor (TRF) from the hypothalamus stimulates the release of thyroid-stimulating hormone (TSH) from the anterior pituitary gland. In turn, TSH stimulates the thyroid gland. Diminished TSH response to administered TRF is observed in approximately 25 percent of depressed persons. This laboratory test has potential for identifying clients at high risk for affective illness.

Physiological Influences

Depressive symptoms that occur as a consequence of a non-mood disorder or as an adverse effect of certain medications are called a *secondary* depression. Secondary depression may be related to medication side effects, neurological disorders, electrolyte or hormonal disturbances, nutritional deficiencies, and other physiological or psychological conditions.

Medication Side Effects

A number of drugs, either alone or in combination with other medications, can produce a depressive syndrome. Most common among these drugs are those that have a direct effect on the central nervous system (CNS). Examples of these include the anxiolytics, antipsychotics, and sedative-hypnotics. Certain antihypertensive medications, such as propranolol and reserpine, have been known to produce depressive symptoms. One research study has found a statistically significant association between the acne medication isotretinoin (Accutane) and depression (Azoulay, Blais, Koren, LeLorier, & Berard, 2008). Depressed mood may also occur with any of the following medications, although the list is by no means all-inclusive (Sadock & Sadock, 2007):

- Steroids: prednisone and cortisone
- Hormones: estrogen and progesterone
- Sedatives: barbiturates and benzodiazepines
- Antibacterial and antifungal drugs: ampicillin, cycloserine, tetracycline, and sulfonamides
- Antineoplastics: vincristine and zidovudine
- Analgesics and anti-inflammatory drugs: opiates, ibuprofen, and phenylbutazone
- Antiulcer: cimetidine

Neurological Disorders

An individual who has suffered a cardiovascular accident (CVA) may experience a despondency unrelated to the severity of the CVA. These are true mood disorders, and antidepressant drug therapy may be indicated. Brain tumors, particularly in the area of the temporal lobe, often cause symptoms of depression. Agitated depression may be part of the clinical picture associated with Alzheimer's disease, Parkinson's disease, and Huntington's disease. Agitation and restlessness may also represent an underlying depression in the individual with multiple sclerosis.

Electrolyte Disturbances

Excessive levels of sodium bicarbonate or calcium can produce symptoms of depression, as can deficits in magnesium and sodium. Potassium is also implicated in the syndrome of depression. Symptoms have been observed with excesses of potassium in the body, as well as in instances of potassium depletion.

Hormonal Disturbances

Depression is associated with dysfunction of the adrenal cortex and is commonly observed in both Addison's disease and Cushing's syndrome. Other endocrine conditions that may result in symptoms of depression include hypoparathyroidism, hyperparathyroidism, hypothyroidism, and hyperthyroidism.

An imbalance of the hormones estrogen and progesterone has been implicated in the predisposition to premenstrual dysphoric disorder. It is postulated that excess estrogen or a high estrogen-to-progesterone ratio during the luteal phase of the menstrual cycle is responsible for the symptoms associated with premenstrual syndrome, although the exact etiology is unknown (Sadock & Sadock, 2007).

Nutritional Deficiencies

Deficiencies in vitamin B_1 (thiamine), vitamin B_6 (pyridoxine), vitamin B_{12}, niacin, vitamin C, iron, folic acid, zinc, calcium, and potassium may produce symptoms of depression (Schimelpfening, 2009).

A number of nutritional alterations have also been indicated in the etiology of premenstrual dysphoric disorder. They include deficiencies in the B vitamins, calcium, magnesium, manganese, vitamin E, and linolenic acid (Frackiewicz & Shiovitz, 2001). Glucose tolerance fluctuations, abnormal fatty acid metabolism, and sensitivity to caffeine and alcohol may also play a role in bringing about the symptoms associated with this disorder. No definitive evidence exists to support any specific nutritional alteration in the etiology of these symptoms.

Other Physiological Conditions

Other conditions that have been associated with secondary depression include collagen disorders, such as systemic lupus erythematosus (SLE) and polyarteritis nodosa; cardiovascular disease, such as cardiomyopathy, congestive heart failure, myocardial infarction, and cerebrovascular accident (stroke); infections, such as encephalitis, hepatitis, mononucleosis, pneumonia, and syphilis; and metabolic disorders, such as diabetes mellitus and porphyria.

Psychosocial Theories

Psychoanalytical Theory

Freud (1957) presented his classic paper "Mourning and Melancholia" in 1917. He defined the distinguishing features of melancholia as:

> . . . a profoundly painful dejection, cessation of interest in the outside world, loss of the capacity to love, inhibition of all activity, and a lowering of the self-regarding feelings to a degree that finds utterances in self-reproaches and self-revilings, and culminates in a delusional expectation of punishment.

He observed that melancholia occurs after the loss of a loved object, either actually by death or emotionally by rejection, or the loss of some other abstraction of value to the individual. Freud indicated that, in melancholia, the depressed patient's rage is internally directed because of identification with the lost object (Sadock & Sadock, 2007).

Freud believed that the individual predisposed to melancholia experienced ambivalence in love relationships. He postulated, therefore, that once the loss had been incorporated into the self (ego), the hostile part of the ambivalence that had been felt for the lost object is then turned inward against the ego.

Learning Theory

The model of "learned helplessness" arises out of Seligman's (1973) experiments with dogs. The animals were exposed to electrical stimulation from which they could not escape. Later, when they were given the opportunity to avoid the traumatic experience, they reacted with helplessness and made no attempt to escape. A similar state of helplessness exists in humans who have experienced numerous failures (either real or perceived). The individual abandons any further attempt to succeed. Seligman theorized that learned helplessness predisposes individuals to depression by imposing a feeling of lack of control over their life situation. They become depressed because they feel helpless; they have learned that whatever they do is futile. This can be especially damaging very early in life, because the sense of mastery over one's environment is an important foundation for future emotional development.

Object Loss Theory

The theory of object loss suggests that depressive illness occurs as a result of having been abandoned by or otherwise separated from a significant other during the first 6 months of life. Because during this period the mother represents the child's main source of security, she is considered to be the "object." This absence of attachment, which may be either physical or emotional, leads to feelings of helplessness and despair that contribute to lifelong patterns of depression in response to loss.

The concept of "anaclitic depression" was introduced in 1946 by psychiatrist René Spitz to refer to children who became depressed after being separated from their mothers for an extended period of time during the first year of life (Cartwright, 2004). The condition included behaviors such as excessive crying, anorexia, withdrawal, **psychomotor retardation,** stupor, and a generalized impairment in the normal process of growth and development. Some researchers suggest that loss in adult life afflicts people much more severely in the form of depression if the subjects have suffered early childhood loss.

Cognitive Theory

Beck and colleagues (1979) proposed a theory suggesting that the primary disturbance in depression is cognitive rather than affective. The underlying cause of the depressive affect is seen as cognitive distortions that result in negative, defeated attitudes. Beck and colleagues identified three cognitive distortions that they believe serve as the basis for depression:

1. Negative expectations of the environment
2. Negative expectations of the self
3. Negative expectations of the future

These cognitive distortions arise out of a defect in cognitive development, and the individual feels inadequate, worthless, and rejected by others. Outlook for the future is one of pessimism and hopelessness.

Cognitive theorists believe that depression is the product of negative thinking. This is in contrast to the other theorists, who suggest that negative thinking occurs when an individual is depressed. **Cognitive therapy** focuses on helping the individual to alter mood by changing the way he or she thinks. The individual is taught to control negative thought distortions that lead to pessimism, lethargy, procrastination, and low self-esteem (see Chapter 20).

The Transactional Model

As is clearly evident, no single theory or hypothesis exists to substantiate a clear-cut explanation for depressive disorder. Evidence continues to mount in support of multiple causation. The transactional model recognizes the combined effects of genetic, biochemical, and psychosocial influences on an individual's susceptibility to depression. The dynamics of depression using the Transactional Model of Stress/Adaptation are presented in Figure 27–2.

Developmental Implications

Childhood

Only in recent years has a consensus developed among investigators identifying major depressive disorder as an entity in children and adolescents that can be identified using criteria similar to those used for adults (APA, 2000; Dubovsky et al., 2003). It is not uncommon, however, for the symptoms of depression to be manifested differently in childhood, and the picture changes with age (Harvard Medical School, 2002; Joska & Stein, 2008; Tempfer, 2006):

1. **Up to age 3:** Signs may include feeding problems, tantrums, lack of playfulness and emotional expressiveness, failure to thrive, or delays in speech and gross motor development.

2. **From ages 3 to 5:** Common symptoms may include accident proneness, phobias, aggressiveness, and excessive self-reproach for minor infractions.

3. **From ages 6 to 8:** There may be vague physical complaints and aggressive behavior. They may cling to parents and avoid new people and challenges. They may lag behind their classmates in social skills and academic competence.

4. **At ages 9 to 12:** Common symptoms include morbid thoughts and excessive worrying. They may reason that they are depressed because they have disappointed their parents in some way. There may be lack of interest in playing with friends.

Other symptoms of childhood depression may include hyperactivity, delinquency, school problems, psychosomatic complaints, sleeping and eating disturbances, social isolation, delusional thinking, and suicidal thoughts or actions.

Children may become depressed for various reasons. In many depressed children, there is a genetic predisposition toward the condition, which is then precipitated by a stressful situation. Common precipitating factors include physical or emotional detachment by the primary caregiver, parental separation or divorce, death of a loved one (person or pet), a move, academic failure, or physical illness. In any event, the common denominator is loss.

The focus of therapy with depressed children is to alleviate the child's symptoms and strengthen the child's coping and adaptive skills, with the hope of possibly preventing future psychological problems. Some studies have shown that untreated childhood depression may lead to subsequent problems in adolescence and adult life. Most children are treated on an outpatient basis. Hospitalization of the depressed child usually occurs only if he or she is actively suicidal, when the home environment precludes adherence to a treatment regimen, or if the child needs to be separated from the home because of psychosocial deprivation.

Parental and family therapy are commonly used to help the younger depressed child. Recovery is facilitated by emotional support and guidance to family members. Children older than age 8 years usually participate in family therapy. In some situations, individual treatment may be appropriate for older children. Medications, such as antidepressants, can be important in the treatment of children, especially for the more serious and recurrent forms of depression. The selective serotonin reuptake inhibitors (SSRIs) have been used with success, particularly in combination with psychosocial therapies. However, because there has been some concern that the use of antidepressant medications may cause suicidal behavior in young people, the U.S. Food and Drug Administration (FDA) has applied a "black-box" label warning (described in the next section) to all antidepressant medications.

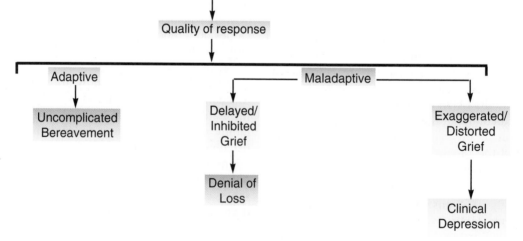

FIGURE 27–2 The dynamics of depression using the Transactional Model of Stress/Adaptation.

The National Institute of Mental Health (2010) stated:

> Those who are prescribed an [antidepressant] medication should receive ongoing medical monitoring. Children already taking an [antidepressant] should remain on the medication if it has been helpful, but should be carefully monitored by a doctor for side effects. Parents should promptly seek medical advice and evaluation if their child or adolescent experiences suicidal thinking or behavior, nervousness, agitation, irritability, mood instability, or sleeplessness that either emerges or worsens during treatment with [antidepressant] medications.

Adolescence

Depression may be even harder to recognize in an adolescent than in a younger child. Feelings of sadness, loneliness, anxiety, and hopelessness associated with depression may be perceived as the normal emotional stresses of growing up. Therefore, many young people whose symptoms are attributed to the "normal adjustments" of adolescence do not get the help they need. Depression is a major cause of suicide among teens, and suicide is the third leading cause of death in the 15- to 24-year-old age group (National Center for Health Statistics [NCHS], 2010b).

Common symptoms of depression in the adolescent are inappropriately expressed anger, aggressiveness, running away, delinquency, social withdrawal, sexual acting out, substance abuse, restlessness, and apathy. Loss of self-esteem, sleeping and eating disturbances, and psychosomatic complaints are also common.

What, then, is the indicator that differentiates mood disorder from the typical stormy behavior of adolescence? A visible manifestation of *behavioral change that lasts for several weeks* is the best clue for a mood disorder. Examples include the normally outgoing and extroverted adolescent who has become withdrawn and antisocial, the good student who previously received consistently high marks but is now failing and skipping classes, and the usually self-confident teenager who is now inappropriately irritable and defensive with others.

Adolescents become depressed for all the same reasons that were discussed under childhood depression. In adolescence, however, depression is a common manifestation of the stress and independence conflicts associated with the normal maturation process. Depression may also be the response to death of a parent, other relative, or friend, or to a breakup with a boyfriend or girlfriend. This perception of abandonment by parents or closest peer relationship is thought to be the most frequent immediate precipitant to adolescent suicide.

Treatment of the depressed adolescent is often conducted on an outpatient basis. Hospitalization may be required in cases of severe depression or threat of imminent suicide, when a family situation is such that treatment cannot be carried out in the home, when the physical condition precludes self-care of biological needs, or when the adolescent has indicated possible harm to self or others in the family.

In addition to supportive psychosocial intervention, antidepressant therapy may be part of the treatment of adolescent mood disorders. However, as mentioned previously, the FDA has issued a public health advisory warning the public about the increased risk of suicidal thoughts and behavior in children and adolescents being treated with antidepressant medications. The black-box warning label on all antidepressant medications describes this risk and emphasizes the need for close monitoring of clients started on these mediation. The advisory language does not prohibit the use of antidepressants in children and adolescents. Rather, it warns of the risk of suicidality and encourages prescribers to balance this risk with clinical need.

Fluoxetine (Prozac) has been approved by the FDA to treat depression in children and adolescents, and escitalopram (Lexapro) was approved in 2009 for treatment of MDD in adolescents ages 12 to 17 years. The other SSRI medications, such as sertraline, citalopram, and paroxetine, and the serotonin-norepinephrine reuptake inhibitor (SNRI) antidepressant venlafaxine, have not been approved for treatment of depression in children or adolescents, although they have been prescribed to children by physicians in "off-label use"—a use other than the FDA-approved use. In June 2003, the FDA recommended that paroxetine not be used in children and adolescents for the treatment of major depressive disorder.

Senescence

Depression is the most common psychiatric disorder of the elderly, who make up 12.9 percent of the general population of the United States (Administration on Aging, 2011). This is not surprising considering the disproportionate value our society places on youth, vigor, and uninterrupted productivity. These societal attitudes continually nurture the feelings of low self-esteem, helplessness, and hopelessness that become more pervasive and intensive with advanced age. Further, the aging individual's adaptive coping strategies may be seriously challenged by major stressors, such as financial problems, physical illness, changes in bodily functioning, and an increasing awareness of approaching death. The problem is often intensified by the numerous losses individuals experience during this period in life, such as spouse, friends, children, home, and independence. A phenomenon called *bereavement overload* occurs when individuals experience so many losses in their lives that they are not able to resolve one grief response before another one begins. Bereavement overload predisposes elderly individuals to depressive illness.

Although they make up less than 13 percent of the population, the elderly account for about 16 percent of the suicides in the United States (NCHS, 2010a). The highest number of suicides is among white men 85 years of age and older, at more than four times the national rate.

Symptoms of depression in the elderly are not very different from those in younger adults. However, depressive syndromes are often confused by other illnesses associated with the aging process. Symptoms of depression are often misdiagnosed as senile dementia, when in fact the memory loss, confused thinking, or apathy symptomatic of dementia actually may be the result of depression. The early awakening and reduced appetite typical of depression are common among many older people who are not depressed. Compounding this situation is the fact that many medical conditions, such as endocrinological, neurological, nutritional, and metabolic disorders, often present with classic symptoms of depression. Many medications commonly used by the elderly, such as antihypertensives, corticosteroids, and analgesics, can also produce a depressant effect.

Depression does accompany many of the illnesses that afflict older people, such as Parkinson's disease, cancer, arthritis, and the early stages of Alzheimer's disease. Treating depression in these situations can reduce unnecessary suffering and help afflicted individuals cope with their medical problems.

The most effective treatment of depression in the elderly individual is thought to be a combination of psychosocial and biological approaches. Antidepressant medications are administered with consideration for age-related physiological changes in absorption, distribution, elimination, and brain receptor sensitivity. Because of these changes, plasma concentrations of these medications can reach very high levels despite moderate oral doses.

Electroconvulsive therapy (ECT) remains one of the safest and most effective treatments for major depression in the elderly. The response to ECT appears to be slower with advancing age, and the therapeutic effects are of limited duration. However, it may be considered the treatment of choice for the elderly individual who is an acute suicidal risk or is unable to tolerate antidepressant medications.

Other therapeutic approaches include interpersonal, behavioral, cognitive, group, and family psychotherapies. Appropriate treatment of the depressed elderly individual can bring relief from suffering and offer a new lease on life with a feeling of renewed productivity.

Postpartum Depression

The severity of depression in the postpartum period varies from a feeling of the "blues," to moderate depression, to psychotic depression or melancholia. Of women who give birth, approximately 50 to 85 percent experience the "blues" following delivery (Mehta & Sheth, 2006). The incidence of moderate depression is 10 to 20 percent. Severe, or psychotic, depression occurs rarely, in about 1 or 2 out of 1,000 postpartum women.

Symptoms of the "maternity blues" include tearfulness, despondency, anxiety, and subjectively impaired concentration appearing in the early puerperium. The symptoms usually begin within 48 hours of delivery, peak at about 3 to 5 days, and last approximately 2 weeks (Mehta & Sheth, 2006).

Symptoms of moderate **postpartum depression** have been described as depressed mood varying from day to day, with more bad days than good, tending to be worse toward evening and associated with fatigue, irritability, loss of appetite, sleep disturbances, and loss of libido. In addition, the new mother expresses a great deal of concern about her inability to care for her baby. These symptoms begin somewhat later than those described in the "maternity blues," and take from a few weeks to several months to abate.

Postpartum melancholia, or depressive psychosis, is characterized by depressed mood, agitation, indecision, lack of concentration, guilt, and an abnormal attitude toward bodily functions. There may be lack of interest in, or rejection of, the baby, or a morbid fear that the baby may be harmed. Risks of suicide and infanticide should not be overlooked. These symptoms usually develop during the first few days following birth, but may occur later (Mehta & Sheth, 2006).

The etiology of postpartum depression remains unclear. "Maternity blues" may be associated with hormonal changes, tryptophan metabolism, or alterations in membrane transport during the early postpartum period. Besides being exposed to these same somatic changes, the woman who experiences moderate to severe symptoms probably possesses a vulnerability to depression related to heredity, upbringing, early life experiences, personality, or social circumstances. Some women with this disorder complain of lack of support from their husbands and dissatisfaction with their marriage. The etiology of postpartum depression may very likely be a combination of hormonal, metabolic, and psychosocial influences.

Treatment of postpartum depression varies with the severity of the illness. Psychotic depression may be treated with antidepressant medication, along with supportive psychotherapy, group therapy, and possibly family therapy. Moderate depression may be relieved with supportive psychotherapy and continuing assistance with home management until the symptoms subside. "Maternity blues" usually needs no treatment beyond a word of reassurance from the physician or nurse that these feelings are common and will soon pass. Extra support and comfort from significant others also is important.

Application of the Nursing Process

Background Assessment Data

Symptomatology of depression can be viewed on a continuum according to severity of the illness. All individuals become depressed from time to time. These are the transient symptoms that accompany the everyday disappointments of life. Examples of the disappointments include failing an examination or breaking up with a boyfriend or girlfriend. Transient symptoms of depression subside relatively quickly as the individual advances toward other goals and achievements.

Mild depressive episodes occur when the grief process is triggered in response to the loss of a valued object. This can occur with the loss of a loved one, pet, friend, home, or significant other. As one is able to work through the stages of grief, the loss is accepted, symptoms subside, and activities of daily living are resumed within a few weeks. If this does not occur, grief is prolonged or exaggerated, and symptoms intensify.

Moderate depression occurs when grief is prolonged or exaggerated. The individual becomes fixed in the anger stage of the grief response, and the anger is turned inward on the self. All of the feelings associated with normal grieving are exaggerated out of proportion, and the individual is unable to function without assistance. Dysthymic disorder is an example of moderate depression.

Severe depression is an intensification of the symptoms associated with the moderate level. The individual who is severely depressed may also demonstrate a loss of contact with reality. This level is associated with a complete lack of pleasure in all activities, and ruminations about suicide are common. Major depressive disorder is an example of severe depression. A continuum of depression is presented in Figure 27–3.

A number of assessment rating scales are available for measuring severity of depressive symptoms. Some are meant to be clinician administered, whereas others may be self-administered. Examples of self-rating scales include the Zung Self-Rating Depression Scale and the Beck Depression Inventory. One of the most widely used clinician-administered scales is the Hamilton Depression Rating Scale (HDRS). It has been reviewed and revised over the years, and exists today in several versions. The original version (see Box 27-4) contains 17 items and is designed to measure mood, guilty feelings, suicidal ideation, sleep disturbances, anxiety levels, and weight loss.

Symptoms of depression can be described as alterations in four spheres of human functioning: (1) affective, (2) behavioral, (3) cognitive, and (4) physiological. Alterations within these spheres differ according to degree of severity of symptomatology.

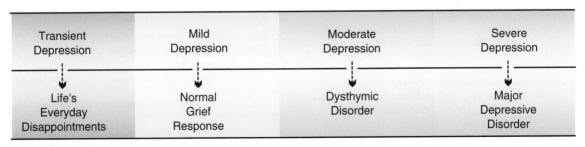

FIGURE 27–3 A continuum of depression.

BOX 27-4 Hamilton Depression Rating Scale (HDRS)

Instructions: For each item, circle the number to select the one "cue" that best characterizes the patient.

1. **Depressed Mood** (sadness, hopeless, helpless, worthless)
   0 = Absent
   1 = These feeling states indicated only on questioning.
   2 = These feeling states spontaneously reported verbally.
   3 = Communicates feeling states nonverbally, i.e., through facial expression, posture, voice, tendency to weep.
   4 = Patient reports virtually only these feeling states in spontaneous verbal and nonverbal communication.

2. **Feelings of Guilt**
   0 = Absent.
   1 = Self reproach; feels he/she has let people down.
   2 = Ideas of guilt or rumination over past errors or sinful deeds.
   3 = Present illness is a punishment. Delusions of guilt.
   4 = Hears accusatory or denunciatory voices and/or experiences threatening visual hallucinations.

3. **Suicide**
   0 = Absent.
   1 = Feels life is not worth living.
   2 = Wishes he/she were dead or any thoughts of possible death to self.
   3 = Suicidal ideas or gesture.
   4 = Attempts at suicide (any serious attempt rates 4).

4. **Insomnia: Early in the Night**
   0 = No difficulty falling asleep.
   1 = Complains of occasional difficulty falling asleep, i.e., more than ½ hour.
   2 = Complains of nightly difficulty falling asleep.

5. **Insomnia: Middle of the Night**
   0 = No difficulty.
   1 = Complains of being restless and disturbed during the night.
   2 = Waking during the night—any getting out of bed rates 2 (except for purposes of voiding).

6. **Insomnia: Early Hours of the Morning**
   0 = No difficulty.
   1 = Waking in early hours of the morning, but goes back to sleep.
   2 = Unable to fall asleep again if he/she gets out of bed.

7. **Work and Activities**
   0 = No difficulty.
   1 = Thoughts and feelings of incapacity, fatigue, or weakness related to activities, work, or hobbies.
   2 = Loss of interest in activity, hobbies, or work—either directly reported by patient, or indirectly in listlessness, indecision, and vacillation (feels he/she has to push self to work or activities).
   3 = Decrease in actual time spent in activities or decrease in productivity. Rate 3 if patient does not spend at least 3 hours a day in activities (job or hobbies), excluding routine chores.
   4 = Stopped working because of present illness. Rate 4 if patient engages in no activities except routine chores, or if does not perform routine chores unassisted.

8. **Psychomotor Retardation** (slowness of thought and speech, impaired ability to concentrate, decreased motor activity)
   0 = Normal speech and thought.
   1 = Slight retardation during the interview.
   2 = Obvious retardation during the interview.
   3 = Interview difficult.
   4 = Complete stupor.

9. **Agitation**
   0 = None.
   1 = Fidgetiness.
   2 = Playing with hands, hair, etc.
   3 = Moving about, can't sit still.
   4 = Hand wringing, nail biting, hair pulling, biting of lips.

10. **Anxiety (Psychic)**
    0 = No difficulty.
    1 = Subjective tension and irritability.
    2 = Worrying about minor matters.
    3 = Apprehensive attitude apparent in face or speech.
    4 = Fears expressed without questioning.

11. **Anxiety (Somatic):** Physiological concomitants of anxiety (e.g., dry mouth, indigestion, diarrhea, cramps, belching, palpitations, headache, tremor, hyperventilation, sighing, urinary frequency, sweating, flushing)
    0 = Absent.   3 = Severe.
    1 = Mild.   4 = Incapacitating.
    2 = Moderate.

12. **Somatic Symptoms (Gastrointestinal)**
    0 = None.
    1 = Loss of appetite, but eating without encouragement. Heavy feelings in abdomen.
    2 = Difficulty eating without urging from others. Requests or requires medication for constipation or gastrointestinal symptoms.

13. **Somatic Symptoms (General)**
    0 = None.
    1 = Heaviness in limbs, back or head. Backaches, headache, muscle aches. Loss of energy and fatigability.
    2 = Any clear-cut symptom rates 2.

14. **Genital Symptoms** (e.g., loss of libido, impaired sexual performance, menstrual disturbances)
    0 = Absent.
    1 = Mild.
    2 = Severe.

15. **Hypochondriasis**
    0 = Not present.
    1 = Self-absorption (bodily).
    2 = Preoccupation with health.
    3 = Frequent complaints, requests for help, etc.
    4 = Hypochondriacal delusions.

16. **Loss of Weight** (Rate *either* A *or* B)
    A. According to subjective patient history:
        0 = No weight loss.
        1 = Probably weight loss associated with present illness.
        2 = Definite weight loss associated with present illness.

BOX 27-4 **Hamilton Depression Rating Scale (HDRS)—cont'd**

B. According to objective weekly measurements:
0 = Less than 1 lb. weight loss in week.
1 = Greater than 1 lb. weight loss in week.
2 = Greater than 2 lb. weight loss in week.

17. **Insight**
0 = Acknowledges being depressed and ill.
1 = Acknowledges illness but attributes cause to bad food, climate, overwork, virus, need for rest, etc.
2 = Denies being ill at all.

SCORING:
0–6 = No evidence of depressive illness
7–17 = Mild depression
18–24 = Moderate depression
> 24 = Severe depression

TOTAL SCORE_____

From Hamilton, M. (1960). A rating scale for depression. Journal of Neurology, Neurosurgery, & Psychiatry, 23, 56–62. The HDRS is in the public domain.

Transient Depression

Symptoms at this level of the continuum are not necessarily dysfunctional. Alterations include the following:

■ **Affective:** sadness, dejection, feeling downhearted, having the "blues."

■ **Behavioral:** some crying possible.

■ **Cognitive:** some difficulty getting mind off of one's disappointment.

■ **Physiological:** feeling tired and listless.

Mild Depression

Symptoms at the mild level of depression are identified by those associated with normal grieving. Alterations at the mild level include the following:

■ **Affective:** denial of feelings, anger, anxiety, guilt, helplessness, hopelessness, sadness, despondency.

■ **Behavioral:** tearfulness, regression, restlessness, agitation, withdrawal.

■ **Cognitive:** preoccupation with the loss, self-blame, ambivalence, blaming others.

■ **Physiological:** anorexia or overeating, insomnia or hypersomnia, headache, backache, chest pain, or other symptoms associated with the loss of a significant other.

Moderate Depression

Dysthymic disorder, which is an example of moderate depression, represents a more problematic disturbance. Symptoms associated with this disorder include the following:

■ **Affective:** feelings of sadness, dejection, helplessness, powerlessness, hopelessness; gloomy and pessimistic outlook; low self-esteem; difficulty experiencing pleasure in activities.

■ **Behavioral:** slowed physical movements (i.e., psychomotor retardation); slumped posture; slowed speech; limited verbalizations, possibly consisting of ruminations about life's failures or regrets; social isolation with a focus on the self; increased use of substances possible; self-destructive behavior possible; decreased interest in personal hygiene and grooming.

■ **Cognitive:** retarded thinking processes; difficulty concentrating and directing attention; obsessive and repetitive thoughts, generally portraying pessimism and negativism; verbalizations and behavior reflecting suicidal ideation.

■ **Physiological:** anorexia or overeating; insomnia or hypersomnia; sleep disturbances; amenorrhea; decreased libido; headaches; backaches; chest pain; abdominal pain; low energy level; fatigue and listlessness; feeling best early in the morning and continually worse as the day progresses. This may be related to the diurnal variation in the level of neurotransmitters that affect mood and level of activity.

Severe Depression

Severe depression is characterized by an intensification of the symptoms described for moderate depression. Examples of severe depression include major depressive disorder and bipolar depression. Symptoms at the severe level of depression include the following:

■ **Affective:** feelings of total despair, hopelessness, and worthlessness; flat (unchanging) affect, appearing devoid of emotional tone; prevalent feelings of nothingness and emptiness; apathy; loneliness; sadness; inability to feel pleasure.

■ **Behavioral:** psychomotor retardation so severe that physical movement may literally come to a standstill, or psychomotor behavior manifested by rapid, agitated, purposeless movements; slumped posture; sitting in a curled-up position; walking slowly and rigidly; virtually nonexistent communication (when verbalizations do occur, they may reflect delusional thinking); no personal hygiene and grooming; social isolation is common, with virtually no inclination toward interaction with others.

■ **Cognitive:** prevalent delusional thinking, with delusions of persecution and somatic delusions being most common; confusion, indecisiveness, and an inability to concentrate; hallucinations reflecting misinterpretations of the environment; excessive self-deprecation, self-blame, and thoughts of suicide.

NOTE: Because of the low energy level and retarded thought processes, the individual may be unable to follow through on suicidal ideas. However, the desire is strong at this level.

■ **Physiological:** a general slowdown of the entire body, reflected in sluggish digestion, constipation, and urinary retention; amenorrhea; impotence; diminished libido; anorexia; weight loss; difficulty falling asleep and awakening very early in the morning; feeling worse early in the morning and somewhat better as the day progresses. As with moderate depression, this may reflect the diurnal variation in the level of neurotransmitters that affect mood and activity.

Diagnosis/Outcome Identification

Using information collected during the assessment, the nurse completes the client database, from which the selection of appropriate nursing diagnoses is determined. Table 27-1 presents a list of client behaviors and the NANDA nursing diagnoses that correspond to those behaviors, which may be used in planning care for the depressed client.

TABLE 27-1 Assigning Nursing Diagnoses to Behaviors Commonly Associated With Depression

BEHAVIORS	NURSING DIAGNOSES
Depressed mood; feelings of hopelessness and worthlessness; anger turned inward on the self; misinterpretations of reality; suicidal ideation, plan, and available means	**Risk for suicide**
Depression, preoccupation with thoughts of loss, self-blame, grief avoidance, inappropriate expression of anger, decreased functioning in life roles	**Complicated grieving**
Expressions of helplessness, uselessness, guilt, and shame; hypersensitivity to slight or criticism; negative, pessimistic outlook; lack of eye contact; self-negating verbalizations	**Low self-esteem**
Apathy, verbal expressions of having no control, dependence on others to fulfill needs	**Powerlessness**
Expresses anger toward God, expresses lack of meaning in life, sudden changes in spiritual practices, refuses interactions with significant others or with spiritual leaders	**Spiritual distress**
Withdrawn, uncommunicative, seeks to be alone, dysfunctional interaction with others, discomfort in social situations	**Social isolation/Impaired social interaction**
Inappropriate thinking, confusion, difficulty concentrating, impaired problem-solving ability, inaccurate interpretation of environment, memory deficit	**Disturbed thought processes**
Weight loss, poor muscle tone, pale conjunctiva and mucous membranes, poor skin turgor, weakness	**Imbalanced nutrition: Less than body requirements**
Difficulty falling asleep, difficulty staying asleep, lack of energy, difficulty concentrating, verbal reports of not feeling well rested	**Insomnia**
Uncombed hair, disheveled clothing, offensive body odor	**Self-care deficit (hygiene, grooming)**

Outcome Criteria

The following criteria may be used for measurement of outcomes in the care of the depressed client.

The Client:

- Has experienced no physical harm to self.
- Discusses the loss with staff and family members.
- No longer idealizes or obsesses about the lost entity/concept.
- Sets realistic goals for self.
- Is no longer afraid to attempt new activities.
- Is able to identify aspects of self-control over life situation.
- Expresses personal satisfaction and support from spiritual practices.
- Interacts willingly and appropriately with others.
- Is able to maintain reality orientation.
- Is able to concentrate, reason, and solve problems.
- Eats a well-balanced diet with snacks, to prevent weight loss and maintain nutritional status.
- Sleeps 6 to 8 hours per night and reports feeling well rested.
- Bathes, washes and combs hair, and dresses in clean clothing without assistance.

Planning/Implementation

The following section presents a group of selected nursing diagnoses, with short- and long-term goals and nursing interventions for each.

Some institutions are using a case management model to coordinate care (see Chapter 9 for more detailed explanation). In case management models, the plan of care may take the form of a critical pathway.

Risk for Suicide

Risk for suicide is defined as "at risk for self-inflicted, life-threatening injury" (NANDA-International [NANDA-I], 2009, p. 330). For additional interventions and to view this nursing diagnosis in care plan format, please see Chapter 18.

Client Goals

Outcome criteria include short- and long-term goals. Timelines are individually determined.

Short-Term Goals

- Client will seek out staff when feeling urge to harm self.

- Client will make short-term verbal (or written) contract with nurse not to harm self.
- Client will not harm self.

Long-Term Goal

- Client will not harm self.

Interventions

- Create a safe environment for the client. Remove all potentially harmful objects from client's access (sharp objects, straps, belts, ties, glass items, alcohol). Supervise closely during meals and medication administration. Perform room searches as deemed necessary.

> **CLINICAL PEARL**
>
> Ask the client directly, "Have you thought about killing yourself" or "Have you thought about harming yourself in any way?" "If so, what do you plan to do? Do you have the means to carry out this plan?" The risk of suicide is greatly increased if the client has developed a plan and particularly if means exist for the client to execute the plan.

- Formulate a short-term verbal or written contract with the client that he or she will not harm self during a specific time period. When that contract expires, make another. Repeat this process for as long as required. Discussion of suicidal feelings with a trusted individual provides some relief to the client. A contract gets the subject out in the open and some of the responsibility for his or her safety is given to the client. An attitude of unconditional acceptance of the client as a worthwhile individual is conveyed.

- Secure a promise from the client that he or she will seek out a staff member or support person if thoughts of suicide emerge. Suicidal clients are often very ambivalent about their feelings. Discussion of feelings with a trusted individual may provide assistance before the client experiences a crisis situation.

> **CLINICAL PEARL** Be direct. Talk openly and matter-of-factly about suicide. Listen actively and encourage expression of feelings, including anger. Accept the client's feelings in a nonjudgmental manner.

- Maintain close observation of client. Depending on level of suicide precaution, provide one-to-one contact, constant visual observation, or every-15-minute checks. Place in room close to nurse's station; do not assign to private room. Accompany to off-ward activities if attendance is indicated. May need to accompany to bathroom. Close observation is necessary to ensure that client does not harm self in any way. Being alert for suicidal and escape attempts facilitates being able to prevent or interrupt harmful behavior.

■ Maintain special care in administration of medications. This prevents saving up to overdose or discarding and not taking.

■ Make rounds at frequent, *irregular* intervals (especially at night, toward early morning, at change of shift, or other predictably busy times for staff). This prevents staff surveillance from becoming predictable. To be aware of client's location is important, especially when staff is busy, unavailable, or less observable.

■ Encourage verbalizations of honest feelings. Through exploration and discussion, help the client to identify symbols of hope in his or her life.

■ Encourage the client to express angry feelings within appropriate limits. Provide a safe method of hostility release. Help the client to identify the true source of anger and to work on adaptive coping skills for use outside the treatment setting. Depression and suicidal behaviors may be viewed as anger turned inward on the self. If this anger can be verbalized in a nonthreatening environment, the client may be able to eventually resolve these feelings.

■ Identify community resources that the client may use as a support system and from whom he or she may request help if feeling suicidal. Having a concrete plan for seeking assistance during a crisis may discourage or prevent self-destructive behaviors.

■ Orient the client to reality, as required. Point out sensory misperceptions or misinterpretations of the environment. Take care not to belittle the client's fears or indicate disapproval of verbal expressions.

■ Most important, spend time with client. This provides a feeling of safety and security, while also conveying the message, "I want to spend time with you because I think you are a worthwhile person."

Complicated Grieving

Complicated grieving is defined as "a disorder that occurs after the death of a significant other [or any other loss of significance to the individual], in which the experience of distress accompanying bereavement fails to follow normative expectations and manifests in functional impairment" (NANDA-I, 2009, p. 265). Table 27-2 presents this nursing diagnosis in care plan format.

Client Goals

Outcome criteria include short- and long-term goals. Timelines are individually determined.

Short-Term Goals

■ Client will express anger about the loss.

■ Client will verbalize behaviors associated with normal grieving.

Table 27-2 CARE PLAN FOR THE DEPRESSED CLIENT

NURSING DIAGNOSIS: COMPLICATED GRIEVING
RELATED TO: Real or perceived loss, bereavement overload
EVIDENCED BY: Denial of loss, inappropriate expression of anger, idealization of or obsession with lost object, inability to carry out activities of daily living.

OUTCOME CRITERIA	NURSING INTERVENTIONS	RATIONALE
Short-Term Goals • Client will express anger about the loss. • Client will verbalize behaviors associated with normal grieving. **Long-Term Goal** • Client will be able to recognize his or her own position in the grief process, while progressing at own pace toward resolution	1. Determine the stage of grief in which the client is fixed. Identify behaviors associated with this stage. 2. Develop a trusting relationship with the client. Show empathy, concern, and unconditional positive regard. Be honest and keep all promises. 3. Convey an accepting attitude, and enable the client to express feelings openly.	1. Accurate baseline assessment data are necessary to effectively plan care for the grieving client. 2. Trust is the basis for a therapeutic relationship. 3. An accepting attitude conveys to the client that you believe he or she is a worthwhile person. Trust is enhanced.

Table 27-2 CARE PLAN FOR THE DEPRESSED CLIENT—cont'd

OUTCOME CRITERIA	NURSING INTERVENTIONS	RATIONALE
	4. Encourage the client to express anger. Do not become defensive if the initial expression of anger is displaced on the nurse or therapist. Help the client explore angry feelings so that they may be directed toward the actual intended person or situation.	4. Verbalization of feelings in a non-threatening environment may help the client come to terms with unresolved issues.
	5. Help the client to discharge pent-up anger through participation in large-motor activities (e.g., brisk walks, jogging, physical exercises, volleyball, punching bag, exercise bike).	5. Physical exercise provides a safe and effective method for discharging pent-up tension.
	6. Teach the normal stages of grief and behaviors associated with each stage. Help the client to understand that feelings such as guilt and anger toward the lost concept/entity are appropriate and acceptable during the grief process and should be expressed rather than held inside.	6. Knowledge of acceptability of the feelings associated with normal grieving may help to relieve some of the guilt that these responses generate.
	7. Encourage the client to review the relationship with the lost concept/entity. With support and sensitivity, point out the reality of the situation in areas where misrepresentations are expressed.	7. The client must give up an idealized perception and be able to accept both positive and negative aspects about the lost concept/entity before the grief process is complete.
	8. Communicate to the client that crying is acceptable. Use of touch may also be therapeutic.	8. Some cultures believe it is important to remain stoic and refrain from crying openly. Individuals from certain cultures are uncomfortable with touch. It is important to be aware of cultural influences before employing these interventions.
	9. Encourage the client to reach out for spiritual support during this time in whatever form is desirable to him or her. Assess spiritual needs of the client (see Chapter 6) and assist as necessary in the fulfillment of those needs.	9. Client may find comfort in religious rituals with which he or she is familiar.

Long-Term Goal

■ Client will be able to recognize his or her own position in the grief process, while progressing at own pace toward resolution.

Interventions

■ Determine the stage of grief in which the client is fixed. Identify behaviors associated with this stage. It is important to obtain accurate baseline assessment data to effectively plan care for the grieving client.

■ Develop a trusting relationship with the client. Show empathy, concern, and unconditional positive regard. Be honest and keep all promises. Convey an accepting attitude, and encourage the client to express feelings openly.

■ Encourage the client to express anger. Do not become defensive if the initial expression of anger is displaced on the nurse or therapist. Help the client to explore angry feelings so that they may be directed toward the actual intended person or situation.

■ Help the client to discharge pent-up anger through participation in large-motor activities (e.g., brisk walks, jogging, physical exercises, volleyball, punching bag, exercise bike). Physical exercise provides a safe and effective method for discharging pent-up tension.

■ Teach the normal stages of grief and behaviors associated with each stage. Help the client to understand that feelings such as guilt and anger toward the lost concept/entity are appropriate and acceptable during the grief process, and should be expressed rather than held inside. Knowledge of acceptability of the feelings associated with normal grieving may help to relieve some of the guilt that these responses generate.

■ Encourage the client to review the relationship with the lost concept/entity. With support and sensitivity, point out the reality of the situation in areas where misrepresentations are expressed. The client must give up an idealized perception and be able to accept both positive and negative aspects about the lost concept/entity before the grief process is complete.

■ Communicate to the client that crying is acceptable. The use of touch is therapeutic and appropriate with most clients. Knowledge of cultural influences specific to the client is important before using this technique.

■ Assist the client in problem solving as he or she attempts to determine methods for more adaptive coping with the experienced loss. Provide positive feedback for strategies identified and decisions made.

■ Encourage the client to reach out for spiritual support during this time in whatever form is desirable to him or her. Assess spiritual needs of the client (see Chapter 6) and assist as necessary in the fulfillment of those needs.

■ Encourage the client to attend a support group of individuals who are experiencing life situations similar to his or her own. Help the client to locate a group of this type.

Low Self-Esteem/Self-Care Deficit

Low self-esteem is defined as "negative self-evaluating/feelings about self or self-capabilities [either long-standing or in response to a current situation]" (NANDA-I, pp. 193–194). *Self-care deficit* is defined as "impaired ability to perform or complete [activities of daily living (ADLs)] for self" (NANDA-I, 2009, pp. 153–156).

Client Goals
Short-Term Goals

■ Client will verbalize attributes he or she likes about self.

■ Client will participate in ADLs with assistance from health-care provider.

Long-Term Goals

■ By time of discharge from treatment, the client will exhibit increased feelings of self-worth as evidenced by verbal expression of positive aspects of self, past accomplishments, and future prospects.

■ By time of discharge from treatment, the client will exhibit increased feelings of self-worth by setting realistic goals and trying to reach them, thereby demonstrating a decrease in fear of failure.

■ By time of discharge from treatment, the client will satisfactorily accomplish ADLs independently.

Interventions

■ Be accepting of the client and spend time with him or her even though pessimism and negativism may seem objectionable. Focus on strengths and accomplishments and minimize failures.

■ Promote attendance in therapy groups that offer client simple methods of accomplishment. Encourage client to be as independent as possible.

■ Encourage the client to recognize areas of change and provide assistance toward this effort.

■ Teach assertiveness techniques: the ability to recognize the differences among passive, assertive, and aggressive behaviors, and the importance of respecting the human rights of others while protecting one's own basic human rights. Self-esteem is enhanced by the ability to interact with others in an assertive manner.

■ Teach effective communication techniques, such as the use of "I" messages. Emphasize ways to avoid making judgmental statements (see Chapter 15).

■ Encourage independence in the performance of ADLs, but intervene when client is unable to perform.

CLINICAL PEARL

Offer recognition and positive reinforcement for independent accomplishments (e.g., "Mrs. J., I see you have put on a clean dress and combed your hair.").

■ Show the client how to perform activities with which he or she is having difficulty. When a client is depressed, he or she may require simple, concrete demonstrations of activities that would be performed without difficulty under normal conditions.

■ Keep strict records of food and fluid intake. Offer nutritious snacks and fluids between meals. The client may be unable to tolerate large amounts of food at mealtimes and may therefore require additional nourishment at other times during the day to receive adequate nutrition.

■ Before bedtime, provide nursing measures that promote sleep, such as back rub; warm bath; warm, nonstimulating drinks; soft music; and relaxation exercises.

Powerlessness

Powerlessness is defined as "perception that one's own action will not significantly affect an outcome; a perceived lack of control over a current situation or immediate happening" (NANDA-I, 2009, p. 190).

Client Goals
   Short-Term Goal

■ Client will participate in decision making regarding own care within 5 days.

   Long-Term Goal

■ Client will be able to effectively problem-solve ways to take control of his or her life situation by time of discharge from treatment, thereby decreasing feelings of powerlessness.

Interventions
■ Encourage the client to take as much responsibility as possible for his or her own self-care practices. Providing the client with choices will increase feelings of control.

EXAMPLES
■ Include the client in setting the goals of care he or she wishes to achieve.

■ Allow the client to establish own schedule for self-care activities.

■ Provide the client with privacy as need is determined.

■ Provide positive feedback for decisions made. Respect the client's right to make

those decisions independently, and refrain from attempting to influence him or her toward those that may seem more logical.

■ Help the client set realistic goals. Unrealistic goals set the client up for failure and reinforce feelings of powerlessness.

■ Help the client identify areas of his or her life situation that can be controlled. The client's emotional condition interferes with his or her ability to solve problems. Assistance is required to perceive the benefits and consequences of available alternatives accurately.

■ Discuss with the client areas of life that are not within his or her ability to control. Encourage verbalization of feelings related to this inability in an effort to deal with unresolved issues and accept what cannot be changed.

Concept Care Mapping

The concept map care plan is an innovative approach to planning and organizing nursing care (see Chapter 9). It is a diagrammatic teaching and learning strategy that allows visualization of interrelationships between medical diagnoses, nursing diagnoses, assessment data, and treatments. An example of a concept map care plan for a client with depression is presented in Figure 27–4.

Client/Family Education

The role of client teacher is important in the psychiatric area, as it is in all areas of nursing. A list of topics for client/family education relevant to depression is presented in Box 27-5. Sample client teaching guides are presented in Appendix G.

Evaluation of Care for the Depressed Client

In the final step of the nursing process, a reassessment is conducted to determine if the nursing actions have been successful in achieving the objectives of care. Evaluation of the nursing actions for the depressed client may be facilitated by gathering information using the following types of questions:

■ Has self-harm to the individual been avoided?

■ Have suicidal ideations subsided?

■ Does the individual know where to seek assistance outside the hospital when suicidal thoughts occur?

■ Has the client discussed the recent loss with staff and family members?

■ Is he or she able to verbalize feelings and behaviors associated with each stage of the

Clinical Vignette: Judith, age 56, has been despondent since her husband of 30 years left her 3 months ago to live with a 26-year-old secretary from his office. She has lost weight and rarely goes out of the house. Today the divorce was finalized. When Judith's daughter, Cathy, went to her mother's house, she found Judith going through her medication saying she was going to "take enough to put me to sleep for good." Cathy convinced her mother to go to the hospital, and Judith was admitted to the psychiatric unit with a diagnosis of Major Depression. Judith tells the nurse, "I'm so angry at my husband...I could just kill him! How could he do this to me? I guess it's my fault. I'm not as pretty as his girlfriend." Then she says, "What's the use of going on? No one would want me now. I'm old...and I don't have anything to live for." The nurse develops the following concept map care plan for Judith.

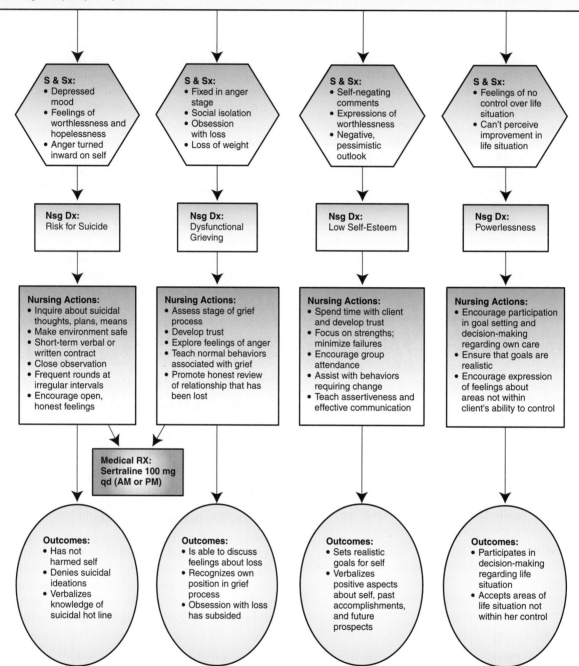

S & Sx:
- Depressed mood
- Feelings of worthlessness and hopelessness
- Anger turned inward on self

S & Sx:
- Fixed in anger stage
- Social isolation
- Obsession with loss
- Loss of weight

S & Sx:
- Self-negating comments
- Expressions of worthlessness
- Negative, pessimistic outlook

S & Sx:
- Feelings of no control over life situation
- Can't perceive improvement in life situation

Nsg Dx:
Risk for Suicide

Nsg Dx:
Dysfunctional Grieving

Nsg Dx:
Low Self-Esteem

Nsg Dx:
Powerlessness

Nursing Actions:
- Inquire about suicidal thoughts, plans, means
- Make environment safe
- Short-term verbal or written contract
- Close observation
- Frequent rounds at irregular intervals
- Encourage open, honest feelings

Nursing Actions:
- Assess stage of grief process
- Develop trust
- Explore feelings of anger
- Teach normal behaviors associated with grief
- Promote honest review of relationship that has been lost

Nursing Actions:
- Spend time with client and develop trust
- Focus on strengths; minimize failures
- Encourage group attendance
- Assist with behaviors requiring change
- Teach assertiveness and effective communication

Nursing Actions:
- Encourage participation in goal setting and decision-making regarding own care
- Ensure that goals are realistic
- Encourage expression of feelings about areas not within client's ability to control

Medical RX:
Sertraline 100 mg qd (AM or PM)

Outcomes:
- Has not harmed self
- Denies suicidal ideations
- Verbalizes knowledge of suicidal hot line

Outcomes:
- Is able to discuss feelings about loss
- Recognizes own position in grief process
- Obsession with loss has subsided

Outcomes:
- Sets realistic goals for self
- Verbalizes positive aspects about self, past accomplishments, and future prospects

Outcomes:
- Participates in decision-making regarding life situation
- Accepts areas of life situation not within her control

FIGURE 27–4   Concept map care plan for a client with depression.

BOX 27-5 Topics for Client/Family Education Related to Depression

NATURE OF THE ILLNESS
1. Stages of grief and symptoms associated with each stage.
2. What is depression?
3. Why do people get depressed?
4. What are the symptoms of depression?

MANAGEMENT OF THE ILLNESS
1. Medication management
   a. Nuisance side effects
   b. Side effects to report to physician
   c. Importance of taking regularly
   d. Length of time to take effect
   e. Diet (related to MAO inhibitors)
2. Assertiveness techniques
3. Stress-management techniques
4. Ways to increase self-esteem
5. Electroconvulsive therapy

SUPPORT SERVICES
1. Suicide hotline
2. Support groups
3. Legal/financial assistance

■ Can the client identify areas of life situation over which he or she has control?

■ Is the client able to participate in usual religious practices and feel satisfaction and support from them?

■ Is the client seeking out interaction with others in an appropriate manner?

■ Does the client maintain reality orientation with no evidence of delusional thinking?

■ Is he or she able to concentrate and make decisions concerning own self-care?

■ Is the client selecting and consuming foods sufficiently high in nutrients and calories to maintain weight and nutritional status?

■ Does the client sleep without difficulty and wake feeling rested?

■ Does the client show pride in appearance by attending to personal hygiene and grooming?

■ Have somatic complaints subsided?

Quality and Safety Education for Nurses (QSEN)

The Institute of Medicine (IOM), in its 2003 report, *Health Professions Education: A Bridge to Quality*, challenged faculties of medicine, nursing, and other health professions to ensure that their graduates have achieved a core set of competencies in order to meet the needs of the 21st century health-care system. These competencies include *providing patient-centered care, working in interdisciplinary teams, employing evidence-based practice, applying quality improvement,* and *utilizing informatics.* A QSEN teaching strategy is included in Box 27-6. The use of this type of activity is

grieving process and recognize own position in the process?

■ Have obsession with and idealization of the lost object subsided?

■ Is anger toward the lost object expressed appropriately?

■ Does the client set realistic goals for self?

■ Is he or she able to verbalize positive aspects about self, past accomplishments, and future prospects?

BOX 27-6 QSEN TEACHING STRATEGY

Assignment: Staff Work-Arounds
Placing a Client on Suicide Precautions

Competency Domains: Evidence-based Practice; Patient-centered Care; Quality Improvement; Safety; Teamwork and Collaboration

Learning Objectives: Student will:
• Demonstrate skills in identifying gaps between practice on the unit and what has been identified as best practice.
• Demonstrate skills at finding professional practice standards and research literature related to placing a client on suicide precautions.
• Demonstrate skills in accounting for patient preferences within the boundaries of safe and therapeutic practice.
• Demonstrate attitudes and behaviors that show that he or she values teamwork and want to contribute to maintaining standards of safe and effective care.

Continued

BOX 27-6 QSEN TEACHING STRATEGY—cont'd

Strategy Overview:

This assignment is meant to familiarize the student with standardized nursing policies, procedures, standards of care, and other evidence-based nursing practice guidelines, and to encourage students to observe actual nursing practice on the units to note compliance with, deviations from, or "work arounds" by RNs when implementing nursing procedures. The following aspects of the assignment can guide students in preparation for clinical conference discussion, in writing a paper, or in putting together a poster presentation.

1. Identify a need to place a client on suicide precautions.
2. Find the current written nursing policy or procedure in place for your institution/unit and answer these questions:
   a. How easy/difficult was it to find the policy/procedure?
   b. Did the RNs know where to find the written policy/procedure?
   c. How was the policy/procedure originally disseminated to the staff?
   d. Is the policy/procedure evidence-based?
      (Review the current practice standards from professional organizations and/or oversight and accreditation groups [e.g.: The Joint Commission, CDC], and/or the research literature.)
3. Observe RNs on the unit putting a client on suicide precautions and describe:
   a. What steps the RN took
   b. In what ways the RN deviated from the written policy/procedure
   c. What prompted the RN to make the deviations she/he did
   d. As many details as you can recollect
4. Discuss why RNs may or may not follow the institution's written policies and procedures. Reflect on the opportunities and challenges of evidence-based practice and the implementation into actual bedside nursing practice.
5. Discuss what the proper response should be when you as an RN discover unsafe practice that deviates from standards, policies, or procedures.

Adapted from teaching strategy submitted by Lisa Day, Assistant Clinical Professor, UCSF, School of Nursing, San Francisco, CA. © 2009 QSEN; http://qsen.org, with permission.

intended to arm the instructor and the student with guidelines for attaining the knowledge, skills, and attitudes necessary for achievement of quality and safety competencies in nursing.

Treatment Modalities for Depression

Individual Psychotherapy

Research has documented both the importance of close and satisfactory attachments in the prevention of depression and the role of disrupted attachments in the development of depression. With this concept in mind, interpersonal psychotherapy focuses on the client's current interpersonal relations. Interpersonal psychotherapy with the depressed person proceeds through the following phases and interventions.

Phase I

During the first phase, the client is assessed to determine the extent of the illness. Complete information is then given to the individual regarding the nature of depression, symptom pattern, frequency, clinical course, and alternative treatments. If the level of depression is severe, interpersonal psychotherapy has been shown to be more effective if conducted in combination with antidepressant medication. The client is encouraged to continue working and participating in regular activities during therapy. A mutually agreeable therapeutic contract is negotiated.

Phase II

Treatment at this phase focuses on helping the client resolve complicated grief reactions. This may include resolving the ambivalence with a lost relationship, serving as a temporary substitute for the lost relationship, and assistance with establishing new relationships. Other areas of treatment focus may include interpersonal disputes between the client and a significant other, difficult role transitions at various developmental life cycles, and correction of interpersonal deficits that may interfere with the client's ability to initiate or sustain interpersonal relationships.

Phase III

During the final phase of interpersonal psychotherapy, the therapeutic alliance is terminated. With emphasis on reassurance, clarification of emotional states, improvement of interpersonal communication, testing of perceptions, and performance in interpersonal settings, interpersonal psychotherapy has been successful in helping depressed persons recover enhanced social functioning.

Group Therapy

Group therapy forms an important dimension of multimodal treatment for the depressed client. Once an acute phase of the illness is passed, groups can provide an atmosphere in which individuals may discuss issues in their lives that cause, maintain, or arise out of having a serious affective disorder. The element of peer support provides a feeling of security, as troublesome or embarrassing issues are discussed and resolved. Some groups have other specific purposes, such as helping to monitor medication-related issues or serving as an avenue for promoting education related to the affective disorder and its treatment.

Support groups help members gain a sense of perspective on their condition and tangibly encourage them to link up with others who have common problems. A sense of hope is conveyed when the individual is able to see that he or she is not alone or unique in experiencing affective illness.

Self-help groups offer another avenue of support for the depressed client. These groups are usually peer led and are not meant to substitute for, or compete with, professional therapy. They offer supplementary support that frequently enhances compliance with the medical regimen. Examples of self-help groups are the Depression and Bipolar Support Alliance (DBSA), Depressives Anonymous, Recovery International, and GriefShare (grief recovery support groups). Although self-help groups are not psychotherapy groups, they do provide important adjunctive support experiences, which often have therapeutic benefit for participants.

Family Therapy

The ultimate objectives in working with families of clients with mood disorders are to resolve the symptoms and initiate or restore adaptive family functioning. As with group therapy, the most effective approach appears to be with a combination of psychotherapeutic and pharmacotherapeutic treatments. Sadock and Sadock, (2007) stated:

Family therapy is indicated if the disorder jeopardizes the patient's marriage or family functioning or if the mood disorder is promoted or maintained by the family situation. Family therapy examines the role of the mood-disordered member in the overall psychological well-being of the whole family; it also examines the role of the entire family in the maintenance of the patient's symptoms. (p. 565)

Cognitive Therapy

In cognitive therapy, the individual is taught to control thought distortions that are considered to be a factor in the development and maintenance of mood disorders. In the cognitive model, depression is characterized by a triad of negative distortions related to expectations of the environment, self, and future. The environment and activities within it are viewed as unsatisfying, the self is unrealistically devalued, and the future is perceived as hopeless.

The general goals in cognitive therapy are to obtain symptom relief as quickly as possible, to assist the client in identifying dysfunctional patterns of thinking and behaving, and to guide the client to evidence and logic that effectively test the validity of the dysfunctional thinking (see Chapter 20). Therapy focuses on changing "automatic thoughts" that occur spontaneously and contribute to the distorted affect. Examples of automatic thoughts in depression include:

- **Personalizing:** "I'm the only one who failed."
- **All or nothing:** "I'm a complete failure."
- **Mind reading:** "He thinks I'm foolish."
- **Discounting positives:** "The other questions were so easy. Any dummy could have gotten them right."

The client is asked to describe evidence that both supports and disputes the automatic thought. The logic underlying the inferences is then reviewed with the client. Another technique involves evaluating what would most likely happen if the client's automatic thoughts were true. Implications of the consequences are then discussed.

Clients should not become discouraged if one technique seems not to be working. No single technique works with all clients. He or she should be reassured that any of a number of techniques may be used, and both therapist and client may explore these possibilities.

Cognitive therapy has offered encouraging results in the treatment of depression. In fact, the results of several studies with depressed clients show that in some cases cognitive therapy may be equally or even more effective than antidepressant medication (Rupke, Blecke, & Renfrow, 2006).

Electroconvulsive Therapy

Electroconvulsive therapy (ECT) is the induction of a grand mal (generalized) seizure through the application of electrical current to the brain. ECT is effective with clients who are acutely suicidal and in the treatment of severe depression, particularly in those clients who are also experiencing psychotic symptoms and those with psychomotor retardation and neurovegetative changes, such as disturbances in sleep, appetite, and energy. It is often considered for treatment only after a trial of therapy with antidepressant medication has proved ineffective (see Chapter 21 for a detailed discussion of ECT).

Transcranial Magnetic Stimulation

Transcranial magnetic stimulation (TMS) is a procedure that is used to treat depression by stimulating nerve cells in the brain. TMS involves the use of very short pulses of magnetic energy to stimulate nerve cells in the brain, similar to the electrical activity observed with ECT. However, unlike ECT, the electrical waves generated by TMS do not result in generalized seizure activity (DeNoon, 2008). The waves are passed through a coil placed on the scalp to areas of the brain involved in mood regulation. Some clinicians believe that TMS holds a great deal of promise in the treatment of depression, whereas others remain skeptical. In rare instances, seizures have been triggered with the use of TMS therapy (Lanocha, 2010). In a study at King's College in London, researchers compared the efficacy of TMS with ECT in the treatment of severe depression (Eranti et al., 2007). They concluded that ECT was substantially more effective for the short-term treatment of depression, and they indicated the need for further intense clinical evaluation of TMS.

Light Therapy

Between 15 and 25 percent of people with recurrent depressive disorder exhibit a seasonal pattern whereby symptoms are exacerbated during the winter months and subside during the spring and summer (Thase, 2007). The *DSM-IV-TR* identifies this disorder as Major Depressive Disorder With Seasonal Pattern. It has commonly been known as seasonal affective disorder (SAD). Bright light therapy has been suggested as a first-line treatment for winter "blues" and as an adjunct in chronic major depressive disorder or dysthymia with seasonal exacerbations (Karasu, Gelenberg, Merriam, & Wang, 2006).

SAD is thought to be related to the presence of the hormone melatonin, which is produced by the pineal gland. Melatonin plays a role in the regulation of biological rhythms for sleep and activation. It is produced during the cycle of darkness and shuts off in the light of day. During the months of longer darkness hours, there is increased production of melatonin, which seems to trigger the symptoms of SAD in susceptible people.

Light therapy, or exposure to light, has been shown to be an effective treatment for SAD. The light therapy is administered by a 10,000-lux light box, which contains white fluorescent light tubes covered with a plastic screen that blocks ultraviolet rays. The individual sits in front of the box with the eyes open (although they should not look directly into the light). Therapy usually begins with 10- to 15-minute sessions, and gradually progresses to 30 to 45 minutes. Some people notice improvement rapidly, within a few days, whereas others may take several weeks to feel better. Side effects appear to be dosage related, and include headache, eyestrain, nausea, irritability, photophobia (eye sensitivity to light), insomnia (when light therapy is used late in the day), and (rarely) hypomania (Terman & Terman, 2005). Light therapy and antidepressants have shown comparable efficacy in studies of SAD treatment. One study compared the efficacy of light therapy for SAD to daily treatment with 20 mg of fluoxetine (Lam et al., 2006). The authors concluded that, "Light treatment showed earlier response onset and lower rate of some adverse events relative to fluoxetine, but there were no other significant differences in outcome between light therapy and antidepressant medication" (p. 805).

Psychopharmacology

Historical Aspects

Antidepressant medication had a serendipitous beginning. In the early 1950s, patients with tuberculosis were being treated with the monoamine oxidase inhibitor (MAOI) iproniazid. Although the drug proved ineffective for tuberculosis, it was found that patients exhibited a sustained elevation of mood while taking the medication (Schatzberg, Cole, & DeBattista, 2010). Following the initial enthusiasm about MAOIs, they fell into relative disuse for nearly 2 decades because of a perceived poor risk-to-benefit ratio.

The tricyclic antidepressants (TCAs) had a similar introduction. In the late 1950s, imipramine was being investigated as a treatment for schizophrenia, and although it did not relieve psychotic symptoms, it appeared to elevate mood. For almost 50 years, the tricyclic antidepressants (TCAs) have been widely used to treat depression. Since the initial discovery of their antidepressant properties, they have been subjected to hundreds of controlled trials, and their efficacy in treating depressive illness is now firmly established.

The success of these first two groups of antidepressants led the pharmaceutical industry to search for compounds with similar efficacy and fewer side effects than the MAOIs and the TCAs. Examples of commonly used antidepressant medications are presented in Table 27-3. A detailed description of these medications follows.

TABLE 27-3 Medications Used in the Treatment of Depression				
CHEMICAL CLASS	GENERIC (TRADE) NAME*	PREGNANCY CATEGORIES/ HALF-LIFE (hr)	DAILY ADULT DOSAGE RANGE (mg)†	THERAPEUTIC PLASMA RANGES
Tricyclics	Amitriptyline	D/ 31–46	50–300	110–250 (including metabolite)
	Amoxapine	C/ 8	50–300	200–500
	Clomipramine (Anafranil)	C/ 19–37	25–250	80–100
	Desipramine (Norpramin)	C/ 12–24	25–300	125–300
	Doxepin (Sinequan)	C/ 8–24	25–300	100–200 (including metabolite)
	Imipramine (Tofranil)	D/ 11–25	30–300	200–350 (including metabolite)
	Nortriptyline (Aventyl; Pamelor)	D/ 18–44	30–100	50–150
	Protriptyline (Vivactil)	C/ 67–89	15–60	100–200
	Trimipramine (Surmontil)	C/ 7–30	50–300	180 (including metabolite)
Selective Serotonin Reuptake Inhibitors (SSRIs)	Citalopram (Celexa)	C/ ~35	20–40	Not well established
	Escitalopram (Lexapro)	C/ 27–32	10–20	Not well established
	Fluoxetine (Prozac; Serafem)	C/ 1–16 days (including metabolite)	20–80	Not well established
	Fluvoxamine (Luvox)	C/ 13.6–15.6	50–300	Not well established
	Paroxetine (Paxil)	D/ 21 (CR: 15–20)	10–50 (CR: 12.5–75)	Not well established
	Sertraline (Zoloft)	C/ 26–104 (including metabolite)	25–200	Not well established
	Vilazodone (Viibryd) (also acts as a partial serotonergic agonist)	C/ 25	40	Not well established
Monoamine Oxidase Inhibitors	Isocarboxazid (Marplan)	C/ Not established	20–60	Not well established
	Phenelzine (Nardil)	C/ 2–3	45–90	Not well established
	Tranylcypromine (Parnate)	C/ 2.4–2.8	30–60	Not well established
	Selegiline Transdermal System (Emsam)	C/ 18–25 (including metabolites)	6/24 hr – 12/24 hr patch	Not well established

Continued

TABLE 27-3 Medications Used in the Treatment of Depression—cont'd

CHEMICAL CLASS	GENERIC (TRADE) NAME*	PREGNANCY CATEGORIES/ HALF-LIFE (hr)	DAILY ADULT DOSAGE RANGE (mg)†	THERAPEUTIC PLASMA RANGES
Heterocyclics	Bupropion (Wellbutrin)	C/ 8–24	200–450	Not well established
	Maprotiline	B/ 21–25	25–225	200–300 (including metabolite)
	Mirtazapine (Remeron)	C/ 20–40	15–45	Not well established
	Nefazodone‡	C/ 2–4	200–600	Not well established
	Trazodone	C/ 4–9	150–600	800–1600
Serotonin-Norepinephrine Reuptake Inhibitors (SNRIs)	Desvenlafaxine (Pristiq)	C/ 11	50–400	Not well established
	Duloxetine (Cymbalta)	C/ 8–17	40–60	Not well established
	Venlafaxine (Effexor)	C/ 5–11 (including metabolite)	75–375	Not well established
Psychotherapeutic Combinations	Olanzapine and fluoxetine (Symbyax)	C/ (see individual drugs)	6/25–12/50	Not well established
	Chlordiazepoxide and fluoxetine (Limbitrol)	D/ (see individual drugs)	20/50–40/100	Not well established
	Perphenazine and amitriptyline (Etrafon)	C–D/ (see individual drugs)	6/30–16/200	Not well established

*Drugs without trade names are available in generic form only.
†Dosage requires slow titration; onset of therapeutic response may be 1 to 4 weeks.
‡Bristol Myers Squibb voluntarily removed their brand of nefazodone (Serzone) from the market in 2004. The generic equivalent is currently available through various other manufacturers.

Indications

Antidepressant medications are used in the treatment of dysthymic disorder; major depression with melancholia or psychotic symptoms; depression associated with organic disease, alcoholism, schizophrenia, or mental retardation; depressive phase of bipolar disorder; and depression accompanied by anxiety. These drugs elevate mood and alleviate other symptoms associated with moderate to severe depression. Selected agents are also used to treat anxiety disorders, bulimia nervosa, and premenstrual dysphoric disorder.

Action

These drugs ultimately work to increase the concentration of norepinephrine, serotonin, and/or dopamine in the body. This is accomplished in the brain by blocking the reuptake of these neurotransmitters by the neurons (TCAs, heterocyclics, SSRIs, and SNRIs). It also occurs when an enzyme, monoamine oxidase, that is known to inactivate norepinephrine, serotonin, and dopamine, is inhibited at various sites in the nervous system (MAOIs).

Contraindications/Precautions

Antidepressant medications are contraindicated in individuals with hypersensitivity. TCAs are contraindicated in the acute recovery phase following myocardial infarction and in individuals with angle-closure glaucoma. TCAs, heterocyclics, SSRIs, and SNRIs are contraindicated with concomitant use of MAOIs.

> **CLINICAL PEARL** All antidepressants carry an FDA black-box warning for increased risk of suicidality in children and adolescents.

Caution should be used in administering these medications to elderly or debilitated clients and those with hepatic, renal, or cardiac insufficiency. (The dosage usually must be decreased.) Caution is also required with psychotic clients, with clients who have benign prostatic hypertrophy, and with individuals who have a history of seizures (may decrease seizure threshold).

> **CLINICAL PEARL** As these drugs take effect, and mood begins to lift, the individual may have increased energy with which to implement a suicide plan. Suicide potential often increases as level of depression decreases. The nurse should be particularly alert to sudden lifts in mood.

Interactions

Tricyclic Antidepressants

■ Increased effects of tricyclic antidepressants may occur with bupropion, cimetidine, haloperidol, SSRIs, and valproic acid.

■ Decreased effects of tricyclic antidepressants may occur with carbamazepine, barbiturates, and rifamycins.

■ Hyperpyretic crisis, convulsions, and death may occur with MAOIs.

■ Coadministration with clonidine may produce hypertensive crisis.

■ Decreased effects of levodopa and guanethidine may occur with tricyclic antidepressants.

■ Potentiation of pressor response may occur with direct-acting sympathomimetics.

■ Increased anticoagulation effects may occur with dicumarol.

■ Increased serum levels of carbamazepine occur with concomitant use of tricyclics.

■ There is an increased risk of seizures with concomitant use of maprotiline and phenothiazines.

Monoamine Oxidase Inhibitors

■ Serious, potentially fatal adverse reactions may occur with concurrent use of all other antidepressants, carbamazepine, cyclobenzaprine, buspirone, sympathomimetics, tryptophan, dextromethorphan, anesthetic agents, CNS depressants, and amphetamines. Avoid using within 2 weeks of each other (5 weeks after therapy with fluoxetine).

■ Hypertensive crisis may occur with amphetamines, methyldopa, levodopa, dopamine, epinephrine, norepinephrine, guanethidine, guanadrel, reserpine, or vasoconstrictors.

■ Hypertension or hypotension, coma, convulsions, and death may occur with opioids (avoid use of meperidine within 14 to 21 days of MAOI therapy).

■ Excess CNS stimulation and hypertension may occur with methylphenidate.

■ Additive hypotension may occur with antihypertensives, thiazide diuretics, or spinal anesthesia.

■ Additive hypoglycemia may occur with insulins or oral hypoglycemic agents.

■ Doxapram may increase pressor response.

■ Serotonin syndrome may occur with concomitant use of St. John's wort.

■ Hypertensive crisis may occur with ingestion of foods or other products containing high concentrations of **tyramine** (Table 27-4).

■ Consumption of foods or beverages with high caffeine content increases the risk of hypertension and arrhythmias.

TABLE 27-4 Diet and Drug Restrictions for Clients on MAOI Therapy
FOODS CONTAINING TYRAMINE

High Tyramine Content (Avoid while on MAOI therapy)	Moderate Tyramine Content (May eat occasionally while on MAOI therapy)	Low Tyramine Content (Limited quantities permissible while on MAOI therapy)
Aged cheeses (cheddar, Swiss, Camembert, blue cheese, Parmesan, provolone, Romano, brie)	Gouda cheese, processed American cheese, mozzarella	Pasteurized cheeses (cream cheese, cottage cheese, ricotta)
Raisins, fava beans, flat Italian beans, Chinese pea pods	Yogurt, sour cream	Figs
Red wines (Chianti, burgundy, cabernet sauvignon)	Avocados, bananas	Distilled spirits (in moderation)

Continued

TABLE 27-4 Diet and Drug Restrictions for Clients on MAOI Therapy—cont'd

FOODS CONTAINING TYRAMINE

High Tyramine Content (Avoid while on MAOI therapy)	Moderate Tyramine Content (May eat occasionally while on MAOI therapy)	Low Tyramine Content (Limited quantities permissible while on MAOI therapy)
Smoked and processed meats (salami, bologna, pepperoni, summer sausage)	Beer, white wine, coffee, colas, tea, hot chocolate	
Caviar, pickled herring, corned beef, chicken or beef liver	Meat extracts, such as bouillon	
Soy sauce, brewer's yeast, meat tenderizer (MSG)	Chocolate	

DRUG RESTRICTIONS

Ingestion of the following substances while on MAOI therapy could result in life-threatening hypertensive crisis. A 14-day interval is recommended between use of these drugs and an MAOI.
- All other antidepressant medications (e.g., SSRIs, TCAs, SNRIs, heterocyclics)
- Sympathomimetics: (epinephrine, dopamine, norepinephrine, ephedrine, pseudoephedrine, phenylephrine, phenylpropanolamine, over-the-counter cough and cold preparations)
- Stimulants (amphetamines, cocaine, diet drugs)
- Antihypertensives (methyldopa, guanethidine, reserpine)
- Meperidine and (possibly) other opioid narcotics (morphine, codeine)
- Antiparkinsonian agents (levodopa)

SOURCES: Black and Andreasen (2010); Martinez, Marangell, and Martinez (2008); and Sadock and Sadock (2007).

■ Bradycardia may occur with concurrent use of MAOIs and beta blockers.

■ There is a risk of toxicity from the 5-hydroxytryptamine (5-HT) receptor agonists with concurrent use of MAOIs.

Selective Serotonin Reuptake Inhibitors (SSRIs)

■ Toxic, sometimes fatal, reactions have occurred with concomitant use of MAOIs.

■ Increased effects of SSRIs may occur with cimetidine, L-tryptophan, lithium, linezolid, and St. John's wort.

■ Serotonin syndrome may occur with concomitant use of SSRIs and metoclopramide, sibutramine, tramadol, or 5-HT receptor agonists (triptans).

■ Concomitant use of SSRIs may increase effects of hydantoins, tricyclic antidepressants, cyclosporine, benzodiazepines, beta blockers, methadone, carbamazepine, clozapine, olanzapine, pimozide, haloperidol, phenothiazines, St. John's wort, sumatriptan, sympathomimetics, tacrine, theophylline, and warfarin.

■ Concomitant use of SSRIs may decrease effects of buspirone and digoxin.

■ Lithium levels may be increased or decreased by concomitant use of SSRIs.

■ There may be decreased effects of SSRIs with concomitant use of carbamazepine and cyproheptadine.

Others (Heterocyclics and SNRIs)

■ Concomitant use with MAOIs results in serious, sometimes fatal, effects resembling neuroleptic malignant syndrome. Coadministration is contraindicated.

■ Serotonin syndrome may occur when any of the following are used together: St. John's wort, sibutramine, trazodone, nefazodone, venlafaxine, desvenlafaxine, duloxetine, SSRIs, 5-HT receptor agonists (triptans).

■ Increased effects of haloperidol, clozapine, and desipramine may occur when used concomitantly with venlafaxine.

■ Increased effects of venlafaxine may occur with cimetidine.

■ Increased effects of duloxetine may occur with cytochrome P450 (CYP)1A2 inhibitors (e.g., fluvoxamine, quinolone antibiotics) and CYP2D6 inhibitors (e.g., fluoxetine, quinidine, paroxetine).

■ Increased risk of liver injury occurs with concomitant use of alcohol and duloxetine.

■ There is an increased risk of toxicity or adverse effects from drugs extensively metabolized by CYP2D6 (e.g., flecainide, phenothiazines, propafenone, tricyclic antidepressants, thioridazine) when used concomitantly with duloxetine, desvenlafaxine, or bupropion.

■ Decreased effects of bupropion and trazodone may occur with carbamazepine.

■ Altered anticoagulant effect of warfarin may occur with bupropion, venlafaxine, desvenlafaxine, duloxetine, or trazodone.

Side Effects

The plan of care should include monitoring for the following side effects from antidepressant medications. Nursing implications related to each side effect are designated by an asterisk (*).

May Occur With All Chemical Classes
■ Dry mouth
*Offer the client sugarless candy, ice, frequent sips of water.
*Strict oral hygiene is very important.

■ Sedation
*Request an order from the physician for the drug to be given at bedtime.
*Request that the physician decrease the dosage or perhaps order a less sedating drug.
*Instruct the client not to drive or use dangerous equipment while experiencing sedation.

■ Nausea
*Medication may be taken with food to minimize GI distress.

■ Discontinuation syndrome
*All classes of antidepressants have varying potentials to cause discontinuation syndromes. Abrupt withdrawal following long-term therapy with SSRIs, venlafaxine, desvenlafaxine, or duloxetine may result in dizziness, lethargy, headache, and nausea. Fluoxetine is less likely to result in withdrawal symptoms because of its long half-life. Abrupt withdrawal from tricyclics may produce hypomania, akathisia, cardiac arrhythmias, gastrointestinal upset, and panic attacks. The discontinuation syndrome associated with MAOIs includes flu-like symptoms, confusion, hypomania, and worsening of depressive symptoms. All antidepressant medication should be tapered gradually to prevent withdrawal symptoms (Schatzberg et al., 2010).

Most Commonly Occur With Tricyclics and Heterocyclics
■ Blurred vision
*Offer reassurance that this symptom should subside after a few weeks.
*Instruct the client not to drive until vision is clear.
*Clear small items from routine pathway to prevent falls.

■ Constipation
*Order foods high in fiber; increase fluid intake if not contraindicated; and encourage the client to increase physical exercise, if possible.

■ Urinary retention
*Instruct the client to report hesitancy or inability to urinate.
*Monitor intake and output.
*Try various methods to stimulate urination, such as running water in the bathroom or pouring water over the perineal area.

■ Orthostatic hypotension
*Instruct the client to rise slowly from a lying or sitting position.
*Monitor blood pressure (lying and standing) frequently, and document and report significant changes.
*Avoid long hot showers or tub baths.

■ Reduction of seizure threshold
*Observe clients with history of seizures closely.
*Institute seizure precautions as specified in hospital procedure manual.
*Bupropion (Wellbutrin) should be administered in doses of no more than 150 mg and should be given at least 4 hours apart. Bupropion has been associated with a relatively high incidence of seizure activity in anorexic and cachectic clients.

■ Tachycardia; arrhythmias
*Carefully monitor blood pressure and pulse rate and rhythm, and report any significant change to the physician.

■ Photosensitivity
*Ensure that client wears sunblock lotion, protective clothing, and sunglasses while outdoors.

■ Weight gain
*Provide instructions for reduced-calorie diet.
*Encourage increased level of activity, if appropriate.

Most Commonly Occur With SSRIs and SNRIs

■ Insomnia; agitation
*Administer or instruct client to take dose early in the day.
*Instruct client to avoid caffeinated food and drinks.
*Teach relaxation techniques to use before bedtime.

■ Headache
*Administer analgesics, as prescribed.
*If relief is not achieved, physician may order another antidepressant.

■ Weight loss (may occur early in therapy)
*Ensure that client is provided with caloric intake sufficient to maintain desired weight.
*Caution should be taken in prescribing these drugs for anorectic clients.
*Weigh client daily or every other day, at the same time, and on the same scale, if possible.
*After prolonged use, some clients may gain weight on these drugs.

■ Sexual dysfunction
*Men may report abnormal ejaculation or impotence.
*Women may experience delay or loss of orgasm.
*If side effect becomes intolerable, a switch to another antidepressant may be necessary.

■ Serotonin syndrome (may occur when two drugs that potentiate serotonergic neurotransmission are used concurrently [see "Interactions"])
*Most frequent symptoms include changes in mental status, restlessness, myoclonus, hyperreflexia, tachycardia, labile blood pressure, diaphoresis, shivering, and tremors.
*Discontinue the offending agent immediately.
*The physician may prescribe medications to block serotonin receptors, relieve hyperthermia and muscle rigidity, and prevent seizures. In severe cases, artificial ventilation may be required. The histamine$_1$ receptor antagonist cyproheptadine is commonly used to treat the symptoms of serotonin syndrome.
*Supportive nursing measures include monitoring vital signs, providing safety measures to prevent injury when muscle rigidity and changes in mental status are present, cooling blankets and tepid baths to assist with temperature regulation, and monitoring intake and output (Prator, 2006).

*The condition will usually resolve on its own once the offending medication has been discontinued. However, if left untreated, the condition may progress to life-threatening complications such as seizures, coma, hypotension, ventricular arrhythmias, disseminated intravascular coagulation, rhabdomyolysis, metabolic acidosis, and renal failure (Prator, 2006).

Most Commonly Occur With MAOIs

■ Hypertensive crisis
*Hypertensive crisis occurs if the individual consumes foods containing tyramine while receiving MAOI therapy (see Table 27-4).

NOTE: Hypertensive crisis has not shown to be a problem with the selegiline transdermal system at the 6 mg/24 hr dosage, and dietary restrictions at this dose are not recommended. Dietary modifications are recommended, however, at the 9 mg/24 hr and 12 mg/24 hr dosages.

*Symptoms of hypertensive crisis include severe occipital headache, palpitations, nausea/vomiting, nuchal rigidity, fever, sweating, marked increase in blood pressure, chest pain, and coma.
*Treatment of hypertensive crisis includes discontinuing the drug immediately; monitoring vital signs; administering short-acting antihypertensive medication, as ordered by the physician; and using external cooling measures to control hyperpyrexia.

■ Application site reactions (with selegiline transdermal system [Emsam])
*The most common reactions include rash, itching, erythema, irritation, swelling, or urticarial lesions. Most reactions resolve spontaneously, requiring no treatment. However, if a reaction becomes problematic, it should be reported to the physician. Topical corticosteroids have been used in treatment.

Miscellaneous Side Effects

■ Priapism (with trazodone)
*Priapism is a rare side effect, but it has occurred in some men taking trazodone.
*If prolonged or inappropriate penile erection occurs, the medication should be withheld and the physician notified immediately.
*Priapism can become very problematic, requiring surgical intervention, and, if not treated successfully, can result in impotence.

■ Hepatic failure (with nefazodone)
  *Cases of life-threatening hepatic failure have been reported in clients treated with nefazodone.
  *Advise clients to be alert for signs or symptoms suggestive of liver dysfunction (e.g., jaundice, anorexia, GI complaints, or malaise) and to report them to the physician immediately.

Client/Family Education Related to Antidepressants

The Client Should:

■ Continue to take the medication even though the symptoms have not subsided. The therapeutic effect may not be seen for as long as 4 weeks. If after this length of time no improvement is noted, the physician may prescribe a different medication.

■ Use caution when driving or operating dangerous machinery. Drowsiness and dizziness can occur. If these side effects become persistent or interfere with activities of daily living, the client should report them to the physician. Dosage adjustment may be necessary.

■ Not discontinue use of the drug abruptly. To do so might produce withdrawal symptoms, such as nausea, vertigo, insomnia, headache, malaise, nightmares, and return of symptoms for which the medication was prescribed.

■ Use sunblock lotion and wear protective clothing when spending time outdoors. The skin may be sensitive to sunburn.

■ Report occurrence of any of the following symptoms to the physician immediately: sore throat, fever, malaise, yellowish skin, unusual bleeding, easy bruising, persistent nausea/vomiting, severe headache, rapid heart rate, difficulty urinating, anorexia/weight loss, seizure activity, stiff or sore neck, and chest pain.

■ Rise slowly from a sitting or lying position to prevent a sudden drop in blood pressure.

■ Take frequent sips of water, chew sugarless gum, or suck on hard candy if dry mouth is a problem. Good oral care (frequent brushing, flossing) is very important.

■ Not consume the following foods or medications while taking MAOIs: aged cheese, wine (especially Chianti), beer, chocolate, colas, coffee, tea, sour cream, smoked and processed meats, beef or chicken liver, canned figs, soy sauce, overripe and fermented foods, pickled herring, raisins, caviar, yogurt, yeast products, broad beans, cold remedies, diet pills. To do so could cause a life-threatening hypertensive crisis.

■ Avoid smoking while receiving tricyclic therapy. Smoking increases the metabolism of tricyclics, requiring an adjustment in dosage to achieve the therapeutic effect.

■ Avoid drinking alcohol while taking antidepressant therapy. These drugs potentiate the effects of each other.

■ Avoid use of other medications (including over-the-counter medications) without the physician's approval while receiving antidepressant therapy. Many medications contain substances that, in combination with antidepressant medication, could precipitate a life-threatening hypertensive crisis.

■ Notify physician immediately if inappropriate or prolonged penile erections occur while taking trazodone. If the erection persists longer than 1 hour, seek emergency department treatment. This condition is rare, but has occurred in some men who have taken trazodone. If measures are not instituted immediately, impotence can result.

■ Not "double up" on medication if a dose of bupropion (Wellbutrin) is missed, unless advised to do so by the physician. Taking bupropion in divided doses will decrease the risk of seizures and other adverse effects.

■ Follow the correct procedure for applying the selegiline transdermal patch:
  • Apply to dry, intact skin on upper torso, upper thigh, or outer surface of upper arm.
  • Apply approximately same time each day to new spot on skin, after removing and discarding old patch.
  • Wash hands thoroughly after applying the patch.
  • Avoid exposing application site to direct heat (e.g., heating pads, electric blankets, heat lamps, hot tub, or prolonged direct sunlight).
  • If patch falls off, apply new patch to a new site and resume previous schedule.

■ Be aware of possible risks of taking antidepressants during pregnancy. Safe use during pregnancy and lactation has not been fully established. These drugs are believed to readily cross the placental barrier; if so, the fetus could experience adverse effects of the drug. Inform the physician immediately if pregnancy occurs, is suspected, or is planned.

■ Be aware of the side effects of antidepressants. Refer to written materials furnished by health-care providers for safe self-administration.

■ Carry a card or other identification at all times describing the medications being taken.

CASE STUDY AND SAMPLE CARE PLAN

NURSING HISTORY AND ASSESSMENT

Sam is a 45-year-old white male admitted to the psychiatric unit of a general medical center by his family physician, Dr. Jones, who reported that Sam had become increasingly despondent over the past month. His wife reported that he had made statements such as, "Life is not worth living," and "I think I could just take all those pills Dr. Jones prescribed at one time; then it would all be over." Sam says he loves his wife and children and does not want to hurt them, but feels they no longer need him. He states, "They would probably be better off without me." His wife appears to be very concerned about his condition, although in his despondency, he seems oblivious to her feelings. His mother (a widow) lives in a neighboring state, and he sees her infrequently. His father was an alcoholic and physically abused Sam and his siblings. He admits that he is somewhat bitter toward his mother for allowing him and his siblings to "suffer from the physical and emotional brutality of their father." His siblings and their families live in distant states, and he sees them rarely, during holiday gatherings.

Sam earned a college degree working full-time at night to pay his way. He is employed in the administration department of a large corporation. Over the past 12 years, Sam has watched while a number of his peers were promoted to management positions. Sam has been considered for several of these positions but has never been selected. Last month a management position became available for which Sam felt he was qualified. He applied for this position, believing he had a good chance of being promoted. However, when the announcement was made, the position had been given to a younger man who had been with the company only 5 years. Sam seemed to accept the decision, but over the past few weeks he has become more and more withdrawn. He speaks to very few people at the office and is becoming more and more behind in his work. At home, he eats very little, talks to family members only when they ask a direct question, withdraws to his bedroom very early in the evening, and does not come out until time to leave for work the next morning. Today, he refused to get out of bed or to go to work. His wife convinced him to talk to their family doctor, who admitted him to the hospital. The referring psychiatrist diagnosed Sam with Major Depressive Disorder.

NURSING DIAGNOSES/OUTCOME IDENTIFICATION

From the assessment data, the nurse develops the following nursing diagnoses for Sam:

1. **Risk for suicide** related to depressed mood and expressions of having nothing to live for.
   a. **Short-Term Goals:**
      • Sam will seek out staff when ideas of suicide occur.

   • Sam will maintain a short-term contract not to harm himself.
   b. **Long-Term Goal:**
      • Sam will not harm himself during his hospitalization.

2. **Complicated grieving** related to unresolved losses (job promotion and unsatisfactory parent-child relationships) evidenced by anger turned inward on self and desire to end his life.
   a. **Short-Term Goal:**
      • Sam will verbalize anger toward boss and parents within 1 week.
   b. **Long-Term Goal:**
      • Sam will verbalize his position in the grief process and begin movement in the progression toward resolution by time of discharge from treatment.

PLANNING/IMPLEMENTATION

Risk for Suicide

The following nursing interventions have been identified for Sam:

1. Ask Sam directly, "Have you thought about killing yourself? If so, what do you plan to do? Do you have the means to carry out this plan?"

2. Create a safe environment. Remove all potentially harmful objects from immediate access (sharp objects, straps, belts, ties, glass items).

3. Formulate a short-term verbal contract with Sam that he will not harm himself during the next 24 hours. When that contract expires, make another. Continue with this intervention until Sam is discharged.

4. Secure a promise from Sam that he will seek out a staff member if thoughts of suicide emerge.

5. Encourage verbalizations of honest feelings. Through exploration and discussion, help him to identify symbols of hope in his life (participating in activities he finds satisfying outside of his job).

6. Allow Sam to express angry feelings within appropriate limits. Encourage use of the exercise room and punching bag each day. Help him to identify the true source of his anger, and work on adaptive coping skills for use outside the hospital (e.g., jogging, exercise club available to employees of his company).

7. Identify community resources that he may use as a support system and from whom he may request help if feeling suicidal (e.g., suicidal or crisis hotline; psychiatrist or social worker at community mental health center; hospital "HELP" line).

8. Introduce Sam to support and education groups for adult children of alcoholics (ACOA).

CASE STUDY AND SAMPLE CARE PLAN — cont'd

9. Spend time with Sam. This will help him to feel safe and secure while conveying the message that he is a worthwhile person.

Complicated Grieving

The following nursing interventions have been identified for Sam:

1. Sam is fixed in the anger stage of the grieving process. Discuss with him behaviors associated with this stage, so that he may come to realize why he is feeling this way.

2. Develop a trusting relationship with Sam. Show empathy and caring. Be honest and keep all promises.

3. Convey an accepting attitude—one in which he is not afraid to express feelings openly.

4. Allow him to verbalize feelings of anger. The initial expression of anger may be displaced on to the healthcare provider. Do not become defensive if this should occur. Assist him to explore these angry feelings so that they may be directed toward the intended persons (boss, parents).

5. Have Sam write letters (not to be mailed) to his boss and to his parents stating his true feelings toward them. Discuss these feelings with him; then destroy the letters.

6. Assist Sam to discharge pent-up anger through participation in large-motor activities (brisk walks, jogging, physical exercises, volleyball, punching bag, exercise bike, or other equipment).

7. Explain normal stages of grief, and the behaviors associated with each stage. Help Sam to understand that feelings such as guilt and anger toward his boss and parents are appropriate and acceptable during this stage of the grieving process. Help him also to understand that he must work through these feelings and move past this stage in order to eventually feel better. Knowledge of acceptability of the feelings associated with normal grieving may help to relieve some of the guilt that these responses generate. Knowing why he is experiencing these feelings may also help to resolve them.

8. Encourage Sam to review the relationship with his parents. With support and sensitivity, point out the reality of the situation in areas in which misrepresentations are expressed. Explain common roles and behaviors of members in an alcoholic family. Sam must give up the desire for an idealized family and accept the reality of his childhood situation and the effect it has had on his adult life, before the grief process can be completed.

9. Assist Sam in problem solving as he attempts to determine methods for more adaptive coping. Suggest alternatives to anger turned inward on the self when negative thinking sets in (e.g., thought-stopping techniques). Provide positive feedback for strategies identified and decisions made.

10. Encourage Sam to reach out for spiritual support during this time in whatever form is desirable to him. Assess spiritual needs (see Chapter 6), and assist as necessary in the fulfillment of those needs. Sam may find comfort in religious rituals with which he is familiar.

EVALUATION

The outcome criteria identified for Sam have been met. He sought out staff when feelings of suicide surfaced. He maintained an active no-suicide contract. He has not harmed himself in any way. He verbalizes no further thought of suicide and expresses hope for the future. He is able to verbalize names of resources outside the hospital from whom he may request help if thoughts of suicide return. He is able to verbalize normal stages of the grief process and behaviors associated with each stage. He is able to identify his own position in the grief process and express honest feelings related to the loss of his job promotion and satisfactory parent-child relationships. He is no longer manifesting exaggerated emotions and behaviors related to complicated grieving, and is able to carry out self-care activities independently.

Summary and Key Points

■ Depression is one of the oldest recognized psychiatric illnesses that is still prevalent today. It is so common, in fact, that it has been referred to as the "common cold of psychiatric disorders."

■ The cause of depressive disorders is not entirely known. A number of factors, including genetics, biochemical influences, and psychosocial experiences, likely enter into the development of the disorder.

■ Secondary depression occurs in response to other physiological disorders.

■ Symptoms of depression occur along a continuum according to the degree of severity from transient to severe.

■ The disorder occurs in all developmental levels, including childhood, adolescence, senescence, and during the puerperium.

■ Treatment of depression includes individual therapy, group and family therapy, cognitive therapy, electroconvulsive therapy, light therapy, transcranial magnetic stimulation, and psychopharmacology.

■ Nursing care of the depressed client is provided using the six steps of the nursing process.

 DavisPlus

Additional info available @ davisplus.fadavis.com

Review Questions
Self-Examination/Learning Exercise

*Select the answer that is **most** appropriate for each of the following questions:*

1. Margaret, age 68, is a widow of 6 months. Since her husband died, her sister reports that Margaret has become socially withdrawn, has lost weight, and does little more each day than visit the cemetery where her husband was buried. She told her sister today that she "didn't have anything more to live for." She has been hospitalized with Major Depressive Disorder. The *priority* nursing diagnosis for Margaret would be:
   a. Imbalanced nutrition: less than body requirements.
   b. Complicated grieving.
   c. Risk for suicide.
   d. Social isolation.

2. The physician orders sertraline (Zoloft) 50 mg bid for Margaret, a 68-year-old woman with Major Depressive Disorder. After 3 days of taking the medication, Margaret says to the nurse, "I don't think this medicine is doing any good. I don't feel a bit better." What is the most appropriate response by the nurse?
   a. "Cheer up, Margaret. You have so much to be happy about."
   b. "Sometimes it takes a few weeks for the medicine to bring about an improvement in symptoms."
   c. "I'll report that to the physician, Margaret. Maybe he will order something different."
   d. "Try not to dwell on your symptoms, Margaret. Why don't you join the others down in the dayroom?"

3. The goal of cognitive therapy with depressed clients is to:
   a. Identify and change dysfunctional patterns of thinking.
   b. Resolve the symptoms and initiate or restore adaptive family functioning.
   c. Alter the neurotransmitters that are creating the depressed mood.
   d. Provide feedback from peers who are having similar experiences.

4. Education for the client who is taking MAOIs should include which of the following?
   a. Fluid and sodium replacement when appropriate, frequent drug blood levels, signs and symptoms of toxicity.
   b. Lifetime of continuous use, possible tardive dyskinesia, advantages of an injection every 2 to 4 weeks.
   c. Short-term use, possible tolerance to beneficial effects, careful tapering of the drug at end of treatment.
   d. Tyramine-restricted diet, prohibitive concurrent use of over-the-counter medications without physician notification.

5. In teaching a client about his antidepressant medication, fluoxetine, which of the following would the nurse include? (Select all that apply.)
   a. Don't eat chocolate while taking this medication.
   b. Keep taking this medication, even if you don't feel it is helping. It sometimes takes a while to take effect.
   c. Don't take this medication with the migraine drugs "triptans."
   d. Go to the lab each week to have your blood drawn for therapeutic level of this drug.
   e. This drug causes a high degree of sedation, so take it just before bedtime.

6. A client has just been admitted to the psychiatric unit with a diagnosis of Major Depressive Disorder. Which of the following behavioral manifestations might the nurse expect to assess? (Select all that apply.)
   a. Slumped posture.
   b. Delusional thinking.
   c. Feelings of despair.
   d. Feels best early in the morning and worse as the day progresses.
   e. Anorexia.

7. A client with depression has just be prescribed the antidepressant phenelzine (Nardil). She says to the nurse, "The doctor says I will need to watch my diet while I'm on this medication. What foods should I avoid?" Which of the following is the correct response by the nurse?
   a. Blue cheese, red wine, raisins.
   b. Black beans, garlic, pears.
   c. Pork, shellfish, egg yolks.
   d. Milk, peanuts, tomatoes.

8. A client whose husband died 6 months ago is diagnosed with Major Depressive Disorder. She says to the nurse, "I start feeling angry that Harold died and left me all alone; he should have stopped smoking years ago! But then I start feeling guilty for feeling that way." What is an appropriate response by the nurse?
   a. "Yes, he should have stopped smoking. Then he probably wouldn't have gotten lung cancer."
   b. "I can understand how you must feel."
   c. "Those feelings are a normal part of the grief response."
   d. "Just think about the good times that you had while he was alive."

9. A newly admitted depressed client isolates herself in her room and just sits and stares into space. How best might the nurse begin an therapeutic relationship with this client?
   a. Say, "Come with me. I will go with you to group therapy."
   b. Make frequent short visits to her room and sit with her.
   c. Offer to introduce her to the other clients.
   d. Help her to identify stressors in her life that precipitate crises.

10. John is a client at the mental health clinic. He is depressed, has been expressing suicidal ideations, and has been seeing the psychiatric nurse every 3 days. He has been taking 100 mg of sertraline daily for about a month, receiving small amounts of the medication from his nurse at each visit. Today he comes to the clinic in a cheerful mood, much different than he seemed just 3 days ago. How might the nurse assess this behavioral change?
    a. The sertraline is finally taking effect.
    b. He is no longer in need of antidepressant medication.
    c. He has completed the grief response over loss of his wife.
    d. He may have decided to carry out his suicide plan.

TEST YOUR CRITICAL THINKING SKILLS

Carol is a 17-year-old high school senior. She will graduate in 1 month and has plans to attend the state university a few hours from her home. Carol has always made good grades in school, has participated in many activities, and has been a pep squad cheerleader. She had been dating the star quarterback, Alan, since last summer, and they had spoken a number of times about going to the senior prom together. About a month before the prom, Alan broke up with Carol and began dating Sally, whom he subsequently took to the prom. Since that time, Carol has become despondent. She doesn't go out with her friends; she dropped out of the pep squad; her grades have fallen; and she has lost 10 pounds. She attends classes most of the time, but evenings and weekends she spends in her room alone listening to her music, crying, and sleeping. Her parents have become very concerned and contacted the family physician, who has had Carol admitted to the psychiatric unit of the local hospital. The admitting psychiatrist has made the diagnosis of Major Depressive Disorder. Carol tells the nurse, "Sometimes I drive around and try to find Alan and Sally. I don't know why he broke up with me. I hate myself! I just want to die!"

Answer the following questions related to Alice:

1. What is the primary nursing diagnosis that is identified for Carol?

2. To determine the seriousness of this problem, what are important nursing assessments that must be made?

3. What medication might the physician order for Carol?

4. What concern has the FDA identified that is associated with this medication?

References

Administration on Aging. (2011). *A profile of older Americans: 2010.* Washington, DC: U.S. Department of Health and Human Services.

American Psychiatric Association. (2000). *Diagnostic and statistical manual of mental disorders* (4th ed.). Text Revision. Washington, DC: American Psychiatric Publishing.

Azoulay, L., Blais, L., Koren, G., LeLorier, J., & Berard, A. (2008). Isotretinoin and the risk of depression in patients with acne vulgaris: A case-crossover study. *The Journal of Clinical Psychiatry, 69,* 526–532.

Black, D. W., & Andreasen, N. C. (2010). *Introductory textbook of psychiatry* (5th ed.). Washington, DC: American Psychiatric Publishing.

Cartwright, L. (2004). Emergencies of survival: Moral spectatorship and the new vision of the child in postwar child psychoanalysis. *Journal of Visual Culture, 3*(1), 35–49.

Davidson, L. (2005). *Suicide and season.* New York: American Foundation for Suicide Prevention.

DeNoon, D. J. (2008). *FDA approves first transcranial magnetic stimulation device for depression.* Retrieved September 14, 2010, from http://www.medscape.com/viewarticle/581830

Dubovsky, S. L., Davies, R., & Dubovsky, A. M. (2003). Mood disorders. In R. E. Hales & S. C. Yudofsky (Eds.). *Textbook of clinical psychiatry* (4th ed., pp. 439–542). Washington, DC: American Psychiatric Publishing.

Eranti, S., Mogg, A., Pluck, G., Landau, S., Purvis, R., Brown, R.G., et al. (2007). A randomized, controlled trial with 6-month follow-up of repetitive transcranial magnetic stimulation and electroconvulsive therapy for severe depression. *American Journal of Psychiatry, 164,* 73–81.

Frackiewicz, E. J., & Shiovitz, T. M. (2001). Evaluation and management of premenstrual syndrome. *Journal of the American Pharmaceutical Association, 41,* 437–447.

George, L. K. (1992). Social factors and depression. In K. W. Schaie, D. Blazer, & J. S. House (Eds.), *Aging, health behaviors, and health outcomes.* Hillsdale, NJ: Lawrence Erlbaum Associates.

Hakko, H. (2000). *Seasonal variation of suicides and homicides in Finland.* Oulu, Finland: University of Oulu.

Harvard Medical School. (2002, February). Depression in Children—Part I. *The Harvard Mental Health Letter.* Boston, MA: Harvard Medical School Publications Group.

Hudson, C. G. (2005). Socioeconomic status and mental illness: Tests of the social causation and selection hypotheses. *American Journal of Orthopsychiatry, 75,* 3–18.

Institute of Medicine. (2003). *Health professions education: A bridge to quality.* Washington, DC: Author.

Joska, J. A., & Stein, D. J. (2008). Mood disorders. In R. E. Hales, S. C. Yudofsky, & G. O. Gabbard (Eds.), *Textbook of psychiatry* (5th ed., pp. 457–503). Washington, DC: American Psychiatric Publishing.

Karasu, T. B., Gelenberg, A., Merriam, A., & Wang, P. (2006). Practice guideline for the treatment of patients with major depressive disorder (2nd ed.). *American Psychiatric Association Practice Guidelines for the Treatment of Psychiatric Disorders, Compendium 2006.* Washington, DC: American Psychiatric Publishing.

Kornstein, S. G. (2006). Gender and depression. *MedscapeCME.* Retrieved September 12, 2010, from http://cme.medscape.com/viewarticle/527494.

Lam, R. W., Levitt, A. J., Levitan, R. D., Enns, M. W., Morehouse, R., Michalak, E. E., et al. (2006). The Can-SAD Study: A randomized controlled trial of the effectiveness of light therapy and fluoxetine in patients with winter seasonal affective disorder. *The American Journal of Psychiatry, 163,* 805–812.

Lanocha, K. (2010). Presenting TMS to patients. *Current Psychiatry, 9*(12), S7–S8.

LaPierre, T. A. (2004). *An investigation of the role of age and life stage in the moderation and mediation of the effect of marital status on depression.* Paper presented at the annual meeting of the American Sociological Association, Hilton San Francisco & Renaissance Parc 55 Hotel, San Francisco, CA, August 14, 2004. Retrieved September 12, 2010, from http://www.allacademic.com/meta/p109917_index.html

Martinez, M., Marangell, L. B., & Martinez, J. M. (2008). Psychopharmacology. In R. E. Hales, S. C. Yudofsky, & G. O. Gabbard (Eds.), *Textbook of psychiatry* (5th ed., pp. 1053–1131). Washington, DC: American Psychiatric Publishing.

Mehta, A., & Sheth, S. (2006). Postpartum depression: How to recognize and treat this common condition. *Medscape Psychiatry & Mental Health, 11*(1). Retrieved September 13, 2010, from http://www.medscape.com/viewarticle/529390

NANDA International. (2009). *Nursing diagnoses: Definitions and classification 2009–2011.* Hoboken, NJ: Wiley-Blackwell.

National Center for Health Statistics. (2010a, May). Deaths: Final data for 2007. *National Vital Statistics Reports, 58*(19). Hyattsville, MD: Author.

National Center for Health Statistics. (2010b). *Health, United States, 2009.* DHS Publication No. 2010-1232. Hyattsville, MD: Author.

National Institute of Mental Health. (2010). *Antidepressant medications for children and adolescents: Information for parents and caregivers.* Retrieved September 13, 2010, from http://www.nimh.nih.gov/

Prator, B. C. (2006). Serotonin syndrome. *Journal of Neuroscience Nursing, 38*(2), 102–105.

Rupke, S. J., Blecke, D., & Renfrow, M. (2006). Cognitive therapy for depression. *American Family Physician, 73,* 83–86.

Sadock, B. J., & Sadock, V. A. (2007). *Synopsis of psychiatry: Behavioral sciences/clinical psychiatry* (10th ed.). Philadelphia: Lippincott Williams & Wilkins.

Schatzberg, A. F., Cole, J. O., & DeBattista, C. (2010). *Manual of clinical psychopharmacology* (7th ed.). Washington, DC: American Psychiatric Publishing.

Schimelpfening, N. (2009). *A good vitamin supplement could be just what the doctor ordered.* Retrieved September 12, 2010, from http://depression.about.com/cs/diet/a/vitamin.htm

Slattery, D. A., Hudson, A. L., & Nutt, D. J. (2004). Invited review: The evolution of antidepressant mechanisms. *Fundamental & Clinical Pharmacology, 18*(1), 1–21.

Substance Abuse and Mental Health Services Administration. (2009). *2008 National Survey on Drug Use & Health.* Retrieved September 12, 2010, from http://www.oas.samhsa.gov

Tempfer, T. C. (2006). *Identifying childhood depression.* Highlights of the National Association of Pediatric Nurse Practitioners 27th Annual Conference. Retrieved September 15, 2010, from http://www.medscape.com/viewprogram/5458

Terman, M., & Terman, J. S. (2005). Light therapy for seasonal and nonseasonal depression: Efficacy, protocol, safety, and side effects. *CNS Spectrums, 10,* 647–663.

Thase, M. E. (2007). The new "blue light" intervention for seasonal affective disorder (SAD). *Medscape Psychiatry & Mental Health.* Retrieved September 14, 2010, from http://cme.medscape.com/viewarticle/550845

Williams, D. R., Gonzalez, H. M., Neighbors, H., Nesse, R., Abelson, J. M., Sweetman, J., et al. (2007). Prevalence and distribution of major depressive disorder in African Americans, Caribbean Blacks, and Non-Hispanic Whites: Results from the National Survey of American Life. *Archives of General Psychiatry, 64,* 305–315.

Classical References

Beck, A. T., Rush, A. J., Shaw, B. F., & Emery, G. (1979). *Cognitive theory of depression.* New York: Guilford Press.

Freud, S. (1957). *Mourning and melancholia,* Vol. 14 (standard ed.). London: Hogarth Press. (Original work published 1917.)

Seligman, M. E. P. (1973). Fall into helplessness. *Psychology Today, 7,* 43–48.

@ INTERNET REFERENCES

- Additional information about depression, including psychosocial and pharmacological treatment of these disorders, may be located at the following websites:
  - http://www.pslgroup.com/depression.htm
  - http://www.ndmda.org/
  - http://www.fadavis.com/townsend
  - http://www.mentalhealth.com/
  - http://www.cmellc.com/topics/depress.html
  - http://www.mental-health-matters.com/
  - http://www.mentalhelp.net/
  - http://www.nlm.nih.gov/medlineplus
  - http://nami.org/

MOVIE CONNECTIONS

Prozac Nation (depression) • *The Butcher Boy* (depression) • *Night, Mother* (depression) • *The Prince of Tides* (depression/suicide)

Mood Disorders—Bipolar Disorder

KEY TERMS

bipolar disorder

cyclothymic disorder

delirious mania

hypomania

OBJECTIVES

After reading this chapter, the student will be able to:

1. Recount historical perspectives of bipolar disorder.
2. Discuss epidemiological statistics related to bipolar disorder.
3. Describe various types of bipolar disorders.
4. Identify predisposing factors in the development of bipolar disorder.
5. Discuss implications of bipolar disorder related to developmental stage.
6. Identify symptomatology associated with bipolar disorder and use this information in client assessment.
7. Formulate nursing diagnoses and goals of care for clients with bipolar mania.
8. Identify topics for client and family teaching relevant to bipolar disorder.
9. Describe appropriate nursing interventions for behaviors associated with bipolar mania.
10. Describe relevant criteria for evaluating nursing care of clients with bipolar mania.
11. Discuss various modalities relevant to treatment of bipolar disorder.

HOMEWORK ASSIGNMENT

Please read the chapter and answer the following questions:

1. What is the most common medication that has been known to trigger manic episodes?
2. What is the speech pattern of a person experiencing a manic episode?
3. What is the difference between cyclothymic disorder and bipolar disorder?
4. Why should a person on lithium therapy have blood levels drawn regularly?

Mood was defined in the previous chapter as a pervasive and sustained emotion that may have a major influence on a person's perception of the world. Examples of mood include depression, joy, elation, anger, and anxiety. *Affect* is described as the emotional reaction associated with an experience.

The previous chapter focused on the consequences of complicated grieving as it is manifested by depressive disorders. This chapter looks at mood disorders as they are manifested by cycles of mania and depression—called **bipolar disorder.** A historical perspective and epidemiological statistics related to bipolar disorder are presented. Predisposing factors that have been implicated in the etiology of bipolar disorder provide a framework for studying the dynamics of the disorder.

The implications of bipolar disorder relevant to children and adolescents are discussed. An explanation of the symptomatology is presented as background knowledge for assessing the client with bipolar disorder. Nursing care is described in the context of the six steps of the nursing process. Various medical treatment modalities are explored.

CORE CONCEPT

Mania

An alteration in mood that is expressed by feelings of elation, inflated self-esteem, grandiosity, hyperactivity, agitation, and accelerated thinking and speaking. Mania can occur as a biological (organic) or psychological disorder, or as a response to substance use or a general medical condition.

Historical Perspective

Documentation of the symptoms associated with bipolar disorder dates back to about the second century in ancient Greece. Aretaeus of Cappadocia, a Greek physician, is credited with associating these extremes of mood as part of the same illness. It was not until much later, however, that his view gained some acceptance.

In early writings, mania was categorized with all forms of "severe madness." In 1025, the Persian physician Avicenna wrote *The Canon of Medicine,* in which he described mania as "bestial madness characterized by rapid onset and remission, with agitation and irritability. He considered rabies as a kind of mania" (Youssef, Youssef, & Dening, 1996, p. 57).

The modern concept of manic-depressive illness began to emerge in the 19th century. In 1854, Jules Baillarger presented information to the French Imperial Academy of Medicine in which he used the term *dual-form insanity* to describe the illness. In the same year, Jean-Pierre Falret described the same disorder, which he termed "circular insanity" (Nakate, 2009).

Contemporary thinking has been shaped a great deal by the works of Emil Kraepelin, who first coined the term *manic-depressive* in 1913. His approach became the most widely accepted theory of the early 1930s (Guadiz, 2008). In 1980, the American Psychiatric Association (APA) adopted the term *bipolar disorder* as the diagnostic category for manic-depressive illness in the third edition of the *Diagnostic and Statistical Manual of Mental Disorders* (DSM-III).

Epidemiology

Bipolar disorder affects approximately 5.7 million American adults, or about 2.6 percent of the U.S. population ages 18 and older, in a given year (National Institute of Mental Health [NIMH], 2010). In terms of gender, the incidence of bipolar disorder is roughly equal, with a ratio of women to men of about 1.2 to 1. The average age of onset for bipolar disorder is the early 20s, and following the first manic episode, the disorder tends to be recurrent. As with depression, bipolar disorder appears to be more common in unmarried than in married persons (Joska & Stein, 2008). Unlike depressive disorders, bipolar disorder appears to occur more frequently among the higher socioeconomic classes (Sadock & Sadock, 2007). Bipolar disorder is the sixth leading cause of disability in the middle age group, and the loss of earnings and productivity attributable to mood disorders (depression and bipolar disorder) may amount to about $33 billion per year in the United States (Joska & Stein, 2008).

Types of Bipolar Disorders

A bipolar disorder is characterized by mood swings from profound depression to extreme euphoria (mania), with intervening periods of normalcy. Delusions or hallucinations may or may not be a part of the clinical picture, and onset of symptoms may reflect a seasonal pattern.

During a manic episode, the mood is elevated, expansive, or irritable. The disturbance is sufficiently severe to cause marked impairment in occupational functioning or in usual social activities or relationships with others or to require hospitalization to prevent harm to self or others. Motor activity is excessive and frenzied. Psychotic features may be present.

A somewhat milder degree of this clinical symptom picture is called **hypomania.** Hypomania is not severe enough to cause marked impairment in social or occupational functioning or to require hospitalization, and it does not include psychotic features. The *Diagnostic and Statistical Manual of Mental Disorders, Fourth Edition, Text Revision* (DSM-IV-TR) (APA, 2000) diagnostic criteria for a manic episode are presented in Box 28-1.

BOX 28-1 Diagnostic Criteria for Manic Episode

A. A distinct period of abnormally and persistently elevated, expansive, or irritable mood, lasting 1 week (or any duration if hospitalization is necessary).

B. During the period of mood disturbance, three (or more) of the following symptoms have persisted (four if the mood is only irritable) and have been present to a significant degree:

  1. Inflated self-esteem or grandiosity.
  2. Decreased need for sleep (e.g., feels rested after only 3 hours of sleep).
  3. More talkative than usual or pressure to keep talking.
  4. Flight of ideas or subjective experience that thoughts are racing.
  5. Distractibility (i.e., attention too easily drawn to unimportant or irrelevant external stimuli).
  6. Increase in goal-directed activity (either socially, at work or school, or sexually) or psychomotor agitation.
  7. Excessive involvement in pleasurable activities that have a high potential for painful consequences (e.g., engaging in unrestrained buying sprees, sexual indiscretions, or foolish business investments).

C. The mood disturbance is sufficiently severe to cause marked impairment in occupational functioning or in usual social activities or relationships with others, or to necessitate hospitalization to prevent harm to self or others, or there are psychotic features.

D. The symptoms are not due to the direct physiological effects of a substance (e.g., a drug of abuse, a medication, or other treatment) or a general medical condition (e.g., hyperthyroidism).

From American Psychiatric Association. (2000). Diagnostic and statistical manual of mental disorders (4th ed.). Text revision. Washington, DC: American Psychiatric Publishing, with permission.

The diagnostic picture for depression associated with bipolar disorder is similar to that described for major depressive disorder, with one major distinction: the client must have a history of one or more manic episodes.

When the symptom presentation includes rapidly alternating moods (sadness, irritability, euphoria) accompanied by symptoms associated with both depression and mania, the individual is given a diagnosis of *bipolar disorder, mixed.* This disturbance is severe enough to cause marked impairment in social or occupational functioning or to require hospitalization. Psychotic features may be evident.

Bipolar I Disorder

Bipolar I disorder is the diagnosis given to an individual who is experiencing, or has experienced, a full syndrome of manic or mixed symptoms. The client may also have experienced episodes of depression. This diagnosis is further specified by the current or most recent behavioral episode experienced. For example, the specifier might be "single manic episode" (to describe individuals having a first episode of mania). For individuals who have had recurrent mood episodes, the current (or most recent) episode may be identified as manic, hypomanic, mixed, or depressed.

Bipolar II Disorder

The bipolar II disorder diagnostic category is characterized by recurrent bouts of major depression with episodic occurrence of hypomania. The individual who is assigned this diagnosis may present with symptoms (or history) of depression or hypomania. The client has never experienced an episode that meets the full criteria for mania or mixed symptomatology.

Cyclothymic Disorder

The essential feature of **cyclothymic disorder** is a chronic mood disturbance of at least 2 years' duration, involving numerous episodes of hypomania and depressed mood of insufficient severity or duration to meet the criteria for either bipolar I or II disorder. The individual is never without hypomanic or depressive symptoms for more than 2 months. The *DSM-IV-TR* criteria for cyclothymic disorder are presented in Box 28-2.

Other Bipolar Disorders

Bipolar Disorder due to a General Medical Condition

This disorder is characterized by a prominent and persistent disturbance in mood that is judged to be the result of direct physiological effects of a general medical condition (APA, 2000). The mood disturbance may involve depression or elevated, expansive, or irritable mood, and causes clinically significant distress or impairment in social, occupational, or other important areas of functioning. Types of physiological influences are included in the discussion of predisposing factors associated with bipolar disorders.

BOX 28-2 **Diagnostic Criteria for Cyclothymic Disorder**

A. For at least 2 years, the presence of numerous periods with hypomanic symptoms and numerous periods with depressive symptoms that do not meet the criteria for major depressive disorder. In children and adolescents, the duration must be at least 1 year.

B. During the 2-year period (1 year in children and adolescents), the person has not been without the symptoms in criterion A for more than 2 months at a time.

C. No major depressive episode, manic episode, or mixed episode has been present during the first 2 years of the disturbance.

D. The symptoms in criterion A are not better accounted for by schizoaffective disorder and are not superimposed on schizophrenia, schizophreniform disorder, delusional disorder, or psychotic disorder not otherwise specified.

E. The symptoms are not due to the direct physiological effects of a substance (e.g., a drug of abuse, a medication) or a general medical condition (e.g., hyperthyroidism).

F. The symptoms cause clinically significant distress or impairment in social, occupational, or other important areas of functioning.

From American Psychiatric Association. (2000). Diagnostic and statistical manual of mental disorders (4th ed.). Text revision. Washington, DC: American Psychiatric Publishing, with permission.

Substance-Induced Bipolar Disorder

The disturbance of mood associated with this disorder is considered to be the direct result of physiological effects of a substance (e.g., a drug of abuse, a medication, or toxin exposure). The mood disturbance may involve depression or elevated, expansive, or irritable mood, and causes clinically significant distress or impairment in social, occupational, or other important areas of functioning.

Mood disturbances are associated with *intoxication* from substances such as alcohol, amphetamines, cocaine, hallucinogens, inhalants, opioids, phencyclidine, sedatives, hypnotics, and anxiolytics. Symptoms can occur with *withdrawal* from substances such as alcohol, amphetamines, cocaine, sedatives, hypnotics, and anxiolytics. Heavy metals and toxins, such as gasoline, paint, organophosphate insecticides, nerve gases, carbon monoxide, and carbon dioxide, may also cause mood symptoms (APA, 2000).

A number of medications have been known to evoke mood symptoms. Classifications include anesthetics, analgesics, anticholinergics, anticonvulsants, antihypertensives, antiparkinsonian agents, antiulcer agents, cardiac medications, oral contraceptives, psychotropic medications, muscle relaxants, steroids, and sulfonamides. Some specific examples are included in the discussion of predisposing factors associated with bipolar disorders.

Predisposing Factors

The exact etiology of bipolar disorder has yet to be determined. Scientific evidence supports a chemical imbalance in the brain, although the cause of the imbalance remains unclear. Theories that consider a combination of hereditary factors and environmental triggers (stressful life events) appear to hold the most credibility.

Biological Theories

Genetics

Research suggests that bipolar disorder strongly reflects an underlying genetic vulnerability. Evidence from family, twin, and adoption studies exists to support this observation.

Twin Studies

Twin studies have indicated a concordance rate for bipolar disorder among monozygotic twins at 60 to 80 percent compared to 10 to 20 percent in dizygotic twins. Because monozygotic twins have identical genes and dizygotic twins share only approximately half their genes, this is strong evidence that genes play a major role in the etiology.

Family Studies

Family studies have shown that, if one parent has bipolar disorder, the risk that a child will have the disorder is around 28 percent (Dubovsky, Davies, & Dubovsky, 2003). If both parents have the disorder, the risk is two to three times as great. This has also been shown to be the case in studies of children born to parents with bipolar disorder who were adopted at birth and reared by adoptive parents without evidence of the disorder. These results strongly indicate that genes play a role separate from that of the environment.

Other Genetic Studies

Soreff and McInnes (2010) stated:

Four genome-wide association studies of large samples of subjects with bipolar disorder have now been published, and a collaborative analysis of 3 of the studies give combined support for two particular genes, *ANK3* (ankyrin G) and *CACNA1C* (alpha 1C subunit of the L-type voltage-gated calcium channel).

The ANK3 protein is located on the first part of the axon and is involved in making the determination of whether a neuron will fire. Studies have shown that lithium carbonate, the most common medication used to prevent manic episodes, reduces expression of *ANK3* (NIMH, 2008). The CACNA1C protein regulates the influx and outflow of calcium from the cells, and is the site of action of the calcium channel blockers sometimes used in the treatment of bipolar disorder.

Biochemical Influences

Biogenic Amines

Early studies have associated symptoms of depression with a functional deficiency of norepinephrine and dopamine and mania with a functional excess of these amines. The neurotransmitter serotonin appears to remain low in both states. One study at the University of Michigan using a presynaptic marker and positron emission tomography revealed an increased density in the amine-releasing cells in the brains of people with bipolar disorder compared to control subjects (Zubieta et al., 2000). It was hypothesized that these excess cells result in the altered brain chemistry that is associated with the symptoms of bipolar disorder. Some support of this neurotransmitter hypothesis has been demonstrated by the effects of neuroleptic drugs that influence the levels of these biogenic amines to produce the desired effect.

More recently, the biogenic amine hypothesis has been expanded to include another neurotransmitter, acetylcholine. Because cholinergic agents do have profound effects on mood, electroencephalograms, sleep, and neuroendocrine function, it has been suggested that the problem in depression and mania may be an imbalance between the biogenic amines and acetylcholine. Cholinergic transmission is thought to be excessive in depression and inadequate in mania (Dubovsky et al., 2003)

Physiological Influences

Neuroanatomical Factors

Right-sided lesions in the limbic system, temporobasal areas, basal ganglia, and thalamus have been shown to induce secondary mania. Magnetic resonance imaging studies have revealed enlarged third ventricles and subcortical white matter and periventricular hyperintensities in clients with bipolar disorder (Dubovsky et al., 2003).

Medication Side Effects

Certain medications used to treat somatic illnesses have been known to trigger a manic response. The most common of these are the steroids frequently used to treat chronic illnesses such as multiple sclerosis and systemic lupus erythematosus (SLE). Some clients whose first episode of mania occurred during steroid therapy have reported spontaneous recurrence of manic symptoms years later. Amphetamines, antidepressants, and high doses of anticonvulsants and narcotics also have the potential for initiating a manic episode (Dubovsky et al., 2003).

Psychosocial Theories

The credibility of psychosocial theories has declined in recent years. Conditions such as schizophrenia and bipolar disorder are being viewed as diseases of the brain with biological etiologies. The etiology of these illnesses remains unclear, however, and it is possible that both biological and psychosocial factors (such as environmental stressors) are influential (Soreff & McInnes, 2010).

The Transactional Model

Bipolar disorder most likely results from an interaction between genetic, biological and psychosocial determinants. Soreff and McInnes (2010) stated, "The cycle may be directly linked to external stresses or the external pressures may serve to exacerbate some underlying genetic or biochemical predisposition." The transactional model takes into consideration these various etiological influences, as well as those associated with past experiences, existing conditions, and the individual's perception of the event. Figure 28–1 depicts the dynamics of bipolar mania using the Transactional Model of Stress/Adaptation.

Developmental Implications

Childhood and Adolescence

The lifetime prevalence of pediatric and adolescent bipolar disorders is estimated to be about 1 percent, but children and adolescents are often difficult to diagnose (Nandagopal & DelBello, 2008). The developmental courses and symptom profiles of psychiatric disorders in children are unique from those of adults; therefore, approaches to diagnosis and treatment

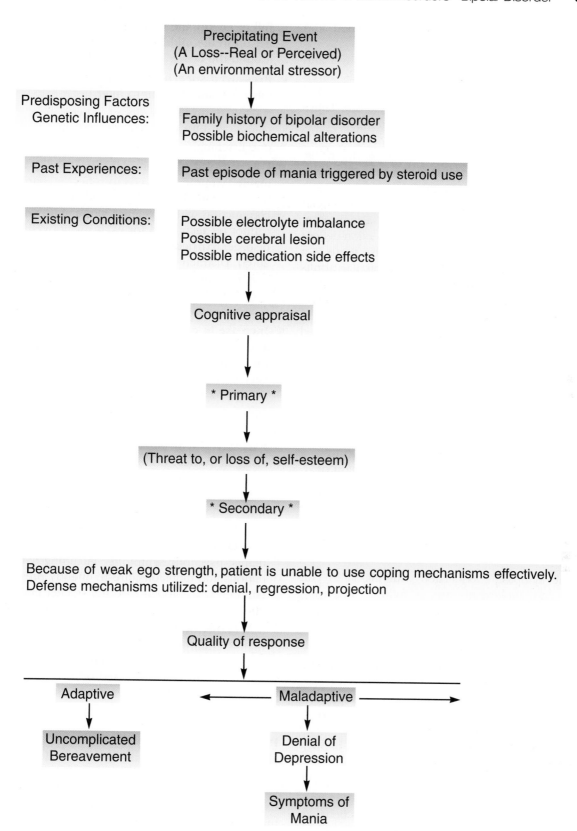

FIGURE 28–1 The dynamics of bipolar disorder, mania, using the Transactional Model of Stress/Adaptation.

cannot merely rely on strategies examined and implemented in a typical adult population.

A working group sponsored by the Child and Adolescent Bipolar Foundation (CABF) has developed consensus guidelines for the diagnosis and treatment of children with bipolar disorder. These guidelines were presented in the March 2005 issue of the *Journal of the American Academy of Child and Adolescent Psychiatry* and address diagnosis, comorbidity, acute treatment, and maintenance treatment (Kowatch et al., 2005).

Symptoms of bipolar disorder are often difficult to assess in children, and they may also present with comorbid conduct disorders or attention-deficit/hyperactivity disorder (ADHD). Because there is a genetic component and children of bipolar adults are at higher risk, family history may be particularly important (Nandagopal & DelBello, 2008). To differentiate between occasional spontaneous behaviors of childhood and behaviors associated with bipolar disorder, the Consensus Group recommends that clinicians use the FIND (frequency, intensity, number, and duration) strategy (Kowatch et al., 2005):

■ **Frequency:** Symptoms occur most days in a week.

■ **Intensity:** Symptoms are severe enough to cause extreme disturbance in one domain or moderate disturbance in two or more domains.

■ **Number:** Symptoms occur three or four times a day.

■ **Duration:** Symptoms occur 4 or more hours a day.

The symptoms associated with mania in children and adolescents are as follows. Regarding these symptoms, Kowatch and associates (2005) stated:

> For any of these symptoms to be counted as a manic symptom, they must exceed the FIND threshold. Additionally, they must occur in concert with other manic symptoms because no one symptom is diagnostic of mania. (p. 215)

■ **Euphoric/expansive mood.** Extremely happy, silly, or giddy.

■ **Irritable mood.** Hostility and rage, often over trivial matters. The irritability may be accompanied by aggressive and/or self-injurious behavior.

■ **Grandiosity.** Believing that his or her abilities are better than everyone else's.

■ **Decreased need for sleep.** May sleep only 4 or 5 hours per night and wake up fresh and full of energy the next day. Or he or she may get up in the middle of the night and wander around the house looking for things to do.

■ **Pressured speech.** Rapid speech that is loud, intrusive, and difficult to interrupt.

■ **Racing thoughts.** Topics of conversation change rapidly, in a manner confusing to anyone listening.

■ **Distractibility.** To consider distractibility a manic symptom, it needs to reflect a change from baseline functioning, needs to occur in conjunction with a "manic" mood shift, and cannot be accounted for exclusively by another disorder, particularly ADHD (Kowatch et al., 2005). Distractibility during a manic episode may be reflected in a child who is normally a B or C student and is unable to focus on any school lessons.

■ **Increase in goal-directed activity/psychomotor agitation.** A child who is not usually highly productive, during a manic episode becomes very project oriented, increasing goal-directed activity to an obsessive level. Psychomotor agitation represents a distinct change from baseline behavior.

■ **Excessive involvement in pleasurable or risky activities.** Children with bipolar disorder are often hypersexual, exhibiting behavior that has an erotic, pleasure-seeking quality about it (Kowatch et al., 2005). Adolescents may seek out sexual activity multiple times in a day.

■ **Psychosis.** In addition to core symptoms of mania, psychotic symptoms, including hallucinations and delusions, are frequently present in children with bipolar disorder (Geller et al., 2002; Kafantaris, Dicker, Coletti, & Kane, 2001).

■ **Suicidality.** Although not a core symptom of mania, children with bipolar disorder are at risk of suicidal ideation, intent, plans, and attempts during a depressed or mixed episode or when psychotic (Geller et al., 2002).

Treatment Strategies

Psychopharmacology

Monotherapy with the traditional mood stabilizers (e.g., lithium, divalproex, carbamazepine) or atypical antipsychotics (e.g., olanzapine, quetiapine, risperidone, aripiprazole, ziprasidone) was determined to be the first-line treatment (Kowatch et al., 2005). In the event of inadequate response to initial monotherapy, an alternate monotherapeutic agent is suggested. Augmentation with a second medication is indicated when monotherapy fails.

ADHD has been identified as the most common comorbid condition in children and adolescents with bipolar disorder. Because stimulants can exacerbate mania, it is suggested that medication for ADHD be initiated only after bipolar symptoms have been controlled with a mood stabilizer (Kowatch et al., 2005). Nonstimulant medications indicated for ADHD (e.g., atomoxetine, bupropion, the tricyclic antidepressants) may also induce switches to mania or hypomania.

Bipolar disorder in children and adolescents appears to be a chronic condition with a high risk of relapse (Kowatch et al., 2005). Maintenance therapy is with the same medications used to treat acute symptoms, although few research studies exist that deal with long-term maintenance of bipolar disorder in children. The Consensus Group recommends that medication tapering or discontinuation be considered after remission has been achieved for a minimum of 12 to 24 consecutive months. It was acknowledged, however, that some clients may require long-term or even lifelong pharmacotherapy (Kowatch et al., 2005).

Family Interventions

Although pharmacological treatment is acknowledged as the primary method of stabilizing an acutely ill bipolar client, adjunctive psychotherapy has been recognized as playing an important role in preventing relapses and improving adjustment. Allen (2003) suggested that involving the family in post-episode stabilization of bipolar disorder is important and helps family members:

■ Integrate their experience of the mood disorder.

■ Know the symptoms of bipolar disorder and what precipitates episodes.

■ Understand the client's vulnerability to future episodes.

Family support is also important in helping the client accept the necessity of ongoing medication administration. Family dynamics and attitudes can play a crucial role in the outcome of a client's recovery. Interventions with family members must include education that promotes understanding that at least part of the client's negative behaviors are attributable to an illness that must be managed, as opposed to being willful and deliberate.

Studies show that family-focused psychoeducational treatment (FFT) is an effective method of reducing relapses and increasing medication adherence in bipolar clients (Miklowitz, George, Richards, Simoneau, & Suddath, 2003). FFT includes sessions that deal with psychoeducation about bipolar disorder (i.e., symptoms, early recognition, etiology, treatment, self-management), communication training, and problem-solving skills training. Allen (2003) stated:

> There are several important goals of FFT, which include: improving communication within the family, teaching the family to recognize the early warning signs of a relapse, teaching the family how to respond to these warning signs, and educating them regarding the necessary treatments. This education helps families gain some control over the conflict that occurs in the post-episode phases.

There is evidence to suggest that the addition of psychosocial therapy enhances the effectiveness of psychopharmacological therapy in the maintenance of bipolar disorder in children and adolescents.

Application of the Nursing Process to Bipolar Disorder (Mania)

Background Assessment Data

Symptoms of manic states can be described according to three stages: hypomania, acute mania, and **delirious mania.** Symptoms of mood, cognition and perception, and activity and behavior are presented for each stage.

Stage I: Hypomania

At this stage the disturbance is not sufficiently severe to cause marked impairment in social or occupational functioning or to require hospitalization (APA, 2000).

Mood

The mood of a hypomanic person is cheerful and expansive. There is an underlying irritability that surfaces rapidly when the person's wishes and desires go unfulfilled, however. The nature of the hypomanic person is very volatile and fluctuating.

Cognition and Perception

Perceptions of the self are exalted—ideas of great worth and ability. Thinking is flighty, with a rapid flow of ideas. Perception of the environment is heightened, but the individual is so easily distracted by irrelevant stimuli that goal-directed activities are difficult.

Activity and Behavior

Hypomanic individuals exhibit increased motor activity. They are perceived as being very extroverted and sociable, and because of this they attract numerous acquaintances. However, they lack the depth of personality and warmth to formulate close friendships. They talk and laugh a great deal, usually very loudly and often inappropriately. Increased libido is common. Some individuals experience anorexia and weight loss. The exalted self-perception leads some hypomanic individuals to engage in inappropriate behaviors, such as phoning the President of the United States, or buying huge amounts on a credit card without having the resources to pay.

Stage II: Acute Mania

Symptoms of acute mania may be a progression in intensification of those experienced in hypomania, or they may be manifested directly. Most individuals experience marked impairment in functioning and require hospitalization.

Mood

Acute mania is characterized by euphoria and elation. The person appears to be on a continuous "high." However, the mood is always subject to frequent variation, easily changing to irritability and anger or even to sadness and crying.

Cognition and Perception

Cognition and perception become fragmented and often psychotic in acute mania. Rapid thinking proceeds to racing and disjointed thinking (flight of ideas) and may be manifested by a continuous flow of accelerated, pressured speech (loquaciousness), with abrupt changes from topic to topic. When flight of ideas is severe, speech may be disorganized and incoherent. Distractibility becomes all-pervasive. Attention can be diverted by even the smallest of stimuli. Hallucinations and delusions (usually paranoid and grandiose) are common.

Activity and Behavior

Psychomotor activity is excessive. Sexual interest is increased. There is poor impulse control, and the individual who is normally discreet may become socially and sexually uninhibited. Excessive spending is common. Individuals with acute mania have the ability to manipulate others to carry out their wishes, and if things go wrong, they can skillfully project responsibility for the failure onto others. Energy seems inexhaustible, and the need for sleep is diminished. They may go for many days without sleep and still not feel tired. Hygiene and grooming may be neglected. Dress may be disorganized, flamboyant, or bizarre, and the use of excessive makeup or jewelry is common.

Stage III: Delirious Mania

Delirious mania is a grave form of the disorder characterized by severe clouding of consciousness and an intensification of the symptoms associated with acute mania. This condition has become relatively rare since the availability of antipsychotic medication.

Mood

The mood of the delirious person is very labile. He or she may exhibit feelings of despair, quickly converting to unrestrained merriment and ecstasy or becoming irritable or totally indifferent to the environment. Panic anxiety may be evident.

Cognition and Perception

Cognition and perception are characterized by a clouding of consciousness, with accompanying confusion, disorientation, and sometimes stupor. Other common manifestations include religiosity, delusions of grandeur or persecution, and auditory or visual hallucinations. The individual is extremely distractible and incoherent.

Activity and Behavior

Psychomotor activity is frenzied and characterized by agitated, purposeless movements. The safety of these individuals is at stake unless this activity is curtailed. Exhaustion, injury to self or others, and eventually death could occur without intervention.

Diagnosis/Outcome Identification

Using information collected during the assessment, the nurse completes the client database, from which the selection of appropriate nursing diagnoses is determined. Table 28-1 presents a list of client behaviors and the NANDA nursing diagnoses that correspond to those behaviors, which may be used in planning care for the client with bipolar mania.

Outcome Criteria

The following criteria may be used for measuring outcomes in the care of the manic client.

The client:

■ Exhibits no evidence of physical injury.

■ Has not harmed self or others.

■ Is no longer exhibiting signs of physical agitation.

■ Eats a well-balanced diet with snacks to prevent weight loss and maintain nutritional status.

■ Verbalizes an accurate interpretation of the environment.

■ Verbalizes that hallucinatory activity has ceased and demonstrates no outward behavior indicating hallucinations.

■ Accepts responsibility for own behaviors.

■ Does not manipulate others for gratification of own needs.

TABLE 28-1 Assigning Nursing Diagnoses to Behaviors Commonly Associated with Bipolar Mania

BEHAVIORS	NURSING DIAGNOSES
Extreme hyperactivity; increased agitation and lack of control over purposeless and potentially injurious movements	**Risk for injury**
Manic excitement, delusional thinking, hallucinations, impulsivity	**Risk for violence: Self-directed or other-directed**
Loss of weight, amenorrhea, refusal or inability to sit still long enough to eat	**Imbalanced nutrition: Less than body requirements**
Delusions of grandeur and persecution; inaccurate interpretation of the environment	**Disturbed thought processes**
Auditory and visual hallucinations; disorientation	**Disturbed sensory perception**
Inability to develop satisfying relationships, manipulation of others for own desires, use of unsuccessful social interaction behaviors	**Impaired social interaction**
Difficulty falling asleep, sleeping only short periods	**Insomnia**

■ Interacts appropriately with others.

■ Is able to fall asleep within 30 minutes of retiring.

■ Is able to sleep 6 to 8 hours per night without medication.

Planning/Implementation

The following section presents a group of selected nursing diagnoses, with short- and long-term goals and nursing interventions for each.

Some institutions are using a case management model to coordinate care (see Chapter 9 for a more detailed explanation). In case management models, the plan of care may take the form of a critical pathway.

Risk for Violence: Self-Directed or Other-Directed

Risk for self- or other-directed violence is defined as "at risk for behaviors in which an individual demonstrates that he or she can be physically, emotionally, and/or sexually harmful to [self or to others]" (NANDA International [NANDA-I], 2009, pp. 332–333).

> **NOTE:** Please refer to Chapter 17 for additional concepts related to anger and aggression management.

Client Goals

Outcome criteria include short- and long-term goals. Timelines are individually determined.

Short-Term Goals

■ Within [a specified time], client will recognize signs of increasing anxiety and agitation and report to staff (or other care provider) for assistance with intervention.

■ Client will not harm self or others.

Long-Term Goal

■ Client will not harm self or others.

Interventions

■ Maintain a low level of stimuli in the client's environment (low lighting, few people, simple decor, low noise level). Anxiety level rises in a stimulating environment. A suspicious, agitated client may perceive individuals as threatening.

■ Observe the client's behavior frequently. Do this while carrying out routine activities so as to avoid creating suspiciousness in the individual. Close observation is necessary so that intervention can occur if required to ensure client's (and others') safety.

■ Remove all dangerous objects from the client's environment so that, in his or her agitated, confused state, the client may not use them to harm self or others.

■ Intervene at the first sign of increased anxiety, agitation, or verbal or behavioral aggression. Offer empathetic response to client's feelings: "You seem anxious (or frustrated, or angry) about this situation. How can I help?" Validation of the client's feelings conveys a caring attitude and offering assistance reinforces trust.

■ It is important to maintain a calm attitude toward the client. As the client's anxiety increases, offer some alternatives: participating in a physical activity (e.g., punching bag, physical exercise), talking about the situation, taking some antianxiety medication. Offering alternatives to the client gives him or her a feeling of some control over the situation.

■ Have sufficient staff available to indicate a show of strength to the client if it becomes necessary. This shows the client evidence of control over the situation and provides some physical security for staff.

■ If the client is not calmed by "talking down" or by medication, use of mechanical restraints may be necessary.

> **CLINICAL PEARL** The avenue of the "least restrictive alternative" must be selected when planning interventions for a violent client. Restraints should be used only as a last resort, after all other interventions have been unsuccessful, and the client is clearly at risk of harm to self or others.

■ If restraint is deemed necessary, ensure that sufficient staff is available to assist. Follow protocol established by the institution. The Joint Commission (formerly the Joint Commission on Accreditation of Healthcare Organizations [JCAHO]) requires that an in-person evaluation by a physician or other licensed independent practitioner (LIP) be conducted within 1 hour of the initiation of the restraint or seclusion (The Joint Commission, 2010). The physician or LIP must reissue a new order for restraints every 4 hours for adults and every 1 to 2 hours for children and adolescents.

■ The Joint Commission requires that the client in restraints be observed at least every 15 minutes to ensure that circulation to extremities is not compromised (check temperature, color, pulses); to assist the client with needs related to nutrition, hydration, and elimination; and to position the client so that comfort is facilitated and aspiration can be prevented. Some institutions may require continuous one-to-one monitoring of restrained clients, particularly those who are highly agitated, and for whom there is a high risk of self- or accidental injury.

■ As agitation decreases, assess the client's readiness for restraint removal or reduction. Remove one restraint at a time while assessing the client's response. This minimizes the risk of injury to client and staff.

Impaired Social Interaction

Impaired social interaction is defined as "insufficient or excessive quantity or ineffective quality of social exchange" (NANDA-I, 2009, p. 223). Table 28-2 presents this nursing diagnosis in care plan format.

Client Goals

Outcome criteria include short- and long-term goals. Timelines are individually determined.

Short-Term Goal

■ Client will verbalize which of his or her interaction behaviors are appropriate and which are inappropriate within 1 week.

Table 28-2 CARE PLAN FOR THE CLIENT EXPERIENCING A MANIC EPISODE

NURSING DIAGNOSIS: IMPAIRED SOCIAL INTERACTION
RELATED TO: Delusional thought processes (grandeur and/or persecution); underdeveloped ego and low self-esteem
EVIDENCED BY: Inability to develop satisfying relationships and manipulation of others for own desires

OUTCOME CRITERIA	NURSING INTERVENTIONS	RATIONALE
Short-Term Goal • Client will verbalize which of his or her interaction behaviors are appropriate and which are inappropriate within 1 week. **Long-Term Goal** • Client will demonstrate use of appropriate interaction skills as evidenced by lack of, or marked decrease in, manipulation of others to fulfill own desires.	1. Recognize the purpose manipulative behaviors serve for the client: to reduce feelings of insecurity by increasing feelings of power and control. 2. Set limits on manipulative behaviors. Explain to the client what is expected and what the consequences are if the limits are violated. Terms of the limitations must be agreed on by all staff who will be working with the client.	1. Understanding the motivation behind the manipulation may facilitate acceptance of the individual and his or her behavior. 2. The client is unable to establish own limits, so this must be done for him or her. Unless administration of consequences for violation of limits is consistent, manipulative behavior will not be eliminated.

Table 28-2 CARE PLAN FOR THE CLIENT EXPERIENCING A MANIC EPISODE—cont'd

OUTCOME CRITERIA	NURSING INTERVENTIONS	RATIONALE
	3. Do not argue, bargain, or try to reason with the client. Merely state the limits and expectations. Confront the client as soon as possible when interactions with others are manipulative or exploitative. Follow through with established consequences for unacceptable behavior.	3. Because of the strong id influence on client's behavior, he or she should receive immediate feedback when behavior is unacceptable. Consistency in enforcing the consequences is essential if positive outcomes are to be achieved. Inconsistency creates confusion and encourages testing of limits.
	4. Provide positive reinforcement for non-manipulative behaviors. Explore feelings and help the client seek more appropriate ways of dealing with them.	4. Positive reinforcement enhances self-esteem and promotes repetition of desirable behaviors.
	5. Help the client recognize that he or she must accept the consequences of own behaviors and refrain from attributing them to others.	5. The client must accept responsibility for own behaviors before adaptive change can occur.
	6. Help the client identify positive aspects about self, recognize accomplishments, and feel good about them.	6. As self-esteem is increased, client will feel less need to manipulate others for own gratification.

Long-Term Goal

■ Client will demonstrate use of appropriate interaction skills as evidenced by lack of, or marked decrease in, manipulation of others to fulfill own desires.

Interventions

■ Recognize the purpose these behaviors serve for the client: to reduce feelings of insecurity by increasing feelings of power and control. Understanding the motivation behind the manipulation may help to facilitate acceptance of the individual and his or her behavior.

■ Set limits on manipulative behaviors. Explain to the client what is expected and what the consequences are if the limits are violated. Terms of the limitations must be agreed on by all staff who will be working with the client. The client is unable to establish own limits, so this must be done for him or her. Unless administration of consequences for violation of limits is consistent, manipulative behavior will not be eliminated.

■ Do not argue, bargain, or try to reason with the client. Merely state the limits and expectations. Individuals with mania can be very charming in their efforts to fulfill their own desires. Confront the client as soon as possible when interactions with others are manipulative or exploitative. Follow through with established consequences for unacceptable behavior. Because of the strong id influence on the client's behavior, he or she should receive immediate feedback when behavior is unacceptable. Consistency in enforcing the consequences is essential if positive outcomes are to be achieved. Inconsistency creates confusion and encourages testing of limits.

■ Provide positive reinforcement for nonmanipulative behaviors. Explore feelings, and help the client seek more appropriate ways of dealing with them.

■ Help the client recognize that he or she must accept the consequences of own behaviors and refrain from attributing them to others. The client must accept responsibility for own behaviors before adaptive change can occur.

■ Help the client identify positive aspects about self, recognize accomplishments, and feel good about them. As self-esteem is increased, the client will feel less need to manipulate others for own gratification.

Imbalanced Nutrition: Less Than Body Requirements/Insomnia

Imbalanced nutrition: Less than body requirements is defined as "intake of nutrients insufficient to meet metabolic needs" (NANDA-I, 2009, p. 74). *Insomnia* is defined as "a disruption in amount and quality of sleep that impairs functioning" (NANDA-I, 2009, p. 115).

Client Goal

Outcome criteria include short- and long-term goals. Timelines are individually determined.

Short-Term Goals

■ Client will consume sufficient finger foods and between-meal snacks to meet recommended daily allowances of nutrients.

■ Within 3 days, with the aid of a sleeping medication, client will sleep 4 to 6 hours without awakening.

Long-Term Goals

■ Client will exhibit no signs or symptoms of malnutrition.

■ By time of discharge from treatment, client will be able to acquire 6 to 8 hours of uninterrupted sleep without medication.

Interventions

■ In collaboration with the dietitian, determine the number of calories required to provide adequate nutrition for maintenance or realistic (according to body structure and height) weight gain. Determine client's likes and dislikes, and try to provide favorite foods, if possible. The client is more likely to eat foods that he or she particularly enjoys.

■ Provide the client with high-protein, high-calorie, nutritious finger foods and drinks that can be consumed "on the run." Because of the hyperactive state, the client has difficulty sitting still long enough to eat a meal. The likelihood is greater that he or she will consume food and drinks that can be carried around and eaten with little effort. Have juice and snacks available on the unit at all times. Nutritious intake is required on a regular basis to compensate for increased caloric requirements due to the hyperactivity.

■ Maintain an accurate record of intake, output, and calorie count. Weigh the client daily. Administer vitamin and mineral supplements, as ordered by the physician. Monitor laboratory values, and report significant changes to the physician. It is important to carefully monitor the data that provide an objective assessment of the client's nutritional status.

■ Assess the client's activity level. He or she may ignore or be unaware of feelings of fatigue. Observe for signs such as increasing restlessness; fine tremors; slurred speech; and puffy, dark circles under eyes. The client could collapse from exhaustion if hyperactivity is uninterrupted and rest is not achieved.

■ Monitor sleep patterns. Provide a structured schedule of activities that includes established times for naps or rest. Accurate baseline data are important in planning care to help the client with this problem. A structured schedule, including time for short naps, will help the hyperactive client achieve much-needed rest.

■ Client should avoid intake of caffeinated drinks, such as tea, coffee, and colas. Caffeine is a CNS stimulant and may interfere with the client's achievement of rest and sleep.

■ Before bedtime, provide nursing measures that promote sleep, such as back rub; warm bath; warm, nonstimulating drinks; soft music; and relaxation exercises.

■ Administer sedative medications, as ordered, to assist client to achieve sleep until normal sleep pattern is restored.

Concept Care Mapping

The concept map care plan is an innovative approach to planning and organizing nursing care (see Chapter 9). It is a diagrammatic teaching and learning strategy that allows visualization of interrelationships between medical diagnoses, nursing diagnoses, assessment data, and treatments. An example of a concept map care plan for a client with bipolar disorder, mania, is presented in Figure 28–2.

Client/Family Education

The role of client teacher is important in the psychiatric area, as it is in all areas of nursing. A list of topics for client/family education relevant to bipolar disorder is presented in Box 28-3. Sample client teaching guides are presented in Appendix G.

Evaluation of Care for the Manic Client

In the final step of the nursing process, a reassessment is conducted to determine if the nursing actions have been successful in achieving the objectives of care. Evaluation of the nursing actions for the manic client may be facilitated by

Clinical Vignette: Sam and Janet had been engaged for a year. Three months ago, Sam called Janet and told her he didn't want to get married, and he was leaving to take a job transfer in Japan. Janet became hysterical, then depressed, and then seemed to be accepting the situation. She got a new hairstyle, bought lots of new clothes, and started going to lots of parties with her roommate, Nancy. She started losing weight, exercising excessively, and sleeping very little. She became quite promiscuous. She stopped menstruating and said to Nancy, "I wonder if I'm pregnant!" Tonight she and Nancy went to a bar. Janet started buying drinks "for the house." She became quite loud and disruptive, climbing on the bar, and announcing to the crowd that she had received a "message" that she would be the winner of tonight's multimillion-dollar lottery. When the bar owner eventually asked her to leave, she became violent, striking out at him, and destroying bar property. He called 911, and Janet was taken to the emergency department of the hospital. She has been admitted to the psychiatric unit with Bipolar I disorder, manic episode. She is agitated and restless. The nurse develops the following concept map care plan for Janet.

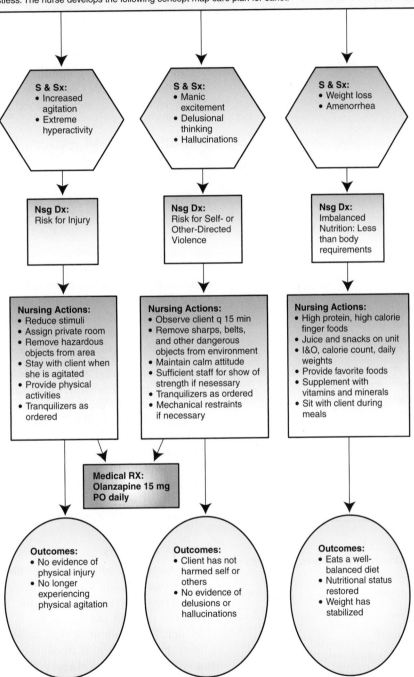

S & Sx:
- Increased agitation
- Extreme hyperactivity

S & Sx:
- Manic excitement
- Delusional thinking
- Hallucinations

S & Sx:
- Weight loss
- Amenorrhea

Nsg Dx:
Risk for Injury

Nsg Dx:
Risk for Self- or Other-Directed Violence

Nsg Dx:
Imbalanced Nutrition: Less than body requirements

Nursing Actions:
- Reduce stimuli
- Assign private room
- Remove hazardous objects from area
- Stay with client when she is agitated
- Provide physical activities
- Tranquilizers as ordered

Nursing Actions:
- Observe client q 15 min
- Remove sharps, belts, and other dangerous objects from environment
- Maintain calm attitude
- Sufficient staff for show of strength if nesessary
- Tranquilizers as ordered
- Mechanical restraints if necessary

Nursing Actions:
- High protein, high calorie finger foods
- Juice and snacks on unit
- I&O, calorie count, daily weights
- Provide favorite foods
- Supplement with vitamins and minerals
- Sit with client during meals

Medical RX:
Olanzapine 15 mg PO daily

Outcomes:
- No evidence of physical injury
- No longer experiencing physical agitation

Outcomes:
- Client has not harmed self or others
- No evidence of delusions or hallucinations

Outcomes:
- Eats a well-balanced diet
- Nutritional status restored
- Weight has stabilized

FIGURE 28–2   Concept map care plan for a client with bipolar mania.

BOX 28-3 Topics for Client/Family Education Related to Bipolar Disorder

NATURE OF THE ILLNESS
1. Causes of bipolar disorder
2. Cyclic nature of the illness
3. Symptoms of depression
4. Symptoms of mania

MANAGEMENT OF THE ILLNESS
1. Medication management
   a. Lithium
   b. Others
      1) Carbamazepine
      2) Valproic acid
      3) Clonazepam
      4) Verapamil
      5) Lamotrigine
      6) Gabapentin
      7) Topiramate
      8) Oxcarbazepine
      9) Olanzapine
      10) Risperidone
      11) Chlorpromazine
      12) Aripiprazole
      13) Quetiapine
      14) Ziprasidone
      15) Asenapine
   c. Side effects
   d. Symptoms of lithium toxicity
   e. Importance of regular blood tests
   f. Adverse effects
   g. Importance of not stopping medication, even when feeling well
2. Assertive techniques
3. Anger management

SUPPORT SERVICES
1. Crisis hotline
2. Support groups
3. Individual psychotherapy
4. Legal and/or financial assistance

gathering information using the following types of questions:

■ Has the individual avoided personal injury?

■ Has violence to client or others been prevented?

■ Has agitation subsided?

■ Have nutritional status and weight been stabilized? Is the client able to select foods to maintain adequate nutrition?

■ Have delusions and hallucinations ceased? Is the client able to interpret the environment correctly?

■ Is the client able to make decisions about own self-care? Has hygiene and grooming improved?

■ Is behavior socially acceptable? Is client able to interact with others in a satisfactory manner? Has the client stopped manipulating others to fulfill own desires?

■ Is the client able to sleep 6 to 8 hours per night and awaken feeling rested?

■ Does the client understand the importance of maintenance medication therapy? Does he or she understand that symptoms may return if medication is discontinued?

■ Can the client taking lithium verbalize early signs of lithium toxicity? Does he or she understand the necessity for monthly blood level checks?

Treatment Modalities for Bipolar Disorder (Mania)

Individual Psychotherapy

Manic clients traditionally have been difficult candidates for psychotherapy. They form a therapeutic relationship easily because they are eager to please and grateful for the therapist's interest. However, the relationship often tends to remain shallow and rigid. Some reports have indicated that psychotherapy (in conjunction with medication maintenance treatment) and counseling may indeed be useful with these individuals. Goldberg and Hoop (2004) stated:

> Interpersonal and social rhythm therapy is a form of interpersonal therapy tailored to bipolar patients. In addition to focusing on grief, role conflicts, role transitions, and interpersonal deficiencies, [it] includes psychoeducation about bipolar disorder and encourages treatment adherence. [Studies have] suggested that bipolar patients receiving the treatment were more often euthymic [stable mood] than patients receiving only clinical management.

Group Therapy

Once an acute phase of the illness is passed, groups can provide an atmosphere in which individuals may discuss issues in their lives that cause, maintain, or arise out of having a serious affective disorder. The element of peer support may provide a feeling of security, as troublesome or embarrassing issues are discussed and resolved. Some groups have other specific purposes, such as helping to monitor medication-related issues or serving as an avenue for promoting education related to the affective disorder and its treatment.

Support groups help members gain a sense of perspective on their condition and tangibly encourage them to link up with others who have common problems. A sense of hope is conveyed when the individual is able to see that he or she is not alone or unique in experiencing affective illness.

Self-help groups offer another avenue of support for the individual with bipolar disorder. These groups are usually peer led and are not meant to substitute for, or compete with, professional therapy. They offer supplementary support that frequently enhances compliance with the medical regimen. The Depression and Bipolar Support Alliance (DBSA) and the Child and Adolescent Bipolar Foundation put individuals in touch with their local support groups. Although self-help groups are not psychotherapy groups, they do provide important adjunctive support experiences, which often have therapeutic benefit for participants.

Family Therapy

The ultimate objectives in working with families of clients with mood disorders are to resolve the symptoms and initiate or restore adaptive family functioning. As with group therapy, the most effective approach appears to be with a combination of psychotherapeutic and pharmacotherapeutic treatments. Some studies with bipolar disorder have shown that behavioral family treatment combined with medication substantially reduces relapse rate compared with medication therapy alone.

Sadock and Sadock (2007) stated:

Family therapy is indicated if the disorder jeopardizes the patient's marriage or family functioning or if the mood disorder is promoted or maintained by the family situation. Family therapy examines the role of the mood-disordered member in the overall psychological well-being of the whole family; it also examines the role of the entire family in the maintenance of the patient's symptoms. (p. 555)

IMPLICATIONS OF RESEARCH FOR EVIDENCE–BASED PRACTICE

Zauszniewski, J. A., Bekhet, A. K., & Suresky, M. J. (2008). Factors associated with perceived burden, resourcefulness, and quality of life in female family members of adults with serious mental illness. *Journal of the American Psychiatric Association, 14,* 125–135.

DESCRIPTION OF THE STUDY: About 10 to 17.5 million persons experience serious mental illness (SMI) each year. Most of their caregivers are female family members. The authors stated, "Caregiver burden is affected by disruptive behaviors of the mentally ill person, changes in household routines, strained social relationships, lack of social support, deteriorating finances, diminished opportunity for leisure, exhaustion, and the stigma associated with mental illness, termed *stigma by association*" (p. 125). Depression is not uncommon among caregivers, who are largely female. The purpose of this study was to examine the associations between characteristics of female family members (age, race, education), adults with serious burden, stigma, depressive cognitions, resourcefulness, and quality of life (mental and physical health) of caregivers of the mentally ill. The sample consisted of 60 female family members of adults with SMI (i.e., schizophrenia, bipolar disorder, major depressive disorder, and anxiety disorders). Thirty were Caucasian and 30 were African American. Age range was 18 to 65. The majority of the women lived in the same household and provided care for their mentally ill family members. Most had some college education.

RESULTS OF THE STUDY: Age and level of education were not associated with burden, stigma, depressive

cognitions, resourcefulness, or quality of life. However, Caucasian women reported greater burden than did African American women. Perceived burden was inversely associated with length of caregiving time, suggesting that women adapt over time to having a mentally ill family member. A greater burden and stigma by association was expressed by caregivers of adults with bipolar disorder than those with schizophrenia. Mothers of adults with SMI expressed greater feelings of burden and stigma than other female family members (e.g., sisters, daughters, wives). The authors suggest that this may be related to mothers' feelings of being in some way responsible for the mental illness in their offspring. In-home caregivers expressed greater burden than out-of-home caregivers. The characteristics that related to lowest personal resourcefulness of caregivers included Caucasian race, relationship of mother, younger age of the mentally ill person, and diagnosis of bipolar disorder.

IMPLICATIONS FOR NURSING PRACTICE: These findings have direct implications for psychiatric nursing of female caregivers of family members with SMI. The authors suggested that teaching personal resourcefulness skills in a systematic way to women with newly diagnosed family members may be beneficial in maintaining their optimal quality of life. The population at highest risk was suggested by this study to be Caucasian mothers of younger aged offspring with bipolar disorder. The authors stated, "These women may benefit from programs that teach the cognitive-behavioral, self-help skills that constitute personal resourcefulness, because such skills have been associated with optimal quality of life" (p. 133).

Cognitive Therapy

In cognitive therapy, the individual is taught to control thought distortions that are considered to be a factor in the development and maintenance of mood disorders. In the cognitive model, depression is characterized by a triad of negative distortions related to expectations of the environment, self, and future. The environment and activities within it are viewed as unsatisfying, the self is unrealistically devalued, and the future is perceived as hopeless. In the same model, mania is characterized by exaggeratedly positive cognitions and perceptions. The individual perceives the self as highly valued and powerful. Life is experienced with overstated self-assurance, and the future is viewed with unrealistic optimism.

The general goals in cognitive therapy are to obtain symptom relief as quickly as possible, to assist the client in identifying dysfunctional patterns of thinking and behaving, and to guide the client to evidence and logic that effectively test the validity of the dysfunctional thinking (see Chapter 20). Therapy focuses on changing "automatic thoughts" that occur spontaneously and contribute to the distorted affect. Examples of automatic thoughts in bipolar mania include:

- **Personalizing:** "She's this happy only when she's with me."

- **All or nothing:** "Everything I do is great."

- **Mind reading:** "She thinks I'm wonderful."

- **Discounting negatives:** "None of those mistakes are really important."

The client is asked to describe evidence that both supports and disputes the automatic thought. The logic underlying the inferences is then reviewed with the client. Another technique involves evaluating what would most likely happen if the client's automatic thoughts were true. Implications of the consequences are then discussed.

Clients should not become discouraged if one technique seems not to be working. No single technique works with all clients. He or she should be reassured that any of a number of techniques may be used, and both therapist and client may explore these possibilities.

Finally, the use of cognitive therapy does not preclude the value of administering medication. Particularly in the treatment of bipolar mania, cognitive therapy should be considered a secondary treatment to pharmacological treatment.

Electroconvulsive Therapy

Episodes of acute mania are occasionally treated with electroconvulsive therapy (ECT), particularly when the client does not tolerate or fails to respond to lithium or other drug treatment, or when life is threatened by dangerous behavior or exhaustion (see Chapter 21 for a detailed discussion of ECT).

The Recovery Model

The concept of recovery is not new. It originally began in the addictions field, referring to a person recovering from a substance-related disorder. The term has recently been adopted by mental health professionals who believe that recovery from mental illness is also possible.

A number of definitions of recovery as it applies to mental illness have been proposed. The Substance Abuse and Mental Health Services Administration (SAMHSA) suggested the following:

> Mental health recovery is a journey of healing and transformation enabling a person with a mental health problem to live a meaningful life in a community of his or her choice while striving to achieve his or her full potential. (U.S. Department of Health and Human Services [USDHHS], 2010)

William A. Anthony, Executive Director of the Center for Psychiatric Rehabilitation at Boston University, offered this definition:

> Recovery is described as a deeply personal, unique process of changing one's attitudes, values, feelings, goals, skills, and/or roles. It is a way of living a satisfying, hopeful, and contributing life even with limitations caused by illness. Recovery involves the development of new meaning and purpose in one's life as one grows beyond the catastrophic effects of mental illness. (Anthony, 1993, p. 13)

The President's New Freedom Commission on Mental Health (2003) has proposed to transform the mental health system by shifting the paradigm of care of persons with serious mental illness from traditional medical psychiatric treatment toward the concept of recovery, and the American Psychiatric Association has endorsed a recovery model from a psychiatric services perspective (Sharfstein, 2005).

The basic concept of a recovery model is empowerment of the consumer. The recovery model is designed to allow consumers primary control over decisions about their own care. The National Association of Social Workers (NASW, 2010) suggested that this means, "Consumers need to be as fully informed as possible about the potential benefits and consequences of each decision. They also need to know the possible results if they become a danger to themselves or others."

The USDHHS (2010) outlined the following 10 fundamental components of the recovery model:

1. **Self-direction.** Consumers lead, control, exercise choice over, and determine their own path of recovery by optimizing autonomy, independence, and control of resources to achieve a self-determined life.

2. **Individualized and person-centered.** Multiple pathways to recovery exist and are based on an individual's unique strengths, needs, preferences, experiences, and cultural background. Recovery is identified as an ongoing journey and an end result as well as an overall paradigm for achieving wellness and optimal mental health.

3. **Empowerment.** Through empowerment, individuals gain control of their own destiny and influence the organizational and societal structures in their lives. They have the authority to choose from a range of options and to participate in all decisions—including the allocation of resources—that will affect their lives, and are educated and supported in doing so.

4. **Holistic.** Recovery encompasses an individual's whole life, including mind, body, spirit, and community. Recovery embraces all aspects of life, including housing, employment, education, mental health and health-care treatment and services, complementary and naturalistic services, additions treatment, spirituality, creativity, social networks, community participation, and family supports as determined by the person.

5. **Nonlinear.** Recovery is not a step-by-step process, but one based on continual growth, occasional setbacks, and learning from experience. It begins with an initial stage of awareness in which a person recognizes that positive change is possible, and progresses to full engagement in the work of recovery.

6. **Strengths-based.** Recovery builds on the multiple capacities, resiliencies, talents, coping abilities, and inherent worth of the individual, encouraging consumers to leave stymied life roles behind and engage in new life roles (e.g., partner, caregiver, friend, student, employee). The process of recovery moves forward through interaction with others in supportive, trust-based relationships.

7. **Peer support.** Mutual support—including the sharing of experiential knowledge and skills and social learning—plays an invaluable role in recovery. Individuals provide each other with a sense of belonging, supportive relationships, valued roles, and community.

8. **Respect.** Community, systems, and societal acceptance and appreciation of consumers—including protecting their rights and eliminating discrimination and stigma—are crucial in achieving recovery. Self-acceptance and regaining belief in one's self are particularly vital. Respect ensures the inclusion and full participation of consumers in all aspects of their lives.

9. **Responsibility.** Consumers have a personal responsibility for their own self-care and journeys of recovery. They must strive to understand and give meaning to their experiences and identify coping strategies and healing processes to promote their own wellness.

10. **Hope.** Recovery provides the essential and motivating message of a better future—that people can and do overcome the barriers and obstacles that confront them. Hope is internalized; but can be fostered by peers, families, friends, providers, and others. Hope is the catalyst of the recovery process.

The recovery model integrates services provided by professionals (e.g., medication, therapy, case management), services provided by consumers (e.g., advocacy, peer support programs, hotlines, mentoring), and services provided in collaboration (e.g., recovery education, crisis planning, community integration, consumer rights education) (Jacobson & Greenley, 2001). Jacobson and Greenley (2001) stated,

> Although many of these services may sound similar to services currently being offered in many mental health systems, it is important to recognize that no service is recovery-oriented unless it incorporates the attitude that recovery is possible and has the goal of promoting hope, healing, empowerment, and connection. (p. 485)

Psychopharmacology With Mood-Stabilizing Agents

For many years, the drug of choice for treatment and management of bipolar mania was lithium carbonate. However, in recent years, a number of investigators and clinicians in practice have achieved satisfactory results with several other medications, either alone or in combination with lithium. Table 28-3 provides information about the indications, actions, and contraindications and precautions of various medications being used as mood stabilizers. Drug interactions associated with mood stabilizers are presented in Table 28-4.

TABLE 28-3 Mood-Stabilizing Agents

CLASSIFICATION: GENERIC (TRADE)	PREGNANCY CATEGORY/ HALF-LIFE/ INDICATIONS	MECHANISM OF ACTION	CONTRAINDICATIONS/ PRECAUTIONS	DAILY ADULT DOSAGE RANGE/ THERAPEUTIC PLASMA RANGE
Antimanic:				
Lithium carbonate (Eskalith, Lithobid)	D/ 24 hr/ ■ Prevention and treatment of manic episodes of bipolar disorder. *Unlabeled uses:* ■ Neutropenia ■ Cluster headaches (prophylaxis) ■ Alcohol dependence ■ Bulimia ■ Postpartum affective psychosis ■ Corticosteroid-induced psychosis	Not fully understood, but may modulate the effects of various neurotransmitters such as norepinephrine, serotonin, dopamine, glutamate, and GABA, that are thought to play a role in the symptomatology of bipolar disorder (may take 1–3 weeks for symptoms to subside).	Hypersensitivity. Cardiac or renal disease, dehydration; sodium depletion; brain damage; pregnancy and lactation. Caution with thyroid disorders, diabetes, urinary retention, history of seizures, and with the elderly.	Acute mania: 1800–2400 mg Maintenance: 900–1200 mg/ Acute mania: 1.0–1.5 mEq/L Maintenance: 0.6–1.2 mEq/L
Anticonvulsants:				
Carbamazepine (Tegretol)	D/ 25–65 hr (initial); 12–17 hr (repeated doses)/ ■ Epilepsy ■ Trigeminal neuralgia *Unlabeled uses:* ■ Bipolar disorder ■ Resistant schizophrenia ■ Management of alcohol withdrawal ■ Restless legs syndrome ■ Postherpetic neuralgia	Action in the treatment of bipolar disorder is unclear.	Hypersensitivity. With MAOIs, lactation. Caution with elderly, liver/renal/cardiac disease, pregnancy.	200–1600 mg/ 4–12 mcg/mL
Clonazepam (Klonopin)	C/ 18–60 hr/ ■ Petit mal, akinetic, and myoclonic seizures ■ Panic disorder *Unlabeled uses:* ■ Acute manic episodes ■ Uncontrolled leg movements during sleep ■ Neuralgias	Action in the treatment of bipolar disorder is unclear.	Hypersensitivity, glaucoma, liver disease, lactation. Caution in elderly, liver/renal disease, pregnancy.	0.5–20 mg/ 20–80 ng/mL

Drug	Uses	Action	Contraindications/Precautions	Daily Dosage Range/Therapeutic Plasma Level
Valproic acid (Depakene; Depakote)	D/ 5–20 hr/ ■ Epilepsy ■ Manic episodes ■ Migraine prophylaxis ■ Adjunct therapy in schizophrenia	Action in the treatment of bipolar disorder is unclear.	Hypersensitivity; liver disease. Caution in elderly, renal/cardiac diseases, pregnancy and lactation.	5 mg/kg to 60 mg/kg/ 50–150 mcg/mL
Lamotrigine (Lamictal)	C/ ~33 hr/ ■ Epilepsy *Unlabeled use:* ■ Bipolar disorder	Action in the treatment of bipolar disorder is unclear.	Hypersensitivity. Caution in renal and hepatic insufficiency, pregnancy, lactation, and children < 16 years old.	100–200 mg/ Not established
Gabapentin (Neurontin; Gabarone)	C/ 5–7 hr/ ■ Epilepsy ■ Postherpetic neuralgia *Unlabeled uses:* ■ Bipolar disorder ■ Migraine prophylaxis ■ Neuropathic pain ■ Tremors associated with multiple sclerosis	Action in the treatment of bipolar disorder is unclear.	Hypersensitivity and children < 3 years. Caution in renal insufficiency, pregnancy, lactation, children, and the elderly.	900–1800 mg/ Not established
Topiramate (Topamax)	C/ 21 hr/ ■ Epilepsy ■ Migraine prophylaxis *Unlabeled uses:* ■ Bipolar disorder ■ Cluster headaches ■ Bulimia ■ Binge eating disorder ■ Weight loss in obesity	Action in the treatment of bipolar disorder is unclear.	Hypersensitivity. Caution in renal and hepatic impairment, pregnancy, lactation, children, and the elderly.	50–400 mg/ Not established

Continued

TABLE 28-3 Mood-Stabilizing Agents—cont'd

CLASSIFICATION: GENERIC (TRADE)	PREGNANCY CATEGORY/ HALF-LIFE/ INDICATIONS	MECHANISM OF ACTION	CONTRAINDICATIONS/ PRECAUTIONS	DAILY ADULT DOSAGE RANGE/ THERAPEUTIC PLASMA RANGE
Oxcarbazepine (Trileptal)	C/ 2–9 hr/ ■ Epilepsy *Unlabeled uses:* ■ Bipolar disorder ■ Diabetic neuropathy ■ Neuralgia	Action in the treatment of bipolar disorder is unclear.	Hypersensitivity. Caution in renal and hepatic impairment, pregnancy, lactation, children, and the elderly.	600–2400 mg/ Not established
Calcium Channel Blocker:				
Verapamil (Calan; Isoptin)	C/ 3–7 hr (initially); 4.5–12 hr (repeated dosing)/ ■ Angina ■ Arrhythmias ■ Hypertension *Unlabeled uses:* ■ Bipolar mania ■ Migraine headache prophylaxis	Action in the treatment of bipolar disorder is unclear.	Hypersensitivity; severe left ventricular dysfunction, heart block, hypotension, cardiogenic shock, congestive heart failure. Caution in liver or renal disease, cardiomyopathy, increased intracranial pressure, elderly patients, pregnancy and lactation.	80–320 mg/ Not established
Antipsychotics:				
Olanzapine (Zyprexa)	C/ 21–54 hr/ ■ Schizophrenia ■ Acute manic episodes ■ Management of bipolar disorder ■ Agitation associated with schizophrenia or mania *Unlabeled uses:* ■ Obsessive-compulsive disorder	**All antipsychotics:** Efficacy in schizophrenia is achieved through a combination of dopamine and serotonin type 2 (5-HT$_2$) antagonism. Mechanism of action in the treatment of mania is unknown.	**All antipsychotics:** Hypersensitivity, children, lactation. Caution with hepatic or cardiovascular disease, history of seizures, comatose or other CNS depression, prostatic hypertrophy, narrow-angle glaucoma, diabetes or risk factors for diabetes, pregnancy, elderly and debilitated patients.	10–20 mg/ Not established

Drug	Pregnancy Category/Half-life/Pediatric dosage	Adult dosage	Uses
Olanzapine and fluoxetine (Symbyax)	C/ (see individual drugs)/ Not established	6/25–12/50 mg/	■ For the treatment of depressive episodes associated with bipolar disorder
Aripiprazole (Abilify)	C/ 50–80 hr/ Not established	10–30 mg/	■ Bipolar mania ■ Schizophrenia
Chlorpromazine	C/ 24 hr/ Not established	75–400 mg/	■ Bipolar mania ■ Schizophrenia ■ Emesis/hiccoughs ■ Acute intermittent porphyria ■ Preoperative apprehension *Unlabeled uses:* ■ Migraine headaches
Quetiapine (Seroquel)	C/ 6 hr/ Not established	100–800 mg/	■ Schizophrenia ■ Acute manic episodes
Risperidone (Risperdal)	C/ 3–20 hr/ Not established	1–6 mg/	■ Bipolar mania ■ Schizophrenia *Unlabeled uses:* ■ Severe behavioral problems in children ■ Behavioral problems associated with autism ■ Obsessive-compulsive disorder
Ziprasidone (Geodon)	C/ 7 hr (oral)/ Not established	40–160 mg/	■ Bipolar mania ■ Schizophrenia ■ Acute agitation in schizophrenia
Asenapine (Saphris)	C/ 24 hr/ Not established	10–20 mg/	■ Schizophrenia ■ Bipolar mania

TABLE 28-4 Interactions of Mood-Stabilizing Agents

THE EFFECTS OF:	ARE INCREASED BY:	ARE DECREASED BY:	CONCURRENT USE MAY RESULT IN:
Antimanic: Lithium	Carbamazepine, fluoxetine, haloperidol, loop diuretics, methyldopa, NSAIDs, and thiazide diuretics	Acetazolamide, osmotic diuretics, theophylline, and urinary alkalinizers	Increased effects of neuromuscular blocking agents and tricyclic antidepressants; decreased pressor sensitivity of sympathomimetics; neurotoxicity may occur with phenothiazines or calcium channel blockers
Anticonvulsants: Clonazepam	CNS depressants, cimetidine, hormonal contraceptives, disulfiram, fluoxetine, isoniazid, ketoconazole, metoprolol, propranolol, valproic acid, and probenecid	Rifampin, theophylline (↓ sedative effects), and phenytoin	Increased phenytoin levels; decreased efficacy of levodopa
Carbamazepine	Verapamil, diltiazem, erythromycin, clarithromycin, SSRIs, antidepressants, cimetidine, isoniazid, danazol, lamotrigine, niacin, acetazolamide, dalfopristin, valproate, and nefazodone	Cisplatin, doxorubicin, felbamate, rifampin, barbiturates, hydantoins, primidone, and theophylline	Decreased levels of corticosteroids, doxycycline, felbamate, quinidine, warfarin, estrogen-containing contraceptives, cyclosporine, benzodiazepines, theophylline, lamotrigine, valproic acid, bupropion, haloperidol, olanzapine, tiagabine, topiramate, voriconazole, ziprasidone, felbamate, levothyroxine, or antidepressants; increased levels of lithium; life-threatening hypertensive reaction with MAOIs
Valproic acid	Chlorpromazine, cimetidine, erythromycin, felbamate, and salicylates	Rifampin, carbamazepine, cholestyramine, lamotrigine, phenobarbital, phenytoin, ethosuximide, and hydantoins	Increased effects of tricyclic antidepressants, carbamazepine, CNS depressants, ethosuximide, lamotrigine, phenobarbital, warfarin, zidovudine, hydantoins
Gabapentin	Cimetidine, hydrocodone, and morphine	Antacids	Decreased effects of hydrocodone

TABLE 28-4 Interactions of Mood-Stabilizing Agents—cont'd

THE EFFECTS OF:	ARE INCREASED BY:	ARE DECREASED BY:	CONCURRENT USE MAY RESULT IN:
Lamotrigine	Valproic acid	Primidone, phenobarbital, phenytoin, rifamycin, succinimides, oral contraceptives, oxcarbazepine, carbamazepine, and acetaminophen	Decreased levels of valproic acid; increased levels of carbamazepine and topiramate
Topiramate	Metformin and hydrochlorothiazide	Phenytoin, carbamazepine, valproic acid, and lamotrigine	Increased risk of CNS depression with alcohol or other CNS depressants; increased risk of kidney stones with carbonic anhydrase inhibitors; increased effects of phenytoin, metformin, amitriptyline; decreased effects of oral contraceptives, digoxin, lithium, riseridone, and valproic acid
Oxcarbazepine		Carbamazepine, phenobarbital, phenytoin, valproic acid, and verapamil	Increased concentrations of phenobarbital and phenytoin; decreased effects of oral contraceptives, felodipine, and lamotrigine
Calcium Channel Blocker: Verapamil	Amiodarone, beta blockers, cimetidine, ranitidine, and grapefruit juice	Barbiturates, calcium salts, hydantoins, rifampin, and antineoplastics	Increased effects of beta blockers, disopyramide, flecainide, doxorubicin, benzodiazepines, buspirone, carbamazepine, digoxin, dofetilide, ethanol, imipramine, nondepolarizing muscle relaxants, prazosin, quinidine, sirolimus, tacrolimus, and theophylline; altered serum lithium levels

Continued

TABLE 28-4 Interactions of Mood-Stabilizing Agents—cont'd

THE EFFECTS OF:	ARE INCREASED BY:	ARE DECREASED BY:	CONCURRENT USE MAY RESULT IN:
Antipsychotics: Olanzapine	Fluvoxamine and other CYP1A2 inhibitors, and fluoxetine	Carbamazepine and other CYP1A2 inducers, omeprazole, and rifampin	Decreased effects of levodopa and dopamine agonists; increased hypotension with antihypertensives; increased CNS depression with alcohol or other CNS depressants
Aripiprazole	Ketoconazole and other CYP3A4 inhibitors; quinidine, fluoxetine, paroxetine, or other potential CYP2D6 inhibitors	Carbamazepine, famotidine, and valproate	Increased CNS depression with alcohol or other CNS depressants; increased hypotension with antihypertensives
Chlorpromazine	Beta-blockers and paroxetine	Centrally acting anticholinergics	Increased effects of beta blockers; excessive sedation and hypotension with meperidine; decreased hypotensive effect of guanethidine; decreased effect of oral anticoagulants; decreased or increased phenytoin levels; increased orthostatic hypotension with thiazide diuretics; increased CNS depression with alcohol or other CNS depressants; increased hypotension with antihypertensives; increased anticholinergic effects with anticholinergic agents
Quetiapine	Cimetidine; ketoconazole, itraconazole, fluconazole, erythromycin, or other CYP3A4 inhibitors	Phenytoin and thioridazine	Decreased effects of levodopa and dopamine agonists; increased CNS depression with alcohol or other CNS depressants; increased hypotension with antihypertensives

TABLE 28-4 Interactions of Mood-Stabilizing Agents—cont'd

THE EFFECTS OF:	ARE INCREASED BY:	ARE DECREASED BY:	CONCURRENT USE MAY RESULT IN:
Risperidone	Clozapine, fluoxetine, paroxetine, or ritonavir	Carbamazepine	Decreased effects of levodopa and dopamine agonists; increased effects of clozapine and valproate; increased CNS depression with alcohol or other CNS depressants; increased hypotension with antihypertensives
Ziprasidone	Ketoconazole and other CYP3A4 inhibitors	Carbamazepine	Life-threatening prolongation of QT interval with quinidine, dofetilide, other class Ia and III antiarrhythmics, pimozide, sotalol, thioridazine, chlorpromazine, floquine, pentamadine, arsenic trioxide, mefloquine, dolasetron, tacrolimus, droperidol, gatifloxacin, or moxifloxacin; decreased effects of levodopa and dopamine agonists; increased CNS depression with alcohol or other CNS depressants; increased hypotension with antihypertensives
Asenapine	Fluvoxamine, imipramine, and valproate	Carbamazepine, cimetidine, and paroxetine	Increased effects of paroxetine and dextromethorphan; increased CNS depression with alcohol or other CNS depressants; increased hypotention with antihypertensives; additive effects on QT interval prolongation with quinidine, dofetilide, other class Ia and III antiarrhythmics, pimozide, sotalol, thioridazine, chlorpromazine, floquine, pentamadine, arsenic trioxide, mefloquine, dolasetron, tacrolimus, droperidol, gatifloxacin, or moxifloxacin

Side Effects

The plan of care should include monitoring for side effects of therapy with mood-stabilizing agents and intervening when required to prevent the occurrence of adverse events related to medication administration. Side effects and nursing implications for mood-stabilizing agents are presented in Table 28-5.

TABLE 28-5 Side Effects and Nursing Implications of Mood-Stabilizing Agents		
MEDICATION	**SIDE EFFECTS**	**NURSING IMPLICATIONS**
Antimanic: Lithium carbonate (Eskalith, Lithane, Lithobid)	1. Drowsiness, dizziness, headache	1. Ensure that client does not participate in activities that require alertness, or operate dangerous machinery.
	2. Dry mouth; thirst	2. Provide sugarless candy, ice, frequent sips of water. Ensure that strict oral hygiene is maintained.
	3. GI upset; nausea/vomiting	3. Administer medications with meals to minimize GI upset.
	4. Fine hand tremors	4. Report to physician, who may decrease dosage. Some physicians prescribe a small dose of the beta blocker propranolol to counteract this effect.
	5. Hypotension; arrhythmias; pulse irregularities	5. Monitor vital signs two or three times a day. Physician may decrease dose of medication.
	6. Polyuria; dehydration	6. May subside after initial week or two. Monitor daily intake and output and weight. Monitor skin turgor daily.
	7. Weight gain	7. Provide instructions for reduced-calorie diet. Emphasize importance of maintaining adequate intake of sodium.
Anticonvulsants: Clonazepam (Klonopin) Carbamazepine (Tegretol) Valproic acid (Depakene; Depakote) Gabapentin (Neurontin) Lamotrigine (Lamictal) Topiramate (Topamax) Oxcarbazepine (Trileptal)	1. Nausea/vomiting	1. May give with food or milk to minimize GI upset.
	2. Drowsiness; dizziness	2. Ensure that client does not operate dangerous machinery or participate in activities that require alertness.
	3. Blood dyscrasias	3. Ensure that client understands the importance of regular blood tests while receiving anticonvulsant therapy.
	4. Prolonged bleeding time (with valproic acid)	4. Ensure that platelet counts and bleeding time are determined before initiation of therapy with valproic acid. Monitor for spontaneous bleeding or bruising
	5. Risk of severe rash (with lamotrigine)	5. Ensure that client is informed that he or she must report evidence of skin rash to physician immediately.
	6. Decreased efficacy with oral contraceptives (with topiramate)	6. Ensure that client is aware of decreased efficacy of oral contraceptives with concomitant use.
	7. Risk of suicide with all antiepileptic drugs (warning by FDA, December 2008).	7. Monitor for worsening of depression, suicidal thoughts or behavior, or any unusual changes in mood or behavior.

TABLE 28-5 Side Effects and Nursing Implications of Mood-Stabilizing Agents—cont'd

MEDICATION	SIDE EFFECTS	NURSING IMPLICATIONS
Calcium Channel Blocker: Verapamil (Calan; Isoptin)	1. Drowsiness; dizziness	1. Ensure that client does not operate dangerous machinery or participate in activities that require alertness.
	2. Hypotension; bradycardia	2. Take vital signs just before initiation of therapy and before daily administration of the medication. Physician will provide acceptable parameters for administration. Report marked changes immediately.
	3. Nausea	3. May give with food to minimize GI upset.
	4. Constipation	4. Encourage increased fluid (if not contraindicated) and fiber in the diet.
Antipsychotics: Olanzapine (Zyprexa) Aripiprazole (Abilify) Chlorpromazine Quetiapine (Seroquel) Risperidone (Risperdal) Ziprasidone (Geodon) Asenapine (Saphris)	1. Drowsiness, dizziness	1. Ensure that client does not operate dangerous machinery or participate in activities that require alertness.
	2. Dry mouth, constipation	2. Provide sugarless candy or gum, ice, and frequent sips of water. Provide foods high in fiber. Encourage physical activity and fluid if not contraindicated.
	3. Increased appetite, weight gain	3. Provide calorie-controlled diet; provide opportunity for physical exercise; provide diet and exercise instruction.
	4. ECG changes	4. Monitor vital signs. Observe for symptoms of dizziness, palpitations, syncope, or weakness.
	5. Extrapyramidal symptoms	5. Monitor for symptoms. Administer prn medications at first sign.
	6. Hyperglycemia and diabetes	6. Monitor blood glucose regularly. Observe for the appearance of symptoms of polydipsia, polyuria, polyphagia, and weakness at any time during therapy.

Lithium Toxicity

The margin between the therapeutic and toxic levels of lithium carbonate is very narrow. The usual ranges of therapeutic serum concentrations are:

■ For acute mania: 1.0 to 1.5 mEq/L
■ For maintenance: 0.6 to 1.2 mEq/L

Serum lithium levels should be monitored once or twice a week after initial treatment until dosage and serum levels are stable, then monthly during maintenance therapy. Blood samples should be drawn 12 hours after the last dose.

Symptoms of lithium toxicity begin to appear at blood levels greater than 1.5 mEq/L and are dosage determinate. Symptoms include the following:

■ **At serum levels of 1.5 to 2.0 mEq/L:** blurred vision, ataxia, tinnitus, persistent nausea and vomiting, severe diarrhea.

■ **At serum levels of 2.0 to 3.5 mEq/L:** excessive output of dilute urine, increasing tremors, muscular irritability, psychomotor retardation, mental confusion, giddiness.

■ **At serum levels above 3.5 mEq/L:** impaired consciousness, nystagmus, seizures, coma, oliguria/anuria, arrhythmias, myocardial infarction, cardiovascular collapse.

Lithium levels should be monitored prior to medication administration. The dosage should be withheld and the physician notified if the level reaches 1.5 mEq/L or at the earliest observation or report by the client of even the mildest symptom. If left untreated, lithium toxicity can be life threatening.

Lithium is similar in chemical structure to sodium, behaving in the body in much the same manner and competing at various sites in the body with sodium. If sodium intake is reduced or the body is depleted of its normal sodium (e.g., due to excessive sweating, fever, or diuresis), lithium is reabsorbed by the kidneys, increasing the possibility of toxicity. Therefore, the client must consume a diet adequate in sodium as well as 2,500 to 3,000 mL of fluid per day. Accurate records of intake, output, and client's weight should be kept on a daily basis.

Client/Family Education for Lithium

The Client Should:

■ Take medication on a regular basis, even when feeling well. Discontinuation can result in return of symptoms.

■ Not drive or operate dangerous machinery until lithium levels are stabilized. Drowsiness and dizziness can occur.

■ Not skimp on dietary sodium intake. He or she should eat a variety of healthy foods and avoid "junk" foods. The client should drink 6 to 8 large glasses of water each day and avoid excessive use of beverages containing caffeine (coffee, tea, colas), which promote increased urine output.

■ Notify the physician if vomiting or diarrhea occurs. These symptoms can result in sodium loss and an increased risk of toxicity.

■ Carry card or other identification noting that he or she is taking lithium.

■ Be aware of appropriate diet should weight gain become a problem. Include adequate sodium and other nutrients while decreasing number of calories.

■ Be aware of risks of becoming pregnant while receiving lithium therapy. Use information furnished by health-care providers regarding methods of contraception. Notify the physician as soon as possible if pregnancy is suspected or planned.

■ Be aware of side effects and symptoms associated with toxicity. Notify the physician if any of the following symptoms occur: persistent nausea and vomiting, severe diarrhea, ataxia, blurred vision, tinnitus, excessive output of urine, increasing tremors, or mental confusion.

■ Refer to written materials furnished by health-care providers while receiving self-administered maintenance therapy. Keep appointments for outpatient follow-up; have serum lithium level checked every 1 to 2 months, or as advised by physician.

Client/Family Education for Anticonvulsants

The Client Should:

■ Refrain from discontinuing the drug abruptly. Physician will administer orders for tapering the drug when therapy is to be discontinued.

■ Report the following symptoms to the physician immediately: skin rash, unusual bleeding, spontaneous bruising, sore throat, fever, malaise, dark urine, and yellow skin or eyes.

■ Not drive or operate dangerous machinery until reaction to the medication has been established.

■ Avoid consuming alcoholic beverages and nonprescription medications without approval from physician.

■ Carry card at all times identifying the names of medications being taken.

CLINICAL PEARL The U.S. Food and Drug Administration requires that all antiepileptic (anticonvulsant) drugs carry a warning label indicating that use of the drugs increases risk for suicidal thoughts and behaviors. Patients being treated with these medications should be monitored for the emergence or worsening of depression, suicidal thoughts or behavior, or any unusual changes in mood or behavior.

Client/Family Education for Calcium Channel Blocker

The Client Should:

■ Take medication with meals if gastrointestinal (GI) upset occurs.

■ Use caution when driving or when operating dangerous machinery. Dizziness, drowsiness, and blurred vision can occur.

■ Refrain from discontinuing the drug abruptly. To do so may precipitate cardiovascular problems. Physician will administer orders for tapering the drug when therapy is to be discontinued.

■ Report occurrence of any of the following symptoms to physician immediately: irregular heartbeat, shortness of breath, swelling of the hands and feet, pronounced dizziness, chest pain, profound mood swings, severe and persistent headache.

■ Rise slowly from a sitting or lying position to prevent a sudden drop in blood pressure.

■ Avoid taking other medications (including over-the-counter medications) without physician's approval.

■ Carry card at all times describing medications being taken.

Client/Family Education for Antipsychotics

The Client Should:

■ Use caution when driving or operating dangerous machinery. Drowsiness and dizziness can occur.

■ Refrain from discontinuing the drug abruptly after long-term use. To do so might produce withdrawal symptoms, such as nausea, vomiting, dizziness, gastritis, headache, tachycardia, insomnia, and tremulousness. Physician will administer orders for tapering the drug when therapy is to be discontinued.

■ Use sunblock lotion and wear protective clothing when spending time outdoors. Skin is more susceptible to sunburn, which can occur in as little as 30 minutes.

■ Report the occurrence of any of the following symptoms to the physician immediately: sore throat, fever, malaise, unusual bleeding, easy bruising, persistent nausea and vomiting, severe headache, rapid heart rate, difficulty urinating, muscle twitching, tremors, darkly colored urine, excessive urination, excessive thirst, excessive hunger, weakness, pale stools, yellow skin or eyes, muscular incoordination, or skin rash.

■ Rise slowly from a sitting or lying position to prevent a sudden drop in blood pressure.

■ Take frequent sips of water, chew sugarless gum, or suck on hard candy, if dry mouth is a problem. Good oral care (frequent brushing, flossing) is very important.

■ Consult the physician regarding smoking while on antipsychotic therapy. Smoking increases the metabolism of these drugs, requiring an adjustment in dosage to achieve a therapeutic effect.

■ Dress warmly in cold weather, and avoid extended exposure to very high or low temperatures. Body temperature is harder to maintain with this medication.

■ Avoid drinking alcohol while on antipsychotic therapy. These drugs potentiate each other's effects.

■ Avoid taking other medications (including over-the-counter products) without the physician's approval. Many medications contain substances that interact with antipsychotic medications in a way that may be harmful.

■ Be aware of possible risks of taking antipsychotics during pregnancy. Safe use during pregnancy has not been established. Antipsychotics are thought to readily cross the placental barrier; if so, a fetus could experience adverse effects of the drug. Inform the physician immediately if pregnancy occurs, is suspected, or is planned.

■ Be aware of side effects of antipsychotic medications. Refer to written materials furnished by health-care providers for safe self-administration.

■ Continue to take the medication, even if feeling well and as though it is not needed. Symptoms may return if medication is discontinued.

■ Carry a card or other identification at all times describing medications being taken.

CASE STUDY AND SAMPLE CARE PLAN

NURSING HISTORY AND ASSESSMENT

Candace, age 32, recently moved to New York City from Omaha, Nebraska, where she had been working as a television reporter. She felt that Omaha had become "too boring" and wanted to experience the big city life. Candace has a history of Bipolar I Disorder, and has been maintained on lithium since she was 23 years old. Since she arrived in New York City, she has run out of her medication and has not found a doctor to have her prescription renewed. She has been staying in an inexpensive apartment, using her

savings to live on. She has been seeking employment in her chosen line of work, but it has been 2 months now, and she has been unable to find a job. She is becoming anxious, because her savings are becoming depleted. She has lost weight and has trouble sleeping.

Today, after two failed interviews, Candace went to a bar and began drinking. She ordered several rounds of drinks for everyone in the bar, and told the bartender to "put it on my tab." The bartender called the police when Candace refused to pay her tab and became loud and belligerent.

Continued

CASE STUDY AND SAMPLE CARE PLAN — cont'd

He said she began shouting that she knew the mayor, and he was going to help her find a job, and if they didn't leave her alone, she would tell the mayor how they were treating her. She took out her cell phone and said she was calling the mayor. When others in the room began laughing at her, she began cursing and saying that "they would be sorry one day that they laughed at her." When the police arrived, Candace was resistant and had to be physically restrained. The police took Candace to the emergency department of the community hospital, where she was admitted with a diagnosis of Bipolar Disorder, Manic Episode. The psychiatrist ordered olanzapine 10 mg IM STAT, olanzapine 10 mg PO qd, lithium carbonate 600 mg PO bid, and vitamin supplement daily. He ordered lithium level to be drawn prior to first dose of lithium.

NURSING DIAGNOSES/OUTCOME IDENTIFICATION

From the assessment data, the admitting nurse develops the following nursing diagnoses for Candace:

1. **Risk for self- or other-directed violence** related to manic hyperactivity, delusional thinking, impulsivity

   a. **Short-Term Goal:**
   - Agitation and hyperactivity will be maintained at manageable level with the administration of tranquilizing medication.

   b. **Long-Term Goal:**
   - Candace will not harm self or others during hospitalization.

2. **Imbalanced nutrition: Less than body requirements** related to lack of appetite and excessive physical agitation, evidenced by loss of weight.

   a. **Short-Term Goal:**
   - Candace will consume sufficient finger foods and between-meal snacks to meet recommended daily allowances of nutrients.

   b. **Long-Term Goal:**
   - Candace will begin to regain weight and exhibit no signs or symptoms of malnutrition.

PLANNING/IMPLEMENTATION

Risk for Self- or Other-Directed Violence

The following nursing interventions have been identified for Candace:

1. Place Candace in a private room near the nurse's station. Observe her behavior frequently.
2. Remove all dangerous objects from her environment.

3. Plan some physical activities for Candace (e.g., treadmill, punching bag) and regular rest periods during the day.
4. Administer tranquilizing medication as ordered by physician.
5. Monitor lithium levels 3 times during first week of therapy. Monitor for signs and symptoms of toxicity (e.g., ataxia, blurred vision, severe diarrhea, persistent nausea and vomiting, tinnitus).
6. Ensure that sufficient staff is available to intervene should Candace become agitated and aggressive.

Imbalanced Nutrition: Less Than Body Requirements

The following nursing interventions have been identified for Candace:

1. Consult dietitian to determine appropriate diet for Candace to restore nutrition and gain weight. Ensure that her diet includes foods that she particularly likes.
2. Ensure that Candace has access to "finger foods" and between-meal snacks if she cannot or will not sit still to eat off a meal tray.
3. Maintain an accurate record of intake, output, and calorie count.
4. Obtain daily weights.
5. Administer vitamin supplement, as ordered by physician.
6. Sit with Candace during mealtime.

EVALUATION

The outcome criteria identified for Candace have been met. She has not harmed herself or others in any way. She is able to verbalize names of resources outside the hospital from whom she may request help if needed. With help from the social worker, she has applied for unemployment assistance, and will begin receiving help within 2 weeks. She has gained 3 pounds in the hospital, and verbalizes understanding of the importance of maintaining good nutrition. She is taking her medication regularly, and has a follow-up appointment with the psychiatric nurse practitioner who will see Candace biweekly and ensure that Candace is compliant with medication and laboratory requirements. Candace verbalizes understanding of the importance of taking her medication on a continuing basis. She has a hopeful, but realistic, attitude about finding work in New York City, and states that she will give herself a deadline, after which she plans to return to her home in Omaha, where she may be near family and friends.

Summary and Key Points

■ Bipolar disorder is manifested by mood swings from profound depression to extreme elation and euphoria.

■ Genetic influences have been strongly implicated in the development of bipolar disorder. Various other physiological factors, such as biochemical and electrolyte alterations, as well as cerebral structural changes, have been implicated. Side effects of certain medications may also induce symptoms of mania. No single theory can explain the etiology of bipolar disorder, and it is likely that the illness is caused by a combination of factors.

■ Symptoms of mania may be observed on a continuum of three phases, each identified by the degree of severity: phase I, hypomania; phase II, acute mania; and phase III, delirious mania.

■ The symptoms of bipolar disorder may occur in children and adolescents, as well as adults.

■ Treatment of bipolar disorders includes individual therapy, group and family therapy, cognitive therapy, electroconvulsive therapy, and psychopharmacology. For the majority of clients, the most effective treatment appears to be a combination of psychotropic medication and psychosocial therapy.

■ Some clinicians are choosing a course of therapy based on a model of recovery, somewhat like that which has been used for many years with problems of addiction. The basic premise of a recovery model is empowerment of the consumer. The recovery model is designed to allow consumers primary control over decisions about their own care, and to enable a person with a mental health problem to live a meaningful life in a community of his or her choice while striving to achieve his or her full potential.

■ For many years, the pharmacological treatment of choice for bipolar mania was lithium carbonate. A number of other medications are now being used with satisfactory results, including anticonvulsants and antipsychotics.

■ There is a narrow margin between the therapeutic and toxic levels of lithium. Serum lithium levels must be monitored regularly while on maintenance therapy.

Additional info available @
davisplus.fadavis.com

Review Questions
Self-Examination/Learning Exercise

*Select the answer that is **most** appropriate for each of the following questions:*

1. Margaret, a 68-year-old widow, is brought to the emergency department by her sister-in-law. Margaret has a history of bipolar disorder and has been maintained on medication for many years. Her sister-in-law reports that Margaret quit taking her medication a few months ago, thinking she didn't need it anymore. She is agitated, pacing, demanding, and speaking very loudly. Her sister-in-law reports that Margaret eats very little, is losing weight, and almost never sleeps: "I'm afraid she's going to just collapse!" Margaret is admitted to the psychiatric unit. The *priority* nursing diagnosis for Margaret is:
   a. Imbalanced nutrition: less than body requirements related to not eating.
   b. Risk for injury related to hyperactivity.
   c. Disturbed sleep pattern related to agitation.
   d. Ineffective coping related to denial of depression.

2. Margaret, age 68, is diagnosed with Bipolar Disorder, Manic Episode. She is extremely hyperactive and has lost weight. One way to promote adequate nutritional intake for Margaret is to:
   a. Sit with her during meals to ensure that she eats everything on her tray.
   b. Have her sister-in-law bring all her food from home because she knows Margaret's likes and dislikes.
   c. Provide high-calorie, nutritious finger foods and snacks that Margaret can eat "on the run."
   d. Tell Margaret that she will be on room restriction until she starts gaining weight.

Continued

Review Questions—cont'd
Self-Examination/Learning Exercise

3. The physician orders lithium carbonate 600 mg tid for a newly diagnosed client with Bipolar I Disorder. There is a narrow margin between the therapeutic and toxic levels of lithium. Therapeutic range for acute mania is:
   a. 1.0 to 1.5 mEq/L.
   b. 10 to 15 mEq/L.
   c. 0.5 to 1.0 mEq/L.
   d. 5 to 10 mEq/L.

4. Although historically lithium has been the drug of choice for mania, several other drugs have been used with good results. Which of the following are used in the treatment of bipolar disorder? (Select all that apply.)
   a. Olanzepine (Zyprexa).
   b. Paroxetine (Paxil).
   c. Carbamazepine (Tegretol).
   d. Gabapentin (Neurontin).
   e. Tranylcypromine (Parnate).

5. Margaret, a 68-year-old widow with bipolar mania, is admitted to the psychiatric unit after being brought to the emergency department by her sister-in-law. Margaret yells, "My sister-in-law is just jealous of me! She's trying to make it look like I'm insane!" This behavior is an example of:
   a. A delusion of grandeur.
   b. A delusion of persecution.
   c. A delusion of reference.
   d. A delusion of control or influence.

6. The most common comorbid condition in children with bipolar disorder is:
   a. Schizophrenia.
   b. Substance disorders.
   c. Oppositional defiant disorder.
   d. Attention-deficit/hyperactivity disorder.

7. A nurse is educating a client about his lithium therapy. She is explaining signs and symptoms of lithium toxicity. For which of the following would she instruct the client to be on the alert?
   a. Fever, sore throat, malaise.
   b. Tinnitus, severe diarrhea, ataxia.
   c. Occipital headache, palpitations, chest pain.
   d. Skin rash, marked rise in blood pressure, bradycardia.

8. A client diagnosed with bipolar mania enters the milieu area dressed in a provocative and physically revealing outfit. Which of the following is the most appropriate intervention by the nurse?
   a. Tell the client she cannot wear this outfit while she is in the hospital.
   b. Do nothing and allow her to learn from the responses of her peers.
   c. Quietly walk with her back to her room and help her change into something more appropriate.
   d. Explain to her that, if she wears this outfit, she must remain in her room.

Review Questions—cont'd
Self-Examination/Learning Exercise

9. The nurse is prioritizing nursing diagnoses in the plan of care for a client with bipolar mania. Number the diagnoses in order of the appropriate priority.
    ____a. Disturbed sleep pattern evidenced by sleeping only 4 to 5 hours per night.
    ____b. Risk for injury related to manic hyperactivity.
    ____c. Impaired social interaction evidenced by manipulation of others.
    ____d. Imbalanced nutrition: Less than body requirements evidenced by loss of weight and poor skin turgor.

10. A child with bipolar disorder also has attention-deficit/hyperactivity disorder (ADHD). How would these comorbid conditions most likely be treated?
    a. No medication would be given for either condition.
    b. Medication would be given for both conditions simultaneously.
    c. The bipolar condition would be stabilized first before medication for the ADHD would be given.
    d. The ADHD would be treated before consideration of the bipolar disorder.

TEST YOUR CRITICAL THINKING SKILLS

Alice, age 29, had been working in the typing pool of a large corporation for 6 years. Her immediate supervisor recently retired and Alice was promoted to supervisor, in charge of 20 people in the department. Alice was flattered by the promotion but anxious about the additional responsibility of the position. Shortly after the promotion, she overheard two of her former coworkers saying, "Why in the world did they choose her? She's not the best one for the job. I know *I* certainly won't be able to respect her as a boss!" Hearing these comments added to Alice's anxiety and self-doubt.

Shortly after Alice began her new duties, her friends and coworkers noticed a change. She had a great deal of energy and worked long hours on her job. She began to speak very loudly and rapidly. Her roommate noticed that Alice slept very little, yet seldom appeared tired. Every night she would go out to bars and dances. Sometimes she brought men she had just met home to the apartment, something she had never done before. She bought lots of clothes and makeup and had her hair restyled in a more youthful look. She failed to pay her share of the rent and bills but came home with a brand new convertible. She lost her temper and screamed at her roommate to "Mind your own business!" when asked to pay her share.

She became irritable at work, and several of her subordinates reported her behavior to the corporate manager. When the manager confronted Alice about her behavior, she lost control, shouting, cursing, and striking out at anyone and anything that happened to be within her reach. The security officers restrained her and took her to the emergency department of the hospital, where she was admitted to the psychiatric unit. She had no previous history of psychiatric illness.

The psychiatrist assigned a diagnosis of Bipolar I Disorder and wrote orders for olanzapine (Zyprexa) 10 mg IM STAT, olanzapine 15 mg PO daily, and lithium carbonate 600 mg qid.

Answer the following questions related to Alice:

1. What are the most important considerations with which the nurse who is taking care of Alice should be concerned?
2. Why was Alice given the diagnosis of Bipolar I Disorder?
3. The doctor should order a lithium level drawn after 4 to 6 days. For what symptoms should the nurse be on the alert?
4. Why did the physician order olanzapine in addition to the lithium carbonate?

References

Allen, M. H. (2003). Approaches to the treatment of mania. *Medscape Psychiatry.* Retrieved September 15, 2010, from http://cme.medscape.com/viewprogram/2639

American Psychiatric Association. (2000). *Diagnostic and statistical manual of mental disorders* (4th ed.). *Text revision.* Washington, DC: American Psychiatric Publishing.

Anthony, W. A. (1993). Recovery from mental illness: The guiding vision of the mental health service system in the 1990s. *Psychosocial Rehabilitation Journal, 16*(4), 11–23.

Dubovsky, S. L., Davies, R., & Dubovsky, A. M. (2003). Mood disorders. In R. E. Hales & S. C. Yudofsky (Eds.), *Textbook of clinical psychiatry* (4th ed., pp. 439–542). Washington, DC: American Psychiatric Publishing.

Geller, B., Zimerman, B., Williams, M., Delbello, M. P., Frazier, J., & Beringer, L. (2002). Phenomenology of prepubertal and early adolescent bipolar disorder: Examples of elated mood, grandiose behaviors, decreased need for sleep, racing thoughts, and hypersexuality. *Journal of Child and Adolescent Psychopharmacology, 12,* 3–9.

Goldberg, J. F., & Hoop, J. (2004). Bipolar depression: Long-term challenges for the clinician. *Medscape Psychiatry.* Retrieved September 15, 2010, from http://cme.medscape.com/viewprogram/3350

Guadiz, B. (2008). *History of bipolar disorder: Bipolar disorder already existed centuries ago.* Retrieved September 15, 2010, from http://ezinearticles.com/?History-of-Bipolar-Disorder-Bipolar-Disorder-Already-Existed-Centuries-Ago&id=1147777

Jacobson, N., & Greenley, D. (2001). What is recovery? A conceptual model and explication. *Psychiatric Services, 52*(4), 482–485.

Joska, J. A., & Stein, D. J. (2008). Mood disorders. In R. E. Hales, S. C. Yudofsky, & G. O. Gabbard (Eds.), *Textbook of Psychiatry* (5th ed., pp. 457–503). Washington, DC: American Psychiatric Publishing.

Kafantaris, V., Dicker, R., Coletti, D. J., & Kane, J. M. (2001). Adjunctive antipsychotic treatment is necessary for adolescents with psychotic mania. *Journal of Child and Adolescent Psychopharmacology, 11,* 409–413.

Kowatch, R. A., Fristad, M., Birmaher, B., Wagner, K. D., Findling, R. L., & Hellander, M. (2005). Treatment guidelines for children and adolescents with bipolar disorder. *Journal of the American Academy of Child and Adolescent Psychiatry, 44,* 213–235.

Miklowitz, D. J., George, E. L., Richards, J. A., Simoneau, T. L., & Suddath, R. L. (2003). A randomized study of family-focused psychoeducation and pharmacotherapy in the outpatient management of bipolar disorder. *Archives of General Psychiatry, 60,* 904–912.

Nakate, S. (2009). *History of bipolar disorder (manic depression).* Retrieved September 15, 2010, from http://www.buzzle.com/articles/history-of-bipolar-disorder-manic-depression.html

NANDA International. (2009). *Nursing diagnoses: Definitions and classification 2009–2011.* Hoboken, NJ: Wiley-Blackwell.

Nandagopal, J. J., & DelBello, M. P. (2008). Diagnosis and treatment of pediatric bipolar disorder. *Medscape Psychiatry.* Retrieved September 15, 2010, from http://cme.medscape.com/viewprogram/15741

National Association of Social Workers. (2010). *NASW practice snapshot: The mental health recovery model.* Retrieved September 8, 2010, from http://www.socialworkers.org/practice/behavioral_health/0206snapshot.asp?

National Institute of Mental Health. (2008). Bipolar disorder and gene abnormalities: Sodium, calcium imbalances linked to manic depressive episodes. *ScienceDaily.* Retrieved September 15, 2010, from http://www.sciencedaily.com/releases/2008/08/080817223548.htm

National Institute of Mental Health. (2010). *Mental disorders in America: The numbers count.* Bethesda, MD: National Institutes of Health.

Sadock, B. J., and Sadock, V. A. (2007). *Synopsis of psychiatry: Behavioral sciences/clinical psychiatry* (10th ed.). Philadelphia: Lippincott Williams & Wilkins.

Sharfstein, S. (2005). Recovery model will strengthen psychiatrist-patient relationship. *Psychiatric News, 40*(20), 3.

Soreff, S., & McInnes, L. A. (2010). Bipolar affective disorder. *E-medicine: Psychiatry.* Retrieved September 15, 2010, from http://www.emedicine.medscape.com/article/286342-overview

The Joint Commission. (2010, January). *The comprehensive accreditation manual for hospitals: The official handbook.* Oakbrook Terrace, IL: Joint Commission Resources.

U.S. Department of Health and Human Services, Substance Abuse and Mental Health Services Administration, Center for Mental Health Services. (2010). *National concensus statement on mental health recovery.* Retrieved September 8, 2010, from http://www.samhsa.gov

Youssef, H. A., Youssef, F. A., & Dening, T. R. (1996). Evidence for the existence of schizophrenia in medieval Islamic society. *History of Psychiatry, 7*(25), 55–62.

Zubieta, J. K., Huguelet, P., Koeppe, R. A., Kilbourn, M. R., Carr, J. M., Giordani, B. J., et al. (2000). High vesicular monoamine transporter binding in asymptomatic bipolar I disorder: Sex differences and cognitive correlates. *American Journal of Psychiatry, 157,* 1619–1628.

@ INTERNET REFERENCES

- Additional information about bipolar disorders, including psychosocial and pharmacological treatment of these disorders, may be located at the following websites:
  - http://www.ndmda.org/
  - http://www.fadavis.com/townsend
  - http://www.mentalhealth.com/
  - http://www.cmellc.com/topics/bipolar.html
  - http://nami.org/
  - http://www.mental-health-matters.com/
  - http://www.mentalhelp.net/
  - http://www.nlm.nih.gov/medlineplus

MOVIE CONNECTIONS

Lust for Life (bipolar disorder) • Call Me Anna (bipolar disorder) • Blue Sky (bipolar disorder) • A Woman Under the Influence (bipolar disorder)

Anxiety Disorders CHAPTER

29

CORE CONCEPTS

anxiety

compulsions

obsessions

panic

phobia

KEY TERMS

agoraphobia

flooding

generalized anxiety disorder

implosion therapy

obsessive-compulsive disorder

panic disorder

posttraumatic stress disorder

social phobia

specific phobia

systematic desensitization

OBJECTIVES

After reading this chapter, the student will be able to:

1. Differentiate among the terms *stress, anxiety,* and *fear.*
2. Discuss historical aspects and epidemiological statistics related to anxiety disorders.
3. Differentiate between normal anxiety and psychoneurotic anxiety.
4. Describe various types of anxiety disorders, identify symptomatology associated with each, and use this information in client assessment.
5. Identify predisposing factors in the development of anxiety disorders.
6. Formulate nursing diagnoses and outcome criteria for clients with anxiety disorders.
7. Describe appropriate nursing interventions for behaviors associated with anxiety disorders.
8. Identify topics for client and family teaching relevant to anxiety disorders.
9. Evaluate nursing care of clients with anxiety disorders.
10. Discuss various modalities relevant to treatment of anxiety disorders.

HOMEWORK ASSIGNMENT

Please read the chapter and answer the following questions:

1. What are the symptoms of a person with agoraphobia?
2. What neurotransmitter has been implicated in the development of obsessive-compulsive disorder?
3. What two variables are considered to be the best predictors of PTSD according to the psychosocial theory?
4. What is the primary nursing intervention for a person in panic anxiety?

The following is an account by singer-songwriter Michael Johnson (1994) relating his experience with performance anxiety:

> You've got your Jolly Roger clothes on, you've got the microphone, the lights are on you, the owner has just told the crowd to shut up, and you are getting that kind of "show and tell" sickness that you used to get at grade school pageants or college recitals. Suddenly your mouth is so dry that your lips are sticking to your teeth and you find yourself gesturing oddly with your shoulder and wondering if they think that maybe something unfortunate happened to you. And

they're trying to cope with the whole thing. It is now, of course, it hits you that you started with the second verse, you're doing a live rewrite, and you have no idea how this song is going to end. Your vocal range has shrunk and your heartbeat is interfering with your vibrato. Your palms are wet and your mouth is dry—a great combination!

CORE CONCEPT

Anxiety

An emotional response (e.g., apprehension, tension, uneasiness) to anticipation of danger, the source of which is largely unknown or unrecognized. Anxiety may be regarded as pathologic when it interferes with effectiveness in living, achievement of desired goals or satisfaction, or reasonable emotional comfort (Shahrokh & Hales, 2003).

Individuals face anxiety on a daily basis. Anxiety, which provides the motivation for achievement, is a necessary force for survival. The term *anxiety* is often used interchangeably with the word *stress;* however, they are not the same. Stress, or more properly, a *stressor,* is an external pressure that is brought to bear on the individual. Anxiety is the subjective emotional response to that stressor. (See Chapter 2 for an overview of anxiety as a psychological response to stress.)

Anxiety may be distinguished from *fear* in that the former is an emotional process, whereas fear is a cognitive one. Fear involves the intellectual appraisal of a threatening stimulus; anxiety involves the emotional response to that appraisal.

This chapter focuses on disorders that are characterized by exaggerated and often disabling anxiety reactions. Historical aspects and epidemiological statistics are presented. Predisposing factors that have been implicated in the etiology of anxiety disorders provide a framework for studying the dynamics of phobias, obsessive-compulsive disorder (OCD), generalized anxiety disorder, panic disorder, posttraumatic stress disorder (PTSD), and other anxiety disorders. Various theories of causation are presented, although it is most likely that a combination of factors contribute to the etiology of anxiety disorders. The neurobiology of anxiety disorders is presented in Figure 29–1.

An explanation of the symptomatology is presented as background knowledge for assessing the client with an anxiety disorder. Nursing care is described in the context of the nursing process. Various treatment modalities are explored.

Historical Aspects

Individuals have experienced anxiety throughout the ages. Yet anxiety, like fear, was not clearly defined or isolated as a separate entity by psychiatrists or psychologists until the 19th and 20th centuries. In fact, what we now know as anxiety was once solely identified by its physiological symptoms, focusing largely on the cardiovascular system. Clinicians used a myriad of diagnostic terms in attempting to identify these symptoms. For example, cardiac neurosis, DaCosta's syndrome, irritable heart, nervous tachycardia, neurocirculatory asthenia, soldier's heart, vasomotor neurosis, and vasoregulatory asthenia are just a few of the names under which anxiety has been concealed over the years (Sadock & Sadock, 2007).

Freud first introduced the term *anxiety neurosis* in 1895. Freud wrote, "I call this syndrome 'anxiety neurosis' because all its components can be grouped round the chief symptom of anxiety" (Freud, 1959). This notion attempted to negate the previous concept of the problem as strictly physical, although it was some time before physicians of internal medicine were ready to accept the psychological implications for the symptoms. In fact, it was not until the years during World War II that the psychological dimensions of these various functional heart conditions were recognized.

For many years, anxiety disorders were viewed as purely psychological or purely biological in nature. Researchers have begun to focus on the interrelatedness of mind and body, and anxiety disorders provide an excellent example of this complex relationship. It is likely that various factors, including genetic, developmental, environmental, and psychological, play a role in the etiology of anxiety disorders.

Epidemiological Statistics

Anxiety disorders are the most common of all psychiatric illnesses and result in considerable functional impairment and distress (Hollander & Simeon, 2008). Statistics vary widely, but most

FIGURE 29–1   Neurobiology of anxiety disorders

Neurotransmitters

Although other neurotransmitters have also been implicated in the pathophysiology of anxiety disorders, disturbances in serotonin, norepinephrine, and gamma-aminobutyric acid (GABA) appear to be most significant.

Cell bodies of origin for the serotonin pathways lie within the raphe nuclei located in the brainstem. Serotonin is thought to be decreased in anxiety disorders. Cell bodies for norepinephrine originate in the locus ceruleus. Norepinephrine is thought to be increased in anxiety disorders. GABA is the major inhibitory neurotransmitter in the brain. It is involved in the reduction and slowing of cellular activity. It is synthesized from glutamic acid, with vitamin B_6 as a cofactor. It is found in almost every region of the brain. GABA is thought to be decreased in anxiety disorders (allowing for increased cellular excitability).

Areas of the Brain Affected

Areas of the brain affected by anxiety disorders and the symptoms that they mediate include the following:
- Amygdala: Fear; particularly important in panic and phobic disorders
- Hippocampus: Associated with memory related to fear responses
- Locus ceruleus: Arousal
- Brainstem: Respiratory activation; heart rate
- Hypothalamus: Activation of stress response
- Frontal cortex: Cognitive interpretations
- Thalamus: Integration of sensory stimuli
- Basal ganglia: Tremor

ANXIOLYTIC MEDICATIONS

Type	Action	Side Effects
Benzodiazepines	Increases the affinity of the $GABA_A$ receptor for GABA	Sedation, dizziness, weakness, ataxia, decreased motor performance, dependence, withdrawal
SSRIs; SNRIs	SSRIs block reuptake of serotonin into the presynaptic nerve terminal, increasing synaptic concentration of serotonin	SSRIs: Nausea, diarrhea, headache, insomnia, somnolence, sexual dysfunction
	SNRIs inhibit reuptake of neuronal serotonin and norepinephrine; mild reuptake of dopamine	SNRIs: Headache, dry mouth, nausea, somnolence, dizziness, insomnia, asthenia, constipation, diarrhea
Noradrenergic agents (e.g., propranolol, clonidine)	Propranolol: blocks beta-adrenergic receptor activity	Propranolol: bradycardia, hypotension, weakness, fatigue, impotence, GI upset, bronchospasm

Continued

ANXIOLYTIC MEDICATIONS—cont'd

Type	Action	Side Effects
	Clonidine: stimulates alpha-adrenergic receptors	Clonidine: dry mouth, sedation, fatigue, hypotension
Barbiturates	CNS depression. Also produce effects in the hepatic and cardiovascular systems	Somnolence, agitation, confusion, ataxia, dizziness, bradycardia, hypotension, constipation
Buspirone	Partial agonist of 5-HT_{1A} receptor	Dizziness, drowsiness, dry mouth, headache, nervousness, nausea, insomnia

agree that anxiety disorders are more common in women than in men by at least 2 to 1. Prevalence rates for anxiety disorders within the general population have been given at 3 to 5 percent for generalized anxiety disorder and panic disorder, 2 to 3 percent for OCD, 8 percent for PTSD, 13 percent for social anxiety disorder, and 25 percent for phobias (Rowney, Hermida, & Malone, 2010). A review of the literature reveals a wide range of reports regarding the prevalence of anxiety disorders in children (2 percent to 43 percent). Epidemiological studies suggest that the symptoms are more prevalent among girls than boys (American Psychiatric Association [APA], 2000) and that minority children and children from low socioeconomic environments may be at greater risk for all emotional illness (National Mental Health Association [NMHA], 2005). Studies of familial patterns suggest that a familial predisposition to anxiety disorders probably exists.

IMPLICATIONS OF RESEARCH FOR EVIDENCE-BASED PRACTICE

Johnson, J. G., Cohen, P., Pine, D. S., Klein, D. F., Kasen, S., & Brook, J. S. (2000, November 8). Association between cigarette smoking and anxiety disorders during adolescence and early adulthood. *Journal of the American Medical Association, 284,* 2348–2351.

DESCRIPTION OF THE STUDY: The main objective of this study was to investigate the longitudinal association between cigarette smoking and anxiety disorders among adolescents and young adults. The study sample included 688 teenagers (51 percent female and 49 percent male) from upstate New York. The youths were interviewed at a mean age of 16 years, during the years 1985 to 1986, and again at a mean age of 22 years, during the years 1991 to 1993. At age 16, 6 percent of the participants smoked 20 or more cigarettes a day. The number increased to 15 percent by age 22.

RESULTS OF THE STUDY: Of the participants who smoked 20 cigarettes or more a day during adolescence, a significant number developed an anxiety disorder during young adulthood: 20.5 percent developed generalized anxiety disorder, 10.3 percent developed agoraphobia, and 7.7 percent developed panic disorder. According to the researchers, cigarette smoking does not appear to increase the risk of developing OCD or social anxiety disorder.

IMPLICATIONS FOR NURSING PRACTICE: The results of this study present just one more reason why adolescents should be encouraged not to smoke or not to begin smoking. The implications for nursing practice are serious. Nurses can initiate and become involved in educational programs to discourage cigarette smoking. Many negative health concerns are related to smoking, and this study provides additional information to include in educational programs designed specifically for adolescents.

How Much Is Too Much?

Anxiety is usually considered a normal reaction to a realistic danger or threat to biological integrity or self-concept. Normal anxiety dissipates when the danger or threat is no longer present.

It is difficult to draw a precise line between normal and abnormal anxiety. Normality is determined by societal standards; what is considered normal in Chicago, Illinois, may not be considered so in Cairo, Egypt. There may even be regional differences within a country or cultural differences within a region. So what criteria can be used to determine if an individual's anxious response is normal? Anxiety can be considered abnormal or pathological if:

1. *It is out of proportion to the situation that is creating it.*

EXAMPLE

Mrs. K witnessed a serious automobile accident 4 weeks ago when she was out driving in her car, and since that time refuses to drive even to the grocery store a few miles from her house. When he is available, her husband must take her wherever she needs to go.

2. *The anxiety interferes with social, occupational, or other important areas of functioning.*

EXAMPLE

Because of the anxiety associated with driving her car, Mrs. K has been forced to quit her job in a downtown bank for lack of transportation.

Application of the Nursing Process

CORE CONCEPT

Panic

A sudden overwhelming feeling of terror or impending doom. This most severe form of emotional anxiety is usually accompanied by behavioral, cognitive, and physiological signs and symptoms considered to be outside the expected range of normalcy.

Panic Disorder

Background Assessment Data

Panic disorder is characterized by recurrent panic attacks, the onset of which is unpredictable, and manifested by intense apprehension, fear, or terror, often associated with feelings of impending doom and accompanied by intense physical discomfort. The symptoms come on unexpectedly; that is, they do not occur immediately before or on exposure to a situation that usually causes anxiety (as in specific phobia). They are not triggered by situations in which the person is the focus of others' attention (as in social phobia). A role for organic factors in the etiology has been ruled out.

At least four of the following symptoms must be present to identify the presence of a panic attack. When fewer than four symptoms are present, the individual is diagnosed as having a limited-symptom attack.

- Palpitations, pounding heart, or accelerated heart rate
- Sweating
- Trembling or shaking
- Sensations of shortness of breath or smothering
- Feeling of choking
- Chest pain or discomfort
- Nausea or abdominal distress
- Feeling dizzy, unsteady, lightheaded, or faint
- Derealization (feelings of unreality) or depersonalization (feelings of being detached from oneself)
- Fear of losing control or going crazy
- Fear of dying
- Paresthesias (numbness or tingling sensations)
- Chills or hot flashes

The attacks usually last minutes, or more rarely, hours. The individual often experiences varying degrees of nervousness and apprehension between attacks. Symptoms of depression are common.

The average age of onset of panic disorder is the late 20s. Frequency and severity of the panic attacks vary widely (APA, 2000). Some individuals may have attacks of moderate severity weekly; others may have less severe or limited-symptom attacks several times a week. Still others may experience panic attacks that are separated by weeks or months. The disorder may last for a few weeks or months or for a number of years. Sometimes the individual experiences periods of remission and exacerbation. In times of remission, the person may have recurrent limited-symptom attacks. Panic disorder may or may not be accompanied by agoraphobia.

Panic Disorder With Agoraphobia

Panic disorder with **agoraphobia** is characterized by the symptoms described for panic disorder. In addition, the individual experiences a fear of being in places or situations from which escape might be difficult (or embarrassing) or in which help might not be available in the event that a panic attack should occur (APA, 2000). This fear severely restricts travel, and the individual may become nearly or completely housebound or unable to leave the house unaccompanied. Common agoraphobic situations include being outside the home alone; being in a crowd or standing in a line; being on a bridge; and traveling in a bus, train, or car.

Generalized Anxiety Disorder

Background Assessment Data

Generalized anxiety disorder is characterized by chronic, unrealistic, and excessive anxiety and worry. The symptoms have existed for 6 months or longer and cannot be attributed to specific organic factors, such as caffeine intoxication or hyperthyroidism.

The *Diagnostic and Statistical Manual of Mental Disorders, Fourth Edition, Text Revision* (DSM-IV-TR) (APA, 2000) identifies the following symptoms associated with generalized anxiety disorder. The symptoms must have occurred more days than not for at least 6 months and must cause clinically significant distress or impairment in social, occupational, or other important areas of functioning.

■ Excessive anxiety and worry about a number of events that the individual finds difficult to control

■ Restlessness or feeling keyed up or on edge

■ Being easily fatigued

■ Difficulty concentrating or mind "going blank"

■ Irritability

■ Muscle tension

■ Sleep disturbance (difficulty falling or staying asleep, or restless unsatisfying sleep)

The disorder may begin in childhood or adolescence, but onset is not uncommon after age 20. Depressive symptoms are common, and numerous somatic complaints may also be a part of the clinical picture. Generalized anxiety disorder tends to be chronic, with frequent stress-related exacerbations and fluctuations in the course of the illness.

Predisposing Factors for Panic and Generalized Anxiety Disorders

Psychodynamic Theory

The psychodynamic view focuses on the inability of the ego to intervene when conflict occurs between the id and the superego, producing anxiety. For various reasons (unsatisfactory parent-child relationship; conditional love or provisional gratification), ego development is delayed. When developmental defects in ego functions compromise the capacity to modulate anxiety, the individual resorts to unconscious mechanisms to resolve the conflict. Overuse or ineffective use of ego defense mechanisms results in maladaptive responses to anxiety.

Cognitive Theory

The main thesis of the cognitive view is that faulty, distorted, or counterproductive thinking patterns accompany or precede maladaptive behaviors and emotional disorders (Sadock & Sadock, 2007). When there is a disturbance in this central mechanism of cognition, there is a consequent disturbance in feeling and behavior. Because of distorted thinking, anxiety is maintained by erroneous or dysfunctional appraisal of a situation. There is a loss of ability to reason regarding the problem, whether it is physical or interpersonal. The individual feels vulnerable in a given situation, and the distorted thinking results in an irrational appraisal, fostering a negative outcome.

Biological Aspects

Research investigations into the psychobiological correlation of panic and generalized anxiety disorders have implicated a number of possibilities.

Genetics Panic disorder has a strong genetic element (Harvard Medical School, 2006). The concordance rate for identical twins is 30 percent, and the risk for the disorder in a close relative is 10 to 20 percent. Hollander and Simeon (2008) reported on research findings of an association between panic disorder and a variant of the gene that controls the manufacture of the protein cholecystokinin, which has been known to induce panic attacks when it is injected.

Neuroanatomical Modern theory on the physiology of emotional states places the key to these disorders in the lower brain centers, including the limbic system, the diencephalon (thalamus and hypothalamus), and the reticular formation. Structural brain imaging studies in patients with panic disorder have implicated pathological involvement in the temporal lobes, particularly the hippocampus (Sadock & Sadock, 2007).

Biochemical Abnormal elevations of blood lactate have been noted in clients with panic disorder. Likewise, infusion of sodium lactate into clients with anxiety neuroses produced symptoms of panic disorder. Although several laboratories have replicated these findings of increased lactate sensitivity in panic-prone individuals, no specific mechanism that triggers the panic symptoms can be explained (Hollander & Simeon, 2008).

Neurochemical Stronger evidence exists for the involvement of the neurotransmitter norepinephrine in the etiology of panic disorder. Norepinephrine is known to mediate arousal, and it causes hyperarousal and anxiety. This fact has been demonstrated by a notable increase in anxiety following the administration of drugs that increase the synaptic availability of norepinephrine, such as yohimbine. The neurotransmitters serotonin and gamma-aminobutyric acid (GABA) are thought to be decreased in anxiety disorders (Harvard Medical School, 2006).

Medical Conditions The following medical conditions have been associated to a greater degree with individuals who suffer panic and generalized anxiety disorders than with individuals in the general population:

■ Abnormalities in the hypothalamic-pituitary-adrenal and hypothalamic-pituitary-thyroid axes

■ Acute myocardial infarction

■ Pheochromocytomas

■ Substance intoxication and withdrawal (cocaine, alcohol, marijuana, opioids)

■ Hypoglycemia

■ Caffeine intoxication

■ Mitral valve prolapse

■ Complex partial seizures

Transactional Model of Stress/Adaptation

Panic and generalized anxiety disorders are most likely caused by multiple factors. In Figure 29–2, a graphic depiction of this theory of multiple causation is presented in the Transactional Model of Stress/Adaptation.

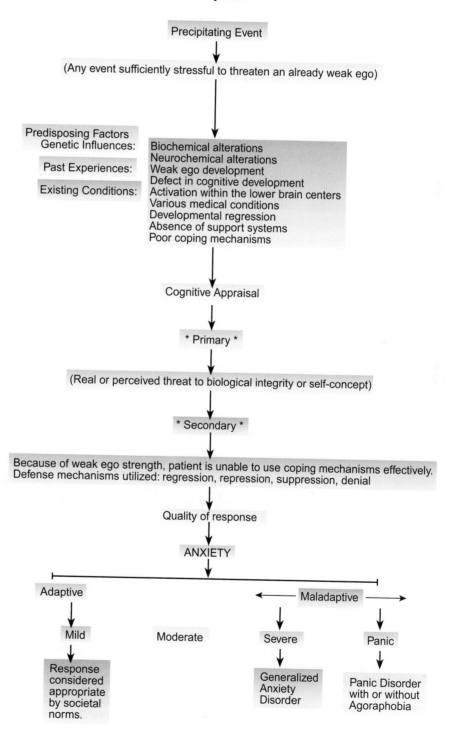

FIGURE 29–2 The dynamics of panic and generalized anxiety disorders using the Transactional Model of Stress/Adaptation.

CORE CONCEPT

Phobia

Fear cued by the presence or anticipation of a specific object or situation, exposure to which almost invariably provokes an immediate *anxiety* response or *panic attack* even though the subject recognizes that the fear is excessive or unreasonable. The phobic stimulus is avoided or endured with marked distress (Shahrokh & Hales, 2003).

Phobias

Background Assessment Data

Agoraphobia Without History of Panic Disorder

Agoraphobia without accompanying panic disorder is less common than the type that precipitates panic attacks. In this disorder, there is a fear of being in places or situations from which escape might be difficult, or in which help might not be available if a limited-symptom attack or panic-like symptoms (rather than full panic attacks) should occur (APA, 2000). It is possible that the individual may have experienced the symptom(s) in the past and is preoccupied with fears of their recurrence. The *DSM-IV-TR* diagnostic criteria for agoraphobia without history of panic disorder are presented in Box 29-1.

Onset of symptoms most commonly occurs in the 20s and 30s and persists for many years. It is diagnosed more commonly in women than in men. Impairment can be severe. In extreme cases the individual is unable to leave his or her home without being accompanied by a friend or relative. If this is not possible, the person may become totally confined to his or her home.

Social Phobia

Social phobia is an excessive fear of situations in which a person might do something embarrassing or be evaluated negatively by others. The individual has extreme concerns about being exposed to possible scrutiny by others and fears social or performance situations in which embarrassment may occur (APA, 2000). In some instances, the fear may be quite defined, such as the fear of speaking or eating in a public place, fear of using a public restroom, or fear of writing in the presence of others. In other cases, the social phobia may involve general social situations, such as saying things or answering questions in a manner that would provoke laughter on the part of others. Exposure to the phobic situation usually results in feelings of panic anxiety, with sweating, tachycardia, and dyspnea.

Onset of symptoms of this disorder often begins in late childhood or early adolescence and runs a chronic, sometimes lifelong, course. It appears to be equally common among men and women (APA, 2000). Impairment interferes with social or occupational functioning, or causes marked distress. The *DSM-IV-TR* diagnostic criteria for social phobia are presented in Box 29-2.

Specific Phobia

Specific phobia was formerly called simple phobia. The essential feature of this disorder is a marked, persistent, and excessive or unreasonable fear when in the presence of, or when anticipating an encounter with, a specific object or situation (APA, 2000).

Specific phobias frequently occur concurrently with other anxiety disorders, but are rarely the focus of clinical attention in these situations (APA, 2000). Treatment is generally aimed at the primary diagnosis because it usually produces the greatest

---

BOX 29-1 Diagnostic Criteria for Agoraphobia Without History of Panic Disorder

A. The presence of agoraphobia related to fear of developing panic-like symptoms. Agoraphobia is the fear of being in places or situations from which escape might be difficult (or embarrassing) or in which help might not be available in the event of suddenly developing a symptom(s) that could be incapacitating or extremely embarrassing. Examples include: dizziness or falling, depersonalization or derealization, loss of bladder or bowel control, vomiting, or cardiac distress. As a result of this fear, the person either restricts travel or needs a companion when away from home, or else endures agoraphobic situations despite intense anxiety. Common agoraphobic situations include being outside the home alone, being in a crowd or standing in a line, being on a bridge, and traveling in a bus, train, or car.

B. Criteria for panic disorder have never been met.

C. The disturbance is not due to the direct physiological effects of a substance (e.g., a drug of abuse, a medication) or a general medical condition.

D. If an associated general medical condition is present, the fear is clearly in excess of that usually associated with the condition.

BOX 29-2 Diagnostic Criteria for Social Phobia

A. A marked and persistent fear of one or more social or performance situations in which the person is exposed to unfamiliar people or to possible scrutiny by others. The individual fears that he or she will act in a way (or show anxiety symptoms) that will be humiliating or embarrassing. In children, there must be evidence of the capacity for age-appropriate social relationships with familiar people and the anxiety must occur in peer settings, not just in interactions with adults.

B. Exposure to the feared social situation almost invariably provokes anxiety, which may take the form of a situationally bound or situationally predisposed panic attack. In children, the anxiety may be expressed by crying, tantrums, freezing, or shrinking from social situations with unfamiliar people.

C. The person recognizes that the fear is excessive or unreasonable. In children, this feature may be absent.

D. The feared social or performance situations are avoided or else are endured with intense anxiety or distress.

E. The avoidance, anxious anticipation, or distress in the feared social or performance situation(s) interferes significantly with the person's normal routine, occupational (academic) functioning, or social activities or relationships, or there is marked distress about having the phobia.

F. In individuals under age 18 years, the duration is at least 6 months.

G. The fear or avoidance is not due to the direct physiological effects of a substance (e.g., a drug of abuse, a medication) or a general medical condition and is not better accounted for by another mental disorder (e.g., panic disorder with or without agoraphobia, separation anxiety disorder, body dysmorphic disorder, a pervasive developmental disorder, or schizoid personality disorder).

H. If a general medical condition or another mental disorder is present, the fear in criterion A is unrelated to it (e.g., the fear is not of stuttering, trembling in Parkinson's disease, or exhibiting abnormal eating behavior in anorexia nervosa or bulimia nervosa).

The diagnosis is further specified as *generalized* if the fears include most social situations.

From the American Psychiatric Association. (2000). Diagnostic and statistical manual of mental disorders (4th ed.). Text revision. Washington, DC: American Psychiatric Publishing, with permission.

distress and interferes with functioning more so than does a specific phobia.

The phobic person may be no more (or less) anxious than anyone else until exposed to the phobic object or situation. Exposure to the phobic stimulus produces overwhelming symptoms of panic, including palpitations, sweating, dizziness, and difficulty breathing. In fact, these symptoms may occur in response to the individual's merely *thinking* about the phobic stimulus. Invariably the person recognizes that his or her fear is excessive or unreasonable, but is powerless to change, even though the individual may occasionally endure the phobic stimulus when experiencing intense anxiety.

Phobias may begin at almost any age. Those that begin in childhood often disappear without treatment, but those that begin or persist into adulthood usually require assistance with therapy. The disorder is diagnosed more often in women than in men.

Even though the disorder is common among the general population, people seldom seek treatment unless the phobia interferes with ability to function. Obviously the individual who has a fear of snakes, but who lives on the 23rd floor of an urban, high-rise apartment building, is not likely to

be bothered by the phobia unless he or she decides to move to an area where snakes are prevalent. On the other hand, a fear of elevators may very well interfere with this individual's daily functioning.

Specific phobias have been classified according to the phobic stimulus. A list of some of the more common ones appears in Table 29-1. This list is by no means all-inclusive. People can become phobic about almost any object or situation, and anyone with a little knowledge of Greek or Latin can produce a phobia classification, thereby making possibilities for the list almost infinite.

The *DSM-IV-TR* identifies subtypes of the most common specific phobias. They include the following:

■ **Animal type.** This subtype would be identified as part of the diagnosis if the fear is of animals or insects.

■ **Natural environment type.** Examples of this subtype include objects or situations that occur within the natural environment, such as heights, storms, or water.

■ **Blood-injection-injury type.** This diagnosis should be specified if the fear is of seeing

TABLE 29-1 Classifications of Specific Phobias

CLASSIFICATION	FEAR
Acrophobia	Height
Ailurophobia	Cats
Algophobia	Pain
Anthophobia	Flowers
Anthropophobia	People
Aquaphobia	Water
Arachnophobia	Spiders
Astraphobia	Lightning
Belonephobia	Needles
Brontophobia	Thunder
Claustrophobia	Closed spaces
Cynophobia	Dogs
Dementophobia	Insanity
Equinophobia	Horses
Gamophobia	Marriage
Herpetophobia	Lizards, reptiles
Homophobia	Homosexuality
Murophobia	Mice
Mysophobia	Dirt, germs, contamination
Numerophobia	Numbers
Nyctophobia	Darkness
Ochophobia	Riding in a car
Ophidiophobia	Snakes
Pyrophobia	Fire
Scoleciphobia	Worms
Siderodromophobia	Railroads or train travel
Taphophobia	Being buried alive
Thanatophobia	Death
Trichophobia	Hair
Triskaidekaphobia	The number 13
Xenophobia	Strangers
Zoophobia	Animals

blood or an injury or of receiving an injection or other invasive medical or dental procedure.

■ **Situational type.** This subtype is designated if the fear is of a specific situation, such as public transportation, tunnels, bridges, elevators, flying, driving, or enclosed places.

■ **Other type.** This category covers all other excessive or irrational fears. It may include fear of contracting a serious illness, fear of situations that might lead to vomiting or choking, fear of loud noises, or fear of driving.

The *DSM-IV-TR* diagnostic criteria for specific phobia are presented in Box 29-3.

Predisposing Factors to Phobias

The cause of phobias is unknown. However, various theories exist that may offer insight into the etiology.

Psychoanalytic Theory

Freud believed that phobias developed when a child experiences normal incestual feelings toward the opposite-gender parent (Oedipal/Electra complex) and fears aggression from the same-gender parent (castration anxiety). To protect themselves, these children *repress* this fear of hostility from the same-gender parent, and *displace* it onto something safer and more neutral, which becomes the phobic stimulus. The phobic stimulus becomes the symbol for the parent, but the child does not realize this.

Modern-day psychoanalysts believe in the same concept of phobic development, but believe that castration anxiety is not the sole source of phobias. They believe that other unconscious fears may also be expressed in a symbolic manner as phobias. For example, a female child who was sexually abused by an adult male family friend when he was taking her for a ride in his boat grew up with an intense, irrational fear of all water vessels. Psychoanalytic theory postulates that fear of the man was repressed and displaced on to boats. Boats became an unconscious symbol for the feared person, but one that the young girl viewed as safer since her fear of boats prevented her from having to confront the real fear.

Learning Theory

Classic conditioning in the case of phobias may be explained as follows: a stressful stimulus produces an "unconditioned" response of fear. When the stressful stimulus is repeatedly paired with a

BOX 29-3 Diagnostic Criteria for Specific Phobia

A. Marked and persistent fear that is excessive or unreasonable, cued by the presence or anticipation of a specific object or situation (e.g., flying, heights, animals, receiving an injection, seeing blood).
B. Exposure to the phobic stimulus almost invariably provokes an immediate anxiety response, which may take the form of a situationally bound or situationally predisposed panic attack. In children, the anxiety may be expressed by crying, tantrums, freezing, or clinging.
C. The person recognizes that the fear is excessive or unreasonable. In children, this feature may be absent.
D. The phobic situation(s) is avoided or else is endured with intense anxiety or distress.
E. The avoidance, anxious anticipation, or distress in the feared situation(s) interferes significantly with the person's normal routine, occupational (academic)

functioning, or social activities or relationships, or there is marked distress about having the phobia.
F. In individuals under 18 years, the duration is at least 6 months.
G. The anxiety, panic attacks, or phobic avoidance associated with the specific object or situation are not better accounted for by another mental disorder.

The diagnosis may be further specified as:

Animal type

Natural environment type (e.g., heights, storms, water)

Blood-injection-injury type

Situational type (e.g., airplanes, elevators, enclosed places)

Other type

From the American Psychiatric Association. (2000). Diagnostic and statistical manual of mental disorders (4th ed.). Text revision. Washington, DC: American Psychiatric Publishing, with permission.

harmless object, eventually the harmless object alone produces a "conditioned" response: fear. This becomes a phobia when the individual consciously avoids the harmless object to escape fear.

Some learning theorists hold that fears are conditioned responses and, thus, they are learned by imposing rewards for certain behaviors. In the instance of phobias, when the individual avoids the phobic object, he or she escapes fear, which is indeed a powerful reward.

Phobias also may be acquired by direct learning or imitation (modeling) (e.g., a mother who exhibits fear toward an object will provide a model for the child, who may also develop a phobia of the same object).

Cognitive Theory

Cognitive theorists espouse that anxiety is the product of faulty cognitions or anxiety-inducing self-instructions. Two types of faulty thinking have been investigated: negative self-statements and irrational beliefs. Cognitive theorists believe that some individuals engage in negative and irrational thinking that produces anxiety reactions. The individual begins to seek out avoidance behaviors to prevent the anxiety reactions, and phobias result.

Somewhat related to the cognitive theory is the involvement of locus of control. Johnson and Sarason (1978) suggested that individuals with internal locus of control and those with external locus of control might respond differently to life change. These researchers proposed that locus of

control orientation may be an important variable in the development of phobias. Individuals with an external control orientation experiencing anxiety attacks in a stressful period are likely to mislabel the anxiety and attribute it to external sources (e.g., crowded areas) or to a disease (e.g., heart attack). They may perceive the experienced anxiety as being outside of their control. Figure 29–3 depicts a graphic model of the relationship between locus of control and the development of phobias.

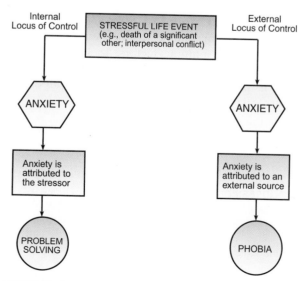

FIGURE 29–3 Locus of control as a variable in the etiology of phobias.

Biological Aspects

Temperament Children experience fears as a part of normal development. Most infants are afraid of loud noises. Common fears of toddlers and preschoolers include strangers, animals, darkness, and fears of being separated from parents or attachment figures. During the school-age years, there is fear of death and anxiety about school achievement. Fears of social rejection and sexual anxieties are common among adolescents.

Innate fears represent a part of the overall characteristics or tendencies with which one is born that influence how he or she responds throughout life to specific situations. Innate fears usually do not reach phobic intensity but may have the capacity for such development if reinforced by events in later life. For example, a 4-year-old girl is afraid of dogs. By age 5, however, she has overcome her fear and plays with her own dog and the neighbors' dogs without fear. Then, when she is 19, she is bitten by a stray dog and develops a dog phobia.

Life Experiences

Certain early experiences may set the stage for phobic reactions later in life. Some researchers believe that phobias, particularly specific phobias, are symbolic of original anxiety-producing objects or situations that have been repressed. Examples include:

■ A child who is punished by being locked in a closet develops a phobia for elevators or other closed places.

■ A child who falls down a flight of stairs develops a phobia for high places.

■ A young woman who, as a child, survived a plane crash in which both her parents were killed has a phobia of airplanes.

Transactional Model of Stress/Adaptation

The etiology of phobic disorders is most likely influenced by multiple factors. In Figure 29–4, a graphic depiction of this theory of multiple causation is presented in the Transactional Model of Stress/Adaptation.

CORE CONCEPT

Obsessions

Unwanted, intrusive, persistent ideas, thoughts, impulses, or images that cause marked anxiety or distress. The most common ones include repeated thoughts about contamination, repeated doubts, a need to have things in a particular order, aggressive or horrific impulses, and sexual imagery (APA, 2000).

CORE CONCEPT

Compulsions

Unwanted repetitive behavior patterns or mental acts (e.g., praying, counting, repeating words silently) that are intended to reduce anxiety, not to provide pleasure or gratification (APA, 2000). They may be performed in response to an obsession or in a stereotyped fashion.

Obsessive-Compulsive Disorder

Background Assessment Data

The *DSM-IV-TR* describes **obsessive-compulsive disorder** (OCD) as recurrent obsessions or compulsions that are severe enough to be time consuming or to cause marked distress or significant impairment (APA, 2000). The individual recognizes that the behavior is excessive or unreasonable but, because of the feeling of relief from discomfort that it promotes, is compelled to continue the act. The most common compulsions involve washing and cleaning, counting, checking, requesting or demanding assurances, repeating actions, and ordering (APA, 2000).

The disorder is equally common among men and women. It may begin in childhood, but more often begins in adolescence or early adulthood. The course is usually chronic, and may be complicated by depression or substance abuse. Single people are affected by OCD more often than are married people (Sadock & Sadock, 2007). The *DSM-IV-TR* diagnostic criteria for OCD are presented in Box 29-4.

Predisposing Factors to Obsessive-Compulsive Disorder

Psychoanalytic Theory

Psychoanalytic theorists propose that individuals with OCD have weak, underdeveloped egos (for any of a variety of reasons: unsatisfactory parent-child relationship, conditional love, or provisional gratification). The psychoanalytic concept views clients with OCD as having regressed to earlier developmental stages of the infantile superego—the harsh, exacting, punitive characteristics that now reappear as part of the psychopathology. Regression to the pre-Oedipal anal-sadistic phase, combined with use of specific ego defense mechanisms (isolation, undoing, displacement, reaction formation), produces the clinical symptoms of obsessions and compulsions (Sadock & Sadock, 2007). Aggressive impulses (common during the anal-sadistic developmental phase) are channeled into thoughts and behaviors that prevent the feelings of

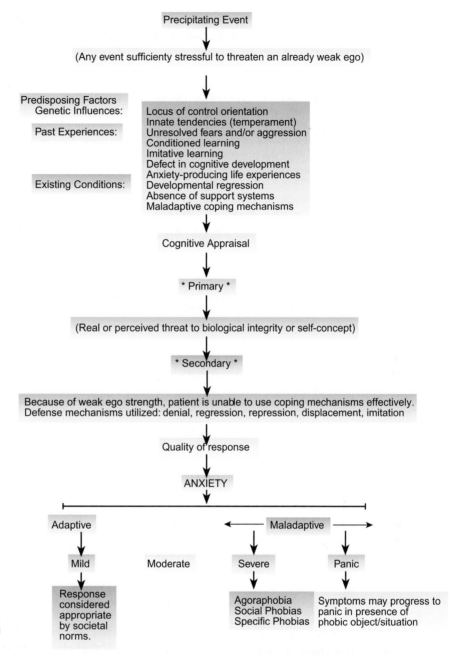

FIGURE 29–4 The dynamics of phobic disorder using the Transactional Model of Stress/Adaptation.

BOX 29-4 Diagnostic Criteria for Obsessive-Compulsive Disorder

A. Either obsessions or compulsions:

Obsessions as defined by 1, 2, 3, and 4:

1. Recurrent and persistent thoughts, impulses, or images that are experienced at some time during the disturbance as intrusive and inappropriate and that cause marked anxiety or distress.

2. The thoughts, impulses, or images are not simply excessive worries about real-life problems.

3. The person attempts to ignore or suppress such thoughts, impulses, or images, or to neutralize them with some other thought or action.

4. The person recognizes that the obsessional thoughts, impulses, or images are a product of his or her own mind (not imposed from without as in thought insertion).

Compulsions as defined by 1 and 2:

1. Repetitive behaviors (e.g., hand washing, ordering, checking) or mental acts (e.g., praying, counting, repeating words silently) that the person feels driven to perform in response to an obsession, or according to rules that must be applied rigidly.

Continued

BOX 29-4 **Diagnostic Criteria for Obsessive-Compulsive Disorder—cont'd**

2. The behaviors or mental acts are aimed at preventing or reducing distress or preventing some dreaded event or situation; however, these behaviors or mental acts either are not connected in a realistic way with what they are designed to neutralize or prevent or are clearly excessive.

B. At some point during the course of the disorder, the person has recognized that the obsessions or compulsions are excessive or unreasonable. This does not apply to children.

C. The obsessions or compulsions cause marked distress, are time consuming (take more than 1 hour a day), or significantly interfere with the person's normal routine, occupational (or academic) functioning, or usual social activities or relationships.

D. If another axis I disorder is present, the content of the obsessions or compulsions is not restricted to it (e.g., preoccupation with food in the presence of an eating disorder; hair pulling in the presence of trichotillomania; concern with appearance in the presence of body dysmorphic disorder; preoccupation with having a serious illness in the presence of hypochondriasis; preoccupation with sexual urges or fantasies in the presence of a paraphilia; or guilty ruminations in the presence of major depressive disorder).

E. This disturbance is not due to the direct physiological effects of a substance (e.g., drug of abuse, a medication) or a general medical condition.

From the American Psychiatric Association. (2000). Diagnostic and statistical manual of mental disorders (4th ed.). Text revision. Washington, DC: American Psychiatric Publishing, with permission.

---

aggression from surfacing and producing intense anxiety fraught with guilt (generated by the punitive superego).

Learning Theory

Learning theorists explain obsessive-compulsive behavior as a conditioned response to a traumatic event. The traumatic event produces anxiety and discomfort, and the individual learns to prevent the anxiety and discomfort by avoiding the situation with which they are associated. This type of learning is called *passive avoidance* (staying away from the source). When passive avoidance is not possible, the individual learns to engage in behaviors that provide relief from the anxiety and discomfort associated with the traumatic situation. This type of learning is called *active avoidance* and describes the behavior pattern of the individual with OCD (Sadock & Sadock, 2007).

According to this classic conditioning interpretation, a traumatic event should mark the beginning of the obsessive-compulsive behaviors. However, in a significant number of cases, the onset of the behavior is gradual and the clients relate the onset of their problems to life stress in general rather than to one or more traumatic events.

Biological Aspects

Recent findings suggest that neurobiological disturbances may play a role in the pathogenesis and maintenance of OCD.

Neuroanatomy Abnormalities in various regions of the brain have been implicated in the neurobiology of OCD. Functional neuroimaging techniques have shown abnormal metabolic rates in the basal ganglia and orbital-frontal cortex of individuals with the disorder (Hollander & Simeon, 2008).

Physiology Electrophysiological studies, sleep electroencephalogram studies, and neuroendocrine studies have suggested that there are commonalities between depressive disorders and OCD (Sadock & Sadock, 2007). Neuroendocrine commonalities were suggested in studies in which about one third of OCD clients show nonsuppression on the dexamethasone suppression test and decreased growth hormone secretion with clonidine infusions.

Biochemical Factors A number of studies have implicated the neurotransmitter serotonin as influential in the etiology of obsessive-compulsive behaviors. Drugs that have been used successfully in alleviating the symptoms of OCD are clomipramine and the selective serotonin reuptake inhibitors (SSRIs), all of which are believed to block the neuronal reuptake of serotonin, thereby potentiating serotoninergic activity in the central nervous system (see Figure 29–1).

Transactional Model of Stress/Adaptation

The etiology of obsessive-compulsive disorder is most likely influenced by multiple factors. In Figure 29–5, a graphic depiction of this theory of multiple causation is presented in the Transactional Model of Stress/Adaptation.

Posttraumatic Stress Disorder

Background Assessment Data

Posttraumatic stress disorder (PTSD) is described by the *DSM-IV-TR* as the development of characteristic symptoms following exposure to an extreme

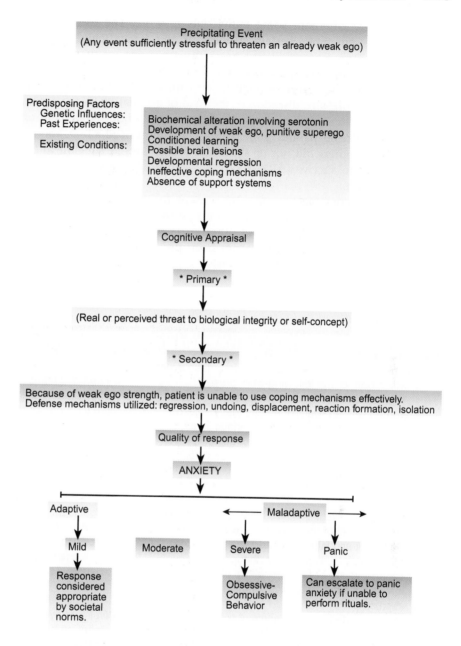

FIGURE 29–5 The dynamics of obsessive-compulsive disorder using the Transactional Model of Stress/Adaptation.

traumatic stressor involving a personal threat to physical integrity or to the physical integrity of others. The symptoms may occur after learning about unexpected or violent death, serious harm, or threat of death or injury of a family member or other close associate (APA, 2000). These symptoms are not related to common experiences such as uncomplicated bereavement, marital conflict, or chronic illness, but are associated with events that would be markedly distressing to almost anyone. The individual may experience the trauma alone or in the presence of others. Examples of some

experiences that may produce this type of response include participation in military combat, experiencing violent personal assault, being kidnapped or taken hostage, being tortured, being incarcerated as a prisoner of war, experiencing natural or man-made disasters, surviving severe automobile accidents, or being diagnosed with a life-threatening illness (APA, 2000).

Characteristic symptoms include re-experiencing the traumatic event and a sustained high level of anxiety or arousal or a general numbing of responsiveness. Intrusive recollections or nightmares of the event are common. Some individuals may be unable to remember certain aspects of the trauma.

Symptoms of depression are common with this disorder and may be severe enough to warrant a diagnosis of a depressive disorder. In the case of a life-threatening trauma shared with others, survivors often describe painful guilt feelings about surviving when others did not or about the things they had to do to survive (APA, 2000). Substance abuse is common.

The full symptom picture must be present for more than 1 month and cause significant interference with social, occupational, and other areas of functioning. If the symptoms have not been present for more than 1 month, the diagnosis assigned is acute stress disorder (APA, 2000).

The disorder can occur at any age. Symptoms may begin within the first 3 months after the trauma, or there may be a delay of several months or even years. Studies reveal a lifetime prevalence for PTSD of approximately 8 percent of the adult population in the United States (Rowney et al., 2010). About 30 percent of Vietnam veterans have experienced PTSD, and an additional 25 percent encountered subclinical forms of the disorder (Sadock & Sadock, 2007). The *DSM-IV-TR* diagnostic criteria for PTSD are presented in Box 29-5.

Predisposing Factors to Posttraumatic Stress Disorder

Reports of symptoms and syndromes with PTSD-like features have existed in writing throughout the centuries. In the early part of the 20th century,

---

BOX 29-5 Diagnostic Criteria for Posttraumatic Stress Disorder

A. The person has been exposed to a traumatic event in which both of the following were present:
   1. The person experienced, witnessed, or was confronted with an event or events that involved actual or threatened death or serious injury, or a threat to the physical integrity of self or others.
   2. The person's response involved intense fear, helplessness, or horror. In children, this may be expressed instead by disorganized or agitated behavior.

B. The traumatic event is persistently re-experienced in one (or more) of the following ways:
   1. Recurrent and intrusive distressing recollections of the event, including images, thoughts, or perceptions. In young children, repetitive play may occur in which themes or aspects of the trauma are expressed.
   2. Recurrent distressing dreams of the event. In children, there may be frightening dreams without recognizable content.
   3. Acting or feeling as if the traumatic event were recurring (includ**es a** sense of reliving the experience, illusions, hallucinations, and dissociative flashback episodes, including those that occur on awakening or when intoxicated). In young children, trauma-specific reenactment may occur.
   4. Intense psychological distress at exposure to internal or external cues that symbolize or resemble an aspect of the traumatic event.
   5. Physiological reactivity on exposure to internal or external cues that symbolize or resemble an aspect of the traumatic event.

C. Persistent avoidance of stimuli associated with the trauma and numbing of general responsiveness (not present before the trauma), as indicated by three (or more) of the following:
   1. Efforts to avoid thoughts or feelings associated with the trauma.
   2. Efforts to avoid activities, places, or people that arouse recollections of the trauma.
   3. Inability to recall an important aspect of the trauma.
   4. Markedly diminished interest or participation in significant activities.
   5. Feeling of detachment or estrangement from others.
   6. Restricted range of affect (e.g., unable to have loving feelings).
   7. Sense of a foreshortened future (e.g., does not expect to have a career, marriage, children, or a normal life span).

D. Persistent symptoms of increased arousal (not present before the trauma), as indicated by two (or more) of the following:
   1. Difficulty falling or staying asleep.
   2. Irritability or outbursts of anger.
   3. Difficulty concentrating.
   4. Hypervigilance.
   5. Exaggerated startle response.

E. Duration of the disturbance more than 1 month

F. Disturbance that causes clinically significant distress or impairment in social, occupational, or other important areas of functioning

Specify if acute (symptoms less than 3 months), chronic (symptoms 3 months or more), or delayed onset (onset of symptoms at least 6 months after the stressor).

From the American Psychiatric Association. (2000). Diagnostic and statistical manual of mental disorders (4th ed.). Text revision. Washington, DC: American Psychiatric Publishing, with permission.

traumatic neurosis was viewed as the ego's inability to master the degree of disorganization brought about by a traumatic experience. Very little was written about post-traumatic neurosis during the years between 1950 and 1970. This absence was followed in the 1970s and 1980s with an explosion in the amount of research and writing on the subject. Many of the papers written during this time were about Vietnam veterans. Clearly, the renewed interest in PTSD was linked to the psychological casualties of the Vietnam War.

The diagnostic category of PTSD did not appear until the third edition of the *Diagnostic and Statistical Manual of Mental Disorders* (*DSM-III*) in 1980, after a need was indicated by increasing numbers of problems with Vietnam veterans and victims of multiple disasters.

Psychosocial Theory

One psychosocial model that has become widely accepted seeks to explain why certain persons exposed to massive trauma develop PTSD and others do not. Variables include characteristics that relate to (1) the traumatic experience, (2) the individual, and (3) the recovery environment.

The Traumatic Experience Specific characteristics relating to the trauma have been identified as crucial elements in the determination of an individual's long-term response to stress. They include:

■ Severity and duration of the stressor

■ Extent of anticipatory preparation for the event

■ Exposure to death

■ Numbers affected by life threat

■ Amount of control over recurrence

■ Location where the trauma was experienced (e.g., familiar surroundings, at home, in a foreign country)

The Individual Variables that are considered important in determining an individual's response to trauma include:

■ Degree of ego strength

■ Effectiveness of coping resources

■ Presence of preexisting psychopathology

■ Outcomes of previous experiences with stress/trauma

■ Behavioral tendencies (temperament)

■ Current psychosocial developmental stage

■ Demographic factors (e.g., age, socioeconomic status, education)

The Recovery Environment It has been suggested that the quality of the environment in which the individual attempts to work through the traumatic experience is correlated with the outcome. Environmental variables include:

■ Availability of social supports

■ The cohesiveness and protectiveness of family and friends

■ The attitudes of society regarding the experience

■ Cultural and subcultural influences

In research with Vietnam veterans, it was shown that the best predictors of PTSD were the severity of the stressor and the degree of psychosocial isolation in the recovery environment.

Learning Theory

Learning theorists view negative reinforcement as behavior that leads to a reduction in an aversive experience, thereby reinforcing and resulting in repetition of the behavior. The avoidance behaviors and psychic numbing in response to a trauma are mediated by negative reinforcement (behaviors that decrease the emotional pain of the trauma). Behavioral disturbances, such as anger and aggression and drug and alcohol abuse, are the behavior patterns that are reinforced by their capacity to reduce objectionable feelings.

Cognitive Theory

These models take into consideration the cognitive appraisal of an event and focus on assumptions that an individual makes about the world. Epstein (1991) outlined three fundamental beliefs that most people construct within a personal theory of reality. They include:

■ The world is benevolent and a source of joy.

■ The world is meaningful and controllable.

■ The self is worthy (e.g., lovable, good, and competent).

As life situations occur, some disequilibrium is expected to occur until accommodation for the change has been made and it has become assimilated into one's personal theory of reality. An individual is vulnerable to PTSD when the fundamental beliefs are invalidated by a trauma that cannot be comprehended and a sense of helplessness and hopelessness prevail. One's appraisal of the environment can be drastically altered.

Biological Aspects

It has been suggested that an individual who has experienced previous trauma is more likely to develop symptoms after a stressful life event (Hollander & Simeon, 2008). These individuals with previous traumatic experiences may be more likely to become exposed to future traumas, as they can be inclined to reactivate the behaviors associated with the original trauma.

Hollander and Simeon (2008) also reported on studies that suggest an endogenous opioid peptide response may assist in the maintenance of chronic PTSD. The hypothesis supports a type of "addiction to the trauma," which is explained in the following manner.

Opioids, including endogenous opioid peptides, have the following psychoactive properties:

■ Tranquilizing action

■ Reduction of rage/aggression

■ Reduction of paranoia

■ Reduction of feelings of inadequacy

■ Antidepressant action

These studies suggest that physiological arousal initiated by reexposure to trauma-like situations enhances production of endogenous opioid peptides and results in increased feelings of comfort and control. When the stressor terminates, the individual may experience opioid withdrawal, the symptoms of which bear strong resemblance to those of PTSD.

Other biological systems have also been implicated in the symptomatology of PTSD. Hageman and associates (2001) stated:

> It is reasonable to suggest that any disorder such as PTSD that can persist for decades (e.g., Holocaust survivors and Vietnam veterans) is associated with measurable biological features. Evidence suggests that biological dysregulation of the opioid, glutamatergic, noradrenergic, serotonergic, and neuroendocrine pathways are involved in the pathophysiology of PTSD. (p. 412)

Transactional Model of Stress/Adaptation

The etiology of PTSD is most likely influenced by multiple factors. In Figure 29–6, a graphic depiction of this theory of multiple causation is presented in the Transactional Model of Stress/Adaptation.

Anxiety Disorder due to a General Medical Condition

Background Assessment Data

The symptoms of this disorder are judged to be the direct physiological consequence of a general medical condition. Symptoms may include prominent generalized anxiety symptoms, panic attacks, or obsessions or compulsions (APA, 2000). History, physical examination, or laboratory findings must be evident to substantiate the diagnosis.

The *DSM-IV-TR* (APA, 2000) lists the following types and examples of medical conditions that may cause anxiety symptoms:

■ *Endocrine conditions:* Hyperthyroidism and hypothyroidism, pheochromocytoma, hypoglycemia, hyperadrenocorticism

■ *Cardiovascular conditions:* Congestive heart failure, pulmonary embolism, arrhythmia

■ *Respiratory conditions:* Chronic obstructive pulmonary disease, pneumonia, hyperventilation

■ *Metabolic conditions:* Vitamin B_{12} deficiency, porphyria

■ *Neurological conditions:* Neoplasms, vestibular dysfunction, encephalitis

Care of clients with this disorder must take into consideration the underlying cause of the anxiety. Holistic nursing care is essential to ensure that the client's physiological and psychosocial needs are met. Nursing actions appropriate for the specific medical condition must be considered.

Substance-Induced Anxiety Disorder

Background Assessment Data

The *DSM-IV-TR* (APA, 2000) describes the essential features of this disorder as prominent anxiety symptoms that are judged to be due to the direct physiological effects of a substance (i.e., a drug of abuse, a medication, or toxin exposure). The symptoms may occur during substance intoxication or withdrawal, and may involve prominent anxiety, panic attacks, phobias, or obsessions or compulsions. Diagnosis of this disorder is made only if the anxiety symptoms are in excess of those usually associated with the intoxication or withdrawal syndrome and warrant independent clinical attention. Evidence of intoxication or withdrawal must be available from history, physical examination, or laboratory findings to substantiate the diagnosis. See Chapter 25 for a discussion of the types of substances that may produce these symptoms.

Nursing care of the client with substance-induced anxiety disorder must take into consideration the nature of the substance and the context in which the symptoms occur; that is, intoxication or withdrawal (see Chapter 25).

Assessment Scales

A number of assessment rating scales are available for measuring severity of anxiety symptoms. Some are meant to be clinician administered, whereas others may be self-administered. Examples of self-rating scales include the Beck Anxiety Inventory and the Zung Self-Rated Anxiety Scale. One of the most widely used clinician-administered scales is the Hamilton Anxiety Rating Scale (HAM-A), which is

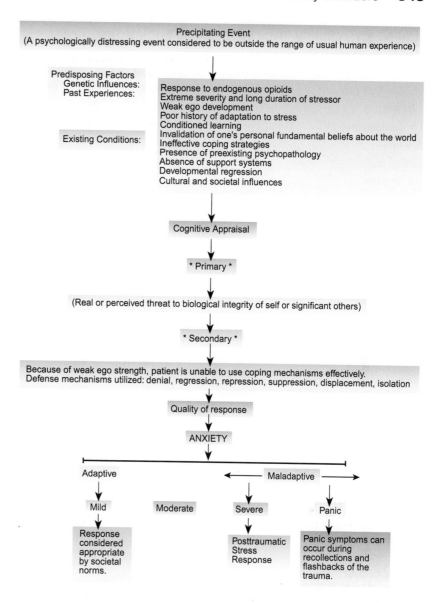

FIGURE 29–6 The dynamics of posttraumatic stress disorder using the Transactional Model of Stress/Adaptation.

used in both clinical and research settings. The scale consists of 14 items and measures both psychic and somatic anxiety symptoms (psychological distress and physical complaints associated with anxiety). A copy of the HAM-A is presented in Box 29-6.

Diagnosis/Outcome Identification

Nursing diagnoses are formulated from the data gathered during the assessment phase and with background knowledge regarding predisposing factors to the disorder. Table 29-2 presents a list of client behaviors and the NANDA nursing diagnoses that correspond to those behaviors, which may be used in planning care for clients with anxiety disorders.

Outcome Criteria

The following criteria may be used for measurement of outcomes in the care of the client with anxiety disorders.

The client:

■ Is able to recognize signs of escalating anxiety and intervene before reaching panic level (*panic and generalized anxiety disorders*).

■ Is able to maintain anxiety at manageable level and make independent decisions about life situation (*panic and generalized anxiety disorders*).

■ Functions adaptively in the presence of the phobic object or situation without experiencing panic anxiety (*phobic disorder*).

■ Verbalizes a future plan of action for responding in the presence of the phobic object or situation without developing panic anxiety (*phobic disorder*).

■ Is able to maintain anxiety at a manageable level without resorting to the use of ritualistic behavior (*OCD*).

BOX 29-6 Hamilton Anxiety Rating Scale (HAM-A)

Below are descriptions of symptoms commonly associated with anxiety. Assign the client the rating between 0 and 4 (for each of the 14 items) that best describes the extent to which he/she has these symptoms.

0 = Not present   1 = Mild   2 = Moderate   3 = Severe   4 = Very severe

Rating

1. Anxious mood

_____

Worries, anticipation of the worst, fearful anticipation, irritability

2. Tension

_____

Feelings of tension, fatigability, startle response, moved to tears easily, trembling, feelings of restlessness, inability to relax

3. Fears

_____

Of dark, of strangers, of being left alone, of animals, of traffic, of crowds

4. Insomnia

_____

Difficulty in falling asleep, broken sleep, unsatisfying sleep and fatigue on waking, dreams, nightmares, night terrors

5. Intellectual

_____

Difficulty in concentration, poor memory

6. Depressed mood

_____

Loss of interest, lack of pleasure in hobbies, depression, early waking, diurnal swing

7. Somatic (muscular)

_____

Pains and aches, twitching, stiffness, myoclonic jerks, grinding of teeth, unsteady voice, increased muscular tone

Rating

8. Somatic (sensory)

_____

Tinnitus, blurred vision, hot/cold flushes, feelings of weakness, tingling sensation

9. Cardiovascular symptoms

_____

Tachycardia, palpitations, pain in chest, throbbing of vessels, feeling faint

10. Respiratory symptoms

_____

Pressure or constriction in chest, choking feelings, sighing, dyspnea

11. Gastrointestinal symptoms

_____

Difficulty swallowing, flatulence, abdominal pain and fullness, burning sensations, nausea/vomiting, borborygmi, diarrhea, constipation, weight loss

12. Genitourinary symptoms

_____

Urinary frequency, urinary urgency, amenorrhea, menorrhagia, loss of libido, premature ejaculation, impotence

13. Autonomic symptoms

_____

Dry mouth, flushing, pallor, tendency to sweat, giddiness, tension headache

14. Behavior at interview

_____

Fidgeting, restlessness or pacing, tremor of hands, furrowed brow, strained face, sighing or rapid respiration, facial pallor, swallowing, clearing throat

Client's Total Score _____

SCORING:
14 – 17 = Mild Anxiety
18 – 24 = Moderate Anxiety
25 – 30 = Severe Anxiety

From Hamilton, M. (1959). The assessment of anxiety states by rating. *British Journal of Medical Psychology, 32,* 50–55. The HAM-A is in the public domain.

TABLE 29-2 Assigning Nursing Diagnoses to Behaviors Commonly Associated with Anxiety Disorders

BEHAVIORS	NURSING DIAGNOSES
Palpitations, trembling, sweating, chest pain, shortness of breath, fear of going crazy, fear of dying (*panic disorder*). Excessive worry, difficulty concentrating, sleep disturbance (*generalized anxiety disorder*).	**Panic anxiety**
Verbal expressions of having no control over life situation; nonparticipation in decision making related to own care or life situation; expressions of doubt regarding role performance (*panic and generalized anxiety disorders*).	**Powerlessness**
Behavior directed toward avoidance of a feared object or situation (*phobic disorder*)	**Fear**
Stays at home alone, afraid to venture out alone (*phobic disorder*)	**Social isolation**

TABLE 29-2 Assigning Nursing Diagnoses to Behaviors Commonly Associated with Anxiety Disorders—cont'd

BEHAVIORS	NURSING DIAGNOSES
Ritualistic behavior; obsessive thoughts, inability to meet basic needs; severe level of anxiety (*OCD*)	**Ineffective coping**
Inability to fulfill usual patterns of responsibility because of need to perform rituals (*OCD*).	**Ineffective role performance**
Flashbacks, intrusive recollections, nightmares, psychological numbness related to the event, dissociation, amnesia, anxiety, anger (*PTSD*).	**Post-trauma syndrome**
Irritability, explosiveness, self-destructiveness, substance abuse, verbalization of survival guilt or guilt about behavior required for survival (*PTSD*).	**Complicated grieving**

- Demonstrates more adaptive coping strategies for dealing with anxiety than ritualistic behaviors (*OCD*).
- Is experiencing fewer flashbacks, intrusive recollections, and nightmares (*PTSD*).
- Demonstrates adaptive coping strategies and verbalizes desire to put the trauma in the past and progress with his or her life (*PTSD*).

Planning/Implementation

The following section presents a group of selected nursing diagnoses, with short- and long-term goals and nursing interventions for each.

Some institutions are using a case management model to coordinate care (see Chapter 9 for more detailed explanation). In case management models, the plan of care may take the form of a critical pathway.

Anxiety (Panic)

Anxiety is defined as a "vague uneasy feeling of discomfort or dread accompanied by an autonomic response (the source often nonspecific or unknown to the individual); a feeling of apprehension caused by anticipation of danger. It is an alerting signal that warns of impending danger and enables the individual to take measures to deal with threat" (NANDA International [NANDA-I], 2009, p. 242).

Client Goals

Outcome criteria include short- and long-term goals. Timelines are individually determined.

Short-Term Goal

- The client will verbalize ways to intervene in escalating anxiety within 1 week.

Long-Term Goal

- By time of discharge from treatment, client will be able to recognize symptoms of onset of anxiety and intervene before reaching panic stage.

Interventions

- Do not leave a client who is experiencing panic anxiety alone. Stay with him or her and offer reassurance of safety and security. At this level of anxiety, clients often express a fear of dying or of "going crazy." They need the presence and assurance of their safety from a trusted individual.
- Maintain a calm, nonthreatening, matter-of-fact approach. Anxiety is contagious and can be transferred from staff to client or vice versa. The presence of a calm person provides a feeling of security to an anxious client.
- Use simple words and brief messages, spoken calmly and clearly, to explain hospital experiences to the client. In an intensely anxious situation, the client is unable to comprehend anything but the most elementary communication.
- Hyperventilation may occur during periods of extreme anxiety. Hyperventilation causes the amount of carbon dioxide (CO_2) in the blood to decrease, possibly resulting in lightheadedness, rapid heart rate, shortness of breath, numbness or tingling in the hands or feet, and syncope. If hyperventilation occurs, assist the client to breathe into a small paper bag held over the mouth and nose. Six to 12 natural breaths should be taken, alternating with short periods of diaphragmatic breathing. This technique should not be used with clients who have coronary or respiratory disorders, such as coronary artery disease, asthma, or chronic obstructive pulmonary disease.
- Keep the immediate surroundings low in stimuli (dim lighting, few people, simple decor). A stimulating environment may increase the level of anxiety.
- Administer tranquilizing medication, as ordered by the physician. Assess the medication for effectiveness and for adverse side effects.

■ When the level of anxiety has been reduced, explore with the client possible reasons for its occurrence. If the client is going to learn to interrupt escalating anxiety, he or she must first learn to recognize the factors that precipitate its onset.

■ Teach the client the signs and symptoms of escalating anxiety. Discuss ways to interrupt its progression, such as relaxation techniques, deep-breathing exercises, physical exercises, brisk walks, jogging, and meditation. The client will determine which method is most appropriate for him or her. Relaxation techniques result in a physiological response opposite that of the anxiety response, and physical activities discharge excess energy in a healthful manner.

Fear

Fear is defined as the "response to perceived threat that is consciously recognized as a danger" (NANDA-I, 2009, p. 261).

Client Goals

Outcome criteria include short- and long-term goals. Timelines are individually determined.

Short-Term Goal

■ Client will discuss the phobic object or situation with the health-care provider within (time specified).

Long-Term Goal

■ By time of discharge from treatment, client will be able to function in the presence of the phobic object or situation without experiencing panic anxiety.

Interventions

■ Explore the client's perception of threat to physical integrity or threat to self-concept. Reassure the client of his or her safety and security. It is important to understand the client's perception of the phobic object or situation in order to assist with the desensitization process.

■ Discuss the reality of the situation with the client in order to recognize aspects that can be changed and those that cannot. The client must accept the reality of the situation (aspects that cannot change) before the work of reducing the fear can progress. For example, a man who has a fear of flying and whose employment position requires long-distance air travel must accept that he needs to conquer the fear of flying if he is going to stay in this particular job.

■ Include the client in making decisions related to the selection of alternative coping strategies. For example, the client may choose either to avoid the phobic stimulus or to attempt to eliminate the fear associated with it. Encouraging the client to make choices promotes feelings of empowerment and serves to increase feelings of self-worth.

■ If the client elects to work on elimination of the fear, the techniques of systematic desensitization or implosion therapy may be employed. (See the explanation of these techniques under "Treatment Modalities" at the end of this chapter.) Systematic desensitization is a plan of behavior modification designed to expose the individual gradually to the situation or object (either in reality or through fantasizing) until the fear is no longer experienced. With implosion therapy, the individual is "flooded" with stimuli related to the phobic situation or object (rather than in gradual steps) until anxiety associated with the object or situation is no longer experienced. Fear is decreased as the physical and psychological sensations diminish in response to repeated exposure to the phobic stimulus under nonthreatening conditions.

■ Encourage the client to explore underlying feelings that may be contributing to irrational fears, and to face them rather than suppress them. Exploring underlying feelings may help the client to confront unresolved conflicts and develop more adaptive coping abilities.

Ineffective Coping

Ineffective coping is defined as the "inability to form a valid appraisal of the stressors, inadequate choices of practiced responses, and/or inability to use available resources" (NANDA-I, 2009, p. 254).

Client Goals

Outcome criteria include short- and long-term goals. Timelines are individually determined.

Short-Term Goal

■ Within 1 week, the client will decrease participation in ritualistic behavior by half.

Long-Term Goal

■ By the time of discharge from treatment, the client will demonstrate the ability to cope effectively without resorting to obsessive-compulsive behaviors or increased dependency.

Interventions

■ Work with the client to determine the types of situations that increase anxiety and result in ritualistic behaviors. If the client is going to learn to interrupt escalating anxiety, he or she must first learn to recognize the factors that precipitate its onset.

■ Initially meet the client's dependency needs as required. To suddenly and completely eliminate all avenues for dependency would create intense anxiety on the part of the client. Encourage independence and give positive reinforcement for independent behaviors. Positive reinforcement enhances self-esteem and may encourage repetition of the desired behaviors.

■ In the beginning of treatment, allow plenty of time for rituals. Do not be judgmental or verbalize disapproval of the behavior. To deny the client this activity may precipitate a panic level of anxiety.

■ Support the client's efforts to explore the meaning and purpose of the behavior. He or she is most likely unaware of the relationship between emotional problems and compulsive behaviors. Knowledge and recognition of this fact are important before change can occur.

■ Provide a structured schedule of activities for the client, including adequate time for the completion of rituals. The anxious individual needs a great deal of structure in his or her life. Assistance is needed with decision making, and structure provides a sense of security and comfort to deal with activities of daily living.

■ Gradually begin to limit the amount of time allotted for ritualistic behavior as the client becomes more involved in other activities. Anxiety is minimized when the client is able to replace ritualistic behaviors with more adaptive ones. Give positive reinforcement for nonritualistic behaviors.

■ Help the client learn ways of interrupting obsessive thoughts and ritualistic behaviors with techniques such as thought-stopping (see Chapter 15), relaxation techniques (see Chapter 14), physical exercise, or other constructive activity with which the client feels comfortable. Knowledge and practice of coping techniques that are more adaptive will help the client change and let go of maladaptive responses to anxiety.

Post-trauma Syndrome

Post-trauma syndrome is defined as a "sustained maladaptive response to a traumatic, overwhelming event" (NANDA-I, 2009, p. 237). Table 29-3 presents this nursing diagnosis in care plan format.

Client Goals

Outcome criteria include short- and long-term goals. Timelines are individually determined.

Table 29-3 CARE PLAN FOR THE CLIENT WITH POSTTRAUMATIC STRESS DISORDER

NURSING DIAGNOSIS: POST-TRAUMA SYNDROME′
RELATED TO: Distressing event considered to be outside the range of usual human experience
EVIDENCED BY: Flashbacks, intrusive recollections, nightmares, psychological numbness related to the event, dissociation, or amnesia

OUTCOME CRITERIA	NURSING INTERVENTIONS	RATIONALE
Short-Term Goals • Client will begin a healthy grief resolution, initiating the process of psychological healing (within time frame specific to individual). • Client will demonstrate ability to deal with emotional reactions in an individually appropriate manner.	1. a. Assign the same staff as often as possible. b. Use a nonthreatening, matter-of-fact, but friendly approach. c. Respect client's wishes regarding interaction with individuals of opposite sex at this time (especially important if the trauma was rape). d. Be consistent; keep all promises; convey acceptance; spend time with client. 2. Stay with client during periods of flashbacks and nightmares. Offer reassurance of safety and security and that these symptoms are not uncommon following a trauma of the magnitude he or she has experienced.	1. A post-trauma client may be suspicious of others in his or her environment. All of these interventions serve to facilitate a trusting relationship. 2. Presence of a trusted individual may calm fears for personal safety and reassure the anxious client that he or she is not "going crazy."

Continued

Table 29-3 CARE PLAN FOR THE CLIENT WITH POSTTRAUMATIC STRESS DISORDER—cont'd

OUTCOME CRITERIA	NURSING INTERVENTIONS	RATIONALE
Long-Term Goal • Client will integrate the traumatic experience into his or her persona, renew significant relationships, and establish meaningful goals for the future.	3. Obtain accurate history from significant others about the trauma and the client's specific response.	3. Various types of traumas elicit different responses in clients (e.g., human-engendered traumas often generate a greater degree of humiliation and guilt in victims than trauma associated with natural disasters).
	4. Encourage the client to talk about the trauma at his or her own pace. Provide a nonthreatening, private environment, and include a significant other if the client wishes. Acknowledge and validate client's feelings as they are expressed.	4. This debriefing process is the first step in the progression toward resolution.
	5. Discuss coping strategies used in response to the trauma, as well as those used during stressful situations in the past. Determine those that have been most helpful, and discuss alternative strategies for the future. Include available support systems, including religious and cultural influences. Identify maladaptive coping strategies (e.g., substance use, psychosomatic responses) and practice more adaptive coping strategies for possible future post-trauma responses.	5. Resolution of the post-trauma response is largely dependent on the effectiveness of the coping strategies employed.
	6. Assist the individual to try to comprehend the trauma if possible. Discuss feelings of vulnerability and the individual's "place" in the world following the trauma.	6. Post-trauma response is largely a function of the shattering of basic beliefs the victim holds about self and world. Assimilation of the event into one's persona requires that some degree of meaning associated with the event be incorporated into the basic beliefs, which will affect how the individual eventually comes to reappraise self and world (Epstein, 1991).

Short-Term Goals

■ The client will begin a healthy grief resolution, initiating the process of psychological healing (within time frame specific to individual).

■ The client will demonstrate ability to deal with emotional reactions in an individually appropriate manner.

Long-Term Goal

■ The client will integrate the traumatic experience into his or her persona, renew significant relationships, and establish meaningful goals for the future.

Interventions

■ A post-trauma client may be suspicious of others in his or her environment. Establishing a trusting relationship with this individual is essential before care can be given. To do this, assign the same staff as often as possible. Use a nonthreatening, matter-of-fact, but friendly approach. Respect the client's wishes regarding interaction with individuals of opposite sex at this time (especially important if the trauma was rape). Be consistent and keep all promises, and convey an attitude of unconditional acceptance.

■ Stay with the client during periods of flashbacks and nightmares. Offer reassurance of safety and security and that these symptoms are not uncommon following a trauma of the magnitude he or she has experienced. The presence of a trusted individual may help to calm fears for personal safety and reassure the anxious client that he or she is not "going crazy."

■ Obtain an accurate history from significant others about the trauma and the client's specific response. Various types of traumas elicit different responses in clients. For example, human-engendered traumas often generate a greater degree of humiliation and guilt in victims than trauma associated with natural disasters.

■ Encourage the client to talk about the trauma at his or her own pace. Provide a nonthreatening, private environment, and include a significant other if the client wishes. Acknowledge and validate the client's feelings as they are expressed. This debriefing process is the first step in the progression toward resolution.

■ Discuss coping strategies used in response to the trauma, as well as those used during stressful situations in the past. Determine those that have been most helpful, and discuss alternative strategies for the future. Include available support systems, including religious and cultural influences. Identify maladaptive coping strategies, such as substance use or psychosomatic responses, and practice more adaptive coping strategies for possible future post-trauma responses. Resolution of the post-trauma response is largely dependent on the effectiveness of the coping strategies employed.

■ Assist the individual to try to comprehend the trauma if possible. Discuss feelings of vulnerability and the individual's "place" in the world following the trauma. Post-trauma response is largely a function of the shattering of basic beliefs the victim holds about self and world. Assimilation of the event into one's persona requires that some degree of meaning associated with the event be incorporated into the basic beliefs, which will affect how the individual eventually comes to reappraise self and world (Epstein, 1991).

Concept Care Mapping

The concept map care plan is an innovative approach to planning and organizing nursing care (see Chapter 9). It is a diagrammatic teaching and learning strategy that allows visualization of interrelationships between medical diagnoses, nursing diagnoses, assessment data, and treatments. An example of a concept map care plan for the client with an anxiety disorder is presented in Figure 29–7.

Client/Family Education

The role of client teacher is important in the psychiatric area, as it is in all areas of nursing. A list of topics for client/family education relevant to anxiety disorders is presented in Box 29-7. Sample client teaching guides are presented in Appendix G.

Evaluation

In the final step of the nursing process, a reassessment is conducted in order to determine if the nursing actions have been successful in achieving the objectives of care. Evaluation of the nursing actions for the client with an anxiety disorder may be facilitated by gathering information utilizing the following types of questions:

■ Can the client recognize signs and symptoms of escalating anxiety?

■ Can the client use skills learned to interrupt the escalating anxiety before it reaches the panic level?

■ Can the client demonstrate the activities most appropriate for him or her that can be used to maintain anxiety at a manageable level (e.g., relaxation techniques; physical exercise)?

■ Can the client maintain anxiety at a manageable level without medication?

■ Can the client verbalize a long-term plan for preventing panic anxiety in the face of a stressful situation?

■ Can the client discuss the phobic object or situation without becoming anxious?

■ Can the client function in the presence of the phobic object or situation without experiencing panic anxiety?

■ Can the OCD client refrain from performing rituals when anxiety level rises?

■ Can the OCD client demonstrate substitute behaviors to maintain anxiety at a manageable level?

■ Does the OCD client recognize the relationship between escalating anxiety and the dependence on ritualistic behaviors for relief?

■ Can the PTSD client discuss the traumatic event without experiencing panic anxiety?

■ Can the PTSD client discuss changes that have occurred in his or her life because of the traumatic event?

■ Has the PTSD client learned new, adaptive coping strategies for assistance with recovery?

Clinical Vignette: During her senior year in college, Candice, now age 24, begun having panic attacks. All during her college years, she had experienced high anxiety, and spent time with a counselor because of severe test anxiety. The college physician prescribed buspirone 15 mg/day, which has been helpful and eased some of her symptoms. She married shortly after graduation and works as a website designer from her computer at home. She must visit clients in their offices several times a week. Lately, she has started having panic attacks when it is time to make her client visits. She tells the Psychiatric Nurse Practitioner at the mental health clinic, "Just thinking about leaving my house causes me panic. I have chest pains. I have trouble breathing. I get dizzy and feel like I'm going to pass out! My clients are getting upset with me for not keeping my appointments. I don't know what to do!" The nurse develops the following concept map care plan for Candice.

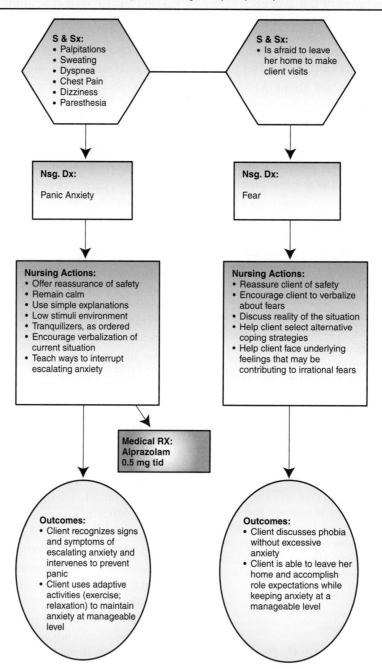

FIGURE 29–7 Concept map care plan for client with panic disorder with agoraphobia.

Treatment Modalities

Individual Psychotherapy

Most clients experience a marked lessening of anxiety when given the opportunity to discuss their difficulties with a concerned and sympathetic therapist. Sadock and Sadock (2007) stated:

[Insight-oriented psychotherapy] focuses on helping patients understand the hypothesized unconscious meaning of the anxiety,

---

BOX 29-7 Topics for Client/Family Education Related to Anxiety Disorders

NATURE OF THE ILLNESS
1. What is anxiety?
2. To what might it be related?
3. What is OCD?
4. What is PTSD?
5. Symptoms of anxiety disorders.

MANAGEMENT OF THE ILLNESS
1. Medication management:
   • Possible adverse effects
   • Length of time to take effect
   • What to expect from the medication
   a. For panic disorder and generalized anxiety disorder
      (1) Benzodiazepines
      (2) Buspirone (Buspar)
      (3) Tricyclics
      (4) SSRIs
      (5) SNRIs
      (6) Propranolol
      (7) Clonidine
   b. For phobic disorders
      (1) Benzodiazepines
      (2) Tricyclics
      (3) Propranolol
      (4) SSRIs
   c. For OCD
      (1) SSRIs
      (2) Clomipramine
   d. For PTSD
      (1) Tricyclics
      (2) SSRIs
      (3) MAOIs
      (4) Trazodone
      (5) Propranolol
      (6) Carbamazepine
      (7) Valproic acid
      (8) Lithium carbonate
2. Stress management
   a. Teach ways to interrupt escalating anxiety
      (1) Relaxation techniques (see Chapter 14)
         (a) Progressive muscle relaxation
         (b) Imagery
         (c) Music
         (d) Meditation
         (e) Yoga
         (f) Physical exercise

SUPPORT SERVICES
1. Crisis hotline
2. Support groups
3. Individual psychotherapy

---

the symbolism of the avoided situation, the need to repress impulses, and the secondary gains of the symptoms. (p. 596)

With continuous and regular contact with an interested, sympathetic, and encouraging professional person, patients may be able to function by virtue of this help, without which their symptoms would incapacitate them. (p. 612)

The psychotherapist also can use logical and rational explanations to increase the client's understanding about various situations that create anxiety in his or her life. Psychoeducational information may also be presented in individual psychotherapy.

Cognitive Therapy

The cognitive model relates how individuals respond in stressful situations to their subjective cognitive appraisal of the event. Anxiety is experienced when the cognitive appraisal is one of danger with which the individual perceives that he or she is unable to cope. Impaired cognition can contribute to anxiety disorders when the individual's appraisals are chronically negative. Automatic negative appraisals provoke self-doubts, negative evaluations, and negative predictions. Anxiety is maintained by this dysfunctional appraisal of a situation.

Cognitive therapy strives to assist the individual to reduce anxiety responses by altering cognitive distortions. Anxiety is described as being the result of exaggerated, *automatic* thinking.

Cognitive therapy for anxiety is brief and time limited, usually lasting from 5 to 20 sessions. Brief therapy discourages the client's dependency on the therapist, which is prevalent in anxiety disorders, and encourages the client's self-sufficiency.

A sound therapeutic relationship is a necessary condition for effective cognitive therapy. For the therapeutic process to occur, the client must be able to talk openly about fears and feelings. A major part of treatment consists of encouraging the client to face frightening situations to be able to view them realistically, and talking about them is one way of achieving this. Treatment is a collaborative effort between client and therapist.

Rather than offering suggestions and explanations, the therapist uses questions to encourage the client to correct his or her anxiety-producing thoughts. The client is encouraged to become aware of the thoughts, examine them for cognitive distortions, substitute more balanced thoughts, and eventually develop new patterns of thinking.

Cognitive therapy is very structured and orderly, which is important for the anxious client who is often confused and lacks self-assurance. The focus is on solving current problems. Together, the client and therapist work to identify and correct maladaptive thoughts and behaviors that maintain a problem and block its solution.

Cognitive therapy is based on education. The premise is that one develops anxiety because he or she has learned inappropriate ways of handling life experiences. The belief is that, with practice, individuals can learn more effective ways of responding to these experiences. Homework assignments, a central feature of cognitive therapy, provide an experimental, problem-solving approach to overcoming long-held anxieties. Through fulfillment of these personal "experiments," the effectiveness of specific strategies and techniques is determined.

Behavior Therapy

Two common forms of behavior therapy include **systematic desensitization** and **implosion therapy (flooding)**. They are commonly used to treat clients with phobic disorders and to modify stereotyped behavior of clients with PTSD. They have also been shown to be effective in a variety of other anxiety-producing situations.

Systematic Desensitization

In systematic desensitization, the client is gradually exposed to the phobic stimulus, either in a real or in an imagined situation. The concept was introduced by Joseph Wolpe in 1958, and is based on behavioral conditioning principles. Emphasis is placed on reciprocal inhibition or counterconditioning.

Reciprocal inhibition is described as the restriction of anxiety prior to the effort of reducing avoidance behavior. The rationale behind this concept is that, because relaxation is antagonistic to anxiety, individuals cannot be anxious and relaxed at the same time.

Systematic desensitization with reciprocal inhibition involves two main elements:

1. Training in relaxation techniques.
2. Progressive exposure to a hierarchy of fear stimuli while in the relaxed state.

The individual is instructed in the art of relaxation using techniques most effective for him or her (e.g., progressive relaxation, mental imagery, tense and relax, meditation). When the individual has mastered the relaxation technique, exposure to the phobic stimulus is initiated. He or she is asked to present a hierarchal arrangement of situations pertaining to the phobic stimulus in order from most disturbing to least disturbing. While in a state of maximum relaxation, the client may be asked to imagine the phobic stimulus. Initial exposure is focused on a concept of the phobic stimulus that produces the least amount of fear or anxiety. In subsequent sessions, the individual is gradually exposed to stimuli that are more fearful. Sessions may be executed in fantasy, in real-life *(in vivo)* situations, or sometimes in a combination of both. Following is a case study describing systematic desensitization.

CASE STUDY: SYSTEMATIC DESENSITIZATION

John was afraid to ride on elevators. He had been known to climb 24 flights of stairs in an office building to avoid riding the elevator. John's own insurance office had plans for moving the company to a high-rise building soon, with offices on the 32nd floor. John sought assistance from a therapist for help to treat this fear. He was taught to achieve a sense of calmness and well-being by using a combination of mental imagery and progressive relaxation techniques. In the relaxed state, John was initially instructed to imagine the entry level of his office building, with a clear image of the bank of elevators. In subsequent sessions, and always in the relaxed state, John progressed to images of walking onto an elevator, having the elevator door close after he had entered, riding the elevator to the 32nd floor, and emerging from the elevator once the doors were opened. The progression included being accompanied in the activities by the therapist and eventually accomplishing them alone.

Therapy for John also included *in vivo* sessions in which he was exposed to the phobic stimulus in real-life situations (always after achieving a state of relaxation). This technique, combining imagined and *in vivo* procedures, proved successful for John, and his employment in the high-rise complex was no longer in jeopardy because of his fear of elevators.

Implosion Therapy (Flooding)

Implosion therapy, or *flooding,* is a therapeutic process in which the client must imagine situations or participate in real-life situations that he or she finds extremely frightening, for a prolonged period of time. Relaxation training is not a part of this technique. Plenty of time must be allowed for these sessions because brief periods may be ineffective or even harmful. A session is terminated when the client responds with considerably less anxiety than at the beginning of the session.

In flooding, the therapist "floods" the client with information concerning situations that trigger anxiety in him or her. The therapist describes anxiety-provoking situations in vivid detail and is guided by the client's response; the more anxiety provoked, the more expedient is the therapeutic endeavor. The same theme is continued as long as it arouses anxiety. The therapy is continued until a topic no longer elicits inappropriate anxiety on the part of the client. Sadock and Sadock (2007) stated:

> Many patients refuse flooding because of the psychological discomfort involved. It is also contraindicated when intense anxiety would be hazardous to a patient (e.g., those with heart disease or fragile psychological adaptation). The technique works best with specific phobias. (p. 955)

A similar therapy, called *Prolonged Exposure Therapy* (PE) is also used in treatment of PTSD. It has four main parts: (1) education about the treatment, (2) breathing retraining for relaxation, (3) exposure to real-world situations related to the trauma, and (4) imagined exposure through repeated discussion about the trauma with a therapist.

Eye Movement Desensitization and Reprocessing

Eye movement desensitization and reprocessing (EMDR) is a type of psychotherapy that was developed in 1989 by psychologist Francine Shapiro. It "has evolved from a simple technique into an integrative psychotherapy approach with a theoretical model that emphasizes the brain's information processing system and memories of disturbing experiences as the basis of pathology" (Shapiro, 2007, p. 3). EMDR has been shown to be an effective therapy for PTSD and other trauma-related disorders. It has been used with other disorders, including depression, adjustment disorder, phobias, addictions, generalized anxiety disorder, and panic disorder. However, at present, EMDR has only been empirically validated for trauma-related disorders such as PTSD and acute stress disorder (Aetna Healthcare, 2011). EMDR is contraindicated in clients who have neurological impairments (e.g., seizure disorders), clients who are suicidal or experiencing psychosis, those with severe dissociative disorders or unstabile substance abuse, and those with detached retina or glaucoma (Center for Integrative Medicine, 2011).

The exact biological mechanisms by which EMDR achieves its therapeutic effects are unknown. Some studies have indicated that eye movements cause a decrease in imagery vividness and distress, as well as an increase in memory access. The process, which involves rapid eye movements while processing painful emotions, is thought to "relieve the anxiety associated with the trauma so that the original event can be examined from a more detached perspective, somewhat like watching a movie of what happened" (Bartson, Smith, & Corcoran, 2011). While concentrating on a particular emotion or physical sensation surrounding the traumatic event, the client is asked to focus his or her eye movements on the therapist's fingers as the therapist moves them from left to right and back again. Although some individuals report rapid results with this therapy, research has indicated that from 5 to 12 sessions are required to achieve lasting treatment effects. The treatment encompasses the following eight-phase process.

Phase 1: History and Treatment Planning In the first phase, the therapist takes a thorough history and develops a treatment plan. The problem for which the client is seeking treatment and current symptoms are discussed. However, the client is not required to discuss the traumatic event in detail, unless he or she chooses to do so. Instead, emphasis is placed on the emotions and physical sensations surrounding the traumatic event.

Phase 2: Preparation During this phase, the therapist teaches the client certain self-care techniques (e.g., relaxation techniques) for dealing with emotional disturbances that may arise during or between sessions. Self-care is an important component of EMDR. It is important for the client to develop a sense of trust in the therapist during this phase.

Phase 3: Assessment During this phase, the therapist asks the client to identify a specific scene or picture from the target event identified in phase 1 that best represents the memory. The client is then directed to express a negative self-belief associated with the memory (e.g., "I am bad" or "I'm in danger"). The next step is to identify a self-statement that he or she would *rather* believe (e.g., "I am good" or "I'm safe now"). When the self-statements have been identified, the client is asked to rate the validity of each of the statements on the Validity of Cognition (VOC) scale from "completely false" (a score of 1) to "completely true" (a score of 7). In this phase, the client is also asked to rank the disturbing emotions on the 0-to-10 Subjective Units of Disturbance (SUD) scale (with 0 meaning the disturbance is not disturbing at all and 10 meaning it is the worst feeling he or she has ever had).

Phase 4: Densensitization During this phase, the client gives attention to the negative beliefs and disturbing emotions associated with the traumatic event while focusing his or her vision on the back-and-forth motion of the therapist's finger. All personal feelings and physical reactions experienced during this time are noted. Following each set of rapid eye movements, the therapist reassesses the level of disturbance associated with the feelings, images, and beliefs. This desensitization process continues until the distress level (as measured by the SUD scale) is reduced to 0 or 1.

Phase 5: Installation In phase 5, the client gives attention to the positive belief that he or she has identified to replace the negative belief associated with the trauma. This is accomplished while simultaneously visually tracking the therapist's finger. Following each set of rapid eye movements, the client is asked to rate the positive belief on the VOC scale. The goal is to strengthen the positive belief or self-statement until it is accepted as completely true (a score of 7 on the VOC scale).

Phase 6: Body Scan When the positive cognition has been strengthened, the therapist asks the client to concentrate on any lingering physical sensations. While focusing on the traumatic event, the client is asked to identify any areas of the body where residual tension is experienced. Because positive self-beliefs must be believed on more than just an intellectual level, phase 6 is not complete until the client is able to think about or discuss the traumatic event (or the feelings associated with it) without experiencing bodily tension.

Phase 7: Closure Closure ensures that the client leaves each session feeling better than he or she felt at the beginning. If the processing that took place during the session is not complete, the therapist will direct the client through a variety of self-calming relaxation techniques to help him or her regain emotional equilibrium. The client is briefed about what to expect between sessions. Until processing of the trauma is complete, disturbing images, thoughts, and emotions may arise between

therapy sessions. The therapist instructs the client to record these experiences in a journal so that they may be used as targets for processing in future therapy sessions.

Phase 8: Reevaluation Reevaluation begins each new therapy session. The therapist assesses whether the positive changes have been maintained, determines if previous target areas need reprocessing, and identifies any new target areas that need attention.

Clients often feel relief quite rapidly with EMDR. However, to achieve lasting results, it is important that each of the eight phases be completed. Treatment is not complete until "EMDR therapy has focused on the past memories that are contributing to the problem, the present situations that are disturbing, and what skills the client may need for the future" (EMDR Network, 2011).

Group/Family Therapy

Group therapy has been strongly advocated for clients with PTSD. It has proved especially effective with military veterans (Sadock & Sadock, 2007). The importance of being able to share their experiences with empathetic fellow veterans, to talk about problems in social adaptation, and to discuss options for managing their aggression toward others has been emphasized. Some PTSD groups are informal and leaderless, such as self-help or support groups, and some are led by experienced group therapists who may have had some first-hand experience with the trauma. Some groups involve family members, thereby recognizing that the symptoms of PTSD may also severely affect them. Hollander and Simeon (2008) stated:

> Because of past experiences, [clients with PTSD] are often mistrustful and reluctant to depend on authority figures, whereas the identification, support, and hopefulness of peer settings can facilitate therapeutic change. (p. 579)

Psychopharmacology

Antianxiety Agents

Antianxiety drugs are also called *anxiolytics* and *minor tranquilizers*. Examples of commonly used antianxiety agents are presented in Table 29-4.

Indications

Antianxiety agents are used in the treatment of anxiety disorders, anxiety symptoms, acute alcohol withdrawal, skeletal muscle spasms, convulsive

TABLE 29-4 Antianxiety Agents

CHEMICAL CLASS	GENERIC NAME (TRADE)	CONTROLLED CATEGORIES	PREGNANCY CATEGORIES/ HALF-LIFE (HR)	DAILY ADULT DOSAGE RANGE (MG)	COMMON SIDE EFFECTS OF ANTIANXIETY AGENTS
Antihistamines	Hydroxyzine (Vistaril)		C (3)	100–400	■ Drowsiness, confusion, lethargy
Benzodiazepines	Alprazolam (Xanax)	C IV	D (6.3–26.9)	0.75–4	■ Tolerance; physical and psychological dependence (does not apply to Buspirone). Client should be tapered off long-term use.
	Chlordia- zepoxide (Librium)	C IV	D (5–30)	15–100	
	Clonazepam (Klonopin)	C IV	C (18–50)	1.5–20	■ Potentiates the effects of other CNS depressants. Client should not take alco- hol or other CNS depressants with the medication.
	Clorazepate (Tranxene)	C IV	D (40–50)	15–60	
	Diazepam (Valium)	C IV	D (20–80)	4–40	
	Lorazepam (Ativan)	C IV	D (10–20)	2–6	
	Oxazepam	C IV	D (5–20)	30–120	
Carbamate derivative	Meprobamate	C IV	D (6-17)	400–1600	■ May aggravate symp- toms of depression.
Azaspirodecanedione	Buspirone (BuSpar)		B (2–3)	15–60	■ Orthostatic hypoten- sion. Client should rise slowly from lying or sitting position.

Continuation of side effects column for Buspirone:

■ Paradoxical excite- ment. If symptoms opposite of desired effect occur, notify physician immediately.

■ Dry mouth

■ Nausea and vomit- ing. May be taken with food or milk.

■ Blood dyscrasias. Symptoms of sore throat, fever, malaise, easy bruising, or unusual bleeding should be reported to the physician immediately.

■ Delayed onset (with Buspirone). Lag time of 10 to 14 days for anxiety symptoms to diminish with bus- pirone. Buspirone is not recommended for prn administration disorders, status epilepticus, and preoperative sedation. Their use and efficacy for periods greater than 4 months have not been evaluated.

Action

Antianxiety drugs depress subcortical levels of the CNS, particularly the limbic system and reticular formation. They may potentiate the effects of the powerful inhibitory neurotransmitter gamma-aminobutyric acid (GABA) in the brain, thereby producing a calmative effect. All levels of CNS depression can be affected, from mild sedation to hypnosis to coma.

> **NOTE:** Buspirone (BuSpar) does not depress the CNS. Although its action is unknown, the drug is believed to produce the desired effects through interactions with serotonin, dopamine, and other neurotransmitter receptors.

Contraindications/Precautions

Antianxiety drugs are contraindicated in individuals with known hypersensitivity to any of the drugs within the classification (e.g., benzodiazepines). They should not be taken in combination with other CNS depressants and are contraindicated in pregnancy and lactation, narrow-angle glaucoma, shock, and coma.

Caution should be taken in administering these drugs to elderly or debilitated clients and clients with hepatic or renal dysfunction. (The dosage usually has to be decreased.) Caution is also required with individuals who have a history of drug abuse or addiction and with those who are depressed or suicidal. In depressed clients, CNS depressants can exacerbate symptoms.

Interactions

Increased effects of antianxiety agents can occur when taken concomitantly with alcohol, barbiturates, narcotics, antipsychotics, antidepressants, antihistamines, neuromuscular blocking agents, cimetidine, or disulfiram. Increased effects can also occur with herbal depressants (e.g., kava kava; valerian). Decreased effects can be noted with cigarette smoking and caffeine consumption.

Medications for Specific Disorders

For Panic and Generalized Anxiety Disorders

Anxiolytics The benzodiazepines have been used with success in the treatment of generalized anxiety disorder. They can be prescribed on an as-needed basis when the client is feeling particularly anxious. Alprazolam, lorazepam, and clonazepam have been particularly effective in the treatment of panic disorder. The major risks with benzodiazepine therapy are physical dependence and tolerance, which may

encourage abuse. Because withdrawal symptoms can be life threatening, clients must be warned against abrupt discontinuation of the drug and should be tapered off the medication at the end of therapy. Because of this addiction potential, the benzodiazepines have been surpassed as first-line choice of treatment by the selective serotonin reuptake inhibitors (SSRIs), the serotonin and norepinephrine reuptake inhibitors (SNRIs), and buspirone.

The antianxiety agent buspirone (BuSpar) is effective in about 60 to 80 percent of clients with generalized anxiety disorder (Sadock & Sadock, 2007). One disadvantage of buspirone is its 10- to 14-day delay in alleviating symptoms. However, the benefit of lack of physical dependence and tolerance with buspirone may make it the drug of choice in the treatment of generalized anxiety disorder.

Antidepressants Several antidepressants are effective as major antianxiety agents. The tricyclic antidepressants clomipramine and imipramine have been used with success in clients experiencing panic disorder. However, since the advent of SSRIs, the tricyclics are less widely used because of their tendency to produce severe side effects at the high doses required to relieve symptoms of panic disorder.

The SSRIs have been effective in the treatment of panic disorder. Paroxetine, fluoxetine, and sertraline have been approved by the U.S. Food and Drug Administration (FDA) for this purpose. The dosage of these drugs must be titrated slowly because clients with panic disorder appear to be sensitive to the overstimulation caused by SSRIs.

The use of antidepressants in the treatment of generalized anxiety disorder is still being investigated. Some success has been reported with the tricyclic imipramine and with the SSRIs. The FDA has approved paroxetine, escitalopram, duloxetine, and extended-release venlafaxine in the treatment of generalized anxiety disorder. Complete information about antidepressants is presented in Chapter 27.

Antihypertensive Agents Several studies have called attention to the effectiveness of beta blockers (e.g., propranolol) and alpha$_2$-adrenoreceptor agonists (e.g., clonidine) in the amelioration of anxiety symptoms (Hollander & Simeon, 2008). Propranolol has potent effects on the somatic manifestations of anxiety (e.g., palpitations, tremors), with less dramatic effects on the psychic component of anxiety. It appears to be most effective in the treatment of acute situational anxiety (e.g., performance anxiety; test anxiety), but it is not the first-line drug of choice in the treatment of panic disorder and generalized anxiety disorder.

Clonidine is effective in blocking the acute anxiety effects in conditions such as opioid and nicotine withdrawal. However, it has had limited usefulness in the long-term treatment of panic and generalized anxiety disorders, particularly because of the development of tolerance to its antianxiety effects.

For Phobic Disorders

Anxiolytics The benzodiazepines have been successful in the treatment of social phobia (Hollander & Simeon, 2008). Controlled studies have shown the efficacy of alprazolam and clonazepam in reducing symptoms of social anxiety. Both are well tolerated and have a rapid onset of action. However, because of their potential for abuse and dependence, they are not considered the first-line choice of treatment for social phobia.

Antidepressants The tricyclic imipramine and the monoamine oxidase inhibitor (MAOI) phenelzine have been effective in diminishing symptoms of agoraphobia and social phobia. In recent years, the SSRIs have become the first-line treatment of choice for social phobia. The SSRIs paroxetine and sertraline have been approved by the FDA for the treatment of social anxiety disorder. Additional clinical trials have also indicated efficacy with other antidepressants, including nefazodone, venlafaxine, and bupropion. Specific phobias are generally not treated with medication unless panic attacks accompany the phobia.

Antihypertensive Agents The beta blockers propranolol and atenolol have been tried with success in clients experiencing anticipatory performance anxiety or "stage fright" (Hollander & Simeon, 2008). This type of phobic response produces symptoms such as sweaty palms, racing pulse, trembling hands, dry mouth, labored breathing, nausea, and memory loss. The beta blockers appear to be quite effective in reducing these symptoms in some individuals.

For Obsessive-Compulsive Disorder

Antidepressants The SSRIs fluoxetine, paroxetine, sertraline, and fluvoxamine have been approved by the FDA for the treatment of OCD. Doses in excess of what is effective for treating depression may be required for OCD. Common side effects include sleep disturbances, headache, and restlessness. These effects are often transient, and

are less troublesome than those of the tricyclics.

The tricyclic antidepressant clomipramine was the first drug approved by the FDA in the treatment of OCD. Clomipramine is more selective for serotonin reuptake than any of the other tricyclics. Its efficacy in the treatment of OCD is well established, although the adverse effects, such as those associated with all the tricyclics, may make it less desirable than the SSRIs.

For Posttraumatic Stress Disorder

Antidepressants The SSRIs are now considered the first-line treatment of choice for PTSD because of their efficacy, tolerability, and safety ratings (Sadock & Sadock, 2007). Paroxetine and sertraline have been approved by the FDA for this purpose. The tricyclic antidepressants (e.g., amitriptyline and imipramine), the MAO inhibitors (e.g., phenelzine), and trazodone have also been effective in the treatment of PTSD.

Anxiolytics Alprazolam has been prescribed for PTSD clients for its antidepressant and antipanic effects. Other benzodiazepines have also been used, despite the absence of controlled studies demonstrating their efficacy in PTSD. Their addictive properties make them less desirable than some of the other medications in the treatment of posttrauma patients.

Buspirone, which has serotonergic properties similar to the SSRIs, may also be useful. Further controlled trials with this drug are needed to validate its efficacy in treating PTSD.

Antihypertensives The beta blocker propranolol and the alpha$_2$-adrenoreceptor agonist clonidine have been successful in alleviating some of the symptoms associated with PTSD. In clinical trials, marked reductions in nightmares, intrusive recollections, hypervigilance, insomnia, startle responses, and angry outbursts were reported with the use of these drugs (Hollander & Simeon, 2008).

Other Medications Carbamazepine, valproic acid, and lithium carbonate have been reported to alleviate symptoms of intrusive recollections, flashbacks, nightmares, impulsivity, irritability, and violent behavior in PTSD clients. Sadock and Sadock (2007) reported that little positive evidence exists concerning the use of antipsychotics in PTSD. They suggested that these drugs "should be reserved for the short-term control of severe aggression and agitation" (p. 621).

CASE STUDY AND SAMPLE CARE PLAN

NURSING HISTORY AND ASSESSMENT

Karen is a 34-year-old mother of a 7-year-old girl named April. Karen's husband, Jake, brought her to the emergency department when she began complaining of chest pain and shortness of breath. Diagnostic testing ruled out cardiac problems, and Karen was referred for psychiatric evaluation. Jake is present at the admission interview. He explained to the nurse that Karen has become increasingly "nervous and high-strung" over the past few years. Four years ago, April, then 3 years old, was attending nursery school 2 days a week. April came down with a very severe case of influenza that developed into pneumonia. She was hospitalized and her prognosis was questionable for a short while, although she eventually made a complete recovery. Since that time, however, Karen has been extremely anxious about her family's health. She is fastidious about housekeeping, and scrubs her floors three times a week. She launders the bedclothes daily, and uses bleach on all the countertops and door handles several times a day. She washes the woodwork twice a week. She washes her hands incessantly, and they are red and noticeably chapped. Jake explained that Karen becomes very upset if she is not able to perform all of her cleaning "chores" according to her self-assigned schedule. This afternoon, April came home from school with a note from the teacher saying that a child in April's class had been diagnosed with a case of meningitis. Jake told the nurse, "Karen just lost it. She got all upset and started crying and had trouble breathing. Then she got those pains in her chest. That's when I brought her to the hospital." Karen is admitted to the psychiatric unit with a diagnosis of Obsessive-Compulsive Disorder. The physician orders alprazolam 0.5 mg tid and paroxetine 20 mg every morning.

The night nurse finds her up at 2 a.m. scrubbing the shower with a hand towel. She refuses to sleep in the bed, stating that it must certainly be contaminated. When the day nurse makes morning rounds, she finds Karen in the bathroom washing her hands.

NURSING DIAGNOSES/OUTCOME IDENTIFICATION

From the assessment data, the nurse develops the following nursing diagnoses for Karen:

1. **Panic anxiety** related to perceived threat to biological integrity evidenced by chest pain and shortness of breath.
   a. **Short-Term Goal:** Client will be able to relax with effects of medication.
   b. **Long-Term Goal:** Client will be able to maintain anxiety at manageable level.

2. **Ineffective coping** related to panic anxiety and weak ego strength evidenced by compulsive cleaning and washing hands.
   a. **Short-Term Goal:** Client will reduce amount of time performing rituals within 3 days.
   b. **Long-Term Goal:** Client will demonstrate ability to cope effectively without resorting to ritualistic behavior.

PLANNING/IMPLEMENTATION

Panic Anxiety

The following nursing interventions have been identified for Karen.

1. Stay with Karen and reassure her that she is safe and that she is not going to die.
2. Maintain a calm, nonthreatening manner with Karen.
3. Speak very clearly and calmly, and use simple words and messages to communicate with Karen.
4. Keep the lights low, the noise level down as much as possible, and as few people in her environment as is necessary.
5. Administer the alprazolam and paroxetine as ordered by the physician. Monitor for effectiveness and side effects.
6. After several days, when the anxiety has subsided, discuss with her the reasons that precipitated this attack.
7. Teach her the signs that indicate her anxiety level is rising.
8. Teach strategies that she may employ to interrupt the escalation of the anxiety. She could choose which is best for her: relaxation exercises, physical exercise, meditation.

Ineffective Coping

The following nursing interventions have been identified for Karen.

1. Initially, allow Karen all the time she needs to wash her hands, straighten up her room, change her own sheets, etc. To deny her these rituals would result in panic anxiety.
2. Initiate discussions with Karen about her behavior. She ultimately must come to understand that these rituals are her way of keeping her anxiety under control.
3. Within a couple of days, begin to limit the amount of time Karen may spend on her rituals. Assign her to groups and activities that take up her time and distract her from her obsessions.

CASE STUDY AND SAMPLE CARE PLAN—cont'd

4. Explore with Karen the types of situations that cause her anxiety to rise. Help her to correlate these times of increased anxiety to initiation of the ritualistic behavior.

5. Help her with problem solving and with making decisions about more adaptive ways to respond to situations that cause her anxiety to rise.

6. Explore her fears surrounding the health of her daughter. Help her to recognize which fears are legitimate and which are irrational.

7. Discuss possible activities in which she may participate that may distract from obsessions about contamination. Make suggestions, and encourage her to follow through. Examples may include enrollment in classes at the local community college, volunteer work at the local hospital, or part-time employment.

8. Explain to her that she will likely be discharged from the hospital with a prescription for paroxetine. Teach her about the medication, how it should be taken,

possible side effects, and what to report to the physician.

9. Suggest that she may benefit from attendance in an anxiety disorder support group. If she is interested, help locate one that would be convenient and appropriate for her.

EVALUATION

The outcome criteria for Karen have been met. She has remained calm during her hospital stay with the use of the medication. The use of ritualistic behavior in the hospital setting diminished rapidly. She has discussed situations that she knows cause her anxiety to rise. She has learned relaxation exercises and practices them daily. She plans to start jogging and has the phone number for an anxiety support group that she plans to call. She says that she hopes the support group will help her maintain rationality about her daughter's health. She knows about paroxetine and plans to take it every morning.

Summary and Key Points

■ Anxiety is a necessary force for survival and has been experienced by humanity throughout the ages.

■ Anxiety was first described as a physiological disorder and identified by its physical symptoms, particularly the cardiac symptoms. The psychological implications for the symptoms were not recognized until the early 1900s.

■ Anxiety is considered a normal reaction to a realistic danger or threat to biological integrity or self-concept.

■ Normality of the anxiety experienced in response to a stressor is defined by societal and cultural standards.

■ Anxiety disorders are more common in women than in men by at least 2 to 1.

■ Studies of familial patterns suggest that a familial predisposition to anxiety disorders probably exists.

■ The *DSM-IV-TR* identifies several broad categories of anxiety disorders. They include panic and generalized anxiety disorders, phobic disorders, OCD, PTSD, anxiety disorder due to a general medical condition, and substance-induced anxiety disorder.

■ Panic disorder is characterized by recurrent panic attacks, the onsets of which are unpredictable and manifested by intense apprehension, fear, and physical discomfort.

■ Generalized anxiety disorder is characterized by chronic, unrealistic, and excessive anxiety and worry.

■ Social phobia is an excessive fear of situations in which a person might do something embarrassing or be evaluated negatively by others.

■ Specific phobia is a marked, persistent, and excessive or unreasonable fear when in the presence of, or when anticipating an encounter with, a specific object or situation.

■ Agoraphobia is a fear of being in places or situations from which escape might be difficult or in which help might not be available in the event that the person becomes anxious.

■ OCD involves recurrent obsessions or compulsions that are severe enough to interfere with social and occupational functioning.

■ PTSD is the development of characteristic symptoms following exposure to an extreme traumatic stressor involving a personal threat to physical integrity or to the integrity of others.

■ A number of elements, including psychosocial factors, biological influences, and learning experiences, most likely contribute to the development of these disorders.

■ Treatment of anxiety disorders include individual psychotherapy, cognitive therapy, behavior therapy, group and family therapy, and psychopharmacology

■ Common behavior therapies include systematic desensitization and implosion therapy (flooding).

■ Nurses can help clients with anxiety disorders gain insight and increase self-awareness in relation to their illness.

■ Intervention focuses on assisting clients to learn techniques with which they may interrupt the escalation of anxiety before it reaches unmanageable proportions, and to replace maladaptive behavior patterns with new, more adaptive, coping skills.

 Additional info available @ davisplus.fadavis.com

Review Questions
Self-Examination/Learning Exercise

*Select the answer that is **most** appropriate for each of the following questions:*

1. Ms. T. has been diagnosed with agoraphobia. Which behavior would be most characteristic of this disorder?
   a. Ms. T. experiences panic anxiety when she encounters snakes.
   b. Ms. T. refuses to fly in an airplane.
   c. Ms. T. will not eat in a public place.
   d. Ms. T. stays in her home for fear of being in a place from which she cannot escape.

2. Which of the following is the most appropriate therapy for a client with agoraphobia?
   a. 10 mg Valium qid.
   b. Group therapy with other agoraphobics.
   c. Facing her fear in gradual step progression.
   d. Hypnosis.

3. With implosion therapy, a client with phobic anxiety would be:
   a. Taught relaxation exercises.
   b. Subjected to graded intensities of the fear.
   c. Instructed to stop the therapeutic session as soon as anxiety is experienced.
   d. Presented with massive exposure to a variety of stimuli associated with the phobic object/ situation.

4. A client with OCD spends many hours each day washing her hands. The most likely reason she washes her hands so much is that it:
   a. Relieves her anxiety.
   b. Reduces the probability of infection.
   c. Gives her a feeling of control over her life.
   d. Increases her self-concept.

5. The *initial* care plan for a client with OCD who washes her hands obsessively would include which of the following nursing interventions?
   a. Keep the client's bathroom locked so she cannot wash her hands all the time.
   b. Structure the client's schedule so that she has plenty of time for washing her hands.
   c. Place the client in isolation until she promises to stop washing her hands so much.
   d. Explain the client's behavior to her, since she is probably unaware that it is maladaptive.

6. Sandy, a client with OCD, says to the nurse, "I've been here 4 days now, and I'm feeling better. I feel comfortable on this unit, and I'm not ill-at-ease with the staff or other patients anymore." In light of this change, which nursing intervention is most appropriate?
   a. Give attention to the ritualistic behaviors each time they occur and point out their inappropriateness.
   b. Ignore the ritualistic behaviors, and they will be eliminated for lack of reinforcement.
   c. Set limits on the amount of time Sandy may engage in the ritualistic behavior.
   d. Continue to allow Sandy all the time she wants to carry out the ritualistic behavior.

7. John, a veteran of the war in Iraq, is diagnosed with PTSD. He says to the nurse, "I can't figure out why God took my buddy instead of me." From this statement, the nurse assesses which of the following in John?
   a. Repressed anger.
   b. Survivor's guilt.
   c. Intrusive thoughts.
   d. Spiritual distress.

8. John, a veteran of the war in Iraq, is diagnosed with PTSD. He experiences a nightmare during his first night in the hospital. He explains to the nurse that he was dreaming about gunfire all around and people being killed. The nurse's most appropriate *initial* intervention is to:
   a. Administer alprazolam as ordered prn for anxiety.
   b. Call the physician and report the incident.
   c. Stay with John and reassure him of his safety.
   d. Have John listen to a tape of relaxation exercises.

9. John, a veteran of the war in Iraq, is diagnosed with PTSD. Which of the following therapy regimens would most appropriately be ordered for John?
   a. Paroxetine and group therapy.
   b. Diazepam and implosion therapy.
   c. Alprazolam and behavior therapy.
   d. Carbamazepine and cognitive therapy.

10. Which of the following may be influential in the predisposition to PTSD?
    a. Unsatisfactory parent-child relationship.
    b. Excess of the neurotransmitter serotonin.
    c. Distorted, negative cognitions.
    d. Severity of the stressor and availability of support systems.

TEST YOUR CRITICAL THINKING SKILLS

Susan, age 29, was taken to the emergency department by her friends. They were at a dinner party when Susan suddenly clasped her chest and started having difficulty breathing. She complained of nausea and was perspiring profusely. She had calmed down some by the time they reached the hospital. She denied any pain, and electrocardiogram and laboratory results were unremarkable.

Susan told the admitting nurse that she had a history of these "attacks." She began having them in her sophomore year of college. She knew her parents had expectations that she should follow in their footsteps and become an attorney. They also expected her to earn grades that would promote acceptance by a top Ivy League university. Susan experienced her first attack when she made a "B" in English during her third semester of college. Since that time, she has experienced these symptoms sporadically, often in conjunction with her perception of the need to excel. She graduated with top honors from Harvard.

Last week Susan was promoted within her law firm. She was assigned her first solo case of representing a couple whose baby had died at birth and who were suing the physician for malpractice. She has experienced these panic symptoms daily for the past week, stating, "I feel like I'm going crazy!"

Susan is transferred to the psychiatric unit. The psychiatrist diagnoses Panic Disorder Without Agoraphobia.

Answer the following questions related to Susan:

1. What would be the priority nursing diagnosis for Susan?

2. What is the priority nursing intervention with Susan?

3. What medical treatment might you expect the physician to prescribe?

References

Aetna Healthcare. (2011). *Clinical policy bulletin: Eye movement desensitization and Reprocessing (EMDR) therapy.* Retrieved May 3, 2011, from http://www.aetna.com/cpb/medical/data/500_599/0583.html

American Psychiatric Association. (2000). *Diagnostic and statistical manual of mental disorders* (4th ed.). *Text revision.* Washington, DC: American Psychiatric Publishing.

Bartson, S., Smith, M., & Corcoran, C. (2011). *EMDR therapy: A guide to making an informed choice.* Retrieved May 3, 2011, from http://www.helpguide.org/mental/pdf/emdr.pdf

@ INTERNET REFERENCES

- Additional information about anxiety disorders and medications to treat these disorders may be located at the following websites:
  - http://www.adaa.org/
  - http://www.mentalhealth.com/
  - http://www.nami.org/
  - http://www.nimh.nih.gov/
  - http://www.anxietynetwork.com/pdhome.html
  - http://www.psychiatrymatters.md/
  - http://www.fadavis.com/townsend

Center for Integrative Medicine. (2011). *Eye movement desensitization and reprocessing.* Retrieved May 3, 2011, from http://www.upmc.com/Services/integrative-medicine/outpatient-services/Pages/eye-movement.aspx

EMDR Network. (2011). *A brief description of EMDR therapy: Eight phases of treatment.* Retrieved May 3, 2011, from http://www.emdrnetwork.org/description.html

Epstein, S. (1991). Beliefs and symptoms in maladaptive resolutions of the traumatic neurosis. In D. Ozer, J. M. Healy, Jr., & A. J. Stewart (Eds.), *Perspectives on personality* (Vol. 3). London: Jessica Kingsley.

Hageman, I., Anderson, H. S., & Jergensen, M. B. (2001). Post-traumatic stress disorder: A review of psychobiology and pharmacotherapy. *Acta Psychiatrica Scandinavica, 104,* 411–422.

Harvard Medical School. (2006). *Coping with anxiety and phobias.* Boston, MA: Harvard Health Publications.

Hollander, E., & Simeon, D. (2008). Anxiety disorders. In R. E. Hales, S. C. Yudofsky, & G. O. Gabbard (Eds.), *Textbook of psychiatry* (5th ed., pp. 505–607). Washington, DC: American Psychiatric Publishing.

Johnson, M. (1994, May/June). Stage fright. From *Performing Songwriter 1*(6). Retrieved September 17, 2010, from http://www.mjblue.com/pfright.html

NANDA International. (2009). *Nursing diagnoses: Definitions and classification 2009–2011.* Hoboken, NJ: Wiley-Blackwell.

National Mental Health Association. (2005). *Children with emotional disorders in the juvenile justice system.* Alexandria, VA: Author.

Rowney, J., Hermida, T., & Malone, D. (2010). Anxiety disorders. In W. D. Carey (Ed.), *Current clinical medicine* (2nd ed., pp. 944–948). Philadelphia: Saunders Elsevier.

Sadock, B. J., & Sadock, V. A. (2007). *Synopsis of psychiatry: Behavioral sciences/clinical psychiatry* (10th ed.). Philadelphia: Lippincott Williams & Wilkins.

Shahrokh, N. C., & Hales, R. E. (2003). *American psychiatric glossary.* Washington, DC: American Psychiatric Publishing.

Shapiro, F. (2007). EMDR and case conceptualization from an adaptive information processing perspective. In F. Shapiro, F. W. Kaslow, & L. Maxfield (Eds.), *Handbook of EMDR and family therapy processes* (pp. 3–34). Hoboken, NJ: John Wiley & Sons.

Classical References

Freud, S. (1959). On the grounds for detaching a particular syndrome from neurasthenia under the description 'anxiety neurosis.' In *The standard edition of the complete psychological works of Sigmund Freud* (Vol. 3). London: Hogarth Press.

Johnson, J. H., & Sarason, I. B. (1978). Life stress, depression and anxiety: Internal-external control as moderator variable. *Journal of Psychosomatic Research, 22,* 205–208.

MOVIE CONNECTIONS

As Good As It Gets (OCD) • *The Aviator* (OCD) • *What About Bob?* (phobias) • *Copycat* (agoraphobia) • *Analyze This* (panic disorder) • *Vertigo* (specific phobia) • *Born on the Fourth of July* (PTSD) • *The Deer Hunter* (PTSD)

Somatoform and Dissociative Disorders

CORE CONCEPTS

amnesia
dissociation
hysteria
somatization

KEY TERMS

abreaction
anosmia
aphonia
depersonalization
derealization

fugue
hypochondriasis
integration
la belle indifference
primary gain

pseudocyesis
secondary gain
tertiary gain

OBJECTIVES

After reading this chapter, the student will be able to:

1. Discuss historical aspects and epidemiological statistics related to somatoform and dissociative disorders.
2. Describe various types of somatoform and dissociative disorders and identify symptomatology associated with each; use this information in client assessment.
3. Identify predisposing factors in the development of somatoform and dissociative disorders.
4. Formulate nursing diagnoses and goals of care for clients with somatoform and dissociative disorders.
5. Describe appropriate nursing interventions for behaviors associated with somatoform and dissociative disorders.
6. Evaluate the nursing care of clients with somatoform and dissociative disorders.
7. Discuss various modalities relevant to treatment of somatoform and dissociative disorders.

HOMEWORK ASSIGNMENT

Please read the chapter and answer the following questions:

1. Past experience with serious or life-threatening physical illness, either personal or that of a close family member, can predispose an individual to what somatoform disorder?
2. In an individual with dissociative identity disorder, what most commonly precipitates transition from one personality to another?
3. Conversion symptoms most commonly occur in an individual for what reason?
4. Somatoform and dissociative disorders are the physical/behavioral responses to what unconscious phenomenon?

Somatoform disorders are characterized by physical symptoms suggesting medical disease, but without demonstrable organic pathology or a known pathophysiological mechanism to account for them. They are classified as mental disorders because pathophysiological processes are not demonstrable or understandable by existing laboratory procedures, and there is either evidence or

669

strong presumption that psychological factors are the major cause of the symptoms. It is now well documented that a large proportion of clients in general medical outpatient clinics and private medical offices do not have organic disease requiring medical treatment. It is likely that many of these clients have somatoform disorders, but they do not perceive themselves as having a psychiatric problem and thus do not seek treatment from psychiatrists.

Dissociative disorders are defined by a disruption in the usually integrated functions of consciousness, memory, identity, or perception (American Psychiatric Association [APA], 2000). Dissociative responses occur when anxiety becomes overwhelming and the personality becomes disorganized. Defense mechanisms that normally govern consciousness, identity, and memory break down, and behavior occurs with little or no participation on the part of the conscious personality. Four types of dissociative disorders are described by the *Diagnostic and Statistical Manual of Mental Disorders* (DSM-IV-TR): dissociative amnesia, dissociative fugue, dissociative identity disorder, and depersonalization disorder.

This chapter focuses on disorders characterized by severe anxiety that has been repressed and is being expressed in the form of physiological symptoms and dissociative behaviors. Historical and epidemiological statistics are presented. Predisposing factors that have been implicated in the etiology of these responses provide a framework for studying the dynamics of somatoform and dissociative disorders. An explanation of the symptomatology of these disorders is presented as background knowledge for assessing the client, and nursing care is described in the context of the nursing process. Additional treatment modalities are explored.

Historical Aspects

> ### CORE CONCEPT
>
> #### Hysteria
>
> A polysymptomatic disorder that usually begins in adolescence (rarely after the 20s), chiefly affects women, and is characterized by recurrent multiple somatic complaints that are unexplained by organic pathology. It is thought to be associated with repressed anxiety.

Historically, somatoform disorders have been identified as *hysterical neuroses*. The concept of hysteria is at least 4,000 years old and probably originated in Egypt. The name has been in use since the time of Hippocrates.

Over the years, symptoms of hysterical neuroses have been associated with witchcraft, demonology, and sorcery; dysfunction of the nervous system; and unexpressed emotion. Somatoform disorders are thought to occur in response to repressed severe anxiety. Freud observed that, under hypnosis, clients with hysterical neurosis could recall past memories and emotional experiences that would relieve their symptoms. This led to his proposal that unexpressed emotion can be "converted" into physical symptoms.

> ### CORE CONCEPT
>
> #### Dissociation
>
> The splitting off of clusters of mental contents from conscious awareness, a mechanism central to hysterical conversion and dissociative disorder (Shahrokh & Hales, 2003).

Freud (1962) viewed dissociation as a type of repression, an active defense mechanism used to remove threatening or unacceptable mental contents from conscious awareness. He also described the defense of splitting of the ego in the management of incompatible mental contents. Despite the fact that the study of dissociative processes dates back to the 19th century, scientists still know remarkably little about the phenomena. Questions still remain unanswered: Are dissociative disorders psychopathological processes or ego-protective devices? Are dissociative processes under voluntary control, or are they a totally unconscious effort? Maldonado and Spiegel (2008) stated,

> [These disorders] have much to teach us about the way humans adapt to traumatic stress, and about information processing in the brain. (p. 665)

Epidemiological Statistics

The lifetime prevalence of somatization disorder in the general population is estimated to be 0.2 to 2 percent in women and 0.2 percent in men (Sadock & Sadock, 2007). Tendencies toward somatization are apparently more common in those who are poorly educated and from the lower socioeconomic classes.

Lifetime prevalence rates of conversion disorder vary widely. Statistics within the general population have ranged from 5 to 30 percent. The disorder occurs more frequently in women than in men and more frequently in adolescents and young adults than in other age groups. A higher prevalence exists in lower socioeconomic groups, in rural populations, and among those with less education (Sadock & Sadock, 2007).

Hypochondriasis affects 1 to 5 percent of the general population (APA, 2000). The disorder is equally common among men and women, and the most common age of onset is in early adulthood.

Pain is likely the most frequent presenting complaint in medical practice today. Pain disorder (previously called *somatoform pain disorder*) is diagnosed more frequently in women than in men by about 2 to 1. Its onset can occur at any age, with the peak ages of onset in the 40s and 50s. It is commonly associated with other psychiatric disorders, particularly affective and anxiety disorders (Sadock & Sadock, 2007).

Body dysmorphic disorder is rare, although it may be more common than once believed. In the practices of plastic surgery and dermatology, reported rates of body dysmorphic disorder range from 6 to 15 percent (APA, 2000). Psychiatrists see only a small fraction of the cases. A profile of these clients reveals that they are usually in the late teens or 20s and unmarried. Comorbidity with another psychiatric disorder, such as major depression, anxiety disorder, or even a psychotic disorder, is not uncommon with body dysmorphic disorder.

Dissociative syndromes are statistically quite rare, but when they do occur they may present very dramatic clinical pictures of severe disturbances in normal personality functioning. Dissociative amnesia is relatively rare, occurring most frequently under conditions of war or during natural disasters. However, in recent years, there has been an increase in the number of reported cases, possibly attributed to increased awareness of the phenomenon, and identification of cases that were previously undiagnosed (APA, 2000). It appears to be more common in women than in men. Dissociative amnesia can occur at any age but is difficult to diagnose in children because it is easily confused with inattention or oppositional behavior.

Dissociative fugue is also rare and occurs most often under conditions of war, natural disasters, or intense psychosocial stress. Information regarding gender distribution and familial patterns of occurrence is not available.

Estimates of the prevalence of dissociative identity disorder (DID) vary widely. Historically, it was thought to be quite rare; however, the number of reported cases has grown rapidly in the past few decades. The disorder occurs from three to nine times more frequently in women than in men, and onset likely occurs in childhood, although manifestations of the disorder may not be recognized until much later (APA, 2000). Clinical symptoms usually are not recognized until late adolescence or early adulthood, although they have probably existed for a number of years prior to diagnosis. There appears to be some evidence that the disorder is more common in first-degree biological relatives of people with the disorder than in the general population.

The prevalence of severe episodes of depersonalization disorder is unknown, although single brief episodes of depersonalization may occur at some time in as many as half of all adults, particularly in the event of severe psychosocial stress (APA, 2000). Symptoms usually begin in adolescence or early adulthood. The disorder is chronic, with periods of remission and exacerbation. The incidence of depersonalization disorder is high under conditions of sustained traumatization, such as in military combat or prisoner-of-war camps. It has also been reported in many individuals who endure near-death experiences.

Application of the Nursing Process

Background Assessment Data: Types of Somatoform Disorders

Somatization Disorder

> **CORE CONCEPT**
> *Somatization*
> The process by which psychological needs are expressed in the form of physical symptoms. Somatization is thought to be associated with repressed anxiety.

Somatization disorder is a syndrome of multiple somatic symptoms that cannot be explained medically and are associated with psychosocial distress and long-term seeking of assistance from healthcare professionals. Symptoms may be vague, dramatized, or exaggerated in their presentation. The disorder is chronic, with symptoms beginning before age 30. The symptoms are identified as pain (in at least four different sites), gastrointestinal symptoms (e.g., nausea, vomiting, diarrhea), sexual symptoms (e.g., irregular menses, erectile or ejaculatory dysfunction), and symptoms suggestive of a neurological condition (e.g., paralysis, blindness, deafness) (APA, 2000). Anxiety and depression are frequently manifested, and suicidal threats and attempts are not uncommon.

The disorder usually runs a fluctuating course, with periods of remission and exacerbation. Clients often receive medical care from several physicians, sometimes concurrently, leading to the possibility of dangerous combinations of treatments (APA, 2000). They have a tendency to seek relief through overmedicating with prescribed analgesics or antianxiety agents. Drug abuse and dependence are common complications of somatization disorder. When suicide results, it is usually in association with substance abuse (Sadock & Sadock, 2007).

It has been suggested that, in somatization disorder, there may be some overlapping of personality characteristics and features associated with histrionic personality disorder. These symptoms include heightened emotionality, impressionistic thought and speech, seductiveness, strong dependency needs, and a preoccupation with symptoms and oneself.

The *DSM-IV-TR* diagnostic criteria for somatization disorder are presented in Box 30-1.

Pain Disorder

The essential feature of pain disorder is severe and prolonged pain that causes clinically significant distress or impairment in social, occupational, or other important areas of functioning (APA, 2000). This diagnosis is made when psychological factors have been judged to have a major role in the onset, severity, exacerbation, or maintenance of the pain, even when the physical examination reveals pathology that is associated with the pain. Psychological implications in the etiology of the pain complaint may be evidenced by the correlation of a stressful situation with the onset of the symptom. Additional psychological implications may be supported by the facts that (1) appearance of the pain enables the client to avoid some unpleasant activity (**primary gain**) and (2) the pain promotes emotional support or attention that the client might not otherwise receive (**secondary gain**).

BOX 30-1 Diagnostic Criteria for Somatization Disorder

A. A history of many physical complaints beginning before age 30 years that occur over a period of several years and result in treatment being sought or significant impairment in social, occupational, or other important areas of functioning.

B. Each of the following criteria must have been met, with individual symptoms occurring at any time during the course of the disturbance:

1. *Four Pain Symptoms:* A history of pain related to at least four different sites or functions (e.g., head, abdomen, back, joints, extremities, chest, rectum, during menstruation, during sexual intercourse, or during urination).

2. *Two Gastrointestinal Symptoms:* A history of at least two gastrointestinal symptoms other than pain (e.g., nausea, bloating, vomiting other than during pregnancy, diarrhea, or intolerance of several different foods).

3. *One Sexual Symptom:* A history of at least one sexual or reproductive symptom other than pain (e.g., sexual indifference, erectile or ejaculatory dysfunction, irregular menses, excessive menstrual bleeding, vomiting throughout pregnancy).

4. *One Pseudoneurological Symptom:* A history of at least one symptom of deficit suggesting a neurological condition not limited to pain (e.g., conversion symptoms such as impaired coordination or balance, paralysis or localized weakness, difficulty swallowing or lump in throat, aphonia, urinary retention, hallucinations, loss of touch or pain sensation, double vision, blindness, deafness, seizures; dissociative symptoms such as amnesia; or loss of consciousness other than fainting).

C. Either 1 or 2:

1. After appropriate investigation, each of the symptoms in criterion B cannot be fully explained by a known general medical condition or the direct effects of a substance (e.g., a drug or abuse, a medication).

2. When there is a related general medical condition, the physical complaints or resulting social or occupational impairment are in excess of what would be expected from the history, physical examination, or laboratory findings.

D. The symptoms are not intentionally produced or feigned (as in factitious disorder or malingering).

From American Psychiatric Association. (2000). Diagnostic and statistical manual of mental disorders (4th ed.). Text revision. Washington, DC: American Psychiatric Publishing, with permission.

Characteristic behaviors include frequent visits to physicians in an effort to obtain relief, excessive use of analgesics, and requests for surgery. Symptoms of depression are common and often severe enough to warrant a diagnosis of major depression. Dependence on addictive substances is a common complication of pain disorder. The *DSM-IV-TR* diagnostic criteria for this disorder are presented in Box 30-2.

Hypochondriasis

Hypochondriasis may be defined as an unrealistic or inaccurate interpretation of physical symptoms or sensations, leading to preoccupation and fear of having a serious disease. The fear becomes disabling and persists despite appropriate reassurance that no organic pathology can be detected. Occasionally medical disease may be present, but in the individual with hypochondriasis, the symptoms are excessive in relation to the degree of pathology.

The preoccupation may be with a specific organ or disease (e.g., cardiac disease), with bodily functions (e.g., peristalsis or heartbeat), or even with minor physical alterations (e.g., a small sore or an occasional cough) (APA, 2000). Individuals with hypochondriasis may become convinced that a rapid heart rate indicates they have heart disease or that the small sore is skin cancer. They are profoundly preoccupied with their bodies and are totally aware of even the slightest change in feeling or sensation. Their response to these small changes, however, is usually unrealistic and exaggerated.

Individuals with hypochondriasis often have a long history of "doctor shopping" and are convinced that they are not receiving the proper care. Anxiety and depression are common, and obsessive-compulsive traits frequently accompany the disorder. Preoccupation with the fear of serious disease may interfere with social or occupational functioning. Some individuals are able to function appropriately on the job, however, while limiting their physical complaints to non-work time.

Individuals with hypochondriasis are so totally convinced that their symptoms are related to organic pathology that they adamantly reject, and are often irritated by, any implication that stress or psychosocial factors play any role in their condition. They are so apprehensive and fearful that they become alarmed at the slightest intimation of serious illness. Even reading about a disease

---

BOX 30-2 Diagnostic Criteria for Pain Disorder

A. Pain in one or more anatomical sites is the predominant focus of the clinical presentation and is of sufficient severity to warrant clinical attention.

B. The pain causes clinically significant distress or impairment in social, occupational, or other important areas of functioning.

C. Psychological factors are judged to have an important role in the onset, severity, exacerbation, or maintenance of the pain.

D. The symptom or deficit is not intentionally produced or feigned (as in factitious disorder or malingering).

E. The pain is not better accounted for by a mood, anxiety, or psychotic disorder and does not meet criteria for dyspareunia.

May be coded as:

- **Pain Disorder Associated with Psychological Factors**
  Psychological factors are judged to have the major role in the onset, severity, exacerbation, or maintenance of the pain.
  Acute: Duration of less than 6 months.
  Chronic: Duration of 6 months or longer.

- **Pain Disorder Associated with Both Psychological Factors and a General Medical Condition**
  Both psychological factors and a general medical condition are judged to have important roles in the onset, severity, exacerbation, or maintenance of the pain.
  Acute: Duration of less than 6 months.
  Chronic: Duration of 6 months or longer.

- **Pain Disorder Associated with a General Medical Condition**
  A general medical condition has a major role in the onset, severity, exacerbation, or maintenance of the pain.

From American Psychiatric Association. (2000). Diagnostic and statistical manual of mental disorders (4th ed.). Text revision. Washington, DC: American Psychiatric Publishing, with permission.

or hearing that someone they know has been diagnosed with an illness precipitates alarm on their part.

The *DSM-IV-TR* diagnostic criteria for hypochondriasis are presented in Box 30-3.

Conversion Disorder

Conversion disorder is a loss of or change in body function resulting from a psychological conflict, the physical symptoms of which cannot be explained by any known medical disorder or pathophysiological mechanism. Clients are unaware of the psychological basis and are therefore unable to control their symptoms.

Conversion symptoms affect voluntary motor or sensory functioning suggestive of neurological disease and are therefore sometimes called "pseudoneurological" (APA, 2000). Examples include paralysis, **aphonia,** seizures, coordination disturbance, difficulty swallowing, urinary retention, akinesia, blindness, deafness, double vision, **anosmia,** loss of pain sensation, and hallucinations. **Pseudocyesis** (false pregnancy) is a conversion symptom and may represent a strong desire to be pregnant.

Precipitation of conversion symptoms must be explained by psychological factors, and this may be evidenced by the presence of primary or secondary gain. When an individual achieves *primary gain,* the conversion symptoms enable the individual to avoid difficult situations or unpleasant activities about which he or she is anxious. Conversion symptoms promote *secondary gain* for the individual as a way to obtain attention or support that might not otherwise be forthcoming.

The symptom usually occurs after a situation that produces extreme psychological stress for the individual. The symptom appears suddenly, and often the person expresses a relative lack of

concern that is out of keeping with the severity of the impairment (APA, 2000). This lack of concern is identified as **la belle indifference** and is often a clue to the physician that the problem may be psychological rather than physical. Other individuals, however, may present symptoms in a dramatic or histrionic fashion (APA, 2000).

Most symptoms of conversion disorder resolve within a few weeks. About 20 to 25 percent of clients will experience a recurrence of symptoms within 1 year of the first episode (Sadock & Sadock, 2007). Symptoms of blindness, aphonia, and paralysis are associated with good prognosis, whereas seizures and tremor are associated with poorer prognosis (APA, 2000). The *DSM-IV-TR* diagnostic criteria for conversion disorder are presented in Box 30-4.

Body Dysmorphic Disorder

This disorder, formerly called dysmorphophobia, is characterized by the exaggerated belief that the body is deformed or defective in some specific way. The most common complaints involve imagined or slight flaws of the face or head, such as thinning hair, acne, wrinkles, scars, vascular markings, facial swelling or asymmetry, or excessive facial hair (APA, 2000). Other complaints may have to do with some aspect of the nose, ears, eyes, mouth, lips, or teeth. Some clients may present with complaints involving other parts of the body, and in some instances a true defect is present. The significance of the defect is unrealistically exaggerated, however, and the person's concern is grossly excessive.

Symptoms of depression and characteristics associated with obsessive-compulsive personality are common in individuals with body dysmorphic disorder. Social and occupational impairment may occur because of the excessive anxiety experienced

---

BOX 30-3 Diagnostic Criteria for Hypochondriasis

A. Preoccupation with fears of having, or the idea that one has, a serious disease, based on the person's misinterpretation of bodily symptoms.

B. The preoccupation persists despite appropriate medical evaluation and reassurance.

C. The belief in criterion A is not of delusional intensity (as in delusional disorder, somatic type) and is not restricted to a circumscribed concern about appearance (as in body dysmorphic disorder).

D. The preoccupation causes clinically significant distress or impairment in social, occupational, or other important areas of functioning.

E. The duration of the disturbance is at least 6 months.

F. The preoccupation is not better accounted for by generalized anxiety disorder, obsessive-compulsive disorder, panic disorder, a major depressive episode, separation anxiety, or another somatoform disorder.

From American Psychiatric Association. (2000). Diagnostic and statistical manual of mental disorders (4th ed.). Text revision. Washington, DC: American Psychiatric Publishing, with permission.

BOX 30-4 Diagnostic Criteria for Conversion Disorder

A. One or more symptoms or deficits affecting voluntary motor or sensory function that suggest a neurological or other general medical condition.

B. Psychological factors are judged to be associated with the symptom or deficit because the initiation or exacerbation of the symptom or deficit is preceded by conflicts or other stressors.

C. The symptom or deficit is not intentionally produced or feigned (as in factitious disorder or malingering).

D. The symptom or deficit cannot, after appropriate investigation, be fully explained by a general medical condition, by the direct effects of a substance, or as a culturally sanctioned behavior or experience.

E. The symptom or deficit causes clinically significant distress or impairment in social, occupational, or other important areas of functioning or warrants medical evaluation.

F. The symptom or deficit is not limited to pain or sexual dysfunction, does not occur exclusively during the course of somatization disorder, and is not better accounted for by another mental disorder.

Specify type of symptom or deficit:

With motor symptom or deficit.

With sensory symptom or deficit.

With seizures or convulsions.

With mixed presentation..

From American Psychiatric Association. (2000). Diagnostic and statistical manual of mental disorders (4th ed.). Text revision. Washington, DC: American Psychiatric Publishing, with permission

by the individual in relation to the imagined defect. The person's medical history may reflect numerous visits to plastic surgeons and dermatologists in an unrelenting drive to correct the imagined defect. He or she may undergo unnecessary surgical procedures toward this effort.

This disorder has been closely associated with delusional thinking, and the *DSM-IV-TR* suggests that, if the perceived body defect is in fact of delusional intensity, the appropriate diagnosis would be delusional disorder, somatic type (APA, 2000). Traits associated with schizoid, obsessive-compulsive, and narcissistic personality disorders are not uncommon. The *DSM-IV-TR* diagnostic criteria for body dysmorphic disorder are presented in Box 30-5.

The etiology of body dysmorphic disorder is unknown. In some clients the belief is due to another more pervasive psychiatric disorder,

such as schizophrenia. A high incidence of comorbidity with major mood disorder and anxiety disorder and the responsiveness of the condition to the serotonin-specific drugs may indicate some involvement of the serotonergic system.

Body dysmorphic disorder has been classified as one of several *monosymptomatic hypochondriacal syndromes*. Each of these syndromes is characterized by a single hypochondriacal belief about one's body. Body dysmorphic disorder is one of the most common such syndromes. Others include delusions of parasitosis (i.e., false belief that one is infested with some parasite or vermin) and of bromosis (i.e., false belief that one is emitting an offensive body odor).

Body dysmorphic disorder has also been defined as the fear of some physical defect thought to be noticeable to others, although the client appears normal. These interpretations suggest that

BOX 30-5 Diagnostic Criteria for Body Dysmorphic Disorder

A. Preoccupation with an imagined defect in appearance. If a slight physical anomaly is present, the person's concern is markedly excessive.

B. The preoccupation causes clinically significant distress or impairment in social, occupational, or other important areas of functioning.

C. The preoccupation is not better accounted for by another mental disorder (e.g., dissatisfaction with body shape and size in anorexia nervosa).

From American Psychiatric Association. (2000). Diagnostic and statistical manual of mental disorders (4th ed.). Text revision. Washington, DC: American Psychiatric Publishing, with permission.

the disorder may be related to predisposing factors similar to those associated with hypochondriasis or phobias. Repression of morbid anxiety is undoubtedly an underlying factor, and it is very likely that multiple factors are involved in the predisposition to body dysmorphic disorder.

Predisposing Factors Associated With Somatoform Disorders

Genetic

Studies have shown an increased incidence of somatization disorder, conversion disorder, and hypochondriasis in first-degree relatives, implying a possible inheritable predisposition (Sadock & Sadock, 2007; Soares & Grossman, 2010; Yutzy & Parish, 2008).

Biochemical

Decreased levels of serotonin and endorphins may play a role in the etiology of pain disorder. Serotonin is probably the main neurotransmitter involved in inhibiting the firing of afferent pain fibers (Parcell, 2008). The deficiency of endorphins seems to correlate with an increase of incoming sensory (pain) stimuli (Wootton, 2008).

Psychodynamic

Some psychodynamicists view hypochondriasis as an ego defense mechanism. Physical complaints are the expression of low self-esteem and feelings of worthlessness, because it is easier to feel something is wrong with the body than to feel something is wrong with the self. Another view of hypochondriasis (as well as pain disorder) is related to a defense against guilt. The individual views the self as "bad," based on real or imagined past misconduct, and views physical suffering as the deserved punishment required for atonement.

The psychodynamic theory of conversion disorder proposes that emotions associated with a traumatic event that the individual cannot express because of moral or ethical unacceptability are "converted" into physical symptoms. The unacceptable emotions are repressed and converted to a somatic hysterical symptom that is symbolic in some way of the original emotional trauma.

Family Dynamics

Some families have difficulty expressing emotions openly and resolving conflicts verbally. When this occurs, the child may become ill, and a shift in focus is made from the open conflict to the child's illness, leaving unresolved the underlying issues that the family cannot confront openly. Thus, somatization by the child brings some stability to the family, as harmony replaces discord and the child's welfare becomes the common concern. The child in turn receives positive reinforcement for the illness. This shift in focus from family discord to concern for the child is sometimes called **tertiary gain.**

Learning Theory

Somatic complaints are often reinforced when the sick role relieves the individual from the need to deal with a stressful situation, whether it be within society or within the family. The sick person learns that he or she may avoid stressful obligations, may postpone unwelcome challenges, and is excused from troublesome duties (primary gain); becomes the prominent focus of attention because of the illness (secondary gain); or relieves conflict within the family as concern is shifted to the ill person and away from the real issue (tertiary gain). These types of positive reinforcements virtually guarantee repetition of the response.

Past experience with serious or life-threatening physical illness, either personal or that of close family members, can predispose an individual to hypochondriasis. Once an individual has experienced a threat to biological integrity, he or she may develop a fear of recurrence. The fear of recurring illness generates an exaggerated response to minor physical changes, leading to hypochondriacal behaviors.

Transactional Model of Stress/Adaptation

The etiology of somatoform disorders is most likely influenced by multiple factors. In Figure 30–1, a graphic depiction of this theory of multiple causation is presented in the Transactional Model of Stress/Adaptation.

Background Assessment Data: Types of Dissociative Disorders

Dissociative Amnesia

> **CORE CONCEPT**
>
> *Amnesia*
>
> Pathologic loss of memory; a phenomenon in which an area of experience becomes inaccessible to conscious recall. The loss in memory may be organic, emotional, dissociative, or of mixed origin, and may be permanent or limited to a sharply circumscribed period of time (Shahrokh & Hales, 2003).

Dissociative amnesia is an inability to recall important personal information, usually of a traumatic or stressful nature, that is too extensive to be explained by ordinary forgetfulness and is not due to the direct effects of substance use or a neurological or

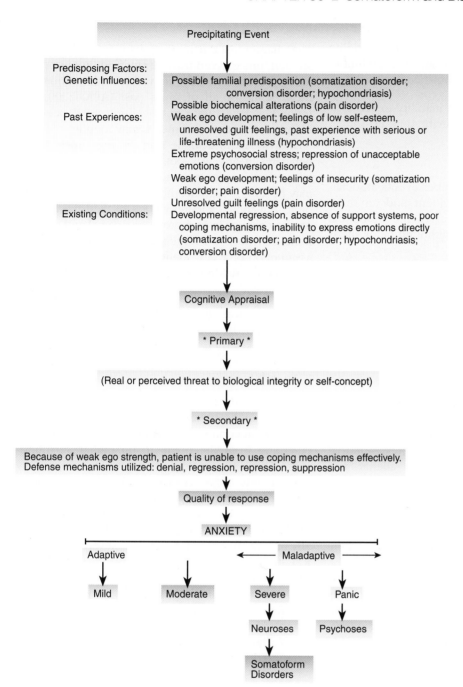

FIGURE 30–1 The dynamics of somatoform disorders using the Transactional Model of Stress/Adaptation.

other general medical condition (APA, 2000). Five types of disturbance in recall have been described. In the following examples, the individual is involved in a traumatic automobile accident in which a loved one is killed.

1. **Localized Amnesia.** The inability to recall all incidents associated with the traumatic event for a specific time period following the event (usually a few hours to a few days).

EXAMPLE

The individual cannot recall events of the automobile accident and events occurring during a period after the accident (a few hours to a few days).

2. **Selective Amnesia.** The inability to recall only certain incidents associated with a traumatic event for a specific period after the event.

EXAMPLE

The individual may not remember events leading to the impact of the accident but may remember being taken away in the ambulance.

3. **Continuous Amnesia.** The inability to recall events occurring after a specific time up to and including the present.

EXAMPLE

The individual cannot remember events associated with the automobile accident and anything that has occurred since. That is, the individual cannot form new memories, although he or she is apparently alert and aware.

4. **Generalized Amnesia.** The rare phenomenon of not being able to recall anything that has happened during the individual's entire lifetime, including his or her personal identity.

5. **Systematized Amnesia.** With this type of amnesia, the individual cannot remember events that relate to a specific category of information (e.g., one's family) or to one particular person or event.

The individual with amnesia usually appears alert and may give no indication to observers that anything is wrong, although some clients may present with alterations in consciousness, with conversion symptoms, or in trance states. Clients suffering from amnesia are often brought to general hospital emergency departments by police who have found them wandering confusedly around the streets.

Onset of an amnestic episode usually follows severe psychosocial stress. Termination is typically abrupt and followed by complete recovery. Recurrences are unusual. The *DSM-IV-TR* diagnostic criteria for dissociative amnesia are presented in Box 30-6.

Dissociative Fugue

The characteristic feature of dissociative **fugue** is a sudden, unexpected travel away from home or customary place of daily activities, with inability to recall some or all of one's past (APA, 2000). An individual in a fugue state cannot recall personal identity and often assumes a new identity.

Individuals in a fugue state do not appear to be behaving in any way out of the ordinary. Contacts with other people are minimal. The assumed identity may be simple and incomplete or complex and elaborate. If a complex identity is established, the individual may engage in intricate interpersonal and occupational activities. A divergent perception regarding the assumption of a new identity in dissociative fugue is reported by Maldonado and Spiegel (2008):

> It was thought that the assumption of a new identity was typical of dissociative fugue. However, [studies have] documented that in most cases there is a loss of personal identity but no clear assumption of a new identity. (p. 678)

Clients with dissociative fugue often are picked up by the police when they are found wandering in a somewhat confused and frightened condition after emerging from the fugue in unfamiliar surroundings. They are usually presented to emergency departments of general hospitals. On assessment, they are able to provide details of their earlier life situation but have no recall from the beginning of the fugue state. Information from other sources usually reveals that the occurrence of severe psychological stress or excessive alcohol use precipitated the fugue behavior.

Duration is usually brief—that is, hours to days or, more rarely, months—and recovery is rapid and complete. Recurrences are not common. The *DSM-IV-TR* diagnostic criteria for dissociative fugue are presented in Box 30-7.

BOX 30-6 Diagnostic Criteria for Dissociative Amnesia

A. The predominant disturbance is one or more episodes of inability to recall important personal information, usually of a traumatic or stressful nature, that is too extensive to be explained by ordinary forgetfulness.

B. The disturbance does not occur exclusively during the course of dissociative identity disorder, dissociative fugue, posttraumatic stress disorder, acute stress disorder, or somatization disorder and is not due to the direct physiological effect of a substance (e.g., a drug of abuse, a medication) or a neurological or other general medical condition (e.g., amnestic disorder due to head trauma).

C. The symptoms cause clinically significant distress or impairment in social, occupational, or other important areas of functioning.

From American Psychiatric Association. (2000). Diagnostic and statistical manual of mental disorders (4th ed.). Text revision. Washington, DC: American Psychiatric Publishing, with permission.

BOX 30-7 Diagnostic Criteria for Dissociative Fugue

A. The predominant disturbance is sudden, unexpected travel away from home or one's customary place of work, with inability to recall one's past.
B. Confusion about personal identity or assumption of a new identity (partial or complete).
C. The disturbance does not occur exclusively during the course of dissociative identity disorder and is not due to the direct physiological effects of a substance (e.g., a drug of abuse, a medication) or a general medical condition (e.g., temporal lobe epilepsy).
D. The symptoms cause clinically significant distress or impairment in social, occupational, or other important areas of functioning.

From American Psychiatric Association. (2000). Diagnostic and statistical manual of mental disorders (4th ed.). Text revision. Washington, DC: American Psychiatric Publishing, with permission.

Dissociative Identity Disorder

Dissociative identity disorder (DID) was formerly called multiple personality disorder. This disorder is characterized by the existence of two or more personalities in a single individual. Only one of the personalities is evident at any given moment, and one of them is dominant most of the time over the course of the disorder. Each personality is unique and composed of a complex set of memories, behavior patterns, and social relationships that surface during the dominant interval. The transition from one personality to another is usually sudden, often dramatic, and usually precipitated by stress. The *DSM-IV-TR* (APA, 2000) states:

> The time required to switch from one identity to another is usually a matter of seconds but, less frequently, may be gradual. Behavior that may be frequently associated with identity switches include rapid blinking, facial changes, changes in voice or demeanor, or disruption in the individual's train of thought. (p. 527)

Before therapy, the original personality usually has no knowledge of the other personalities, but when there are two or more subpersonalities, they are usually aware of each other's existence. Most often, the various subpersonalities have different names, but they may be unnamed and may be of a different gender, race, and age. The various personalities are almost always quite disparate and may even appear to be the exact opposite of the original personality. For example, a normally shy, socially withdrawn, faithful husband may become a gregarious womanizer and heavy drinker with the emergence of another personality.

Generally, there is amnesia for the events that took place when another personality was in the dominant position, and clients report "gaps" in autobiographical histories. Sometimes, however, one personality does not experience such amnesia and retains complete awareness of the existence, qualities, and activities of the other personalities. Subpersonalities that are amnestic for the other subpersonalities experience the periods when others are dominant as "lost time" or blackouts. They may "wake up" in unfamiliar situations with no idea where they are, how they got there, or who the people around them are. They may frequently be accused of lying when they deny remembering or being responsible for events or actions that occurred while another personality controlled the body.

Dissociative identity disorder is not always incapacitating. Some individuals with DID maintain responsible positions, complete graduate degrees, and are successful spouses and parents before diagnosis and while in treatment. Before they are diagnosed with DID, many individuals are misdiagnosed with depression, borderline and antisocial personality disorders, schizophrenia, epilepsy, or bipolar disorder. The *DSM-IV-TR* diagnostic criteria for DID are presented in Box 30-8.

Depersonalization Disorder

Depersonalization disorder is characterized by a temporary change in the quality of self-awareness, which often takes the form of feelings of unreality, changes in body image, feelings of detachment from the environment, or a sense of observing oneself from outside the body. Depersonalization (a disturbance in the perception of oneself) is differentiated from **derealization,** which describes an alteration in the perception of the external environment. Both of these phenomena also occur in a variety of psychiatric illnesses such as schizophrenia, depression, anxiety states, and organic mental disorders. As previously stated, the symptom of depersonalization is very common. It is estimated

---

BOX 30-8 Diagnostic Criteria for Dissociative Identity Disorder

A. The presence of two or more distinct personality states (each with its own relatively enduring pattern of perceiving, relating to, and thinking about the environment and self).

B. At least two of these identities or personality states recurrently take control of the person's behavior.

C. Inability to recall important personal information that is too extensive to be explained by ordinary forgetfulness.

D. The disturbance is not due to the direct physiological effects of a substance (e.g., blackouts or chaotic behavior during alcohol intoxication) or a general medical condition (e.g., complex partial seizures). In children, the symptoms are not attributable to imaginary playmates or other fantasy play.

From American Psychiatric Association. (2000). Diagnostic and statistical manual of mental disorders (4th ed.) Text revision. Washington, DC: American Psychiatric Publishing, with permission.

---

that approximately half of all adults experience transient episodes of depersonalization (APA, 2000). The diagnosis of depersonalization disorder is made only if the symptom causes significant distress or impairment in functioning.

The *DSM-IV-TR* describes this disorder as the persistence or recurrence of episodes of depersonalization characterized by a feeling of detachment or estrangement from one's self (APA, 2000). There may be a mechanical or dreamlike feeling or a belief that the body's physical characteristics have changed. If derealization is present, objects in the environment are perceived as altered in size or shape. Other people in the environment may seem automated or mechanical.

These altered perceptions are experienced as disturbing, and are often accompanied by anxiety, depression, fear of going insane, obsessive thoughts, somatic complaints, and a disturbance in the subjective sense of time (APA, 2000). The disorder occurs more often in women than it does in men and is a disorder of younger people, rarely occurring in individuals older than 40 years of age (Black & Andreasen, 2011). The *DSM-IV-TR* diagnostic criteria for depersonalization disorder are presented in Box 30-9.

Predisposing Factors Associated With Dissociative Disorders

Genetics

The *DSM-IV-TR* suggests that DID is more common in first-degree relatives of people with the disorder than in the general population. The disorder is often seen in more than one generation of a family.

Neurobiological

Some clinicians have suggested a possible correlation between neurological alterations and dissociative disorders. Although available information is inadequate, it is possible that dissociative amnesia and dissociative fugue may be related to neurophysiological dysfunction. Areas of the brain that have been associated with memory include the hippocampus, amydala, fornix, mammillary bodies, thalamus, and frontal cortex. Brunet, Holowka, and Laurence (2003) stated:

> Given the intimate relationship between dissociation, memory, and trauma, researchers have begun to investigate the brain structures and neurochemical systems that mediate functions. Several substances such as sodium-lactate, yohimbine, and metachlorophenylpiper-azine have been shown to elicit dissociative

---

BOX 30-9 Diagnostic Criteria for Depersonalization Disorder

A. Persistent or recurrent experiences of feeling detached from, and as if one is an outside observer of, one's mental processes or body (e.g., feeling like one is in a dream).

B. During the depersonalization experience, reality testing remains intact.

C. The depersonalization causes clinically significant distress or impairment in social, occupational, or other important areas of functioning.

D. The depersonalization experience does not occur exclusively during the course of another mental disorder, such as schizophrenia, panic disorder, acute stress disorder, or another dissociative disorder, and is not due to the direct physiological effects of a substance (e.g., a drug of abuse, a medication) or a general medical condition (e.g., temporal lobe epilepsy).

From American Psychiatric Association. (2000). Diagnostic and statistical manual of mental disorders (4th ed.). Text revision. Washington, DC: American Psychiatric Publishing, with permission.

symptoms in patients with PTSD or panic disorder, but not in normal controls. Such findings suggest a role for the locus coeruleus/noradrenergic system, which is implicated in fear and arousal regulation and influence a number of cortical structures such as the prefrontal, sensory and parietal cortex, the hippocampus, the hypothalamus, the amygdala, and the spinal cord. Still the relationship between trauma exposure, cortisol, hippocampus damage, memory, and dissociation is tentative at best, and remains to be thoroughly investigated. (p. 26)

Some studies have suggested a possible link between DID and certain neurological conditions, such as temporal lobe epilepsy and severe migraine headaches. Electroencephalographic abnormalities have been observed in some clients with DID.

Psychodynamic Theory

Freud (1962) believed that dissociative behaviors occurred when individuals repressed distressing mental contents from conscious awareness. He believed that the unconscious was a dynamic entity in which repressed mental contents were stored and unavailable to conscious recall. Current psychodynamic explanations of dissociation are based on Freud's concepts. The repression of mental contents is perceived as a coping mechanism for protecting the client from emotional pain that has arisen from either disturbing external circumstances or anxiety-provoking internal urges and feelings (Maldonado & Spiegel, 2008). In the case of depersonalization, the pain and anxiety are expressed as feelings of unreality or detachment from the environment of the painful situation.

Psychological Trauma

A growing body of evidence points to the etiology of DID as a set of traumatic experiences that overwhelms the individual's capacity to cope by any means other than dissociation. These experiences usually take the form of severe physical, sexual, or psychological abuse by a parent or significant other in the child's life. The most widely accepted explanation for DID is that it begins as a survival strategy that serves to help children cope with the horrifying sexual, physical, or psychological abuse. In this traumatic environment, the child uses dissociation to become a passive victim of the cruel and unwanted experience. He or she creates a new being who is able to endure the overwhelming pain of the cruel reality, while the primary self can then escape awareness of the pain. Each new personality has as its nucleus a means of responding without anxiety and distress to various painful or dangerous stimuli.

IMPLICATIONS OF RESEARCH FOR EVIDENCE-BASED PRACTICE

Brunner, R., Parzer, P., Schuld, V., & Resch, F. (2000, February). Dissociative symptomatology and traumatogenic factors in adolescent psychiatric patients. *The Journal of Nervous and Mental Disease, 188,* **71–77.**

DESCRIPTION OF THE STUDY: This study describes the relationship between different types of childhood trauma and the degree of dissociative experiences. Subjects were 198 consecutively admitted adolescent psychiatric patients, 11 to 19 years old (89 inpatients and 109 outpatients). All patients completed the Adolescent Dissociative Experiences Scale (ADES), a self-administered questionnaire with 30 items that quantifies the frequency of dissociative experiences on an 11-point scale ranging from 0 (never) to 10 (always). The instrument has been shown to discriminate patients with dissociative disorders from patients in several other diagnostic categories, as well as from adolescents in the general population. Subjects' therapists were asked to complete the Checklist of Traumatic Childhood Events, based on assessments, client self-reports, and reports by caregivers and custodial and social services. The checklist covered four main areas of traumatic experiences: sexual abuse, physical abuse, neglect, and stressful life events. Each area was further categorized by experiences considered from minor to severe. Examples of these abuse extremes included:

- Sexual: From sexualized communication to fondling to masturbation to penetration
- Physical: From being hit with a hand to punching, kicking, lacerations, burns, fractures
- Neglect: From physical and educational neglect to social/environmental neglect to emotional and psychological involvement (rejection; hostility)
- Stressful life events: From loss related to family members to physical/mental illness of family members to "others" (e.g., personal physical illness, witnessing an accident or violence, institutional placement)

Continued

IMPLICATIONS OF RESEARCH FOR EVIDENCE-BASED PRACTICE—cont'd

RESULTS OF THE STUDY: All mean scores by traumatized adolescents were elevated in comparison to those of the control (nontraumatized) group. Increased dissociative symptomatology was unrelated to the degree of severity of sexual abuse experiences. Interestingly, the study found an increased amount of dissociative symptomatology associated with minor forms of physical abuse, as compared to the severe forms. Only severe forms of stressful life events contributed significantly to a higher degree of dissociative experiences. The study revealed that emotional neglect appears to be the best predictor of dissociative symptoms.

IMPLICATIONS FOR NURSING PRACTICE: The authors stated: "In contrast to the current psychopathogenic model of dissociation which maintains that particularly severe traumatic events lead to dissociative symptomatology, moderate but chronic emotional stress may be equal or even more important in the development of dissociation." (p. 76) This is important information for the nursing database. Nurses should be aware that even less severe forms of abuse and neglect may have a significant impact on the development of dissociative psychopathology in adolescents.

Transactional Model of Stress/Adaptation

The etiology of dissociative disorders is most likely influenced by multiple factors. In Figure 30–2, a graphic depiction of this theory of multiple causation is presented in the Transactional Model of Stress/Adaptation.

Diagnosis/Outcome Identification

Nursing diagnoses are formulated from the data gathered during the assessment phase and with background knowledge regarding predisposing factors to the disorder. Table 30-1 presents a list of client behaviors and the NANDA nursing diagnoses that correspond to those behaviors, which may be used in planning care for clients with somatoform and dissociative disorders.

Outcome Criteria

The following criteria may be used for measurement of outcomes in the care of the client with somatoform and dissociative disorders.

The client:

■ Effectively uses adaptive coping strategies during stressful situations without resorting to physical symptoms (*somatoform and pain disorders*).

■ Verbalizes relief from pain and demonstrates adaptive coping strategies during stressful situations to prevent the onset of pain (*pain disorder*).

■ Interprets bodily sensations rationally; verbalizes understanding of the significance the irrational fear held for him or her; and has decreased the number and frequency of physical complaints (*hypochondriasis*).

■ Is free of physical disability and is able to verbalize understanding of the correlation

between the loss of or alteration in function and extreme emotional stress (*conversion disorder*).

■ Verbalizes a realistic perception of his or her appearance and expresses feelings that reflect a positive body image (*body dysmorphic disorder*).

■ Can recall events associated with a traumatic or stressful situation (*dissociative amnesia*).

■ Can recall all events of past life (*dissociative amnesia and dissociative fugue*).

■ Can verbalize the extreme anxiety that precipitated the dissociation (*dissociative disorders*).

■ Can demonstrate more adaptive coping strategies to avert dissociative behaviors in the face of severe anxiety (*dissociative disorders*).

■ Verbalizes understanding of the existence of multiple personalities and the purposes they serve (*dissociative identity disorder*).

■ Is able to maintain a sense of reality during stressful situations (*dissociative disorders*).

Planning/Implementation

The following section presents a group of selected nursing diagnoses, with short- and long-term goals and nursing interventions for each.

Ineffective Coping

Ineffective coping is defined as the "inability to form a valid appraisal of the stressors, inadequate choices of practiced responses, and/or inability to use available resources" (NANDA International [NANDA-I], 2009, p. 254).

Client Goals

Outcome criteria include short- and long-term goals. Timelines are individually determined.

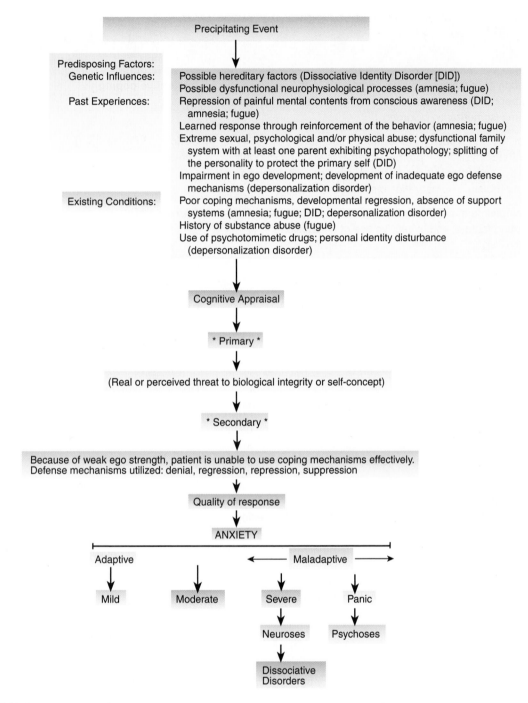

FIGURE 30–2 The dynamics of dissociative disorders using the Transactional Model of Stress/Adaptation.

Short-Term Goal

■ Within 2 weeks, client will verbalize understanding of correlation between physical symptoms and psychological problems.

Long-Term Goal

■ By time of discharge from treatment, client will demonstrate ability to cope with stress by means other than preoccupation with physical symptoms.

Interventions

■ Monitor the physician's ongoing assessments, laboratory reports, and other data to maintain assurance that the possibility of organic pathology is clearly ruled out. Review findings with the client. Accurate medical assessment is vital

TABLE 30-1 Assigning Nursing Diagnoses to Behaviors Commonly Associated With Somatoform and Dissociative Disorders

BEHAVIORS	NURSING DIAGNOSES
Verbalization of numerous physical complaints in the absence of any pathophysiological evidence; focus on the self and physical symptoms (*somatization disorder*)	**Ineffective coping**
History of "doctor shopping" for evidence of organic pathology to substantiate physical symptoms; statements such as, "I don't know why the doctor put me on the psychiatric unit. I have a physical problem." (*somatization disorder*)	**Deficient knowledge (psychological causes for physical symptoms)**
Verbal complaints of pain, with evidence of psychological contributing factors, and excessive use of analgesics (*pain disorder*)	**Chronic pain**
Seeking to be alone; refusal to participate in therapeutic activities (*pain disorder*)	**Social isolation**
Preoccupation with and unrealistic interpretation of bodily signs and sensations (*hypochondriasis*)	**Fear (of having a serious disease)**
Transformation of internalized anger into physical complaints and hostility toward others (*hypochondriasis*)	**Chronic low self-esteem**
Loss or alteration in physical functioning without evidence of organic pathology; "la belle indifference" (*conversion disorder*)	**Disturbed sensory perception**
Need for assistance to carry out self-care activities such as eating, dressing, maintaining hygiene, and toileting due to alteration in physical functioning (*conversion disorder*)	**Self-care deficit**
Preoccupation with imagined defect; verbalizations that are out of proportion to any actual physical abnormality that may exist; numerous visits to plastic surgeons or dermatologists seeking relief (*body dysmorphic disorder*)	**Disturbed body image**
Loss of memory (*dissociative amnesia*)	**Disturbed thought processes; Impaired memory**
Verbalizations of frustration over lack of control and dependence on others (*dissociative amnesia*)	**Powerlessness**
Fear of unknown circumstances surrounding emergence from the fugue state (*dissociative fugue*)	**Risk for other-directed violence**
Sudden travel away from home with inability to recall previous identity (*dissociative fugue*)	**Ineffective coping**
Unresolved grief; depression; self-blame associated with childhood abuse (*DID*)	**Risk for suicide**
Presence of more than one personality within the individual (*DID*)	**Disturbed personality identity**
Alteration in the perception or experience of the self or the environment (*depersonalization disorder*)	**Disturbed sensory perception (visual and kinesthetic)**

for the provision of adequate and appropriate care. Honest explanation may help the client understand the psychological implications.

■ Recognize and accept that the physical complaint is real to the client, even though no organic etiology can be identified. Denial of the client's feelings is nontherapeutic and interferes with establishment of a trusting relationship.

■ Identify gains that the physical symptoms are providing for the client: increased dependency, attention, and distraction from other problems. Identification of underlying motivation is important in assisting the client with problem resolution.

■ Initially, fulfill the client's most urgent dependency needs, but gradually withdraw attention to physical symptoms. Minimize time given in response to physical complaints. Anxiety and maladaptive behaviors will increase if dependency needs are ignored initially. Gradual withdrawal of positive reinforcement will discourage repetition of maladaptive behaviors.

■ Explain to the client that any new physical complaints will be referred to the physician and give no further attention to them. Follow up on the physician's assessment of the complaint. The possibility of organic pathology must always be considered. Failure to do so could jeopardize client safety.

■ Encourage the client to verbalize fears and anxieties. Explain that attention will be withdrawn if rumination about physical complaints begins. Follow through. Without consistency of limit setting, change will not occur.

■ Help the client recognize that physical symptoms often occur because of, or are exacerbated by, specific stressors. Discuss alternative coping responses to these stressors. The client may need help with problem solving. Give positive reinforcement for adaptive coping strategies.

■ Have the client keep a diary of appearance, duration, and intensity of physical symptoms. A separate record of situations that the client finds especially stressful should also be kept. Comparison of these records may provide objective data from which to observe the relationship between physical symptoms and stress.

■ Help the client identify ways to achieve recognition from others without resorting to physical complaints. Positive recognition from others enhances self-esteem and minimizes the need for attention through maladaptive behaviors.

■ Discuss how interpersonal relationships are affected by the client's narcissistic behavior. Explain how this behavior alienates others. The client may not realize how he or she is perceived by others.

■ Provide instruction in relaxation techniques and assertiveness skills. These approaches decrease anxiety and increase self-esteem, which facilitates adaptive responses to stressful situations.

Fear (of Having a Serious Disease)

Fear is defined as the "response to perceived threat that is consciously recognized as a danger" (NANDA-I, 2009, p. 261).

Client Goals

Outcome criteria include short- and long-term goals. Timelines are individually determined.

Short-Term Goal

■ Client will verbalize that fears associated with bodily sensations are irrational (within time limit deemed appropriate for specific individual).

Long-Term Goal

■ Client interprets bodily sensations correctly.

Interventions

■ Monitor the physician's ongoing assessments and laboratory reports. Organic pathology must be clearly ruled out.

■ Refer all new physical complaints to the physician. To assume that all physical complaints are hypochondriacal would place the client's safety in jeopardy.

■ Assess what function the client's illness is fulfilling for him or her (e.g., unfulfilled needs for dependency, nurturing, caring, attention, or control). This information may provide insight into reasons for maladaptive behavior and provide direction for planning client care.

■ Identify times during which the preoccupation with physical symptoms is worse. Determine the extent of correlation of physical complaints with times of increased anxiety. The client is most likely unaware of the psychosocial implications of the physical complaints. Knowledge of the relationship is the first step in the process for creating change.

■ Convey empathy. Let the client know that you understand how a specific symptom may conjure up fears of previous life-threatening illness. Unconditional acceptance and empathy promote a therapeutic nurse-client relationship.

■ Initially allow the client a limited amount of time (e.g., 10 minutes each hour) to discuss physical symptoms. Because this has been his or her primary method of coping for so long, complete prohibition of this activity would likely raise the client's anxiety level significantly, further exacerbating the hypochondriacal behavior.

■ Help the client determine what techniques may be most useful for him or her to implement when fear and anxiety are exacerbated (e.g., relaxation techniques; mental imagery; thought-stopping techniques; physical exercise). All of these techniques are effective in reducing anxiety and may assist the client in the transition from focusing on fear of physical illness to the discussion of honest feelings.

■ Gradually increase the limit on amount of time spent each hour in discussing physical symptoms. If the client violates the limits, withdraw

attention. Lack of positive reinforcement may help to extinguish the maladaptive behavior.

■ Encourage the client to discuss feelings associated with fear of serious illness. Verbalization of feelings in a nonthreatening environment facilitates expression and resolution of disturbing emotional issues. When the client can express feelings directly, there is less need to express them through physical symptoms.

■ Role-play the client's plan for dealing with the fear the next time it assumes control and before it becomes disabling through the exacerbation of physical symptoms. Anxiety and fears are minimized when the client has achieved a degree of comfort through practicing a plan for dealing with stressful situations in the future.

Disturbed Sensory Perception

Disturbed sensory perception is defined as a "change in the amount or patterning of incoming stimuli accompanied by a diminished, exaggerated, distorted, or impaired response to such stimuli" (NANDA-I, 2009, p. 163). Table 30-2 presents this nursing diagnosis in care plan format.

Table 30-2 CARE PLAN FOR THE CLIENT WITH CONVERSION DISORDER

NURSING DIAGNOSIS: DISTURBED SENSORY PERCEPTION
RELATED TO: Repressed severe anxiety
EVIDENCED BY: Loss or alteration in physical functioning, without evidence of organic pathology; "la belle indifference"

OUTCOME CRITERIA	NURSING INTERVENTIONS	RATIONALE
Short-Term Goal • Client will verbalize understanding of emotional problems as a contributing factor to the alteration in physical functioning (within time limit appropriate for specific individual). **Long-Term Goal** • Client will demonstrate recovery of lost or altered function.	1. Monitor physician's ongoing assessments, laboratory reports, and other data to ensure that possibility of organic pathology is clearly ruled out. 2. Identify primary or secondary gains that the physical symptom is providing for the client (e.g., increased dependency, attention, protection from experiencing a stressful event). 3. Do not focus on the disability, and encourage client to be as independent as possible. Intervene only when client requires assistance. 4. Maintain nonjudgmental attitude when providing assistance to the client. The physical symptom is not within the client's conscious control and is very real to him or her.	1. Failure to do so may jeopardize client safety. 2. Primary and secondary gains are etiological factors and may be used to assist in problem resolution. 3. Positive reinforcement would encourage continual use of the maladaptive response for secondary gains, such as dependency. 4. A judgmental attitude interferes with the nurse's ability to provide therapeutic care for the client.

Table 30-2 CARE PLAN FOR THE CLIENT WITH CONVERSION DISORDER—cont'd

OUTCOME CRITERIA	NURSING INTERVENTIONS	RATIONALE
	5. Do not allow the client to use the disability as a manipulative tool to avoid participation in therapeutic activities. Withdraw attention if client continues to focus on physical limitation.	5. Lack of reinforcement may help to extinguish the maladaptive response.
	6. Encourage the client to verbalize fears and anxieties. Help identify physical symptoms as a coping mechanism that is used in times of extreme stress.	6. Clients with conversion disorder are usually unaware of the psychological implications of their illness.
	7. Help client identify coping mechanisms that he or she could use when faced with stressful situations, rather than retreating from reality with a physical disability.	7. Client needs assistance with problem solving at this severe level of anxiety.
	8. Give positive reinforcement for identification or demonstration of alternative, more adaptive coping strategies.	8. Positive reinforcement enhances self-esteem and encourages repetition of desirable behaviors.

Client Goals

Outcome criteria include short- and long-term goals. Timelines are individually determined.

Short-Term Goal

■ The client will verbalize understanding of emotional problems as a contributing factor to the alteration in physical functioning (within time limit appropriate for specific individual).

Long-Term Goal

■ The client will demonstrate recovery of lost or altered function.

Interventions

■ Monitor the physician's ongoing assessments, laboratory reports, and other data to ensure that the possibility of organic pathology is clearly ruled out. Failure to do so may jeopardize the client's safety.

■ Identify primary or secondary gains that the physical symptom is providing for the client (e.g., increased dependency, attention, protection from experiencing a stressful event). These are considered to be etiological factors and will be used to assist in problem resolution.

■ Do not focus on the disability, and encourage the client to be as independent as possible. Intervene only when the client requires assistance. Positive reinforcement would encourage continued use of the maladaptive response for secondary gains, such as dependency.

■ Maintain a nonjudgmental attitude when providing assistance with self-care activities to the client. The physical symptom is not within the client's conscious control and is very real to him or her.

■ Do not allow the client to use the disability as a manipulative tool to avoid participating in therapeutic activities. Withdraw attention if the client continues to focus on the physical limitation. Lack of reinforcement may help to extinguish the maladaptive response.

■ Encourage the client to verbalize fears and anxieties. Help identify physical symptoms as a coping mechanism that is used in times of extreme stress. Clients with conversion disorder are usually unaware of the psychological implications of their illness.

■ Help the client identify coping mechanisms that he or she could use when faced with stressful situations, rather than retreating from reality with a physical disability. The client needs assistance with problem solving at this severe level of anxiety.

■ Give positive reinforcement for identification or demonstration of alternative, more adaptive coping strategies.

Disturbed Thought Processes/Impaired Memory

Disturbed thought processes is defined as a "disruption in cognitive operations and activities" (NANDA-I, 2009, p. 408). *Impaired memory* is defined as an "inability to remember or recall bits of information or behavioral skills" (p. 173).

Client Goals

Outcome criteria include short- and long-term goals. Timelines are individually determined.

Short-Term Goal

■ The client will verbalize understanding that the loss of memory is related to a stressful situation and begin discussing the stressful situation with nurse or therapist.

Long-Term Goal

■ The client will recover deficits in memory and develop more adaptive coping mechanisms to deal with stressful situations.

Interventions

■ Obtain as much information as possible about the client from family and significant others. Consider likes, dislikes, important people, activities, music, and pets. A comprehensive baseline assessment is necessary for the development of an effective plan of care.

■ Do not flood the client with data regarding his or her past life. Individuals who are exposed to painful information from which the amnesia is providing protection may decompensate even further into a psychotic state.

■ Instead, expose the client to stimuli that represent pleasant experiences from the past, such as smells associated with enjoyable activities, beloved pets, and music known to have been pleasurable to the client. As memory begins to return, engage the client in activities that may provide additional stimulation. Recall often occurs during activities such as these that simulate life experiences.

■ Encourage the client to discuss situations that have been especially stressful and to explore the feelings associated with those times. Verbalization of feelings in a nonthreatening environment may help the client come to terms with unresolved issues that may be contributing to the dissociative process.

■ Identify specific conflicts that remain unresolved and help the client identify possible solutions. Provide instruction regarding more adaptive ways to respond to anxiety. Unless these underlying conflicts are resolved, any improvement in coping behaviors must be viewed as only temporary.

■ Provide positive feedback for decisions made. Respect the client's right to make those decisions independently, and refrain from attempting to influence him or her toward those that may seem more logical. Independent choice provides a feeling of control, decreases feelings of powerlessness, and increases self-esteem.

Disturbed Personal Identity

Disturbed personal identity is defined as the "inability to maintain an integrated and complete perception of self" (NANDA-I, 2009, p. 185).

Client Goals

Outcome criteria include short- and long-term goals. Timelines are individually determined.

Short-Term Goals

■ The client will verbalize understanding of the existence of multiple personalities within the self.

■ The client will be able to recognize stressful situations that precipitate transition from one personality to another.

Long-Term Goals

■ The client will verbalize understanding of the reason for existence of each personality and the role each plays for the individual.

■ The client will enter into and cooperate with long-term therapy, with the ultimate goal being integration into one personality.

Interventions

■ The nurse must develop a trusting relationship with the original personality and with each of the subpersonalities. Trust is the basis of a therapeutic relationship. Each of the personalities views itself as a separate entity and initially must be treated as such.

■ Help the client understand the existence of the subpersonalities and the need each serves in the personal identity of the individual. The client may initially be unaware of the dissociative response. Knowledge of the needs each personality fulfills is the first step in the integration process and the client's ability to face unresolved issues without dissociation.

■ Help the client identify stressful situations that precipitate transition from one personality to another. Carefully observe and record these transitions. Identification of stressors is required to assist the client in responding more adaptively and to eliminate the need for transition to another personality.

■ Use nursing interventions necessary to deal with maladaptive behaviors associated with individual subpersonalities. For example, if one personality is suicidal, precautions must be taken to guard against the client's self-harm. If another personality has a tendency toward physical hostility, precautions must be taken to protect others.

> **CLINICAL PEARL** It may be possible to seek assistance from one of the personalities. For example, a strong-willed personality may help to control the behaviors of a "suicidal" personality.

■ Help subpersonalities understand that their "being" will not be destroyed, but rather integrated into a unified identity within the individual. Because the subpersonalities function as separate entities, the idea of total elimination generates fear and defensiveness.

■ Provide support during disclosure of painful experiences and reassurance when the client becomes discouraged with lengthy treatment.

Concept Care Mapping

The concept map care plan is an innovative approach to planning and organizing nursing care (see Chapter 9). It is a diagrammatic teaching and learning strategy that allows visualization of interrelationships between medical diagnoses, nursing diagnoses, assessment data, and treatments. Examples of concept map care plans for clients with somatoform and dissociative disorders are presented in Figures 30–3 and 30–4.

Evaluation

Reassessment is conducted to determine if the nursing actions have been successful in achieving the objectives of care. Evaluation of the nursing actions for the client with a somatoform disorder may be facilitated by gathering information using the following types of questions:

■ Can the client recognize signs and symptoms of escalating anxiety?

■ Can the client intervene with adaptive coping strategies to interrupt the escalating anxiety before physical symptoms are exacerbated?

■ Can the client verbalize an understanding of the correlation between physical symptoms and times of escalating anxiety?

■ Does the client have a plan for dealing with increased stress to prevent exacerbation of physical symptoms?

■ Does the client demonstrate a decrease in ruminations about physical symptoms?

■ Have fears of serious illness diminished?

■ Does the client demonstrate full recovery from previous loss or alteration of physical functioning?

■ Does the client verbalize a realistic perception and satisfactory acceptance of personal appearance?

Evaluation of the nursing actions for the client with a dissociative disorder may be facilitated by gathering information using the following types of questions:

■ Has the client's memory been restored?

■ Can the client connect occurrence of psychological stress to loss of memory?

■ Does the client discuss fears and anxieties with members of the staff in an effort toward resolution?

■ Can the client discuss the presence of various personalities within the self?

■ Can he or she verbalize why these personalities exist?

■ Can the client verbalize situations that precipitate transition from one personality to another?

■ Can the client maintain a sense of reality during stressful situations?

■ Can the client verbalize a correlation between stressful situations and the onset of depersonalization behaviors?

■ Can the client demonstrate more adaptive coping strategies for dealing with stress without resorting to dissociation?

Treatment Modalities

Somatoform Disorders

Individual Psychotherapy

The goal of psychotherapy is to help clients develop healthy and adaptive behaviors, encourage them to move beyond their somatization, and manage their lives more effectively. The focus is on personal and social difficulties that the client is experiencing in daily life as well as the achievement of practical solutions for these difficulties.

Clinical Vignette: Veronica, age 51, has a long history of "doctor shopping" for numerous complaints of gastrointestinal distress, daily headaches, and abdominal pain. She has undergone numerous tests that show no evidence of pathophysiology. Her husband of 25 years recently died of a myocardial infarction (MI). Yesterday, she began having chest pains and was certain she was having a heart attack. Her daughter called 911, and Veronica was transported to the emergency department. The staff performed diagnostic studies and laboratory tests, which were all negative for pathophysiology. She was admitted to the psychiatric unit with a diagnosis of Somatization Disorder. The nurse develops the following concept map care plan for Veronica.

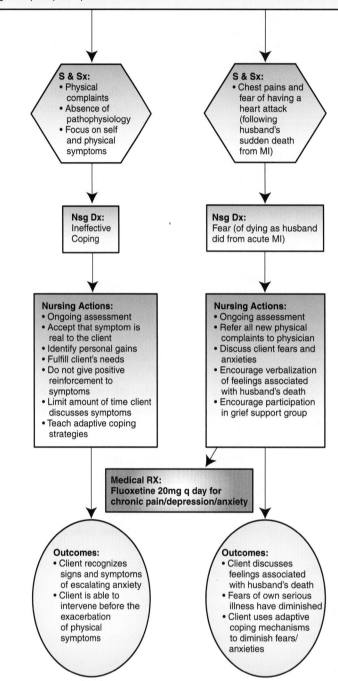

FIGURE 30–3 Concept map care plan for a client with somatization disorder.

Clinical Vignette: Wanda, age 32, was diagnosed 5 years ago with Dissociative Identity Disorder. History revealed severe childhood physical and sexual abuse by both parents. Several personalities have surfaced during years of therapy: an aggressive personality (Jamie), a suicidal personality (Ida), and a 4-year-old child (Anna). Yesterday, following a particularly intense session with her therapist, the personality "Ida" surfaced and swallowed an undisclosed number of sertraline tablets. Wanda's group-home leader called 911, and Wanda was transported to the emergency department (ED). Following stabilization in the ED, Wanda was admitted to the psychiatric unit. The nurse develops the following concept map care plan for Wanda.

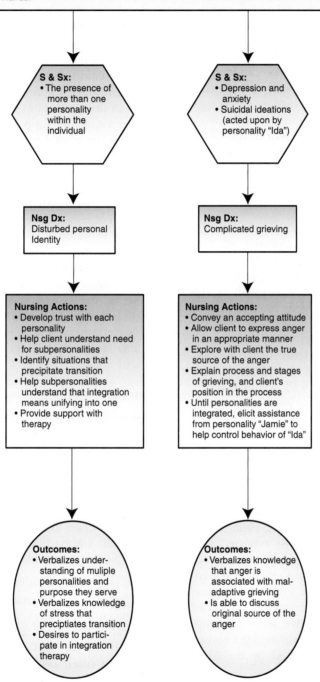

S & Sx:
• The presence of more than one personality within the individual

S & Sx:
• Depression and anxiety
• Suicidal ideations (acted upon by personality "Ida")

Nsg Dx:
Disturbed personal Identity

Nsg Dx:
Complicated grieving

Nursing Actions:
• Develop trust with each personality
• Help client understand need for subpersonalities
• Identify situations that precipitate transition
• Help subpersonalities understand that integration means unifying into one
• Provide support with therapy

Nursing Actions:
• Convey an accepting attitude
• Allow client to express anger in an appropriate manner
• Explore with client the true source of the anger
• Explain process and stages of grieving, and client's position in the process
• Until personalities are integrated, elicit assistance from personality "Jamie" to help control behavior of "Ida"

Outcomes:
• Verbalizes understanding of muliple personalities and purpose they serve
• Verbalizes knowledge of stress that preciptiates transition
• Desires to participate in integration therapy

Outcomes:
• Verbalizes knowledge that anger is associated with mal-adaptive grieving
• Is able to discuss original source of the anger

FIGURE 30–4   Concept map care plan for a client with dissociative identity disorder.

Treatment is initiated with a complete physical examination to rule out organic pathology. Once this has been ensured, the physician turns his or her attention to the client's social and personal problems and away from the somatic complaints.

Group Psychotherapy

Group therapy may be helpful for somatoform disorders because it provides a setting where clients can share their experiences of illness, can learn to verbalize thoughts and feelings, and can be confronted by group members and leaders when they reject responsibility for maladaptive behaviors. It has been reported to be the treatment of choice for both somatization disorder and hypochondriasis, in part because it provides the social support and social interaction that these clients need.

Behavior Therapy

Behavior therapy is more likely to be successful in instances when secondary gain is prominent. This may involve working with the client's family or other significant others who may be perpetuating the physical symptoms by rewarding passivity and dependency and by being overly solicitous and helpful. Behavior therapy focuses on teaching these individuals to reward the client's autonomy, self-sufficiency, and independence. This process becomes more difficult when the client is very regressed and the sick role is well established.

Psychopharmacology

Antidepressants are often used with somatoform pain disorder. They have been shown to be effective in relieving pain, independent of influences on mood. The tricyclic antidepressants (TCAs) have been used extensively, and their efficacy in relieving pain has been demonstrated. Adverse effects with TCAs, however, make their use problematic with some individuals. Leo (2008) reported that "the serotonin and norepinephrine reuptake inhibitors (SNRIs) venlafaxine and duloxetine have demonstrated utility as analgesic agents and bypass several of the untoward effects commonly associated with the TCAs" (p. 1038). Selective serotonin reuptake inhibitors (SSRIs) have not exhibited the consistent analgesic efficacy demonstrated by the TCAs and SNRIs (Leo, 2008).

Anticonvulsants such as phenytoin (Dilantin), carbamazepine (Tegregol), and clonazepam (Klonopin) have been reported to be effective in treating neuropathic and neuralgic pain, at least for short periods. Their efficacy in other somatoform pain disorders is less clear.

Pharmacological therapy also seems to be effective in the treatment of body dysmorphic disorder. The most positive results have been with clomipramine (Anafranil) and fluoxetine (Prozac), which have been shown to reduce symptoms in more than 50 percent of clients with body dysmorphic disorder (Sadock & Sadock, 2007).

Dissociative Amnesia

Many cases of dissociative amnesia resolve spontaneously when the individual is removed from the stressful situation. For other, more refractory conditions, intravenous administration of amobarbital is useful in the retrieval of lost memories. Most clinicians recommend supportive psychotherapy as well to reinforce adjustment to the psychological impact of the retrieved memories and the emotions associated with them.

In some instances, psychotherapy is used as the primary treatment. Techniques of persuasion and free or directed association are used to help the client remember. In other cases, hypnosis may be required to mobilize the memories. Hypnosis is sometimes facilitated by the use of pharmacological agents, such as sodium amobarbital. Once the memories have been obtained through hypnosis, supportive psychotherapy or group psychotherapy may be employed to help the client integrate the memories into his or her conscious state.

Dissociative Fugue

Recovery from dissociative fugue is usually rapid, spontaneous, and complete. In some instances, manipulation of the environment or psychotherapeutic support may help to diminish stress or help the client adapt to stress in the future. When the fugue is prolonged, techniques of gentle encouragement, persuasion, or directed association may be helpful, either alone or in combination with hypnosis or amobarbital interviews. Maldonado and Spiegel (2008) stated:

> Once reorientation is established and the overt aspects of the fugue have been resolved, it is important to work through interpersonal or intrapsychic issues that underlie the dissociative defenses. Individuals with dissociative fugue are often relatively unaware of their reactions to stress because they so effectively can dissociate them. (p. 679)

Cognitive therapy may be useful in helping the client attempt a change in inappropriate or irrational thinking patterns. Creative therapies, such as art and music, allow clients to express and explore thoughts and emotions in "safe" ways. Group therapy can be helpful in providing the client with ongoing support from supportive peers. Family therapy sessions may be used to explore the trauma that precipitated the fugue episode and to educate family members about the dissociative disorder.

Dissociative Identity Disorder

The goal of therapy for the client with DID is to optimize the client's function and potential. The achievement of **integration** (a blending of all the personalities into one) is usually considered desirable, but some clients choose not to pursue this lengthy therapeutic regimen. In these cases resolution, or a smooth collaboration among the subpersonalities, may be all that is realistic.

Intensive, long-term psychotherapy with the DID client is directed toward uncovering the underlying psychological conflicts, helping him or her gain insight into these conflicts, and striving to synthesize the various identities into one integrated personality. Clients are assisted to recall past traumas in detail. They must mentally re-experience the abuse that caused their illness. This process, called **abreaction,** or "remembering with feeling," is so painful that clients may actually cry, scream, and feel the pain that they felt at the time of the abuse.

During therapy, each personality is actively explored and encouraged to become aware of the others across previously amnestic barriers. Traumatic memories associated with the different personality manifestations, especially those related to childhood abuse, are examined. The course of treatment is often difficult and anxiety provoking to client and therapist alike, especially when aggressive or suicidal personalities are in the dominant role. In these instances, brief periods of hospitalization may be necessary as an interim supportive measure.

When integration is achieved, the individual becomes a total of all the feelings, experiences, memories, skills, and talents that were previously in the command of the various personalities. He or she learns how to function effectively without the necessity for creating new personalities to cope with life. This is possible only after years of intense psychotherapy, and even then, recovery is often incomplete.

Depersonalization Disorder

Information about the treatment of depersonalization disorder is sparse and inconclusive. Various psychiatric medications have been tried, both singly and in combination: antidepressants, mood stabilizers, anticonvulsants, and antipsychotics. Results have been sporadic at best. If other psychiatric disorders, such as schizophrenia, are evident, they too may be treated pharmacologically. A study by Simeon, Stein, and Hollander (1998) found the antidepressant clomipramine (Anafranil) to be a promising pharmacological treatment for primary depersonalization disorder. For clients with evident intrapsychic conflict, analytically oriented insight psychotherapy may be useful. Specific recommendations for the management of depersonalization disorder must await more extensive clinical investigation.

CASE STUDY AND SAMPLE CARE PLAN

NURSING HISTORY AND ASSESSMENT

Jake is a 54-year-old client of the psychiatric outpatient department of the VA Medical Center. At age 42, Jake was diagnosed with colon cancer and underwent a colon resection. Since that time, he has had regular follow-up examinations, with no recurrence of the cancer and no residual effects. He did not require follow-up chemotherapy or radiation therapy. For 10 years, Jake has had yearly physical and laboratory examinations. He regularly complains to his family physician of mild abdominal pain, sensations of "fullness," "bowel rumblings," and what he calls a "firm mass," which he says he can sometimes feel in his lower left quadrant. The physician has performed x-rays of the entire gastrointestinal (GI) tract, an esophagoscopy, gastroscopy, and colonoscopy. All results were negative for organic pathology. Rather than being relieved, Jake appears to be resentful and disappointed that the physician has not been able to reveal a pathological problem. Jake's job is in jeopardy because of excessive use of sick leave. The family physician has referred Jake for psychiatric evaluation. Jake was admitted as an outpatient with the diagnosis of hypochondriasis. He has been assigned to Lisa, a psychiatric nurse practitioner.

In her assessment, Lisa learns that Jake has pretty much lived his adult life in isolation. He was never close to his parents, who worked and seldom had time for Jake or his sister. Jake told Lisa that, "My parents really didn't care about me. They were too busy taking care of the farm. Dad wanted me to take over the farm, but I was never interested. I liked working on cars, and went to vocational school to learn how to be a mechanic. I thought they would be proud of me, but they never cared. I think they only had kids so

Continued

CASE STUDY AND SAMPLE CARE PLAN — cont'd

they would have some help on the farm. When I left home, they really didn't care if they ever saw me again." He has never been married nor had a really serious relationship. "Women don't like me much. I spend most of my time alone. I guess I don't really like people, and they don't really like me."

NURSING DIAGNOSES/OUTCOME IDENTIFICATION

From the assessment data, the nurse develops the following nursing diagnoses for Jake:

1. **Fear** (of cancer recurrence) related to history of colon cancer evidenced by numerous complaints of the GI tract and insistence that something is wrong despite objective tests that rule out pathophysiology.

    a. **Short-Term Goal:** Client will verbalize that fears associated with bodily sensations are irrational.

    b. **Long-Term Goal:** Client interprets bodily sensations correctly.

2. **Chronic low self-esteem** related to unfulfilled childhood needs for nurturing and caring evidenced by transformation of internalized anger into physical complaints and hostility toward others.

    a. **Short-Term Goal:** Within 2 weeks, client will verbalize aspects about self that he likes.

    b. **Long-Term Goal:** By discharge from treatment, client will demonstrate acceptance of self as a person of worth, as evidenced by setting realistic goals, limiting physical complaints and hostility toward others, and verbalizing positive prospects for the future.

PLANNING/IMPLEMENTATION

Fear (of Cancer Recurrence)

The following nursing interventions have been identified for Jake.

1. Monitor the physician's ongoing assessments and laboratory reports to ensure that pathology is clearly ruled out.

2. Refer any new physical complaints to the physician.

3. Assess what function these physical complaints are fulfilling for Jake. Is it a way for him to get attention that he can't get in any other way?

4. Show empathy for his feelings. Let him know that you understand how GI symptoms may bring about fears of the colon cancer.

5. Encourage Jake to talk about his fears of cancer recurrence. What feelings did he have when it was first diagnosed? How did he deal with those feelings? What are his fears at this time?

6. Have Jake keep a diary of the appearance of the symptoms. In a separate diary, have Jake keep a record of situations that create stress for him. Compare these two records. Correlate whether symptoms appear at times of increased anxiety.

7. Help Jake determine what techniques may be useful for him to implement when fear and anxiety are exacerbated (e.g., relaxation techniques; mental imagery; thought-stopping techniques; physical exercise).

8. Offer positive feedback when Jake responds to stressful situations with coping strategies other than physical complaints.

Chronic Low Self-esteem

The following nursing interventions have been identified for Jake.

1. Convey acceptance and unconditional positive regard, and remain nonjudgmental at all times.

2. Encourage Jake to participate in decision making regarding his care, as well as in life situations.

3. Help Jake to recognize and focus on strengths and accomplishments. Minimize attention given to past (real or perceived) failures.

4. Encourage Jake to talk about feelings related to his unsatisfactory relationship with his parents.

5. Discuss things in his life that Jake would like to change. Help him determine what *can* be changed and what changes are not realistic.

6. Encourage participation in group activities and in therapy groups that offer simple methods of achievement. Give recognition and positive feedback for actual accomplishments.

7. Teach assertiveness techniques and effective communication techniques.

8. Offer positive feedback for appropriate social interactions with others. Role-play with Jake situations that he finds particularly stressful. Help him to understand that ruminations about himself and his health may cause others to reject him socially.

9. Help Jake to set realistic goals for his future.

EVALUATION

Some of the outcome criteria for Jake have been met, and some are ongoing. He has come to realize that the fears about his "symptoms" are not rational. He understands that the physician has performed adequate diagnostic procedures to rule out illness. He still has fears of cancer occurrence, and discusses these fears with the

CASE STUDY AND SAMPLE CARE PLAN—cont'd

nurse practitioner on a weekly basis. He has kept his symptoms/stressful situations diary, and has correlated the appearance of some of the symptoms to times of increased anxiety. He has started running, and tries to use this as a strategy to keep the anxiety from escalating out of proportion and bringing on new physical symptoms. He continues to discuss feelings associated with his childhood, and the nurse has helped him see

that he has had numerous accomplishments in his life, even though they were not recognized by his parents or others. He has joined a support group for depressed persons, and states that he "has made a few friends." He has made a long-term goal of joining a church with the hope of meeting new people. He is missing fewer workdays because of illness, and his job is no longer in jeopardy.

Summary and Key Points

- Somatoform disorders and dissociative disorders are associated with anxiety that occurs at the severe level. The anxiety is repressed and manifested in the form of symptoms and behaviors associated with these disorders.

- Somatoform disorders, known historically as hysteria, affect about 1 or 2 percent of the female population. Types of somatoform disorders include somatization disorder, pain disorder, hypochondriasis, conversion disorder, and body dysmorphic disorder.

- Somatization disorder is manifested by physical symptoms that may be vague, dramatized, or exaggerated in their presentation. No evidence of organic pathology can be identified.

- In pain disorder, the predominant symptom is pain, for which either there is no medical explanation or the symptom is exaggerated out of proportion to what would be the expected reaction.

- Hypochondriasis is an unrealistic preoccupation with fear of having a serious illness. This disorder may follow a personal experience, or the experience of a close family member, with serious or life-threatening illness.

- The individual with conversion disorder experiences a loss of or alteration in bodily functioning, unsubstantiated by medical or pathophysiological explanation. Psychological factors are evident by the primary or secondary gains the individual achieves from experiencing the physiological manifestation. A relative lack of concern regarding the symptom is identified as "la belle indifference."

- Body dysmorphic disorder, formerly called dysmorphophobia, is the exaggerated belief that the body is deformed or defective in some way. It may be related to more serious psychiatric illness.

- A dissociative response has been described as a defense mechanism to protect the ego in the face of overwhelming anxiety.

- Dissociative responses result in an alteration in the normally integrative functions of identity, memory, or consciousness.

- Classification of dissociative disorders includes dissociative amnesia, dissociative fugue, dissociative identity disorder (DID), and depersonalization disorder.

- The individual with dissociative amnesia has an inability to recall important personal information that is too extensive to be explained by ordinary forgetfulness.

- Dissociative fugue is characterized by a sudden, unexpected travel away from home with an inability to recall the past, including personal identity. Duration of the fugue is usually brief, and once it is over the individual recovers memory of the past life but is amnestic for the time period covered by the fugue.

- The prominent feature of DID is the existence of two or more personalities within a single individual. An individual may have many personalities, each of which serves a purpose for that individual of enduring painful stimuli that the original personality is too weak to face.

- Depersonalization disorder is characterized by an alteration in the perception of oneself (sometimes described as a feeling of having separated from the body and watching the activities of the self from a distance).

■ Individuals with somatoform and dissociative disorders often receive health care initially in areas other than psychiatry.

■ Nurses can assist clients with these disorders by helping them to understand their problem and identify and establish new, more adaptive behavior patterns.

 Additional info available @ davisplus.fadavis.com

Review Questions
Self-Examination/Learning Exercise

*Select the answer that is **most** appropriate for each of the following questions:*

1. Lorraine has been diagnosed with Somatization Disorder. Which of the following symptom profiles would you expect when assessing Lorraine?
   a. Multiple somatic symptoms in several body systems.
   b. Fear of having a serious disease.
   c. Loss or alteration in sensorimotor functioning.
   d. Belief that her body is deformed or defective in some way.

2. Which of the following ego defense mechanisms describes the underlying dynamics of somatization disorder?
   a. Denial of depression.
   b. Repression of anxiety.
   c. Suppression of grief.
   d. Displacement of anger.

3. Nursing care for a client with somatization disorder would focus on helping her to:
   a. Eliminate the stress in her life.
   b. Discontinue her numerous physical complaints.
   c. Take her medication only as prescribed.
   d. Learn more adaptive coping strategies.

4. Lorraine, a client diagnosed with Somatization Disorder, states, "My doctor thinks I should see a psychiatrist. I can't imagine why he would make such a suggestion!" What is the basis for Lorraine's statement?
   a. She thinks her doctor wants to get rid of her as a client.
   b. She does not understand the correlation of symptoms and stress.
   c. She thinks psychiatrists are only for "crazy" people.
   d. She thinks her doctor has made an error in diagnosis.

5. Lorraine, a client diagnosed with Somatization Disorder, tells the nurse about a pain in her side. She says she has not experienced it before. Which is the most appropriate response by the nurse?
   a. "I don't want to hear about another physical complaint. You know they are all in your head. It's time for group therapy now."
   b. "Let's sit down here together and you can tell me about this new pain you are experiencing. You'll just have to miss group therapy today."
   c. "I will report this pain to your physician. In the meantime, group therapy starts in 5 minutes. You must leave now to be on time."
   d. "I will call your physician and see if he will order a new pain medication for your side. The one you have now doesn't seem to provide relief. Why don't you get some rest for now?"

Review Questions—cont'd
Self-Examination/Learning Exercise

6. Ellen has a history of childhood physical and sexual abuse. She was diagnosed with Dissociative Identity Disorder (DID) 6 years ago. She has been admitted to the psychiatric unit following a suicide attempt. The primary nursing diagnosis for Ellen would be:
   a. Disturbed personal identity related to childhood abuse.
   b. Disturbed sensory perception related to repressed anxiety.
   c. Disturbed thought processes related to memory deficit.
   d. Risk for suicide related to unresolved grief.

7. In establishing trust with Ellen, a client with the diagnosis of DID, the nurse must:
   a. Try to relate to Ellen as though she did not have multiple personalities.
   b. Establish a relationship with each of the personalities separately.
   c. Ignore behaviors that Ellen attributes to Beth.
   d. Explain to Ellen that he or she will work with her only if she maintains the status of the primary personality.

8. The ultimate goal of therapy for a client with DID is:
   a. Integration of the personalities into one.
   b. For the client to have the ability to switch from one personality to another voluntarily.
   c. For the client to select which personality he or she wants to be the dominant self.
   d. For the client to recognize that the various personalities exist.

9. The ultimate goal of therapy for a client with DID is most likely achieved through:
   a. Crisis intervention and directed association.
   b. Psychotherapy and hypnosis.
   c. Psychoanalysis and free association.
   d. Insight psychotherapy and dextroamphetamines.

10. A nurse on the psychiatric unit has the understanding that which of the following would describe a client with "la belle indifference"?
    a. A client with somatization disorder who is demanding narcotics.
    b. A client with depersonalization disorder who believes he has died.
    c. A client with DID who is threatening suicide.
    d. A client with conversion disorder showing lack of concern for an altered body function.

TEST YOUR CRITICAL THINKING SKILLS

Tom was admitted to the psychiatric unit from the emergency department of a general hospital in the Midwest. The owner of a local bar called the police when Tom suddenly seemed to "lose control. He just went ballistic." The police reported that Tom did not know where he was or how he got there. He kept saying, "My name is John Brown, and I live in Philadelphia." When the police ran an identity check on Tom, they found that he was indeed John Brown from Philadelphia and his wife had reported him missing a month ago. Mrs. Brown explained that, about 12 months before his disappearance, her husband, who was a shop foreman at a large manufacturing plant, had been having considerable difficulty at work. He had been passed over for a promotion, and his supervisor had been very critical of his work. Several of his staff had left

the company for other jobs, and without enough help, Tom had been unable to meet shop deadlines. Work stress made him very difficult to live with at home. Previously an easygoing, extroverted individual, he became withdrawn and extremely critical of his wife and children. Immediately preceding his disappearance, he had had a violent argument with his 18-year-old son, who called Tom a "loser" and stormed out of the house to stay with some friends. It was the day after this argument that Tom disappeared. The psychiatrist assigns a diagnosis of Dissociative Fugue.
Answer the following questions related to Tom:

1. Describe the *priority* nursing intervention with Tom as he is admitted to the psychiatric unit.

2. What approach should be taken to help Tom with his problem?

3. What is the long-term goal of therapy for Tom?

References

American Psychiatric Association. (2000). *Diagnostic and statistical manual of mental disorders* (4th ed.). *Text revision.* Washington, DC: American Psychiatric Publishing.

Black, D. W., & Andreasen, N. C. (2011). *Introductory textbook of psychiatry* (5th ed.). Washington, DC: American Psychiatric Publishing.

Brunet, A., Holowka, D. W., & Laurence, J. R. (2003). Dissociation. In M. J. Aminoff & R. B. Daroff (Eds.), *Encyclopedia of the neurological sciences* (Vol. 2). New York: Elsevier.

Leo, R. J. (2008). Pain disorders. In R. E. Hales, S. C. Yudofsky, & G. O. Gabbard (Eds.), *Textbook of psychiatry* (5th ed., pp. 1025–1050). Washington, DC: American Psychiatric Publishing.

Maldonado, J. R., & Spiegel, D. (2008). Dissociative disorders. In R. E. Hales, S. C. Yudofsky, & G. O. Gabbard (Eds.), *Textbook of psychiatry* (5th ed., pp. 665–710). Washington, DC: American Psychiatric Publishing.

NANDA International. (2009). *Nursing diagnoses: Definitions and classification 2009-2011.* Hoboken, NJ: Wiley-Blackwell.

Parcell, S. (2008). Biochemical and nutritional influences on pain. In J. F. Audette & A. Bailey (Eds.), *Integrative pain medicine* (pp. 133–172). New York: Springer-Verlag.

Sadock, B. J., & Sadock, V. A. (2007). *Synopsis of psychiatriy: Behavioral sciences/clinical psychiatry* (10th ed.). Philadelphia: Lippincott Williams & Wilkins.

Shahrokh, N. C., & Hales, R. E. (2003). *American psychiatric glossary* (8th ed.). Washington, DC: American Psychiatric Publishing.

Simeon, D., Stein, D. J., & Hollander, E. (1998). Treatment of depersonalization disorder with clomipramine. *Biological Psychiatry, 44,* 302–303.

Soares, N., & Grossman, L. (2010, February 10). Conversion disorder. *Emedicine Pediatrics.* Retrieved September 21, 2010, from http://emedicine.medscape.com/article/917864-overview

Wootton, J. (2008). Meditation and chronic pain. In J. F. Audette & A. Bailey (Eds.), *Integrative pain medicine* (pp. 195–210). New York: Springer-Verlag.

Yutzy, S. H., & Parish, B. S. (2008). Somatoform disorders. In R. E. Hales, S. C. Yudofsky, & G. O. Gabbard (Eds.), *Textbook of psychiatry* (5th ed., pp. 609–664). Washington, DC: American Psychiatric Publishing.

Classical References

Freud, S. (1962). The neuro-psychoses of defense. In J. Strachey (Ed.), *Standard edition of the complete psychological works of Sigmund Freud,* (Vol. 3). London: Hogarth Press. (Original work published 1894).

@ INTERNET REFERENCES

- Additional information about somatoform disorders may be located at the following websites:
  - http://www.psyweb.com/Mdisord/somatd.html
  - http://www.uib.no/med/avd/med_a/gastro/wilhelms/hypochon.html
  - http://emedicine.medscape.com/article/805361-overview
  - http://www.findarticles.com/p/articles/mi_g2601/is_0012/ai_2601001276

- Additional information about dissociative disorders may be located at the following websites:
  - http://www.human-nature.com/odmh/dissociative.html
  - http://www.nami.org/helpline/dissoc.htm
  - http://www.isst-d.org/
  - http://findarticles.com/p/articles/mi_g2601/ is_0004/ai_2601000438/
  - http://www.mental-health-matters.com/disorders/
  - http://www.emedicine.com/med/topic3484.htm

MOVIE CONNECTIONS

Bandits (hypochondriasis) • *Hanna and Her Sisters* (hypochondriasis) • *Send Me No Flowers* (hypochondriasis) • *Dead Again* (amnesia) • *Mirage* (amnesia) • *Suddenly Last Summer* (amnesia) • *The Three Lives of Karen* (fugue) • *Sybil* (DID) • *The Three Faces of Eve* (DID) • *Identity* (DID)

Issues Related to Human Sexuality and Gender Identity

CHAPTER OUTLINE

CORE CONCEPTS

gender

sexuality

KEY TERMS

anorgasmia

dyspareunia

exhibitionism

fetishism

frotteurism

homosexuality

lesbianism

masochism

orgasm

paraphilia

pedophilia

premature ejaculation

retarded ejaculation

sadism

sensate focus

transgenderism

transvestic fetishism

vaginismus

voyeurism

OBJECTIVES

After reading this chapter, the student will be able to:

1. Describe developmental processes associated with human sexuality.
2. Discuss historical and epidemiological aspects of paraphilias and sexual dysfunction disorders.
3. Identify various types of paraphilias, sexual dysfunction disorders, and gender identity disorders.
4. Discuss predisposing factors associated with the etiology of paraphilias, sexual dysfunction disorders, and gender identity disorders.
5. Describe the physiology of the human sexual response.
6. Conduct a sexual history.
7. Formulate nursing diagnoses and goals of care for clients with sexual and gender identity disorders.
8. Identify appropriate nursing interventions for clients with sexual and gender identity disorders.
9. Identify topics for client/family education relevant to sexual disorders.
10. Evaluate care of clients with sexual and gender identity disorders.
11. Describe various treatment modalities for clients with sexual disorders.
12. Discuss variations in sexual orientation.
13. Identify various types of sexually transmitted diseases and discuss the consequences of each.

HOMEWORK ASSIGNMENT
Please read the chapter and answer the following questions:

1. At about what age do children become aware of their own gender?
2. What types of psychosocial factors may predispose individuals to sexual desire disorders?
3. What is *dyspareunia?*
4. To disturbances in what physiological mechanism are sexual dysfunctions related?

Humans are sexual beings. Sexuality is a basic human need and an innate part of the total personality. It influences our thoughts, actions, and interactions, and is involved in aspects of physical and mental health.

Society's attitude toward sexuality is changing. Clients are more open to seeking assistance in matters that pertain to sexuality. Although not all nurses need to be educated as sex therapists, they can readily integrate information on sexuality into the care they give by focusing on preventive, therapeutic, and educational interventions to assist individuals to attain, regain, or maintain sexual wellness.

This chapter focuses on disorders associated with sexual functioning and gender identity. Primary consideration is given to the categories of **paraphilias** and sexual dysfunction as classified in the *Diagnostic and Statistical Manual of Mental Disorders, Fourth Edition, Text Revision* (DSM-IV-TR) (American Psychiatric Association [APA], 2000). An overview of human sexual development throughout the life span is presented. Historical and epidemiological information associated with sexual disorders is included. Predisposing factors that have been implicated in the etiology of sexual disorders and gender identity disorders provide a framework for studying the dynamics of these disorders. Various medical treatment modalities are explored. A discussion of variations in sexual orientation is included. Various types of sexually transmitted diseases (STDs) are described, and an explanation of the consequences of each is presented.

Symptomatology of each disorder is presented as background knowledge for assessing clients with sexual and gender identity disorders. A tool for acquiring a sexual history is included. Nursing care is described in the context of the nursing process.

CORE CONCEPT

Sexuality
Sexuality is the constitution and life of an individual relative to characteristics regarding intimacy. It reflects the totality of the person and does not relate exclusively to the sex organs or sexual behavior.

Development of Human Sexuality

Birth Through Age 12

Although the sexual identity of an infant is determined before birth by chromosomal factors and physical appearance of the genitals, postnatal factors can greatly influence the way developing children perceive themselves sexually. Masculinity and femininity, as well as gender roles, are for the most part culturally defined. For example, differentiation of roles may be initiated at birth by painting a child's room pink or blue and by clothing the child in frilly, delicate dresses or tough, sturdy rompers.

It is not uncommon for infants to touch and explore their genitals. In fact, research on infantile sexuality indicates that both male and female infants are capable of sexual arousal and **orgasm** (Berman & Berman, 2001).

By age 2 or 2½ years, children know what gender they are. They know that they are like the parent of the same gender and different from the parent of the opposite gender and from other children of the opposite gender. They become acutely aware of anatomical gender differences during this time.

By age 4 or 5, children engage in heterosexual play. "Playing doctor" can be a popular game at this age. Through heterosexual play, children form a concept of marriage to a member of the opposite gender.

Children increasingly gain experience with masturbation during childhood, although certainly not all children masturbate during this period. Most children begin self-exploration and genital self-stimulation as soon as they are able to gain sufficient control over their physical movements (King, 2009).

Late childhood and preadolescence may be characterized by heterosexual or homosexual play. Generally the activity involves no more than touching the other's genitals, but may include a wide range of sexual behaviors (Masters, Johnson, & Kolodny, 1995). Girls at this age become interested in menstruation, and both sexes are interested in learning about fertility, pregnancy, and birth. Interest in the opposite gender increases. Children of this age become self-conscious about their bodies and are concerned with physical attractiveness.

Children ages 10 to 12 are preoccupied with pubertal changes and the beginnings of romantic sexual attraction. Prepubescent boys may engage in group sexual activities such as genital exhibition or group masturbation. Homosexual sex play is not uncommon. Prepubescent girls may engage in some genital exhibition, but they are usually not as preoccupied with the genitalia as are boys of this age.

Adolescence

Adolescence represents an acceleration in terms of biological changes and psychosocial and sexual development. This time of turmoil is nurtured by awakening endocrine forces and a new set of psychosocial tasks to undertake. Included in these tasks are issues relating to sexuality, such as how to deal with new or more powerful sexual feelings, whether to participate in various types of sexual behavior, how to recognize love, how to prevent unwanted pregnancy, and how to define age-appropriate sex roles.

Biologically, puberty begins for the female adolescent with breast enlargement, widening of the hips, and growth of pubic and ancillary hair. The onset of menstruation usually occurs between the ages of 11 and 13 years. In the male adolescent, growth of pubic hair and enlargement of the testicles begin at 12 to 16 years of age. Penile growth and the ability to ejaculate usually occur from the ages of 13 to 17. There is a marked growth of the body between ages 11 and 17, accompanied by the growth of body and facial hair, increased muscle mass, and a deeper voice.

Sexuality is slower to develop in the female than in the male adolescent. Women show steady increases in sexual responsiveness that peak in their middle 20s or early 30s. Sexual maturity for men is usually reached in the late teens, but their sexual drive remains high through young adulthood (Murray, Zentner, & Yakimo, 2009). Masturbation is a common sexual activity among male and female adolescents.

Many individuals have their first experience with sexual intercourse during the adolescent years. Although studies indicate a variety of statistics related to incidence of adolescent coitus, three notable trends have become evident during the past three decades:

1. More adolescents are engaging in premarital intercourse.

2. The incidence of premarital intercourse for girls has increased.

3. The average age of first intercourse has decreased.

The most recent data collected on this topic by the Centers for Disease Control and Prevention (CDC) indicated that there is a trend toward safer sex among adolescents. The survey revealed that, among those who reported being sexually active, there has been a trend toward increased condom use since 1991 (CDC, 2010b).

The American culture has ambivalent feelings about adolescent sexuality. Psychosexual development is desired, but most parents want to avoid anything that may encourage teenage sex. The rise in number of cases of STDs, some of which are life threatening, also contributes to fears associated with unprotected sexual activity in all age groups.

In June 2006, the U.S. Food and Drug Administration (FDA) licensed Gardasil, the first vaccine developed to prevent cervical cancer and other diseases caused by certain strains of human papillomavirus (HPV). A second vaccine, Cervarix, was approved by the FDA in October 2009. If administered prior to exposure to the sexually transmitted virus, these vaccines can protect women from ultimately developing cervical cancer caused by these specific strains. The CDC recommends routine administration of the vaccine to all girls ages 11 or 12 years (CDC, 2010a). The vaccine is also recommended for girls and women ages 13 through 26 years who have not already received the vaccine or have not completed all booster shots. In October 2009, the CDC's Advisory Committee on Immunization Practices (ACIP) provided guidance that males ages 9 through 26 years may also be given the HPV vaccine, Gardasil, to reduce their likelihood of acquiring genital warts (CDC, 2010a). The ACIP does not recommend the vaccine for routine use among males. Some state legislatures have proposed making administration of the HPV vaccine mandatory for girls ages 9 to 12 years. However, some parents believe these types of laws circumvent their rights, and may send the message that these young women are protected and therefore promote promiscuity. Currently the controversy is ongoing, with supporters of a mandate saying that states have a rare opportunity to fight a cancer that kills 3,700 American women every year, and it must be given before a woman has been infected with the virus to be effective. But opponents say states—and parents—should be trying to prevent premarital sex instead of requiring a vaccination with the assumption that it is going to happen.

Adulthood

This period of the life cycle begins at approximately 20 years of age and continues to age 65. Sexuality associated with ages 65 and older is discussed in Chapter 35.

Marital Sex

Choosing a marital partner or developing a sexual relationship with another individual is one of the major tasks in the early years of this life-cycle stage. Current cultural perspective reflects that the institution of marriage has survived. About 80 to 90 percent of all people in the United States marry, and of those who divorce, a high percentage remarries. Intimacy in marriage is one of the most common forms of sexual expression for adults. The average American couple has coitus about two or three times per week when they are in their 20s, with the frequency gradually declining to about once weekly for those 45 years of age and over. Many adults continue to masturbate even though they are married and have ready access to heterosexual sex. This behavior is perfectly normal, although it often evokes feelings of guilt and may be kept secret.

Extramarital Sex

A number of studies present various results for surveys of extramarital sex. The estimates are that about a third of married men and a fourth of married women have engaged in extramarital sex at some time during their marriages (King, 2009). Although the incidence of extramarital sex for men seems to be holding constant, some evidence exists to suggest that the incidence for women may be increasing.

Although attitudes toward premarital sex have changed substantially during the last several decades, attitudes toward extramarital sex have remained relatively stable. Most women and men say they believe sexual exclusivity should be a goal in marriage, although they were less certain about what would happen if their partner did not live up to that ideal. Some studies place the incidence of divorce caused by infidelity or adultery at around 20 percent of all divorce cases.

Sex and the Single Person

Attitudes about sexual intimacy among singles—never married, divorced, or widowed—vary from individual to individual. Some single people will settle for any kind of relationship, casual or committed, that they believe will enrich their lives. Others deny any desire for marriage or sexual intimacy, cherishing instead the independence they retain by being "unattached." Still others may search desperately for a spouse, with the desperation increasing as the years wear on.

Most divorced men and women return to having an active sex life following separation from their spouse. More widowed men than widowed women return to an active sex life after the loss of their partner. This may have in part to do with the fact that men choose women partners younger than themselves, and because widows outnumber widowers by more than 4 to 1 (Administration on Aging, 2011).

The "Middle" Years—40 to 65

With the advent of the middle years, a decrease in hormonal production initiates a number of changes in the sex organs, as well as the rest of the body. The average age of onset of menopause for the woman is around 50, although changes can be noted from about 40 to 60 years of age. Approximately 1 percent of women experience symptoms as early as age 35 (Murray et al., 2009). The decrease in the amount of estrogen can result in loss of vaginal lubrication, making intercourse painful. Other symptoms may include insomnia, "hot flashes," headaches, heart palpitations, and depression. Hormonal supplements may alleviate some of these symptoms, although controversy currently exists within the medical community regarding the safety of hormone replacement therapy.

With the decrease of androgen production during these years, men also experience sexual changes. The amount of ejaculate may decrease, and ejaculation may be less forceful. The testes decrease in size, and erections may be less frequent and less rigid. By age 50, the refractory period increases, and men may require 8 to 24 hours after orgasm before another erection can be achieved.

Biological drives decrease, and interest in sexual activity may decrease during these "middle" years. Although men need longer stimulation to reach orgasm and intensity of pleasure may decrease, women stabilize at the same level of sexual activity as at the previous stage in the life cycle and often have a greater capacity for orgasm in middle adulthood than in young adulthood (Sadock & Sadock, 2007). Murray and associates (2009) stated,

> The enjoyment of sexual relations in younger years, rather than the frequency, is a key factor for maintenance of desire and activity in females, whereas frequency of relations and enjoyment are important factors for males. (p. 561)

Sexual Disorders

Paraphilias

The term *paraphilia* is used to identify repetitive or preferred sexual fantasies or behaviors that involve any of the following:

■ The preference for use of a nonhuman object

■ Repetitive sexual activity with humans that involves real or simulated suffering or humiliation

■ Repetitive sexual activity with nonconsenting partners

The *DSM-IV-TR* specifies that these sexual fantasies or behaviors are recurrent over a period of at least 6 months and cause the individual clinically significant distress or impairment in social, occupational, or other important areas of functioning (APA, 2000).

Historical Aspects

Historically, some restrictions on human sexual expression have always existed. Under the code of Orthodox Judaism, masturbation was punishable by death. In ancient Catholicism it was considered a carnal sin. In the late 19th century, masturbation was viewed as a major cause of insanity.

The sexual exploitation of children was condemned in ancient cultures, as it continues to be today. Incest remains the one taboo that crosses cultural barriers. It was punishable by death in Babylonia, Judea, and ancient China, and offenders were given the death penalty as late as 1650 in England.

Oral-genital, anal, homosexual, and animal sexual contacts were viewed by the early Christian church as unnatural and, in fact, were considered greater transgressions than extramarital sexual activity because they did not lead to biological reproduction. Today, of these church-condemned behaviors, only sex with animals (zoophilia) retains its classification as a paraphilia in the *DSM-IV-TR*.

Epidemiological Statistics

Relatively limited data exist on the prevalence or course of the paraphilias. Most available information has been obtained from studies of incarcerated sex offenders. Another source of information has been from outpatient psychiatric services for paraphiliacs outside the criminal justice system.

Because few paraphiliacs experience personal distress from their behavior, most individuals come for treatment because of pressure from their partners or the authorities (Becker & Johnson, 2008). Data suggest that most people with paraphilias who seek outpatient treatment do so for **pedophilia** (45 percent), **exhibitionism** (25 percent), or **voyeurism** (12 percent).

Most individuals with paraphilias are men, and the behavior is generally established in adolescence (Black & Andreasen, 2011). The behavior peaks between ages 15 and 25 and gradually declines so that, by age 50, the occurrence of paraphilic acts is very low, except for those paraphilic behaviors that occur in isolation or with a cooperative partner. Some individuals with these disorders experience multiple paraphilias.

Types of Paraphilias

The following types of paraphilias are identified by the *DSM-IV-TR*.

Exhibitionism

Exhibitionism is characterized by recurrent, intense, sexual urges, behaviors, or sexually arousing fantasies, of at least a 6-month duration, involving the exposure of one's genitals to an unsuspecting stranger (APA, 2000). Masturbation may occur during the exhibitionism. In almost 100 percent of cases of exhibitionism, the perpetrators are men and the victims are women (King, 2009).

The urges for genital exposure intensify when the exhibitionist has excessive free time or is under significant stress. Most people who engage in exhibitionism have rewarding sexual relationships with adult partners but concomitantly expose themselves to others.

Fetishism

Fetishism involves recurrent, intense, sexual urges or behaviors, or sexually arousing fantasies, of at least a 6-month duration, involving the use of non-living objects (APA, 2000). The sexual focus is commonly on objects intimately associated with the human body (e.g., shoes, gloves, stockings). The fetish object is usually used during masturbation or incorporated into sexual activity with another person in order to produce sexual excitation.

When the fetish involves cross-dressing, the disorder is called **transvestic fetishism.** The individual is a heterosexual man who keeps a collection of women's clothing that he intermittently uses to dress in when alone. The sexual arousal may be produced by an accompanying fantasy of the individual as a woman with female genitalia, or merely by the view of himself fully clothed as a woman without attention to the genitalia (APA, 2000).

Requirement of the fetish object for sexual arousal may become so intense in some individuals that to be without it may result in impotence. Onset of the disorder usually occurs during adolescence.

The disorder is chronic, and the complication arises when the individual becomes progressively more intensely aroused by sexual behaviors that exclude a sexual partner. The person with the fetish and his partner may become so distant that the partner eventually terminates the relationship.

Frotteurism

Frotteurism is the recurrent preoccupation with intense sexual urges, behaviors, or fantasies, of at least a 6-month duration, involving touching and rubbing against a nonconsenting person (APA, 2000). Sexual excitement is derived from the actual touching or rubbing, not from the coercive nature of the act. Almost without exception, the gender of the frotteur is male.

The individual usually chooses to commit the act in crowded places, such as on buses or subways during rush hour. In this way, he can provide rationalization for his behavior, should someone complain, and can more easily escape arrest. The frotteur waits in a crowd until he identifies a victim, then he follows her and allows the rush of the crowd to push him against her. He fantasizes a relationship with his victim while rubbing his genitals against her thighs and buttocks or touching her genitalia or breasts with his hands. He often escapes detection because of the victim's initial shock and denial that such an act has been committed in this public place.

Pedophilia

The *DSM-IV-TR* describes the essential feature of pedophilia as recurrent sexual urges, behaviors, or sexually arousing fantasies, of at least a 6-month duration, involving sexual activity with a prepubescent child. The age of the molester is at least 16, and he or she is at least 5 years older than the child. This category of paraphilia is the most common of sexual assaults.

Most child molestations involve genital fondling or oral sex. Vaginal or anal penetration of the child is most common in cases of incest. Others may limit their activity to undressing the child and looking, exposing themselves, masturbating in the presence of the child, or gently touching and fondling of the child (APA, 2000). Onset usually occurs during adolescence, and the disorder often runs a chronic course.

Sexual Masochism

The identifying feature of sexual **masochism** is recurrent, intense, sexual urges, behaviors, or sexually arousing fantasies, of at least a 6-month duration, involving the act (real, not simulated) of being humiliated, beaten, bound, or otherwise made to suffer (APA, 2000). These masochistic activities may be fantasized (e.g., being raped) and may be performed alone (e.g., self-inflicted pain) or with a partner (e.g., being restrained, spanked, or beaten by the partner). Some masochistic activities have resulted in death, in particular those that involve sexual arousal by oxygen deprivation. The disorder is usually chronic and can progress to the point at which the individual cannot achieve sexual satisfaction without masochistic fantasies or activities.

Sexual Sadism

The *DSM-IV-TR* identifies the essential feature of sexual **sadism** as recurrent, intense, sexual urges, behaviors, or sexually arousing fantasies, of at least a 6-month duration, involving acts (real, not simulated) in which the psychological or physical suffering (including humiliation) of the victim is sexually exciting to the person (APA, 2000). The sadistic activities may be fantasized or acted on with a consenting or nonconsenting partner. In all instances, sexual excitation occurs in response to the suffering of the victim. Examples of sadistic acts include restraint, beating, burning, rape, cutting, torture, and even killing.

The course of the disorder is usually chronic, with the severity of the sadistic acts often increasing over time. Activities with nonconsenting partners are usually terminated by legal apprehension.

Voyeurism

This disorder is identified by recurrent, intense, sexual urges, behaviors, or sexually arousing fantasies, of at least a 6-month duration, involving the act of observing an unsuspecting person who is naked, in the process of disrobing, or engaging in sexual activity (APA, 2000). Sexual excitement is achieved through the act of looking, and no contact with the person is attempted. Masturbation usually accompanies the "window peeping" but may occur later as the individual fantasizes about the voyeuristic act.

Onset of voyeuristic behavior is usually before age 15, and the disorder is often chronic. Most voyeurs enjoy satisfying sexual relationships with an adult partner. Few apprehensions occur because most targets of voyeurism are unaware that they are being observed.

Predisposing Factors to Paraphilias

Biological Factors

Various studies have implicated several organic factors in the etiology of paraphilias. Destruction of parts of the limbic system in animals has been shown to cause hypersexual behavior (Becker & Johnson, 2008). Temporal lobe diseases, such as psychomotor seizures or temporal lobe tumors, have been implicated in some individuals with paraphilias. Abnormal levels of androgens also may contribute to inappropriate sexual arousal. The majority of studies have involved violent sex offenders, and the results cannot accurately be generalized.

Psychoanalytic Theory

The psychoanalytic approach defines a paraphiliac as one who has failed the normal developmental process toward heterosexual adjustment (Sadock & Sadock, 2007). This occurs when the individual fails to resolve the Oedipal crisis and either identifies with the parent of the opposite gender or selects an inappropriate object for libido cathexis. Becker and Johnson (2008) offered the following explanation:

> Severe castration anxiety during the Oedipal phase of development leads to the substitution of a symbolic object (inanimate or an anatomic part) for the mother, as in fetishism and transvestitism. Similarly, anxiety over arousal to the mother can lead to the choice of "safe," inappropriate sexual partners, as in pedophilia and zoophilia, or safe sexual behaviors in which there is no sexual contact, as in exhibitionism and voyeurism. (p. 740)

Behavioral Theory

The behavioral model hypothesizes that whether or not an individual engages in paraphiliac behavior depends on the type of reinforcement he or she receives following the behavior. The initial act may be committed for various reasons. Some examples include recalling memories of experiences from an individual's early life (especially the first shared sexual experience), modeling behavior of others who have carried out paraphilic acts, mimicking sexual behavior depicted in the media, and recalling past trauma such as one's own molestation (Sadock & Sadock, 2007).

Once the initial act has been committed, the paraphiliac consciously evaluates the behavior and decides whether to repeat it. A fear of punishment or perceived harm or injury to the victim, or a lack of pleasure derived from the experience, may extinguish the behavior. However, when negative consequences do not occur, when the act itself is highly pleasurable, or when the person with the paraphilia immediately escapes and thereby avoids seeing any negative consequences experienced by the victim, the activity is more likely to be repeated.

Transactional Model of Stress/Adaptation

One model alone is probably not sufficient to explain the etiology of paraphilias. It is most likely that the integration of learning experiences, sociocultural factors, and biological processes must occur to account for these deviant sexual behaviors. A combination of biological, psychosocial, and cultural factors, along with aspects of the learning paradigm previously described, probably provides the most comprehensive etiological explanation for paraphilias to date. In Figure 31–1, a graphic depiction of the theory of multiple causation is presented in the Transactional Model of Stress/Adaptation.

Treatment Modalities for Paraphilias

Biological Treatment

Biological treatment of individuals with paraphilias has focused on blocking or decreasing the level of circulating androgens. The most extensively used of the antiandrogenic medications are the progestin derivatives that block testosterone synthesis or block androgen receptors. They do not influence the direction of sexual drive toward appropriate adult partners. Instead they act to decrease libido, and thus break the individual's pattern of compulsive deviant sexual behavior (Becker & Johnson, 2008). They are not meant to be the sole source of treatment and work best when given in conjunction with participation in individual or group psychotherapy.

Psychoanalytic Therapy

Psychoanalytic approaches have been tried in the treatment of paraphilias. In this type of therapy, the therapist helps the client to identify unresolved conflicts and traumas from early childhood. The therapy focuses on helping the individual resolve these early conflicts, thus relieving the anxiety that prevents him or her from forming appropriate sexual relationships. In turn the individual has no further need for paraphilic fantasies.

Behavior Therapy

Aversion techniques have been used to modify undesirable behavior. Aversion therapy methods in the treatment of paraphilias involve pairing noxious stimuli, such as electric shocks and bad odors, with the impulse, which then diminishes. Behavior therapy also includes skills training and cognitive restructuring in an effort to change the individual's maladaptive beliefs.

Other behavioral approaches to decreasing inappropriate sexual arousal have included covert sensitization and satiation. With covert

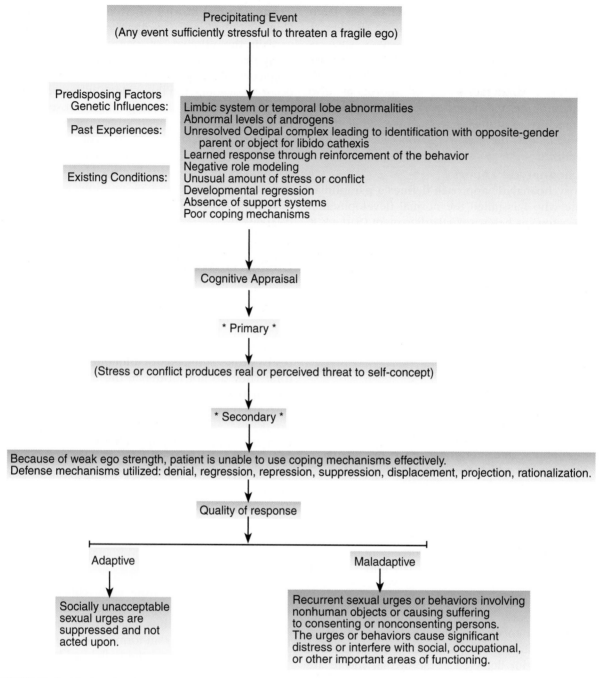

FIGURE 31–1 The dynamics of paraphilia using the Transactional Model of Stress/Adaptation.

sensitization, the individual combines inappropriate sexual fantasies with aversive, anxiety-provoking scenes under the guidance of the therapist (Becker & Johnson, 2008). Satiation is a technique in which the postorgasmic individual repeatedly fantasizes deviant behaviors to the point of saturation with the deviant stimuli, consequently making the fantasies and behavior unexciting.

Role of the Nurse

Treatment of the person with a paraphilia is often very frustrating for both the client and the therapist. Most individuals with paraphilias deny that they have a problem and seek psychiatric care only after their inappropriate behavior comes to the attention of others. In secondary prevention, the focus is to diagnose and treat the problem as early as possible to minimize difficulties. These individuals should be referred to specialists who are accustomed to working with this special population.

Nursing may best become involved in the primary prevention process. The focus of primary prevention in sexual disorders is to intervene in home life or other facets of childhood in an effort to prevent problems from developing. An additional concern of primary prevention is to assist in the development of adaptive coping strategies to deal with stressful life situations.

Three major components of sexual development have been identified: (1) gender identity (one's sense of maleness or femaleness), (2) sexual responsiveness (arousal to appropriate stimuli), and (3) the ability to establish relationships with others. A disturbance in one or more of these components may lead to a variety of sexual deviations.

Different developmental components seem to be disturbed in the various sexual deviations. For example, gender identity may be disturbed in transvestitism or **transgenderism.** The second component, sexual responsiveness to appropriate stimuli, is disturbed in the case of the fetishist. In the case of the exhibitionist or the frotteur, the ability to form relationships may be disturbed.

Nurses can participate in the regular evaluation of these developmental components to ensure that, as children mature, their development in each of these three components is healthy, thereby preventing deviant sexual behaviors. Nurses who work in pediatrics, psychiatry, public health, ambulatory clinics, schools, and any other facility requiring contact with children must be knowledgeable about human sexual development. Accurate assessment and early intervention by these nurses can contribute a great deal toward primary prevention of sexual disorders.

Sexual Dysfunctions

The Sexual Response Cycle

Because sexual dysfunctions occur as disturbances in any of the phases of the sexual response cycle, an understanding of anatomy and physiology is a prerequisite to considerations of pathology and treatment.

■ **Phase I—Desire:** During this phase, the desire to have sexual activity occurs in response to verbal, physical, or visual stimulation. Sexual fantasies can also bring about this desire.

■ **Phase II—Excitement:** This is the phase of sexual arousal and erotic pleasure. Physiological changes occur. The male responds with penile tumescence and erection.

Female changes include vasocongestion in the pelvis, vaginal lubrication and expansion, and swelling of the external genitalia (APA, 2000).

■ **Phase III—Orgasm:** Orgasm is identified as a peaking of sexual pleasure, with release of sexual tension and rhythmic contraction of the perineal muscles and reproductive organs (APA, 2000). Orgasm in women is marked by simultaneous rhythmic contractions of the uterus, the lower third of the vagina, and the anal sphincter. In the man, a forceful emission of semen occurs in response to rhythmic spasms of the prostate, seminal vesicles, vas, and urethra (APA, 2000; King, 2009).

■ **Phase IV—Resolution:** If orgasm has occurred, this phase is characterized by disgorgement of blood from the genitalia, creating a sense of general relaxation and well-being. If orgasm is not achieved, resolution may take several hours, producing pelvic discomfort and a feeling of irritability.

After orgasm, men experience a refractory period that may last from a few minutes to many hours, during which time they cannot be stimulated to further orgasm. Commonly, the length of the refractory period increases with age. Women experience no refractory period and may be able to respond to additional stimulation almost immediately (APA, 2000).

Historical and Epidemiological Aspects Related to Sexual Dysfunction

Concurrent with the cultural changes occurring during the sexual revolution of the 1960s and 1970s came an increase in scientific research into sexual physiology and sexual dysfunctions. Masters and Johnson (1966, 1970) pioneered this work with their studies on human sexual response and the treatment of sexual dysfunctions. Spear (2001) reported:

Sex therapy, the treatment of sexual disorders, has evolved from early studies on sexual behavior made over 50 years ago. During these 50 years, the approach to sex therapy has changed immensely. When William Masters and Virginia Johnson published *Human Sexual Inadequacy* in 1970, the sexual revolution, born in the 1960s, was not yet in full force. Due in part to the development of the oral contraceptive known as 'the pill' and the rise in the politics of feminism, society began to take a different, more open view of sexuality. The rise in sex therapy addressed [sexual] issues as they had never been addressed before, in the privacy of a doctor's office.

Sexual dysfunction consists of an impairment or disturbance in any of the phases of the sexual response cycle. No one knows exactly how many people experience sexual dysfunctions. Knowledge exists only about those who seek some kind of treatment for the problem, and they may be few in number compared with those who have a dysfunction but suffer quietly and never seek therapy.

In 1970, Masters and Johnson reported that 50 percent of all American couples suffered from some type of sexual dysfunction. In 1984, Robins and coworkers estimated that 24 percent of the U.S. population would experience a sexual dysfunction at some time in their lives. Data related to prevalence of sexual problems in the United States based on a recent survey are presented in Table 31-1. This survey included a total of 1,491 men and women ages 40 to 80, and less than 25 percent of the individuals had sought help for their sexual problem(s) from a health professional (Laumann, Glasser, Neves, & Moreira, 2009).

Types of Sexual Dysfunction

Sexual Desire Disorders

Hypoactive Sexual Desire Disorder This disorder is defined by the *DSM-IV-TR* (APA, 2000) as a persistent or recurrent deficiency or absence of sexual fantasies and desire for sexual activity. In making the judgment of deficiency or absence, the clinician considers factors that affect sexual functioning, such as age and the context of the person's life.

An individual's absolute level of sexual desire may not be the problem; rather, the problem may be a discrepancy between the partners' levels. The conflict may occur if one partner wants to have sexual relations more often than the other does. Care must be taken not to label one partner as pathological when the problem actually lies in the discrepancy of sexual desire between the partners. The complaint is more common in women than in men.

Sexual Aversion Disorder This disorder is characterized by a persistent or recurrent extreme aversion to, and avoidance of, all (or almost all) genital sexual contact with a sexual partner (APA, 2000). Whereas individuals displaying hypoactive desire are often neutral or indifferent toward sexual interaction, sexual aversion implies anxiety, fear, or disgust in sexual situations.

Sexual Arousal Disorders

Female Sexual Arousal Disorder Female sexual arousal disorder is identified in the *DSM-IV-TR* as a persistent or recurrent inability to attain, or to maintain until completion of the sexual activity, an adequate lubrication/swelling response of sexual excitement.

Male Erectile Disorder Male erectile disorder is characterized by persistent or recurrent inability to attain, or to maintain until completion of the sexual activity, an adequate erection (APA, 2000). *Primary erectile dysfunction* refers to cases in which the man has never been able to have intercourse; *secondary erectile dysfunction* refers to cases in which the man has difficulty getting or maintaining an erection but has been able to have vaginal or anal intercourse at least once.

Orgasmic Disorders

Female Orgasmic Disorder Female orgasmic disorder is defined by the *DSM-IV-TR* as persistent or recurrent delay in, or absence of, orgasm following a normal sexual excitement phase. This condition is sometimes referred to as **anorgasmia.** Women who can achieve orgasm through noncoital clitoral stimulation but are not able to experience it during coitus in the absence of manual clitoral stimulation are not necessarily categorized as anorgasmic.

A woman is considered to have *primary orgasmic dysfunction* when she has never experienced orgasm by any kind of stimulation. *Secondary orgasmic dysfunction* exists if the woman has experienced at least one orgasm, regardless of the means of stimulation, but no longer does so.

Male Orgasmic Disorder Male orgasmic disorder, sometimes referred to as **retarded ejaculation,** is characterized by persistent or recurrent delay in, or absence of, orgasm following a normal sexual excitement phase during sexual activity that the clinician,

TABLE 31-1	Prevalence of Sexual Problems in Sexually Active Men and Women in the United States	
DISORDER	**MEN (%)**	**WOMEN (%)**
Lack of sexual interest	18.1	33.2
Inability to reach orgasm	12.4	20.7
Pain during sex	3.1	12.7
Premature ejaculation	26.2	—
Erectile difficulties	22.5	—
Lubrication difficulties	—	21.5

Adapted from Laumann, E. O., Glasser, D. B., Neves, R. C. S., & Moreira, E. D. (2009). A population-based survey of sexual activity, sexual problems, and associated help-seeking behavior patterns in mature adults in the United States of America. International Journal of Impotence Research, 21, 171–178.

taking into account the person's age, judges to be adequate in focus, intensity, and duration (APA, 2000). With this disorder, the man is unable to ejaculate, even though he has a firm erection and has had more than adequate stimulation. The severity of the problem may range from only occasional problems ejaculating (*secondary disorder*) to a history of never having experienced an orgasm (*primary disorder*). In the most common version, the man cannot ejaculate during coitus but may be able to ejaculate as a result of other types of stimulation.

Premature Ejaculation The *DSM-IV-TR* describes **premature ejaculation** as persistent or recurrent ejaculation with minimal sexual stimulation before, on, or shortly after penetration and before the person wishes it. Diagnosis should take into account factors that affect duration of the excitement phase, such as age, novelty of the sexual partner or situation, and recent frequency of sexual activity (APA, 2000).

Premature ejaculation is the most common sexual disorder for which men seek treatment. It is particularly common among young men who have a very high sex drive and have not yet learned to control ejaculation.

Sexual Pain Disorders

Dyspareunia **Dyspareunia** is recurrent or persistent genital pain associated with sexual intercourse in either a man or a woman (APA, 2000). It is not caused by **vaginismus,** lack of lubrication, other general medical condition, or physiological effects of substance use. In women, the pain may be felt in the vagina, around the vaginal entrance and clitoris, or deep in the pelvis. In men, the pain is felt in the penis. Dyspareunia makes intercourse very unpleasant and may even lead to abstention from sexual activity. Dyspareunia in men is often associated with urinary tract infection, with pain being experienced during urination as well as during ejaculation.

Vaginismus Vaginismus is an involuntary constriction of the outer one third of the vagina that prevents penile insertion and intercourse (APA, 2000). Vaginismus is less prevalent than female orgasmic disorder, and occurs in about 2 percent of all women (King, 2009). It is estimated that 12 to 17 percent of women presenting to sexual therapy clinics do so with the complaint of vaginismus (Pukall, Lahaie, & Binik, 2006).

Sexual Dysfunction due to a General Medical Condition and Substance-Induced Sexual Dysfunction

With these disorders, the sexual dysfunction is judged to be caused by the direct physiological effects of a general medical condition or use of a substance. The dysfunction may involve pain, impaired desire, impaired arousal, or impaired orgasm. Types of medical conditions that are associated with sexual dysfunction include neurological (e.g., multiple sclerosis, neuropathy), endocrine (e.g., diabetes mellitus, thyroid dysfunctions), vascular (e.g., atherosclerosis), and genitourinary (e.g., testicular disease, urethral or vaginal infections). Some substances that can interfere with sexual functioning include alcohol, amphetamines, cocaine, opioids, sedatives, hypnotics, anxiolytics, antidepressants, antipsychotics, and antihypertensives.

Predisposing Factors to Sexual Dysfunction

Biological Factors

Sexual Desire Disorders Studies have correlated decreased levels of serum testosterone with hypoactive sexual desire disorder in men. Evidence also exists that suggests a relationship between serum testosterone and increased female libido (Traish & Kim, 2006). Diminished libido has been observed in both men and women with elevated levels of serum prolactin (Nappi, Ferdeghini, & Polatti, 2006). Various medications have also been implicated in the etiology of hypoactive sexual desire disorder. Some examples include antihypertensives, antipsychotics, antidepressants, anxiolytics, and anticonvulsants. Alcohol and cocaine have also been associated with impaired desire, especially after chronic use.

Sexual Arousal Disorders Postmenopausal women require a longer period of stimulation for lubrication to occur, and there is generally less vaginal transudate after menopause (Altman & Hanfling, 2003). Various medications, particularly those with antihistaminic and anticholinergic properties, may also contribute to decreased ability for arousal in women. Arteriosclerosis is a common cause of male erectile disorder as a result of arterial insufficiency (King, 2009). Various neurological disorders can contribute to erectile dysfunctions as well. The most common neurologically based cause may be diabetes, which places men at high risk for neuropathy (Kim & Brosman, 2011). Others include temporal lobe epilepsy and multiple sclerosis. Trauma (e.g., spinal cord injury, pelvic cancer surgery) can also result in erectile dysfunction. Several medications have been implicated in the etiology of this disorder, including antihypertensives, antipsychotics, antidepressants, and anxiolytics. Chronic use of alcohol has also been shown to be a contributing factor.

IMPLICATIONS OF RESEARCH FOR EVIDENCE-BASED PRACTICE

Bacon, C. G., Mittleman, M. A., Kawachi, I., Glovannucci, E., Glasser, D. B., & Rimm, E. B. (2003). Sexual function in men older than 50 years of age: Results from the Health Professionals Follow-up Study. *Annals of Internal Medicine, 139,* 161–168.

DESCRIPTION OF THE STUDY: The purpose of the Health Professionals Follow-up Study was to describe the association between age and several aspects of sexual functioning in men older than 50 years of age. Participants included 31,742 male dentists, optometrists, osteopaths, podiatrists, pharmacists, and veterinarians in the United States. The participants were mailed questionnaires every 2 years between 1986 and 2000. Age range of participants was 53 to 90 years. Measures of sexual function included ability to have and maintain an erection adequate for intercourse, sexual desire, and ability to reach orgasm. Independent modifiable health behaviors included physical activity, smoking, obesity, alcohol consumption, and sedentary lifestyle (measured by hours of TV viewing).

RESULTS OF THE STUDY: The results of this study reinforced those of previous studies that linked

sexual dysfunction to increasing age, certain disease processes (e.g., diabetes, cancer, stroke, and hypertension), and medications (e.g., antidepressants; beta blockers). This study also addressed more specifically the correlation between sexual dysfunction and independent, modifiable risk factors. A higher risk for sexual dysfunction was associated with obesity, sedentary lifestyle, smoking, and excess alcohol consumption. Regular physical exercise (>32 metabolic equivalent hours per week), leanness, moderate alcohol consumption, and not smoking were statistically significantly correlated with decreased risk.

IMPLICATIONS FOR NURSING PRACTICE: This study has strong implications for nursing in terms of educating men over age 50 about contributing factors to sexual dysfunction. Establishing and conducting classes for weight reduction (including programs of regular exercise) and smoking cessation are well within the scope of nursing practice. Nurses can intervene to assist clients with behavior modification to achieve and/or maintain sexual wellness.

Orgasmic Disorders Some women report decreased ability to achieve orgasm following hysterectomy. Conversely, some report increased sexual activity and decreased sexual dysfunction following hysterectomy (Rhodes, Kjerulff, Langenberg, & Guzinski, 1999). Studies of the use of transdermal testosterone for sexual dysfunction in women after hysterectomy have revealed mixed results (Nappi et al., 2005). Some medications (e.g., selective serotonin reuptake inhibitors) may inhibit orgasm. Medical conditions, such as depression, hypothyroidism, and diabetes mellitus, may cause decreased sexual arousal and orgasm.

Biological factors associated with inhibited male orgasm include surgery of the genitourinary tract (e.g., prostatectomy), various neurological disorders (e.g., Parkinson's disease), and other diseases (e.g., diabetes mellitus). Medications that have been implicated include opioids, antihypertensives, antidepressants, and antipsychotics (Altman & Hanfling, 2003). Transient cases of the disorder may occur with excessive alcohol intake.

Although premature ejaculation is commonly caused by psychological factors, general medical conditions or substance use may also be contributing influences. Particularly in cases of secondary dysfunction, in which a man at one time had ejaculatory control but later lost it, physical factors

may be involved. Examples include a local infection such as prostatitis or a degenerative neural disorder such as multiple sclerosis.

Sexual Pain Disorders A number of organic factors can contribute to painful intercourse in women, including intact hymen, episiotomy scar, vaginal or urinary tract infection, ligament injuries, endometriosis, or ovarian cysts or tumors. Painful intercourse in men may also be caused by various organic factors. For example, infection caused by poor hygiene under the foreskin of an uncircumsized man can cause pain. Phimosis, a condition in which the foreskin cannot be pulled back, can also cause painful intercourse. An allergic reaction to various vaginal spermicides or irritation caused by vaginal infections may be a contributing factor. Finally, various prostate problems may cause pain on ejaculation.

Psychosocial Factors

Sexual Desire Disorders Phillips (2000) has identified a number of individual and relationship factors that may contribute to hypoactive sexual desire disorder. Individual causes include religious orthodoxy; sexual identity conflicts; past sexual abuse; financial, family, or job problems; depression; and aging-related concerns (e.g., changes in physical appearance). Among the relationship causes are interpersonal conflicts; current physical, verbal, or sexual abuse; extramarital affairs; and desire or practices that differ from those of the partner.

Sexual aversion disorder is sometimes referred to as sexual phobia; however, the word *aversion* connotes revulsion and disgust, rather than fear. Common etiological implications for sexual aversion disorder are sexual abuse in women and performance anxiety in men (Janata & Kingsberg, 2005).

Sexual Arousal Disorders A number of psychological factors have been cited as possible impediments to female arousal. They include doubt, guilt, fear, anxiety, shame, conflict, embarrassment, tension, disgust, irritation, resentment, grief, hostility toward partner, and a puritanical or moralistic upbringing. Sexual abuse has been identified as a significant risk factor for desire and arousal disorders in women.

Problems with male sexual arousal may be related to chronic stress, anxiety, or depression. Developmental factors that hinder the ability to be intimate, that lead to a feeling of inadequacy or distrust, or that develop a sense of being unloving or unlovable may also result in impotence. Relationship factors that may affect erectile functioning include lack of attraction to one's partner, anger toward one's partner, or being in a relationship that is not characterized by trust (Altman & Hanfling, 2003). Unfortunately, regardless of the etiology of the impotence, once it occurs, the man may become increasingly anxious about his next sexual encounter. This anticipatory anxiety about achieving and maintaining an erection may then perpetuate the problem.

Orgasmic Disorders Numerous psychological factors are associated with inhibited female orgasm. They include fears of becoming pregnant, rejection by the sexual partner, damage to the vagina, hostility toward men, and feelings of guilt regarding sexual impulses (Sadock & Sadock, 2007). Negative cultural conditioning ("nice girls don't enjoy sex") may also influence the adult female's sexual response. Various developmental factors also have relevance to orgasmic dysfunction. Examples include childhood exposure to rigid religious orthodoxy, negative family attitudes toward nudity and sex, and traumatic sexual experiences during childhood or adolescence, such as incest or rape (Clayton, 2002; Phillips, 2000).

Psychological factors are also associated with inhibited male orgasm. In the primary disorder (in which the man has never experienced orgasm), the man often comes from a rigid, puritanical

background. He perceives sex as sinful and the genitals as dirty, and he may have conscious or unconscious incest wishes and guilt (Sadock & Sadock, 2007). In the case of secondary disorder (previously experienced orgasms that have now stopped), interpersonal difficulties are usually implicated. There may be some ambivalence about commitment, fear of pregnancy, or unexpressed hostility.

Premature ejaculation may be related to a lack of physical awareness on the part of a sexually inexperienced man. The ability to control ejaculation occurs as a gradual maturing process with a sexual partner in which foreplay becomes more give-and-take "pleasuring," rather than strictly goal oriented. The man becomes aware of the sensations and learns to delay the point of ejaculatory inevitability. Relationship problems such as a stressful marriage, negative cultural conditioning, anxiety over intimacy, and lack of comfort in the sexual relationship may also contribute to this disorder.

Sexual Pain Disorders Vaginismus may occur in response to having experienced dyspareunia (painful intercourse) for various organic reasons stated in the "Biological Factors" section. Involuntary constriction within the vagina occurs in response to anticipatory pain, making intercourse impossible. The diagnosis does not apply if the cause of the vaginismus is determined to be organic. A variety of psychosocial factors have been implicated, including negative childhood conditioning of sex as dirty, sinful, and shameful. Early traumatic sexual experiences (e.g., rape or incest) may also cause vaginismus. Other factors that may be important in the etiology of vaginismus include homosexual orientation, traumatic experience with an early pelvic examination, pregnancy phobia, STD phobia, or cancer phobia (Dreyfus, 1998; King, 2009; Leiblum, 1999; Phillips, 2000; Sadock & Sadock, 2007).

Transactional Model of Stress/Adaptation
The etiology of sexual dysfunction is most likely influenced by multiple factors. In Figure 31–2, a graphic depiction of the theory of multiple causation is presented in the Transactional Model of Stress/Adaptation.

Application of the Nursing Process to Sexual Disorders

Assessment

Most assessment tools for taking a general nursing history contain some questions devoted to sexuality. Many nurses feel uncomfortable obtaining information about the subject. However, accurate data

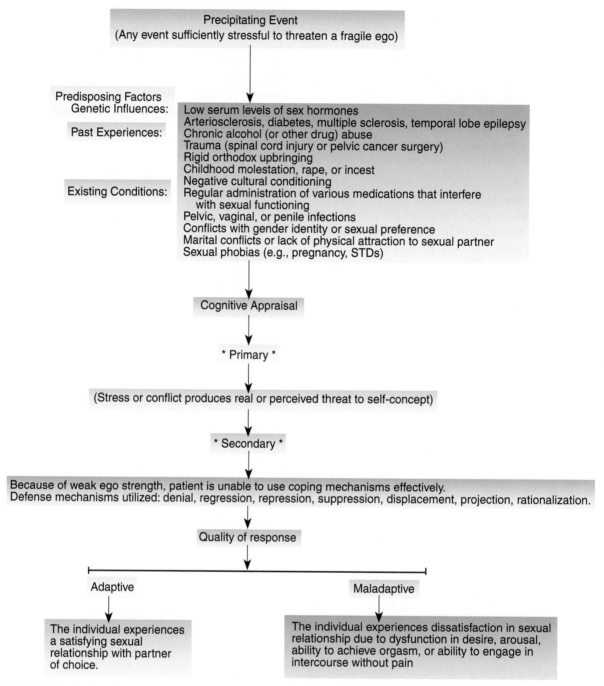

FIGURE 31–2 The dynamics of sexual dysfunction using the transactional model of stress/adaptation.

must be collected if problems are to be identified and resolutions attempted. Sexual health is an integral part of physical and emotional well-being. The nursing history is incomplete if items directed toward sexuality are not included.

Indeed, most nurses are not required to obtain a sexual history as in depth as the one presented in this chapter. However, for certain clients a more extensive sexual history is required than that which is included in the general nursing history. These

include clients who have medical or surgical conditions that may affect their sexuality; clients with infertility problems, STDs, or complaints of sexual inadequacy; clients who are pregnant, or have gynecological problems; those seeking information on abortion or family planning; and individuals in premarital, marital, and psychiatric counseling.

The best approach for taking a sexual history is a nondirective one; that is, it is best to use the sexual history outline as a guideline but allow the interview to progress in a less restrictive manner than the outline permits (with one question immediately following the other). The order of the questions should be adjusted according to the client's needs as they are identified during the interview. A nondirective approach allows time for the client to interject information related to feelings or concerns about his or her sexuality.

The language used should be understandable to the client. If he or she uses terminology that is unfamiliar, ask for clarification. Take level of education and cultural influences into consideration.

The nurse's attitude must convey warmth, openness, honesty, and objectivity. Personal feelings, attitudes, and values should be clarified and should not interfere with acceptance of the client. The nurse must remain nonjudgmental. This is conveyed by listening in an interested matter-of-fact manner without overreacting to any information the client may present.

The content outline for a sexual history presented in Box 31-1 is not intended to be used as a rigid questionnaire but as a guideline from which the nurse may select appropriate topics for gathering

---

BOX 31-1 Sexual History: Content Outline

I. Identify data
A. Client
    1. Age
    2. Gender
    3. Marital status
B. Parents
    1. Ages
    2. Dates of death and ages at death
    3. Birthplace
    4. Marital status
    5. Religion
    6. Education
    7. Occupation
    8. Congeniality
    9. Demonstration of affection
    10. Feelings toward parents
C. Siblings (same information as above)
D. Marital partner (same information as above)
E. Children
    1. Ages
    2. Gender
    3. Strengths
    4. Identified problems

II. Childhood sexuality
A. Family attitudes about sex
    1. Parents' openness about sex
    2. Parents' attitudes about nudity
B. Learning about sex
    1. Asking parents about sex
    2. Information volunteered by parents
    3. At what age and how did client learn about: pregnancy, birth, intercourse, masturbation, nocturnal emissions, menstruation, homosexuality, STDs
C. Childhood sex activity
    1. First sight of nude body
        a. Same gender
        b. Opposite gender
    2. First genital self-stimulation
        a. Age
        b. Feelings
        c. Consequences
    3. First sexual exploration at play with another child
        a. Age (of self and other child)
        b. Gender of other child
        c. Nature of the activity
        d. Feelings and consequences

    4. Sexual activity with older persons
        a. Age (of self and other person)
        b. Gender of other person
        c. Nature of the activity
        d. Client willingness to participate
        e. Feelings and consequences
D. Did you ever see your parents (or others) having intercourse? Describe your feelings.
E. Childhood sexual theories or myths:
    1. Thoughts about conception and birth.
    2. Roles of male/female genitals and other body parts in sexuality.

III. Onset of adolescence
A. In girls
    1. Information about menstruation
        a. How received; from whom
        b. Age received
        c. Feelings
    2. Age
        a. Of first period
        b. When breasts began to develop
        c. At appearance of ancillary and pubic hair
    3. Menstruation
        a. Regularity; discomfort; duration
        b. Feelings about first period
B. In boys
    1. Information about puberty
        a. How received; from whom
        b. Age received
        c. Feelings
    2. Age
        a. Of appearance of ancillary and pubic hair
        b. Change of voice
        c. First orgasm (with or without ejaculation); emotional reaction

IV. Orgastic experiences
A. Nocturnal emissions (male) or orgasms (female) during sleep.
    1. Frequency
B. Masturbation
    1. Age begun; ever punished?
    2. Frequency; methods used
    3. Marital partner's knowledge
    4. Practiced with others? Spouse?
    5. Emotional reactions
    6. Accompanying fantasies

Continued

BOX 31-1 Sexual History: Content Outline—cont'd

C. Necking and petting ("making out")
1. Age when begun
2. Frequency
3. Number of partners
4. Types of activity
D. Premarital intercourse
1. Frequency
2. Relationship with and number of partners
3. Contraceptives used
4. Feelings
E. Orgasmic frequency
1. Past
2. Present

V. Feelings about self as masculine/feminine
A. The male client
1. Does he feel masculine?
2. Accepted by peers?
3. Sexually adequate?
4. Feelings/concerns about body
   a. Size
   b. Appearance
   c. Function
B. The female client
1. Does she feel feminine?
2. Accepted by peers?
3. Sexually adequate?
4. Feelings/concerns about body
   a. Size
   b. Appearance
   c. Function

VI. Sexual fantasies and dreams
A. Nature of sex dreams
B. Nature of fantasies
1. During masturbation
2. During intercourse

VII. Dating
A. Age and feelings about
1. First date
2. First kissing
3. First petting or "making out"
4. First going steady

VIII. Engagement
A. Age
B. Sex activity during engagement period
1. With fiancée
2. With others

IX. Marriage
A. Date of marriage
B. Age at marriage: Spouse:
C. Spouse's occupation
D. Previous marriages: Spouse:
E. Reason for termination of previous marriages
   Client: Spouse:
F. Children from previous marriages
   Client: Spouse:
G. Wedding trip (honeymoon)
1. Where? How long?
2. Pleasant or unpleasant?
3. Sexual considerations?
H. Sex in marriage
1. General satisfaction/dissatisfaction.
2. Thoughts about spouse's general satisfaction/dissatisfaction

I. Pregnancies
1. Number: Ages of couple:
2. Results (normal birth; cesarean delivery; miscarriage; abortion)
3. Planned or unplanned
4. Effects on sexual adjustment
5. Sex of child wanted or unwanted

X. Extramarital sex
A. Emotional attachments
1. Number; frequency; feelings
B. Sexual intercourse
1. Number; frequency; feelings
C. Postmarital masturbation
1. Frequency; feelings
D. Postmarital homosexuality
1. Frequency; feelings
E. Multiple sex ("swinging")
1. Frequency; feelings

XI. Sex after widowhood, separation, or divorce
A. Outlet
1. Orgasms in sleep
2. Masturbation
3. Petting
4. Intercourse
5. Homosexuality
6. Other
B. Frequency; feelings

XII. Variation in sexual orientation
A. Homosexuality
1. First experience; describe circumstances.
2. Frequency since adolescence

XIII. Paraphilias
A. Sexual contact with animals
1. First experience; describe nature of contact
2. Frequency and recent contact
3. Feelings
B. Voyeurism
1. Describe types of observation experienced
2. Feelings
C. Exhibitionism
1. To whom? When?
2. Feelings
D. Fetishes; transvestitism
1. Nature of fetish
2. Nature of transvestite activity
3. Feelings
E. Sadomasochism
1. Nature of activity
2. Sexual response
3. Frequency; recency
4. Consequences
F. Seduction and rape
1. Has client seduced/raped another?
2. Has client ever been seduced/raped?
G. Incest
1. Nature of the sexual activity
2. With whom?
3. When occurred? Frequency; recency.
4. Consequences

XIV. Prostitution
   A. Has client ever accepted/paid money for sex?
   B. Type of sexual activity engaged in
   C. Feelings about prostitution

XV. Certain effects of sex activities
   A. STDs
      1. Age at learning about STDs
      2. Type of STD contracted
      3. Age and treatment received
   B. Illegitimate pregnancy
      1. At what age(s)
      2. Outcome of the pregnancy(ies)
      3. Feelings
   C. Abortion
      1. Why performed?
      2. At what age(s)?

   3. How often?
   4. Before or after marriage?
   5. Circumstance: who, where, how?
   6. Feelings about abortion: at the time; in retrospect; anniversary reaction

XVI. Use of erotic material
   A. Personal response to erotic material
      1. Sexual pleasure—arousal
      2. Mild pleasure
      3. Disinterest; disgust
   B. Use in connection with sexual activity
      1. Type and frequency of use
      2. To accompany what type of sexual activity

Adapted from an outline prepared by the Group for Advancement of Psychiatry, based on the Sexual Performance Evaluation Questionnaire of the Marriage Council of Philadelphia; used with permission.

information about the client's sexuality. The outline should be individualized according to client needs.

Diagnosis/Outcome Identification

Nursing diagnoses are formulated from the data gathered during the assessment phase and with background knowledge regarding predisposing factors to the disorder. The following nursing diagnoses may be used for the client with sexual disorders:

■ Sexual dysfunction related to depression and conflict in relationship or certain biological or psychological contributing factors to the disorder evidenced by loss of sexual desire or ability to perform.

■ Ineffective sexuality pattern related to conflicts with sexual orientation or variant preferences, evidenced by expressed dissatisfaction with sexual behaviors (e.g., voyeurism, transvestitism).

Outcome Criteria

The following criteria may be used for measurement of outcomes in the care of the client with sexual disorders.

The Client:

■ Can correlate stressful situations that decrease sexual desire.

■ Can communicate with partner about sexual situation without discomfort.

■ Can verbalize ways to enhance sexual desire.

■ Verbalizes resumption of sexual activity at level satisfactory to self and partner.

■ Can correlate variant behaviors with times of stress.

■ Can verbalize fears about abnormality and inappropriateness of sexual behaviors.

■ Expresses desire to change variant sexual behavior.

■ Participates and cooperates with extended plan of behavior modification.

■ Expresses satisfaction with own sexuality pattern.

Planning/Implementation

Following are nursing diagnoses commonly used with individuals experiencing alterations in sexual functioning. Short- and long-term goals and nursing interventions are presented for each.

Sexual Dysfunction

Sexual dysfunction is defined as "the state in which an individual experiences a change in sexual function during the sexual response phases of desire, excitation, and/or orgasm, which is viewed as unsatisfying, unrewarding, or inadequate" (NANDA International [NANDA-I], 2009, p. 227).

Client Goals

Outcome criteria include short- and long-term goals. Timelines are individually determined.

Short-Term Goals

■ Client will identify stressors that may contribute to loss of sexual function within 1 week *OR*

■ Client will discuss pathophysiology of disease process that contributes to sexual dysfunction within 1 week.

■ (*For the client with permanent dysfunction due to disease process*): Client will verbalize willingness to seek professional assistance from a sex therapist in order to learn alternative ways of achieving sexual satisfaction with partner by (time is individually determined).

Long-Term Goal

■ Client will resume sexual activity at level satisfactory to self and partner by (time is individually determined).

Interventions

■ Assess the client's sexual history and previous level of satisfaction in his or her sexual relationship. This history establishes a database from which to work and provides a foundation for goal setting.

■ Assess the client's perception of the problem. The client's idea of what constitutes a problem may differ from that of the nurse. It is the client's perception on which the goals of care must be established.

■ Help the client determine the timeline associated with the onset of the problem, and discuss what was happening in his or her life situation at that time. Stress in all areas of life will affect sexual functioning. The client may be unaware of the correlation between stress and sexual dysfunction.

■ Assess the client's mood and level of energy. Depression and fatigue decrease desire and enthusiasm for participation in sexual activity.

■ Review medication regimen; observe for side effects. Many medications can affect sexual functioning. Evaluation of the drug and the individual's response is important to ascertain whether the drug may be contributing to the problem.

■ Encourage the client to discuss the disease process that may be contributing to sexual dysfunction. Ensure that the client is aware that alternative methods of achieving sexual satisfaction exist and can be learned through sex counseling if he or she and the partner desire to do so.

■ Provide information regarding sexuality and sexual functioning. Increasing knowledge and correcting misconceptions can decrease feelings of powerlessness and anxiety and facilitate problem resolution.

■ Make a referral for additional counseling or sex therapy, if required. Complex problems are likely to require assistance from an individual who is specially trained to treat problems related to sexuality. The client and partner may be somewhat embarrassed to seek this kind of

assistance. Support from a trusted nurse can provide the impetus for them to pursue the help they need.

Ineffective Sexuality Pattern

Ineffective sexuality pattern is defined as "expressions of concern regarding own sexuality" (NANDA-I, 2009, p. 229).

Client Goals

Outcome criteria include short- and long-term goals. Timelines are individually determined.

Short-Term Goals

■ Client will verbalize aspects about sexuality that he or she would like to change.

■ Client and partner will communicate with each other ways in which each believes their sexual relationship could be improved.

Long-Term Goals

■ Client will express satisfaction with own sexuality pattern.

■ Client and partner will express satisfaction with sexual relationship.

Interventions

■ Take a sexual history, noting the client's expression of areas of dissatisfaction with his or her sexual pattern. Knowledge of what the client perceives as the problem is essential for providing the type of assistance he or she may need.

■ Assess areas of stress in the client's life and examine the relationship with his or her sexual partner. Variant sexual behaviors are often associated with added stress in the client's life. The relationship with his or her partner may deteriorate as the individual eventually gains sexual satisfaction only from variant practices.

■ Note cultural, social, ethnic, racial, and religious factors that may contribute to conflicts regarding variant sexual practices. The client may be unaware of the influence these factors exert in creating feelings of discomfort, shame, and guilt regarding sexual attitudes and behavior.

■ Be accepting and nonjudgmental. Sexuality is a very personal and sensitive subject. The client is more likely to share this information if he or she does not fear being judged by the nurse.

■ Assist the therapist in a plan of behavior modification to help the client who desires to decrease variant sexual behaviors. Individuals with paraphilias are treated by specialists who have experience in modifying variant sexual behaviors. Nurses can intervene by providing assistance with implementation of the plan for behavior modification.

■ If altered sexuality patterns are related to illness or medical treatment, provide information to the client and partner regarding the correlation between the illness and the sexual alteration. Explain possible modifications in usual sexual patterns that the client and partner may try in an effort to achieve a satisfying sexual experience in spite of the limitation. The client and his or her partner may be unaware of alternate possibilities for achieving sexual satisfaction, or anxiety associated with the limitation may interfere with rational problem solving.

■ Teach the client that sexuality is a normal human response and is not synonymous with any one sexual act; that it reflects the totality of the person and does not relate exclusively to the sex organs or sexual behavior. The client must understand that *sexual* feelings are *human* feelings.

■ If the client feels abnormal or very unlike everyone else, the self-concept is likely to be very low—even worthless. Helping him or her to understand that, even though the behavior is variant, the feelings and motivations are common may help to increase feelings of self-worth and desire to change behavior.

Concept Care Mapping

The concept map care plan is an innovative approach to planning and organizing nursing care (see Chapter 9). It is a diagrammatic teaching and learning strategy that allows visualization of interrelationships between medical diagnoses, nursing diagnoses, assessment data, and treatments. An example of a concept map care plan for a client with a sexual disorder is presented in Figure 31–3.

Client/Family Education

The role of client teacher is important in the psychiatric area, as it is in all areas of nursing. A list of topics for client/family education relevant to sexual disorders is presented in Box 31-2. Sample client teaching guides are presented in Appendix G.

Evaluation

Reassessment is necessary to determine if selected interventions have been successful in helping the client overcome problems with sexual functioning. Evaluation may be facilitated by gathering information using the following types of questions.

For the Client with Sexual Dysfunction:

■ Has the client identified life situations that promote feelings of depression and decreased sexual desire?

■ Can he or she verbalize ways to deal with this stress?

■ Can the client satisfactorily communicate with his or her sexual partner about the problem?

■ Have the client and sexual partner identified ways to enhance sexual desire and the achievement of sexual satisfaction for both?

■ Are the client and partner seeking assistance with relationship conflict?

■ Do both partners agree on what the major problem is? Do they have the motivation to attempt change?

■ Do the client and partner verbalize an increase in sexual satisfaction?

For the Client with Variant Sexual Behaviors:

■ Can the client correlate an increase in variant sexual behavior to times of severe stress?

■ Has the client been able to identify those stressful situations and verbalize alternative ways to deal with them?

■ Does the client express a desire to change variant sexual behavior and a willingness to cooperate with extended therapy to do so?

■ Does the client express an understanding about the normalcy of sexual feelings, aside from the inappropriateness of his or her behavior?

■ Are expressions of increased self-worth evident?

Quality and Safety Education for Nurses (QSEN)

The Institute of Medicine (IOM), in its 2003 report, *Health Professions Education: A Bridge to Quality,* challenged faculties of medicine, nursing, and other health professions to ensure that their graduates have achieved a core set of competencies in order to meet the needs of the 21st century health-care system. These competencies include *providing patient-centered care, working in interdisciplinary teams, employing evidence-based practice, applying quality improvement,* and *utilizing informatics.* A QSEN teaching strategy is included in Box 31-3. The use of this type of activity is intended to arm the instructor and the student with guidelines for attaining the knowledge, skills, and attitudes necessary for achievement of quality and safety competencies in nursing.

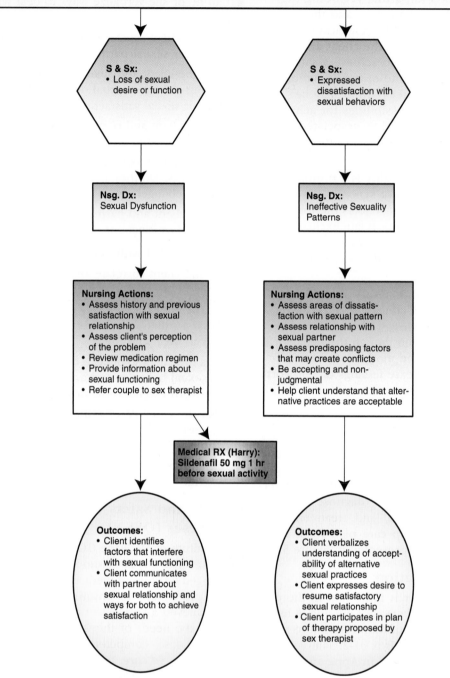

Clinical Vignette: Harry (age 60) and Sally (age 58) have been married 35 years. They have come to the mental health clinic for couple's therapy because they are having problems in their sexual relationship. They tell the Psychiatric Nurse Practitioner that they once had an active, satisfying sexual relationship, but Sally admits that although she still loves Harry, she no longer has a desire for sex. She states that she must create sexual fantasies or view sexual videos to become aroused, and that this makes her feel uncomfortable and "dirty." Harry desires sex with Sally, but has lately developed some difficulties with erectile dysfunction. The nurse develops the following concept map care plan for Harry and Sally.

S & Sx:
• Loss of sexual desire or function

S & Sx:
• Expressed dissatisfaction with sexual behaviors

Nsg. Dx:
Sexual Dysfunction

Nsg. Dx:
Ineffective Sexuality Patterns

Nursing Actions:
• Assess history and previous satisfaction with sexual relationship
• Assess client's perception of the problem
• Review medication regimen
• Provide information about sexual functioning
• Refer couple to sex therapist

Nursing Actions:
• Assess areas of dissatisfaction with sexual pattern
• Assess relationship with sexual partner
• Assess predisposing factors that may create conflicts
• Be accepting and non-judgmental
• Help client understand that alternative practices are acceptable

Medical RX (Harry):
Sildenafil 50 mg 1 hr before sexual activity

Outcomes:
• Client identifies factors that interfere with sexual functioning
• Client communicates with partner about sexual relationship and ways for both to achieve satisfaction

Outcomes:
• Client verbalizes understanding of acceptability of alternative sexual practices
• Client expresses desire to resume satisfactory sexual relationship
• Client participates in plan of therapy proposed by sex therapist

FIGURE 31–3 Concept map care plan for clients with sexual disorders.

BOX 31-2 **Topics for Client/Family Education Related to Sexual Disorders**

NATURE OF THE ILLNESS

1. The human sexual response cycle
2. What is "normal" and "abnormal?"
3. Types of sexual dysfunctions
4. Causes of sexual dysfunctions
5. Types of paraphilias
6. Causes of paraphilias
7. Symptoms associated with sexual dysfunctions and paraphilias

MANAGEMENT OF THE DISORDER

1. Teach practices and ways of sexual expression.
2. Teach relaxation techniques.
3. Teach side effects of medications that may be contributing to sexual dysfunction.
4. Teach effects of alcohol consumption on sexual functioning.
5. Teach about STDs (see Table 31-2).

SUPPORT SERVICES

1. Provide appropriate referral for assistance from sex therapist.
2. One national association to which many qualified sex therapists belong is:

American Association of Sexuality Educators, Counselors and Therapists

1444 I Street NW, Suite 700
Washington, D.C. 20005
(202) 449-1099
http://www.aasect.org

Treatment Modalities for Sexual Dysfunctions

Sexual Desire Disorders

Hypoactive Sexual Desire Disorder

Hypoactive sexual desire disorder has been treated in both men and women with the administration of testosterone. The masculinizing side effects make this approach unacceptable to women, and the evidence that it increases libido in men is inconclusive. Becker and Stinson (2008) described the most effective treatment as a combination of cognitive therapy to deal with maladaptive beliefs; behavioral treatment, such as exercises to enhance sexual pleasuring and communication; and relationship therapy to deal with the individual's use of sex as a method of control.

Low sexual desire is often the result of partner incompatibility. If this is the case, the therapist may choose to shift from the sexual issue to helping a couple identify and deal with their incompatibility.

Sexual Aversion Disorder

Systematic desensitization (see Chapter 29) is often the treatment of choice for sexual aversion disorder, to reduce the client's fear and avoidance of sex (Becker & Stinson, 2008). Gradual exposure, under relaxed conditions, to imagined and actual sexual situations decreases the amount of anxiety generated by these experiences. Successful treatment of sexual phobias has also been reported using tricyclic medications and psychosexual therapy aimed at developing insight into unconscious conflicts.

BOX 31-3 QSEN TEACHING STRATEGY

Assignment: Using a Capstone Cultural Diversity Paper for Program Outcomes Evaluation

Intervening with a Client of an Alternative Sexual Orientation

Competency Domain: Patient-Centered Care

Learning Objectives: Student will:

• Identify dimensions of the client's sexual orientation identified through the nursing interview.
• Discuss common problems/concerns for the diverse group.
• Plan potential patient-centered interventions that promote wellness and demonstrate respect for the client's diversity.
• Identify how knowledge gained from this assignment will influence his/her future nursing care of clients with diverse sexual orientations.
• Recognize and analyze how culturally based attitudes, values, and beliefs impact nursing care.

Strategy Overview:

• **Part I. Client Interview Data**
   1. Using the Sexual History assessment tool in Chapter 31 of the textbook, conduct a sexual history of a client with a diverse sexual orientation.

Continued

QSEN TEACHING STRATEGY—cont'd

2. During the interview, identify the client's values, beliefs, practices, preferences, and expressed needs related to health care, communication, and sexual expression.

• **Part II. Cultural Analysis and Health Care Needs Identification**

Submit a typed analysis of the client's diversity supported with in-text reference citations (minimum 3–4 pages). The paper should include the following information:

1. Using the client interview data and current literature, describe the traditional cultural health-care beliefs and practices, including interpersonal relationships and worldview beliefs for this diverse group.

2. Discuss any differences between what you have read in the literature and what your client told you. Include possible explanations for these differences.

3. Identify actual or potential health-care problems/concerns for the client and his or her diverse group.

4. Discuss potential therapeutic interventions for the client that promote wellness; that demonstrate respect for the client's diversity, rights, beliefs, values, and life experiences; and that incorporate professional values and practice standards.

5. Record your observations from the interview regarding verbal and nonverbal communication (such as eye contact, rate of speech, personal space, and touch) demonstrated by you and the client.

• **Part III. Personal Reflections**

Submit a paper describing personal reflections of how this knowledge might influence your nursing care of persons with diverse sexual orientations (minimum 2 pages). The paper should include the following information:

1. To what extent do your beliefs, prejudices, or bias influence your thinking and nursing care? Give several examples.

2. Discuss specifically how the knowledge from this assignment will influence your future nursing care of clients with different sexual orientations. Discuss several examples.

Adapted from teaching strategy submitted by Lisa Sue Flood, Associate Professor, Northern Michigan University, Marquette, MI.
© 2009 QSEN; http://qsen.org, with permission.

Sexual Arousal Disorders

Female Sexual Arousal Disorder

The goal of treatment for female sexual arousal disorder is to reduce the anxiety associated with sexual activity. Masters and Johnson (1970) reported successful results using their behaviorally oriented **sensate focus** exercises to treat this disorder. The objective is to reduce the goal-oriented demands of intercourse on both the man and the woman, thus reducing performance pressures and anxiety associated with possible failure. Altman and Hanfling (2003) stated:

The cornerstone of sex therapy is a series of behavioral exercises called sensate focus exercises. These highly structured touching activities are designed to help overcome performance anxiety and increase comfort with physical intimacy. Initially, the couple agrees to refrain from intercourse or genital stimulation until the later stages of treatment. This helps dispel anxiety that's built up around sexual performance and allows establishment of new patterns of relating. (pp. 38–39)

The couple is instructed to take turns caressing each other's bodies. Initially, they are to avoid touching breasts and genitals, and to focus on the sensations of being touched. The caressing progresses to include touching of the breasts and genitals, to touching each other simultaneously, and eventually to include intercourse. These non–goal-oriented exercises promote the sensual side of sexual interaction in a nonpressured, nonevaluative way (Masters et al., 1995).

Male Erectile Disorder

Sensate focus has been used effectively for male erectile disorder as well. Clinicians widely agree that, even when significant organic factors have been identified, psychological factors may also be present and must be considered in treatment.

Group therapy, hypnotherapy, and systematic desensitization have also been used successfully in reducing the anxiety that may contribute to erectile difficulties. Psychodynamic interventions may help alleviate intrapsychic conflicts contributing to performance anxiety (Becker & Stinson, 2008).

Various medications, including testosterone and yohimbine, have been used to treat male erectile dysfunction. Penile injections of papaverine or prostaglandin have been used to produce an erection lasting from 1 to 4 hours. However, this treatment is unacceptable to many men because of pain of the injection and side effects, such as priapism and fibrotic nodules in the penis (Becker & Stinson, 2008).

Several other medications have been approved by the U.S. Food and Drug Administration (FDA) for the treatment of erectile dysfunction. They include sildenafil (Viagra), tadalafil (Cialis), and vardenafil (Levitra). These newer impotence agents block the action of phosphodiesterase-5 (PDE5), an enzyme that breaks down cyclic guanosine monophosphate (cGMP), a compound that is required to produce an erection. This action only occurs, however, in the presence of nitric oxide (NO), which is released during sexual arousal. PDE5 inhibitors do not result in sexual arousal. They work to achieve penile erection in the presence of sexual arousal. Adverse effects include headache, facial flushing, indigestion, nasal congestion, dizziness, and visual changes (mild color tinges and blurred vision) (Kim & Brosman, 2011). In 2005, the FDA ordered that the manufacturers of these medications add a warning to their labels. This action was taken in response to 43 cases of sudden vision loss by individuals taking the drugs. It is not possible to ascertain whether the medications are responsible for nonarteritic ischemic optic neuropathy (NAION), a condition in which blood flow to the optic nerve is blocked. PDE5 inhibitors are contraindicated in concurrent use with nitrates.

Two other oral medications, apomorphine and phentolamine, are currently being investigated for use with erectile dysfunction. Phentolamine has been used in combination with papaverine in an injectable form. Both of these medications increase blood flow to the penis, resulting in an erection.

For erectile dysfunction refractory to other treatment methods, penile prostheses may be implanted. Two basic types are currently available: a bendable silicone implant and an inflatable device. The bendable variety requires a relatively simple surgical technique for insertion of silicone rods into the erectile areas of the penis. This results in a perpetual state of semierection for the client. The inflatable penile prosthesis produces an erection only when it is desired, and the appearance of the penis in both the flaccid and erect states is completely normal. Potential candidates for penile implantation should undergo careful psychological and physical screening. Although penile implants do not enable the client to recover the ability to ejaculate or to have an orgasm, men with prosthetic devices have generally reported satisfaction with their subsequent sexual functioning.

Orgasmic Disorders

Female Orgasmic Disorder

Because anxiety may contribute to the lack of orgasmic ability in women, sensate focus is often advised to reduce anxiety, increase awareness of physical sensations, and transfer communication skills from the verbal to the nonverbal domain. Phillips (2000) provided the following description of therapy for the anorgasmic woman:

> Treatment relies on maximizing stimulation and minimizing inhibition. Stimulation may include masturbation with prolonged stimulation (initially up to one hour) and/or the use of a vibrator as needed, and muscular control of sexual tension (alternating contraction and relaxation of the pelvic muscles during high sexual arousal). The latter is similar to [Kegel] exercises. Methods to minimize inhibition include distraction by "spectatoring" (observing oneself from a third-party perspective), fantasizing, or listening to music (p. 135).

Treatment for secondary anorgasmia (in which the client has had orgasms in the past, but is now unable to achieve them) focuses on the couple and their relationship. Therapy with both partners is essential to the success of this disorder.

Male Orgasmic Disorder

Treatment for male orgasmic disorder is very similar to that described for the anorgasmic woman. A combination of sensate focus and masturbatory training has been used with a high degree of success in the Masters and Johnson clinic. Treatment for male orgasmic disorder almost always includes the sexual partner.

Premature Ejaculation

Masters and associates (1995) advocated what they suggested is a highly successful technique for the treatment of premature ejaculation. Sensate focus is used, with progression to genital stimulation. When the man reaches the point of imminent ejaculation, the woman is instructed to apply the "squeeze" technique: applying pressure at the base of the glans penis with her thumb and first two fingers. Pressure is held for about 4 seconds and then released. This technique is continued until the man is no longer on the verge of ejaculating. This technique is practiced during subsequent periods of sexual stimulation.

No medication has been approved by the FDA for the treatment of premature ejaculation, but a number of studies have shown efficacy for this disorder with the selective serotonin reuptake inhibitors (SSRIs) (Benson & Ost, 2009). Some individuals may achieve positive results with single dosing prior to sexual relations, while others may require regular daily dosing to achieve an adequate blood level.

Sexual Pain Disorders

Dyspareunia

Treatment for the pain of intercourse begins with a thorough physical and gynecological examination. When organic pathology has been eliminated, the client's fears and anxieties underlying sexual functioning are investigated (Becker & Stinson, 2008). Systematic desensitization has been used successfully to decrease fears and anxieties associated with painful intercourse.

Vaginismus

Treatment of this disorder begins with education of the woman and her sexual partner regarding the anatomy and physiology of the disorder (i.e., what exactly is occurring during the vaginismus reflex and possible etiologies). The involuntary nature of the disorder is stressed in an effort to alleviate the sexual partner's perception that this occurrence is an act of willful withholding by the woman.

The second phase of treatment involves systematic desensitization. The client is taught a series of tensing and relaxing exercises aimed at relaxation of the pelvic musculature. Relaxation of the pelvic muscles is followed by a procedure involving the systematic insertion of dilators of graduated sizes until the woman is able to accept the penis into the vagina without discomfort. This physical therapy, combined with treatment of any identified relationship problems, has been used by the Masters and Johnson clinic with considerable success (Masters et al., 1995).

Gender Identity Disorder

> **CORE CONCEPT**
>
> *Gender*
> The condition of being either male or female.

Gender identity is the sense of knowing whether one is male or female—that is, the awareness of one's masculinity or femininity. Gender identity disorder (GID) occurs when there is incongruence between anatomical sex and gender identity. The *DSM-IV-TR* categorizes diagnosis of the

disorder according to the client's current age: gender identity disorder in children and gender identity disorder in adolescents or adults. Although most cases of the disorder begin in childhood, persons who present clinically with gender identity problems may be of any age. It is for this reason that they are categorized together.

For purposes of this text, differentiation between the age groups will be discussed, but the major focus will be on the disorder as it emerges in childhood. Nurses who work in areas of primary prevention with children can have the greatest effect in terms of treating this disorder. Treatment aimed at reversal in behavior is considered cautiously optimistic if initiated in childhood. After establishment of a core gender identity, it is difficult later in life to instill attributes of an opposite identity.

The fifth edition of the *Diagnostic and Statistical Manual of Mental Disorders* is currently in production, with a target date of 2013 for publication. One of the topics for which there has been much controversy is that of GID. The transgender community has expressed a great deal of concern about the inclusion of the diagnosis in the new edition, protesting to the psychiatric working group that, "different is not a disease." The working group has attempted to address some of the concerns of the transgender community, taking into consideration the stigma associated with inclusion of the diagnosis, but also the need for inclusion in terms of access to adequate treatment and care. One of the proposals currently under consideration is to change the name Gender Identity Disorder to *Gender Incongruence,* thereby emphasizing the incongruence between one's expressed and assigned genders. Other proposals for changes are also under consideration.

Course and Epidemiology

The prevalence of GID is estimated at 1 in 30,000 men and 1 in 100,000 women (Black & Andreasen, 2011). Most (approximately 75 percent) are biological males desiring reassignment to female gender (MTF), and the remaining 25 percent are females desiring to be male (FTM) (Martin, 2007). Some individuals with GID choose to find ways of living with their cross-gender identity without altering their bodies. Others have a strong desire to change their physical body to reflect their core gender identity. Meston and Frohlich (2002) reported on studies suggesting that childhood GID may predict adult GID. The American Psychiatric Association (2000) states:

> Only a very small number of children with Gender Identity Disorder will continue to

have symptoms that meet criteria for Gender Identity Disorder in adolescence or adulthood (p. 579).

By late adolescence or adulthood, about three-quarters of boys who had a childhood history of Gender Identity Disorder report a homosexual or bisexual orientation, but without concurrent Gender Identity Disorder (p. 580).

Predisposing Factors

Biological Influences

Becker and Johnson (2008) reported that studies of females with congenital adrenal hyperplasia (CAH) as a result of high levels of prenatal androgens suggest that there may be a relation between CAH and gender identity disorders. The data are still inconclusive, and further research in this area is indicated.

Several studies have been conducted to determine if sex hormone levels are abnormal in individuals with gender dysphoria. In some studies, decreased levels of testosterone were found in male transgendered individuals, and abnormally high levels of testosterone were found in female transgendered individuals, but the results have been inconsistent (Becker & Johnson, 2008). A recent large-scale study of cross-gender behavior in twins revealed that the similarity for cross-gender behavior was greater in monozygotic (identical) than in dizygotic (nonidentical) twin pairs, suggesting a possible genetic link in transgenderism (Beijsterveldt, Hudziak, & Boomsma, 2006).

An additional study reports on possible effects of testosterone on brain differentiation (Zhou et al., 1995). The researchers found that the red nucleus of the stria terminalis (a region of the hypothalamus) in male-to-female transsexuals corresponded to that of typical females, rather than of typical males. This was the case whether the individual was heterosexual or homosexual, and was not accounted for by hormone therapy.

Family Dynamics

It appears that family dynamics may play an influential role in the etiology of gender disorders. Sadock and Sadock (2007) stated, "Children usually develop a gender identity consonant with their sex of rearing (also known as *assigned sex*)" (p. 718). Gender roles are culturally determined, and parents encourage masculine or feminine behaviors in their children. Although "temperament" may play a role, with certain behavioral characteristics being present at birth, mothers usually foster a child's

pride in their gender. Sadock and Sadock (2007) stated:

> The father's role is also important in the early years, and his presence normally helps the separation-individuation process. Without a father, mother and child may remain overly close. For a girl, the father is normally the prototype of future love objects; for a boy, the father is a model for male identification. (p. 719)

Psychoanalytic Theory

The psychoanalytic theory suggests that gender identity problems begin during the struggle of the Oedipal conflict. Problems may reflect both real family events and those created in the child's imagination. These conflicts, whether real or imagined, interfere with the child's loving of the opposite-gender parent and identifying with the same-gender parent, and ultimately with normal gender identity.

Application of the Nursing Process to Gender Identity Disorders

Background Assessment Data (Symptomatology)

Gender Identity Disorder in Children

The *DSM-IV-TR* (APA, 2000) describes the manifestations of this disorder as the presence of four (or more) of the following:

1. Repeatedly stated desire to be, or insistence that he or she is, the opposite gender.

2. In boys, preference for cross-dressing or simulating female attire; in girls, insistence on wearing only stereotypical masculine clothing.

3. Strong and persistent preferences for cross-gender roles in make-believe play or persistent fantasies of being the opposite gender.

4. Intense desire to participate in the stereotypical games and pastimes of the opposite gender.

5. Strong preference for playmates of the opposite gender.

They may be subjected to teasing and rejection by their peers and disapproval from family members. This occurs early in childhood for boys, but often does not occur before adolescence in girls. Because of this rejection, interpersonal relationships are hampered. The disorder is not common but occurs more frequently in boys than in girls.

Gender Identity Disorder in Adolescents and Adults

The *DSM-IV-TR* describes this disorder as one in which there is a strong and persistent cross-gender identification (not merely a desire for any perceived cultural advantages of being the opposite gender) (APA, 2000). Symptomatic manifestations include a stated desire to be of the opposite gender, frequently passing as the opposite gender, a desire to live or be treated as the opposite gender, or the conviction that he or she has the typical feelings and reactions of the opposite gender (APA, 2000). These symptoms are accompanied by a persistent discomfort with or sense of inappropriateness in the assigned gender role. Some individuals are so convinced they were born the wrong gender that they become preoccupied with methods to eliminate the sex characteristics of the assigned gender, such as requesting opposite gender hormones or surgery to alter sexual characteristics.

Diagnosis/Outcome Identification

Intervention with adolescents and adults with GID is complex. Adolescents commonly act out and rarely have the motivation required to alter their cross-gender roles (Sadock & Sadock, 2007). Some adults seek therapy to learn how to cope with their altered sexual identity, while others have direct and immediate request for hormonal therapy and surgical sex reassignment. Becker and Johnson (2008) stated,

> Treatment [of gender identity disorder in the child] has three goals: increasing peer support and acceptance, treating co-occurring mental health concerns, and reducing the likelihood of transsexualism in adulthood. (p. 737)

Most of the treatment of children with GID has been in outpatient clinics. Nurses working in these settings may encounter these clients from time to time, although the disorder is not common. One-to-one nursing intervention may be provided by a psychiatric clinical nurse specialist Nurse Practitioner.

Based on the data collected during the nursing assessment, possible nursing diagnoses for the client with GID in children may include the following:

■ Disturbed personal identity related to biological factors or parenting patterns that encourage culturally unacceptable behaviors for assigned gender

■ Impaired social interaction related to socially and culturally unacceptable behaviors

■ Low self-esteem related to rejection by peers

The following criteria may be used for measurement of outcomes in the care of the client with gender identity disorder in children.

The Client:

■ Demonstrates trust in a therapist of the same gender.

■ Demonstrates development of a close relationship with the parent of the same gender.

■ Demonstrates a diminishment in the excessively close relationship with the parent of the opposite gender.

■ Demonstrates behaviors that are culturally appropriate for assigned gender.

■ Verbalizes and demonstrates comfort in, and satisfaction with, assigned gender role.

■ Interacts appropriately with others demonstrating culturally acceptable behaviors.

■ Verbalizes and demonstrates self-satisfaction with assigned gender role.

Planning/Implementation

Following are nursing diagnoses commonly used with individuals experiencing alterations in sexual functioning. Short- and long-term goals and nursing interventions are presented for each.

Disturbed Personal Identity

Disturbed personal identity is defined as the "inability to maintain an integrated and complete perception of self" (NANDA-I, 2009, p. 185).

Client Goals

Outcome criteria include short- and long-term goals. Timelines are individually determined.

Short-Term Goals

■ Client will verbalize knowledge of behaviors that are appropriate and culturally acceptable for assigned gender.

■ Client will verbalize desire for congruence between personal feelings and behavior and assigned gender.

Long-Term Goals

■ Client will demonstrate behaviors that are appropriate and culturally acceptable for assigned gender.

■ Client will express personal satisfaction and feelings of being comfortable in assigned gender.

Interventions

■ Spend time with the client and show positive regard. Trust and unconditional acceptance are essential to the establishment of a therapeutic nurse-client relationship.

■ Be aware of personal feelings and attitudes toward this client and his or her behavior. Attitudes influence behavior. The nurse must not allow negative attitudes to interfere with the effectiveness of interventions.

■ Allow the client to describe his or her perception of the problem. It is important to know how the client perceives the problem before attempting to correct misperceptions.

■ Discuss with the client the types of behaviors that are more culturally acceptable. Practice these behaviors through role-playing or with play therapy strategies (e.g., male and female dolls). Positive reinforcement or social attention may be given for use of appropriate behaviors. No response is given for stereotypical opposite-gender behaviors.

> **CLINICAL PEARL** The objective in working for behavioral change in a child who has GID is to enhance culturally appropriate same-gender behaviors, but not necessarily to extinguish all coexisting opposite-gender behaviors.

Impaired Social Interaction

Impaired social interaction is defined as "insufficient or excessive quantity or ineffective quality of social exchange" (NANDA-I, 2009, p. 223).

Client Goals
Outcome criteria include short- and long-term goals. Timelines are individually determined.

Short-Term Goal

■ Client will verbalize possible reasons for ineffective interactions with others.

Long-Term Goal

■ Client will interact with others using culturally acceptable behaviors.

Interventions
■ Once the client feels comfortable with the new behaviors in role-playing or one-to-one nurse-client interactions, the new behaviors may be tried in group situations. If possible, remain with the client during initial interactions with others. The presence of a trusted individual provides security for the client in a new situation, and also provides the potential for feedback to the client about his or her behavior.

■ Observe client behaviors and the responses he or she elicits from others. Give social attention (e.g., smile, nod) to desired behaviors. Follow up these "practice" sessions with one-to-one processing of the interaction. Give positive

reinforcement for efforts. Positive reinforcement encourages repetition of desirable behaviors. One-to-one processing provides time for discussing the appropriateness of specific behaviors and why they should or should not be repeated.

■ Offer support if client is feeling hurt from peer ridicule. Matter-of-factly discuss the behaviors that elicited the ridicule. Offer no personal reaction to the behavior. Personal reaction from the nurse would be considered judgmental. Validation of the client's feelings is important, yet it is also important that client understand why his or her behavior was the subject of ridicule and how to avoid it in the future.

■ The goal is to create a trusting, nonthreatening atmosphere for the client in an attempt to change behavior and improve social interactions. Long-term studies have not yet revealed the significance of therapy with these children for psychosexual relationship development in adolescence or adulthood. One variable that must be considered is the evidence of psychopathology within the families of many of these children.

Low Self-Esteem

Low self-esteem is defined as "negative self-evaluating/feelings about self or self-capabilities" (NANDA-I, 2009, pp. 193–194).

Client Goals
Outcome criteria include short- and long-term goals. Timelines are individually determined.

Short-Term Goal

■ Client will verbalize positive statements about self, including past accomplishments and future prospects.

Long-Term Goal

■ Client will verbalize and demonstrate behaviors that indicate self-satisfaction with assigned gender, ability to interact with others, and a sense of self as a worthwhile person.

Interventions
■ In an effort to enhance the child's self-esteem, encourage him or her to engage in activities in which he or she is likely to achieve success.

■ Help the child to focus on aspects of his or her life for which positive feelings exist. Discourage rumination about situations that are perceived as failures or over which the client has no control. Give positive feedback for these behaviors.

■ Help the client identify behaviors or aspects of life he or she would like to change. If realistic, assist the child in problem-solving ways to bring about the change. Having some control over his or her life may decrease feelings of powerlessness and increase feelings of self-worth.

■ Offer to be available for support to the child when he or she is feeling rejected by peers. Having an available support person who does not judge the child's behavior and who provides unconditional acceptance assists the child to progress toward acceptance of self as a worthwhile person.

Evaluation

The final step of the nursing process is to determine if the nursing interventions have been effective in achieving the intended outcomes. This evaluation process requires that the nurse reassess the client's behaviors and determine if the changes at which the interventions had been directed have occurred. For the child with gender identity disorder, this may be accomplished by using the following types of questions:

■ Does the client perceive that a problem existed that requires a change in behavior for resolution?

■ Does the client demonstrate use of behaviors that are culturally accepted for his or her assigned gender?

■ Can the client use these culturally accepted behaviors in interactions with others?

■ Is the client accepted by peers when same-gender behaviors are used?

■ If the client is refusing to change behaviors, what is the peer reaction?

■ What is the client's response to negative peer reaction?

■ Can the client verbalize positive statements about self?

■ Can the client discuss past accomplishments without dwelling on the perceived failures?

■ Has the client shown progress toward accepting self as a worthwhile person regardless of others' responses to his or her behavior?

Variations in Sexual Orientation

Homosexuality

Homosexual activity occurs under some circumstances in probably all known human cultures and all mammalian species for which it has been studied. The term **homosexuality** is derived from the Greek root *homo,* meaning "same," and refers to sexual preference for individuals of the same gender. It may be applied in a general way to homosexuals of both genders but is often used to specifically denote male homosexuality. The term **lesbianism,** used to identify female homosexuality, is traced to the Greek poet Sappho, who lived on the island of Lesbos and is famous for the love poems she wrote to other women. Most homosexuals prefer the term "gay" because it is less derogatory in its lack of emphasis on the sexual aspects of the orientation. A heterosexual is referred to as "straight."

The psychiatric community in general does not consider consensual homosexuality to be a mental disturbance. The concept of homosexuality as a disturbance in sexual orientation no longer appears in the *DSM.* Instead, the *DSM-IV-TR* (APA, 2000) is concerned only with the individual who experiences "persistent and marked distress about his or her sexual orientation" (p. 582).

A recent Gallup poll showed that Americans are closely divided in their belief on the morality of homosexuality. In this poll, 52 percent considered homosexual relations morally acceptable and 43 percent stated they believed them to be morally wrong (Gallup, 2010). Some experts believe that many Americans' attitudes toward homosexuals can best be described as homophobic. *Homophobia* is defined as a negative attitude toward or fear of homosexuality or homosexuals (King, 2009). It may be indicative of a deep-seated insecurity about one's own gender identity. Homophobic behaviors include extreme prejudice against, abhorrence of, and discomfort around homosexuals. These behaviors are usually rationalized by religious, moral, or legal considerations.

Relationship patterns are as varied among homosexuals as they are among heterosexuals. Some homosexuals may remain with one partner for an extended period of time, even for a lifetime, whereas others prefer not to make a commitment, and "play the field" instead.

No one knows for sure why people become homosexual or heterosexual. Various theories have been proposed regarding the issue, but no single etiological factor has consistently emerged. Many contributing factors likely influence the development of sexual orientation.

Predisposing Factors

Biological Theories

A study by Bailey and Pillard (1991) revealed a 52 percent concordance for homosexual orientation in monozygotic twins and 22 percent in dizygotic twins. Other studies have produced similar results (Kendler, Thornton, Gilman, & Kessler, 2000; Whitam, Diamond, & Martin, 1993). These data were significant to suggest the possibility of a heritable trait. Sadock and Sadock (2007) stated:

> Gay men show a familial distribution; they have more brothers who are gay than do heterosexual men. One study found that 33 out of 40 pairs of gay brothers shared a genetic marker on the bottom half of the X chromosome. (p. 686)

A number of studies have been conducted to determine whether or not there is a hormonal influence in the etiology of homosexuality. It has been hypothesized that levels of testosterone may be lower and levels of estrogen higher in homosexual men than in heterosexual men. Results have been inconsistent. It has also been suggested that exposure to inappropriate levels of androgens during the critical fetal period of sexual differentiation may contribute to homosexual orientation. This hypothesis lacks definitive evidence, and conclusions regarding its validity remain tentative.

Psychosocial Theories

Freud (1930) believed that all humans are inherently bisexual, with the capacity for both heterosexual and homosexual behavior. He theorized all individuals go through a homoerotic phase as children. Thus, if homosexuality occurs later in life, it is due to arrest of normal psychosexual development. He also believed homosexuality could occur as a result of pathological family relationships in which the child adopts a negative Oedipal position; that is, there is sexualized attachment to the parent of the same gender and identification with the parent of the opposite gender.

Some theories suggest that a dysfunctional family pattern may have an etiological influence in the development of homosexuality. These "nurture" theories focus on the parent-child relationship, and most specifically, the relationship with the same-gender parent. They suggest that gay men often have a dominant, supportive mother and a weak, remote, or hostile father. Lesbians may have had a dysfunctional mother-daughter relationship. Both subsequently try to meet their unmet same-gender needs through sexual relationships.

These theories of family dynamics have been disputed by some clinicians who believe that parents have very little influence on the outcome of their children's sexual-partner orientation. Others suggest there may not be one single answer—that sexual orientation may result from a complex interaction between environmental, cognitive, and anatomical factors, shaping the individual at an early age.

Special Concerns

People with homosexual preferences have problems that are similar to those of their heterosexual counterparts. Considerations of attractiveness, finding a partner, and concerns about sexual adequacy are common to both. STDs are epidemic among sexually active individuals of all sexual orientations. Of particular concern is acquired immunodeficiency syndrome (AIDS), which was considered a "gay disease" for the first few years of the epidemic. AIDS is a fatal viral illness that, initially in the Western world, was indeed largely transmitted by male homosexual activity. Although AIDS is now known to spread through contaminated blood products, the sharing of needles by intravenous drug users, and heterosexual contact, some individuals still believe AIDS is God's way of punishing homosexuals. These societal attitudes are considered by many homosexuals to be their greatest burden.

Some homosexuals live in fear of the discovery of their sexual orientation; they fear being rejected by parents and significant others. They experience a great deal of cognitive dissonance related to the disparity between their overt behavior and their inner feelings. Social sanctions still exist in some areas for homosexuals in regard to employment, housing, and public accommodations. The Human Rights Commission protects homosexuals; however, discrimination is still widespread.

Another area of concern to the gay community is the issue of gay marriage. In the United States, gay marriage is legal in Connecticut, Iowa, New Hampshire, New York, Massachusetts, Vermont, and Washington, DC. Same-sex marriage is also legal in Canada, Spain, the Netherlands, Belgium, Norway, Sweden, and South Africa. Other states (e.g., New Jersey, Oregon, Washington, California, Nevada, Illinois, and Rhode Island) and countries (e.g., Denmark, France, Germany, New Zealand, Portugal, Switzerland, United Kingdom) now recognize "civil unions" or "domestic partnerships," which allow same-sex couples various financial, insurance, and family benefits usually restricted to married heterosexual couples.

Opponents of the issue of same-sex marriage define marriage as an institution between one man and one woman. They argue that a gay relationship is not an optimal environment in which to raise children and that it goes against the traditional American value system. In addition, many people oppose homosexuality and gay marriage based on their religious beliefs, including: (1) that homosexuality is wrong because it involves sex that doesn't create life, (2) that homosexuality is "unnatural" (that God created men and women with the innate capacities for sexual relations that are distinctly absent from a same-sex relationship), and (3) that it is discouraged (or forbidden) by the Bible.

Proponents of gay marriage believe that the issue has to do with equality, pure and simple. They believe that all loving, consenting adult couples have the same rights under the law. They cite the real nature of marriage as a binding commitment (legally, socially, and personally) between two people, and they believe that individuals of the same gender have an equal right to make such a commitment to each other as do heterosexual couples. Regarding the rearing of children, research has suggested that having a gay or lesbian parent does not affect a child's social adjustment, school success, or sexual orientation (Wainright, Russell, & Patterson, 2004).

Nurses must examine their personal attitudes and feelings about homosexuality. They must be able to recognize when negative feelings are compromising the care they give. Increasing numbers of homosexuals are being honest about their sexual orientation. Health-care workers must ensure that these individuals receive care with dignity, which is the right of all human beings. Nurses who have come to terms with their own feelings about homosexuality are better able to separate the person from the behavior. Unconditional acceptance of each individual is an essential component of compassionate nursing.

Transgenderism

Transgenderism is a disorder of gender identity or gender dysphoria (unhappiness or dissatisfaction with one's gender) of the most extreme variety. An individual, despite having the anatomical characteristics of a given gender, has the self-perception of being of the opposite gender. Individuals with this disorder do not feel comfortable wearing the clothes of their assigned gender and often engage in cross-dressing. They may find their own genitals repugnant and may repeatedly submit requests to the health-care system for hormonal and surgical gender reassignment. Depression and anxiety are common and are often attributed by the individual to his or her inability to live in the desired gender role.

The *DSM-IV-TR* does not identify transgenderism as a specific disorder, choosing instead to discuss the broader category of *gender identity disorder*. Refer to the previous section on Gender Identity Disorder for predisposing factors to the disorder.

Special Concerns

Treatment is a complex process. The true transgendered individual intensely desires to have the genitalia and physical appearance of the assigned gender changed to conform to his or her gender identity. This change requires a great deal more than surgical alteration of physical features. In most cases, the individual must undergo extensive psychological testing and counseling, as well as live in the role of the desired gender for up to 2 years before surgery.

Hormonal treatment is initiated during this period. Male clients receive estrogen, which results in a redistribution of body fat in a more "feminine" pattern, enlargement of the breasts, a softening of the skin, and reduction in body hair. Women receive testosterone, which also causes a redistribution of body fat, growth of facial and body hair, enlargement of the clitoris, and deepening of the voice (Becker & Johnson, 2008). Amenorrhea occurs within a few months.

Surgical treatment for male-to-female transgender reassignment involves removal of the penis and testes and creation of an artificial vagina. Care is taken to preserve sensory nerves in the area so that the individual may continue to experience sexual stimulation.

Surgical treatment for female-to-male transgender reassignment is more complex. A mastectomy and sometimes a hysterectomy are performed. A penis and scrotum are constructed from tissues in the genital and abdominal area, and the vaginal orifice is closed. A penile implant is used to attain erection.

Both men and women continue to receive maintenance hormone therapy following surgery. Satisfaction with the results is highest among clients who are emotionally healthy, have adequate social support, and attain reasonable cosmetic results (Martin, 2007). Black and Andreasen (2011) stated, "Many patients will continue to benefit from psychotherapy following surgery to assist them in adjusting to their new gender role" (p. 340).

Nursing care of the post–gender-reassignment surgical client is similar to that of most other postsurgical clients. Particular attention is given to maintaining comfort, preventing infection, preserving integrity of the surgical site, maintaining elimination, and meeting nutritional needs. Psychosocial needs may have to do with body image, fears and insecurities about relating to others, and being accepted in the new gender role. Meeting these needs can begin with nursing in a nonthreatening, nonjudgmental healing atmosphere.

Bisexuality

A bisexual person is not exclusively heterosexual or homosexual; he or she engages in sexual activity with members of both genders. Bisexuals are also sometimes referred to as ambisexual.

Bisexuality is more common than exclusive homosexuality. Statistics suggest that approximately 75 percent of all men are exclusively heterosexual and only 2 percent are exclusively homosexual, leaving a relatively large percentage who have engaged in sexual activity with both men and women.

A diversity of sexual preferences exists among bisexuals. Some individuals prefer men and women equally, whereas others have a preference for one gender but also accept sexual activity with the other gender. Some bisexuals may alternate between homosexual and heterosexual activity for long periods; others may have both a male and a female lover at the same time. Whereas some individuals maintain their bisexual orientation throughout their lives, others may become exclusively homosexual or heterosexual.

Predisposing Factors

Little research exists on the etiology of bisexuality. As stated previously, Freud (1930) believed that all humans are inherently bisexual; that is, he believed that all individuals have the capacity for both heterosexual and homosexual interactions.

Much research on the development of homosexuality rests on the assumption that it is somehow determined by pathological conditions in childhood. Many heterosexual individuals, however, have their first homosexual encounter later in life. It is unlikely that an initial homosexual encounter that occurs in the 30s or 40s was determined by a pathological condition that occurred when the individual was 3 or 4 years old. Some encounters, too, are based solely on the situation, such as the heterosexual man who engages in homosexual behavior while in prison, and then returns to heterosexuality following his release. This behavior most likely was determined by circumstances rather than a pathological process that occurred in childhood.

Gender identity (determining whether one is male or female) is usually established by the age of 2 to 3 years. Sexual identity (determining whether one is heterosexual or homosexual or both) may continue to evolve throughout one's lifetime.

Sexually Transmitted Diseases

Sexually transmitted diseases (STDs) refer to infections that are contracted primarily through sexual activities or intimate contact with the genitals, mouth, or rectum of another individual. They may be transmitted from one person to another through heterosexual or homosexual contact, and external genital evidence of pathology may or may not be manifested.

STDs are at epidemic levels in the United States. Individuals are beginning an active sex life at an earlier age. More women are sexually active than ever before. The social changes that may have contributed to the increase in STDs are sometimes referred to as the "three Ps": permissiveness, promiscuity, and the pill. The widespread knowledge that antibiotics were available to cure infections and the availability of oral contraceptives to prevent pregnancy resulted in significant increases in promiscuity and the subsequent exposure to and spread of STDs.

A primary nursing responsibility in STD control is education that is aimed at prevention of the disease. Nurses must know which diseases are most prevalent, how they are transmitted, their signs and symptoms, available treatment, and consequences of avoiding treatment (Table 31-2). They must teach this information to clients in hospitals and clinics and take an active role in programs of education in the community. Early education is important to decrease the spread of STDs.

STDs have a particularly emotive significance because they can be transmitted between sexual partners. Consequently, STDs carry strong connotations of illicit sex and considerable social stigma, as well as potentially disastrous medical consequences. Feelings of guilt in clients with STDs can be overwhelming. These individuals need strong support to overcome not only the physical difficulties but also the social and emotional ones associated with having this type of illness.

Prevention of STDs is the ideal goal, but early detection and appropriate treatment continue to be considered realistic objectives. Nurses are in an excellent position to provide the education required for prevention, as well as the physical treatment and social and emotional support to assist clients with STDs to regain and maintain optimal wellness.

TABLE 31-2 Sexually Transmitted Diseases

DISEASE	ORGANISM OF TRANSMISSION	METHOD OF TRANSMISSION	SIGNS AND SYMPTOMS	TREATMENT	POTENTIAL COMPLICATIONS
Gonorrhea	*Neisseria gonorrhoeae* (bacterium)	Vaginal sex, anal sex, genital-oral sex, via hand moistened with infected secretions and placed in contact with mucous membranes (e.g., the eyes)	Men: urethritis; dysuria, purulent discharge from urethra; proctitis; pharyngitis. Women: initially asymptomatic; progression to infection of cervix, urethra, and fallopian tubes	Ceftriaxone, cefixime, and other cephalosporin antibiotics	Men: sterility from orchitis or epididymitis Women: chronic pelvic inflammatory disease, infertility, ectopic pregnancy, blindness from gonococcal conjunctivitis
Syphilis	*Treponema pallidum* (spirochete)	Vaginal sex, anal sex, genital-oral sex, via contact of infected secretions with intact mucous membranes or abraded skin	Primary stage: painless chancre on penis, vulva, vagina, mouth, anus, or other point of contact with mucous membranes or abraded skin Secondary stage: rash, headache, anorexia, weight loss, fever, sore throat, body aches, anemia	Long-acting penicillin G, tetracycline, erythromycin	Latent stage: lasts many years; no symptoms, but can be passed on to fetus Tertiary stage: blindness; heart disease; insanity; ulcerated lesions on skin, mucous membranes, or internal organs
Chlamydial infection	*Chlamydia trachomatis* (intracellular bacterium)	Vaginal sex, anal sex, via hand moistened with infected secretions and placed in contact with mucous membranes	Men: urethral discharge and dysuria Women: cervicitis (either asymptomatic or may have discharge, dysuria, soreness, bleeding)	Tetracycline; erythromycin; azithromycin	Scarring in the fallopian tubes, ectopic pregnancy, infertility
Genital herpes	Herpes simplex virus, type 1 or type 2	Vaginal sex, anal sex, genital-oral sex; skin-to-skin contact with infected areas, to newborn through vaginal delivery	Blistery lesions in the genital area causing pain, itching, burning; also vaginal or urethral discharge, fever, headache, malaise, and myalgias	No cure; treatment is palliative with acyclovir, valacyclovir, or famciclovir	Recurrences are possible; potential complications include: meningitis, encephalitis, urethral strictures; possible risk of cervical cancer

Condition	Pathogen	Transmission	Symptoms	Treatment	Complications
Genital warts	Condyloma acuminatum (human papillomavirus)	Vaginal sex, anal sex, skin-to-skin contact with infected areas	Cauliflower-like warts that appear on penis or scrotum in men, and labia, vaginal walls, or cervix in women; mild itching may occur	Application of podofilox or podophyllin; cryotherapy; electrocautery; surgical removal	Recurrences possible; potential increased risk of cervical cancer
Hepatitis B	Hepatitis B virus	Vaginal sex, anal sex, genital-oral sex, contact with infectious blood or blood products, contact of infectious secretions with mucous membranes or abraded skin	Malaise, anorexia, nausea/vomiting, fever, headache, mild pain in right upper quadrant of abdomen, jaundice	No cure; treatment involves supportive care, bedrest for extended period; medications generally have not been found to be useful	Chronic hepatitis; cirrhosis; liver cancer
AIDS	Human immunodeficiency virus (HIV)	Exchange of body fluids via anal sex, vaginal sex, genital-oral sex; Shared use of needles during drug use or accidental needle stick with infected needle; Skin-to-skin contact when there are open sores on the skin; Transfusion with contaminated blood; Perinatal transmission: during delivery and through breast milk	May be asymptomatic for 10 years or longer following infection with HIV; Early signs of AIDS include severe weight loss, diarrhea, fever, night sweats, or the presence of a persistent opportunistic infection (e.g., herpes or candidiasis)	No cure; antiretroviral medication used to slow growth of the virus; Other medications given for symptomatic relief and to treat opportunistic infections	Regardless of treatment, AIDS is eventually fatal; new medications have dramatically increased the time from diagnosis to death, and research continues in drug treatments and vaccine development

CASE STUDY AND SAMPLE CARE PLAN

NURSING HISTORY AND ASSESSMENT

Janet's obstetrician/gynecologist (OB/GYN) has referred her to the mental health clinic with what he has diagnosed as Postpartum Depression. Janet (age 30) tells Carol, the psychiatric nurse practitioner, that she and her husband Bert (age 32) have been married for 2 years, and that she gave birth 4 months ago to their first child, a boy they named Jason. Jason has been a difficult baby, was diagnosed with colic, and is wakeful and cries much of the time. Janet is sleep-deprived and continuously fatigued. Janet states, "I'm not depressed. I'm just exhausted! Bert is a computer analyst and is gone from home about 10 hours a day. When he gets home, we do what we can to put some dinner together and take care of Jason at the same time. By 9 o'clock, I'm ready to collapse, and Bert wants to go to bed and make love. I just don't have the energy. It's starting to cause a lot of friction in our marriage. Bert gets so angry when I refuse his advances. He also gets angry when I passively comply with his advances. To be honest, I'm just not interested in sex anymore. I certainly don't want to risk another pregnancy. But I also don't want to risk losing my husband. We used to have such a great sexual relationship, but that seems like another lifetime ago. I don't know what to do!"

NURSING DIAGNOSIS/OUTCOME IDENTIFICATION

From the assessment data, the nurse develops the following nursing diagnosis for Janet:

Sexual dysfunction related to extreme fatigue and depressed mood evidenced by loss of sexual desire.

a. **Short-Term Goals**
   - Client will identify ways to receive respite from child care.
   - Client will identify ways to devote time to regain satisfactory sexual relationship with husband.

b. **Long-Term Goal:** Client will resume sexual activity at a level satisfactory to herself and her husband.

PLANNING/IMPLEMENTATION

Sexual Dysfunction

The following nursing interventions have been identified for Janet.

1. Take Janet's sexual history.
2. Determine the previous level of satisfaction in current sexual relationship.

3. Assess Janet's perception of the problem.
4. Suggest alternative strategies for resolution of the problem. (Because of Janet's fatigue and mild depression, she may not be able to adequately problem-solve the situation without assistance).
   a. Respite from child care (e.g., babysitting service, Mom's Day Out program, sharing babysitting with other mothers, grandparents).
   b. Schedule regular "date nights" with husband.
   c. Schedule periodic weekends away with husband.
5. Provide information regarding sexuality and sexual functioning.
6. Discuss with Janet her fear of pregnancy. Provide information about various methods of contraception.
7. Make referral to sex therapist, if Janet requests this service.

EVALUATION

The outcome criteria for Janet have been met. She was able to identify ways to receive respite from child care. She takes Jason to Mom's Day Out at her church every Friday morning. She now has an agreement with another new mother to trade one afternoon a week of babysitting duties. She inquired at the local community college in the department of early childhood education for names of students who would be interested in babysitting. Gina, a 19-year-old sophomore at the college, now baby-sits for Janet and Bert every Wednesday evening while they have a "date night." And one weekend a month, Bert's widowed mother stays with Jason while Janet and Bert have time away together. Her OB/GYN prescribed oral contraceptives, and Janet's fear of pregnancy has subsided. Janet's mood has lifted and she looks forward to her "free" time, and time alone with her husband. She reports that her sexual desire has increased, and that she and Bert now enjoy a satisfactory sexual relationship. She also states that she feels she is giving more quality care to Jason now that she has the periods of respite to which she looks forward every week.

Summary and Key Points

- The *DSM-IV-TR* identifies two major categories of sexual disorders: paraphilias and sexual dysfunctions.

- Paraphilias are a group of behaviors involving sexual activity with nonhuman objects or with nonconsenting partners or that involve suffering to others.

- Types of paraphilias include exhibitionism, fetishism, frotteurism, pedophilia, sexual masochism or sadism, and voyeurism.

- Sexual dysfunctions are disturbances that occur in any of the phases of the normal human sexual response cycle.

- Types of sexual dysfunctions include sexual desire disorders, sexual arousal disorders, orgasmic disorders, and sexual pain disorders.

- Biological treatment of paraphilias involves decreasing the level of circulating androgens.

- Psychoanalytic treatment of paraphilias focuses on helping the individual resolve early conflicts, thus relieving the anxiety that prevents him or her from forming appropriate sexual relationships.

- Behavior therapy for paraphilias includes use of aversion techniques, covert sensitization, and satiation.

- Nurses may best become involved in the treatment of paraphilias at the primary level of prevention.

- Treatment of sexual dysfunction disorders involves a variety of techniques, including cognitive therapy, systematic desensitization, and sensate focus exercises.

- Several medications are available for the treatment of erectile dysfunction. These include sildenafil (Viagra), tadalafil (Cialis), and vardenafil (Levitra). Others are currently under investigation.

- Gender identity disorders (GIDs) occur when there is an incongruence between anatomical sex and the assigned gender role.

- Individuals with GID experience extreme discomfort in the assigned gender and desire to be, or insist that they are, the opposite gender.

- Variations in sexual orientation include homosexuality, transgenderism, and bisexuality.

- Sexually transmitted diseases (STDs) refer to infections that are contracted primarily through sexual activities or intimate contact with the genitals, mouth, or rectum of another individual.

- STDs are at epidemic levels in the United States. Prevention is the ideal goal, but early detection and appropriate treatment continue to be considered realistic objectives.

- Nurses are in an excellent position to provide the education required for prevention, as well as the physical treatment and social and emotional support to assist clients with STDs to regain and maintain optimal wellness.

- Human sexuality influences all aspects of physical and mental health. Clients are becoming more open to discussing matters pertaining to sexuality, and it is therefore important for nurses to integrate information on sexuality into the care they give. This can be done by focusing on preventive, therapeutic, and educational interventions to assist individuals to attain, regain, or maintain sexual wellness.

 DavisPlus   Additional info available @ davisplus.fadavis.com

Review Questions
Self-Examination/Learning Exercise

*Select the answer that is **most** appropriate for each of the following questions.*

1. Anne, age 24, and her husband are seeking treatment at the sex therapy clinic. They have been married for 3 weeks and have never had sexual intercourse together. Pain and vaginal tightness prevent penile entry. Sexual history reveals Anne was raped when she was 15 years old. The physician would most likely assign which of the following diagnoses to Anne?
   a. Dyspareunia.
   b. Vaginismus.
   c. Anorgasmia.
   d. Sexual aversion disorder.

Continued

2. Anne, age 24, and her husband are seeking treatment at the sex therapy clinic. They have been married for 3 weeks and have never had sexual intercourse together. Pain and vaginal tightness prevent penile entry. Sexual history reveals Anne was raped when she was 15 years old. The most appropriate nursing diagnosis for Anne would be:
   a. Pain related to vaginal constriction.
   b. Ineffective sexuality patterns related to inability to have vaginal intercourse.
   c. Sexual dysfunction related to history of sexual trauma.
   d. Complicated grieving related to loss of self-esteem because of rape.

3. A client comes to the mental health clinic with a complaint of lack of sexual desire. In the initial interview, what assessments would the nurse make? (Select all that apply.)
   a. Mood.
   b. Level of energy.
   c. Medications being taken.
   d. Previous level of sexual activity.

4. Which of the following medications may be prescribed for premature ejaculation?
   a. Paroxetine.
   b. Tadalafil.
   c. Diazepam.
   d. Imipramine.

5. Tom watches his neighbor through her window each night as she undresses for bed. Later he fantasizes about having sex with her. This is an example of which paraphilia?
   a. Exhibitionism.
   b. Voyeurism.
   c. Frotteurism.
   d. Pedophilia.

6. Frank drives his car up to a strange woman, stops, and asks her for directions. As she is explaining, he reveals his erect penis to her. This is an example of which paraphilia?
   a. Sadism.
   b. Masochism.
   c. Frotteurism.
   d. Exhibitionism.

7. Tim, age 17, babysits for his 11-year-old neighbor, Jeff. Six months ago, Tim began fondling Jeff's genitals. They now engage in mutual masturbation each time they are together. This is an example of which paraphilia?
   a. Fetishism.
   b. Pedophilia.
   c. Exhibitionism.
   d. Voyeurism.

8. John is 32 years old. He buys women's clothing at the thrift shop. Sometimes he dresses as a woman and goes to a singles' bar. He becomes sexually excited as he fantasizes about men being attracted to him as a woman. This is an example of which paraphilia?
   a. Masochism.
   b. Voyeurism.
   c. Exhibitionism.
   d. Transvestic fetishism.

Review Questions—cont'd
Self-Examination/Learning Exercise

9. Fred rides a crowded subway every day. He stands beside a woman he views as very attractive. Just as the subway is about to stop, he places his hand on her breast and rubs his genitals against her buttock. As the door opens, he dashes out and away. Later he fantasizes she is in love with him. This is an example of which paraphilia?
   a. Voyeurism.
   b. Sadism.
   c. Frotteurism.
   d. Exhibitionism.

10. A client with erectile dysfunction has a new prescription for sildenafil. The nurse who is providing education about this medication tells the client that which of the following are common side effects of this medication? (Select all that apply.)
   a. Headache.
   b. Facial flushing.
   c. Constipation.
   d. Nasal congestion.
   e. Indigestion.

TEST YOUR CRITICAL THINKING SKILLS

Linda was hospitalized on the psychiatric unit for depression. During her nursing assessment interview, she stated, "According to my husband, I can't do anything right—not even have sex." When asked to explain further, Linda said she and her husband had been married for 17 years. She said that, in the beginning, they had experienced a mutually satisfying sexual relationship and "made love" two or three times a week. Their daughter was born after they had been married 2 years, followed 2 years later by the birth of their son. They now have two teenagers (ages 15 and 13) who, by Linda's admission, require a great deal of her time and energy. She says, "I'm too tired for sex. And, besides, the kids might hear. I would be so embarrassed if they did. I walked in on my parents having sex once when I was a teenager, and I thought I would die! And my parents never mentioned it. It was just like it never happened! It was so awful! But sex is just so important to my husband, though, and we haven't had sex in months. We argue all the time about it. I'm afraid it's going to break us up."
Answer the following questions related to Linda.

1. Regarding her sexual relationship problem, what would be the nursing diagnosis for Linda?

2. What interventions for this problem might the nurse include in the treatment plan for Linda?

3. Regarding this problem, what would be a realistic goal for which Linda might strive?

References

Administration on Aging. (2011). *A profile of older Americans: 2010.* Washington, DC: U.S. Department of Health and Human Services.

Altman, A., & Hanfling, S. (2003). *Sexuality in midlife and beyond.* Boston: Harvard Health Publications.

American Psychiatric Association. (2000). *Diagnostic and statistical manual of mental disorders* (4th ed.). *Text revision.* Washington, DC: American Psychiatric Publishing.

Bailey, J. M., & Pillard, R. C. (1991). A genetic study of male sexual orientation. *Archives of General Psychiatry, 48,* 1089–1096.

Becker, J. V., & Johnson, B. R. (2008). Gender identity disorders and paraphilias. In R. E. Hales, S. C. Yudofsky, & G. O. Gabbard (Eds.), *Textbook of psychiatry* (5th ed., pp. 729–753) Washington, DC: American Psychiatric Publishing.

Becker, J. V., & Stinson, J. D. (2008). Human sexuality and sexual dysfunction. In R. E. Hales, S. C. Yudofsky, & G. O. Gabbard (Eds.), *Textbook of psychiatry* (5th ed., pp. 711–728) Washington, DC: American Psychiatric Publishing.

Beijsterveldt, C. E. M., Hudziak, J. J., & Boomsma, D. I. (2006). Genetic and environmental influences on cross-gender behavior and relation to behavior problems: A study of Dutch twins at ages 7 and 10 years. *Archives of Sexual Behavior, 35,* 647–658.

Benson, A., & Ost, L. B. (2009). Premature ejaculation. *EMedicine Urology.* Retrieved September 24, 2010, from http://emedicine.medscape.com/article/435884-overview

Berman, J., & Berman, L. (2001). *For women only: A revolutionary guide to overcoming sexual dysfunction and reclaiming your sex life.* New York: Henry Holt.

Black, D. W., & Andreasen, N. C. (2011). *Introductory textbook of psychiatry* (5th ed.). Washington, DC: American Psychiatric Publishing.

Centers for Disease Control and Prevention. (2010a). FDA licensure of bivalent human papillomavirus vaccine (HPV2, Cervarix) for use in females and updated HPV vaccination recommendations from the Advisory Committee on Immunization Practices (ACIP). *Morbidity and Mortality Weekly Report, 59*(20), 626–631.

Centers for Disease Control and Prevention. (2010b). *Trends in the prevalence of sexual behaviors: National youth risk behavior survey, 1991–2009.* Retrieved September 22, 2010, from http://www.cdc.gov/HealthyYouth/yrbs/trends.htm

Clayton, A. H. (2002). Sexual dysfunction. In S. G. Kornstein & A. H. Clayton (Eds.), *Women's mental health* (pp. 263–273). New York: Guilford Press.

Dreyfus, E. A. (1998). *Sexuality and sex therapy: When there is sexual dysfunction.* Retrieved September 23, 2010, from http://www.selfhelpmagazine.com/article/node/1065

Gallup. (2010). *Four moral issues sharply divide Americans.* Retrieved September 25, 2010, from http://www.gallup.com/poll/137357/Four-Moral-Issues-Sharply-Divide-Americans.aspx

Institute of Medicine. (2003). *Health professions education: A bridge to quality.* Washington, DC: Author.

Janata, J. W., & Kingsberg, S. A. (2005). Sexual aversion disorder. In R. Balon & R. T. Segraves (Eds.), *Handbook of sexual dysfunction* (pp. 111–122). Boca Raton, FL: Taylor & Francis Group.

Kendler, K. S., Thornton, L. M., Gilman, S. E., & Kessler, R. C. (2000). Sexual orientation in a U.S. national sample of twin and nontwin sibling pairs. *American Journal of Psychiatry, 157,* 1843–1846.

Kim, E. D., & Brosman, S. A. (2011). Erectile dysfunction. Retrieved August 17, 2011, from http://emedicine.medscape.com/article/444220-overview

King, B. M. (2009). *Human sexuality today* (6th ed.). Upper Saddle River, NJ: Pearson Education.

Laumann, E. O., Glasser, D. B., Neves, R. C. S., & Moreira, E. D. (2009). A population-based survey of sexual activity, sexual problems, and associated help-seeking behavior patterns in mature adults in the United States of America. *International Journal of Impotence Research, 21,* 171–178.

Leiblum, S. R. (1999). Sexual problems and dysfunction: Epidemiology, classification, and risk factors. *The Journal of Gender-Specific Medicine, 2*(5), 41–45.

Martin, K. A. (2007). Transsexualism: Clinical guide to gender identity disorder. *Current Psychiatry, 6*(2), 81–91.

Masters, W. H., Johnson, V. E., & Kolodny, R. C. (1995). *Human sexuality* (5th ed.). New York: Addison Wesley Longman.

Meston, C. M., & Frohlich, P. F. (2002). The psychobiology of sexual and gender identity disorders. In H. D'haenen, J. A. denBoer, & P. Willner (Eds.), *Biological psychiatry* (3rd ed., pp. 1099–1113). London: John Wiley & Sons.

Murray, R. B., Zentner, J. P., & Yakimo, R. (2009). *Health promotion strategies through the life span* (8th ed.). Upper Saddle River, NJ: Prentice Hall.

NANDA International. (2009). *Nursing diagnoses: Definitions and classification 2009–2011.* Hoboken, NJ: Wiley-Blackwell.

Nappi, R., Salonia, A., Traish, A. M., vanLunsen, R. H. W., Vardi, Y., Kodiglu, A., et al. (2005). Clinical biologic pathophysiologies of women's sexual dysfunction. *Journal of Sexual Medicine, 2*(1): 4–25.

Nappi, R. E., Ferdeghini, F., & Polatti, F. (2006). Mechanisms involved in desire and arousal. In I. Goldstein, C. M. Meston, S. R. Davis, & A. Traish (Eds.), *Women's sexual function and dysfunction: Study, diagnosis, and treatment.* London: Informa Healthcare.

Phillips, N. A. (2000, July 1). Female sexual dysfunction: Evaluation and treatment. *American Family Physician, 62,* 127–136, 141–142.

Pukall, C. F., Lahaie, M. A., & Binik, Y. M. (2006). Sexual pain disorders: Pathophysiologic factors. In I. Goldstein, C. M. Meston, S. R. Davis, & A. Traish (Eds.), *Women's sexual function and dysfunction: Study, diagnosis, and treatment.* London: Informa Healthcare.

Rhodes, J. C., Kjerulff, K. H., Langenberg, P. W., & Guzinski, G. M. (1999). Hysterectomy and sexual functioning. *Journal of the American Medical Association, 282,* 1934–1941.

Robins, L. N., Helzer, J. E., Weissman, M. M., Orvaschel, H., Gruenberg, E., Burke, J. D., et al. (1984). Lifetime prevalence of specific psychiatric disorders in three sites. *Archives of General Psychiatry, 41,* 949–958.

Sadock, B. J., & Sadock, V. A. (2007). *Synopsis of psychiatry: Behavioral sciences/clinical psychiatry* (10th ed.). Philadelphia: Lippincott Williams & Wilkins.

Spear, J. (2001, April 6). Sex therapies. *Gale encyclopedia of psychology* (2nd ed.). Retrieved September 23, 2010, from http://www.findarticles.com/p/articles/mi_g2699/is_0003/ai_2699000313

Traish, A., & Kim, N. N. (2006). Modulation of female genital sexual arousal by sex steroid hormones. In I. Goldstein, C. M. Meston, S. R. Davis, & A. Traish (Eds.), *Women's sexual function and dysfunction: Study, diagnosis, and treatment.* London: Informa Healthcare.

Wainright, J. L., Russell, S. T., & Patterson, C. J. (2004). Psychosocial adjustment, school outcomes, and romantic relationships of adolescents with same-sex parents. *Child Development, 75,* 1886–1898.

Whitam, F. L., Diamond, M., & Martin, J. (1993). Homosexual orientation in twins: A report on 61 pairs and three triplet sets. *Archives of Sexual Behavior, 22,* 187–205.

Zhou, J., Horman, M. A., Gooren, L. J., & Swaab, D. F. (1995). A sex difference in the human brain and its relation to transsexuality. *Nature, 378,* 68–70.

Classical References

Freud, S. (1930). *Three contributions to the theory of sex* (4th ed.). New York: Nervous and Mental Disease Publishing.

Masters, W. H., & Johnson, V. E. (1966). *Human sexual response.* Boston: Little, Brown.

Masters, W. H., & Johnson, V. E. (1970). *Human sexual inadequacy.* Boston: Little, Brown.

@ INTERNET REFERENCES

- Additional information about sexual and gender identity disorders may be located at the following websites:
  - http://www.sexualhealth.com/
  - http://www.priory.com/sex.htm
  - http://emedicine.medscape.com/article/293890-overview
  - http://www.emedicine.com/med/topic3127.htm

- Additional information about sexually transmitted diseases may be located at the following websites:
  - http://www.cdc.gov/std/
  - http://www3.niaid.nih.gov/topics/sti

MOVIE CONNECTIONS

Mystic River (pedophilia) ● *Blue Velvet (sexual masochism)* ● *Looking for Mr. Goodbar (sadism/masochism)* ● *Normal (transvestitism)* ● *TransAmerica (transvestitism)*

CHAPTER 32 — Eating Disorders

CORE CONCEPTS

anorexia
body image
bulimia

KEY TERMS

amenorrhea
anorexia nervosa
anorexiants

bingeing
bulimia nervosa
emaciated

obesity
purging

OBJECTIVES
After reading this chapter, the student will be able to:

1. Identify and differentiate among the various eating disorders.
2. Discuss epidemiological statistics related to eating disorders.
3. Describe symptomatology associated with anorexia nervosa, bulimia nervosa, and obesity, and use the information in client assessment.
4. Identify predisposing factors in the development of eating disorders.
5. Formulate nursing diagnoses and outcomes of care for clients with eating disorders.
6. Describe appropriate interventions for behaviors associated with eating disorders.
7. Identify topics for client and family teaching relevant to eating disorders.
8. Evaluate the nursing care of clients with eating disorders.
9. Discuss various modalities relevant to treatment of eating disorders.

HOMEWORK ASSIGNMENT
Please read the chapter and answer the following questions:

1. There is some speculation that anorexia nervosa may be associated with a primary dysfunction of which brain structure?
2. What is the level of body mass index (BMI) that is associated with the definition of *obesity?*
3. Individuals with anorexia nervosa have a "distorted body image." What does this mean?
4. What physiological signs may be associated with the excessive vomiting of the purging syndrome?

Nutrition is required to sustain life, and most individuals acquire nutrients from eating food; however, nutrition and life sustenance are not the only reasons most people eat food. Indeed, in an affluent culture, life sustenance may not even be a consideration. It is sometimes difficult to remember that many people within this affluent American culture, as well as all over the world, are starving from lack of food.

The hypothalamus contains the appetite regulation center within the brain. This complex neural system regulates the body's ability to recognize when it is hungry and when it has been sated. Halmi (2008) stated,

Eating behavior is now known to reflect an interaction between an organism's physiological state and environmental conditions. Salient physiological variables include the balance of various neuropeptides and neurotransmitters, metabolic state, metabolic rate, condition of the gastrointestinal tract, amount of storage tissue, and sensory receptors for taste and smell. Environmental conditions include features of the food such as taste, texture, novelty, accessibility, and nutritional composition, and other external conditions such as ambient temperature, presence of other people, and stress. (p. 971)

Society and culture have a great deal of influence on eating behaviors. Eating is a social activity; seldom does an event of any social significance occur without the presence of food. Yet, society and culture also influence how people (and in particular, women) must look. History reveals a regularity of fluctuation in what society has considered desirable in the human female body. Archives and historical paintings from the 16th and 17th centuries reveal that plump, full-figured women were considered fashionable and desirable. In the Victorian era, beauty was characterized by a slender, wan appearance that continued through the flapper era of the 1920s. During the Depression era and World War II, the full-bodied woman was again admired, only to be superseded in the late 1960s by the image of the superthin models propagated by the media, which remains the ideal of today. As it has been said, "A woman can't be too rich or too thin." Eating disorders, as we know them, can refute this concept.

This chapter explores the disorders associated with undereating and overeating. Because psychological or behavioral factors play a potential role in the presentation of these disorders, they fall well within the realm of psychiatry and psychiatric nursing. Epidemiological statistics are presented along with predisposing factors that have been implicated in the etiology of anorexia nervosa, bulimia nervosa, and obesity. An explanation of the symptomatology is presented as background knowledge for assessing the client with an eating disorder. Nursing care is described in the context of the nursing process. Various treatment modalities are explored.

Epidemiological Factors

The incidence of **anorexia nervosa** has increased in the past 30 years both in the United States and in Western Europe (Halmi, 2008). Studies indicate a prevalence rate among young women in the United States of approximately 1 percent (Black & Andreasen, 2011). Anorexia nervosa occurs predominantly in females 12 to 30 years of age. Fewer than 10 percent of the cases are males (American Psychiatric Association [APA], 2000). Anorexia

nervosa was once believed to be more prevalent in the higher socioeconomic classes, but evidence is lacking to support this hypothesis.

Bulimia nervosa is more prevalent than anorexia nervosa, with estimates up to 4 percent of young women (Black & Andreasen, 2011). Onset of bulimia nervosa occurs in late adolescence or early adulthood. Cross-cultural research suggests that bulimia nervosa occurs primarily in societies that place emphasis on thinness as the model of attractiveness for women and where an abundance of food is available.

Obesity has been defined as a body mass index (BMI) (weight/height^2) of 30 or greater. In the United States, statistics indicate that, among adults 20 years of age or older, 68 percent are overweight, with 34 percent of these in the obese range (Centers for Disease Control and Prevention [CDC], 2010a). The percentage of obese individuals is higher in black women than in white women and slightly higher in black men than in white men (CDC, 2010a). The prevalence of obesity is greater among the lower socioeconomic group (Halmi, 2008), and there is an inverse relationship between obesity and level of education (CDC, 2010b). The latest figures from the CDC indicate that 5.7 percent of the U.S. adult population may be categorized as *extremely* obese, which is defined by the National Institutes of Health as a BMI greater than 40 (CDC, 2010a).

Application of the Nursing Process

Background Assessment Data (Anorexia Nervosa)

> **CORE CONCEPT**
> *Anorexia*
> Prolonged loss of appetite.

> **CORE CONCEPT**
> *Body Image*
> A subjective concept of one's physical appearance based on the personal perceptions of self and the reactions of others.

Anorexia nervosa is characterized by a morbid fear of obesity. Symptoms include gross distortion of body image, preoccupation with food, and refusal to eat. The term *anorexia* is actually a misnomer. It was initially believed that anorexics did not experience sensations of hunger. However, research indicates that they do indeed suffer from pangs of hunger, and it is only with food intake of less than 200 calories per day that hunger sensations actually cease.

The distortion in body image is manifested by the individual's perception of being "fat" when he or she is obviously underweight or even **emaciated.** Weight loss is usually accomplished by reduction in food intake and often extensive exercising. Self-induced vomiting and the abuse of laxatives or diuretics also may occur.

Weight loss is marked. For example, the individual may present for health-care services weighing less than 85 percent of expected weight. Other symptoms include hypothermia, bradycardia, hypotension, edema, lanugo, and a variety of metabolic changes. **Amenorrhea** usually follows weight loss but in some instances may precede it (APA, 2000).

Individuals with anorexia nervosa may be obsessed with food. For example, they may hoard or conceal food, talk about food and recipes at great length, or prepare elaborate meals for others, only to restrict themselves to a limited amount of low-calorie food intake. Compulsive behaviors, such as hand washing, may also be present.

Age at onset is usually early to late adolescence, and psychosexual development is often delayed. Feelings of depression and anxiety often accompany the disorder. In fact, some studies have suggested a possible interrelationship between eating disorders and affective disorders. Box 32-1 outlines the

Diagnostic and Statistical Manual of Mental Disorders, Fourth Edition, Text Revision (DSM-IV-TR) (APA, 2000) diagnostic criteria for anorexia nervosa.

Background Assessment Data (Bulimia Nervosa)

> ### CORE CONCEPT
> **Bulimia**
> Excessive, insatiable appetite.

Bulimia nervosa is an episodic, uncontrolled, compulsive, rapid ingestion of large quantities of food over a short period of time (**bingeing**), followed by inappropriate compensatory behaviors to rid the body of the excess calories. The food consumed during a binge often has a high caloric content, a sweet taste, and a soft or smooth texture that can be eaten rapidly, sometimes even without being chewed (Sadock & Sadock, 2007). The bingeing episodes often occur in secret and are usually only terminated by abdominal discomfort, sleep, social interruption, or self-induced vomiting. Although the eating binges may bring pleasure while they are occurring, self-degradation and depressed mood commonly follow.

To rid the body of the excessive calories, the individual may engage in **purging** behaviors (self-induced vomiting, or the misuse of laxatives, diuretics, or enemas) or other inappropriate compensatory behaviors, such as fasting or excessive exercise. There is a persistent overconcern with personal

---

BOX 32-1 Diagnostic Criteria for Anorexia Nervosa

A. Refusal to maintain body weight at or above a minimally normal weight for age and height (e.g., weight loss leading to maintenance of body weight less than 85% of that expected; or failure to make expected weight gain during period of growth, leading to body weight less than 85% of that expected).

B. Intense fear of gaining weight or becoming fat, even though underweight.

C. Disturbance in the way in which one's body weight or shape is experienced, undue influence of body weight or shape on self-evaluation, or denial of the seriousness of the current low body weight.

D. In postmenarcheal females, amenorrhea (i.e., the absence of at least three consecutive menstrual cycles). (A woman is considered to have amenorrhea if her periods occur only following hormone, e.g., estrogen, administration.)

Specify type:

Restricting Type: During the current episode of anorexia nervosa, the person has not regularly engaged in binge-eating or purging behavior (i.e., self-induced vomiting or the misuse of laxatives, diuretics, or enemas).

Binge-Eating/Purging Type: During the current episode of anorexia nervosa, the person has regularly engaged in binge eating or purging behavior (i.e., self-induced vomiting or the misuse of laxatives, diuretics, or enemas).

From American Psychiatric Association. (2000). Diagnostic and statistical manual of mental disorders (4th ed.). Text revision. Washington, DC: American Psychiatric Publishing, with permission.

appearance, particularly regarding how they believe others perceive them. Weight fluctuations are common because of the alternating binges and fasts. However, most individuals with bulimia are within a normal weight range—some slightly underweight, some slightly overweight.

Excessive vomiting and laxative or diuretic abuse may lead to problems with dehydration and electrolyte imbalance. Gastric acid in the vomitus also contributes to the erosion of tooth enamel. In rare instances, the individual may experience tears in the gastric or esophageal mucosa.

Some people with this disorder are subject to mood disorders, anxiety disorders, and substance abuse or dependence, most frequently involving amphetamines or alcohol (APA, 2000). Diagnostic criteria for bulimia nervosa are presented in Box 32-2.

Predisposing Factors to Anorexia Nervosa and Bulimia Nervosa

Biological Influences

Genetics A hereditary predisposition to eating disorders has been hypothesized on the basis of family histories and an apparent association with other disorders for which the likelihood of genetic influences exists. In their study of monozygotic and dizygotic twins, Bulik and associates (2006) concluded that genetic factors account for 56 percent of the risk for developing anorexia nervosa. Other genetics studies have suggested possible linkage sites for anorexia nervosa on chromosomes 1, 2, and 13 (Halmi, 2008). Anorexia nervosa is more

common among sisters and mothers of those with the disorder than among the general population. Several studies have reported a higher than expected frequency of mood disorders among first-degree biological relatives of people with anorexia nervosa and bulimia nervosa and of substance abuse and dependence in relatives of individuals with bulimia nervosa (APA, 2000).

Neuroendocrine Abnormalities Some speculation has occurred regarding a primary hypothalamic dysfunction in anorexia nervosa. Studies consistent with this theory have revealed elevated cerebrospinal fluid cortisol levels and a possible impairment of dopaminergic regulation in individuals with anorexia (Halmi, 2008). Additional evidence in the etiological implication of hypothalamic dysfunction is gathered from the fact that many people with anorexia experience amenorrhea before the onset of starvation and significant weight loss.

Neurochemical Influences Neurochemical influences in bulimia may be associated with the neurotransmitters serotonin and norepinephrine. This hypothesis has been supported by the positive response these individuals have shown to therapy with the selective serotonin reuptake inhibitors (SSRIs). Some studies have found high levels of endogenous opioids in the spinal fluid of clients with anorexia, promoting the speculation that these chemicals may contribute to denial of hunger (Sadock & Sadock, 2007). Some of these

---

BOX 32-2 **Diagnostic Criteria for Bulimia Nervosa**

A. Recurrent episodes of binge eating. An episode of binge eating is characterized by both of the following:
   1. Eating, in a discrete period of time (e.g., within any 2-hour period), an amount of food that is definitely larger than most people would eat during a similar period of time and under similar circumstances.
   2. A sense of lack of control over eating during the episode (e.g., a feeling that one cannot stop eating or control what or how much one is eating).
B. Recurrent inappropriate compensatory behavior in order to prevent weight gain, such as self-induced vomiting; misuse of laxatives, diuretics, enemas, or other medications; fasting; or excessive exercise.
C. The binge eating and inappropriate compensatory behaviors both occur, on average, at least twice a week for 3 months.
D. Self-evaluation is unduly influenced by body shape and weight.
E. The disturbance does not occur exclusively during episodes of anorexia nervosa.

Specify type:

Purging Type: During the current episode of bulimia nervosa, the person has regularly engaged in self-induced vomiting or the misuse of laxatives, diuretics, or enemas.

Nonpurging Type: During the current episode of bulimia nervosa, the person has used other inappropriate compensatory behaviors, such as fasting or excessive exercise, but has not regularly engaged in self-induced vomiting or the misuse of laxatives, diuretics, or enemas.

From American Psychiatric Association. (2000). Diagnostic and statistical manual of mental disorders (4th ed.). Text revision. Washington, DC: American Psychiatric Publishing, with permission.

individuals have been shown to gain weight when given naloxone, an opioid antagonist.

Psychodynamic Influences

Psychodynamic theories suggest that eating disorders result from very early and profound disturbances in mother-infant interactions. The result is retarded ego development in the child and an unfulfilled sense of separation-individuation. This problem is compounded when the mother responds to the child's physical and emotional needs with food. Manifestations include a disturbance in body identity and a distortion in body image. When events occur that threaten the vulnerable ego, feelings of lack of control over one's body (self) emerge. Behaviors associated with food and eating serve to provide feelings of control over one's life.

Family Influences

Conflict Avoidance In the theory of the family as a system, psychosomatic symptoms, including anorexia nervosa, are reinforced in an effort to avoid spousal conflict. Parents are able to deny marital conflict by defining the sick child as the family problem. In these families, there is an unhealthy involvement between the members (enmeshment), the members strive at all costs to maintain "appearances," and the parents endeavor to retain the child in the dependent position. Conflict avoidance may be a strong factor in the interpersonal dynamics of some families in which children develop eating disorders.

Elements of Power and Control The issue of control may become the overriding factor in the family of the client with an eating disorder. These families often consist of a passive father, a domineering mother, and an overly dependent child. A high value is placed on perfectionism in this family, and the child feels he or she must satisfy these standards. Parental criticism promotes an increase in obsessive and perfectionistic behavior on the part of the child, who continues to seek love, approval, and recognition. The child eventually begins to feel helpless and ambivalent toward the parents. In adolescence, these distorted eating patterns may represent a rebellion against the parents, viewed by the child as a means of gaining and remaining in control. The symptoms are often triggered by a stressor that the adolescent perceives as a loss of control in some aspect of his or her life.

Background Assessment Data (Obesity)

Obesity is not classified as a psychiatric disorder in the *DSM-IV-TR*, but because of the strong emotional factors associated with the condition, it may be considered under "Psychological Factors Affecting Medical Condition."

A third category of eating disorder is also being considered by the American Psychiatric Association. Research criteria for binge-eating disorder (BED) are included in the *DSM-IV-TR* (see Box 32-3). Obesity is a factor in BED because the individual binges on

---

BOX 32-3 Research Criteria for Binge-Eating Disorder

A. Recurrent episodes of binge eating. An episode of binge eating is characterized by both of the following:
   (1) eating, in a discrete period of time (e.g., within any 2-hour period), an amount of food that is definitely larger than most people would eat in a similar period of time under similar circumstances
   (2) a sense of lack of control over eating during the episode (e.g., a feeling that one cannot stop eating or control what or how much one is eating)

B. The binge-eating episodes are associated with three (or more) of the following:
   (1) eating much more rapidly than normal
   (2) eating until feeling uncomfortably full
   (3) eating large amounts of food when not feeling physically hungry
   (4) eating alone because of being embarrassed by how much one is eating
   (5) feeling disgusted with oneself, depressed, or very guilty after overeating

C. Marked distress regarding binge eating is present.

D. The binge eating occurs, on average, at least 2 days a week for 6 months.

Note: The method of determining frequency differs from that used for Bulimia Nervosa; future research should address whether the preferred method of setting a frequency threshold is counting the number of days on which binges occur or counting the number of episodes of binge eating.

E. The binge eating is not associated with the regular use of inappropriate compensatory behaviors (e.g., purging, fasting, excessive exercise) and does not occur exclusively during the course of Anorexia Nervosa or Bulimia Nervosa.

From American Psychiatric Association. (2000). Diagnostic and statistical manual of mental disorders (4th ed.). Text revision. Washington, DC: American Psychiatric Publishing, with permission.

large amounts of food (as in bulimia nervosa) but does not engage in behaviors to rid the body of the excess calories. The following formula is used to determine extent of obesity in an individual:

$$\text{Body mass index} = \frac{\text{Weight (kg)}}{\text{Height (m)}^2}$$

The BMI range for normal weight is 20 to 24.9. Studies by the National Center for Health Statistics indicate that *overweight* is defined as a BMI of 25.0 to 29.9 (based on U.S. Dietary Guidelines for Americans). Based on criteria of the World Health Organization, *obesity* is defined as a BMI of 30.0 or greater. These guidelines, which were released by the National Heart, Lung, and Blood Institute in July 1998, markedly increased the number of Americans considered to be overweight. The average American woman has a BMI of 26, and fashion models typically have BMIs of 18. Anorexia nervosa is characterized by a BMI of 17.5 or lower (Black & Andreasen, 2011). Table 32-1 presents an example of some BMIs based on weight (in pounds) and height (in inches).

Individuals who are obese often present with hyperlipidemia, particularly elevated triglyceride and cholesterol levels. They commonly have hyperglycemia and are at risk for developing diabetes mellitus. Osteoarthritis may be evident because of trauma to weight-bearing joints. Workload on the heart and lungs is increased, often leading to symptoms of angina or respiratory insufficiency (CDC, 2009).

Predisposing Factors to Obesity

Biological Influences

Genetics Genetics have been implicated in the development of obesity in that 80 percent of offspring of two obese parents are obese (Halmi, 2008). Studies of twins and adoptees reared by normal and overweight parents have also supported this implication of heredity as a predisposing factor to obesity.

Physiological Factors Lesions in the appetite and satiety centers in the hypothalamus may contribute to overeating and lead to obesity. Hypothyroidism is a problem that interferes with basal metabolism and may lead to weight gain. Weight gain can also occur in response to the decreased insulin production of diabetes mellitus and the increased cortisone production of Cushing's disease.

Lifestyle Factors On a more basic level, obesity can be viewed as the ingestion of a greater number of calories than are expended. Weight gain occurs when caloric intake exceeds caloric output in terms of basal metabolism and physical activity. Many overweight individuals lead sedentary lifestyles, making it very difficult to burn off calories.

IMPLICATIONS OF RESEARCH FOR EVIDENCE-BASED PRACTICE

Long, J. D., & Stevens, K. R. (2004). Using technology to promote self-efficacy for healthy eating in adolescents. *Journal of Nursing Scholarship,* **36(2), 134–139.**

DESCRIPTION OF THE STUDY: Obesity and overweight have reached epidemic proportions and they are risk factors for the development of chronic disease. The purpose of this study was to test the effects of a classroom and World Wide Web (WWW) educational intervention on self-efficacy for healthy eating. The sample consisted of 63 adolescents in the participant group and 58 in the control group. The age range was between 12 and 16 years. The participant group received the intervention that consisted of 10 hours of classroom and 5 hours of Web-based nutrition education endorsed by the American Cancer Society and the National Cancer Institute. Information was included to encourage healthy eating behaviors that reduce the risk of cancer, obesity, heart disease, and diabetes. Participants in the control group received the nutrition education integrated in the health, science, and home economics curriculum. All participants completed six questionnaires to measure dietary knowledge and eating behaviors. Pre- and post-tests were administered to both groups.

RESULTS OF THE STUDY: Although no difference in food consumption was found between groups during the month of intervention, the participant group had significantly higher scores related to knowledge of good nutrition and healthy eating behaviors. The study was limited to individual adolescents and did not attempt to initiate change in the home or school environment.

IMPLICATIONS FOR NURSING PRACTICE: Nurses, and especially school nurses, can become actively involved in nutrition education for children and adolescents. The authors reported that 9 million young people are overweight—a number that more than doubled in the last 20 years. This has serious implications for nursing to assist in the educational process needed to reverse this unhealthy trend.

TABLE 32-1 Body Mass Index (BMI) Chart

BMI	19	20	21	22	23	24	25	26	27	28	29	30	31	32	33	34	35	36	37	38	39	40
Height (inches)									Body Weight (pounds)													
58	91	96	100	105	110	115	119	124	129	134	138	143	148	153	158	162	167	172	177	181	186	191
59	94	99	104	109	114	119	124	128	133	138	143	148	153	158	163	168	173	178	183	188	193	198
60	97	102	107	112	118	123	128	133	138	143	148	153	158	163	168	174	179	184	189	194	199	204
61	100	106	111	116	122	127	132	137	143	148	153	158	164	169	174	180	185	190	195	201	206	211
62	104	109	115	120	126	131	136	142	147	153	158	164	169	175	180	186	191	196	202	207	213	218
63	107	113	118	124	130	135	141	146	152	158	163	169	175	180	186	191	197	203	208	214	220	225
64	110	116	122	128	134	140	145	151	157	163	169	174	180	186	192	197	204	209	215	221	227	232
65	114	120	126	132	138	144	150	156	162	168	174	180	186	192	198	204	210	216	222	228	234	240
66	118	124	130	136	142	148	155	161	167	173	179	186	192	198	204	210	216	223	229	235	241	247
67	121	127	134	140	146	153	159	166	172	178	185	191	198	204	211	217	223	230	236	242	249	255
68	125	131	138	144	151	158	164	171	177	184	190	197	203	210	216	223	230	236	243	249	256	262
69	128	135	142	149	155	162	169	176	182	189	196	203	209	216	223	230	236	243	250	257	263	270
70	132	139	146	153	160	167	174	181	188	195	202	209	216	222	229	236	243	250	257	264	271	278
71	136	143	150	157	165	172	179	186	193	200	208	215	222	229	236	243	250	257	265	272	279	286
72	140	147	154	162	169	177	184	191	199	206	213	221	228	235	242	250	258	265	272	279	287	294
73	144	151	159	166	174	182	189	197	204	212	219	227	235	242	250	257	265	272	280	288	295	302
74	148	155	163	171	179	186	194	202	210	218	225	233	241	249	256	264	272	280	287	295	303	311
75	152	160	168	176	184	192	200	208	216	224	232	240	248	256	264	272	279	287	295	303	311	319
76	156	164	172	180	189	197	205	213	221	230	238	246	254	263	271	279	287	295	304	312	320	328

From National Heart, Lung, and Blood Institute. (2010). Clinical guidelines on the identification, evaluation, and treatment of overweight and obesity in adults: Body mass index tables. Retrieved September 27, 2010, from http://www.nhlbi.nih.gov/guidelines/obesity/bmi_tbl.htm

Psychosocial Influences

The psychoanalytic view of obesity proposes that obese individuals have unresolved dependency needs and are fixed in the oral stage of psychosexual development. The symptoms of obesity are viewed as depressive equivalents, attempts to regain "lost" or frustrated nurturance and caring.

Sadock and Sadock (2007) stated:

> Although psychological factors are evidently crucial to the development of obesity, how such psychological factors result in obesity is not known. Overweight persons may suffer from every conceivable psychiatric disorder and come from a variety of disturbed backgrounds. Many obese patients are emotionally disturbed persons who, because of the availability of the overeating mechanism in their environments, have learned to use hyperphagia as a means of coping with psychological problems. Some patients may show signs of serious mental disorder when they attain normal weight because they no longer have that coping mechanism. (p. 742)

Transactional Model of Stress/Adaptation

The etiology of eating disorders is most likely influenced by multiple factors. In Figure 32–1, a graphic depiction of this theory of multiple causation is presented in the Transactional Model of Stress/Adaptation.

Diagnosis/Outcome Identification

Nursing diagnoses are formulated from the data gathered during the assessment phase and with background knowledge regarding predisposing factors to the disorder. Table 32-2 presents a list of client behaviors and the NANDA nursing diagnoses that correspond to those behaviors, which may be used in planning care for clients with eating disorders.

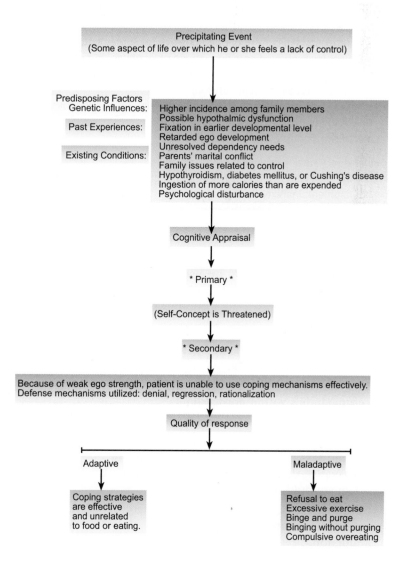

FIGURE 32–1 The dynamics of eating disorders using the Transactional Model of Stress/Adaptation.

TABLE 32-2 Assigning Nursing Diagnoses to Behaviors Commonly Associated with Eating Disorders

BEHAVIORS	NURSING DIAGNOSES
Refusal to eat; abuse of laxatives, diuretics, and/or diet pills; loss of 15 percent of expected body weight; pale conjunctiva and mucous membranes; poor muscle tone; amenorrhea; poor skin turgor; electrolyte imbalances; hypothermia; bradycardia; hypotension; cardiac irregularities; edema	**Imbalanced nutrition: Less than body requirements**
Decreased fluid intake; abnormal fluid loss caused by self-induced vomiting; excessive use of laxatives, enemas, or diuretics; electrolyte imbalance; decreased urine output; increased urine concentration; elevated hematocrit; decreased blood pressure; increased pulse rate; dry skin; decreased skin turgor; weakness	**Deficient fluid volume**
Minimizes symptoms; unable to admit impact of disease on life pattern; does not perceive personal relevance of symptoms; does not perceive personal relevance of danger	**Ineffective denial**
Compulsive eating; excessive intake in relation to metabolic needs; sedentary lifestyle; weight 20 percent over ideal for height and frame; BMI of 30 or more	**Imbalanced nutrition: More than body requirements**
Distorted body image; views self as fat, even in the presence of normal body weight or severe emaciation; denies that problem with low body weight exists; difficulty accepting positive reinforcement; self-destructive behavior (self-induced vomiting, abuse of laxatives or diuretics, refusal to eat); preoccupation with appearance and how others perceive it (anorexia nervosa, bulimia nervosa) Verbalization of negative feelings about the way he or she looks and the desire to lose weight (obesity) Lack of eye contact; depressed mood (all)	**Disturbed body image/Low self-esteem**
Increased tension; increased helplessness; overexcited; apprehensive; fearful; restlessness; poor eye contact; increased difficulty taking oral nourishment; inability to learn	**Anxiety (moderate to severe)**

Outcome Criteria

The following criteria may be used for measurement of outcomes in the care of the client with eating disorders.

The client:

■ Has achieved and maintained at least 80 percent of expected body weight.

■ Has vital signs, blood pressure, and laboratory serum studies within normal limits.

■ Verbalizes importance of adequate nutrition.

■ Verbalizes knowledge regarding consequences of fluid loss caused by self-induced vomiting (or laxative/diuretic abuse) and importance of adequate fluid intake.

■ Verbalizes events that precipitate anxiety and demonstrates techniques for its reduction.

■ Verbalizes ways in which he or she may gain more control of the environment and thereby reduce feelings of helplessness.

■ Expresses interest in welfare of others and less preoccupation with own appearance.

■ Verbalizes that image of body as "fat" was misperception and demonstrates ability to take control of own life without resorting to maladaptive eating behaviors (anorexia nervosa).

■ Has established a healthy pattern of eating for weight control, and weight loss toward a desired goal is progressing.

■ Verbalizes plans for future maintenance of weight control.

Planning/Implementation

In most instances, individuals with eating disorders are treated on an outpatient basis, but in some cases hospitalization becomes necessary. Reasons for hospitalization include the following: malnutrition (less than 85% of expected body weight), dehydration, severe electrolyte imbalance, cardiac arrhythmia, severe bradycardia, hypothermia, hypotension, suicidal ideation, or uncooperative outpatient treatment (Yager et al., 2006).

The following section presents a group of selected nursing diagnoses, with short- and long-term goals and nursing interventions for each.

Imbalanced Nutrition: Less Than Body Requirements/Deficient Fluid Volume (Risk for or Actual)

Imbalanced nutrition: less than body requirements is defined as "intake of nutrients insufficient to meet metabolic needs" (NANDA International [NANDA-I], 2009, p. 74). *Deficient fluid volume* is defined as "decreased intravascular, interstitial, and/or intracellular fluid" (NANDA-I, 2009, p. 84). Table 32-3 presents this nursing diagnosis in care plan format.

Table 32-3 CARE PLAN FOR CLIENT WITH EATING DISORDERS: ANOREXIA NERVOSA AND BULIMIA NERVOSA

NURSING DIAGNOSES: IMBALANCED NUTRITION: LESS THAN BODY REQUIREMENTS DEFICIENT FLUID VOLUME (RISK FOR OR ACTUAL)

RELATED TO: Refusal to eat/drink; self-induced vomiting; abuse of laxatives/diuretics
EVIDENCED BY: Loss of weight; poor muscle tone and skin turgor; lanugo; bradycardia; hypotension; cardiac arrhythmias; pale, dry mucous membranes

OUTCOME CRITERIA	NURSING INTERVENTIONS	RATIONALE
Short-Term Goals • Client will gain ____ pounds per week (amount to be established by client, nurse, and dietitian) • Client will drink 125 mL of fluid each hour during waking hours. **Long-Term Goal** • By time of discharge from treatment, client will exhibit no signs or symptoms of malnutrition or dehydration.	1. Dietitian will determine number of calories required to provide adequate nutrition and realistic weight gain.	1. Adequate calories are required to allow a weight gain of 2–3 pounds per week.
	2. Explain to the client that privileges and restrictions will be based on compliance with treatment and direct weight gain. Do not focus on food and eating.	2. The real issues have little to do with food or eating patterns. Focus on the control issues that have precipitated these behaviors.
	3. Weigh client daily, immediately upon arising and following first voiding. Always use same scale, if possible. Keep strict record of intake and output. Assess skin turgor and integrity regularly. Assess moistness and color of oral mucous membranes.	3. These assessments are important measurements of nutritional status and provide guidelines for treatment.
	4. Stay with client during established time for meals (usually 30 minutes) and for at least 1 hour following meals.	4. Lengthy mealtimes put excessive focus on food and eating and provide client with attention and reinforcement. The hour following meals may be used to discard food stashed from tray or to engage in self-induced vomiting.
	5. If weight loss occurs, enforce restrictions. Client must understand that if nutritional status deteriorates, tube feedings will be initiated. This is implemented in a matter-of-fact, nonpunitive way.	5. Restrictions and limits must be established and carried out consistently to avoid power struggles, to encourage client compliance with therapy, and to ensure client safety.
	6. Encourage the client to explore and identify the true feelings and fears that contribute to maladaptive eating behaviors.	6. Emotional issues must be resolved if these maladaptive responses are to be eliminated.

Client Goals

Outcome criteria include short- and long-term goals. Timelines are individually determined.

Short-Term Goals

■ The client will gain ___ pounds per week (amount to be established by client, nurse, and dietitian).

■ The client will drink 125 mL of fluid each hour during waking hours.

Long-Term Goal

■ By time of discharge from treatment, the client will exhibit no signs or symptoms of malnutrition or dehydration.

Interventions

■ For the client who is emaciated and is unable or unwilling to maintain an adequate oral intake, the physician may order a liquid diet to be administered via nasogastric tube. Without adequate nutrition, a life-threatening situation exists. Nursing care of the individual receiving tube feedings should be administered according to established hospital procedures.

■ For the client who is able and willing to consume an oral diet, the dietitian should determine the appropriate number of calories required to provide adequate nutrition and realistic (according to body structure and height) weight gain.

■ Explain the program of behavior modification to client and family. Explain that privileges and restrictions will be based on compliance with treatment and direct weight gain.

■ Do not focus on food and eating specifically. Instead, focus on the emotional issues that have precipitated these behaviors.

■ Do not discuss food or eating with the client once protocol has been established. Do, however, offer support and positive reinforcement for obvious improvements in eating behaviors.

■ Keep a strict record of intake and output. Weigh the client daily immediately on arising and following first voiding. Always use the same scale, if possible.

■ Assess skin turgor and integrity regularly. Assess moistness and color of oral mucous membranes. The condition of the skin and mucous membranes provides valuable data regarding client hydration. Discourage the client from bathing every day if the skin is very dry.

■ Sit with the client during mealtimes for support and to observe the amount ingested. A limit (usually 30 minutes) should be imposed on time allotted for meals. Without a time limit, meals can become lengthy, drawn-out sessions, providing the client with attention based on food and eating.

■ The client should be observed for at least 1 hour following meals. The client may use this time to discard food that has been stashed from the food tray or to engage in self-induced vomiting. He or she may need to be accompanied to the bathroom if self-induced vomiting is suspected.

■ If weight loss occurs, enforce restrictions. Restrictions and limits must be established and carried out consistently to avoid power struggles and to encourage client compliance with therapy.

■ Ensure that the client and family understand that, if nutritional status deteriorates, tube feedings will be initiated. This is implemented in a matter-of-fact, nonpunitive way, for the client's safety and protection from a life-threatening condition.

■ Encourage the client to explore and identify the true feelings and fears that contribute to maladaptive eating behaviors. Emotional issues must be resolved if these maladaptive responses are to be eliminated.

Ineffective Denial

Ineffective denial is defined as a "conscious or unconscious attempt to disavow the knowledge or meaning of an event to reduce anxiety/fear, but leading to the detriment of health" (NANDA-I, 2009, p. 259).

Client Goals

Outcome criteria include short- and long-term goals. Timelines are individually determined.

Short-Term Goal

■ The client will verbalize understanding of the correlation between emotional issues and maladaptive eating behaviors (within time deemed appropriate for individual client).

Long-Term Goal

■ By discharge from treatment, the client will demonstrate the ability to discontinue use of maladaptive eating behaviors and to cope with emotional issues in a more adaptive manner.

Interventions

■ Establish a trusting relationship with the client by being honest, accepting, and available, and by keeping all promises. Convey unconditional positive regard.

■ Acknowledge the client's anger at feelings of loss of control brought about by the established eating regimen associated with the program of behavior modification.

■ Avoid arguing or bargaining with the client who is resistant to treatment. State matter-of-factly which behaviors are unacceptable and how privileges will be restricted for noncompliance. It is essential that all staff members are consistent with this intervention.

■ Encourage the client to verbalize feelings regarding his or her role within the family and issues related to dependence/independence, the intense need for achievement, and sexuality. Help the client recognize how maladaptive eating behaviors may be related to these emotional issues. Discuss ways in which he or she can gain control over these problematic areas of life without resorting to maladaptive eating behaviors.

Imbalanced Nutrition: More Than Body Requirements

Imbalanced nutrition: more than body requirements is defined as "intake of nutrients that exceeds metabolic needs" (NANDA-I, 2009, p. 75).

Client Goals

Outcome criteria include short- and long-term goals. Timelines are individually determined.

Short-Term Goal

■ Client will verbalize understanding of what must be done to lose weight.

Long-Term Goal

■ Client will demonstrate a change in eating patterns that results in a steady weight loss.

Interventions

■ Encourage the client to keep a diary of food intake. A food diary provides the opportunity for the client to gain a realistic picture of the amount of food ingested and provides a database on which to tailor the dietary program.

■ Discuss feelings and emotions associated with eating. This helps to identify when the client is eating to satisfy an emotional need rather than a physiological one.

■ With input from the client, formulate an eating plan that includes food from the required food groups with emphasis on low-fat intake. It is helpful to keep the plan as similar to the client's usual eating pattern as possible. The diet must eliminate calories while maintaining adequate nutrition. The client is more likely to stay on the eating plan if he or she is able to participate in its creation and it deviates as little as possible from usual types of foods.

■ Identify realistic incremental goals for weekly weight loss. Reasonable weight loss (1 to 2 pounds per week) results in more lasting effects. Excessive, rapid weight loss may result in fatigue and irritability and ultimately lead to failure in meeting goals for weight loss. Motivation is more easily sustained by meeting "stair-step" goals.

■ Plan a progressive exercise program tailored to individual goals and choice. Exercise may enhance weight loss by burning calories and reducing appetite, increasing energy, toning muscles, and enhancing sense of well-being and accomplishment. Walking is an excellent choice for overweight individuals.

■ Discuss the probability of reaching plateaus when weight remains stable for extended periods. The client should know this is likely to happen as changes in metabolism occur. Plateaus cause frustration, and the client may need additional support during these times to remain on the weight-loss program.

■ Provide instruction about medications to assist with weight loss if ordered by the physician. Appetite-suppressant drugs (e.g., phentermine) and others that have weight loss as a side effect (e.g., fluoxetine; topiramate) may be helpful to someone who is severely overweight. They should be used for this purpose for only a short period while the individual attempts to adjust to the new pattern of eating.

Disturbed Body Image/Low Self-esteem

Disturbed body image is defined as "confusion in mental picture of one's physical self" (NANDA-I, 2009, p. 197). *Low self-esteem* is defined as "negative self-evaluating/feelings about self or self-capabilities" (NANDA-I, 2009, p. 194).

Client Goals (for the Client With Anorexia Nervosa or Bulimia Nervosa)

Outcome criteria include short- and long-term goals. Timelines are individually determined.

Short-Term Goal

■ The client will verbally acknowledge misperception of body image as "fat" within specified time (depending on severity and chronicity of condition).

Long-Term Goal

■ By the time of discharge from treatment, client will demonstrate an increase in self-esteem as manifested by verbalizing positive aspects of self and exhibiting less preoccupation with own appearance as a more realistic body image is developed.

Client Goals (for the Client With Obesity)

Outcome criteria include short- and long-term goals. Timelines are individually determined.

Short-Term Goal

■ The client will begin to accept self based on self-attributes rather than on appearance.

Long-Term Goal

■ The client will pursue loss of weight as desired.

Interventions

For the client with anorexia nervosa or bulimia nervosa:

■ Help the client to develop a realistic perception of body image and relationship with food. Compare specific measurement of the client's body with the client's perceived calculations. There may be a large discrepancy between the actual body size and the client's perception of his or her body size. The client needs to recognize that the misperception of body image is unhealthy and that maintaining control through maladaptive eating behaviors is dangerous—even life threatening.

■ Promote feelings of control within the environment through participation and independent decision making. Through positive feedback, help the client learn to accept self as is, including weaknesses as well as strengths. The client must come to understand that he or she is a capable, autonomous individual who can perform outside the family unit and who is not expected to be perfect. Control of his or her life must be achieved in other ways besides dieting and weight loss.

■ Help the client realize that perfection is unrealistic, and explore this need with him or her. As the client begins to feel better about self, identifies positive self-attributes, and develops the ability to accept certain personal inadequacies, the need for unrealistic achievement should diminish.

For the client with obesity:

■ Assess the client's feelings and attitudes about being obese. Obesity and compulsive eating behaviors may have deep-rooted psychological implications, such as compensation for lack of love and nurturing or a defense against intimacy.

■ Ensure that the client has privacy during self-care activities. The obese individual may be sensitive or self-conscious about his or her body.

■ Have the client recall coping patterns related to food in family of origin, and explore how these may affect current situation. Parents are role models for their children. Maladaptive eating behaviors are learned within the family system and are supported through positive reinforcement. Food may be substituted by the parent for affection and love, and eating is associated with a feeling of satisfaction, becoming the primary defense.

■ Determine the client's motivation for weight loss and set goals. The individual may harbor repressed feelings of hostility, which may be expressed inwardly on the self. Because of a poor self-concept, the person often has difficulty with relationships. When the motivation is to lose weight for someone else, successful weight loss is less likely to occur.

■ Help the client identify positive self-attributes. Focus on strengths and past accomplishments unrelated to physical appearance. It is important that self-esteem not be tied solely to size of the body. The client needs to recognize that obesity need not interfere with positive feelings regarding self-concept and self-worth.

■ Refer the client to a support or therapy group. Support groups can provide companionship, increase motivation, decrease loneliness and social ostracism, and give practical solutions to common problems. Group therapy can be helpful in dealing with underlying psychological concerns.

Concept Care Mapping

The concept map care plan is an innovative approach to planning and organizing nursing care (see Chapter 9). It is a diagrammatic teaching and learning strategy that allows visualization of interrelationships between medical diagnoses, nursing diagnoses, assessment data, and treatments. Examples of concept map care plans for clients with eating disorders are presented in Figures 32–2 and 32–3.

Client/Family Education

The role of client teacher is important in the psychiatric area, as it is in all areas of nursing. A list of topics for client/family education relevant to eating

Clinical Vignette: Alice, age 18, graduated from high school 6 months ago. She is 5'10" tall, and had frequently been teased by her peers because of her height. She lived in a rural community and was often ridiculed when she made statements that she planned to become a model after graduation. But Alice was determined, and instead of going to college, she moved to New York City to pursue her dream. However, at the first modeling agency, she was told that she would never be accepted for modeling at her weight (140 pounds), and to come back when she had lost at least 15 pounds. She was devastated, but steadfast in her determination to succeed. She cut her calories to 500 a day, exercised relentlessly, took over-the-counter laxatives and diuretics, and engaged in self-induced vomiting when she ate more than she felt she should. She became weak and chronically fatigued, but persisted, until yesterday when she collapsed at the gym and the owner called 911. She was admitted to the psychiatric unit weighing 118 pounds, with poor skin turgor, blood pressure 75/45, pulse 60 and irregular. She tells the nurse, "I can't be a model unless I get thin! Everyone at home will think I'm a failure!" The nurse develops the following concept map care plan for Alice.

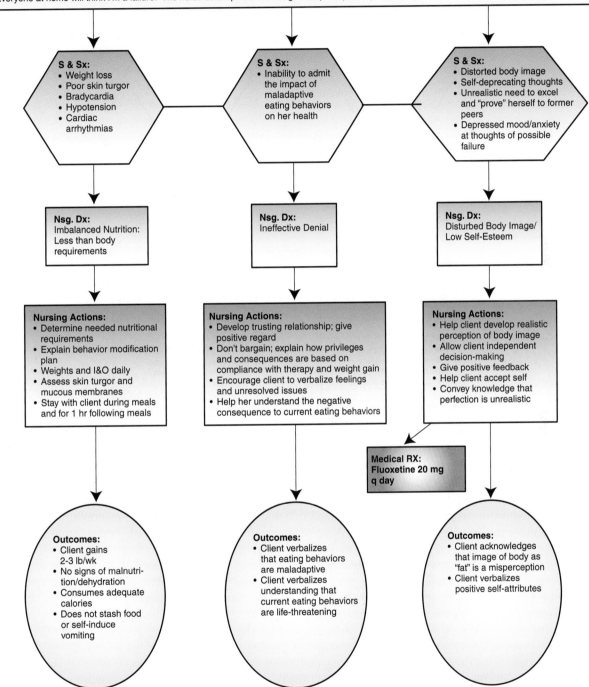

S & Sx:
- Weight loss
- Poor skin turgor
- Bradycardia
- Hypotension
- Cardiac arrhythmias

S & Sx:
- Inability to admit the impact of maladaptive eating behaviors on her health

S & Sx:
- Distorted body image
- Self-deprecating thoughts
- Unrealistic need to excel and "prove" herself to former peers
- Depressed mood/anxiety at thoughts of possible failure

Nsg. Dx:
Imbalanced Nutrition: Less than body requirements

Nsg. Dx:
Ineffective Denial

Nsg. Dx:
Disturbed Body Image/ Low Self-Esteem

Nursing Actions:
- Determine needed nutritional requirements
- Explain behavior modification plan
- Weights and I&O daily
- Assess skin turgor and mucous membranes
- Stay with client during meals and for 1 hr following meals

Nursing Actions:
- Develop trusting relationship; give positive regard
- Don't bargain; explain how privileges and consequences are based on compliance with therapy and weight gain
- Encourage client to verbalize feelings and unresolved issues
- Help her understand the negative consequence to current eating behaviors

Nursing Actions:
- Help client develop realistic perception of body image
- Allow client independent decision-making
- Give positive feedback
- Help client accept self
- Convey knowledge that perfection is unrealistic

Medical RX:
Fluoxetine 20 mg q day

Outcomes:
- Client gains 2-3 lb/wk
- No signs of malnutrition/dehydration
- Consumes adequate calories
- Does not stash food or self-induce vomiting

Outcomes:
- Client verbalizes that eating behaviors are maladaptive
- Client verbalizes understanding that current eating behaviors are life-threatening

Outcomes:
- Client acknowledges that image of body as "fat" is a misperception
- Client verbalizes positive self-attributes

FIGURE 32–2   Concept map care plan for a client with anorexia nervosa.

Clinical Vignette: Harriet, age 20, has been overweight since childhood. Her mother and sister were both of normal weight, but her mother always said, "Harriet took after her dad's side of the family." Through her teens, she tried innumerable times to lose weight, only to lose a few pounds and then gain back more. In college, out from under the watchful eye of her mother, she has gained even more weight. She has never had a date. Her sister is engaged to be married in 6 months and has asked Harriet to be the Maid of Honor. Harriet has come to the university student health center to seek assistance with weight loss. She is 5'4" tall and weighs 204 pounds. She tells the nurse, "I hate the way I look. I can't be in my sister's wedding looking like this!" The nurse develops the following concept map care plan for Harriet.

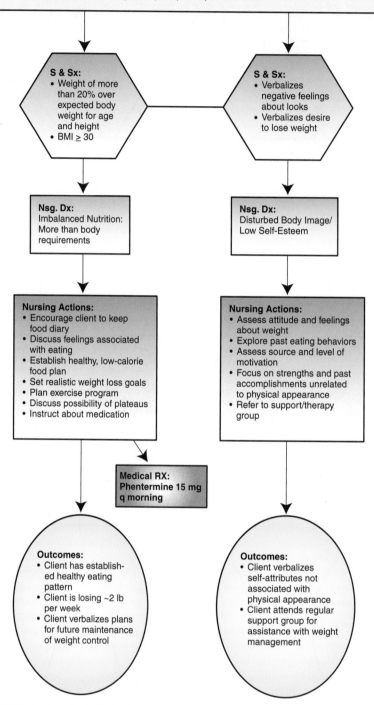

FIGURE 32–3 Concept map care plan for a client with obesity.

disorders is presented in Box 32-4. Sample client teaching guides are presented in Appendix G.

Evaluation

Evaluation of the client with an eating disorder requires a reassessment of the behaviors for which the client sought treatment. Behavioral change will be required on the part of both the client and family members. The following types of questions may provide assistance in gathering data required for evaluating whether the nursing interventions have been effective in achieving the goals of therapy.

BOX 32-4 Topics for Client/Family Education Related to Eating Disorders

NATURE OF THE ILLNESS
1. Symptoms of anorexia nervosa
2. Symptoms of bulimia nervosa
3. What constitutes obesity
4. Causes of eating disorders
5. Effects of the illness or condition on the body

MANAGEMENT OF THE ILLNESS
1. Principles of nutrition (foods for maintenance of wellness)
2. Ways client may feel in control of life (aside from eating)
3. Importance of expressing fears and feelings, rather than holding them inside
4. Alternative coping strategies (to maladaptive eating behaviors)
5. For the obese client:
   a. How to plan a reduced-calorie, nutritious diet
   b. How to read food content labels
   c. How to establish a realistic weight loss plan
   d. How to establish a planned program of physical activity
6. Correct administration of prescribed medications (e.g., antidepressants, anorexiants)
7. Indication for and side effects of prescribed medications
8. Relaxation techniques
9. Problem-solving skills

SUPPORT SERVICES
1. Weight Watchers International
2. Overeaters Anonymous
3. National Association of Anorexia Nervosa and Associated Disorders (ANAD)

   P.O. Box 640

   Naperville, IL 60566

   (630) 577-1330

   http://www.anad.org/

4. National Eating Disorders Association

   603 Stewart Street, Suite 803

   Seattle, WA 98101

   1-800-931-2237

   http://www.nationaleatingdisorders.org/

For the Client With Anorexia Nervosa or Bulimia Nervosa:

■ Has the client steadily gained 2 to 3 pounds per week to at least 80 percent of body weight for age and size?

■ Is the client free of signs and symptoms of malnutrition and dehydration?

■ Does the client consume adequate calories as determined by the dietitian?

■ Have there been any attempts to stash food from the tray to discard later?

■ Have there been any attempts to self-induce vomiting?

■ Has the client admitted that a problem exists and that eating behaviors are maladaptive?

■ Have behaviors aimed at manipulating the environment been discontinued?

■ Is the client willing to discuss the real issues concerning family roles, sexuality, dependence/independence, and the need for achievement?

■ Does the client understand how he or she has used maladaptive eating behaviors in an effort to achieve a feeling of some control over life events?

■ Has the client acknowledged that perception of body image as "fat" is incorrect?

For the Client With Obesity:

■ Has the client shown a steady weight loss since starting the new eating plan?

■ Does the client verbalize a plan to help stay on the new eating plan?

■ Does the client verbalize positive self-attributes not associated with body size or appearance?

For the Client With Anorexia, Bulimia, or Obesity:

■ Has the client been able to develop a more realistic perception of body image?

■ Has the client acknowledged that past self-expectations may have been unrealistic?

■ Does the client accept self as less than perfect?

■ Has the client developed adaptive coping strategies to deal with stress without resorting to maladaptive eating behaviors?

Quality and Safety Education for Nurses (QSEN)

The Institute of Medicine (IOM), in its 2003 report, *Health Professions Education: A Bridge to Quality,* challenged faculties of medicine, nursing, and other health professions to ensure that their graduates have achieved a core set of competencies in order to meet the needs of the 21st century health-care system. These competencies include *providing patient-centered care, working in interdisciplinary teams, employing evidence-based practice, applying quality improvement,* and *utilizing informatics.* A QSEN teaching strategy is included in Box 32-5. The use of this type of activity is intended to arm the instructor and the student with guidelines for attaining the knowledge, skills, and attitudes necessary for achievement of quality and safety competencies in nursing.

Treatment Modalities

The immediate aim of treatment in eating disorders is to restore the client's nutritional status. Complications of emaciation, dehydration, and electrolyte imbalance can lead to death. Once the

---

BOX 32-5 QSEN TEACHING STRATEGY

Assignment: Using Evidence to Address Clinical Problems
Intervention With a Client Who Fears Gaining Weight (Anorexia Nervosa)

Competency Domain: Evidence-Based Practice

Learning Objectives: Student will:
• Differentiate clinical opinion from research and evidence summaries.
• Explain the role of evidence in determining the best clinical practice for intervening with clients who do not want to eat.
• Identify gaps between what is observed in the treatment setting and what has been identified as best practice.
• Discriminate between valid and invalid reasons for modifying evidence-based clinical practice based on clinical expertise or other reasons.
• Participate effectively in appropriate data collection and other research activities.
• Acknowledge own limitations in knowledge and clinical expertise before determining when to deviate from evidence-based best practices.

Strategy Overview:
1. Investigate the research related to intervening with a client who does not want to eat.
2. Identify best practices described in the literature. How were these best practices determined?
3. Compare and contrast staff intervention with best practices described in the literature.
4. Investigate staff perceptions related to intervening with a client who is refusing to eat. How have they developed these perceptions?
5. Do staff members view any problems associated with their practice versus best practice described in the literature? If so, how would they like to see the problem addressed?
6. Describe ethical issues associated with intervening with a client who does not want to eat.
7. What is your personal perception regarding the best evidence available to date related to intervening with an anorexic client? Are there situations that you can think of when you might deviate from the best practice model?
8. What questions do you have about intervening with an anorexic client that are not being addressed by current researchers?

Adapted from teaching strategy submitted by Pamela M. Ironside, Associate Professor, Indiana University School of Nursing, Indianapolis, IN. © 2009 QSEN; http://qsen.org, with permission.

physical condition is no longer life threatening, other treatment modalities may be initiated.

Behavior Modification

Efforts to change the maladaptive eating behaviors of clients with anorexia nervosa and bulimia nervosa have become the widely accepted treatment. The importance of instituting a behavior modification program with these clients is to ensure that the program does not "control" them. Issues of control are central to the etiology of these disorders, and in order for the program to be successful, the client must perceive that he or she is in control of the treatment.

Successes have been observed when the client with anorexia nervosa is allowed to contract for privileges based on weight gain. The client has input into the care plan and can clearly see what the treatment choices are. The client has control over eating, over the amount of exercise pursued, and even over whether or not to induce vomiting. Goals of therapy, along with the responsibilities of each for goal achievement, are agreed on by client and staff.

Staff and client also agree on a system of rewards and privileges that can be earned by the client, who is given ultimate control. He or she has a choice of whether or not to abide by the contract—a choice of whether or not to gain weight—a choice of whether or not to earn the desired privilege.

This method of treatment gives a great deal of autonomy to the client. It must be understood, however, that these behavior modification techniques are helpful for weight restoration only. Concomitant individual and/or family psychotherapy are required to prevent or reduce further morbidity.

Some clinicians incorporate cognitive therapy concepts along with behavior modification techniques. Cognitive therapy helps the client to confront irrational thinking and strive to modify distorted and maladaptive cognitions about body image and eating behaviors. Halmi (2008) stated, "Cognitive techniques such as cognitive restructuring and problem solving help the patient deal with distorted and overvalued beliefs about food and thinness and cope with life's stresses" (p. 981).

IMPLICATIONS OF RESEARCH FOR EVIDENCE-BASED PRACTICE

McIntosh, V. V. W., Jordan, J., Carter, F. A., Luty, S. E., McKenzie, J. M., Bulik, C. M., et al. (2005). Three psychotherapies for anorexia nervosa: A randomized, controlled trial. *American Journal of Psychiatry, 162,* 741–747.

DESCRIPTION OF THE STUDY: The objective of this study was to examine the efficacy of three types of therapies in treatment of anorexia nervosa. Fifty-six women (age range: 17 to 40 years) with anorexia nervosa were randomly assigned to one of three treatments. Two were specialized psychotherapies: cognitive-behavior therapy (CBT) and interpersonal psychotherapy (IPT). The third (the intervention) included treatment combining clinical management and supportive psychotherapy (called "nonspecific supportive clinical management"). The women participated in 20 therapy sessions over a minimum of 20 weeks. The intervention consisted of education, care, and support, fostering a therapeutic relationship that promotes adherence to treatment. Emphasis was placed on resumption of normal eating and restoration of weight. Information on weight maintenance strategies, energy requirements, and relearning to eat normally were included. Outcomes were measured on a global anorexia nervosa measure using a 4-point ordinal scale:

4 = meets full criteria for the anorexia nervosa spectrum
3 = not full anorexia nervosa, but having a number of
   features of eating disorders

2 = few features of eating disorders
1 = no significant features of eating disorders

RESULTS OF THE STUDY: Of the participants who received nonspecific supportive clinical management, 56 percent received a score of 1 or 2 on the final outcome measure, compared with 32 percent and 10 percent of those receiving CBT and IPT, respectively. The authors suggested that IPT may not have been as successful because of the lack of symptom focus and relatively long time taken to decide on the problem area. They hypothesized that CBT may have been less effective because of the large amount of psychoeducational material and extensive skills acquisition associated with this therapy, and the difficulty of anorexia clients to generate alternatives due to cognitive rigidity. These results were in direct opposition to the original hypothesis generated by the researchers in the beginning of the study.

IMPLICATIONS FOR NURSING PRACTICE: Nurses in advanced practice are usually trained to provide CBT and IPT. Often, generalist nurses do not have the theoretical background to perform these therapies. The interventions associated with nonspecific supportive clinical management are within the scope of nursing practice, and the results of this study indicate that they are superior to CBT and IPT in the treatment of anorexia nervosa. Nurses could become instrumental in establishing programs based on this type of treatment for individuals with this type of eating disorder.

Individual Therapy

Although individual psychotherapy is not the therapy of choice for eating disorders, it can be helpful when underlying psychological problems are contributing to the maladaptive behaviors. In supportive psychotherapy, the therapist encourages the client to explore unresolved conflicts and to recognize the maladaptive eating behaviors as defense mechanisms used to ease the emotional pain. The goals are to resolve the personal issues and establish more adaptive coping strategies for dealing with stressful situations.

Family Therapy

Kirkpatrick and Caldwell (2004) stated:

> Eating disorders have a profound effect on families. While these disorders can help bring families together, they always cause some level of distress. Stresses can cause a breakdown of the whole family unit if there isn't some form of intervention. Family therapy aims at finding solutions to help the healing process for everyone in the family. (pp. 159–160)

In many instances, eating disorders may be considered *family* disorders, and resolution cannot be achieved until dynamics within the family have improved. Family therapy deals with education of the members about the disorder's manifestations, possible etiology, and prescribed treatment. Support is given to family members as they deal with feelings of guilt associated with the perception that they may have contributed to the onset of the disorder. Support is also given as they deal with the social stigma of having a family member with emotional problems.

In some instances when the dysfunctional family dynamics are related to conflict avoidance, the family may be noncompliant with therapy, as they attempt to maintain equilibrium by keeping a member in the sick role. When this occurs, it is essential to focus on the functional operations within the family and to help them manage conflict and create change.

Referrals are made to local support groups for families of individuals with eating disorders. Resolution and growth can sometimes be achieved through interaction with others who are experiencing, or have experienced, the numerous problems of living with a family member with an eating disorder.

Psychopharmacology

There are no medications specifically indicated for eating disorders. Various medications have been prescribed for associated symptoms such as anxiety and depression. Halmi (2008) reported on success with fluoxetine (Prozac) and clomipramine (Anafranil) in clients with anorexia nervosa, and particularly those with depression or obsessive-compulsive symptoms. Cyproheptadine (Periactin), in its unlabeled use as an appetite stimulant, and the antipsychotic chlorpromazine (Thorazine) have also been used to treat this disorder in selected clients. Success has been reported in a controlled trial of olanzapine (Zyprexa) with anorexic clients (Bissada, Tasca, Barber, & Bradwejn, 2008).

Fluoxetine (Prozac) has been found to be useful in the treatment of bulimia nervosa (Schatzberg, Cole, & DeBattista, 2010). A dosage of 60 mg/day (triple the usual antidepressant dosage) was found to be most effective with bulimic clients. It is possible that fluoxetine, a selective serotonin reuptake inhibitor, may decrease the craving for carbohydrates, thereby decreasing the incidence of binge eating, which is often associated with consumption of large amounts of carbohydrates. Other antidepressants, such as imipramine (Tofranil), desipramine (Norpramine), amitriptyline (Elavil), nortriptyline (Aventyl), and phenelzine (Nardil), also have been shown to be effective in controlled treatment studies (Halmi, 2008).

One study was conducted with topiramate (Topamax), a novel anticonvulsant, in the long-term treatment of binge-eating disorder with obesity (McElroy et al., 2007). Dosage was titrated to 400 mg/day (or the maximum tolerated dose). Participants experienced a significant decline in mean weekly binge frequency and significant reduction in body weight. Nickel and associates (2005) also reported effective results with topiramate in clients with bulimia nervosa. Episodes of bingeing and purging were decreased. Clients lost weight and reported a significant improvement in health-related quality of life when compared with the placebo group.

Fluoxetine has been successful in treating clients who are overweight, possibly for the same reason that was explained for clients with bulimia. The effective dosage for promoting weight loss is 60 mg/day. Regarding the use of anorexiants, Sadock and Sadock (2007) stated:

> Sympathomimetics are used in the treatment of obesity because of their anorexia-inducing effects. Because tolerance develops for the anorectic effects and because of the drugs' high abuse potential, their use for this indication is limited. (p. 1100)

Withdrawal from **anorexiants** may result in a rebound weight gain and, in some clients, a concomitant lethargy and depression. Two anorexiants that were once widely used, fenfluramine and dexfenfluramine, have been removed from the market because of their association with serious heart and lung disease. Other anorexiants currently on the market include phentermine, diethylpropion, benzphetamine, and phendimetrazine. All are indicated only for short-term weight loss.

A medication for treating obesity, called sibutramine (Meridia), was approved by the U.S. Food and Drug Administration (FDA) in 1998. It was indicated only for individuals who had a significant amount of weight to lose. The mechanism of action in the control of appetite appears to occur by inhibiting the neurotransmitters serotonin and norepinephrine. Some concern was expressed about possible cardiovascular disease associated with the use of sibutramine, and several deaths have been associated with its use by high-risk clients. Based on pressure from the FDA (2010), the manufacturer issued a recall of the drug in October 2010.

CASE STUDY AND SAMPLE CARE PLAN

NURSING HISTORY AND ASSESSMENT

When Connie fainted in history class, she was taken to the university health center by her roommate, Nan. Nan told the nurse that Connie had been taking a lot of over-the-counter laxatives and diuretics. She also said that Connie often self-induced vomiting when she felt that she had eaten too much. After an initial physical assessment, the nurse in the university health center referred Connie to the mental health clinic.

At the mental health clinic, Connie weighed 110 lbs, and measured 5'6" tall. She admitted to the psychiatric nurse, Kathy, that she tried to keep her weight down by dieting, but sometimes she got so hungry that she would overeat, and then she felt the need to self-induce vomiting to get rid of the calories. "I really don't like doing it, but lots of the girls do. In fact, that is where I got the idea. I always thought I was too fat in high school, but the competition wasn't so great there. Here all the girls are so pretty...and so thin!! It's the only way I can keep my weight down!!"

Connie admitted to Kathy that she hoards food in her dorm room and that she eats when she is feeling particularly anxious and depressed (often during the night). She admitted to having eaten several bags of potato chips and whole packages of cookies in a single sitting. She sometimes drives to the local hamburger stand in the middle of the night, orders several hamburgers, fries, and milkshakes, and consumes them as she sits in her car alone. She stated that she feels so much better while she is eating these foods, but then feels panicky after they have been consumed. That is when she self-induces vomiting. "Then I feel more depressed, and the only thing that helps is eating! I feel so out of control!"

NURSING DIAGNOSES/OUTCOME IDENTIFICATION

From the assessment data, the nurse develops the following nursing diagnosis for Connie:
Ineffective coping related to feelings of helplessness, low self-esteem, and lack of control in life situation.

■ **Short-Term Goal:** Client will identify and discuss fears and anxieties with the nurse.

■ **Long-Term Goal:** Client will identify adaptive coping strategies that can be realistically incorporated into her lifestyle, thereby eliminating binging and purging in response to anxiety.

PLANNING/IMPLEMENTATION

Ineffective Coping

The following nursing interventions have been identified for Connie.

1. Establish a trusting relationship with Connie. Be honest and accepting. Show unconditional positive regard.

2. Help Connie identify the situations that produce anxiety and discuss how she coped with these situations before she began binging and purging.

3. Help Connie identify the emotions that precipitate binging (e.g., fear, boredom, anger, loneliness).

4. Once these high-risk situations have been identified, help her identify alternate behaviors, such as exercise, a hobby, or a warm bath.

5. Encourage Connie to express feelings that have been suppressed because they were considered unacceptable. Help her identify healthier ways to express those feelings.

6. Use role-play with Connie to deal with feelings and experiment with new behaviors.

Continued

CASE STUDY AND SAMPLE CARE PLAN— cont'd

7. Explore the dynamics of Connie's family. Intrafamilial conflicts reinforce maladaptive eating behaviors.

8. Teach the concepts of good nutrition, and the importance of healthy eating patterns in overall wellness.

9. Consult with the physician about a prescription for fluoxetine for Connie.

10. Help Connie find a support group for individuals with eating disorders. Encourage regular attendance in this group.

EVALUATION

The outcome criteria for Connie have been met. She discussed with the nurse the feelings that triggered binging episodes and the situations that precipitated those feelings. She has joined a support group of individuals with eating disorders and now has a "buddy" that she may call (even in the middle of the night) when she is feeling like binging. She has started riding her bicycle regularly and goes to the fitness center when she is feeling especially anxious. She still sees the mental health nurse weekly and continues to discuss her fears and anxieties. The urges to binge at stressful times have not disappeared completely. However, they have decreased in frequency, and Connie is now able to choose more adaptive strategies for dealing with stress.

Summary and Key Points

- The incidence of eating disorders has continued to increase over the past 30 years.

- Individuals with anorexia nervosa, a disorder that is characterized by a morbid fear of obesity and a gross distortion of body image, literally can starve themselves to death.

- The individual with anorexia nervosa believes he or she is fat even when emaciated. The disorder is commonly accompanied by depression and anxiety.

- Bulimia nervosa is an eating disorder characterized by the consumption of huge amounts of food, usually in a short period of time, and often in secret.

- With bulimia nervosa, tension is relieved and pleasure felt during the time of the binge, but this is soon followed by feelings of guilt and depression.

- Individuals with bulimia nervosa "purge" themselves of the excessive intake with self-induced vomiting or the misuse of laxatives, diuretics, or enemas. They also are subject to mood and anxiety disorders.

- Compulsive eating can result in obesity, which is defined by the National Institutes of Health as a body mass index (BMI) of 30.

- Obesity predisposes the individual to many health concerns, and at the morbid level (a BMI of 40), the weight alone can contribute to increases in morbidity and mortality.

- Predisposing factors to eating disorders include genetics, physiological factors, family dynamics, and environmental and lifestyle factors.

- Treatment modalities for eating disorders include behavior modification, individual psychotherapy, family therapy, and psychopharmacology.

DavisPlus. Additional info available @ davisplus.fadavis.com

Review Questions
Self-Examination/Learning Exercise

*Select the answer that is **most** appropriate for each of the following questions:*

1. Some obese individuals take amphetamines to suppress appetite and help them lose weight. Which of the following is an adverse effect associated with use of amphetamines that makes this practice undesirable?
   a. Bradycardia.
   b. Amenorrhea.
   c. Tolerance.
   d. Convulsions.

2. Psychoanalytically, the theory of obesity relates to the individual's unconscious equation of food with:
   a. Nurturance and caring.
   b. Power and control.
   c. Autonomy and emotional growth.
   d. Strength and endurance.

3. From a physiological point of view, the *most common* cause of obesity is probably:
   a. Lack of nutritional education.
   b. More calories consumed than expended.
   c. Impaired endocrine functioning.
   d. Low basal metabolic rate.

4. Nancy, age 14, has just been admitted to the psychiatric unit for anorexia nervosa. She is emaciated and refusing to eat. What is the primary nursing diagnosis for Nancy?
   a. Complicated grieving.
   b. Imbalanced nutrition: Less than body requirements.
   c. Interrupted family processes.
   d. Anxiety (severe).

5. Which of the following physical manifestations would you expect to assess in a client suffering from anorexia nervosa?
   a. Tachycardia, hypertension, hyperthermia.
   b. Bradycardia, hypertension, hyperthermia.
   c. Bradycardia, hypotension, hypothermia.
   d. Tachycardia, hypotension, hypothermia.

6. Nurse Jones is caring for a client who has been hospitalized with anorexia nervosa and is severely malnourished. The client continues to refuse to eat. What is the most appropriate response by the nurse?
   a. "You know that if you don't eat, you will die."
   b. "If you continue to refuse to take food orally, you will be fed through a nasogastric tube."
   c. "You might as well leave if you are not going to follow your therapy regimen."
   d. "You don't have to eat if you don't want to. It is your choice."

7. Which medication has been used with some success in clients with anorexia nervosa?
   a. Phentermine (Ionamin).
   b. Diazepam (Valium).
   c. Fluoxetine (Prozac).
   d. arbamazepine (Tegretol).

Continued

Review Questions—cont'd
Self-Examination/Learning Exercise

8. Jane is hospitalized on the psychiatric unit. She has a history and current diagnosis of Bulimia Nervosa. Which of the following symptoms would be congruent with Jane's diagnosis?
   a. Binging, purging, obesity, hyperkalemia.
   b. Binging, purging, normal weight, hypokalemia.
   c. Binging, laxative abuse, amenorrhea, severe weight loss.
   d. Binging, purging, severe weight loss, hyperkalemia.

9. A hospitalized client with bulimia nervosa has stopped vomiting in the hospital and tells the nurse she is afraid she is going to gain weight. Which is the most appropriate response by the nurse?
   a. "Don't worry. The dietitian will ensure you don't get too many calories in your diet."
   b. "Don't worry about your weight. We are going to work on other problems while you are in the hospital."
   c. "I understand that you are concerned about your weight, and we will talk about the importance of good nutrition; but for now I want you to tell me about your recent invitation to join the National Honor Society. That's quite an accomplishment."
   d. "You are not fat, and the staff will ensure that you do not gain weight while you are in the hospital, because we know that is important to you."

10. The binging episode is thought to involve:
    a. A release of tension, followed by feelings of depression.
    b. Feelings of fear, followed by feelings of relief.
    c. Unmet dependency needs and a way to gain attention.
    d. Feelings of euphoria, excitement, and self-gratification.

TEST YOUR CRITICAL THINKING SKILLS

Janice, a high school sophomore, wanted desperately to become a cheerleader. She practiced endlessly before tryouts, but she was not selected. A week later, her boyfriend, Roy, broke up with her to date another girl. Janice, who was 5′3″ tall and weighed 110 pounds, decided it was because she was too fat. She began to exercise at every possible moment. She skipped meals, and tried to keep her daily consumption to no more than 300 calories. She lost a great deal of weight but became very weak. She felt cold all of the time and wore sweaters in the warm weather. She collapsed during her physical education class at school and was rushed to the emergency department. On admission, she weighed 90 pounds. She was emaciated and anemic. The physician admitted her with a diagnosis of Anorexia Nervosa.

Answer the following questions about Janice:

1. What will be the *primary* consideration in her care?

2. How will treatment be directed toward helping her gain weight?

3. How will the nurse know if Janice is using self-induced vomiting to rid herself of food consumed at meals?

References

American Psychiatric Association. (2000). *Diagnostic and statistical manual of mental disorders* (4th ed.). *Text revision.* Washington, DC: American Psychiatric Publishing.

Bissada, H., Tasca, G., Barber, A. M., & Bradwejn, J. (2008). Olanzapine in the treatment of low body weight and obsessive thinking in women with anorexia nervosa: A randomized, double-blind, placebo-controlled trial. *American Journal of Psychiatry, 165,* 1281–1288.

Black, D. W., & Andreasen, N. C. (2011). *Introductory textbook of psychiatry* (5th ed.). Washington, DC: American Psychiatric Publishing.

Bulik, C. M., Sullivan, P. F., Tozzi, F., Furberg, H., Lichtenstein, P., & Pedersen, N. L. (2006). Prevalence, heritability, and prospective risk factors for anorexia nervosa. *Archives of General Psychiatry, 63,* 305–312.

Centers for Disease Control and Prevention. (2009). *Obesity and overweight for professionals: Health consequences.* Retrieved September 27, 2010, from http://www.cdc.gov/obesity/causes/health.html

Centers for Disease Control and Prevention. (2010a). *Prevalence of overweight, obesity, and extreme obesity among U.S. adults.* Retrieved September 27, 2010, from http://www.cdc.gov/NCHS/data/hestat/obesity_adult_07_08/obesity_adult_07_08.pdf

Centers for Disease Control and Prevention. (2010b). Vital signs: State-specific obesity prevalence among adults—United States, 2009. *Morbidity and Mortality Weekly Report, 59* (Early release), 1–5.

Halmi, K. A. (2008). Eating disorders: Anorexia nervosa, bulimia nervosa, and obesity. In R. E. Hales, S. C. Yudofsky, & G. O. Gabbard (Eds.), *Textbook of psychiatry* (5th ed., pp. 971–997). Washington, DC: American Psychiatric Publishing.

Kirkpatrick, J., & Caldwell, P. (2004). *Eating disorders: Everything you need to know.* Buffalo, NY: Firefly Books.

McElroy, S. L., Hudson, J. I., Capece, J. A., Beyers, K., Fisher, A. C., & Rosenthal, N. R. (2007). Topiramate for the treatment of binge-eating disorder associated with obesity: A placebo-controlled study. *Biological Psychiatry 61,* 1039–1048.

NANDA International. (2009). *Nursing diagnoses: Definitions and classification 2009–2011.* Hoboken, NJ: Wiley-Blackwell.

National Heart, Lung, and Blood Institute. (2010). *Clinical guidelines on the identification, evaluation, and treatment of overweight and obesity in adults: Body mass index tables.* Retrieved September 27, 2010, from http://www.nhlbi.nih.gov/guidelines/obesity/bmi_tbl.htm

Nickel, C., Tritt, K., Muehlbacher, M., Pedrosa, F., Mitterlehner, F. O., Kaplan, P., et al. (2005). Topiramate treatment in bulimia nervosa patients: A randomized, double-blind, placebo-controlled trial. *International Journal of Eating Disorders, 38,* 295–300.

Sadock, B. J., & Sadock, V. A. (2007). *Synopsis of psychiatry: Behavioral sciences/clinical psychiatry* (10th ed.). Philadelphia: Lippincott Williams & Wilkins.

Schatzberg, A. F., Cole, J. O., & DeBattista, C. (2010). *Manual of clinical psychopharmacology* (7th ed.). Washington, DC: American Psychiatric Publishing.

U.S. Food and Drug Administration. (2010). *Meridia (sibutramine hydrochloride): Follow-up to an early communication about an ongoing safety review.* Retrieved September 28, 2010, from http://www.fda.gov/Safety/MedWatch/SafetyInformation/SafetyAlertsforHumanMedicalProducts/ucm198221.htm

Yager, J., Devlin, M. J., Halmi, K. A., Herzog, D. B., Mitchell, J. E., Powers, P., et al. (2006). Practice guideline for the treatment of patients with eating disorders. *American Psychiatric Association practice guidelines for the treatment of psychiatric disorders, Compendium 2006.* Washington, DC: American Psychiatric Publishing.

@ INTERNET REFERENCES

- Additional information about anorexia nervosa and bulimia nervosa may be located at the following websites:
  - http://www.anad.org/
  - http://healthyminds.org/
  - http://www.nationaleatingdisorders.org/
  - http://www.mentalhealth.com/dis/p20-et01.html
  - http://www.mentalhealth.com/dis/p20-et02.html
  - http://www.nimh.nih.gov/health/publications/eating-disorders/complete-index.shtml
  - http://medlineplus.nlm.nih.gov/medlineplus/eatingdisorders.html

- Additional information about obesity may be located at the following websites:
  - http://www.shapeup.org/
  - http://www.obesity.org/
  - http://medlineplus.nlm.nih.gov/medlineplus/obesity.html
  - http://www.asbp.org/
  - http://win.niddk.nih.gov/publications/binge.htm

MOVIE CONNECTIONS

The Best Little Girl in the World (anorexia nervosa) • *Kate's Secret (bulimia nervosa)* • *For the Love of Nancy (anorexia nervosa)* • *Super Size Me (obesity)*

Adjustment and Impulse Control Disorders

KEY TERMS

adjustment disorder

Gamblers Anonymous

kleptomania

pathological gambling

pyromania

trichotillomania

OBJECTIVES

After reading this chapter, the student will be able to:

1. Discuss historical aspects and epidemiological statistics related to adjustment and impulse control disorders.
2. Describe various types of adjustment and impulse control disorders and identify symptomatology associated with each; use this information in client assessment.
3. Identify predisposing factors in the development of adjustment and impulse control disorders.
4. Formulate nursing diagnoses and goals of care for clients with adjustment and impulse control disorders.

5. Describe appropriate nursing interventions for behaviors associated with adjustment and impulse control disorders.
6. Identify topics for client and family teaching relevant to adjustment and impulse control disorders.
7. Evaluate nursing care of clients with adjustment and impulse control disorders.
8. Discuss various modalities relevant to treatment of adjustment and impulse control disorders.

HOMEWORK ASSIGNMENT
Please read the chapter and answer the following questions.

1. What neurotransmitter systems have been correlated with a predisposition to pathological gambling?
2. What is associated with the onset of an adjustment disorder?
3. What are the elements that determine one's response (and subsequent adjustment) to a stressful situation?

4. In developing a trusting relationship with an individual who has an impulse control disorder, in what basic way does the nurse show unconditional positive regard?

Although **adjustment disorder** and impulse control disorders are two separate diagnostic categories in the *Diagnostic and Statistical Manual of Mental Disorders, Fourth Edition, Text Revision* (DSM-IV-TR) (American Psychiatric Association [APA], 2000), they do share some common characteristics. It is likely that they are precipitated by a type of psychosocial stress, the severity of which may or may not directly affect the individual response. Conversely, adjustment disorders are quite common, and impulse control disorders are relatively rare.

This chapter focuses on disorders that occur in response to stressful situations with which the individual cannot cope. The behavior may include:

■ Impairment in an individual's usual social and occupational functioning

■ Compulsive acts that may be harmful to the person or others

Historical and epidemiological statistics are presented. Predisposing factors that have been implicated in the etiology of adjustment and impulse control disorders provide a framework for studying the dynamics of these pathological conditions.

An explanation of the symptomatology is presented as background knowledge for assessing the client with an adjustment or impulse control disorder. Nursing care is described in the context of the nursing process. Various medical treatment modalities are explored.

Historical and Epidemiological Factors

Historically, clients with symptoms identified by adjustment or impulse control disorders were classified as having personality disturbances. Problems with these diagnostic categories began after World War II, when, as a result of the lack of a standardized diagnostic system, psychiatrists began to experience difficulties formulating diagnoses for behaviors attributed to combat stress.

The concept of impulse disorders dates back to the 19th century and was identified by the term *instinctive monomania*. The original monomanias included alcoholism, fire setting, homicide, and kleptomania.

A number of studies have indicated that adjustment disorders are probably quite common. Sadock and Sadock (2007) reported,

> Adjustment disorders are one of the most common psychiatric diagnoses for disorders of patients hospitalized for medical and surgical problems. In one study, 5 percent of people admitted to a hospital over a 3-year period were classified as having an adjustment disorder. (p. 786)

Adjustment disorder is more common in women than in men by about 2 to 1 (APA, 2000).

The *DSM-IV-TR* (APA, 2000) identifies five specific categories of impulse control disorders: intermittent explosive disorder, **kleptomania, pathological gambling, pyromania,** and **trichotillomania.** Apparently these disorders are quite rare.

Various sources place the prevalence range at from less than 1 percent to 5 percent of the adult population, with kleptomania being at the higher end of the range. Intermittent explosive disorder, pathological gambling, and pyromania are more common among men, whereas kleptomania and trichotillomania are diagnosed more often in women (Hollander, Berlin, & Stein, 2008).

Adjustment Disorders—Application of the Nursing Process

> ### CORE CONCEPT
>
> ***Adjustment***
> The process of modifying one's behavior in changed circumstances or an altered environment in order to fulfill psychological, physiological, and social needs.

Classifications of Adjustment Disorder: Background Assessment Data

An adjustment disorder is characterized by a maladaptive reaction to an identifiable psychosocial stressor or stressors that results in the development of clinically significant emotional or behavioral symptoms (APA, 2000). The response occurred within 3 months after onset of the stressor and has persisted for no longer than 6 months. An exception to the 6 months' criterion is a situation in which the symptoms occur in response to a chronic stressor, such as a chronic, disabling physical illness.

The individual shows impairment in social and occupational functioning or exhibits symptoms that are in excess of an expected reaction to the stressor. The symptoms are expected to remit soon after the stressor is relieved, or if the stressor persists, when a new level of adaptation is achieved. The DSM-IV-TR diagnostic criteria for adjustment disorders are presented in Box 33-1.

The stressor itself can be almost anything, but an individual's response to any particular stressor cannot be predicted. If an individual is highly predisposed or vulnerable to maladaptive response, a severe form of the disorder may follow what most people would consider only a mild or moderate stressor. In contrast, a less vulnerable individual may develop only a mild form of the disorder in response to what others might consider a severe stressor.

A number of clinical presentations are associated with adjustment disorders. The following categories, identified by the *DSM-IV-TR,* are distinguished by

---

BOX 33-1 Diagnostic Criteria for Adjustment Disorders

A. The development of emotional or behavioral symptoms in response to an identifiable stressor(s) occurring within 3 months of the onset of the stressor(s).

B. These symptoms or behaviors are clinically significant as evidenced by either of the following:
  1. Marked distress that is in excess of what would be expected from exposure to the stressor.
  2. Significant impairment in social or occupational (academic) functioning.

C. The stress-related disturbance does not meet the criteria for another specific axis I disorder and is not merely an exacerbation of a preexisting axis I or axis II disorder.

D. The symptoms do not represent bereavement.

E. Once the stressor (or its consequences) has terminated, the symptoms do not persist for more than an additional 6 months.

Specify if:

Acute: If the disturbance lasts less than 6 months.

Chronic: If the disturbance lasts for 6 months or longer.

From American Psychiatric Association. (2000). *Diagnostic and statistical manual of mental disorders* (4th ed.). Text revision. Washington, DC: American Psychiatric Publishing, with permission.

---

the predominant features of the maladaptive response.

Adjustment Disorder With Anxiety

This category denotes a maladaptive response to a psychosocial stressor in which the predominant manifestation is anxiety. For example, the symptoms may reveal nervousness, worry, and jitteriness. The clinician must differentiate this diagnosis from those of anxiety disorders.

Adjustment Disorder With Depressed Mood

This category is the most commonly diagnosed adjustment disorder. The clinical presentation is one of predominant mood disturbance, although less pronounced than that of major depression. The symptoms, such as depressed mood, tearfulness, and feelings of hopelessness, exceed what is an expected or normative response to an identified psychosocial stressor.

Adjustment Disorder With Disturbance of Conduct

This category is characterized by conduct in which there is violation of the rights of others or of major age-appropriate societal norms and rules. Examples include truancy, vandalism, reckless driving, fighting, and defaulting on legal responsibilities. Differential diagnosis must be made from conduct disorder or antisocial personality disorder.

Adjustment Disorder With Mixed Disturbance of Emotions and Conduct

The predominant features of this category include emotional disturbances (e.g., anxiety or depression) as well as disturbances of conduct in which there is violation of the rights of others or of major age-appropriate societal norms and rules (e.g., truancy, vandalism, fighting).

Adjustment Disorder, Unspecified

This subtype is used when the maladaptive reaction is not consistent with any of the other categories. Manifestations may include physical complaints, social withdrawal, or work or academic inhibition, without significant depressed or anxious mood (APA, 2000).

Predisposing Factors to Adjustment Disorders

Biological Theory

Chronic disorders, such as cognitive disorders or mental retardation, are thought to impair the ability of an individual to adapt to stress, causing increased vulnerability to adjustment disorder. Sadock and Sadock (2007) suggested that genetic factors also may influence individual risks for maladaptive response to stress.

Psychosocial Theories

Some proponents of psychoanalytic theory view adjustment disorder as a maladaptive response to stress that is caused by early childhood trauma, increased dependency, and retarded ego development. Other psychoanalysts put considerable weight on the constitutional factor, or birth characteristics that contribute to the manner in which individuals respond to stress. In many instances, adjustment disorder is precipitated by a specific meaningful stressor having found a point of vulnerability in an individual of otherwise adequate ego strength.

Some studies relate a predisposition to adjustment disorder to factors such as developmental stage, timing of the stressor, and available support systems. When a stressor occurs, and the individual does not have the developmental maturity, available support systems, or adequate coping strategies to adapt, normal functioning is disrupted, resulting in psychological or somatic symptoms. The disorder also may be related to a dysfunctional grieving process. The individual may remain in the denial or anger stage, with inadequate defense mechanisms to complete the grieving process.

Transactional Model of Stress/Adaptation

Why are some individuals able to confront stressful situations adaptively and even gain strength from the experience, whereas others not only fail to cope adaptively, but may even encounter psychopathological dysfunction? The Transactional Model of Stress/Adaptation takes into consideration the interaction between the individual and the environment.

The type of stressor that one experiences may influence one's adaptation. Sudden-shock stressors occur without warning, and continuous stressors are those that an individual is exposed to over an extended period. Although many studies have been directed to individuals' responses to sudden-shock stressors, it has been found that continuous stressors were more commonly cited than sudden-shock stressors as precipitants to maladaptive functioning.

Both situational and intrapersonal factors most likely contribute to an individual's stress response. Situational factors include personal and general economic conditions; occupational and recreational opportunities; and the availability of social supports such as family, friends, neighbors, and cultural or religious support groups.

Intrapersonal factors such as constitutional vulnerability have also been implicated in the predisposition to adjustment disorder. Some studies have indicated that a child with a difficult temperament (defined as one who cries loudly and often; adapts to changes slowly; and has irregular patterns of hunger, sleep, and elimination) is at greater risk of developing a behavior disorder. Freud (1964) theorized that traumatic childhood experiences created points of fixation to which the individual, during times of stress, would be likely to regress. This might also apply to other unresolved conflicts or developmental issues. Other intrapersonal factors that might influence one's ability to adjust to a painful life change include social skills, coping strategies, the presence of psychiatric illness, degree of flexibility, and level of intelligence.

The etiology of adjustment disorder is most likely influenced by multiple factors. A graphic depiction of this theory of multiple causation is presented in Figure 33–1.

Diagnosis/Outcome Identification

Nursing diagnoses are formulated from the data gathered during the assessment phase and with background knowledge regarding predisposing factors to the disorder. Nursing diagnoses that may be used for the client with an adjustment disorder include:

- Complicated grieving related to real or perceived loss of any concept of value to the individual evidenced by interference with life functioning, developmental regression, or somatic complaints.

- Risk-prone health behavior related to change in health status requiring modification in lifestyle (e.g., chronic illness, physical disability) evidenced by inability to problem-solve or set realistic goals for the future.

NOTE: This diagnosis would be appropriate for the person with adjustment disorder if the precipitating stressor was a change in health status.

- Anxiety (moderate to severe) related to situational and/or maturational crisis evidenced by restlessness, increased helplessness, and diminished productivity.

Outcome Criteria

The following criteria may be used for measurement of outcomes in the care of the client with an adjustment disorder.

The client:

- Verbalizes acceptable behaviors associated with each stage of the grief process.

- Demonstrates a reinvestment in the environment.

- Accomplishes activities of daily living independently.

- Demonstrates ability for adequate occupational and social functioning.

- Verbalizes awareness of change in health status and the effect it will have on lifestyle.

- Solves problems and sets realistic goals for the future.

- Demonstrates ability to cope effectively with change in lifestyle.

Planning/Implementation

The following section presents a group of selected nursing diagnoses, with short- and long-term goals and nursing interventions for each.

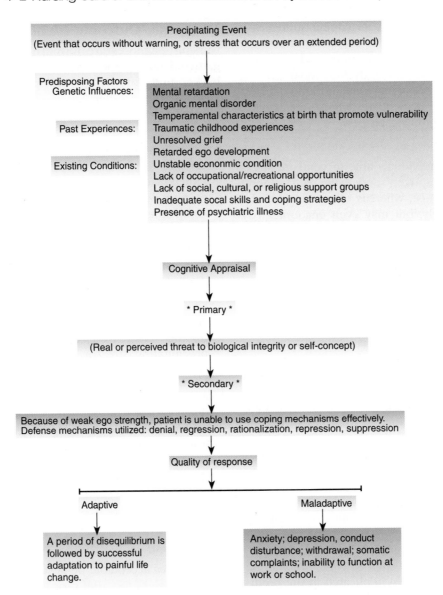

FIGURE 33–1 The dynamics of adjustment disorder using the Transactional Model of Stress/Adaptation.

Complicated Grieving

Complicated grieving is defined as "a disorder that occurs after the death of a significant other [or any other loss of significance to the individual], in which the experience of distress accompanying bereavement fails to follow normative expectations and manifests in functional impairment" (NANDA International [NANDA-I], 2009, p. 265).

Client Goals
Short-Term Goal

■ By end of 1 week, client will express anger toward lost entity.

Long-Term Goal

■ The client will be able to verbalize behaviors associated with the normal stages of grief and identify own position in grief process, while progressing at own pace toward resolution.

Interventions

■ Determine the stage of grief in which client is fixed. Identify behaviors associated with this stage. Accurate baseline assessment data are necessary to plan effective care for the grieving client.

■ Develop a trusting relationship with the client. Show empathy and caring. Be honest and keep all promises. Trust is the basis for a therapeutic relationship.

■ Convey an accepting attitude so that the client is not afraid to express feelings openly. An accepting attitude conveys to the client that you believe he or she is a worthwhile person. Trust is enhanced.

■ Allow the client to express anger. Do not become defensive if the initial expression of anger is displaced on the nurse or therapist. Help the client explore angry feelings so that they may be directed toward the intended object or person. Verbalization of feelings in a nonthreatening environment may help the client come to terms with unresolved issues.

■ Assist the client to discharge pent-up anger through participation in large-motor activities (e.g., brisk walks, jogging, physical exercises, volleyball, punching bag, exercise bike). Physical exercise provides a safe and effective method for discharging pent-up tension.

■ Explain to the client the normal stages of grief and the behaviors associated with each stage. Help the client to understand that feelings such as guilt and anger toward the lost entity/ concept are natural and acceptable during the grief process. Knowledge of the acceptability of the feelings associated with normal grieving may help to relieve some of the guilt that these responses generate.

■ Encourage the client to review his or her perception of the loss or change. With support and sensitivity, point out the reality of the situation in areas where misrepresentations are expressed. The client must give up an idealized perception and be able to accept both positive and negative aspects about the painful life change before the grief process is complete.

■ Communicate to the client that crying is acceptable. The use of touch is therapeutic and appropriate with most clients. Knowledge of cultural influences specific to the client is important before employing this technique. Touch is considered inappropriate in some cultures.

■ Help the client to solve problems as he or she attempts to determine methods for more adaptive coping with the stressor. Provide positive feedback for strategies identified and decisions made. Positive reinforcement enhances self-esteem and encourages repetition of desirable behaviors.

■ Encourage the client to reach out for spiritual support during this time in whatever form is desirable. Assess the client's spiritual needs, and assist as necessary in the fulfillment of those needs. For some individuals, spiritual support can enhance successful adaptation to painful life experiences.

Risk-Prone Health Behavior

Risk-prone health behavior is defined as "impaired ability to modify lifestyle/behaviors in a manner that improves health status" (NANDA-I, 2009, p. 247).

Client Goals
Short-Term Goals

■ The client and primary nurse will discuss the kinds of lifestyle changes that will occur because of the change in health status.

■ With the help of the primary nurse, the client will formulate a plan of action for incorporating those changes into his or her lifestyle.

■ The client will demonstrate movement toward independence, considering the change in health status.

Long-Term Goal

■ The client will demonstrate competence to function independently to his or her optimal ability, considering the change in health status, by the time of discharge from treatment.

Interventions

■ Encourage the client to talk about his or her lifestyle prior to the change in health status. Discuss coping mechanisms that were used at stressful times in the past. It is important to identify the client's strengths so that they may be used to facilitate adaptation to the change or loss that has occurred.

■ Encourage the client to discuss the change or loss and particularly to express anger associated with it. Anger is a normal stage in the grieving process and, if not released in an appropriate manner, may be turned inward on the self, leading to pathological depression.

■ Encourage the client to express fears associated with the change or loss or alteration in lifestyle that it has created. Change often creates a feeling of disequilibrium, and the individual may respond with fears that are irrational or unfounded. The client may benefit from feedback that corrects misperceptions about how life will be with the change in health status.

■ Provide assistance with activities of daily living as required, but encourage independence to the limit that the client's ability will allow. Give positive feedback for activities accomplished independently. Independent accomplishments and positive feedback enhance self-esteem and encourage repetition of desired behaviors. Successes also provide hope that adaptive functioning is possible and decrease feelings of powerlessness.

■ Help the client with decision making regarding incorporation of the change or loss into his or her lifestyle. Identify problems the change or loss is likely to create. Discuss alternative solutions, weighing potential benefits and consequences of each alternative. Support the client's decision in the selection of an alternative. The great amount of anxiety that usually accompanies a major lifestyle change often interferes with an individual's ability to solve problems and to make appropriate decisions. The client may need assistance with this process in an effort to progress toward successful adaptation.

■ Use role-play to practice stressful situations that might occur in relation to the health status change. Role-playing decreases anxiety and provides a feeling of security by providing the client with a plan of action for responding in an appropriate manner when a stressful situation occurs.

■ Ensure that the client and family are fully knowledgeable regarding the physiology of the change in health status and understand the necessity of such knowledge for optimal wellness. Encourage them to ask questions, and provide printed material explaining the change to which they may refer.

■ Ensure that the client can identify resources within the community from which he or she may seek assistance in adapting to the change in health status. Examples include self-help or support groups and a public health nurse, counselor, or social worker. Encourage the client to keep follow-up appointments with his or her physician, or to call the physician's office prior to the follow-up date if problems or concerns arise.

Concept Care Mapping

The concept map care plan is an innovative approach to planning and organizing nursing care. It is a diagrammatic teaching and learning strategy that allows visualization of interrelationships between medical diagnoses, nursing diagnoses, assessment data, and treatments. An example of a concept map care plan for a client with an adjustment disorder is presented in Figure 33–2.

Evaluation

Reassessment is conducted to determine if the nursing actions have been successful in achieving the objectives of care. Evaluation of the nursing actions for the client with adjustment disorder may be facilitated by gathering information using the following types of questions:

■ Does the client verbalize understanding of the grief process and his or her position in the process?

■ Does the client recognize his or her adaptive and maladaptive behaviors associated with the grief response?

■ Does the client demonstrate evidence of progression along the grief response?

■ Can the client accomplish activities of daily living independently?

■ Does the client demonstrate the ability to perform occupational and social activities adequately?

■ Does the client discuss the change in health status and modification of lifestyle it will effect?

■ Does the client demonstrate acceptance of the modification?

■ Can the client participate in decision making and problem solving for his or her future?

■ Does the client set realistic goals for the future?

■ Does the client demonstrate new adaptive coping strategies for dealing with the change in lifestyle?

■ Can the client verbalize available resources to whom he or she may go for support or assistance should it be necessary?

Impulse Control Disorders—Application of the Nursing Process

CORE CONCEPT

Impulsive

The urge or inclination to act without consideration of the possible consequences of one's behavior.

The *DSM-IV-TR* (APA, 2000) describes the essential features of impulse control disorders as follows:

■ Failure to resist an impulse, drive, or temptation to perform an act that is harmful to the person or others.

■ An increasing sense of tension or arousal before committing the act.

■ An experience of pleasure, gratification, or relief at the time of committing the act. Following the act, there may or may not be regret, self-reproach, or guilt.

Clinical Vignette: Hanna, age 16, has just been diagnosed with Celiac disease, and has been placed on a gluten-free diet. Deviation from this diet results in severe abdominal cramping and diarrhea. Hanna is devastated, has refused to follow the diet, and is losing considerable weight. Her mother is concerned and brings Hanna to the community mental health center for counseling. Hanna tells the nurse, "I'm not going to eat that stuff. All the kids will think I'm a freak! We go for hamburgers everyday at noon. I can't even go for pizza! It's not fair!" The nurse develops the following concept care plan for Hanna.

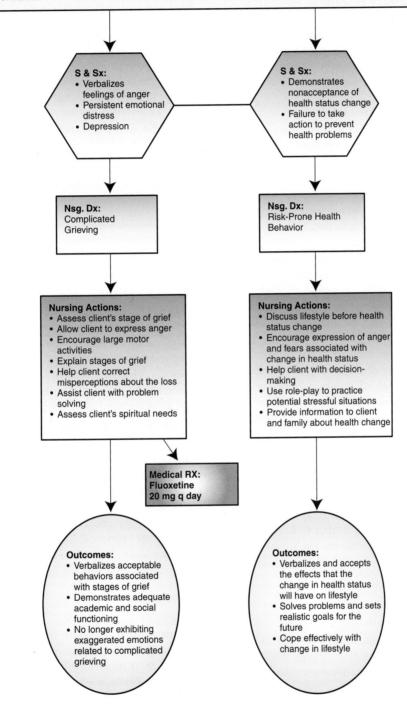

FIGURE 33–2 Concept map care plan for a client with adjustment disorder.

Individuals who suffer from impulse control disorders follow their impulses to behave in a certain manner without regard to the consequences of their behavior. They seldom know why they do what they do or why it is pleasurable. These behaviors have been likened to sexual excitement and orgasmic release. Some authors have noted that many of the behaviors have adverse or even destructive consequences for the person.

Many people with impulse control disorders function fairly well in other areas of their lives. They are merely unable to contain their behavior in the moment when tension builds, and immediate gratification prevails. Some researchers have associated other behaviors, such as substance abuse, obsessive-compulsive behaviors, and self-mutilation, with disorders of impulse control.

Background assessment data (including descriptions of symptomatology and predisposing factors) of the five categories of impulse control disorders identified by the *DSM-IV-TR* (APA, 2000) are presented in the following sections.

Intermittent Explosive Disorder

This disorder is characterized by discrete episodes of failure to resist aggressive impulses resulting in serious assaultive acts or destruction of property (APA, 2000). The individual is not normally an aggressive person between episodes, and the degree of aggressiveness expressed during the episodes is grossly out of proportion to any precipitating psychosocial stressor.

The symptoms appear suddenly, without any apparent provocation, and the violence is usually the result of an irresistible impulse to lash out. Some clients report sensorium changes, such as confusion during episodes or amnesia for events that occurred during episodes (Sadock & Sadock, 2007). Symptoms terminate abruptly, commonly lasting only minutes or at most a few hours, and are followed by feelings of genuine remorse and self-reproach about the inability to control self and the consequences of the aggressive behavior.

Symptoms of the disorder most often begin in adolescence or young adulthood and gradually disappear as the individual approaches middle age. Clients often have histories of learning disabilities, hyperkinesis, and proneness to accidents in childhood. The disorder, which is relatively rare, occurs more often in males than in females (APA, 2000). The *DSM-IV-TR* diagnostic criteria for intermittent explosive disorder are presented in Box 33-2.

Predisposing Factors to Intermittent Explosive Disorder

Biological Influences

Genetic Some studies have suggested that the disorder is more common in first-degree biological relatives of people with the disorder than in the general population. Twin studies have confirmed that the tendencies toward impulsivity and aggression are under substantial genetic influence (Hollander et al., 2008).

Physiological Any central nervous system insult may predispose an individual to the syndrome. Predisposing factors in childhood are thought to include perinatal trauma, infantile seizures, head

BOX 33-2 Diagnostic Criteria for Intermittent Explosive Disorder

A. Several discrete episodes of failure to resist aggressive impulses that result in serious assaultive acts or destruction of property.
B. The degree of aggressiveness expressed during the episodes is grossly out of proportion to any precipitating psychosocial stressors.
C. The aggressive episodes are not better accounted for by another mental disorder (e.g., antisocial personality disorder, borderline personality disorder, a psychotic disorder, a manic episode, conduct disorder, or attention-deficit/hyperactivity disorder) and are not due to the direct physiological effects of a substance (e.g., a drug of abuse, a medication) or a general medical condition (e.g., head trauma, Alzheimer's disease).

From American Psychiatric Association. (2000). Diagnostic and statistical manual of mental disorders (4th ed.). Text revision. Washington, DC: American Psychiatric Publishing, with permission.

trauma, encephalitis, minimal brain dysfunction, and hyperactivity (Sadock & Sadock, 2007). Some studies have indicated a possible role of altered levels of neurotransmitters, such as serotonin, norepinephrine, and dopamine, in the predisposition to episodic violence (Hollander et al., 2008). High concentrations of cerebrospinal fluid (CSF) testosterone in men have also been implicated.

Psychosocial Influences

Family Dynamics Individuals with intermittent explosive disorder often have strong identifications with assaultive parental figures. The typical history includes a chaotic and violent early family milieu with heavy drinking by one or both parents, parental hostility, child abuse, threats to life, and the emotional or physical unavailability of a father figure. The individual often has childhood memories of parental inconsistencies and unpredictability.

Kleptomania

The *DSM-IV-TR* describes kleptomania as "the recurrent failure to resist impulses to steal items even though the items are not needed for personal use or for their monetary value" (p. 667). The stolen items are commonly given away, discarded, covertly returned to the place where they were taken, or kept and hidden from view. The individual usually has enough money to pay for the stolen objects.

The individual with kleptomania steals purely for the sake of stealing and for the sense of relief and gratification that follows an episode. The impulsive stealing is in response to increasing tension, and even though the individual almost always knows that the act is wrong, he or she cannot resist the force of mounting tension and the pursuit of pleasure and relief that follows. Seldom is attention given to the possibility or consequences of being apprehended.

Some individuals, who most often steal without assistance or collaboration from others, may feel shame or remorse following the incident. Others never experience guilt or regret for their behavior. Symptoms of depression and anxiety have been associated with the disorder.

Onset of the disorder is usually in adolescence. It tends to be chronic, with periods of waxing and waning throughout the course of the disorder. The condition is rare but is thought to be more common among women than men. Fewer than 5 percent of arrested shoplifters give a history that is consistent with kleptomania (APA, 2000).

The *DSM-IV-TR* diagnostic criteria for kleptomania are presented in Box 33-3.

Predisposing Factors to Kleptomania

Biological Influences
As with other disorders of impulse control, brain disease and mental retardation have been associated with kleptomania (Sadock & Sadock, 2007). Disinhibition and poor impulse control have been linked with cortical atrophy in the frontal region and enlargement of the lateral ventricles of the brain.

Psychosocial Influences
Cupchik (2002), a Toronto psychologist who has studied and treated theft offenders for almost 30 years, stated that most individuals who steal compulsively do so in response to some personal crisis. He stated,

> We learned that when such essentially honest persons committed their acts of theft,

they were in most cases acting out in response to the recent occurrence of what they have perceived to be unfair, personally meaningful losses. These losses had usually either just happened, or were being anticipated. (p. 73)

In the results of two separate studies, Cupchik (2002) found that almost 75 percent of the cases could be linked to a personal crisis, such as a life-threatening diagnosis or the death of a loved one. Unresolved traumatic childhood losses (or perceived losses) also appeared to be a predisposing factor to acting out theft behaviors.

Pathological Gambling

This disorder is defined by the *DSM-IV-TR* as persistent and recurrent maladaptive gambling behavior (APA, 2000). The preoccupation with and impulse to gamble intensifies when the individual is under stress. Many impulsive gamblers describe a physical sensation of restlessness and anticipation that can only be relieved by placing a bet. Blume (2010) stated:

> In some cases the initial change in gambling behavior leading to pathological gambling begins with a "big win," bringing a rapid development of preoccupation, tolerance, and loss of control. Winning brings feelings of special status, power, and omnipotence. The gambler increasingly depends on this activity to cope with disappointments, problems, and negative emotional states, pulling away from emotional attachment to family and friends.

As the need to gamble increases, the individual is forced to obtain money by any means available. This may include borrowing money from illegal sources or pawning personal items (or items that belong to others). As gambling debts accrue, or out of a need to continue gambling, the individual may desperately resort to forgery, theft, or even embezzlement. Family relationships are disrupted, and impairment in occupational functioning may occur because of absences from work in order to gamble.

Gambling behavior usually begins in adolescence; however, compulsive behaviors rarely occur before young adulthood. The disorder generally runs a chronic course, with periods of waxing and waning, largely dependent on periods of psychosocial stress. Lifetime prevalence rates of pathological gambling range from 0.4 to 6.5 percent in adults and 2.8 to 8 percent among adolescents and college students (APA, 2000). It is more common among men than women.

BOX 33-3 Diagnostic Criteria for Kleptomania

A. Recurrent failure to resist impulses to steal objects not needed for personal use or for their monetary value.

B. Increasing sense of tension immediately before committing the theft.

C. Pleasure, gratification, or relief at the time of committing the theft.

D. The stealing is not committed to express anger or vengeance and is not in response to a delusion or a hallucination.

E. The stealing is not better accounted for by conduct disorder, a manic episode, or antisocial personality disorder.

From American Psychiatric Association. (2000). Diagnostic and statistical manual of mental disorders (4th ed.). Text revision. Washington, DC: American Psychiatric Publishing, with permission.

IMPLICATIONS OF RESEARCH FOR EVIDENCE-BASED PRACTICE

Petry, N. M., & Tawfik, Z. (2001, November). Comparison of problem-gambling and non-problem-gambling youths seeking treatment for marijuana abuse. *Journal of the American Academy of Child and Adolescent Psychiatry, 40,* 1324–1331.

DESCRIPTION OF THE STUDY: The objective of this study was to evaluate the prevalence and parallels of problem gambling in marijuana-abusing adolescents. Data were collected from 255 adolescents entering treatment for marijuana abuse in Philadelphia, PA, and Hartford, CT, between 1998 and 2000. A retrospective analysis was conducted.

RESULTS OF THE STUDY: Twenty-two percent of the 255 participants experienced gambling problems. Comparisons were made between the problem-gamblers (PGs) and the non–problem-gamblers (NPGs) with the following results. PGs were more likely than NPGs to be male, to be of African American ethnicity, and to live in single-parent homes. Other differences emerged between the two groups as well. PGs showed a greater severity of drug and alcohol use than NPGs. PGs were involved in more illegal activity and experienced a higher number of somatization and anxiety symptoms. PGs also reported more recent sexual partners and human immunodeficiency virus risk behaviors.

IMPLICATIONS FOR NURSING PRACTICE: The authors suggested that these data support the need for early identification and treatment of problem gambling in substance-abusing adolescents. This has particularly important implications for nurses who work in the area of substance abuse and addictions. Information about problem gambling should become a routine part of the nursing assessment in these areas.

Various personality traits have been attributed to pathological gamblers. Unwin, Davis, and Leeuw (2000) stated:

Evidence points to the common existence of narcissistic personality characteristics and impulse control problems in pathologic gamblers. High rates of personality disorders (e.g., obsessive-compulsive, avoidant, schizotypal and paranoid) are noted in several studies. Personality profiles of persons who are alcoholics and pathologic gamblers are also similar in some studies. Some experts view pathologic gambling as an addictive disorder, citing as evidence the tolerance and withdrawal symptoms exhibited by pathologic gamblers because of debt escalation behaviors. However, no physical or biochemical markers exist to help physicians make the diagnosis. (p. 744)

The *DSM-IV-TR* diagnostic criteria for pathological gambling are presented in Box 33-4.

BOX 33-4 Diagnostic Criteria for Pathological Gambling

A. Persistent and recurrent maladaptive gambling behavior as indicated by five (or more) of the following:
  1. Is preoccupied with gambling (e.g., preoccupied with reliving past gambling experiences, handicapping or planning the next venture, or thinking of ways to get money with which to gamble).
  2. Needs to gamble with increasing amounts of money in order to achieve the desired excitement.
  3. Has repeated unsuccessful efforts to control, cut back, or stop gambling.
  4. Is restless or irritable when attempting to cut down or stop gambling.
  5. Gambles as a way of escaping from problems or of relieving a dysphoric mood (e.g., feelings of helplessness, guilt, anxiety, depression).
  6. After losing money gambling, often returns another day to get even ("chasing" one's losses).
  7. Lies to family members, therapist, or others to conceal the extent of involvement with gambling.
  8. Has committed illegal acts such as forgery, fraud, theft, or embezzlement to finance gambling.
  9. Has jeopardized or lost a significant relationship, job, or educational or career opportunity because of gambling.
  10. Relies on others to provide money to relieve a desperate financial situation caused by gambling.
B. The gambling behavior is not better accounted for by a manic episode.

From American Psychiatric Association. (2000). Diagnostic and statistical manual of mental disorders (4th ed.). Text revision. Washington, DC: American Psychiatric Publishing, with permission.

Predisposing Factors to Pathological Gambling

Biological Influences

Genetic Familial and twin studies show an increased prevalence of pathological gambling in family members of individuals diagnosed with the disorder. The *DSM-IV-TR* reports that both pathological gambling and alcohol dependence are more common among the parents of individuals of pathological gambling than in the general population (APA, 2000).

Physiological Hollander and associates (2008) suggested a correlation between pathological gambling and abnormalities in the serotonergic, noradrenergic, and dopaminergic neurotransmitter systems. They stated,

> Serotonergic function is linked to behavioral initiation, inhibition, and aggression. Noradrenergic function mediates arousal and detects novel or aversive stimuli. Dopaminergic function is associated with reward and reinforcement mechanisms. Thus, decreased serotonin, increased norepinephrine, and increased dopamine function facilitate addictive or impulsive behavior [such as pathological gambling]. (p. 796)

Other studies have indicated alterations in the electroencephalographic patterns of pathologic gamblers (Regard, Knoch, Gutling, & Landis, 2003).

Psychosocial Influences

Sadock and Sadock (2007) reported that the following may be predisposing factors to the development of pathological gambling: "loss of a parent by death, separation, divorce, or desertion before the child is 15 years of age; inappropriate parental discipline (absence, inconsistency, or harshness); exposure to and availability of gambling activities for the adolescent; a family emphasis on material and financial symbols; and a lack of family emphasis on saving, planning, and budgeting" (p. 779).

The early psychoanalytic view attempted to explain compulsive gambling in terms of psychosexual maturation. In this theory, the gambling is compared to masturbation; both of these activities derive motive force from a buildup of tension that is released through repetitive actions or the anticipation of them. Another view suggests a masochistic component to pathological gambling and the gambler's inherent need for punishment, which is then achieved through losing (Moreyra, Ibanez, Saiz-Ruiz, Nisssenson, & Blanco, 2000).

Pyromania

Pyromania is the inability to resist the impulse to set fires. The act of starting the fire is preceded by tension or affective arousal. The individual experiences intense pleasure, gratification, or relief when setting the fires, witnessing their effects, or participating in their aftermath (APA, 2000). The sole motive for setting the fire is self-gratification, not revenge, insurance collection, or sabotage. They may take precautions to avoid apprehension; however, many individuals with pyromania are totally indifferent to the consequences of their behavior.

The onset of symptoms is usually in childhood. Many individuals with pyromania report early fascination with fire and excitement associated with firefighting equipment and activities. The disorder is relatively rare and is much more common in men than in women. Features associated with pyromania include low intelligence, learning disabilities, alcoholism, psychosexual dysfunction, chronic personal frustrations, resentment of authority figures, and the occurrence of sexual arousal secondary to fires (Sadock & Sadock, 2007).

The *DSM-IV-TR* diagnostic criteria for pyromania are presented in Box 33-5.

Predisposing Factors to Pyromania

Biological Influences

Mild mental retardation and learning disabilities have been associated with fire setting. A biochemical influence has been suggested based on evidence of significantly low cerebrospinal fluid levels of 5-hydroxyindole acetic acid (5-HIAA) and 3-methoxy-4-hydroxyphenylglycol (MHPG) found in a study of individuals with pyromania (Hollander

---

BOX 33-5 Diagnostic Criteria for Pyromania

A. Deliberate and purposeful fire setting on more than one occasion.
B. Tension or affective arousal before the act.
C. Fascination with, interest in, curiosity about, or attraction to fire and its situational contexts (e.g., paraphernalia, uses, consequences).
D. Pleasure, gratification, or relief when setting fires, or when witnessing or participating in their aftermath.
E. The fire setting is not done for monetary gain, as an expression of sociopolitical ideology, to conceal criminal activity, to express anger or vengeance, to improve one's living circumstances, in response to a delusion or hallucination, or as a result of impaired judgment (e.g., in dementia, mental retardation, substance intoxication).
F. The fire setting is not better accounted for by conduct disorder, a manic episode, or antisocial personality disorder.

From American Psychiatric Association. (2000). Diagnostic and statistical manual of mental disorders (4th ed.). Text revision. Washington, DC: American Psychiatric Publishing, with permission.

et al., 2008). The same study showed a possible hypoglycemic tendency in these individuals.

Psychosocial Influences

Three major psychoanalytic issues that have been associated with impulsive fire setting are (1) an association between fire setting and sexual gratification; (2) a feeling of impotence and powerlessness; and (3) poor social skills. This is consistent with Freud's (1964) view of fire as a symbol of sexuality. He suggested that the warmth radiated by fire can be compared to the sensation that accompanies a state of sexual excitation. Several authors have described clients who have masturbated after setting fires and describe the gratification they experience as "orgasmic." Other psychoanalytic writers have suggested that fire may symbolize activities deriving from various levels of libidinal and aggressive development. The act of fire setting is viewed as a means of relieving accumulated rage over the frustration caused by a sense of social, physical, and sexual inferiority (Sadock & Sadock, 2007).

Trichotillomania

The *DSM-IV-TR* defines this disorder as the recurrent pulling out of one's own hair that results in noticeable hair loss (APA, 2000). The impulse is preceded by an increasing sense of tension and results in a sense of release or gratification from pulling out the hair. The most common sites for hair pulling are the scalp, eyebrows, and eyelashes, but it may occur in any area of the body on which hair grows. These areas of hair loss are often found on the opposite side of the body from the dominant hand. Pain is seldom reported to accompany the hair pulling, although tingling and pruritus in the area are not uncommon.

Comorbid psychiatric disorders are common with trichotillomania. Some of these include mood disorders, eating disorders, anxiety disorders, substance abuse disorders, and personality disorders—most commonly histrionic, borderline, and obsessive-compulsive (Hollander et al., 2008).

The disorder usually begins in childhood and may be accompanied by nail biting, head banging, scratching, biting, or other acts of self-mutilation. This relatively rare phenomenon occurs more often in women than in men.

The *DSM-IV-TR* diagnostic criteria for trichotillomania are presented in Box 33-6.

Predisposing Factors to Trichotillomania

Biological Influences

Trichotillomania has commonly been associated with obsessive-compulsive disorders among first-degree relatives, leading researchers to conclude that the disorder has a possible hereditary or

---

> **BOX 33-6 Diagnostic Criteria for Trichotillomania**
>
> A. Recurrent pulling out of one's hair resulting in noticeable hair loss.
> B. An increasing sense of tension immediately before pulling out the hair or when attempting to resist the behavior.
> C. Pleasure, gratification, or relief when pulling out the hair.
> D. The disturbance is not better accounted for by another mental disorder and is not due to a general medical condition (e.g., a dermatological condition).
> E. The disturbance causes clinically significant distress or impairment in social, occupational, or other important areas of functioning.

From American Psychiatric Association. (2000). Diagnostic and statistical manual of mental disorders (4th ed.). Text revision. Washington, DC: American Psychiatric Publishing, with permission.

---

familial predisposition. Structural abnormalities in various areas of the brain, as well as alterations in the serotonin and endogenous opioid systems, have also been noted.

Psychosocial Influences

The onset of trichotillomania can be related to stressful situations in more than one quarter of cases. Additional factors that have been implicated include disturbances in mother-child relationships, fear of abandonment, and recent object loss. Studies also have shown a possible correlation between trichotillomania and a history of childhood abuse (e.g., physical, emotional, or sexual) or emotional neglect (Lochner et al., 2002).

Transactional Model of Stress/Adaptation

The etiology of impulse control disorders is most likely influenced by multiple factors. In Figure 33–3, a graphic depiction of this theory of multiple causation is presented in the Transactional Model of Stress/Adaptation.

Diagnosis/Outcome Identification

Nursing diagnoses are formulated from the data gathered during the assessment phase and with background knowledge regarding predisposing factors to the disorder. The following nursing diagnoses may be used for the client with impulse control disorder:

■ Risk for other-directed violence related to dysfunctional family system; possible genetic or physiological influences evidenced by episodes of violent, aggressive, or assaultive behavior.

■ Ineffective coping related to possible hereditary factors, physiological alterations, dysfunctional

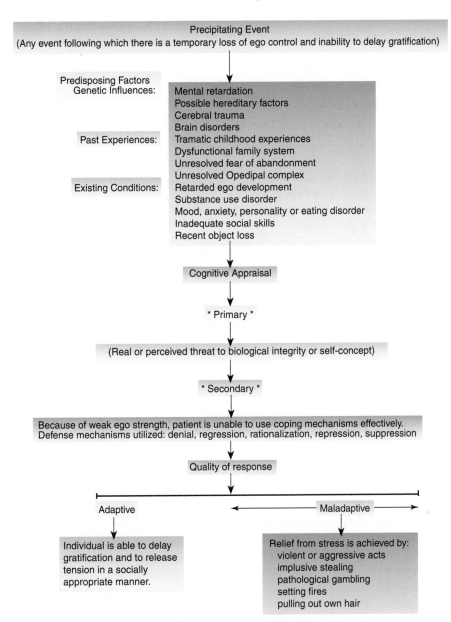

FIGURE 33–3   The dynamics of impulse control disorders using the Transactional Model of Stress/Adaptation.

family, or unresolved developmental issues evidenced by inability to control impulse to gamble, steal, set fires, or pull out own hair.

Outcome Criteria

The following criteria may be used for measurement of outcomes in the care of the client with an impulse control disorder.

The client:

■ Has not caused harm to self or others.

■ Is able to inhibit the impulse for violence and aggression.

■ Verbalizes the symptoms of increasing tension.

■ Verbalizes strategies to avoid becoming violent.

■ Verbalizes actual object at which anger is directed.

■ Continues to work on increasing frustration tolerance.

■ Verbalizes more adaptive strategies for coping with stressful situations.

■ Demonstrates the ability to delay gratification.

■ Verbalizes understanding that the behavior is unacceptable and accepts responsibility for own behavior.

Planning/Implementation

The following section presents selected nursing diagnoses, with short- and long-term goals and nursing interventions for each.

Risk for Other-Directed Violence

Risk for other-directed violence is defined as "at risk for behaviors in which an individual demonstrates that he or she can be physically, emotionally, and/or sexually harmful to others" (NANDA-I, 2009, p. 332).

Client Goals
Short-Term Goal

■ The client will recognize signs of increasing tension, anxiety, and agitation, and report to staff (or others) for assistance with intervention (time dimension to be individually determined).

Long-Term Goal

■ The client will not harm others or the property of others (time dimension to be individually determined).

Interventions

■ Convey an accepting attitude toward the client. Feelings of rejection are undoubtedly familiar to him or her. Work on the development of trust. Be honest, keep all promises, and convey the message that it is not the *person* but the *behavior* that is unacceptable. An attitude of acceptance promotes feelings of self-worth, and trust is the basis of a therapeutic relationship.

■ Maintain low level of stimuli in the client's environment (low lighting, few people, simple decor, low noise level). A stimulating environment may increase agitation and promote aggressive behavior. Make the client's environment as safe as possible by removing all potentially dangerous objects.

■ Help the client identify the true object of his or her hostility. Because of weak ego development, the client may be unable to use ego defense mechanisms correctly. Helping him or her recognize this in a nonthreatening manner may help reveal unresolved issues so that they may be confronted.

■ Staff should maintain and convey a calm attitude. Anxiety is contagious and can be transferred from staff to client. A calm attitude provides the client with a feeling of safety and security.

■ Help the client recognize the signs that tension is increasing and ways in which violence can be averted. Activities that require physical exertion are helpful in relieving pent-up tension.

■ Explain to the client that, should explosive behavior occur, staff will intervene in whatever way is required (e.g., tranquilizing medication, restraints, isolation) to protect the client and others. This conveys to the client evidence of control over the situation and provides a feeling of safety and security.

Ineffective Coping

Ineffective coping is defined as "inability to form a valid appraisal of the stressors, inadequate choices of practiced responses, and/or inability to use available resources" (NANDA-I, 2009, p. 254).

Client Goals
Short-Term Goal

■ The client will verbalize adaptive ways to cope with stress by means other than impulsive behaviors (time dimension to be individually determined).

Long-Term Goal

■ The client will be able to delay gratification and use adaptive coping strategies in response to stress (time dimension to be individually determined).

Interventions

■ Help the client gain insight into his or her behaviors. Often these individuals rationalize to such an extent that they deny that what they have done is wrong. The client must come to understand that certain behaviors will not be tolerated within the society and that severe consequences will be imposed on those individuals who refuse to comply. The client must *want* to become a productive member of society before he or she can be helped.

■ Talk about past behaviors with the client. Discuss behaviors that are acceptable by societal norms and those that are not. Help the client identify ways in which he or she has exploited others. Encourage the client to explore how he or she would feel if the circumstances were reversed. An attempt may be made to enlighten the client to the sensitivity of others by promoting self-awareness in an effort to assist the client to gain insight into his or her own behavior.

■ Throughout the relationship with the client, maintain an attitude of "It is not *you,* but your *behavior,* that is unacceptable." An attitude of acceptance promotes feelings of dignity and self-worth.

■ Work with the client to increase the ability to delay gratification. Reward desirable behaviors, and provide immediate positive feedback. This will serve to enhance self-esteem and encourage repetition of the desirable behaviors.

■ Help the client identify and practice more adaptive strategies for coping with stressful life situations. The impulse to perform the maladaptive behavior may be so great that the client is unable to see any other alternatives to relieve stress. He or she will need assistance with problem solving.

Client/Family Education

Box 33-7 provides topics for client and family education related to adjustment and impulse control disorders. Sample client teaching guides are presented in Appendix G.

Evaluation

Reassessment is conducted in order to determine if the nursing actions have been successful in achieving the objectives of care. Evaluation of the nursing actions for the client with an impulse control disorder may be facilitated by gathering information using the following types of questions:

■ Has violence, aggression, or assaultive behavior been avoided?

■ Have the client and others escaped harm?

■ Does the client verbalize understanding of the unacceptability of his or her behavior?

■ Can the client verbalize and demonstrate more adaptive strategies for coping with stress?

■ Can the client demonstrate the ability to delay gratification?

■ Can the client verbalize the symptoms of tension that precede unacceptable behavior?

■ Can the client demonstrate ways to intervene that inhibit the compulsion for maladaptive behavior when tension rises?

■ Can the client verbalize the types of stress that create the tension?

■ Can the client verbalize a plan to deal with the stress in the future without resorting to behaviors that are socially unacceptable?

Treatment Modalities

Adjustment Disorders

Various treatments are used for clients with adjustment disorder. Strain, Klipstein, and Newcorn (2008)

BOX 33-7 Topics for Client/Family Education Related to Adjustment and Impulse Control Disorders

NATURE OF THE ILLNESS

1. Define adjustment disorder
2. Describe types and symptoms of adjustment disorder
3. Describe types and symptoms of impulse control disorders
4. Discuss possible causes of the disorders

MANAGEMENT OF THE ILLNESS

1. Adjustment disorder
   a. Discuss possible need for lifestyle changes
   b. Discuss ways to identify onset of escalating anxiety
   c. Discuss problem-solving techniques
   d. Teach assertive and relaxation techniques
   e. Ways to increase feelings of control and decrease feelings of powerlessness
   f. Pharmacology: Antianxiety agents and antidepressants. If these medications are given for associated symptoms, teach client about what to expect and possible adverse effects that may occur.
2. Impulse control disorder
   a. Discuss ways to identify onset of escalating anxiety and methods to prevent maladaptive responses
   b. Discuss alternative adaptive coping strategies
   c. Teach assertive and relaxation techniques
   d. Teach ways to increase feelings of control and decrease feelings of powerlessness

e. Pharmacology: The following drugs may be prescribed for impulse control disorders. Ensure that client and family have sufficient knowledge about the medication prior to its administration.
   (1) Intermittent explosive disorder: lithium, anticonvulsants, serotonin-modulating drugs, beta blockers, antipsychotics
   (2) Kleptomania: SSRIs, tricyclic antidepressants, trazodone, lithium, valproate, and naltrexone
   (3) Pathological gambling: clomipramine, SSRIs, lithium, carbamazepine, and naltrexone
   (4) Trichotillomania: chlorpromazine, amitriptyline, lithium, SSRIs/pimozide, olanzapine

SUPPORT SERVICES

1. Support groups:

Gamblers Anonymous
P.O. Box 17173
Los Angeles, CA 90017
(213) 386-8789
www.gamblersanonymous.org/

National Council on
   Problem Gambling
730 11th Street, NW,
   Ste. 601
Washington, DC 20001
(202) 547-9204
www.ncpgambling.org/

2. Individual psychotherapy
3. Crisis intervention
4. Behavior therapy
5. Family therapy

cited the following as major goals of therapy for these individuals:

1. To relieve symptoms associated with a stressor.
2. To enhance coping with stressors that cannot be reduced or removed.
3. To establish support systems that maximize adaptation.

Individual Psychotherapy

Individual psychotherapy is the most common treatment for adjustment disorder. Individual psychotherapy allows the client to examine the stressor that is causing the problem, possibly assign personal meaning to the stressor, and confront unresolved issues that may be exacerbating this crisis. Treatment works to remove these blocks to adaptation so that normal developmental progression can resume. Techniques are used to clarify links between the current stressor and past experiences, and to assist with the development of more adaptive coping strategies.

Family Therapy

The focus of treatment is shifted from the individual to the system of relationships in which the individual is involved. The maladaptive response of the identified client is viewed as symptomatic of a dysfunctional family system. All family members are included in the therapy, and treatment serves to improve the functioning within the family network. Emphasis is placed on communication, family rules, and interaction patterns among the family members.

Behavior Therapy

The goal of behavior therapy is to replace ineffective response patterns with more adaptive ones. The situations that promote ineffective responses are identified, and carefully designed reinforcement schedules, along with role modeling and coaching, are used to alter the maladaptive response patterns. This type of treatment is very effective when implemented in an inpatient setting where the client's behavior and its consequences may be more readily controlled.

Self-Help Groups

Group experiences with or without a professional facilitator provide an arena in which members may consider and compare their responses to those of individuals with similar life experiences. Members benefit from learning that they are not alone in their painful experiences. Hope is derived from knowing that others have survived and even grown from similar experiences. Members of the group exchange advice, share coping strategies, and provide support and encouragement for each other.

Crisis Intervention

In crisis intervention, the therapist, or other intervener, becomes a part of the individual's life situation. Because of increased anxiety, the individual with adjustment disorder is unable to problem-solve, so he or she requires guidance and support from another to help mobilize the resources needed to resolve the crisis. Crisis intervention is short term, and relies heavily on orderly problem-solving techniques and structured activities that are focused on change. The ultimate goal of crisis intervention in the treatment of adjustment disorder is to resolve the immediate crisis, restore adaptive functioning, and promote personal growth.

Psychopharmacology

Adjustment disorder is not commonly treated with medications, for the following reasons: (1) their effect may be temporary and only mask the real problem, interfering with the possibility of finding a more permanent solution, and (2) psychoactive drugs carry the potential for physiological and psychological dependence.

When the client with adjustment disorder has symptoms of anxiety or depression, the physician may prescribe antianxiety or antidepressant medication. These medications are considered only adjuncts to psychotherapy and should not be given as the primary therapy. In these instances they are given to alleviate symptoms so that the individual may more effectively cope while attempting to adapt to the stressful situation.

Impulse Control Disorders

Intermittent Explosive Disorder

Individual psychotherapy with intermittent explosive disorder has not been successful. Group therapy, with its elements of group loyalty, peer pressure, expectation, and confrontation, may be more useful. Family therapy may be helpful when the client is an adolescent or young adult.

Clients with intermittent explosive disorder are commonly treated with psychopharmacological agents. A variety of agents have been tried, including mood stabilizers (e.g., lithium), anticonvulsants (e.g., carbamazepine, gabapentin, phenytoin, valproate), serotonin-modulating drugs (e.g., selective serotonin reuptake inhibitors [SSRIs], buspirone, clomipramine, trazodone), and beta blockers (e.g., propranolol). Although antipsychotics have been used for aggressive behavior, they are often problematic because of adverse side effects. Antianxiety medications, such as the benzodiazepines, may lower inhibitions and self-control, increasing the severity of the disorder. Hollander and associates

(2008) stated that recent studies identify SSRIs and mood stabilizers as first-line treatments.

Kleptomania

Insight-oriented psychodynamic psychotherapy has been successful in the treatment of kleptomania. It has been most helpful with those individuals who experience guilt and shame and are thus motivated to change their behavior.

Sadock and Sadock (2007) reported the following behavioral therapy methods as useful in the treatment of kleptomania: systematic desensitization, aversive conditioning, and a combination of aversive conditioning and altered social contingencies.

Success in the treatment of kleptomania has been achieved with some medications, including the SSRIs, tricyclic antidepressants, trazodone, lithium, and valproate. One research study reported effective results in the treatment of kleptomania with naltrexone (Grant & Kim, 2002). The authors stated:

> As the treatment progressed, many patients expressed that their struggle to resist the urges to steal and thoughts associated with stealing were reduced or abolished altogether. In addition to reducing urges, naltrexone seemed to reduce the subjective experience of pleasure if they engaged in stealing. (p. 355)

Electroconvulsive therapy has also shown to be effective in some cases.

Pathological Gambling

Because most pathological gamblers deny that they have a problem, treatment is difficult. In fact, most gamblers only seek treatment due to legal difficulties, family pressures, or other psychiatric complaints. Behavior therapy, cognitive therapy, and psychoanalysis have been used with pathological gambling, with various degrees of success (Moreyra et al., 2000).

Some medications have been used with effective results in the treatment of pathological gambling. The SSRIs and clomipramine have been used successfully in the treatment of pathological gambling as a form of obsessive-compulsive disorder (Moreyra et al., 2000). Lithium, carbamazepine, and naltrexone have also been shown to be effective.

Possibly the most effective treatment of pathological gambling is participation by the individual in **Gamblers Anonymous** (GA). This organization of inspirational group therapy is modeled after Alcoholics Anonymous. The only requirement for GA membership is an expressed desire to stop gambling. Treatment is based on peer pressure, public confession, and the availability of other reformed gamblers to help individuals resist the urge to gamble. Gam-Anon (for family and spouses of compulsive gamblers) and Gam-a-Teen (for adolescent children of compulsive gamblers) are also important sources of treatment.

Pyromania

Treatment of individuals with pyromania has been difficult because of the lack of motivation for change. Denial of problems, refusal to take responsibility for their behavior, and often the existence of alcoholism interfere with improvement in this disorder. Some behavioral treatments, such as aversive therapy and stimulus satiation, have been tried, but no single treatment has been proved effective. Franklin and associates (2002) initiated a program of prevention for pyromania. The interactive program focused on the medical, financial, legal, and societal impacts of fire-setting behavior. Results of the program showed a dramatic termination in recidivism for most of the study participants.

Trichotillomania

Behavior modification has been used to treat trichotillomania. Various techniques have been tried, including covert desensitization and habit-reversal practices. These include a system of rewards and punishment that are applied in an effort to modify the hair-pulling behaviors.

Psychodynamic intervention has been used in children with trichotillomania. Exploration is conducted into areas of parent-child relationships or other areas of potential conflict that may provide some enlightenment about the problem.

Various psychopharmacological agents, including chlorpromazine, amitriptyline, and lithium carbonate, have been tried in the treatment of trichotillomania, with moderate results. Recent success with SSRIs augmented with pimozide has been reported. One recent study showed olanzapine to be a safe and effective treatment for trichotillomania (Van Ameringen, Mancini, Patterson, Bennett, & Oakman, 2010).

Summary and Key Points

■ This chapter has focused on disorders that occur in response to stressful situations with which the individual cannot cope.

■ Behaviors associated with adjustment disorders include those that impair an individual's usual social and occupational functioning.

- Impulse control disorders involve compulsive acts that may be harmful to the person or others.

- Adjustment disorders are relatively common. In fact, some studies indicate they are the most commonly ascribed psychiatric diagnoses.

- Clinical symptoms include inability to function socially or occupationally in response to a psychosocial stressor.

- Adjustment disorder is distinguished by the predominant features of the maladaptive response. These include anxiety, depression, disturbance of conduct, and mixed disturbance of emotions and conduct.

- Of the two types of stressors discussed (i.e., sudden-shock and continuous), more individuals respond with maladaptive behaviors to long-term continuous stressors.

- Treatment modalities for adjustment disorders include individual psychotherapy, family therapy, behavior therapy, self-help groups, and psychopharmacology.

- Impulse control disorders are quite rare but involve compulsive acts that may be harmful to the individual or to others.

- Individuals with impulse control disorders experience increased tension, followed by the inability to resist committing a specific act, after which the individual feels a sense of release and gratification.

- Impulse control disorders include:
  - *Intermittent explosive disorder:* violent or aggressive behavior that culminates in serious assaultive acts or the destruction of property.
  - *Kleptomania:* inability to resist the impulse to steal.
  - *Pathological gambling:* inability to resist the impulse to gamble.
  - *Pyromania:* inability to resist the impulse to set fires.
  - *Trichotillomania:* inability to resist the impulse to pull out one's own hair.

- Treatment modalities for impulse control disorders include group therapy, family therapy, insight-oriented psychodynamic psychotherapy, behavior therapy, and various types of psychopharmacology. Electroconvulsive therapy has been used successfully with kleptomania. Gamblers Anonymous is an effective treatment for pathological gambling.

- Nursing care of individuals with adjustment and impulse control disorders is accomplished using the steps of the nursing process.

DavisPlus Additional info available @ davisplus.fadavis.com

Review Questions
Self-Examination/Learning Exercise

*Select the answer that is **most** appropriate for each of the following questions:*

1. Linda recently left her husband of 10 years. She was very dependent on her husband and is having difficulty adjusting to an independent lifestyle. She has been hospitalized with a diagnosis of Adjustment Disorder with Depressed Mood. The *priority* nursing diagnosis for Linda would be:
   a. Risk-prone health behavior related to loss of dependency.
   b. Complicated grieving related to break-up of marriage.
   c. Ineffective coping related to problems with dependency.
   d. Social isolation related to depressed mood.

2. Linda, who is depressed following the breakup of a very stormy marriage, says to the nurse, "I feel so bad. I thought I would feel better once I left, but I feel worse!" Which is the *best* response by the nurse?
   a. "Cheer up, Linda. You have a lot to be happy about."
   b. "You are grieving for the marriage you did not have. It's natural for you to feel bad."
   c. "Try not to dwell on how you feel. If you don't think about it, you'll feel better."
   d. "You did the right thing, Linda. Knowing that should make you feel better."

Review Questions—cont'd
Self-Examination/Learning Exercise

3. Linda has been hospitalized with adjustment disorder with depressed mood following the break-up of her marriage. Which of the following is true regarding the diagnosis of adjustment disorder?
   a. Linda will require long-term psychotherapy to achieve relief.
   b. Linda likely inherited a genetic tendency for the disorder.
   c. Linda's symptoms will likely remit once she has accepted the change in her life.
   d. Linda probably would not have experienced adjustment disorder if she had a higher level of intelligence.

4. The physician orders sertraline (Zoloft) for a client who is hospitalized with adjustment disorder with depressed mood. This medication is intended to:
   a. Increase energy and elevate mood.
   b. Stimulate the central nervous system.
   c. Prevent psychotic symptoms.
   d. Produce a calming effect.

5. The category of adjustment disorder with depressed mood identifies the individual who:
   a. Violates the rights of others to feel better.
   b. Expresses symptoms that reveal a high level of anxiety.
   c. Exhibits severe social isolation and withdrawal.
   d. Is experiencing a complicated grieving process.

6. Tony has been fascinated by fire for as long as he can remember. He played with matches as a child. As an adult, he has set numerous fires, always feeling exhilarated and even sexually stimulated afterward. Which of the following impulse control disorders would apply to Tony?
   a. Kleptomania.
   b. Trichotillomania.
   c. Pyromania.
   d. Intermittent explosive disorder.

7. Janet received a great deal of money and property in a divorce settlement. Shortly after the divorce, she experienced an impulse to enter a large department store and steal some inexpensive costume jewelry. Although she had been apprehended twice for shoplifting, she was indifferent to being discovered at this time. Which of the following impulse control disorders would apply to Janet?
   a. Kleptomania.
   b. Trichotillomania.
   c. Pyromania.
   d. Intermittent explosive disorder.

8. Frankie, a 16-year-old boy, had had temper tantrums since age 2. As he matured, the "tantrums" intensified, with explosions of rage, usually without identifiable provocation. He had attempted to molest his 12-year-old sister and went after his father with a butcher knife. He has an abnormal electroencephalogram. Which of the following impulse control disorders would apply to Frankie?
   a. Kleptomania.
   b. Trichotillomania.
   c. Pathological gambling.
   d. Intermittent explosive disorder.

Review Questions—cont'd
Self-Examination/Learning Exercise

9. Callie, a 10-year-old girl, has been pulling her hair out of the crown of her head for several years. She has been referred to psychiatry from the dermatology clinic. Her mother reports the hair pulling usually occurs at night when Callie is tired. Further history reveals Callie's father left her mother when Callie was 4 years old and has never been heard from since. Callie tells the psychiatrist he left because she was a bad girl. Which of the following impulse control disorders would apply to Callie?
   a. Kleptomania.
   b. Trichotillomania.
   c. Pyromania.
   d. Intermittent explosive disorder.

10. Harold has borrowed a great deal of money from an illegal source in an effort to pay back a gambling debt. He has continued to gamble so that he can pay back the loan with his winnings. Last night, the loan sharks threatened harm if he did not pay soon. He withdraws all the money from his joint account with his wife and heads for the racetrack. Which of the following impulse control disorders would apply to Harold?
   a. Pyromania.
   b. Kleptomania.
   c. Pathological gambling.
   d. Intermittent explosive disorder.

11. Which of the following interventions are appropriate for working with a client who has a diagnosis of kleptomania? (Select all that apply.)
   a. Help her to understand that she is a worthwhile person.
   b. Help her to understand that stealing will not be tolerated.
   c. Administer fluoxetine, as ordered by the physician.
   d. Place her in isolation until denial of responsibility has subsided.

12. Carol, age 16, has recently been diagnosed with diabetes mellitus. She must watch her diet and take an oral hypoglycemic medication daily. She has become very depressed, and her mother reports that Carol refuses to change her diet and often skips her medication. Carol has been hospitalized for stabilization of her blood sugar. The psychiatric nurse practitioner has been called in as a consult. Which of the following nursing diagnoses by the psychiatric nurse would be a priority for Carol at this time?
   a. Anxiety related to hospitalization evidenced by noncompliance.
   b. Low self-esteem related to feeling different from her peers evidenced by social isolation.
   c. Risk for suicide related to new diagnosis of diabetes mellitus.
   d. Risk-prone health behavior related to denial of seriousness of her illness evidenced by refusal to follow diet and take medication.

TEST YOUR CRITICAL THINKING SKILLS

Laura, age 48, underwent a mastectomy of the right breast after her mammogram revealed a lump that proved to be malignant when biopsied. Since her surgery 6 weeks ago, Laura has refused to see any of her friends. She stays in her bedroom, speaks to her husband only when he speaks first, is having difficulty sleeping, and eats very little. She refuses to look at the mastectomy scar and has refused to see the Reach to Recovery representative who has tried several times to help fit her with a prosthesis. Her husband has become very worried about her and spoke to the family doctor, who recommended a psychiatrist. She has been admitted to the psychiatric unit with a diagnosis of Adjustment Disorder with Depressed Mood.

Answer the following questions about Laura:

1. What would be the primary nursing diagnosis for Laura?
2. Describe a short-term goal and a long-term goal for Laura.
3. Discuss a priority nursing intervention in working with Laura.

References

American Psychiatric Association. (2000). *Diagnostic and statistical manual of mental disorders* (4th ed.). *Text revision.* Washington, DC: American Psychiatric Publishing.

Blume, S. G. (2010). *Pathological gambling: Recognition and intervention.* Retrieved September 29, 2010, from http://education.iupui.edu/soe/programs/graduate/counselor/readings_n_docs/reading4.pdf

Cupchik, W. (2002). *Why honest people shoplift or commit other acts of theft.* Toronto: Tagami Communications.

Franklin, G. A., Pucci, P. S., Arbabi, S., Brandt, M. M., Wahl, W. L., & Taheri, P. A. (2002). Decreased juvenile arson and firesetting recidivism after implementation of a multidisciplinary prevention program. *Journal of Trauma-Injury Infection & Critical Care, 53,* 260–266.

Grant, J. E., & Kim, S. W. (2002). An open-label study of naltrexone in the treatment of kleptomania. *Journal of Clinical Psychiatry, 63,* 349–356.

Hollander, E., Berlin, H. A., & Stein, D. J. (2008). Impulse-control disorders not elsewhere classified. In R. E. Hales, S. C. Yudofsky, & G. O. Gabbard (Eds.), *Textbook of psychiatry* (5th ed., pp. 777–820). Washington, DC: American Psychiatric Publishing.

Lochner, C., duToit, P. L., Zungu-Dirwayi, N., Marais, A., vanKradenburg, J., Curr, B., et al. (2002). Childhood trauma in obsessive-compulsive disorder, trichotillomania, and controls. *Depression and Anxiety, 15,* 66–68.

Moreyra, P., Ibanez, A., Saiz-Ruiz, J., Nissenson, K., & Blanco, C. (2000). Review of the phenomenology, etiology and treatment of pathological gambling. *German Journal of Psychiatry, 3,* 37–52.

NANDA International. (2009). *Nursing diagnoses: Definitions and classification 2009–2011.* Hoboken, NJ: Wiley-Blackwell.

Regard, M., Knoch, D., Gutling, E., & Landis, T. (2003). Brain damage and addictive behavior: A neuropsychological and electroencephalogram investigation with pathologic gamblers. *Cognitive and Behavioral Neurology, 16*(1), 47–53.

Sadock, B. J., & Sadock, V. A. (2007). *Synopsis of psychiatry: Behavioral sciences/clinical psychiatry* (10th ed.). Philadelphia: Lippincott Williams & Wilkins.

Scott, C. L., Hilty, D. M., & Brook, M. (2003). Impulse-control disorders not elsewhere classified. In R. E. Hales & S. C. Yudofsky (Eds.), *Textbook of clinical psychiatry* (4th ed., pp. 781–802). Washington, DC: American Psychiatric Publishing.

Strain, J. J., Klipstein, K. G., & Newcorn, J. H. (2008). Adjustment disorders. In R. E. Hales, S. C. Yudofsky, & G. O. Gabbard (Eds.), *Textbook of psychiatry* (5th ed., pp. 755–775). Washington, DC: American Psychiatric Publishing.

Unwin, B. K., Davis, M. K., & Leeuw, J. B. (2000). Pathologic gambling. *American Family Physician, 61,* 741–749.

Van Ameringen, M., Mancini, C., Patterson, B., Bennett, M., & Oakman, J. (2010).

A randomized, double-blind, placebo-controlled trial of olanzapine in the treatment of trichotillomania. *Journal of Clinical Psychiatry.* Epub ahead of print, April 20, 2010, doi:10.4088/JCP.09m05114gre.

Classical References

Freud, S. (1964). New introductory lectures on psychoanalysis and other works. In *The standard edition of the complete psychological works of Sigmund Freud* (Vol. 22). London: Hogarth Press.

@ INTERNET REFERENCES

- Additional information about adjustment disorder may be located at the following websites:
  - http://www.mentalhealth.com/rx/p23-aj01.html
  - http://www.findarticles.com/cf_dls/g2601/0000/2601000025/p1/article.jhtml
  - http://www.athealth.com/Consumer/disorders/Adjustment.html
  - http://www.mentalhealth.com/dis/p20-aj01.html
- Additional information about impulse control disorders may be located at the following websites:
  - http://www.ncpgambling.org/
  - http://www.gamblersanonymous.org/
  - http://www.minddisorders.com/Py-Z/Pyromania.html
  - http://www.mayoclinic.com/health/kleptomania/DS01034
  - http://www.mayoclinic.com/health/intermittent-explosive-disorder/DS00730
  - http://www.nmha.org/go/information/get-info/trichotillomania
  - http://www.healthline.com/galecontent/pyromania-1

Personality Disorders

CORE CONCEPT

personality

KEY TERMS

histrionic	passive-aggressive	schizotypal
narcissism	schizoid	splitting
object constancy		

OBJECTIVES

After reading this chapter, the student will be able to:

1. Define *personality*.
2. Compare stages of personality development according to Sullivan, Erikson, and Mahler.
3. Identify various types of personality disorders.
4. Discuss historical and epidemiological statistics related to various personality disorders.
5. Describe symptomatology associated with borderline personality disorder and antisocial personality disorder, and use these data in client assessment.
6. Identify predisposing factors for borderline personality disorder and antisocial personality disorder.
7. Formulate nursing diagnoses and goals of care for clients with borderline personality disorder and antisocial personality disorder.
8. Describe appropriate nursing interventions for behaviors associated with borderline personality disorder and antisocial personality disorder.
9. Evaluate nursing care of clients with borderline personality disorder and antisocial personality disorder.
10. Discuss various modalities relevant to treatment of personality disorder.

HOMEWORK ASSIGNMENT

Please read the chapter and answer the following questions:

1. What are the psychosocial predisposing factors to dependent personality disorder?
2. How are passive-aggressive behaviors manifested?
3. How should a nurse care for the self-inflicted wounds of a client with borderline personality disorder?
4. What are some of the types of family dynamics that may predispose a person to antisocial personality disorder?

CORE CONCEPT

Personality

The totality of emotional and behavioral characteristics that are particular to a specific person and that remain somewhat stable and predictable over time.

The word *personality* is derived from the Greek term *persona*. It was originally used to describe the theatrical mask worn by some dramatic actors at the time. Over the years, it lost its connotation of pretense and illusion and came to represent the person behind the mask—the "real" person.

The *Diagnostic and Statistical Manual of Mental Disorders, Fourth Edition, Text Revision* (DSM-IV-TR) (American Psychiatric Association [APA], 2000) defines personality *traits* as "enduring patterns of perceiving, relating to, and thinking about the environment and oneself that are exhibited in a wide range of social and personal contexts." Personality *disorders* occur when these traits become inflexible and maladaptive and cause either significant functional impairment or subjective distress. These disorders are coded on axis II of the multiaxial diagnostic system used by the APA (see Chapter 2 for an explanation of this system). Virtually all individuals exhibit some behaviors associated with the various personality disorders from time to time. It is only when significant functional impairment occurs in response to these personality characteristics that the individual is thought to have a personality disorder.

Personality development occurs in response to a number of biological and psychological influences. These variables include (but are not limited to) heredity, temperament, experiential learning, and social interaction. A number of theorists have attempted to provide information about personality development. Most suggest that it occurs in an orderly, stepwise fashion. These stages overlap, however, as maturation occurs at different rates in different individuals. The theories of Sullivan (1953), Erikson (1963), and Mahler (Mahler, Pine, & Bergman, 1975) were presented at length in Chapter 3. The stages of personality development according to these three theorists are compared in Table 34-1. The nurse should understand "normal" personality development before learning about what is considered maladaptive.

Historical and epidemiological aspects of personality disorders are discussed in this chapter.

TABLE 34-1 Comparison of Personality Development—Sullivan, Erikson, and Mahler

MAJOR DEVELOPMENTAL TASKS AND DESIGNATED AGES

Sullivan	Erikson	Mahler
Birth to 18 months: Relief from anxiety through oral gratification of needs.	Birth to 18 months: To develop a basic trust in the mothering figure and be able to generalize it to others.	Birth to 1 month: Fulfillment of basic needs for survival and comfort
18 months to 6 years: Learning to experience a delay in personal gratification without undue anxiety.	18 months to 3 years: To gain some self-control and independence within the environment.	1 to 5 months: Developing awareness of external source of need fulfillment.
6 to 9 years: Learning to form satisfactory peer relationships.	3 to 6 years: To develop a sense of purpose and the ability to initiate and direct own activities.	5 to 10 months: Commencement of a primary recognition of separateness from the mothering figure.
9 to 12 years: Learning to form satisfactory relationships with persons of the same gender; the initiation of feelings of affection for another person.	6 to 12 years: To achieve a sense of self-confidence by learning, competing, performing successfully, and receiving recognition from significant others, peers, and acquaintances.	10 to 16 months: Increased independence through locomotor functioning; increased sense of separateness of self.
12 to 14 years: Learning to form satisfactory relationships with persons of the opposite gender; developing a sense of identity.	12 to 20 years: To integrate the tasks mastered in the previous stages into a secure sense of self.	16 to 24 months: Acute awareness of separateness of self; learning to seek "emotional refueling" from mothering figure to maintain feeling of security.

Continued

TABLE 34-1 Comparison of Personality Development—Sullivan, Erikson, and Mahler—cont'd

MAJOR DEVELOPMENTAL TASKS AND DESIGNATED AGES

Sullivan	Erikson	Mahler
14 to 21 years: Establishing self-identity; experiences satisfying relationships; working to develop a lasting, intimate opposite-gender relationship	20 to 30 years: To form an intense, lasting relationship or a commitment to another person, a cause, an institution, or a creative effort.	24 to 36 months: Sense of separateness established; on the way to object constancy: able to internalize a sustained image of loved object/person when it is out of sight; resolution of separation anxiety.
	30 to 65 years: To achieve the life goals established for oneself, while also considering the welfare of future generations.	
	65 years to death: To review one's life and derive meaning from both positive and negative events, while achieving a positive sense of self-worth.	

Predisposing factors that have been implicated in the etiology of personality disorders are presented. Symptomatology is explained to provide background knowledge for assessing clients with personality disorders.

Individuals with personality disorders are not often treated in acute care settings for the personality disorder as their primary psychiatric diagnosis. However, many clients with other psychiatric and medical diagnoses manifest symptoms of personality disorders. Nurses are likely to encounter clients with these personality characteristics frequently in all health-care settings.

Nurses working in psychiatric settings are likely to encounter clients with borderline and antisocial personality characteristics. The behavior of clients with borderline personality disorder is very unstable, and hospitalization is often required as a result of attempts at self-injury. The client with antisocial personality disorder may enter the psychiatric arena as a result of judicially ordered evaluation. Psychiatric intervention may be an alternative to imprisonment for antisocial behavior if it is deemed potentially helpful.

Nursing care of clients with borderline personality disorder or antisocial personality disorder is presented in this chapter in the context of the nursing process. Various medical treatment modalities for personality disorders are explored.

Historical Aspects

The concept of a personality disorder has been described for thousands of years (Skodal & Gunderson, 2008). In the fourth century B.C., Hippocrates concluded that all disease stemmed from an excess of or imbalance among four bodily humors: yellow bile, black bile, blood, and phlegm. Hippocrates identified four fundamental personality styles that he concluded stemmed from excesses in the four humors: the irritable and hostile choleric (yellow bile); the pessimistic melancholic (black bile); the overly optimistic and extroverted sanguine (blood); and the apathetic phlegmatic (phlegm).

The medical profession first recognized that personality disorders, apart from psychosis, were cause for their own special concern in 1801, with the recognition that an individual can behave irrationally even when the powers of intellect are intact. Nineteenth-century psychiatrists embraced the term *moral insanity,* the concept of which defines what we know today as personality disorders.

A major difficulty for psychiatrists has been the establishment of a classification of personality disorders. The *DSM-IV-TR* provides specific criteria for diagnosing these disorders. The *DSM-IV-TR* groups the personality disorders into three clusters. These clusters, and the disorders classified under each, are described as follows:

1. **Cluster A:** Behaviors described as odd or eccentric.
   a. Paranoid personality disorder
   b. Schizoid personality disorder
   c. Schizotypal personality disorder

2. **Cluster B:** Behaviors described as dramatic, emotional, or erratic.
   a. Antisocial personality disorder
   b. Borderline personality disorder
   c. Histrionic personality disorder
   d. Narcissistic personality disorder

3. **Cluster C:** Behaviors described as anxious or fearful.
   a. Avoidant personality disorder
   b. Dependent personality disorder
   c. Obsessive-compulsive personality disorder

NOTE: The third edition of the *DSM* included passive-aggressive personality disorder in cluster C. In the *DSM-IV-TR*, this disorder has been included in the section on "Criteria Provided for Further Study." For purposes of this text, passive-aggressive personality disorder will be described with the cluster C disorders.

Historically, individuals with personality disorders have been labeled as "bad" or "immoral" and as deviants in the range of normal personality dimensions. The events and sequences that result in pathology of the personality are complicated and difficult to unravel. Continued study is needed to facilitate understanding of this complex behavioral phenomenon.

Types of Personality Disorders

Paranoid Personality Disorder

Definition and Epidemiological Statistics

The *DSM-IV-TR* defines *paranoid personality disorder* as "a pervasive distrust and suspiciousness of others such that their motives are interpreted as malevolent, beginning by early adulthood and present in a variety of contexts" (APA, 2000, p. 690). Sadock and Sadock (2007) identified the characteristic feature as a long-standing suspiciousness and mistrust of people in general.

Prevalence is difficult to establish because individuals with the disorder seldom seek assistance for their problem or require hospitalization. When they present for treatment at the insistence of others, they may be able to pull themselves together sufficiently so that their behavior does not appear maladaptive. The disorder is more commonly diagnosed in men than in women.

Clinical Picture

Individuals with paranoid personality disorder are constantly on guard, hypervigilant, and ready for any real or imagined threat. They appear tense and irritable. They have developed a hard exterior and become immune or insensitive to the feelings of others. They avoid interactions with other people, lest they be forced to relinquish some of their own power. They always feel that others are there to take advantage of them.

They are extremely oversensitive and tend to misinterpret even minute cues within the environment, magnifying and distorting them into thoughts of trickery and deception. Because they trust no one, they are constantly "testing" the honesty of others. Their intimidating manner provokes exasperation and anger in almost everyone with whom they come in contact.

Individuals with paranoid personality disorder maintain their self-esteem by attributing their shortcomings to others. They do not accept responsibility for their own behaviors and feelings and project this responsibility on to others. They are envious and hostile toward others who are highly successful and believe the only reason they are not as successful is because they have been treated unfairly. People who are paranoid are extremely vulnerable and constantly on the defensive. Any real or imagined threat can release hostility and anger that is fueled by animosities from the past. The desire for reprisal and vindication is so intense that a possible loss of control can result in aggression and violence. These outbursts are usually brief, and the paranoid person soon regains the external control, rationalizes the behavior, and reconstructs the defenses central to his or her personality pattern.

The *DSM-IV-TR* diagnostic criteria for paranoid personality disorder are presented in Box 34-1.

Predisposing Factors

Research has indicated a possible hereditary link in paranoid personality disorder. Studies have revealed a higher incidence of paranoid personality disorder among relatives of clients with schizophrenia than among control subjects (Sadock & Sadock, 2007).

BOX 34-1 Diagnostic Criteria for Paranoid Personality Disorder

A. A pervasive distrust and suspiciousness of others such that their motives are interpreted as malevolent, beginning by early adulthood and present in a variety of contexts, as indicated by four (or more) of the following:
  1. Suspects, without sufficient basis, that others are exploiting, harming, or deceiving him or her
  2. Is preoccupied with unjustified doubts about the loyalty or trustworthiness of friends or associates
  3. Is reluctant to confide in others because of unwarranted fear that the information will be used maliciously against him or her
  4. Reads hidden demeaning or threatening meanings into benign remarks or events
  5. Persistently bears grudges (i.e., is unforgiving of insults, injuries, or slights)
  6. Perceives attacks on his or her character or reputation that are not apparent to others and is quick to react angrily or to counterattack
  7. Has recurrent suspicions, without justification, regarding fidelity of spouse or sexual partner
B. Does not occur exclusively during the course of schizophrenia, a mood disorder with psychotic features, or another psychotic disorder and is not due to the direct physiological effects of a general medical condition.

From American Psychiatric Association. (2000). Diagnostic and statistical manual of mental disorders (4th ed.). Text revision. Washington, DC: American Psychiatric Publishing, with permission.

Psychosocially, people with paranoid personality disorder may have been subjected to parental antagonism and harassment. They likely served as scapegoats for displaced parental aggression and gradually relinquished all hope of affection and approval. They learned to perceive the world as harsh and unkind, a place calling for protective vigilance and mistrust. They entered the world with a "chip-on-the-shoulder" attitude and were met with many rebuffs and rejections from others. Anticipating humiliation and betrayal by others, the paranoid person learned to attack first.

Schizoid Personality Disorder

Definition and Epidemiological Statistics

Schizoid personality disorder is characterized primarily by a profound defect in the ability to form personal relationships or to respond to others in any meaningful, emotional way (Skodol & Gunderson, 2008). These individuals display a lifelong pattern of social withdrawal, and their discomfort with human interaction is apparent. The prevalence of schizoid personality disorder within the general population has been estimated at between 3 and 7.5 percent. Significant numbers of people with the disorder are never observed in a clinical setting. Gender ratio of the disorder is unknown, although it is diagnosed more frequently in men.

Clinical Picture

People with schizoid personality disorder appear cold, aloof, and indifferent to others. They prefer to work in isolation and are unsociable, with little need or desire for emotional ties. They are able to invest enormous affective energy in intellectual pursuits.

In the presence of others they appear shy, anxious, or uneasy. They are inappropriately serious about everything and have difficulty acting in a lighthearted manner. Their behavior and conversation exhibit little or no spontaneity. Typically they are unable to experience pleasure, and their affect is commonly bland and constricted.

The *DSM-IV-TR* diagnostic criteria for schizoid personality disorder are presented in Box 34-2.

Predisposing Factors

Although the role of heredity in the etiology of schizoid personality disorder is unclear, the feature of introversion appears to be a highly inheritable characteristic. Further studies are required before definitive statements can be made.

Psychosocially, the development of schizoid personality is probably influenced by early interactional patterns that the person found to be cold and unsatisfying. The childhoods of these individuals have often been characterized as bleak, cold, and notably lacking empathy and nurturing. A child brought up with this type of parenting may become a schizoid adult if that child possesses a temperamental disposition that is shy, anxious, and introverted. Skodol and Gunderson (2008) stated,

Clinicians have noted that schizoid personality disorder occurs in adults who experienced cold, neglectful, and ungratifying relationships in early childhood, which leads these persons to assume that relationships are not valuable or worth pursuing. (p. 836)

BOX 34-2 **Diagnostic Criteria for Schizoid Personality Disorder**

A. A pervasive pattern of detachment from social relationships and a restricted range of expression of emotions in interpersonal settings, beginning by early adulthood and present in a variety of contexts, as indicated by four (or more) of the following:
   1. Neither desires nor enjoys close relationships, including being part of a family
   2. Almost always chooses solitary activities
   3. Has little, if any, interest in having sexual experiences with another person
   4. Takes pleasure in few, if any, activities
   5. Lacks close friends or confidants other than first-degree relatives
   6. Appears indifferent to the praise or criticism of others
   7. Shows emotional coldness, detachment, or flattened affectivity
B. Does not occur exclusively during the course of schizophrenia, a mood disorder with psychotic features, another psychotic disorder, or a pervasive development disorder and is not due to the direct physiological effects of a general medical condition.

From American Psychiatric Association. (2000). Diagnostic and statistical manual of mental disorders (4th ed.). Text revision. Washington, DC: American Psychiatric Publishing, with permission.

Schizotypal Personality Disorder

Definition and Epidemiological Statistics

Individuals with **schizotypal** personality disorder were once described as "latent schizophrenics." Their behavior is odd and eccentric but does not decompensate to the level of schizophrenia. Schizotypal personality is a graver form of the pathologically less severe schizoid personality pattern. Studies indicate that approximately 3 percent of the population has this disorder (APA, 2000).

Clinical Picture

Individuals with schizotypal personality disorder are aloof and isolated and behave in a bland and apathetic manner. Magical thinking, ideas of reference, illusions, and depersonalization are part of their everyday world. Examples include superstitiousness; belief in clairvoyance, telepathy, or a "sixth sense"; and beliefs that "others can feel my feelings" (APA, 2000).

The speech pattern is sometimes bizarre. People with this disorder often cannot orient their thoughts logically and become lost in personal irrelevancies and in tangential asides that seem vague, digressive, and not pertinent to the topic at hand. This feature of their personality only further alienates them from others.

Under stress, these individuals may decompensate and demonstrate psychotic symptoms, such as delusional thoughts, hallucinations, or bizarre behaviors, but they are usually of brief duration (Sadock & Sadock, 2007). They often talk or gesture to themselves, as if "living in their own world." Their affect is bland or inappropriate, such as

laughing at their own problems or at a situation that most people would consider sad.

The *DSM-IV-TR* diagnostic criteria for schizotypal personality disorder are presented in Box 34-3.

Predisposing Factors

Some evidence suggests that schizotypal personality disorder is more common among the first-degree biological relatives of people with schizophrenia than among the general population, indicating a possible hereditary factor (APA, 2000). Although speculative, other biogenic factors that may contribute to the development of this disorder include anatomical deficits or neurochemical dysfunctions resulting in diminished activation, minimal pleasure-pain sensibilities, and impaired cognitive functions. These biological etiological factors support the close link between schizotypal personality disorder and schizophrenia and were considered when classifying schizotypal personality disorder with schizophrenia rather than with the personality disorders in the 10th *International Classification of Diseases* (ICD-10) (Skodol & Gunderson, 2008).

The early family dynamics of the individual with schizotypal personality disorder may have been characterized by indifference, impassivity, or formality, leading to a pattern of discomfort with personal affection and closeness. Early on, affective deficits made them unattractive and unrewarding social companions. They were likely shunned, overlooked, rejected, and humiliated by others, resulting in feelings of low self-esteem and a marked distrust of interpersonal relations. Having

---

BOX 34-3 Diagnostic Criteria for Schizotypal Personality Disorder

A. A pervasive pattern of social and interpersonal deficits marked by acute discomfort with, and reduced capacity for, close relationships as well as by cognitive or perceptual distortions and eccentricities of behavior, beginning by early adulthood and present in a variety of contexts, as indicated by five (or more) of the following:

1. Ideas of reference (excluding delusions of reference)
2. Odd beliefs or magical thinking that influences behavior and is inconsistent with subcultural norms (e.g., superstitiousness, belief in clairvoyance, telepathy, or "sixth sense;" in children and adolescents, bizarre fantasies or preoccupations)
3. Unusual perceptual experiences, including bodily illusions
4. Odd thinking and speech (e.g., vague, circumstantial, metaphorical, overelaborate, or stereotyped)
5. Suspiciousness or paranoid ideation
6. Inappropriate or constricted affect
7. Behavior or appearance that is odd, eccentric, or peculiar
8. Lack of close friends or confidants other than first-degree relatives
9. Excessive social anxiety that does not diminish with familiarity and tends to be associated with paranoid fears rather than negative judgments about self

B. Does not occur exclusively during the course of schizophrenia, a mood disorder with psychotic features, another psychotic disorder, or a pervasive developmental disorder.

From American Psychiatric Association. (2000). Diagnostic and statistical manual of mental disorders (4th ed.). Text revision. Washington, DC: American Psychiatric Publishing, with permission.

---

failed repeatedly to cope with these adversities, they began to withdraw and reduce contact with individuals and situations that evoked sadness and humiliation. Their new inner world provided them with a more significant and potentially rewarding existence than the one experienced in reality.

Antisocial Personality Disorder

Definition and Epidemiological Statistics

Antisocial personality disorder is a pattern of socially irresponsible, exploitative, and guiltless behavior that reflects a general disregard for the rights of others. These individuals exploit and manipulate others for personal gain and are unconcerned with obeying the law. They have difficulty sustaining consistent employment and developing stable relationships. It is one of the oldest and best researched of the personality disorders and has been included in all editions of the *Diagnostic and Statistical Manual of Mental Disorders*. In the United States, prevalence estimates range from 3 percent in men to about 1 percent in women (APA, 2000). The disorder is more common among the lower socioeconomic classes, particularly so among highly mobile inhabitants of impoverished urban areas. The *ICD-10* identifies this disorder as *dissocial personality disorder*.

NOTE: The clinical picture, predisposing factors, nursing diagnoses, and interventions for care of clients with antisocial personality disorder are presented later in this chapter.

Borderline Personality Disorder

Definition and Epidemiological Statistics

Borderline personality disorder is characterized by a pattern of intense and chaotic relationships, with affective instability and fluctuating attitudes toward other people. These individuals are impulsive, are directly and indirectly self-destructive, and lack a clear sense of identity. Prevalence of borderline personality disorder is estimated at 1 to 2 percent of the population. It is more common in women than in men, with female-to-male ratios being estimated as high as 4 to 1 (Lubit, 2010). The *ICD-10* identifies this disorder as *emotionally unstable personality disorder*.

NOTE: The clinical picture, predisposing factors, nursing diagnoses, and interventions for care of clients with borderline personality disorder are presented later in this chapter.

Histrionic Personality Disorder

Definition and Epidemiological Statistics

Histrionic personality disorder is characterized by colorful, dramatic, and extroverted behavior in excitable, emotional people. They have difficulty maintaining long-lasting relationships, although they require constant affirmation of approval and acceptance from others. Prevalence of the disorder is thought to be about 2 to 3 percent, and it is more common in women than in men.

Clinical Picture

People with histrionic personality disorder tend to be self-dramatizing, attention seeking, overly gregarious, and seductive. They use manipulative and exhibitionistic behaviors in their demands to be the center of attention. People with histrionic personality disorder often demonstrate, in mild pathological form, what our society tends to foster and admire in its members: to be well liked, successful, popular, extroverted, attractive, and sociable. However, beneath these surface characteristics is a driven quality—an all-consuming need for approval and a desperate striving to be conspicuous and to evoke affection or attract attention at all costs. Failure to evoke the attention and approval they seek often results in feelings of dejection and anxiety.

Individuals with this disorder are highly distractible and flighty by nature. They have difficulty paying attention to detail. They can portray themselves as carefree and sophisticated on the one hand and as inhibited and naive on the other. They tend to be highly suggestible, impressionable, and easily influenced by others. They are strongly dependent.

Interpersonal relationships are fleeting and superficial. The person with histrionic personality disorder, having failed throughout life to develop the richness of inner feelings and lacking resources from which to draw, lacks the ability to provide another with genuinely sustained affection. Somatic complaints are not uncommon in these individuals, and fleeting episodes of psychosis may occur during periods of extreme stress.

The *DSM-IV-TR* diagnostic criteria for histrionic personality disorder are presented in Box 34-4.

Predisposing Factors

Neurobiological correlates have been proposed in the predisposition to histrionic personality disorder. Coccaro and Siever (2000) related the characteristics of enhanced sensitivity and reactivity to environmental stimuli to heightened noradrenergic activity in the individual with histrionic personality disorder. They suggested that the trait of impulsivity may be associated with decreased serotonergic activity.

Heredity also may be a factor because the disorder is apparently more common among first-degree biological relatives of people with the disorder than in the general population. Skodol and Gunderson (2008) reported on research that suggests that the behavioral characteristics of histrionic personality disorder may be associated with a biogenetically determined temperament. From this perspective, histrionic personality disorder would arise out of "an extreme variation of temperamental disposition" (p. 844).

From a psychosocial perspective, learning experiences may contribute to the development of histrionic personality disorder. The child may have learned that positive reinforcement was contingent on the ability to perform parentally approved and admired behaviors. It is likely that the child rarely received either positive or negative feedback. Parental acceptance and approval came inconsistently and only when the behaviors met parental expectations. Millon (2004) stated:

> Because nothing they do works consistently, such children experience frustration in getting their parents' attention and exaggerate behaviors basic to their gender stereotype to secure compliments and affection. Otherwise, they are ignored. Such children enter adolescence with a nearly insatiable thirst for attention and love. (p. 314)

BOX 34-4 **Diagnostic Criteria for Histrionic Personality Disorder**

A pervasive pattern of excessive emotionality and attention seeking, beginning by early adulthood and present in a variety of contexts, as indicated by five (or more) of the following:

1. Is uncomfortable in situations in which he or she is not the center of attention
2. Interaction with others is often characterized by inappropriate sexually seductive or provocative behavior
3. Displays rapidly shifting and shallow expression of emotions
4. Consistently uses physical appearance to draw attention to self
5. Has a style of speech that is excessively impressionistic and lacking in detail
6. Shows self-dramatization, theatricality, and exaggerated expression of emotion
7. Is suggestible, i.e., easily influenced by others or circumstances
8. Considers relationships to be more intimate than they actually are

---

From American Psychiatric Association. (2000). Diagnostic and statistical manual of mental disorders (4th ed.). Text revision. Washington, DC: American Psychiatric Publishing, with permission.

Narcissistic Personality Disorder

Definition and Epidemiological Statistics

Persons with narcissistic personality disorder have an exaggerated sense of self-worth. They lack empathy, and are hypersensitive to the evaluation of others. They believe that they have the inalienable right to receive special consideration and that their desire is sufficient justification for possessing whatever they seek.

This diagnosis appeared for the first time in the third edition of the *Diagnostic and Statistical Manual of Mental Disorders*. However, the concept of **narcissism** has its roots in the 19th century. It was viewed by early psychoanalysts as a normal phase of psychosexual development. The *DSM-IV-TR* (APA, 2000) estimates that the disorder occurs in 2 to 16 percent of the clinical population and less than 1 percent of the general population. It is diagnosed more often in men than in women.

Clinical Picture

Individuals with narcissistic personality disorder appear to lack humility, being overly self-centered and exploiting others to fulfill their own desires. They often do not conceive of their behavior as being inappropriate or objectionable. Because they view themselves as "superior" beings, they believe they are entitled to special rights and privileges.

Although often grounded in grandiose distortions of reality, their mood is usually optimistic, relaxed, cheerful, and carefree. This mood can easily change, however, because of their fragile self-esteem. If they do not meet self-expectations, do not receive the positive feedback they expect from others, or draw criticism from others, they may respond with rage, shame, humiliation, or dejection. They may turn inward and fantasize rationalizations that convince them of their continued stature and perfection.

The exploitation of others for self-gratification results in impaired interpersonal relationships. In selecting a mate, narcissistic individuals frequently choose a person who will provide them with the praise and positive feedback that they require and who will not ask much from their partner in return.

The *DSM-IV-TR* diagnostic criteria for narcissistic personality disorder are presented in Box 34-5.

Predisposing Factors

Several psychodynamic theories exist regarding the predisposition to narcissistic personality disorder. Skodol and Gunderson (2008) suggested that, as children, these individuals had their fears, failures, or dependency needs responded to with criticism, disdain, or neglect. They grow up with contempt for these behaviors in themselves and others and are unable to view others as sources of comfort and support. They project an image of invulnerability and self-sufficiency that conceals their true sense of emptiness and contributes to their inability to feel deeply.

Martinez-Lewi (2008) suggested that the parents of individuals with narcissistic personality disorder were often narcissistic themselves. The parents were demanding, perfectionistic, and critical, and they placed unrealistic expectations on

---

BOX 34-5 Diagnostic Criteria for Narcissistic Personality Disorder

A pervasive pattern of grandiosity (in fantasy or behavior), need for admiration, and lack of empathy, beginning by early adulthood and present in a variety of contexts, as indicated by five (or more) of the following:

1. Has a grandiose sense of self-importance (e.g., exaggerates achievements and talents, expects to be recognized as superior without commensurate achievements)
2. Is preoccupied with fantasies of unlimited success, power, brilliance, beauty, or ideal love
3. Believes that he or she is "special" and unique and can only be understood by, or should associate with, other special or high-status people (or institutions)
4. Requires excessive admiration
5. Has a sense of entitlement (i.e., unreasonable expectations of especially favorable treatment or automatic compliance with his or her expectations)
6. Is interpersonally exploitative (i.e., takes advantage of others to achieve his or her own ends)
7. Lacks empathy: is unwilling to recognize or identify with the feelings and needs of others
8. Is often envious of others or believes that others are envious of him or her
9. Shows arrogant, haughty behaviors or attitudes

From American Psychiatric Association. (2000). Diagnostic and statistical manual of mental disorders (4th ed.). Text revision. Washington, DC: American Psychiatric Publishing, with permission.

the child. Children model their parents' behavior, giving way to the adult narcissist. Some clinicians have suggested that the parents may have subjected the child to physical or emotional abuse or neglect.

Narcissism may also develop from an environment in which parents attempt to live their lives vicariously through their child. They expect the child to achieve the things they did not achieve, possess that which they did not possess, and have life better and easier than they did. The child is not subjected to the requirements and restrictions that may have dominated the parents' lives, and thereby grows up believing he or she is above that which is required for everyone else. Bosson and Prewitt-Freilino (2007) stated:

> Some parents pamper and indulge their youngsters in ways that teach them that their every wish is a command, that they can receive without giving in return, and that they deserve prominence without even minimal effort. Consequently, these youngsters learn to associate the self with positive affect and develop extremely favorable implicit self-representations. [However, because] the world beyond home will not be so benign and accepting, in many cases of parental overindulgence, reality eventually intervenes—in the form of personal failures, humiliations, weaknesses, and the like—and undermines the individual's explicit self-esteem. From this perspective, narcissists' tendencies toward entitlement and exploitativeness reflect the overblown implicit expectations their parents instilled in them, while their shame-proneness reflects their chronic perception of themselves as falling short of these expectations. (p. 414)

Avoidant Personality Disorder

Definition and Epidemiological Statistics

The individual with avoidant personality disorder is extremely sensitive to rejection and because of this may lead a very socially withdrawn life. It is not that he or she is asocial; in fact, there may be a strong desire for companionship. The extreme shyness and fear of rejection, however, create needs for unusually strong assurances of unconditional acceptance. Prevalence of the disorder in the general population is between 0.5 and 1 percent, and it appears to be equally common in men and women (APA, 2000).

Clinical Picture

Individuals with this disorder are awkward and uncomfortable in social situations. From a distance, others may perceive them as timid, withdrawn, or perhaps cold and strange. Those who have closer relationships with them, however, soon learn of their sensitivities, touchiness, evasiveness, and mistrustful qualities.

Their speech is usually slow and constrained, with frequent hesitations, fragmentary thought sequences, and occasional confused and irrelevant digressions. They are often lonely, and express feelings of being unwanted. They view others as critical, betraying, and humiliating. They desire to have close relationships but avoid them because of their fear of being rejected. Depression, anxiety, and anger at oneself for failing to develop social relations are commonly experienced.

The *DSM-IV-TR* diagnostic criteria for avoidant personality disorder are presented in Box 34-6.

Predisposing Factors

It is possible that there is a hereditary influence with avoidant personality disorder because it

---

BOX 34-6 Diagnostic Criteria for Avoidant Personality Disorder

A pervasive pattern of social inhibition, feelings of inadequacy, and hypersensitivity to negative evaluation, beginning by early adulthood and present in a variety of contexts, as indicated by four (or more) of the following:

1. Avoids occupational activities that involve significant interpersonal contact, because of fears of criticism, disapproval, or rejection
2. Is unwilling to get involved with people unless certain of being liked
3. Shows restraint within intimate relationships because of the fear of being shamed or ridiculed
4. Is preoccupied with being criticized or rejected in social situations
5. Is inhibited in new interpersonal situations because of feelings of inadequacy
6. Views self as socially inept, personally unappealing, or inferior to others
7. Is unusually reluctant to take personal risks or to engage in any new activities because they may prove embarrassing

From American Psychiatric Association. (2000). Diagnostic and statistical manual of mental disorders (4th ed.). Text revision. Washington, DC: American Psychiatric Publishing, with permission.

seems to occur more frequently in certain families (Rettew, Jellinek, & Doyle, 2010). Some infants who exhibit traits of hyperirritability, crankiness, tension, and withdrawal behaviors may possess a temperamental disposition toward an avoidant pattern.

The primary psychosocial predisposing influence to avoidant personality disorder is parental rejection and censure, which is often reinforced by peers (Millon, 2004). These children are often reared in families in which they are belittled, abandoned, and criticized, such that any natural optimism is extinguished and replaced with feelings of low self-worth and social alienation. They learn to be suspicious and to view the world as hostile and dangerous.

Dependent Personality Disorder

Definition and Epidemiological Statistics

Dependent personality disorder is characterized by "a pervasive and excessive need to be taken care of that leads to submissive and clinging behavior and fears of separation" (APA, 2000, p. 721). These characteristics are evident in the tendency to allow others to make decisions, to feel helpless when alone, to act submissively, to subordinate needs to others, to tolerate mistreatment by others, to demean oneself to gain acceptance, and to fail to function adequately in situations that require assertive or dominant behavior.

The disorder is relatively common. Sadock and Sadock (2007) discussed the results of one study of personality disorders in which 2.5 percent of the sample were diagnosed with dependent personality disorder. It is more common in women than in

men and more common in the youngest children of a family.

Clinical Picture

Individuals with dependent personality disorder have a notable lack of self-confidence that is often apparent in their posture, voice, and mannerisms. They are typically passive and acquiescent to the desires of others. They are overly generous and thoughtful and underplay their own attractiveness and achievements. They may appear to others to "see the world through rose-colored glasses," but when alone, they may feel pessimistic, discouraged, and dejected. Others are not made aware of these feelings; their "suffering" is done in silence.

Individuals with dependent personality disorder assume the passive and submissive role in relationships. They are willing to let others make their important decisions. Should the dependent relationship end, they feel fearful and vulnerable because they lack confidence in their ability to care for themselves. They may hastily and indiscriminately attempt to establish another relationship with someone they believe can provide them with the nurturance and guidance they need.

They avoid positions of responsibility and become anxious when forced into them. They have feelings of low self-worth and are easily hurt by criticism and disapproval. They will do almost anything, even if it is unpleasant or demeaning, to earn the acceptance of others.

The *DSM-IV-TR* diagnostic criteria for dependent personality disorder are presented in Box 34-7.

BOX 34-7 Diagnostic Criteria for Dependent Personality Disorder

A pervasive and excessive need to be taken care of that leads to submissive and clinging behavior and fears of separation, beginning by early adulthood and present in a variety of contexts, as indicated by five (or more) of the following:

1. Has difficulty making everyday decisions without an excessive amount of advice and reassurance from others
2. Needs others to assume responsibility for most major areas of his or her life
3. Has difficulty expressing disagreement with others because of fear of loss of support or approval.

NOTE: Do not include realistic fears of retribution.

4. Has difficulty initiating projects or doing things on his or her own (because of a lack of self-confidence in judgment or abilities rather than a lack of motivation or energy)
5. Goes to excessive lengths to obtain nurturance and support from others, to the point of volunteering to do things that are unpleasant
6. Feels uncomfortable or helpless when alone because of exaggerated fears of being unable to care for himself or herself
7. Urgently seeks another relationship as a source of care and support when a close relationship ends
8. Is unrealistically preoccupied with fears of being left to take care of himself or herself

---

From American Psychiatric Association. (2000). Diagnostic and statistical manual of mental disorders (4th ed.). Text revision. Washington, DC: American Psychiatric Publishing, with permission.

Predisposing Factors

An infant may be genetically predisposed to a dependent temperament. Twin studies measuring submissiveness have shown a higher correlation between identical twins than fraternal twins.

Psychosocially, dependency is fostered in infancy when stimulation and nurturance are experienced exclusively from one source. The infant becomes attached to one source to the exclusion of all others. If this exclusive attachment continues as the child grows, the dependency is nurtured. A problem may arise when parents become overprotective and discourage independent behaviors on the part of the child. Parents who make new experiences unnecessarily easy for the child and refuse to allow him or her to learn by experience encourage their child to give up efforts at achieving autonomy. Dependent behaviors may be subtly rewarded in this environment, and the child may come to fear a loss of love or attachment from the parental figure if independent behaviors are attempted.

Obsessive-Compulsive Personality Disorder

Definition and Epidemiological Statistics

Individuals with obsessive-compulsive personality disorder are very serious and formal and have difficulty expressing emotions. They are overly disciplined, perfectionistic, and preoccupied with rules. They are inflexible about the way in which things must be done and have a devotion to productivity to the exclusion of personal pleasure. An intense fear of making mistakes leads to difficulty with decision making. The disorder is relatively common and occurs more often in men than in women. Within the family constellation, it appears to be most common in oldest children.

Clinical Picture

Individuals with obsessive-compulsive personality disorder are inflexible and lack spontaneity. They are meticulous and work diligently and patiently at tasks that require accuracy and discipline. They are especially concerned with matters of organization and efficiency and tend to be rigid and unbending about rules and procedures.

Social behavior tends to be polite and formal. They are very "rank conscious," a characteristic that is reflected in their contrasting behaviors with "superiors" as opposed to "inferiors." They tend to be very solicitous to and ingratiating with authority figures. With subordinates, however, the compulsive person can become quite autocratic and condemnatory, often appearing pompous and self-righteous.

People with obsessive-compulsive personality disorder typify the "bureaucratic personality," the so-called company man. They see themselves as conscientious, loyal, dependable, and responsible, and are contemptuous of people whose behavior they consider frivolous and impulsive. Emotional behavior is considered immature and irresponsible.

Although on the surface these individuals appear to be calm and controlled, underneath this exterior lies a great deal of ambivalence, conflict, and hostility. Individuals with this disorder commonly use the defense mechanism of reaction formation. Not daring to expose their true feelings of defiance and anger, they withhold these feelings so strongly that the opposite feelings come forth. The defenses of isolation, intellectualization, rationalization, and undoing are also commonly evident.

The *DSM-IV-TR* diagnostic criteria for obsessive-compulsive personality disorder are presented in Box 34-8.

Predisposing Factors

In the psychoanalytical view, the parenting style in which the individual with obsessive-compulsive personality disorder was reared is one of overcontrol. These parents expect their children to live up to their imposed standards of conduct and condemn them if they do not. Praise for positive behaviors is bestowed on the child with much less frequency than punishment for undesirable behaviors. In this environment, individuals become experts in learning what they must *not* do to avoid punishment and condemnation rather than what they *can* do to achieve attention and praise. They learn to heed rigid restrictions and rules. Positive achievements are expected, taken for granted, and only occasionally acknowledged by their parents, whose comments and judgments are limited to pointing out transgressions and infractions of rules.

Passive-Aggressive Personality Disorder

Definition and Epidemiological Statistics

The *DSM-IV-TR* defines **passive-aggressive** personality disorder as a pervasive pattern of negativistic attitudes and passive resistance to demands for adequate performance in social and occupational situations that begins by early adulthood and occurs in a variety of contexts. The name of the disorder is based on the assumption that such

---

BOX 34-8 Diagnostic Criteria for Obsessive-Compulsive Personality Disorder

A pervasive pattern of preoccupation with orderliness, perfectionism, and mental and interpersonal control, at the expense of flexibility, openness, and efficiency, beginning by early adulthood and present in a variety of contexts, as indicated by four (or more) of the following:

1. Is preoccupied with details, rules, lists, order, organization, or schedules to the extent that the major point of the activity is lost
2. Shows perfectionism that interferes with task completion (e.g., is unable to complete a project because his or her own overly strict standards are not met)
3. Is excessively devoted to work and productivity to the exclusion of leisure activities and friendships (not accounted for by obvious economic necessity)
4. Is overconscientious, scrupulous, and inflexible about matters of morality, ethics, or values (not accounted for by cultural or religious identification)
5. Is unable to discard worn-out or worthless objects even when they have no sentimental value
6. Is reluctant to delegate tasks or to work with others unless they submit to exactly his or her way of doing things
7. Adopts a miserly spending style toward both self and others; money is viewed as something to be hoarded for future catastrophes
8. Shows rigidity and stubbornness

From American Psychiatric Association. (2000). Diagnostic and statistical manual of mental disorders (4th ed.). Text revision. Washington, DC: American Psychiatric Publishing, with permission.

people are passively expressing covert aggression. Passive-aggressive disorder has been included in all editions of the *Diagnostic and Statistical Manual of Mental Disorders,* and although no statistics exist that speak to its prevalence, the syndrome appears to be relatively common.

Clinical Picture

Passive-aggressive individuals feel cheated and unappreciated. They believe that life has been unkind to them, and they express envy and resentment over the "easy life" that they perceive others having. When they feel another person has wronged them, they may go to great lengths to seek retribution, or "get even," but always in a subtle and passive manner rather than discussing their feelings with the offending individual. They demonstrate passive resistance and general obstructiveness in response to the expectations of others. As a tactic of interpersonal behavior, passive-aggressive individuals commonly switch among the roles of the martyr, the affronted, the aggrieved, the misunderstood, the contrite, the guilt-ridden, the sickly, and the overworked. In this way, they are able to vent their anger and resentment subtly, while gaining the attention, reassurance, and dependency they crave.

The *DSM-IV-TR* research criteria for passive-aggressive personality disorder are presented in Box 34-9.

Predisposing Factors

Contradictory parental attitudes and behavior are implicated in the predisposition to passive-aggressive

personality disorder. In the nuclear family dynamics, at any moment and without provocation, these children may receive the kindness and support they crave or hostility and rejection. Parental responses are inconsistent and unpredictable, and these children internalize the conflicting attitudes toward themselves and others. For example, they do not know whether to think of themselves as competent or incompetent and are unsure as to whether they love or hate those on whom they depend. Double-bind communication may also be exhibited in these families. Expressions of concern and affection may be verbalized, only to be negated and undone through subtle and devious behavioral manifestations. This *approach-avoidance* pattern is modeled by the children, who then become equally equivocal and ambivalent in their own thinking and actions.

Through this type of environment, children learn to control their anger for fear of provoking parental withdrawal and not receiving love and support—even on an inconsistent basis. Overtly the child appears polite and undemanding; hostility and inefficiency are manifested only covertly and indirectly.

Application of the Nursing Process

Borderline Personality Disorder (Background Assessment Data)

Historically, there have been a group of clients who did not classically conform to the standard

---

BOX 34-9 Research Criteria for Passive-Aggressive Personality Disorder

A. A pervasive pattern of negativistic attitudes and passive resistance to demands for adequate performance, beginning by early adulthood and present in a variety of contexts, as indicated by four (or more) of the following:

1. Passively resists fulfilling routine social and occupational tasks
2. Complains of being misunderstood and unappreciated by others
3. Is sullen and argumentative
4. Unreasonably criticizes and scorns authority
5. Expresses envy and resentment toward those apparently more fortunate
6. Voices exaggerated and persistent complaints of personal misfortune
7. Alternates between hostile defiance and contrition

B. Does not occur exclusively during major depressive episodes and is not better accounted for by dysthymic disorder.

From American Psychiatric Association. (2000). Diagnostic and statistical manual of mental disorders (4th ed.). Text revision. Washington, DC: American Psychiatric Publishing, with permission.

---

categories of neuroses or psychoses. The designation "borderline" was introduced to identify these clients who seemed to fall on the border between the two categories. Other terminology that has been used in an attempt to identify this disorder includes *ambulatory schizophrenia, pseudoneurotic schizophrenia,* and *emotionally unstable personality.* When the term *borderline* was first proposed for inclusion in the third edition of the *DSM,* some psychiatrists feared it might be used as a "wastebasket" diagnosis for difficult-to-treat clients. However, a specific set of criteria has been established for diagnosing what has been described as "a consistent and stable course of unstable behavior" (Box 34-10).

Clinical Picture

Individuals with borderline personality always seem to be in a state of crisis. Their affect is one of extreme intensity, and their behavior reflects frequent changeability. These changes can occur within days, hours, or even minutes. Often these individuals exhibit a single, dominant affective tone, such as depression, which may give way periodically to anxious agitation or inappropriate outbursts of anger.

Chronic Depression

Depression is so common in clients with this disorder that, before the inclusion of borderline personality disorder in the *DSM,* many of these

---

BOX 34-10 Diagnostic Criteria for Borderline Personality Disorder

A pervasive pattern of instability of interpersonal relationships, self-image, and affects, and marked impulsivity beginning by early adulthood and present in a variety of contexts, as indicated by five (or more) of the following:

1. Frantic efforts to avoid real or imagined abandonment. (Does not include suicidal or self-mutilating behavior covered in criterion 5.)
2. A pattern of unstable and intense interpersonal relationships characterized by alternating between extremes of idealization and devaluation.
3. Identity disturbance: markedly and persistently unstable self-image or sense of self.
4. Impulsivity in at least two areas that are potentially self-damaging (e.g., spending, sex, substance abuse, reckless driving, binge eating). Do not include suicidal or self-mutilating behavior covered in criterion 5.
5. Recurrent suicidal behavior, gestures, or threats, or self-mutilating behavior.
6. Affective instability due to marked reactivity of mood (e.g., intense episodic dysphoria, irritability, or anxiety, usually lasting a few hours and only rarely more than a few days).
7. Chronic feelings of emptiness.
8. Inappropriate, intense anger or difficulty controlling anger (e.g., frequent displays of temper, constant anger, recurrent physical fights).
9. Transient, stress-related paranoid ideation or severe dissociative symptoms.

From American Psychiatric Association. (2000). Diagnostic and statistical manual of mental disorders (4th ed.). Text revision. Washington, DC: American Psychiatric Publishing, with permission.

clients were diagnosed as depressed. Depression occurs in response to feelings of abandonment by the mother in early childhood (see "Predisposing Factors"). Underlying the depression is a sense of rage that is sporadically turned inward on the self and externally on the environment. Seldom is the individual aware of the true source of these feelings until well into long-term therapy.

Inability to Be Alone

Because of this chronic fear of abandonment, clients with borderline personality disorder have little tolerance for being alone. They prefer a frantic search for companionship, no matter how unsatisfactory, to sitting with feelings of loneliness, emptiness, and boredom (Sadock & Sadock, 2007).

Patterns of Interaction

Clinging and Distancing

The client with borderline personality disorder commonly exhibits a pattern of interaction with others that is characterized by clinging and distancing behaviors. When clients are clinging to another individual, they may exhibit helpless, dependent, or even childlike behaviors. They overidealize a single individual with whom they want to spend all their time, with whom they express a frequent need to talk, or from whom they seek constant reassurance. Acting-out behaviors, even self-mutilation, may result when they cannot be with this chosen individual. Distancing behaviors are characterized by hostility, anger, and devaluation of others, arising from a feeling of discomfort with closeness. Distancing behaviors also occur in response to separations, confrontations, or attempts to limit certain behaviors. Devaluation of others is manifested by discrediting or undermining their strengths and personal significance.

Splitting

Splitting is a primitive ego defense mechanism that is common in people with borderline personality disorder. It arises from their lack of achievement of **object constancy** and is manifested by an inability to integrate and accept both positive and negative feelings. In their view, people—including themselves—and life situations are either all good or all bad. For example, if a caregiver is nurturing and supportive, he or she is lovingly idealized. Should the nurturing relationship be threatened in any way (e.g., the caregiver must move because of his or her job), suddenly the individual is devalued, and the idealized image changes from beneficent caregiver to one of hateful and cruel persecutor.

Manipulation

In their efforts to prevent the separation they so desperately fear, clients with this disorder become masters of manipulation. Virtually any behavior becomes an acceptable means of achieving the desired result: relief from separation anxiety. Playing one individual against another is a common ploy to allay these fears of abandonment.

Self-Destructive Behaviors

Repetitive, self-mutilative behaviors are classic manifestations of borderline personality disorder. Although these acts can be fatal, most commonly they are manipulative gestures designed to elicit a rescue response from significant others. Suicide attempts are quite common and result from feelings of abandonment following separation from a significant other. The endeavor is often attempted, however, incorporating a measure of "safety" into the plan (e.g., swallowing pills in an area where the person will surely be discovered by others; or swallowing pills and making a phone call to report the deed to someone).

Other types of destructive behaviors include cutting, scratching, and burning. Various theories abound regarding why these individuals are able to inflict pain on themselves. One hypothesis suggests they may have higher levels of endorphins in their bodies than most people, thereby increasing their threshold for pain. Another theory relates to the individual's personal identity disturbance. It proposes that, since many of the self-mutilating behaviors take place when the individual is in a state of depersonalization and derealization, he or she does not initially feel the pain. The mutilation continues until pain is felt in an attempt to counteract the feelings of unreality. Some clients with borderline personality disorder have reported that "to feel pain is better than to feel nothing." The pain validates their existence.

Impulsivity

Individuals with borderline personality disorder have poor impulse control based on primary process functioning. Impulsive behaviors associated with borderline personality disorder include substance abuse, gambling, promiscuity, reckless driving, and binging and purging (APA, 2000). Many times these acting-out behaviors occur in response to real or perceived feelings of abandonment.

Predisposing Factors to Borderline Personality Disorder

Biological Influences

Biochemical Cummings and Mega (2003) have suggested a possible serotonergic defect in clients with borderline personality disorder. In positron emission tomography using α-[¹¹C] methyl-L-tryptophan (α-[¹¹C]MTrp), which reflects serotonergic synthesis capability, clients with borderline personality demonstrated significantly decreased α-[¹¹C]MTrp in medial frontal, superior temporal, and striatal regions of the brain. Cummings and Mega (2003) stated:

> These functional imaging studies support a medial and orbitofrontal abnormality that may promote the impulsive aggression demonstrated by patients with the borderline personality disorder. (p. 230)

Genetic The decrease in serotonin also may have genetic implications for borderline personality disorder. Sadock and Sadock (2007) reported that depression is common in the family backgrounds of clients with borderline personality disorder. They stated:

> These patients have more relatives with mood disorders than do control groups, and persons with borderline personality disorder often have mood disorder as well. (p. 791)

Psychosocial Influences

Childhood Trauma Studies have shown that many individuals with borderline personality disorder were reared in families with chaotic environments. Lubit (2010) stated, "Risk factors [for borderline personality disorder] include family environments characterized by trauma, neglect, and/or separation; exposure to sexual and physical abuse; and serious parental psychopathology, such as substance abuse and antisocial personality disorder." Forty to 71 percent of borderline personality disorder clients report having been sexually abused, usually by a non-caregiver (National Institute of Mental Health [NIMH], 2010). In some instances, this disorder has been likened to post-traumatic stress disorder (PTSD) in response to childhood trauma and abuse. Oldham and associates (2006) stated:

> Even when full criteria for comorbid PTSD are not present, patients with borderline personality disorder may experience PTSD-like symptoms. For example, symptoms such as intrusion, avoidance, and hyperarousal may emerge during psychotherapy. Awareness of the trauma-related nature of these symptoms can facilitate both psychotherapeutic and pharmacological efforts in symptom relief. (p. 1267)

Developmental Factors

Theory of Object Relations According to Mahler's theory of object relations (Mahler, Pine, & Bergman, 1975), the infant passes through six phases from birth to 36 months, when a sense of separateness from the parenting figure is finally established. These phases are as follows:

■ **Phase 1 (Birth to 1 Month), Autistic Phase.** During this period, the baby spends most of his or her time in a half-waking, half-sleeping state. The main goal is fulfillment of needs for survival and comfort.

■ **Phase 2 (1 to 5 Months), Symbiotic Phase.** At this time, there is a type of psychic fusion of mother and child. The child views the self as an extension of the parenting figure, although there is a developing awareness of external sources of need fulfillment.

■ **Phase 3 (5 to 10 Months), Differentiation Phase.** The child is beginning to recognize that there is a separateness between the self and the parenting figure.

■ **Phase 4 (10 to 16 Months), Practicing Phase.** This phase is characterized by increased locomotor functioning and the ability to explore the environment independently. A sense of separateness of the self is increased.

■ **Phase 5 (16 to 24 Months), Rapprochement Phase.** Awareness of separateness of the self becomes acute. This is frightening to the child, who wants to regain some lost closeness but not return to symbiosis. The child wants the mother there as needed for "emotional refueling" and to maintain feelings of security.

■ **Phase 6 (24 to 36 Months), On the Way to Object Constancy Phase.** In this phase, the child completes the individuation process and learns to relate to objects in an effective, constant manner. A sense of separateness is established, and the child is able to internalize a sustained image of the loved object or person when out of sight. Separation anxiety is resolved.

The individual with borderline personality disorder becomes fixed in the rapprochement phase of development. This occurs when the child shows increasing separation and autonomy. The mother, who feels secure in the relationship as long as the child is dependent, begins to feel threatened by the child's increasing independence. The mother may indeed be experiencing her own fears of abandonment. In response to separation behaviors, the mother withdraws the emotional support or "refueling" that is so vitally needed during this phase for the child to feel secure. Instead, the mother rewards clinging, dependent behaviors, and punishes (withholding emotional support) independent behaviors. With his or her sense of emotional survival at stake, the child learns to behave in a manner that satisfies the parental wishes. An internal conflict develops within the child, based on fear of abandonment. He or she wants to achieve independence common to this stage of development, but fears that the mother will withdraw emotional support as a result. This unresolved fear of abandonment remains with the child into adulthood. Unresolved grief for the nurturing they failed to receive results in internalized rage that manifests itself in the depression so common in people with borderline personality disorder.

Diagnosis/Outcome Identification

Nursing diagnoses are formulated from the data gathered during the assessment phase and with background knowledge regarding predisposing factors to the disorder. Table 34-2 presents a list of client behaviors and the NANDA nursing diagnoses that correspond to these behaviors, which may be used in planning care for clients with borderline personality disorder.

Outcome Criteria

The following criteria may be used for measurement of outcomes in the care of clients with borderline personality disorder.

The client:

■ Has not harmed self.
■ Seeks out staff when desire for self-mutilation is strong.
■ Is able to identify true source of anger.
■ Expresses anger appropriately.
■ Relates to more than one staff member.
■ Completes activities of daily living independently.
■ Does not manipulate one staff member against the other in order to fulfill own desires.

Planning/Implementation

The following section presents a group of selected nursing diagnoses common to clients with borderline personality disorder, with short- and long-term goals and nursing interventions for each.

Risk for Self-Mutilation/Risk for Self-Directed or Other-Directed Violence

Risk for self-mutilation is defined as "at risk for deliberate self-injurious behavior causing tissue damage with the intent of causing nonfatal injury to attain relief of tension" (NANDA International [NANDA-I], 2009, p. 329). *Risk for self-directed or*

TABLE 34-2 Assigning Nursing Diagnoses to Behaviors Commonly Associated with Borderline Personality Disorder	
BEHAVIORS	**NURSING DIAGNOSES**
History of self-injurious behavior; history of inability to plan solutions; impulsivity; irresistible urge to damage self; feels threatened with loss of significant relationship	**Risk for self-mutilation**
History of suicide attempts; suicidal ideation; suicidal plan; impulsiveness; childhood abuse; fears of abandonment; internalized rage	**Risk for self-directed violence; Risk for suicide**
Body language (e.g., rigid posture, clenching of fists and jaw, hyperactivity, pacing, breathlessness, threatening stances); history of childhood abuse; impulsivity; transient psychotic symptomatology	**Risk for other-directed violence**
Depression; persistent emotional distress; rumination; separation distress; traumatic distress; verbalizes feeling empty; inappropriate expression of anger	**Complicated grieving**
Alternating clinging and distancing behaviors; staff splitting; manipulation	**Impaired social interaction**
Feelings of depersonalization and derealization	**Disturbed personal identity**
Transient psychotic symptoms (disorganized thinking; misinterpretation of the environment); increased tension; decreased perceptual field	**Anxiety (severe to panic)**
Dependent on others; excessively seeks reassurance; manipulation of others; inability to tolerate being alone	**Chronic low self-esteem**

other-directed violence is defined as "at risk for behaviors in which an individual demonstrates that he/she can be physically, emotionally, and/or sexually harmful to self or others" (NANDA-I, 2009, pp. 232, 233).

Client Goals

Outcome criteria include short- and long-term goals. Timelines are individually determined.

Short-Term Goals

■ The client will seek out staff member if feelings of harming self or others emerge.

■ The client will not harm self or others.

Long-Term Goal

■ The client will not harm self or others.

Interventions

■ Observe the client's behavior frequently. Do this through routine activities and interactions; avoid appearing watchful and suspicious. Close observation is required so that intervention can occur if required to ensure client's (and others') safety.

■ Secure a verbal contract from the client that he or she will seek out a staff member when the urge for self-mutilation is experienced. Discussing feelings of self-harm with a trusted individual provides some relief to the client. A contract gets the subject out in the open and places some of the responsibility for his or her safety with the client. An attitude of acceptance of the client as a worthwhile individual is conveyed.

■ If self-mutilation occurs, care for the client's wounds in a matter-of-fact manner. Do not give positive reinforcement to this behavior by offering sympathy or additional attention. Lack of attention to the maladaptive behavior may decrease repetition of its use.

■ Encourage the client to talk about feelings he or she was having just before this behavior occurred. To problem-solve the situation with the client, knowledge of the precipitating factors is important.

■ Act as a role model for the appropriate expression of angry feelings, and give positive reinforcement to the client when attempts to conform are made. It is vital that the client expresses angry feelings because suicide and other self-destructive behaviors are often viewed as a result of anger turned inward on the self.

■ Remove all dangerous objects from the client's environment so that he or she may not purposefully or inadvertently use them to inflict harm to self or others.

■ Try to redirect violent behavior with physical outlets for the client's anxiety (e.g., punching bag, jogging). Physical exercise is a safe and effective way of relieving pent-up tension.

■ Have sufficient staff available to indicate a show of strength to the client if it becomes necessary. This conveys to the client evidence of control over the situation and provides some physical security for staff.

■ Administer tranquilizing medications as ordered by the physician or obtain an order if necessary. Monitor the client for effectiveness of the medication and for the appearance of adverse side effects. Tranquilizing medications such as anxiolytics or antipsychotics may have a calming effect on the client and may prevent aggressive behaviors.

■ If client is not calmed by "talking down" or by medication, use of mechanical restraints may be necessary. The avenue of the "least restrictive alternative" must be selected when planning interventions for a violent client. Restraints should be used only as a last resort, after all other interventions have been unsuccessful, and the client is clearly at risk of harm to self or others.

■ If restraint is deemed necessary, ensure that sufficient staff is available to assist. Follow protocol established by the institution. The Joint Commission (formerly the Joint Commission on Accreditation of Healthcare Organizations [JCAHO]) requires that an in-person evaluation by a physician or other licensed independent practitioner (LIP) be conducted within 1 hour of the initiation of the restraint or seclusion (The Joint Commission, 2010). The physician or LIP must reissue a new order for restraints every 4 hours for adults and every 1 to 2 hours for children and adolescents.

■ The Joint Commission requires that the client in restraints be observed at least every 15 minutes to ensure that circulation to extremities is not compromised (check temperature, color, pulses); to assist the client with needs related to nutrition, hydration, and elimination; and to position the client so that comfort is facilitated and aspiration is prevented. Some institutions may require continuous one-to-one monitoring of restrained clients, particularly those who are highly agitated, and for whom there is a high risk of self- or accidental injury.

■ As agitation decreases, assess the client's readiness for restraint removal or reduction. Remove one restraint at a time while assessing the client's response. This minimizes the risk of injury to client and staff.

■ If warranted by high acuity of the situation, staff may need to be assigned on a one-to-one basis. Because of their extreme fear of abandonment, clients with borderline personality disorder should not be left alone at a stressful time as it may cause an acute rise in anxiety and agitation levels.

Complicated Grieving

Complicated grieving is defined as "a disorder that occurs after the death of a significant other [or any other loss of significance to the individual], in which the experience of distress accompanying bereavement fails to follow normative expectations and manifests in functional impairment" (NANDA-I, 2009, p. 265). Table 34-3 presents this nursing diagnosis in care plan format.

Table 34-3 CARE PLAN FOR THE CLIENT WITH BORDERLINE PERSONALITY DISORDER

NURSING DIAGNOSIS: COMPLICATED GRIEVING

RELATED TO: Maternal deprivation during rapprochement phase of development (internalized as a loss, with fixation in anger stage of grieving process)

EVIDENCED BY: Depressed mood, acting-out behaviors

OUTCOME CRITERIA	NURSING INTERVENTIONS	RATIONALE
Short-Term Goal • Within 5 days, the client will discuss with nurse or therapist maladaptive patterns of expressing anger. **Long-Term Goal** • By time of discharge from treatment, the client will be able to identify the true source of angry feelings, accept ownership of these feelings, and express them in a socially acceptable manner, in an effort to satisfactorily progress through the grieving process.	1. Convey an accepting attitude—one that creates a nonthreatening environment for the client to express feelings. Be honest and keep all promises. 2. Identify the function that anger, frustration, and rage serve for the client. Allow him or her to express these feelings within reason. 3. Encourage client to discharge pent-up anger through participation in large-motor activities (e.g., brisk walks, jogging, physical exercises, volleyball, punching bag, exercise bike). 4. Explore with client the true source of the anger. This is a painful therapy that often leads to regression as the client deals with the feelings of early abandonment. 5. As anger is displaced onto the nurse or therapist, caution must be taken to guard against the negative effects of countertransference. These are very difficult clients who have the capacity for eliciting a whole array of negative feelings from the therapist. 6. Explain the behaviors associated with the normal grieving process. Help the client recognize his or her position in this process.	1. An accepting attitude conveys to the client that you believe he or she is a worthwhile person. Trust is enhanced. 2. Verbalization of feelings in a nonthreatening environment may help client come to terms with unresolved issues. 3. Physical exercise provides a safe and effective method for discharging pent-up tension. 4. Reconciliation of the feelings associated with this stage is necessary before progression through the grieving process can continue. 5. The existence of negative feelings by the nurse or therapist must be acknowledged, but they must not be allowed to interfere with the therapeutic process. 6. Knowledge of the acceptability of the feelings associated with normal grieving may help to relieve some of the guilt that these responses generate.

OUTCOME CRITERIA	NURSING INTERVENTIONS	RATIONALE
	7. Help the client to understand appropriate ways to express anger. Give positive reinforcement for behaviors used to express anger appropriately. Act as a role model.	7. Positive reinforcement enhances self-esteem and encourages repetition of desirable behaviors. Role modeling ways to express anger in an appropriate manner is a powerful learning tool.
	8. Set limits on acting-out behaviors and explain consequences of violation of those limits. Be supportive, yet consistent and firm in caring for this client.	8. Client lacks sufficient self-control to limit maladaptive behaviors, so assistance is required from staff. Without consistency on the part of all staff members working with this client, however, a positive outcome will not be achieved.

Table 34-3 CARE PLAN FOR THE CLIENT WITH BORDERLINE PERSONALITY DISORDER—cont'd

Client Goals

Outcome criteria include short- and long-term goals. Timelines are individually determined.

Short-Term Goal

■ Within 5 days, the client will discuss with nurse or therapist maladaptive patterns of expressing anger.

Long-Term Goal

■ By the time of discharge from treatment, the client will be able to identify the true source of angry feelings, accept ownership of these feelings, and express them in a socially acceptable manner, in an effort to satisfactorily progress through the grieving process.

Interventions

■ Convey an accepting attitude—one that creates a nonthreatening environment for the client to express feelings. Be honest and keep all promises. An accepting attitude conveys to the client that you believe he or she is a worthwhile person. Trust is enhanced.

■ Identify the function that anger, frustration, and rage serve for the client. Allow him or her to express these feelings within reason. Verbalization of feelings in a nonthreatening environment may help the client come to terms with unresolved issues.

■ Encourage the client to discharge pent-up anger through participation in large-motor activities (e.g., brisk walks, jogging, physical exercises, volleyball, punching bag, exercise bike). Physical exercise provides a safe and effective method for discharging pent-up tension.

■ Explore with the client the true source of anger. This is painful therapy that often leads to regression as the client deals with feelings of early abandonment. It seems that sometimes the client must "get worse before he or she can get better." Reconciliation of the feelings associated with this stage is necessary before progression through the grieving process can continue.

■ As anger is displaced onto the nurse or therapist, caution must be taken to guard against the negative effects of countertransference (see Chapter 7). These are very difficult clients who have the capacity for eliciting a whole array of negative feelings from the therapist. The existence of negative feelings by the nurse or therapist must be acknowledged, but they must not be allowed to interfere with the therapeutic process.

■ Explain the behaviors associated with the normal grieving process. Help the client recognize his or her position in this process. Knowledge of the acceptability of the feelings associated with normal grieving may help to relieve some of the guilt that these responses generate.

■ Help the client understand appropriate ways of expressing anger. Give positive reinforcement for behaviors used to express anger appropriately. Act as a role model. It is appropriate to let the client know when he or she has done something that has generated angry feelings in you. Role modeling ways to express anger in an appropriate manner is a powerful learning tool.

■ Set limits on acting-out behaviors and explain the consequences of violation of those limits. Be supportive, yet consistent and firm, in caring for this client. The client lacks sufficient self-control to limit maladaptive behaviors, so assistance is required. Without consistency on the part of all staff members working with this client, a positive outcome will not be achieved.

Impaired Social Interaction

Impaired social interaction is defined as "insufficient or excessive quantity or ineffective quality of social exchange" (NANDA-I, 2009, p. 223).

Client Goals

Outcome criteria include short- and long-term goals. Timelines are individually determined.

Short-Term Goal

■ Within 5 days, client will discuss with nurse or therapist behaviors that impede the development of satisfactory interpersonal relationships.

Long-Term Goal

■ By the time of discharge from treatment, client will interact appropriately with others in the therapy setting in both social and therapeutic activities (evidencing a discontinuation of splitting and clinging and distancing behaviors).

Interventions

■ Encourage the client to examine these behaviors (to recognize that they are occurring). He or she may be unaware of splitting or of clinging and distancing pattern of interaction with others. Recognition must take place before change can occur.

■ Help the client understand that you will be available, without reinforcing dependent behaviors. Knowledge of your availability may provide needed security.

■ Rotate staff members who work with the client in order to avoid his or her developing a dependence on particular individuals. The client must learn to relate to more than one staff member in an effort to decrease the use of splitting and to diminish fears of abandonment.

■ With the client, explore feelings that relate to fears of abandonment and engulfment. Help him or her to understand that clinging and distancing behaviors are engendered by these fears. Exploration of feelings with a trusted individual may help the client come to terms with unresolved issues.

■ Help the client understand how these behaviors interfere with satisfactory relationships.

He or she may be unaware of how others perceive these behaviors and why they are not acceptable.

■ Assist the client to work toward achievement of object constancy. Be available, without promoting dependency. Give positive reinforcement for independent behaviors. The client must resolve fears of abandonment in the process toward developing the ability to establish satisfactory intimate relationships.

> **CLINICAL PEARL** Recognize when the client is playing one staff member against another. Remember that splitting is the primary defense mechanism of these individuals, and the impressions they have of others as either "good" or "bad" are a manifestation of this defense. Do not listen as client tries to degrade other staff members. Suggest that the client discuss the problem directly with the staff person involved.

Concept Care Mapping

The concept map care plan is an innovative approach to planning and organizing nursing care (see Chapter 9). It is a diagrammatic teaching and learning strategy that allows visualization of interrelationships between medical diagnoses, nursing diagnoses, assessment data, and treatments. An example of a concept map care plan for a client with borderline personality disorder is presented in Figure 34–1.

Evaluation

Reassessment is conducted to determine if the nursing actions have been successful in achieving the objectives of care. Evaluation of the nursing actions for the client with borderline personality disorder may be facilitated by gathering information using the following types of questions:

■ Has the client been able to seek out staff when feeling the desire for self-harm?

■ Has the client avoided self-harm?

■ Can the client correlate times of desire for self-harm to times of elevation in level of anxiety?

■ Can the client discuss feelings with staff (particularly feelings of depression and anger)?

■ Can the client identify the true source toward which the anger is directed?

■ Can the client verbalize understanding of the basis for his or her anger?

■ Can the client express anger appropriately?

■ Can the client function independently?

Clinical Vignette: Clara, age 37, was diagnosed with Borderline Personality Disorder when she was 22 years old. She has had counseling with the same therapist since the initial diagnosis. She suffers from chronic depression and unstable personality. Two days ago, at her regular counseling session, the therapist told Clara that in one month she was getting married and would be moving across the country with her new husband. She told Clara she would help her find a new therapist. Clara became hysterical and shouted, "You can't leave me! I don't want another therapist!" That evening, Clara's husband, Bill, found her sitting in a pool of blood by the bathtub, having sliced the back of both calves with a razor blade. Bill took Clara to the hospital where she is well known by the staff. Her wounds were treated in the emergency department, and she was transferred to the psychiatric unit. She clings to the admitting nurse saying, "Please don't leave. You're the best nurse here. You're the only one I can talk to." The nurse develops the following concept map care plan for Clara.

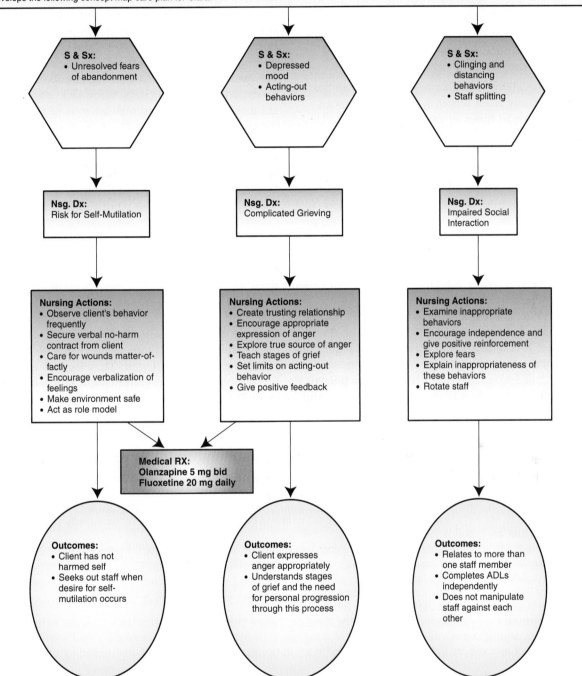

S & Sx:
• Unresolved fears of abandonment

S & Sx:
• Depressed mood
• Acting-out behaviors

S & Sx:
• Clinging and distancing behaviors
• Staff splitting

Nsg. Dx:
Risk for Self-Mutilation

Nsg. Dx:
Complicated Grieving

Nsg. Dx:
Impaired Social Interaction

Nursing Actions:
• Observe client's behavior frequently
• Secure verbal no-harm contract from client
• Care for wounds matter-of-factly
• Encourage verbalization of feelings
• Make environment safe
• Act as role model

Nursing Actions:
• Create trusting relationship
• Encourage appropriate expression of anger
• Explore true source of anger
• Teach stages of grief
• Set limits on acting-out behavior
• Give positive feedback

Nursing Actions:
• Examine inappropriate behaviors
• Encourage independence and give positive reinforcement
• Explore fears
• Explain inappropriateness of these behaviors
• Rotate staff

Medical RX:
Olanzapine 5 mg bid
Fluoxetine 20 mg daily

Outcomes:
• Client has not harmed self
• Seeks out staff when desire for self-mutilation occurs

Outcomes:
• Client expresses anger appropriately
• Understands stages of grief and the need for personal progression through this process

Outcomes:
• Relates to more than one staff member
• Completes ADLs independently
• Does not manipulate staff against each other

FIGURE 34–1   Concept map care plan for a client with borderline personality disorder.

■ Can the client relate to more than one staff member?

■ Can the client verbalize the knowledge that the staff members will return and are not abandoning the client when leaving for the day?

■ Can the client separate from the staff in an appropriate manner?

■ Can the client delay gratification and refrain from manipulating others in order to fulfill own desires?

■ Can the client verbalize resources within the community from whom he or she may seek assistance in times of extreme stress?

Antisocial Personality Disorder (Background Assessment Data)

In the *DSM-I*, antisocial behavior was categorized as a "sociopathic or psychopathic" reaction that was symptomatic of any of several underlying personality disorders. The *DSM-II* represented it as a separate personality type, a distinction that has been retained in subsequent editions. The *DSM-IV-TR* diagnostic criteria for antisocial personality disorder are presented in Box 34-11.

Individuals with antisocial personality disorder are seldom seen in most clinical settings, and when they are, it is commonly a way to avoid legal consequences. Sometimes they are admitted to the health-care system by court order for psychological evaluation. Most frequently, however, these individuals may be encountered in prisons, jails, and rehabilitation services.

Clinical Picture

Antisocial personality disorder is a pattern of socially irresponsible, exploitative, and guiltless behavior that reflects a general disregard for the rights of others. These individuals exploit and manipulate others for personal gain and are unconcerned with obeying the law. They have difficulty sustaining consistent employment and developing stable relationships. They appear cold and callous, often intimidating others with their brusque and belligerent manner. They tend to be argumentative and, at times, cruel and malicious. They lack warmth and compassion and are often suspicious of these qualities in others.

Individuals with antisocial personality have a very low tolerance for frustration, act impetuously, and are unable to delay gratification. They are restless and easily bored, often taking chances and seeking thrills, as if they were immune to danger.

When things go their way, individuals with this disorder act cheerful, even gracious and charming. Because of their low tolerance for frustration, this pleasant exterior can change very quickly. When what they desire at the moment is challenged, they are likely to become furious and vindictive. Easily provoked to attack, their first inclination is to demean and dominate. They believe that "good guys come in last," and show contempt for the weak and underprivileged. They exploit others to fulfill their own desires, showing no trace of shame or guilt for their behavior.

Individuals with antisocial personalities see themselves as victims, using projection as the

---

BOX 34-11 Diagnostic Criteria for Antisocial Personality Disorder

A. There is a pervasive pattern of disregard for and violation of the rights of others occurring since age 15 years, as indicated by three (or more) of the following:
   1. Failure to conform to social norms with respect to lawful behaviors as indicated by repeatedly performing acts that are grounds for arrest.
   2. Deceitfulness, as indicated by repeated lying, use of aliases, or conning others for personal profit or pleasure.
   3. Impulsivity or failure to plan ahead.
   4. Irritability and aggressiveness, as indicated by repeated physical fights or assaults.
   5. Reckless disregard for safety of self or others.
   6. Consistent irresponsibility, as indicated by repeated failure to sustain consistent work behavior or honor financial obligations.
   7. Lack of remorse, as indicated by being indifferent to or rationalizing having hurt, mistreated, or stolen from another.
B. Individual is at least 18 years old.
C. There is evidence of conduct disorder with onset before age 15 years.
D. The occurrence of antisocial behavior is not exclusively during the course of schizophrenia or a manic episode

From American Psychiatric Association. (2000). Diagnostic and statistical manual of mental disorders (4th ed.). Text revision. Washington, DC: American Psychiatric Publishing, with permission.

primary ego defense mechanism. They do not accept responsibility for the consequences of their behavior. Gorman and Sultan (2008) stated:

> Manipulative individuals have come to suspect that any person or institution may try to control them, rendering them powerless and vulnerable to attack. (p. 195)

In their own minds, this perception justifies their malicious behavior, lest they be the recipient of unjust persecution and hostility from others.

Satisfying interpersonal relationships are not possible because individuals with antisocial personalities have learned to place their trust only in themselves. They have a philosophy that "everyone is out to 'help number one' and that one should stop at nothing to avoid being pushed around" (APA, 2000, p. 703).

One of the most distinctive characteristics of antisocial personalities is their tendency to ignore conventional authority and rules. They act as though established social norms and guidelines for self-discipline and cooperative behavior do not apply to them. They are flagrant in their disrespect for the law and for the rights of others.

Predisposing Factors to Antisocial Personality Disorder

Biological Influences

The *DSM-IV-TR* reports that antisocial personality is more common among first-degree biological relatives of those with the disorder than among the general population (APA, 2000). Twin and adoptive studies have implicated the role of genetics in antisocial personality disorder (Skodol & Gunderson, 2008). These studies of families of individuals with antisocial personality show higher numbers of relatives with antisocial personality or alcoholism than are found in the general population. The studies have also shown that children of parents with antisocial behavior are more likely to be diagnosed with antisocial personality, even when they are separated at birth from their biological parents and reared by individuals without the disorder.

Characteristics associated with temperament in the newborn may be significant in the predisposition to antisocial personality. Parents who bring their children with behavior disorders to clinics often report that the child displayed temper tantrums from infancy and would become furious when awaiting a bottle or a diaper change. As these children mature, they commonly develop a bullying attitude toward other children. Parents report that they are undaunted by punishment and generally quite unmanageable. These children are daring and foolhardy in their willingness to chance physical harm, and they seem unaffected by pain.

Fischer and associates (2002) identified attention-deficit/hyperactivity disorder and conduct disorder during childhood and adolescence as predisposing factors to antisocial personality disorder.

Although these biogenetic influences may describe some familial pattern to the development of antisocial personality disorder, no basic pathological process has yet been determined as an etiological factor. Bienenfeld (2010) stated:

> Low levels of behavioral inhibition may be mediated by serotonergic dysregulation in the septohippocampal system. There may also be developmental or acquired abnormalities in the prefrontal brain systems and reduced autonomic activity in antisocial personality disorder. This may underlie the low arousal, poor fear conditioning, and decision-making deficits described in antisocial personality disorder.

Family Dynamics

Antisocial personality disorder frequently arises from a chaotic home environment. Parental deprivation during the first 5 years of life appears to be a critical predisposing factor in the development of antisocial personality disorder. Separation due to parental delinquency appears to be more highly correlated with the disorder than is parental loss from other causes. The presence or intermittent appearance of inconsistent impulsive parents, not the loss of a consistent parent, is environmentally *most* damaging.

Studies have shown that individuals with antisocial personality disorder often have been severely physically abused in childhood. The abuse contributes to the development of antisocial behavior in several ways. First, it provides a model for behavior. Second, it may result in injury to the child's central nervous system, thereby impairing the child's ability to function appropriately. Finally, it engenders rage in the victimized child, which is then displaced onto others in the environment.

IMPLICATIONS OF RESEARCH FOR EVIDENCE-BASED PRACTICE

Dekovic, M., Janssens, J. A. M., & Van As, N. M. C. (2003). Family predictors of antisocial behavior in adolescence. *Family Process, 42,* 223–235.

DESCRIPTION OF THE STUDY: The objective of this study was to examine the combined and unique ability of different aspects of family functioning to predict involvement in antisocial behavior in a large community (nonclinical) sample of adolescents. The aspects of family functioning that were measured included:

1. *Proximal factors:* parental childrearing behaviors and the quality of the parent-adolescent relationship.
2. *Distal factors:* parental characteristics (e.g., depression; parental confidence in his or her competence as a parent)
3. *Contextual factors:* family characteristics (e.g., family cohesion, quality of the marital relationship; involvement between members)
4. *Global factors:* family socioeconomic status; family composition (e.g., single-parent family)

The researchers hypothesized that proximal factors would play a stronger role in future antisocial behavior than the other three variables. The sample included 508 families with an adolescent between 12 and 18 years. There were 254 females and 254 males. The parent sample consisted of 969 parents (502 mothers and 467 fathers). Ninety-one percent of the families were intact families, 7 percent of the parents were divorced or separated, and 2 percent were widowed. There was a wide range of socioeconomic and educational backgrounds, although the parents with low educational and occupational levels were slightly underrepresented. Data were gathered in the subjects' homes through a battery of questionnaires administered individually to adolescents, mothers, and fathers.

RESULTS OF THE STUDY: Results showed that proximal factors were significant predictors of antisocial behavior, independent of their shared variance with other factors. Also consistent with the hypothesized model, the effects of distal and contextual factors appear to be mostly indirect: after their association with proximal factors was taken into account, these factors were no longer significantly related to antisocial behavior. Global indicators of family functioning (socioeconomic status and family composition) were unrelated to adolescent antisocial behavior. This study showed that supportive parents, parents who use more subtle means of guidance (i.e., supervision rather than punitive strategies), and parents who are consistent in their behavior toward adolescents have a lower risk that their child would become involved in antisocial behavior. Adolescents who are exposed to coercive and hostile parenting probably adopt this aggressive style of interacting with others. The parent-adolescent relationship that was characterized by elevated levels of conflict and a lack of closeness and acceptance emerged as a risk factor for involvement in antisocial behavior. Parental depression, conflict in the marital dyad, and lack of cohesion between members were also found to influence adolescent antisocial behavior, but less directly than the proximal factors.

IMPLICATIONS FOR NURSING PRACTICE: Nurses must use this information to design and implement effective parenting programs. Nurses can become actively involved in teaching parents, in inpatient, outpatient, and community education programs. The researchers stated, "The findings of this study suggest that, when designing interventions that focus on family factors, in addition to teaching parents adequate childrearing skills, more attention should be given to finding methods to improve the general *quality* of the parent-adolescent relationship."

A number of factors associated with disordered family functioning have been implicated in the development of antisocial personality (Hill, 2003; Ramsland, 2010; Skodol & Gunderson, 2008). The following circumstances may influence the predisposition to antisocial personality disorder:

■ Absence of parental discipline

■ Extreme poverty

■ Removal from the home

■ Growing up without parental figures of both sexes

■ Erratic and inconsistent methods of discipline

■ Being "rescued" each time they are in trouble (never having to suffer the consequences of one's own behavior)

■ Maternal deprivation

Diagnosis/Outcome Identification

Nursing diagnoses are formulated from the data gathered during the assessment phase and with background knowledge regarding predisposing factors to the disorder. Table 34-4 presents a list of client behaviors and the NANDA nursing diagnoses that correspond to those behaviors, which may be used in planning care for clients with antisocial personality disorder.

TABLE 34-4 Assigning Nursing Diagnoses to Behaviors Commonly Associated with Antisocial Personality Disorder

BEHAVIORS	NURSING DIAGNOSES
Body language (e.g., rigid posture, clenching of fists and jaw, hyperactivity, pacing, breathlessness, threatening stances); cruelty to animals; rage reactions; history of childhood abuse; history of violence against others; impulsivity; substance abuse; negative role modeling; inability to tolerate frustration	Risk for other-directed violence
Disregard for societal norms and laws; absence of guilty feelings; inability to delay gratification; denial of obvious problems; grandiosity; hostile laughter; projection of blame and responsibility; ridicule of others; superior attitude toward others	Defensive coping
Manipulation of others to fulfill own desires; inability to form close, personal relationships; frequent lack of success in life events; passive-aggressiveness; overt aggressiveness (hiding feelings of low self-esteem)	Chronic low-self esteem
Inability to form a satisfactory, enduring, intimate relationship with another; dysfunctional interaction with others; use of unsuccessful social interaction behaviors	Impaired social interaction
Demonstration of inability to take responsibility for meeting basic health practices; history of lack of health-seeking behavior; demonstrated lack of knowledge regarding basic health practices; lack of expressed interest in improving health behaviors	Ineffective health maintenance

Outcome Criteria

The following criteria may be used for measurement of outcomes in the care of the client with antisocial personality disorder.

The client:

■ Discusses angry feelings with staff and in group sessions.

■ Has not harmed self or others.

■ Can rechannel hostility into socially acceptable behaviors.

■ Follows rules and regulations of the therapy environment.

■ Can verbalize which of his or her behaviors are not acceptable.

■ Shows regard for the rights of others by delaying gratification of own desires when appropriate.

■ Does not manipulate others in an attempt to increase feelings of self-worth.

■ Verbalizes understanding of knowledge required to maintain basic health needs.

Planning/Implementation

The following section presents a group of selected nursing diagnoses common to clients with antisocial personality disorder, with short- and long-term goals and nursing interventions for each.

Risk for Other-Directed Violence

Risk for other-directed violence is defined as "at risk for behaviors in which an individual demonstrates that he or she can be physically, emotionally, and/or sexually harmful to others" (NANDA-I, 2009, p. 332).

Client Goals
Outcome criteria include short- and long-term goals. Timelines are individually determined.

Short-Term Goals

■ Within 3 days, client will discuss angry feelings and situations that precipitate hostility.

■ Client will not harm others.

Long-Term Goal

■ Client will not harm others.

Interventions

■ Convey an accepting attitude toward this client. Feelings of rejection are undoubtedly familiar to him or her. Work on development of trust. Be honest, keep all promises, and convey the message to the client that it is not *him* or *her,* but the *behavior,* that is unacceptable. An attitude of acceptance promotes feelings of self-worth. Trust is the basis of a therapeutic relationship.

■ Maintain a low level of stimuli in the client's environment (low lighting, few people, simple decor, low noise level). A stimulating environment may increase agitation and promote aggressive behavior.

■ Observe the client's behavior frequently. Do this through routine activities and interactions; avoid appearing watchful and suspicious. Close observation is required so that intervention can occur if needed to ensure the client's (and others') safety.

■ Remove all dangerous objects from the client's environment so that he or she may not purposefully or inadvertently use them to inflict harm to self or others.

■ Help the client identify the true object of his or her hostility (e.g., "You seem to be upset with . . ."). Because of weak ego development, the client may be misusing the defense mechanism of displacement. Helping him or her recognize this in a nonthreatening manner may help reveal unresolved issues so that they may be confronted.

■ Encourage the client to gradually verbalize hostile feelings. Verbalization of feelings in a nonthreatening environment may help the client come to terms with unresolved issues.

■ Explore with the client alternative ways of handling frustration (e.g., large-motor skills that channel hostile energy into socially acceptable behavior). Physically demanding activities help to relieve pent-up tension.

■ The staff should maintain and convey a calm attitude toward the client. Anxiety is contagious and can be transferred from staff to client. A calm attitude provides the client with a feeling of safety and security.

■ Have sufficient staff available to present a show of strength to the client if necessary. This conveys to the client evidence of control over the situation and provides some physical security for the staff.

■ Administer tranquilizing medications as ordered by the physician or obtain an order if necessary. Monitor the client for effectiveness of the medication as well as for appearance of adverse side effects. Antianxiety agents (e.g., lorazepam, chlordiazepoxide, oxazepam) produce a calming effect and may help to allay hostile behaviors.

NOTE: Medications are not often prescribed for clients with antisocial personality disorder because of these individuals' strong susceptibility to addictions.

■ If client is not calmed by "talking down" or by medication, use of mechanical restraints may be

necessary. The avenue of the "least restrictive alternative" must be selected when planning interventions for a violent client. Restraints should be used only as a last resort, after all other interventions have been unsuccessful, and the client is clearly at risk of harm to self or others.

■ If restraint is deemed necessary, ensure that sufficient staff is available to assist. Follow protocol established by the institution. The Joint Commission (formerly the Joint Commission on Accreditation of Healthcare Organizations [JCAHO]) requires that an in-person evaluation by a physician or other licensed independent practitioner (LIP) be conducted within 1 hour of the initiation of the restraint or seclusion (The Joint Commission, 2010). The physician or LIP must reissue a new order for restraints every 4 hours for adults and every 1 to 2 hours for children and adolescents.

■ The Joint Commission requires that the client in restraints be observed at least every 15 minutes to ensure that circulation to extremities is not compromised (check temperature, color, pulses); to assist the client with needs related to nutrition, hydration, and elimination; and to position the client so that comfort is facilitated and aspiration is prevented. Some institutions may require continuous one-to-one monitoring of restrained clients, particularly those who are highly agitated, and for whom there is a high risk of self- or accidental injury.

■ As agitation decreases, assess the client's readiness for restraint removal or reduction. Remove one restraint at a time while assessing the client's response. This minimizes the risk of injury to client and staff.

Defensive Coping

Defensive coping is defined as "repeated projection of falsely positive self-evaluation based on a self-protective pattern that defends against underlying perceived threats to positive self-regard" (NANDA-I, 2009, p. 251).

Client Goals

Outcome criteria include short- and long-term goals. Timelines are individually determined.

Short-Term Goals

■ Within 24 hours after admission, client will verbalize understanding of treatment setting rules and regulations and the consequences for violation of them.

■ Client will verbalize personal responsibility for difficulties experienced in interpersonal relationships within (time period reasonable for client).

Long-Term Goals

■ By the time of discharge from treatment, the client will be able to cope more adaptively by delaying gratification of own desires and following rules and regulations of the treatment setting.

■ By the time of discharge from treatment, the client will demonstrate ability to interact with others without becoming defensive, rationalizing behaviors, or expressing grandiose ideas.

Interventions

■ From the outset, the client should be made aware of which behaviors are acceptable and which are not. Explain consequences of violation of the limits. Consequences must involve something of value to the client. All staff must be consistent in enforcing these limits. Consequences should be administered in a matter-of-fact manner immediately following the infraction. Because the client cannot (or will not) impose own limits on maladaptive behaviors, these behaviors must be delineated and limits enforced by staff. Undesirable consequences may help to decrease repetition of these behaviors.

■ The ideal goal would be for this client to eventually internalize societal norms, beginning with a step-by-step, "either/or" approach on the unit (*either* you do [don't do] this, *or* this will occur). Explanations must be concise, concrete, and clear, with little or no capacity for misinterpretation.

CLINICAL PEARL 💬

Do not attempt to coax or convince the client to do the "right thing." Do not use the words "You should (or shouldn't) . . ."; instead, use the words "You will be expected to . . ."

■ Provide positive feedback or reward for acceptable behaviors. Positive reinforcement enhances self-esteem and encourages repetition of desirable behaviors.

■ In an attempt to assist the client to delay gratification, begin to increase the length of time requirement for acceptable behavior in order to achieve the reward. For example, 2 hours of acceptable behavior may be exchanged for a phone call; 4 hours of acceptable behavior for 2 hours of television; 1 day of acceptable behavior for a recreational therapy bowling activity; 5 days of acceptable behavior for a weekend pass.

■ A milieu unit provides the appropriate environment for the client with antisocial personality. The democratic approach, with specific rules and regulations, community meetings, and group therapy sessions, emulates the type of societal situation in which the client must learn to live. Feedback from peers is often more effective than confrontation from an authority figure. The client learns to follow the rules of the group as a positive step in the progression toward internalizing the rules of society.

■ Help the client to gain insight into his or her own behavior. Often, these individuals rationalize to such an extent that they deny that their behavior is inappropriate. For example, thinking may be reflected in statements such as: "The owner of this store has so much money, he'll never miss the little bit I take. He has everything, and I have nothing. It's not fair! I deserve to have some of what he has." The client must come to understand that certain behaviors will not be tolerated within the society and that severe consequences will be imposed on those individuals who refuse to comply. The client must *want* to become a productive member of society before he or she can be helped.

■ Talk about past behaviors with the client. Discuss which behaviors are acceptable by societal norms and which are not. Help the client identify ways in which he or she has exploited others. Encourage the client to explore how he or she would feel if the circumstances were reversed. An attempt may be made to enlighten the client to the sensitivity of others by promoting self-awareness in an effort to help the client gain insight into his or her own behavior.

■ Throughout the relationship with the client, maintain an attitude of "It is not *you*, but *your behavior*, that is unacceptable." An attitude of acceptance promotes feelings of dignity and self-worth.

Concept Care Mapping

The concept map care plan is an innovative approach to planning and organizing nursing care (see Chapter 9). It is a diagrammatic teaching and learning strategy that allows visualization of interrelationships between medical diagnoses, nursing diagnoses, assessment data, and treatments. An example of a concept map care plan for a client with antisocial personality disorder is presented in Figure 34–2.

Clinical Vignette: Hank, age 32, is the oldest of 5 children of a single mother, each of whom had a different father. He was physically abused by his mother's boyfriends, did not attend school regularly, and eventually dropped out in 10th grade. He has a history of violence, always carries a weapon (gun or knife) on his person, and threatens to use it if he is challenged in his attempts to fulfill his own desires. He has had numerous skirmishes with the law, from shoplifting, auto theft, possession and sale of heroin and cocaine, and most recently, armed robbery of a liquor store. He was identified by his image on the store's surveillance camera. Because of his long history of criminal behavior, the judge has ordered that Hank undergo psychological testing before handing down his sentence. On the psychiatric unit he says to the nurse, "Why am I here? I'm not crazy! And I've never hurt anybody! I don't belong in this loony bin!" The nurse develops the following concept map care plan for Hank.

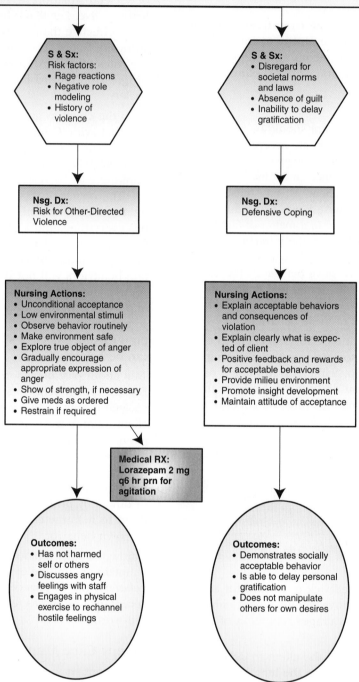

FIGURE 34–2   Concept map care plan for a client with antisocial personality disorder.

Evaluation

Reassessment is conducted to determine if the nursing actions have been successful in achieving the objectives of care. Evaluation of the nursing actions for the client with antisocial personality disorder may be facilitated by gathering information using the following types of questions:

■ Does the client recognize when anger is getting out of control?

■ Can the client seek out staff instead of expressing anger in an inappropriate manner?

■ Can the client use other sources for rechanneling anger (e.g., physical activities)?

■ Has harm to others been avoided?

■ Can the client follow rules and regulations of the therapeutic milieu with little or no reminding?

■ Can the client verbalize which behaviors are appropriate and which are not?

■ Does the client express a desire to change?

■ Can the client delay gratifying own desires in deference to those of others when appropriate?

■ Does the client refrain from manipulating others to fulfill own desires?

■ Does the client fulfill activities of daily living willingly and independently?

■ Can the client verbalize methods of achieving and maintaining optimal wellness?

■ Can the client verbalize community resources from which he or she can seek assistance with daily living and health-care needs when required?

Treatment Modalities

Few would argue that treatment of individuals with personality disorders is difficult and, in some instances, may even seem impossible. Personality characteristics are learned very early in life and perhaps may even be genetic. It is not surprising, then, that these enduring patterns of behavior may take years to change, if change occurs. Skodol and Gunderson (2008) stated,

> Because personality disorders have been thought to consist of deeply ingrained attitudes and behavior patterns that consolidate during development and have endured since early adulthood, they have traditionally been believed to be very resistant to change.

Moreover, treatment efforts are further confounded by the degree to which patients with a personality disorder do not recognize their maladaptive personality traits as undesirable or in need of change. (p. 831)

Most clinicians believe it best to strive for lessening the inflexibility of the maladaptive traits and reducing their interference with everyday functioning and meaningful relationships. Little research exists to guide the decision of which therapy is most appropriate in the treatment of personality disorders. Selection of intervention is generally based on the area of greatest dysfunction, such as cognition, affect, behavior, or interpersonal relations. Following is a brief description of various types of therapies and the disorders to which they are customarily suited.

Interpersonal Psychotherapy

Depending on the therapeutic goals, interpersonal psychotherapy with personality disorders is brief and time-limited, or it may involve long-term exploratory psychotherapy. Interpersonal psychotherapy may be particularly appropriate because personality disorders largely reflect problems in interpersonal style.

Long-term psychotherapy attempts to understand and modify the maladjusted behaviors, cognition, and affects of clients with personality disorders that dominate their personal lives and relationships. The core element of treatment is the establishment of an empathic therapist-client relationship based on collaboration and guided discovery in which the therapist functions as a role model for the client.

Interpersonal psychotherapy is suggested for clients with paranoid, schizoid, schizotypal, borderline, dependent, narcissistic, and obsessive-compulsive personality disorders.

Psychoanalytic Psychotherapy

The treatment of choice for individuals with histrionic personality disorder has been psychoanalytic psychotherapy (Skodol & Gunderson, 2008). Treatment focuses on the unconscious motivation for seeking total satisfaction from others and for being unable to commit oneself to a stable, meaningful relationship.

Milieu or Group Therapy

This treatment is especially appropriate for individuals with antisocial personality disorder, who respond more adaptively to support and feedback from peers. In milieu or group therapy, feedback from peers is more effective than in one-to-one interaction with a therapist. Group therapy—particularly homogeneous supportive groups that emphasize the development of social skills—may be helpful in overcoming social anxiety and developing interpersonal trust and rapport in clients with avoidant personality disorder. Feminist consciousness-raising groups can be useful in helping dependent clients struggling with social-role stereotypes.

Cognitive-Behavioral Therapy

Behavioral strategies offer reinforcement for positive change. Social skills training and assertiveness training teach alternative ways to deal with frustration. Cognitive strategies help the client recognize and correct inaccurate internal mental schemata. This type of therapy may be useful for clients with obsessive-compulsive, passive-aggressive, antisocial, and avoidant personality disorders.

Dialectical Behavior Therapy

Dialectical behavior therapy (DBT) is a type of psychotherapy that was originally developed by Marsha Linehan, Ph.D., as a treatment for the chronic self-injurious and parasuicidal behavior of clients with borderline personality disorder (Sadock & Sadock, 2007). It is a complex, eclectic treatment that combines the concepts of cognitive, behavioral, and interpersonal therapies with Eastern mindfulness practices (Dimeff & Linehan, 2001). Dimeff and Linehan (2001) identified the following five functions of DBT:

1. To enhance behavioral capabilities
2. To improve motivation to change
3. To ensure that new capabilities generalize to the natural environment
4. To structure the treatment environment such that client and therapist capabilities are supported and effective behaviors are reinforced
5. To enhance therapist capabilities and motivation to treat clients effectively

The four primary modes of treatment in DBT are the following:

1. **Group skills training.** In these groups, clients are taught skills considered relevant to the particular problems experienced by people with borderline personality disorder, such as core mindfulness skills, interpersonal effectiveness skills, emotion modulation skills, and distress tolerance skills (Kiehn & Swales, 2010).

2. **Individual psychotherapy.** Weekly sessions in which dysfunctional behavioral patterns, personal motivation, and skills strengthening are addressed.

3. **Telephone contact.** The therapist is available to the client by telephone, usually on a 24-hour per day basis, but according to limits set by the therapist. Kiehn and Swales (2010) stated, "Telephone contact is to give the patient help and support in applying the skills that she is learning to her real life situation between sessions and to help her find ways of avoiding self-injury."

4. **Therapist consultation/team meeting.** Therapists meet regularly to review their work with their clients. These meetings are focused specifically on providing support for each other, keeping the therapists motivated, and providing effective treatment to their clients (Dimeff & Linehan, 2001).

In controlled studies, DBT has been shown to diminish self-destructive behaviors in clients with borderline personality disorder. Additionally, DBT has shown to decrease the drop-out rate from treatment and the number of hospitalizations. Improvement has also been shown in reducing anger and in global and social adjustment scores (Dimeff & Linehan, 2001). This method of treatment is now being used with other disorders, including substance use disorders, eating disorders, schizphrenia, and posttraumatic stress disorder (Sadock & Sadock, 2007).

Psychopharmacology

Psychopharmacology may be helpful in some instances. Although these drugs have no effect in the direct treatment of the disorder itself, some symptomatic relief can be achieved. Antipsychotic medications are helpful in the treatment of psychotic decompensations experienced by clients with paranoid, schizotypal, and borderline personality disorders (Skodol & Gunderson, 2008).

A variety of pharmacological interventions have been used with borderline personality disorder. The selective serotonin reuptake inhibitors (SSRIs) and monoamine oxidase inhibitors (MAOIs) have been successful in decreasing impulsivity and self-destructive acts in these clients. The MAOIs are not commonly used, however, because of concerns about violations of dietary restrictions and the higher risk of fatality with overdose. The combination of an SSRI and an atypical antipsychotic has been successful in treating dysphoria, mood instability, and impulsivity in clients with borderline personality disorder (Schatzberg, Cole, & DeBattista, 2010). Antipsychotics have resulted in

improvement in illusions, ideas of reference, paranoid thinking, anxiety, and hostility in some clients.

IMPLICATIONS OF RESEARCH FOR EVIDENCE-BASED PRACTICE

Nickel, M. K., Muehlbacher, M., Nickel, C., Kettler, C., Gil, F. P., Bachler, E., et al. (2006). Aripiprazole in the treatment of patients with borderline personality disorder: A double-blind, placebo-controlled study. American Journal of Psychiatry, 163, 833–838.

DESCRIPTION OF THE STUDY: The purpose of this study was to determine whether aripiprazole is effective in the treatment of several domains of symptoms of borderline personality disorder (BPD). Subjects included 43 women and 9 men who met the DSM criteria for BPD. Subjects were randomly assigned to 15 mg/day of aripiprazole or placebo for 8 weeks. Outcome measures included changes in scores on the symptom checklist (SCL-90-R), the Hamilton Depression Rating Scale (HAM-D), the Hamilton Anxiety Rating Scale (HAM-A), and the State-Trait Anger Expression Inventory. Test results were assessed weekly, along with side effects and self-injury reports using a nonvalidated questionnaire.

RESULTS OF THE STUDY: Aripiprazole was associated with a significantly greater rate of improvement

than the placebo group on most of the SCL-90-R scales (with the exception of somatization), as well as on the HAM-D and HAM-A, and on all of the State-Trait Anger Expression Inventory scales. Self-injury occurred during the course of the 8-week trial, but only two episodes occurred in the aripiprazole group, compared with seven in the placebo group. The most commonly reported side effects of aripiprazole included headache, insomnia, nausea, numbness, constipation, and anxiety. No significant weight changes were observed, and no serious side effects or suicidal attempts occurred during the study.

IMPLICATIONS FOR NURSING PRACTICE: The authors stated, "Aripiprazole appears to be a safe and effective agent for improving not only the symptoms of borderline personality disorder but also the associated health-related quality of life and interpersonal problems." Nurses who work with individuals who have BPD should be familiar with this medication and understand the nursing implications associated with its administration. The implications of this study are particularly significant for nurses who have prescriptive authority and treat clients with BPD.

Lithium carbonate and propranolol (Inderal) may be useful for the violent episodes observed in clients with antisocial personality disorder (Coccaro & Siever, 2000). Caution must be given to prescribing medications outside the structured setting because of the high risk for substance abuse by these individuals.

For the client with avoidant personality disorder, anxiolytics are sometimes helpful whenever

previously avoided behavior is being attempted. The mere possession of the medication may be reassurance enough to help the client through the stressful period. Antidepressants, such as sertraline (Zoloft) and paroxetine (Paxil), may be useful with these clients if panic disorder develops.

CASE STUDY AND SAMPLE CARE PLAN

NURSING HISTORY AND ASSESSMENT

Anthony, age 34, has been admitted to the psychiatric unit with a diagnosis of Antisocial Personality Disorder. He was recently arrested and convicted for armed robbery of a convenience store, and attempted murder of the store clerk. Due to the actions of the store clerk, who quickly alerted police, and to the store surveillance

camera, Anthony was identified and apprehended within hours of the crime. The judge has ordered physical, neurological, and psychiatric evaluations before sentencing Anthony.

Anthony was physically and psychologically abused as a child by his alcoholic father. He was suspended from high school because of failing grades and habitual truancy.

Continued

CASE STUDY AND SAMPLE CARE PLAN — cont'd

He has a long history of arrests, beginning with shoplifting at age 7, and progressing in adolescence to burglary, auto theft, and sexual assault, and finally to armed robbery, and attempted murder. He was out on probation when he committed his latest crime.

On the psychiatric unit, Anthony is loud, belligerent, and uncooperative. When Carol, his admitting nurse, arrives to work the evening shift on Anthony's second hospital day, he says to her, "I'm so glad you are finally here. You are the best nurse on the unit. I can't talk to anyone but you. These people are nothing but a bunch of loonies around here...and that includes staff as well as patients! Maybe you and I could walk down to the coffee shop together later. Are you married? I'd sure like to get to know you better after I get out of this loony bin!"

NURSING DIAGNOSES/OUTCOME IDENTIFICATION

From the assessment data, the nurse develops the following nursing diagnoses for Anthony:

1. **Risk for other-directed violence** related to history of violence against others and history of childhood abuse.
   a. **Short-Term Goals:** Client will discuss angry feelings and situations that precipitate hostility. Client will not harm others.
   b. **Long-Term Goal:** Client will not harm others.

2. **Defensive coping** related to low self-esteem, dysfunctional nuclear family, underdeveloped ego and superego, evidenced by absence of guilt feelings, disregard for societal laws and norms, inability to delay gratification, superior attitude toward others, denial of problems, and projection of blame and responsibility.
   a. **Short-Term Goal:** Client will verbalize understanding of unit rules and regulations and consequences for violation of them.
   b. **Long-Term Goals:** Client will be able to delay gratification and follow rules and regulations of the unit. Client will verbalize personal responsibility for own actions and behaviors.

PLANNING/IMPLEMENTATION

Risk for Other-Directed Violence

The following nursing interventions have been identified for Anthony.

1. Develop a trusting relationship with Anthony by conveying an accepting attitude. Ensure that he understands it is not *him,* but *his behavior,* that is unacceptable.

2. Try to keep excess stimuli out of the environment. Speak to Anthony in a calm, quiet voice.

3. Observe Anthony's behavior regularly. Do this through routine activity so that he doesn't become suspicious and angry about being watched. This is important so that, if hostile and aggressive behaviors are observed, intervention may prevent harm to Anthony, staff members, and/or other patients.

4. Sit with Anthony and encourage him to talk about his anger and hostile feelings. Help him understand where these feelings originate and who is the true target of the hostility.

5. Help him develop adaptive ways of dealing with frustration, such as exercise and other physical activities.

6. Administer tranquilizing medication, as ordered by the physician.

7. If Anthony should become out of control and mechanical restraints become necessary, ensure that sufficient staff is available to intervene. Do not use restraints as a punishment, but only as a protective measure for Anthony and the other patients.

Defensive Coping

The following nursing interventions have been identified for Anthony.

1. Explain to Anthony which of his behaviors are acceptable on the unit and which are not. Simply state that unacceptable behaviors will not be tolerated.

2. Determine appropriate consequences for violation of these limits (e.g., no TV or movies; no phone calls; time-out room). Ensure that all staff members follow through with these consequences.

3. Don't be taken in by this "charmer." Compliments from Anthony are another form of manipulative behavior. Explain to Anthony that you will not accept these types of comments from him, and if they continue, impose consequences.

4. Encourage Anthony to talk about his past misdeeds. Try to help him understand how he would feel if someone treated him in the manner that he has treated others.

EVALUATION

The outcome criteria for Anthony have only partially been met. Personality characteristics such as those of Anthony's are deep-rooted and enduring. He is not likely to change. Unless testing reveals a serious medical problem, Anthony will no doubt go to prison for most of the rest of his life. During his time on the psychiatric unit, harm to self and others has been avoided. He has

CASE STUDY AND SAMPLE CARE PLAN —cont'd

discussed his anger and hostile feelings with Carol and other staff members. He continues to become belligerent when told that he cannot smoke on the unit and must wait for someone to escort him to the smoking area. He yells at the other patients and calls them "loonies." He refuses to take responsibility for his actions and blames negative behavioral outcomes on others. He has begun a regular exercise program in the fitness room, and receives positive feedback from the staff for this attempt to integrate healthier coping strategies.

Summary and Key Points

■ Clients with personality disorders are undoubtedly some of the most difficult ones health-care workers are likely to encounter.

■ Personality characteristics are formed very early in life and are difficult, if not impossible, to change. In fact, some clinicians believe the therapeutic approach is not to try to change the characteristics but rather to decrease the inflexibility of the maladaptive traits and reduce their interference with everyday functioning and meaningful relationships.

■ The concept of a personality disorder has been present throughout the history of medicine. Problems have arisen in the attempt to establish a classification system for these disorders.

■ The *DSM-IV-TR* groups the personality disorders into three clusters.

■ Cluster A (behaviors described as odd or eccentric) includes paranoid, schizoid, and schizotypal personality disorders.

■ Cluster B (behaviors described as dramatic, emotional, or erratic) includes antisocial, borderline, histrionic, and narcissistic personality disorders.

■ Cluster C (behaviors described as anxious or fearful) includes avoidant, dependent, and obsessive-compulsive disorders.

■ For purposes of this text, passive-aggressive personality disorder, which the *DSM-IV-TR*

includes in "Criteria Provided for Further Study," was included with the cluster C disorders.

■ Nursing care of the client with a personality disorder is accomplished using the steps of the nursing process.

■ Other treatment modalities include interpersonal psychotherapy, psychoanalytic psychotherapy, milieu or group therapy, cognitive-behavioral therapy, dialectical behavior therapy, and psychopharmacology.

■ Individuals with borderline personality disorder may enter the health-care system because of their instability and frequent attempts at self-destructive behavior.

■ The individual with antisocial personality disorder may become part of the health-care system to avoid legal consequences or because of a court order for psychological evaluation.

■ Nurses who work in all types of clinical settings should be familiar with the characteristics associated with personality disorders.

■ Nurses working in psychiatry must be knowledgeable about appropriate intervention with these clients, for it is unlikely that they will encounter a greater professional challenge than these clients present.

 Davis*Plus* Additional info available @ davisplus.fadavis.com

Review Questions
Self-Examination/Learning Exercise

*Select the answer that is **most** appropriate for each of the following questions:*

1. Kim has a diagnosis of Borderline Personality Disorder. She often exhibits alternating clinging and distancing behaviors. The most appropriate nursing intervention with this type of behavior would be to:
   a. Encourage Kim to establish trust in one staff person, with whom all therapeutic interaction should take place.
   b. Secure a verbal contract from Kim that she will discontinue these behaviors.
   c. Withdraw attention if these behaviors continue.
   d. Rotate staff members who work with Kim so that she will learn to relate to more than one person.

2. Kim, a client diagnosed with Borderline Personality Disorder, manipulates the staff in an effort to fulfill her own desires. All of the following may be examples of manipulative behaviors in the borderline client *except:*
   a. Refusal to stay in room alone, stating, "It's so lonely."
   b. Asking Nurse Jones for cigarettes after 30 minutes, knowing the assigned nurse has explained she must wait 1 hour.
   c. Stating to Nurse Jones, "I really like having you for my nurse. You're the best one around here."
   d. Cutting arms with razor blade after discussing dismissal plans with physician.

3. "Splitting" by the client with borderline personality disorder denotes:
   a. Evidence of precocious development.
   b. A primitive defense mechanism in which the client sees objects as all good or all bad.
   c. A brief psychotic episode in which the client loses contact with reality.
   d. Two distinct personalities within the borderline client.

4. According to Margaret Mahler, predisposition to borderline personality disorder occurs when developmental tasks go unfulfilled in which of the following phases?
   a. Autistic phase, during which the child's needs for security and comfort go unfulfilled.
   b. Symbiotic phase, during which the child fails to bond with the mother.
   c. Differentiation phase, during which the child fails to recognize a separateness between self and mother.
   d. Rapprochement phase, during which the mother withdraws emotional support in response to the child's increasing independence.

5. Jack is a new client on the psychiatric unit with a diagnosis of Antisocial Personality Disorder. Which of the following characteristics would you expect to assess in Jack?
   a. Lack of guilt for wrongdoing.
   b. Insight into his own behavior.
   c. Ability to learn from past experiences.
   d. Compliance with authority.

6. Milieu therapy is a good choice for clients with antisocial personality disorder because it:
   a. Provides a system of punishment and rewards for behavior modification.
   b. Emulates a social community in which the client may learn to live harmoniously with others.
   c. Provides mostly one-to-one interaction between the client and therapist.
   d. Provides a very structured setting in which the clients have very little input into the planning of their care.

Review Questions—cont'd
Self-Examination/Learning Exercise

7. In evaluating the progress of Jack, a client diagnosed with Antisocial Personality Disorder, which of the following behaviors would be considered the most significant indication of positive change?
   a. Jack got angry only once in group this week.
   b. Jack was able to wait a whole hour for a cigarette without verbally abusing the staff.
   c. On his own initiative, Jack sent a note of apology to a man he had injured in a recent fight.
   d. Jack stated that he would no longer start any more fights.

8. Donna and Katie work in the secretarial pool of a large organization. It is 30 minutes until quitting time when a supervisor hands Katie a job that will take an hour and says he wants it before she leaves. She then says to Donna, "I can't stay over! I'm meeting Bill at 5 o'clock! Be a doll, Donna. Do this job for me!" Donna agrees, although silently she is furious at Katie because this is the third time this has happened in 2 weeks. Katie leaves and Donna says to herself, "This is crazy. I'm not finishing this job for her. Let's see how she likes getting in trouble for a change." Donna leaves without finishing the job. This is an example of which type of personality characteristic?
   a. Antisocial.
   b. Paranoid.
   c. Passive-aggressive.
   d. Obsessive-compulsive.

9. Carol is a new nursing graduate being oriented on a medical/surgical unit by the head nurse, Mrs. Carey. When Carol describes a new technique she has learned for positioning immobile clients, Mrs. Carey states, "What are you trying to do . . . tell me how to do my job? We have always done it this way on this unit, and we will continue to do it this way until I say differently!" This is an example of which type of personality characteristic?
   a. Antisocial.
   b. Paranoid.
   c. Passive-aggressive.
   d. Obsessive-compulsive.

10. Which of the following behavioral patterns is characteristic of individuals with histrionic personality disorder?
   a. Belittling themselves and their abilities.
   b. Overreacting to minor stimuli.
   c. Suspicious and mistrustful of others.
   d. A lifelong pattern of social withdrawal.

TEST YOUR CRITICAL THINKING SKILLS

Lana, age 32, was diagnosed with borderline personality disorder when she was 26 years old. Her husband took her to the emergency department when he walked into the bathroom and found her cutting her legs with a razor blade. At that time, assessment revealed that Lana had a long history of self-mutilation, which she had carefully hidden from her husband and others. Lana began long-term psychoanalytic psychotherapy on an outpatient basis. Therapy revealed that Lana had been physically and sexually abused as a child by both her mother and her father, both now deceased. She admitted to having chronic depression, and her husband related episodes of rage reactions. Lana has been hospitalized on the psychiatric unit for a week because of suicidal ideations. After making a no-suicide contract with the staff, she is allowed to leave the unit on pass to keep a dental appointment that she made a number of weeks ago. She has just returned to the unit and says to her nurse, "I just took 20 Desyrel while I was sitting in my car in the parking lot."

Answer the following questions related to Lana:

1. The nurse is well acquainted with Lana and believes this is a manipulative gesture. How should the nurse handle this situation?

2. What is the priority nursing diagnosis for Lana?

3. Lana likes to "split" the staff into "good guys" and "bad guys." What is the most important intervention for splitting by a person with borderline personality disorder?

References

American Psychiatric Association. (2000). *Diagnostic and statistical manual of mental disorders* (4th ed.). *Text revision.* Washington, DC: American Psychiatric Publishing.

Bienenfeld, D. (2010). Personality disorders. Retrieved October 4, 2010, from http://emedicine.medscape.com/article/294307-overview

Bosson, J. K., & Prewitt-Freilino, J. L. (2007). Overvalued and ashamed: Considering the roles of self-esteem and self-conscious emotions in covert narcissism. In J. L. Tracy, R. W. Robins, & J. P. Tangney (Eds.), *The self-conscious emotions: Theory and research* (pp. 407–425). New York: Guilford Press.

Coccaro, E. F., & Siever, L. J. (2000). The neuropsychopharmacology of personality disorders. *Psychopharmacology: The fourth generation of progress.* The American College of Neuropsychopharmacology. Retrieved October 1, 2010, from http://www.acnp.org/G4/GN401000152/CH148.html

Cummings, J. L., & Mega, M. S. (2003). *Neuropsychiatry and behavioral neuroscience.* New York: Oxford University Press.

Dimeff, L., & Linehan, M. M. (2001). Dialectical behavior therapy in a nutshell. *The California Psychologist, 34,* 10–13.

Fischer, M., Barkley, R. A., Smallish, L., & Fletcher, K. (2002). Young adult follow-up of hyperactive children: Self-reported psychiatric disorders, comorbidity, and the role of childhood conduct problems and teen CD. *Journal of Abnormal Child Psychology, 30,* 463–475.

Gorman, L., & Sultan, D. F. (2008). *Psychosocial nursing for general patient care* (3rd ed.). Philadelphia: F.A. Davis.

Hill, J. (2003). Early identification of individuals at risk for antisocial personality disorder. *British Journal of Psychiatry, 182*(Suppl. 44), s11–s14.

Kiehn, B., & Swales, M. (2010). An overview of dialectical behaviour therapy in the treatment of borderline personality disorder. *Psychiatry Online.* Retrieved October 4, 2010, from http://www.priory.com/dbt.htm

Lubit, R. H. (2010). Borderline personality disorder. *eMedicine Psychiatry.* Retrieved October 1, 2010, from http://emedicine.medscape.com/article/913575-overview

Martinez-Lewi, L. (2008). *Freeing yourself from the narcissist in your life.* New York: Penguin Group.

Millon, T. (2004). *Personality disorders in modern life* (2nd ed.). Hoboken, NJ: John Wiley and Sons.

NANDA International. (2009). *Nursing diagnoses: Definitions and classification 2009–2011.* Hoboken, NJ: Wiley-Blackwell.

National Institute of Mental Health. (2010). *Borderline personality disorder: Raising questions, finding answers.* Retrieved October 4, 2010, from http://www.nimh.nih.gov/health/publications/borderline-personality-disorder-fact-sheet/index.shtml

Oldham, J. M., Gabbard, G. O., Goin, M. K., Gunderson, J., Soloff, P., Spiegel, D., et al. (2006). Practice guideline for the treatment of patients with borderline personality disorder. In *The American Psychiatric Association Practice Guidelines for the Treatment of Psychiatric Disorders, Compendium 2006.* Washington, DC: American Psychiatric Publishing.

Ramsland, K. (2010). *The childhood psychopath: Bad seed or bad parents?* Retrieved October 4, 2010, from http://www.trutv.com/library/crime/criminal_mind/psychology/psychopath/2.html

Rettew, D. C., Jellinek, M. S., & Doyle, A. C. (2010). *Avoidant personality disorder.* Retrieved August 18, 2011, from http://www.emedicine.medscape.com/article/913360-overview

Sadock, B. J., & Sadock, V. A. (2007). *Synopsis of psychiatry: Behavioral sciences/clinical psychiatry* (10th ed.). Philadelphia: Lippincott Williams & Wilkins.

Skodol, A. E., & Gunderson, J. G. (2008). Personality disorders. In R. E. Hales, S. C. Yudofsky, & G. O. Gabbard (Eds.), *Textbook of psychiatry* (5th ed., pp. 821–859). Washington, DC: American Psychiatric Publishing.

Schatzberg, A. F., Cole, J. O., & DeBattista, C. (2010). *Manual of clinical psychopharmacology* (7th ed.). Washington, DC: American Psychiatric Publishing.

The Joint Commission. (2010, January). *The comprehensive accreditation manual for hospitals: The official handbook.* Oakbrook Terrace, IL: Joint Commission Resources.

Classical References

Erikson, E. (1963). *Childhood and society* (2nd ed.). New York: WW Norton.

Mahler, M., Pine, F., & Bergman, A. (1975). *The psychological birth of the human infant.* New York: Basic Books.

Sullivan, H. S. (1953). *The interpersonal theory of psychiatry.* New York: WW Norton.

@ INTERNET REFERENCES

- Additional information about personality disorders may be located at the following websites:
  - http://www.mentalhealth.com/dis/p20-pe04.html
  - http://www.mentalhealth.com/dis/p20-pe08.html
  - http://www.mentalhealth.com/dis/p20-pe05.html
  - http://www.mentalhealth.com/dis/p20-pe09.html
  - http://www.mentalhealth.com/dis/p20-pe06.html
  - http://www.mentalhealth.com/dis/p20-pe07.html
  - http://www.mentalhealth.com/dis/p20-pe10.html
  - http://www.mentalhealth.com/dis/p20-pe01.html
  - http://www.mentalhealth.com/dis/p20-pe02.html
  - http://www.mentalhealth.com/dis/p20-pe03.html
  - http://www.mentalhealth.com/p13.html#Per

 ## MOVIE CONNECTIONS

Taxi Driver (schizoid personality) • *One Flew Over the Cuckoo's Nest* (antisocial) • *The Boston Strangler* (antisocial) • *Just Cause* (antisocial) • *The Dream Team* (antisocial) • *Goodfellas* (antisocial) • *Fatal Attraction* (borderline) • *Play Misty for Me* (borderline) • *Girl, Interrupted* (borderline) • *Gone With the Wind* (histrionic) • *Wall Street* (narcissistic) • *The Odd Couple* (obsessive-compulsive)

Psychiatric/Mental Health Nursing of Special Populations

The Aging Individual

KEY TERMS

attachment

bereavement overload

disengagement theory

geriatrics

gerontology

geropsychiatry

"granny-bashing"

"granny-dumping"

long-term memory

Medicaid

Medicare

menopause

osteoporosis

reminiscence therapy

short-term memory

OBJECTIVES

After reading this chapter, the student will be able to:

1. Discuss societal perspectives on aging.
2. Describe an epidemiological profile of aging in the United States.
3. Discuss various theories of aging.
4. Describe biological, psychological, socio-cultural, and sexual aspects of the normal aging process.
5. Discuss retirement as a special concern to the aging individual.
6. Explain personal and sociological perspectives of long-term care of the aging individual.
7. Describe the problem of elder abuse as it exists in today's society.
8. Discuss the implications of the increasing number of suicides among the elderly population.
9. Apply the steps of the nursing process to the care of aging individuals.

HOMEWORK ASSIGNMENT

Please read the chapter and answer the following questions:

1. Which theory of aging postulates that life span and longevity changes are predetermined?
2. How is the ability to learn affected by aging?
3. What is the most common cause of psychopathology in the elderly?
4. What are some factors that are thought to contribute to elder abuse?

What is it like to grow old? It is not likely that many people in the American culture would state that it is something they want to do. Most would agree, however, that it is "better than the alternative."

Roberts (1991) told the following often-repeated tale of Supreme Court Justice Oliver Wendell Holmes, Jr. In the year before he retired at age 91

as the oldest justice ever to sit on the Supreme Court of the United States, Holmes and his close friend Justice Louis Brandeis, then a mere 74 years old, were out for one of their frequent walks on Washington's Capitol Hill. On this particular day, the justices spotted a very attractive young woman approaching them. As she passed, Holmes paused, sighed, and said to Brandeis, "Oh, to be 70 again!"

Obviously, being old is relative to the individual experiencing it.

Growing old has not been popular among the youth-oriented American culture. However, with 66 million "baby boomers" reaching their 65th birthdays by the year 2030, greater emphasis is being placed on the needs of an aging population. The disciplines of **gerontology** (the study of the aging process), **geriatrics** (the branch of clinical medicine specializing in problems of the elderly), and **geropsychiatry** (the branch of clinical medicine specializing in psychopathology of the elderly population) are expanding rapidly in response to this predictable demand.

Growing old in a society that has been obsessed with youth may have a critical impact on the mental health of many people. This situation has serious implications for psychiatric nursing.

What is it like to grow old? More and more people will be able to answer this question as the 21st century progresses. Perhaps they will also be asking the question that Roberts (1991) asked: "How did I get here so fast?"

This chapter focuses on physical and psychological changes associated with the aging process, as well as special concerns of the elderly population, such as retirement, long-term care, elder abuse, and high suicide rates. The nursing process is presented as the vehicle for delivery of nursing care to elderly individuals.

How Old Is *Old*?

The concept of "old" has changed drastically over the years. Our prehistoric ancestors probably had a life span of 40 years, with the average individual living around 18 years. As civilization developed, mortality rates remained high as a result of periodic famine and frequent malnutrition. An improvement in the standard of living was not truly evident until about the middle of the 17th century. Since that time, assured food supply, changes in food production, better housing conditions, and more progressive medical and sanitation facilities have contributed to population growth, declining mortality rates, and substantial increases in longevity.

In 1900, the average life expectancy in the United States was 47 years, and only 4 percent of the population was age 65 or over. By 2008, the average life expectancy at birth was 77.8 years (75.3 years for men and 80.3 years for women) (National Center for Health Statistics [NCHS], 2010).

The U.S. Census Bureau has created a system for classification of older Americans:

- Older: 55 through 64 years
- Elderly: 65 through 74 years
- Aged: 75 through 84 years
- Very old: 85 years and older

Some gerontologists have elected to used a simpler classification system:

- Young old: 60 through 74 years
- Middle old: 75 through 84 years
- Old old: 85 years and older

So how old is *old*? Obviously the term cannot be defined by a number. Myths and stereotypes of aging have long obscured our understanding of the aged and the process of aging. Ideas that all elderly individuals are sick, depressed, obsessed with death, senile, and incapable of change affect the way elderly people are treated. They even shape the pattern of aging of the people who believe them. They can become self-fulfilling prophecies—people start to believe they should behave in certain ways and, therefore, act according to those beliefs. Generalized assumptions can be demeaning and interfere with the quality of life for older individuals.

Just as there are many differences in individual adaptation at earlier stages of development, so it is in the elderly population. Erikson (1963) has suggested that the mentally healthy older person possesses a sense of ego integrity and self-acceptance that will help in adapting to the ambiguities of the future with a sense of security and optimism.

Murray, Zentner, and Yakimo (2009) stated:

> [Having accomplished the earlier developmental tasks], the person accepts life as his or her own and as the only life for the self. He or she would wish for none other and would defend the meaning and the dignity of the lifestyle. The person has further refined the characteristics of maturity described for the middle-aged adult, achieving both wisdom and an enriched perspective about life and people. (p. 662)

Everyone, particularly health-care workers, should see aging people as individuals, each with specific needs and abilities, rather than as a stereotypical group. Some individuals may seem "old" at 40, whereas others may not seem "old" at 70. Variables such as attitude, mental health, physical health, and degree of independence strongly influence how an individual perceives himself or herself. Surely, in the final analysis, whether one is considered "old" must be self-determined.

Epidemiological Statistics

The Population

In 1980, Americans 65 years of age or older numbered 25.5 million. By 2009, these numbers had increased to 39.6 million, representing 12.9 percent of the population (Administration on Aging [AoA], 2010). This trend is expected to continue, with a projection for 2030 at about 72.1 million, or 19.3 percent of the population.

Marital Status

In 2008, of individuals ages 65 and older, 72 percent of men and 42 percent of women were married (AoA, 2011). Forty-two percent of all women in this age group were widowed. There were over four times as many widows as widowers, because women live longer than men and tend to marry men older than themselves.

Living Arrangements

The majority of individuals ages 65 or older live alone, with a spouse, or with relatives (AoA, 2011). At any one time, fewer than 5 percent of people in this age group live in institutions. This percentage increases dramatically with age, ranging from 0.9 percent for persons 65 to 74 years, to 3.5 percent for persons 75 to 84 years, and 14.3 percent for persons 85 and older. See Figure 35–1 for a distribution of living arrangements for noninstitutionalized persons ages 65 and older.

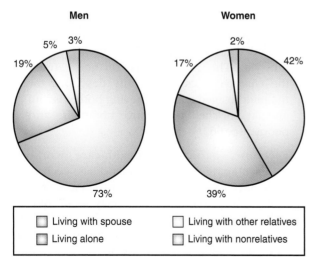

FIGURE 35–1 Living arrangements of noninstitutionalized persons ages 65 and older (NCHS, 2008).

Economic Status

Approximately 3.4 million persons ages 65 or older were below the poverty level in 2009 (AoA, 2011). Older women had a higher poverty rate than older men, and older Hispanic women living alone had the highest poverty rate. Poor people who have worked all their lives can expect to become poorer in old age, and others will become poor only after becoming old. However, there are a substantial number of affluent and middle-income older persons who enjoy a high quality of life.

Of individuals in this age group, 80 percent owned their own homes in 2009 (AoA, 2011). However, the housing of this population of Americans is usually older and less adequate than that of the younger population; therefore, a higher percentage of income must be spent on maintenance and repairs.

Employment

With the passage of the Age Discrimination in Employment Act in 1967, forced retirement has been virtually eliminated in the workplace. Evidence suggests that involvement in purposeful activity is vital to successful adaptation and perhaps even to survival. In 2009, 6.5 million Americans ages 65 and older were in the labor force (working or actively seeking work) (AoA, 2011).

Health Status

The number of days in which usual activities are restricted because of illness or injury increases with age. The Centers for Disease Control and Prevention (CDC, 2010) reported that approximately 80 percent of individuals 65 and older have at least one chronic condition, and 50 percent have at least two. The most commonly occurring conditions among the elderly population are hypertension, arthritis, heart disease, cancer, diabetes, and sinusitis (AoA, 2011).

Emotional and mental illnesses increase over the life cycle. Depression is particularly prevalent, and suicide is a serious problem among elderly Americans. Dementing disorders increase dramatically in old age.

Theories of Aging*

A number of theories related to the aging process have been described. These theories are grouped

---

*This section was adapted from M. Stanley, K. A. Blair, & P. G. Beare (2005). *Gerontological nursing: Promoting successful aging with older adults* (3rd ed.). Philadelphia: F.A. Davis, with permission.

into two broad categories: biological and psychosocial.

Biological Theories

Biological theories attempt to explain the physical process of aging, including molecular and cellular changes in the major organ systems and the body's ability to function adequately and resist disease. They also attempt to explain why people age differently and what factors affect longevity and the body's ability to resist disease.

Genetic Theory

According to genetic theory, aging is an involuntarily inherited process that operates over time to alter cellular or tissue structures. This theory suggests that life span and longevity changes are predetermined. Stanley, Blair, and Beare (2005) stated,

> [Genetic] theories posit that the replication process at the cellular level becomes deranged by inappropriate information provided from the cell nucleus. The DNA molecule becomes cross-linked with another substance that alters the genetic information. This cross-linking results in errors at the cellular level that eventually cause the body's organs and systems to fail. (p. 12)

The development of free radicals, collagen, and lipofuscin in the aging body, and of an increased frequency in the occurrence of cancer and autoimmune disorders, provide some evidence for this theory and the proposition that error or mutation occurs at the molecular and cellular level.

Wear-and-Tear Theory

Proponents of this theory believe that the body wears out on a scheduled basis. Free radicals, which are the waste products of metabolism, accumulate and cause damage to important biological structures. Free radicals are molecules with unpaired electrons that exist normally in the body; they also are produced by ionizing radiation, ozone, and chemical toxins. According to this theory, these free radicals cause DNA damage, cross-linkage of collagen, and the accumulation of age pigments.

Environmental Theory

According to this theory, factors in the environment (e.g., industrial carcinogens, sunlight, trauma, and infection) bring about changes in the aging process. Although these factors are known to accelerate aging, the impact of the environment is a secondary rather than a primary factor in aging.

Science is only beginning to uncover the many environmental factors that affect aging.

Immunity Theory

The immunity theory describes an age-related decline in the immune system. As people age, their ability to defend against foreign organisms decreases, resulting in susceptibility to diseases such as cancer and infection. Along with the diminished immune function, a rise in the body's autoimmune response occurs, leading to the development of autoimmune diseases such as rheumatoid arthritis and allergies to food and environmental agents.

Neuroendocrine Theory

This theory proposes that aging occurs because of a slowing of the secretion of certain hormones that have an impact on reactions regulated by the nervous system. This is most clearly demonstrated in the pituitary gland, thyroid, adrenals, and the glands of reproduction. Although research has given some credence to a predictable biological clock that controls fertility, there is much more to be learned from the study of the neuroendocrine system in relation to a systemic aging process that is controlled by a "clock."

Psychosocial Theories

Psychosocial theories focus on social and psychological changes that accompany advancing age, as opposed to the biological implications of anatomical deterioration. Several theories have attempted to describe how attitudes and behavior in the early phases of life affect people's reactions during the late phase. This work is called the process of "successful aging."

Personality Theory

Personality theories address aspects of psychological growth without delineating specific tasks or expectations of older adults. Some evidence suggests that personality characteristics in old age are highly correlated with early life characteristics. Murray and associates (2009) stated,

> No specific personality changes occur as a result of aging. The older person becomes more of what he or she was. The older person continues to develop emotionally and in personality and adds on characteristics instead of making drastic changes. (p. 663)

In extreme old age, however, people show greater similarity in certain characteristics, probably because of similar declines in biological functioning and societal opportunities.

In a classic study by Reichard, Livson, and Peterson (1962), the personalities of older men were classified into the following five major categories according to their patterns of adjustment to aging.

1. **Mature men.** Mature men are considered well-balanced persons who maintain close personal relationships. They accept both the strengths and weaknesses of their age, finding little to regret about retirement and approaching most problems in a relaxed or convivial manner without continually having to assess blame.

2. **"Rocking chair" personalities.** These are passive-dependent individuals who are content to lean on others for support, to disengage, and to let most of life's activities pass them by.

3. **Armored men.** Armored men have well-integrated defense mechanisms, which serve as adequate protection. Rigid and stable, they present a strong silent front and often rely on activity as an expression of their continuing independence.

4. **Angry men.** This category describes individuals who are bitter about life, themselves, and other people. Aggressiveness is common, as is suspicion of others, especially of minorities or women. With little tolerance for ambiguity or frustration, they have always shown some instability in work and their personal lives, and now feel extremely threatened by old age.

5. **Self-haters.** Self-haters are similar to angry men, except that most of their animosity is turned inward on themselves. Seeing themselves as dismal failures, being old only depresses them all the more.

The investigators identified the mature, "rocking chair," and armored categories as characteristic of healthy, adjusted individuals and the angry and self-hater categories as less successful at aging. In all cases, the evidence suggested that the personalities of the subjects, although distinguished by age-specific criteria, had not changed appreciably throughout most of adulthood.

In a more recent study of personality traits, Srivastava and associates (2003) examined the "big five" personality trait dimensions in a large sample to determine how personality changes over the life span. Age range of the subjects was from 21 to 60. The personality traits tested included conscientiousness, agreeableness, neuroticism, openness, and extroversion. They found that conscientiousness (being organized and disciplined) increased throughout the age range studied, with the biggest increases during the 20s. Agreeableness (being warm, generous, and helpful) increased most during a person's 30s. Neuroticism (being anxious and emotionally labile) declined with age for women, but did not decline for men. Openness (being acceptable to new experiences) showed small declines with age for both men and women. Extroversion (being outwardly expressive and interested in the environment) declined for women but did not show changes in men. This study contradicts the view that personality traits tend to stop changing in early adulthood. These researchers suggested that personality traits change gradually but systematically throughout the life span.

Developmental Task Theory

Developmental tasks are the activities and challenges that one must accomplish at specific stages in life to achieve successful aging. Erikson (1963) described the primary task of old age as being able to see one's life as having been lived with integrity. In the absence of achieving that sense of having lived well, the older adult is at risk for becoming preoccupied with feelings of regret or despair.

Disengagement Theory

Disengagement theory describes the process of withdrawal by older adults from societal roles and responsibilities. According to the theory, this withdrawal process is predictable, systematic, inevitable, and necessary for the proper functioning of a growing society. Older adults were said to be happy when social contacts diminished and responsibilities were assumed by a younger generation. The benefit to the older adult is thought to be in providing time for reflecting on life's accomplishments and for coming to terms with unfulfilled expectations. The benefit to society is thought to be an orderly transfer of power from old to young.

There have been many critics of this theory, and the postulates have been challenged. For many healthy and productive older individuals, the prospect of a slower pace and fewer responsibilities is undesirable.

Activity Theory

In direct opposition to the disengagement theory is the activity theory of aging, which holds that the way to age successfully is to stay active. Multiple studies have validated the positive relationship between maintaining meaningful interaction with others and physical and mental well-being.

Sadock and Sadock (2007) suggested that social integration is the prime factor in determining psychosocial adaptation in later life. Social integration refers to how the aging individual is included and takes part in the life and activities of his or her society. This theory holds that the maintenance of activities is important to most people as a basis for deriving and sustaining satisfaction, self-esteem, and health.

Continuity Theory

This theory, also known as the developmental theory, is a follow-up to the disengagement and activity theories. It emphasizes the individual's previously established coping abilities and personal character traits as a basis for predicting how the person will adjust to the changes of aging. Basic lifestyle characteristics are likely to remain stable in old age, barring physical or other types of complications that necessitate change. A person who has enjoyed the company of others and an active social life will continue to enjoy this lifestyle into old age. One who has preferred solitude and a limited number of activities will probably find satisfaction in a continuation of this lifestyle.

Maintenance of internal continuity is motivated by the need for preservation of self-esteem, ego integrity, cognitive function, and social support. As they age, individuals maintain their self-concept by reinterpreting their current experiences so that old values can take on new meanings in keeping with present circumstances. Internal self-concepts and beliefs are not readily vulnerable to environmental change, and external continuity in skills, activities, roles, and relationships can remain remarkably stable into the 70s. Physical illness or death of friends and loved ones may preclude continued social interaction (Sadock & Sadock, 2007).

The Normal Aging Process

Biological Aspects of Aging

Individuals are unique in their physical and psychological aging processes, as influenced by their predisposition or resistance to illness; the effects of their external environment and behaviors; their exposure to trauma, infections, and past diseases; and the health and illness practices they have adopted during their life span. As the individual ages, there is a quantitative loss of cells and changes in many of the enzymatic activities within cells, resulting in a diminished responsiveness to biological demands made on the body. Age-related changes occur at different rates for different individuals, although in actuality, when growth stops, aging begins. This section presents a brief overview of the normal biological changes that occur with the aging process.

Skin

One of the most dramatic changes that occurs in aging is the loss of elastin in the skin. This effect, as well as changes in collagen, causes aged skin to wrinkle and sag. Excessive exposure to sunlight compounds these changes and increases the risk of developing skin cancer.

Fat redistribution results in a loss of the subcutaneous cushion of adipose tissue. Thus, older people lose "insulation" and are more sensitive to extremes of ambient temperature than are younger people (Stanley et al., 2005). A diminished supply of blood vessels to the skin results in a slower rate of healing.

Cardiovascular System

The age-related decline in the cardiovascular system is thought to be the major determinant of decreased tolerance for exercise and loss of conditioning and the overall decline in energy reserve. The aging heart is characterized by modest hypertrophy with reduced ventricular compliance and diminished cardiac output (Murray et al., 2009; Sadock & Sadock, 2007). This results in a decrease in response to work demands and some diminishment of blood flow to the brain, kidneys, liver, and muscles. Heart rate also slows with time. If arteriosclerosis is present, cardiac function is further compromised.

Respiratory System

Thoracic expansion is diminished by an increase in fibrous tissue and loss of elastin. Pulmonary vital capacity decreases, and the amount of residual air increases. Scattered areas of fibrosis in the alveolar septa interfere with exchange of oxygen and carbon dioxide. These changes are accelerated by the use of cigarettes or other inhaled substances. Cough and laryngeal reflexes are reduced, causing decreased ability to defend the airway. Decreased pulmonary blood flow and diffusion ability result in reduced efficiency in responding to sudden respiratory demands.

Musculoskeletal System

Skeletal aging involving the bones, muscles, ligaments, and tendons probably generates the most frequent limitations on activities of daily living experienced by aging individuals. Loss of muscle mass is significant, although this occurs more slowly in men than in women. Demineralization of the bones occurs at a rate of about 1 percent per year throughout the life span in both men and women. However, this increases to approximately 10 percent in women around **menopause,** making them particularly vulnerable to **osteoporosis.**

Individual muscle fibers become thinner and less elastic with age. Muscles become less flexible following disuse. There is diminished storage of muscle glycogen, resulting in loss of energy reserve for increased activity. These changes are accelerated by nutritional deficiencies and inactivity.

Gastrointestinal System

In the oral cavity, the teeth show a reduction in dentine production, shrinkage and fibrosis of root pulp, gingival retraction, and loss of bone density in the alveolar ridges. There is some loss of peristalsis in the stomach and intestines, and gastric acid production decreases. Levels of intrinsic factor may also decrease, resulting in vitamin B_{12} malabsorption in some aging individuals. A significant decrease in absorptive surface area of the small intestine may be associated with some decline in nutrient absorption. Motility slowdown of the large intestine, combined with poor dietary habits, dehydration, lack of exercise, and some medications, may give rise to problems with constipation.

There is a modest decrease in size and weight of the liver resulting in losses in enzyme activity required to deactivate certain medications by the liver. These age-related changes can influence the metabolism and excretion of these medications. These changes, along with the pharmacokinetics of the drug, must be considered when giving medications to aging individuals.

Endocrine System

A decreased level of thyroid hormones causes a lowered basal metabolic rate. Decreased amounts of adrenocorticotropic hormone may result in less efficient stress response.

Impairments in glucose tolerance are evident in aging individuals. Studies of glucose challenges show that insulin levels are equivalent to or slightly higher than those from younger challenged individuals, although peripheral insulin resistance appears to play a significant role in carbohydrate intolerance. The observed glucose clearance abnormalities and insulin resistance in older people may be related to many factors other than biological aging (e.g., obesity, family history of diabetes) and may be influenced substantially by diet or exercise.

Genitourinary System

Age-related declines in renal function occur because of a steady attrition of nephrons and sclerosis within the glomeruli over time (Stanley et al., 2005). Vascular changes affect blood flow to the kidneys, which results in reduced glomerular filatration and tubular function (Murray et al., 2009).

Elderly people are prone to develop the syndrome of inappropriate antidiuretic hormone secretion, and levels of blood urea nitrogen and creatinine may be elevated slightly. The overall decline in renal functioning has serious implications for physicians who prescribe medications for elderly individuals.

In men, enlargement of the prostate gland is common as aging occurs. Prostatic hypertrophy is associated with an increased risk for urinary retention and may also be a cause of urinary incontinence (Johnston, Harper, & Landefeld, 2009). Loss of muscle and sphincter control, as well as the use of some medications, may cause urinary incontinence in women. Not only is this problem a cause of social stigma, but also, if left untreated, it increases the risk of urinary tract infection and local skin irritation. Normal changes in the genitalia are discussed in the section "Sexual Aspects of Aging."

Immune System

Aging results in changes in both cell-mediated and antibody-mediated immune responses. The size of the thymus gland declines continuously from just beyond puberty to about 15 percent of its original size at age 50. The consequences of these changes include a greater susceptiblity to infections and a diminished inflammatory response that results in delayed healing. There is also evidence of an increase in various autoantibodies as a person ages, increasing the risk of autoimmune disorders, such as rheumatoid arthritis (National Institutes of Health [NIH], 2008).

Because of the overall decrease in efficiency of the immune system, the proliferation of abnormal cells is facilitated in the elderly individual. Cancer is the best example of aberrant cells allowed to proliferate due to the ineffectiveness of the immune system.

Nervous System

With aging, there is an absolute loss of neurons, which correlates with decreases in brain weight of about 10 percent by age 90 (Murray et al., 2009). Gross morphological examination reveals gyral atrophy in the frontal, temporal, and parietal lobes; widening of the sulci; and ventricular enlargement. However, it must be remembered that these changes have been identified in careful study of adults with normal intellectual function.

The brain has enormous reserve, and little cerebral function is lost over time, although greater functional decline is noted in the periphery (Stanley et al., 2005). There appears to be a disproportionately greater loss of cells in the cerebellum, locus ceruleus, substantia nigra, and olfactory bulbs, accounting for some of the more characteristic aging behaviors such as mild gait disturbances, sleep disruptions, and decreased smell and taste perception.

Some of the age-related changes within the nervous system may be due to alterations in neurotransmitter release, uptake, turnover, catabolism, or receptor functions (Beers & Jones, 2004). A great deal of attention is being given to brain biochemistry and in particular to the neurotransmitters acetylcholine, dopamine, norepinephrine, and epinephrine. These biochemical changes may be responsible for the altered responses of many older persons to stressful events and some biological treatments.

Sensory Systems

Vision

Visual acuity begins to decrease in midlife. Presbyopia (blurred near vision) is the standard marker of aging of the eye. It is caused by a loss of elasticity of the crystalline lens, and results in compromised accommodation.

Cataract development is inevitable if the individual lives long enough for the changes to occur. Cataracts occur when the lens of the eye becomes less resilient (due to compression of fibers) and increasingly opaque (as proteins lump together), ultimately resulting in a loss of visual acuity.

The color in the iris may fade, and the pupil may become irregular in shape. A decrease in production of secretions by the lacrimal glands may cause dryness and result in increased irritation and infection. The pupil may become constricted, requiring an increase in the amount of light needed for reading.

Hearing

Hearing changes significantly with the aging process. Gradually over time, the ear loses its sensitivity to discriminate sounds because of damage to the hair cells of the cochlea. The most dramatic decline appears to be in perception of high-frequency sounds.

Although hearing loss is significant in all aging individuals, the decline is more dramatic in men than in women. Men are twice as likely as women to have hearing loss (Murray et al., 2009).

Taste and Smell

Taste sensitivity decreases over the life span. Taste discrimination decreases, and bitter taste sensations predominate. Sensitivity to sweet and salty tastes is diminished.

The deterioration of the olfactory bulbs is accompanied by loss of smell acuity. The aromatic component of taste perception diminishes.

Touch and Pain

Organized sensory nerve receptors on the skin continue to decrease throughout the life span; thus, the touch threshold increases with age (Pietraniec-Shannon, 2007). The ability to feel pain also decreases in response to these changes, and the ability to perceive and interpret painful stimuli changes. These changes have critical implications for the elderly in their potential inability to use sensory warnings to escape serious injury.

Psychological Aspects of Aging

Memory Functioning

Age-related memory deficiencies have been extensively reported in the literature. Although **short-term memory** seems to deteriorate with age, perhaps because of poorer sorting strategies, **long-term memory** does not show similar changes. However, in nearly every instance, well-educated, mentally active people do not exhibit the same decline in memory functioning as their age peers who lack similar opportunities to flex their minds. Nevertheless, with few exceptions, the time required for memory scanning is longer for both recent and remote recall among older people. This can sometimes be attributed to social or health factors (e.g., stress, fatigue, illness), but it can also occur because of certain normal physical changes associated with aging (e.g., decreased blood flow to the brain).

Intellectual Functioning

There appears to be a high degree of regularity in intellectual functioning across the adult age span. Crystallized abilities, or knowledge acquired in the course of the socialization process, tend to remain stable over the adult life span. Fluid abilities, or abilities involved in solving novel problems, tend to decline gradually from young to old adulthood. In other words, intellectual abilities of older people do not decline but do become obsolete. The age of their formal educational experiences is reflected in their intelligence scoring.

Learning Ability

The ability to learn is not diminished by age. Studies, however, have shown that some aspects of learning do change with age. The ordinary slowing of reaction time with age for nearly all tasks or the overarousal of the central nervous system may account for lower performance levels on tests requiring rapid responses. Under conditions that allow for self-pacing by the participant, differences in accuracy of performance diminish. Ability to learn continues throughout life, although strongly influenced by interests, activity, motivation, health, and experience. Adjustments do need to be made in teaching methodology and time allowed for learning.

Adaptation to the Tasks of Aging

Loss and Grief

Individuals experience losses from the very beginning of life. By the time individuals reach their 60s and 70s, they have experienced numerous losses, and mourning has become a lifelong process. Unfortunately, with the aging process comes a convergence of losses, the timing of which makes it impossible for the aging individual to complete the grief process in response to one loss before another occurs. Because grief is cumulative, this can result in **bereavement overload,** which has been implicated in the predisposition to depression in the elderly.

Attachment to Others

Many studies have confirmed the importance of interpersonal relationships at all stages in the life cycle. Murray and associates (2009) stated:

> [Social networks] contribute to well-being of the elder by (a) promoting socialization and companionship, (b) elevating morale and life satisfaction, (c) buffering the effects of stressful events, (d) providing a confidant, and (e) facilitating coping skills and mastery. (p. 620)

This need for **attachment** is consistent with the activity theory of aging that correlates the importance of social integration with successful adaptation in later life.

Maintenance of Self-Identity

Self-concept and self-image appear to remain stable over time. Factors that have been shown to favor good psychosocial adjustment in later life are sustained family relationships, maturity of ego defenses, absence of alcoholism, and absence of

depressive disorder (Vaillant, 2003). Studies show that the elderly have a strong need for and remarkable capability of retaining a persistent self-concept in the face of the many changes that contribute to instability in later life.

Dealing With Death

Death anxiety among the aging is apparently more of a myth than a reality. Studies have not supported the negative view of death as an overriding psychological factor in the aging process. Various investigators who have worked with dying persons report that it is not death itself, but abandonment, pain, and confusion that are feared. What many desire most is someone to talk with, to show them their life's meaning is not shattered merely because they are about to die (Kübler-Ross, 1969; Murray et al., 2009).

Psychiatric Disorders in Later Life

The later years constitute a time of especially high risk for emotional distress. Sadock and Sadock (2007) stated:

> Several psychosocial risk factors predispose older people to mental disorders. These risk factors include loss of social roles, loss of autonomy, the deaths of friends and relatives, declining health, increased isolation, financial constraints, and decreased cognitive functioning. (p. 1353)

Dementia

Dementing disorders are the most common causes of psychopathology in the elderly (Sadock & Sadock, 2007). About half of these disorders are of the Alzheimer's type, which is characterized by an insidious onset and a gradually progressive course of cognitive impairment. No curative treatment is currently available. Symptomatic treatments, including pharmacological interventions, attention to the environment, and family support, can help to maximize the client's level of functioning.

IMPLICATIONS OF RESEARCH FOR EVIDENCE-BASED PRACTICE

Helmes, E., & Wiancko, D. C. (2006). Effects of music in reducing disruptive behavior in a general hospital. *Journal of the American Psychiatric Nurses Association, 12,* 37–44.

DESCRIPTION OF THE STUDY: In settings where cognitively impaired elderly individuals reside, it is not uncommon for loud, disruptive vocalizations such as shouting and the banging of objects to be heard. Studies have shown that music can alleviate the tension and reduce the disruptive vocalizations of some

individuals with dementia. Most reports on the effect of music on these disruptive outbursts have been conducted in residential care facilities. Because there are few studies about the prevalence of disruptive behaviors or the method of dealing with them in the acute care setting, the authors sought to determine if soothing music found to be effective in residential settings could be generalized to acute care environments.

RESULTS OF THE STUDY: The study sample included 7 women and 2 men ranging in age from 68 to 95 years.

IMPLICATIONS OF RESEARCH FOR EVIDENCE-BASED PRACTICE—cont'd

Diagnoses were varied, including diabetes, pneumonia, alcoholic dementia, depression, Alzheimer's disease, Parkinson's dementia, stroke, and congestive heart failure. Length of hospital stays ranged from 1 day to 54 days. All exhibited disruptive behaviors, such as shouting and banging of objects within reach, such as tray tables or bedrails. The intervention included the playing of baroque music in the client's room at a comfortable volume for the listener. Each of the participants was observed for a minimum of four 30-minute periods on a minimum of 3 successive days. Control trials with each participant were also conducted in a randomized order to have at least two observations from each condition. Observations were made unobtrusively, and routine activity of staff and visitors was not minimized during the course of the study. With all participants, the music intervention resulted in a decrease in frequency of noisy disruptive behaviors, with reductions ranging from 30 to 90 percent, when compared with the control trials.

IMPLICATIONS FOR NURSING PRACTICE: The use of music for its soothing and calming effect is a simple intervention well within the scope and capability of nursing practice. This study did not pursue whether the benefits carry over after the music has stopped, and whether more extensive use of music would retain its effectiveness. The authors concluded, "The use of music to reduce disruptive noise in an acute care setting appears to be as effective as other such interventions have been in residential care facilities." One additional benefit was reported. The authors stated, "Nurses on the two units noted positive effects for them in the form of increased pleasant affect that seemed to be independent of the effects of reduced disruptive noise from the participants."

Delirium

Delirium is one of the most common and important forms of psychopathology in later life. A number of factors have been identified that predispose elderly people to delirium, including structural brain disease, reduced capacity for homeostatic regulation, impaired vision and hearing, a high prevalence of chronic disease, reduced resistance to acute stress, and age-related changes in the pharmacokinetics and pharmacodynamics of drugs. Delirium needs to be recognized and the underlying condition treated as soon as possible. A high mortality is associated with this condition.

Depression

Depressive disorders are the most common affective illnesses occurring after the middle years. The incidence of increased depression among elderly people is influenced by the variables of physical illness, functional disability, cognitive impairment, and loss of a spouse (Stanley et al., 2005). Hypochondriacal symptoms are common in the depressed elderly. Symptomatology often mimics that of dementia, a condition that is referred to as *pseudodementia*. (See Table 24-1 for a comparison of the symptoms of dementia and pseudodementia.) Suicide is prevalent in the elderly, with declining health and decreased economic status being considered important influencing factors. Treatment of depression in the elderly individual is with psychotropic medications or electroconvulsive therapy.

Schizophrenia

Schizophrenia and delusional disorders may continue into old age or may manifest themselves for the first time only during senescence (Blazer, 2008). In most instances, individuals who manifest psychotic disorders early in life show a decline in psychopathology as they age. Late-onset schizophrenia (after age 60) is not common, but when it does occur, it often is characterized by delusions or hallucinations of a persecutory nature. The course is chronic, and treatment is with neuroleptics and supportive psychotherapy.

Anxiety Disorders

Most anxiety disorders begin in early to middle adulthood, but some appear for the first time after age 60. Sadock and Sadock (2007) stated:

> The fragility of the autonomic nervous system in older persons may account for the development of anxiety after a major stressor. Because of concurrent physical disability, older persons react more severely to posttraumatic stress disorder than younger persons. (p. 1355)

In older adults, symptoms of anxiety and depression often accompany each other, making it difficult to determine which disorder is dominant.

Personality Disorders

Personality disorders are uncommon in the elderly population. The incidence of personality disorders among individuals over age 65 is less than 5 percent. Most elderly people with personality disorder have likely manifested the symptomatology for many years.

Sleep Disorders

Sleep disorders are very common in the aging individual. Sleep disturbances affect 50 percent of people ages 65 and older who live at home and 66 percent of those who live in long-term care facilities (Stanley et al., 2005). Some common causes of sleep disturbances among elderly people include age-dependent decreases in the ability to sleep ("sleep decay"); increased prevalence of sleep apnea; depression; dementia; anxiety; pain; impaired mobility; medications; and psychosocial factors such as loneliness, inactivity, and boredom. Sedative-hypnotics, along with nonpharmacological approaches, are often used as sleep aids with the elderly. Changes in aging associated with metabolism and elimination must be considered when maintenance medications are administered for chronic insomnia in the aging client.

Sociocultural Aspects of Aging

Old age brings many important socially induced changes, some of which have the potential for negative effect on both the physical and mental well-being of older persons. In American society, old age is defined arbitrarily as being 65 years or older because that is the age when most people have been able to retire with full Social Security and other pension benefits. Recent legislation has increased the age beyond 65 years for full Social Security benefits. Currently, the age increases yearly (based on year of birth) until 2027, when the age for full benefits will be 67 years for all individuals.

Elderly people in virtually all cultures share some basic needs and interests. There is little doubt that most individuals choose to live the most satisfying life possible until their demise. They want protection from hazards and release from the weariness of everyday tasks. They want to be treated with the respect and dignity that is deserving of individuals who have reached this pinnacle in life; and they want to die with the same respect and dignity.

From the beginning of human culture, the aged have had a special status in society. Even today, in some cultures the aged are the most powerful, the most engaged, and the most respected members of the society. This has not been the case in the modern industrial societies, although trends in the status of the aged differ widely between one industrialized country and another. For example, the status and integration of the aged in Japan have remained relatively high when compared with other industrialized nations, such as the United States. There are subcultures in the United States, however, in which the elderly are afforded a higher degree of status than they receive in the mainstream population. Examples include Latino Americans, Asian Americans, and African Americans. The aged are awarded a position of honor in cultures that place emphasis on family cohesiveness. In these cultures, the aged are revered for their knowledge and wisdom gained through their years of life experiences (Purnell & Paulanka, 2008).

Many negative stereotypes color the perspective on aging in the United States. Ideas that elderly individuals are always tired or sick, slow and forgetful, isolated and lonely, unproductive, and angry determine the way younger individuals relate to the elderly in this society. Increasing disregard for the elderly has resulted in a type of segregation, as aging individuals voluntarily seek out or are involuntarily placed in special residences for the aged.

Assisted living centers, retirement apartment complexes, and even entire retirement communities intended solely for individuals over age 50 are becoming more and more common. In 2009, more than half (56.5 percent) of persons ages 65 and older lived in eleven states, with the largest numbers in California, Florida, New York, Texas, and Pennsylvania (AoA, 2011). It is important for elderly individuals to feel part of an integrated group, and they are migrating to these areas in an effort to achieve this integration. This phenomenon provides additional corroboration for the activity theory of aging, and the importance of attachment to others.

Employment is another area in which the elderly experience discrimination. Although compulsory retirement has been virtually eliminated, discrimination still exists in hiring and promotion practices. Many employers are not eager to retain or hire older workers. It is difficult to determine how much of the failure to hire and promote results from discrimination based on age alone and how much of it is related to a realistic and fair appraisal of the aged employee's ability and efficiency. It is true that some elderly individuals are no longer capable of doing as good a job as a younger worker; however, there are many who likely can do a *better* job than their younger counterparts, if given the opportunity. Nevertheless, surveys have shown that some employers accept the negative stereotypes about elderly individuals and believe that older workers are hard to please, set in their ways, less productive, frequently absent, and involved in more accidents.

The status of the elderly may improve with time and as their numbers increase with the aging of the "baby boomers." As older individuals gain political power, the benefits and privileges designed for the elderly will increase. There is power in numbers, and the 21st century promises power for people ages 65 and older.

Sexual Aspects of Aging

Sexuality and the sexual needs of elderly people are frequently misunderstood, condemned, stereotyped, ridiculed, repressed, and ignored. Americans have grown up in a society that has liberated sexual expression for all other age groups, but still retains certain Victorian standards regarding sexual expression by the elderly. Negative stereotyped notions concerning sexual interest and activity of the elderly are common. Some of these include ideas that older people have no sexual interests or desires; that they are sexually undesirable; or that they are too fragile or too ill to engage in sexual activity. Some people even believe it is disgusting or comical to consider elderly individuals as sexual beings.

These cultural stereotypes undoubtedly play a large part in the misperception many people hold regarding sexuality of the aged, and they may be reinforced by the common tendency of the young to deny the inevitability of aging. With reasonable good health and an interesting and interested partner, there is no inherent reason why individuals should not enjoy an active sexual life well into late adulthood (King, 2009).

Physical Changes Associated With Sexuality

Many of the changes in sexuality that occur in later years are related to the physical changes that are taking place at that time of life.

Changes in Women

Menopause may begin anytime during the 40s or early 50s. During this time there is a gradual decline in the functioning of the ovaries and the subsequent production of estrogen, which results in a number of changes. The walls of the vagina become thin and inelastic, the vagina itself shrinks in both width and length, and the amount of vaginal lubrication decreases noticeably. Orgastic uterine contractions may become spastic. All of these changes can result in painful penetration, vaginal burning, pelvic aching, or irritation on urination. In some women, the discomfort may be severe enough to result in an avoidance of intercourse. Paradoxically, these symptoms are more likely to occur with infrequent intercourse of only one time a month or less. Regular and more frequent sexual activity results in a greater capacity for sexual performance (King, 2009). Other symptoms that are associated with menopause in some women

include hot flashes, night sweats, sleeplessness, irritability, mood swings, migraine headaches, urinary incontinence, and weight gain.

Some menopausal women elect to take hormone replacement therapy for relief of these changes and symptoms. With estrogen therapy, the symptoms of menopause are minimized or do not occur at all. However, some women choose not to take the hormone because of an increased risk of breast cancer, and when given alone, an increased risk of endometrial cancer. To combat this latter effect, many women also take a second hormone, progesterone. Taken for 7 to 10 days during the month, progesterone decreases the risk of estrogen-induced endometrial cancer. Some physicians prescribe a low dose of progesterone that is taken, along with estrogen, for the entire month. A combination pill, taken in this manner, is also available.

Results of the Women's Health Initiative (WHI), as reported in the *Journal of the American Medical Association,* indicated that the combination pill is associated with an increased risk of cardiovascular disease and breast cancer. Benefits related to colon cancer and osteoporosis were reported; however, investigators stopped this arm of the study and suggested discontinuation of this type of therapy. In a 3-year follow-up study of the participants, the results showed that the increased risk for cardiovascular disease dissipated with discontinuation of the hormone therapy (Heiss et al., 2008).

Changes in Men

Testosterone production declines gradually over the years, beginning between ages 40 and 60. A major change resulting from this hormone reduction is that erections occur more slowly and require more direct genital stimulation to achieve. There may also be a modest decrease in the firmness of the erection in men older than age 60. The refractory period lengthens with age, increasing the amount of time following orgasm before the man may achieve another erection. The volume of ejaculate gradually decreases, and the force of ejaculation lessens. The testes become somewhat smaller, but most men continue to produce viable sperm well into old age. Prolonged control over ejaculation in middle-aged and elderly men may bring increased sexual satisfaction for both partners.

Sexual Behavior in the Elderly

Coital frequency in early marriage and the overall quantity of sexual activity between age 20 and 40 correlate significantly with frequency patterns of sexual activity during aging (Masters, Johnson, & Kolodny, 1995). Although sexual interest and behavior do appear to decline somewhat with age, studies show that significant numbers of elderly men and women have active and satisfying sex lives well into their 80s. A survey commissioned by the American Association of Retired Persons (AARP) provided some revealing information regarding the sexual attitudes and behavior of senior citizens. Some statistics from the survey are summarized in Table 35-1. The information from this survey clearly indicates that sexual activity can and does continue well past the 70s for healthy

TABLE 35-1 Sexuality at Midlife and Beyond: 2009 Update			
	AGES	**MEN (%)**	**WOMEN (%)**
Have sex at least once a week	45–49	50	26
	50–59	41	32
	60–69	24	24
	70+	15	5
Report very satisfied with physical relationship	45–49	60	48
	50–59	50	40
	60–69	52	41
	70+	26	27
Report very satisfied with emotional relationship	45–49	26	37
	50–59	32	23
	60–69	28	29
	70+	20	24
Report sexual activity is important to their overall quality of life	45–49	69	33
	50–59	65	28
	60–69	55	33
	70+	46	12
Believe non-marital sex is okay	40–49	88	86
	50–59	91	75
	60–69	80	71
	70+	68	61
Describe their partners as physically attractive	45–49	50	60
	50–59	53	48
	60–69	58	58
	70+	51	48
Report always or usually having an orgasm with sexual intercourse	45–49	95	70
	50–59	88	64
	60–69	91	59
	70+	82	61
Report being impotent	45–49	6	
	50–59	16	
	60–69	29	
	70+	48	
Report having used medicine, hormones, or other treatments to improve sexual functioning	45–49	7	9
	50–59	12	16
	60–69	14	14
	70+	13	13
What would most improve your sex life?	All	Better health for self; partner initiates sex more often; less stress	Less stress; better health for self and partner; finding a partner

Adapted from American Association of Retired Persons. 2010. Sex, romance, and relationships: AARP survey of midlife and older adults. Washington, DC: Author.

active individuals who have regular opportunities for sexual expression. King (2009) stated: "For healthy men and women with healthy partners, sexual activity will probably continue throughout life if they had a positive attitude about sex when they were younger" (p. 271).

Special Concerns of the Elderly Population

Retirement

Statistics reflect that a larger percentage of Americans are living longer and that many of them are retiring earlier. Reasons often given for the increasing pattern of early retirement include health problems, Social Security and other pension benefits, attractive "early out" packages offered by companies, and long-held plans (e.g., turning a hobby into a money-making situation).

Sadock and Sadock (2007) reported that, of those people who voluntarily retire, most reenter the work force within 2 years. The reasons they give for doing this include negative reactions to being retired, feelings of being unproductive, economic hardship, and loneliness. Recent downturns in economic conditions have forced many retired people to seek employment to augment dwindling retirement resources.

About 6.5 million older Americans were in the labor force (working or actively seeking work) in 2009. These included 3.6 million men and 2.9 million women, and constituted 4.2 percent of the U.S. labor force (AoA, 2011).

Retirement has both social and economic implications for elderly individuals. The role is fraught with a great deal of ambiguity and is one that requires many adaptations on the part of those involved.

Social Implications

Retirement is often anticipated as an achievement in principle, but met with a great deal of ambiguity when it actually occurs. Our society places a great deal of importance on productivity, making as much money as possible, and doing it at as young an age as possible. These types of values contribute to the ambiguity associated with retirement. Although leisure has been acknowledged as a legitimate reward for workers, leisure during retirement historically has lacked the same social value. Adjustment to this life-cycle event becomes more difficult in the face of societal values that are in direct conflict with the new lifestyle.

Historically, many women have derived a good deal of their self-esteem from their families—birthing them, rearing them, and being a "good

mother." Likewise, many men have achieved self-esteem through work-related activities—creativity, productivity, and earning money. With the termination of these activities may come a loss of self-worth, resulting in depression in some individuals who are unable to adapt satisfactorily. Well-being in retirement is linked to factors such as stable health status and access to health care services, adequate income, the ability to pursue new goals or activities, extended social network of family and friends, and satisfaction with current living arrangements (Murray et al., 2009).

American society often identifies an individual by his or her occupation. This is reflected in the conversation of people who are meeting each other for the first time. Undoubtedly, most everyone has either asked or been asked at some point in time, "What do you do?" or "Where do you work?" Occupation determines status, and retirement represents a significant change in status. The basic ambiguity of retirement occurs in an individual's or society's definition of this change. Is it undertaken voluntarily or involuntarily? Is it desirable or undesirable? Is one's status made better or worse by the change?

In looking at the trend of the past 2 decades, we may presume that retirement is becoming, and will continue to become, more accepted by societal standards. With many individuals retiring earlier and living longer, a growing number of aging people will spend a significantly longer time in retirement. It is a major life event that requires planning and realistic expectations of life changes.

Economic Implications

Because retirement is generally associated with 20 to 40 percent reduction in personal income, the standard of living after retirement may be adversely affected. Most older adults derive post-retirement income from a combination of Social Security benefits, public and private pensions, and income from savings or investments.

In 2009, the median income in households containing families headed by persons 65 or older was $43,702 and 3.4 million elderly people were below the poverty level (AoA, 2011). The rate of those living in poverty was higher among women than men and higher among African Americans and Latino Americans than whites.

The Social Security Act of 1935 promised assistance with financial security for the elderly. Since then, the original legislation has been modified, yet the basic philosophy remains intact. Its effectiveness, however, is now being questioned. Faced with deficits, the program is forced to pay benefits to those currently retired from both the reserve funds and monies being collected at present. There is genuine concern about future generations, when there may be no reserve funds from which to draw. Because many of the programs that benefit older adults depend on contributions from the younger population, the growing ratio of older Americans to younger people may affect society's ability to supply the goods and services necessary to meet this expanding demand.

Medicare and **Medicaid** were established by the government to provide medical care benefits for elderly and indigent Americans. The Medicaid program is jointly funded by state and federal governments, and coverage varies significantly from state to state. Medicare covers only a percentage of health-care costs; therefore, to reduce risk related to out-of-pocket expenditures, many older adults purchase private "medigap" policies designed to cover charges in excess of those approved by Medicare.

The magnitude of retirement earnings depends almost entirely on pre-retirement income. The poor will remain poor and the wealthy are unlikely to lower their status during retirement; however, for many in the middle classes, the relatively fixed income sources may be inadequate, possibly forcing them to face financial hardship for the first time in their lives.

Long-Term Care

Stanley and associates (2005) stated, "The concept of long-term care covers a broad spectrum of comprehensive health care that addresses both illness and wellness and the support services necessary to provide the physical, social, spiritual, and economic needs of persons with chronic illnesses, including disabilities" (p. 94). Long-term care facilities are defined by the level of care they provide. They may be skilled nursing facilities, intermediate care facilities, or a combination of the two. Some institutions provide convalescent care for individuals recovering from acute illness or injury, some provide long-term care for individuals with chronic illness or disabilities, and still others provide both types of assistance.

Most elderly individuals prefer to remain in their own homes or in the homes of family members for as long as this can meet their needs without deterioration of family or social patterns. Many elderly individuals are placed in institutions as a last resort only after heroic efforts have been made to keep them in their own or a relative's home. The increasing emphasis on home health care has extended the period of independence for aging individuals.

Fewer than 5 percent of the population ages 65 and older live in nursing homes. The percentage increases dramatically with age, ranging from 0.9 percent for persons ages 65 to 74, to 3.5 percent for persons ages 75 to 84, to 14.3 percent for persons ages 85 and older (AoA, 2011). A profile of the "typical" elderly nursing home resident is about 80 years of age, white, female, and widowed, with multiple chronic health conditions.

Risk Factors for Institutionalization

In determining who in our society will need long-term care, several factors have been identified that appear to place people at risk. The following risk factors are taken into consideration to predict potential need for services and to estimate future costs.

Age

Because people grow older in very different ways, and the range of differences becomes greater with the passage of time, age is becoming a less relevant characteristic than it was historically. However, because of the high prevalence of chronic health conditions and disabilities, as well as the greater chance of diminishing social supports associated with advancing age, the 65-and-older population is often viewed as an important long-term care target group.

Health

Level of functioning, as determined by ability to perform various behaviors or activities—such as bathing, eating, mobility, meal preparation, handling finances, judgment, and memory—is a measurable risk factor. The need for ongoing assistance from another person is critical in determining the need for long-term care.

Mental Health Status

Mental health problems are risk factors in assessing need for long-term care. Many of the symptoms associated with certain mental disorders (especially the dementias), such as memory loss, impaired judgment, impaired intellect, and disorientation, would render the individual incapable of meeting the demands of daily living independently.

Socioeconomic and Demographic Factors

Low income generally is associated with greater physical and mental health problems among the elderly. Because many elderly individuals have limited finances, they are less able to purchase care resources available outside of institutions (e.g., home health care), although Medicare and Medicaid now contribute a limited amount to this type of noninstitutionalized care.

Women are at greater risk of being institutionalized than men, not because they are less healthy but because they tend to live longer and, thus, reach the age at which more functional and cognitive impairments occur. They are also more likely to be widowed. Whites have a higher rate of institutionalization than nonwhites. This may be related to cultural and financial influences.

Marital Status, Living Arrangement, and the Informal Support Network

Individuals who are married and live with a spouse are the least likely of all disabled people to be institutionalized. Those who live alone without resources for home care and with few or no relatives living nearby to provide informal care are at higher risk for institutionalization.

Attitudinal Factors

Many people dread the thought of even visiting a nursing home, let alone moving to one or placing a relative in one. Negative perceptions exist of nursing homes as "places to go to die." The media picture and subsequent reputation of nursing homes has not been positive. Stories of substandard care and patient abuse have scarred the industry, making it difficult for those facilities that are clean and well managed and provide innovative, quality care to their residents to rise above the stigma.

State and national licensing boards perform periodic inspections to ensure that standards set forth by the federal government are being met. These standards address quality of patient care as well as adequacy of the nursing home facility. Yet, many elderly individuals and their families perceive nursing homes as a place to go to die, and the fact that many of these institutions are poorly equipped, understaffed, and disorganized keeps this societal perception alive. There are, however, many excellent nursing homes that strive to go beyond the minimum federal regulations for Medicaid and Medicare reimbursement. In addition to medical, nursing, rehabilitation, and dental services, social and recreational services are provided to increase the quality of life for elderly people living in nursing homes. These activities include playing cards, bingo, and other games; parties; church activities; books; television; movies; and arts, crafts, and other classes. Some nursing homes provide occupational and professional counseling. These facilities strive to enhance opportunities for improving quality of life and for becoming "places to live," rather than "places to die."

Elder Abuse

Abuse of elderly individuals, which at times has been referred to in the media as "**granny-bashing**," is a serious form of family violence. Sadock and Sadock (2007) estimated that 10 percent of individuals older than age 65 are the victims of abuse or neglect. The abuser is often a relative who lives with the elderly person and may be the assigned caregiver. Typical caregivers who are likely to be abusers of the elderly were described by Murray and associates (2009) as being under economic stress, substance abusers, themselves the victims of previous family violence, and exhausted and frustrated by the caregiver role. Identified risk factors for victims of abuse included being a white female age 70 or older, being mentally or physically impaired, being unable to meet daily self-care needs, and having care needs that exceeded the caregiver's ability.

Abuse of elderly individuals may be psychological, physical, or financial. Neglect may be intentional or unintentional. Psychological abuse includes yelling, insulting, harsh commands, threats, silence, and social isolation. Physical abuse is described as striking, shoving, beating, or restraint. Financial abuse refers to misuse or theft of finances, property, or material possessions. Neglect implies failure to fulfill the physical needs of an individual who cannot do so independently. Unintentional neglect is inadvertent, whereas intentional neglect is deliberate. In addition, elderly individuals may be the victims of sexual abuse, which is sexual intimacy between two persons that occurs without the consent of one of the persons involved. Another type of abuse, which has been called "**granny-dumping**" by the media, involves abandoning elderly individuals at emergency departments, nursing homes, or other facilities—literally leaving them in the hands of others when the strain of caregiving becomes intolerable. Types of elder abuse are summarized in Box 35-1.

Elder victims often minimize the abuse or deny that it has occurred. The elderly person may be unwilling to disclose information because of fear of retaliation, embarrassment about the existence of abuse in the family, protectiveness toward a family member, or unwillingness to institute legal action. Adding to this unwillingness to report is the fact that infirm elders are often isolated, so their mistreatment is less likely to be noticed by those who might be alert to symptoms of abuse. For these reasons, detection of abuse in the elderly is difficult at best.

Factors That Contribute to Abuse

A number of contributing factors have been implicated in the abuse of elderly individuals.

Longer Life

The 65-and-older age group has become the fastest growing segment of the population. Within this segment, the number of elderly older than age 75

BOX 35-1 **Examples of Elder Abuse**	
PHYSICAL ABUSE	Unclean clothes and bedding
Striking, hitting, beating	Lack of needed medication
Shoving	Lack of eyeglasses, hearing aids, false teeth
Bruising	**FINANCIAL ABUSE OR EXPLOITATION**
Cutting	Misuse of the elderly person's income by the caregiver
Restraining	Forcing the elderly person to sign over financial affairs to another person against his or her will or without sufficient knowledge about the transaction
PSYCHOLOGICAL ABUSE	
Yelling	
Insulting, name-calling	**SEXUAL ABUSE**
Harsh commands	Sexual molestation; rape
Threats	Any type of sexual intimacy against the elderly person's will
Ignoring, silence, social isolation	
Withholding of affection	
NEGLECT (INTENTIONAL OR UNINTENTIONAL)	
Withholding food and water	
Inadequate heating	

SOURCES: Murray, Zentner, and Yakimo (2009); Sadock and Sadock (2007); and Stanley, Blair, and Beare (2005).

has increased most rapidly. This trend is expected to continue well into the 21st century. The 75 and older age group is the one most likely to be physically or mentally impaired, requiring assistance and care from family members. This group also is the most vulnerable to abuse from caregivers.

Dependency

Dependency appears to be the most common precondition in domestic abuse. Changes associated with normal aging or induced by chronic illness often result in loss of self-sufficiency in the elderly person, requiring that he or she become dependent on another for assistance with daily functioning. Long life may also consume finances to the point that the elderly individual becomes financially dependent on another as well. This type of dependency also increases the elderly person's vulnerability to abuse.

Stress

The stress inherent in the caregiver role is a factor in most abuse cases. Some clinicians believe that elder abuse results from individual or family psychopathology. Others suggest that even psychologically healthy family members can become abusive as the result of the exhaustion and acute stress caused by overwhelming caregiving responsibilities. This is compounded in an age group that has been dubbed the "sandwich generation"—those individuals who elected to delay childbearing so that they are now at a point in their lives when they are "sandwiched" between providing care for their children and providing care for their aging parents.

Learned Violence

Children who have been abused or witnessed abusive and violent parents are more likely to evolve into abusive adults. Stanley and associates (2005) stated:

> Violence is a learned behavior that is passed down from generation to generation in some families because violence has been modeled as an acceptable coping behavior, with no substantial penalties for the behavior. This model suggests that a child who grows up in a violent family will also become violent. Some believe that elder mistreatment may be related to retribution on the part of an adult offspring who was abused as a child. (p. 290)

Identifying Elder Abuse

Because so many elderly individuals are reluctant to report personal abuse, health-care workers need to be able to detect signs of mistreatment when they are in a position to do so. Box 35-1 listed a number of *types* of elder abuse. The following *manifestations* of the various categories of abuse have been identified (Murray et al., 2009; Stanley et al., 2005):

■ Indicators of psychological abuse include a broad range of behaviors such as the symptoms associated with depression, withdrawal, anxiety, sleep disorders, and increased confusion or agitation.

■ Indicators of physical abuse may include bruises, welts, lacerations, burns, punctures, evidence of hair pulling, and skeletal dislocations and fractures.

■ Neglect may be manifested as consistent hunger, poor hygiene, inappropriate dress, consistent lack of supervision, consistent fatigue or listlessness, unattended physical problems or medical needs, or abandonment.

■ Sexual abuse may be suspected when the elderly person is presented with pain or itching in the genital area; bruising or bleeding in external genitalia, vaginal, or anal areas; or unexplained sexually transmitted disease.

■ Financial abuse may be occurring when there is an obvious disparity between assets and satisfactory living conditions or when the elderly person complains of a sudden lack of sufficient funds for daily living expenses.

Health-care workers often feel intimidated when confronted with cases of elder abuse. In these instances, referral to an individual experienced in management of victims of such abuse may be the most effective approach to evaluation and intervention. Health-care workers are responsible for reporting any suspicions of elder abuse. An investigation is then conducted by regulatory agencies, whose job it is to determine if the suspicions are corroborated. Every effort must be made to ensure the client's safety, but it is important to remember that a competent elderly person has the right to choose his or her health-care options. As inappropriate as it may seem, some elderly individuals choose to return to the abusive situation. In this instance, he or she should be provided with names and phone numbers to call for assistance if needed. A follow-up visit by an adult protective services representative should be conducted.

Increased efforts need to be made to ensure that health-care providers have comprehensive training in the detection of and intervention in elder abuse. More research is needed to increase knowledge and understanding of the phenomenon of elder abuse and ultimately to effect more sophisticated strategies for prevention, intervention, and treatment.

Suicide

Although persons ages 65 and older comprise only 12.9 percent of the population, they represent a disproportionately high percentage of individuals who commit suicide. Of all suicides, 16 percent are committed by this age group (NCHS, 2010). The group especially at risk appears to be white men. Predisposing factors include loneliness, financial problems, physical illness, loss, and depression (Sadock & Sadock, 2007).

IMPLICATIONS OF RESEARCH FOR EVIDENCE-BASED PRACTICE

Turvey, C. L., Conwell, Y., Jones, M. P., Phillips, C., Simonsick, E., Pearson, J. L., et al. (2002). Risk factors for late-life suicide: A prospective, community-based study. *American Journal of Geriatric Psychiatry, 10,* 398–406.

DESCRIPTION OF THE STUDY: Studies have suggested that a negative or depressive mental outlook, being widowed or divorced, sleeping more than 9 hours per day, and drinking more than three alcoholic beverages per day were risk factors for late-life suicide. The primary aim of this study was to examine the relationship between completed suicide in late life and physical health, disability, and social support. The participants were 14,456 individuals selected from a general population of elderly subjects ages 65 and older. Control subjects were a group of 420 individuals who were matched by age and sex. It was a 10-year longitudinal study beginning in 1981. Variables were assessed at baseline, year 3, and year 6, with a 10-year mortality follow-up. Baseline variables included sleep quality, social support, alcohol use, medical illness, physical impairment, cognitive impairment, and depressive symptoms.

RESULTS OF THE STUDY: The 10-year mortality follow-up indicated that 75 percent of the control subjects had died, but none had died from suicide. Twenty-one of the 14,456 participants committed suicide within the follow-up period. Twenty of the 21 suicide victims were male. Average age was 78.6 years, with a range from 67 to 90 years. The most common means was gunshot. Other means included hanging, cutting, overdose, drowning, and carbon monoxide inhalation, and one participant jumped to his death. In this study, presence of friends or relatives to confide in was negatively associated with suicide. Likewise, regular church attendance was more common in control subjects than the participant sample, indicating an even wider range of community support. Those who committed suicide had reported more depressive symptoms than those who did not, but they did not consume more alcohol (inconsistent with previous

Continued

IMPLICATIONS OF RESEARCH FOR EVIDENCE-BASED PRACTICE—cont'd

studies). Poor sleep quality was positively correlated with suicide in this study, but no specific physical illness was identified as a predisposition. The authors identified the small suicide sample as a limitation of this study.

IMPLICATIONS FOR NURSING PRACTICE: This study identified depression, poor sleep quality, and limited social support as important variables in the potential for elderly suicide. Sleep disturbance may be an important indicator of depression, whereas limited social support may be a contributing factor. The study provides reinforcement for the U.S. Department of

Health and Human Services (USDHHS) recommendation in their *National Strategy for Suicide Prevention: Goals and Objectives for Action* (2001). The USDHHS recommended detection and treatment of depression as a strategy to prevent late-life suicide. The authors of this study stated, "Because both depression and social support are amenable to intervention, this study provides further evidence for the possible effectiveness of such strategies to reduce suicides among older adults." Nurses can become actively involved in assessing for these risk factors, as well as planning, implementing, and evaluating the effectiveness of strategies for preventing suicide in the elderly population.

Although the rate of suicide among the elderly remains high, the numbers of suicides among this age group dropped steadily from 1930 to 1980. Investigators who study these trends surmise that this decline was due to increases in services for older people and an understanding of their problems in society. Statistics show that, from 1980 to 1986, the number of suicides among people ages 65 and older increased by 25 percent, which suggests that there are other contributing factors to the problem. However, since 1987, there has been a gradual decline in the number of elderly suicides.

It has been suggested that increased social isolation may be a contributing factor to suicide among the elderly. The number of elderly individuals who are divorced, widowed, or otherwise living alone has increased. Men seem especially vulnerable after the loss of a spouse, with a relative risk three times that of married men (O'Connell, Chin, Cunningham, & Lawlor, 2004).

The National Institute of Mental Health (NIMH) (2010) suggested that major depression is a significant predictor of suicide in older adults. Unfortunately, it is widely underrecognized and undertreated by the medical community. The NIMH (2010) stated:

> Studies show that many older adults who die by suicide—up to 75 percent—visited a physician within a month before death. These findings point to the urgency of improving detection and treatment of depression to reduce suicide risk among older adults.

Many elderly individuals express symptoms associated with depression that are never recognized as

such. Any sign of helplessness or hopelessness should elicit a supportive intervening response. Stanley and associates (2005) suggested that, in assessing suicide intention, while using concern and compassion, direct questions such as the following should be asked:

- Have you thought life is not worth living?
- Have you considered harming yourself?
- Do you have a plan for hurting yourself?
- Have you ever acted on that plan?
- Have you ever attempted suicide?

Components of intervention with a suicidal elderly person should include demonstrations of genuine concern, interest, and caring; indications of empathy for their fears and concerns; and help in identifying, clarifying, and formulating a plan of action to deal with the unresolved issue. If the elderly person's behavior seems particularly lethal, additional family or staff coverage and contact should be arranged to prevent isolation.

Application of the Nursing Process

Assessment

Assessment of the elderly individual may follow the same framework used for all adults, but with consideration of the possible biological, psychological, sociocultural, and sexual changes that occur in the normal aging process described previously in this chapter. In no other area of nursing is it more important for nurses to practice holistic nursing than with the elderly. Older adults are likely to have multiple physical problems that contribute to problems in other areas of their lives. Obviously, these components cannot be addressed as separate entities. Nursing the elderly is a multifaceted, challenging process because of the multiple changes occurring at this time in the life cycle and the way in which each change affects every aspect of the individual.

Several considerations are unique to assessment of the elderly. Assessment of the older person's thought processes is a primary responsibility. Knowledge about the presence and extent of disorientation or confusion will influence the way in which the nurse approaches elder care.

Information about sensory capabilities is also extremely important. Because hearing loss is common, the nurse should lower the pitch and loudness of his or her voice when addressing the older person. Looking directly into the face of the older person when talking facilitates communication. Questions that require a declarative sentence in response should be asked; in this way, the nurse is able to assess the client's ability to use words correctly. Visual acuity can be determined by assessing adaptation to the dark, color matching, and the perception of color contrast. Knowledge about these aspects of sensory functioning is essential in the development of an effective care plan.

The nurse should be familiar with the normal physical changes associated with the aging process. Examples of some of these changes include:

■ Less effective response to changes in environmental temperature, resulting in hypothermia.

■ Decreases in oxygen use and the amount of blood pumped by the heart, resulting in cerebral anoxia or hypoxia.

■ Skeletal muscle wasting and weakness, resulting in difficulty in physical mobility.

■ Limited cough and laryngeal reflexes, resulting in risk of aspiration.

■ Demineralization of bones, resulting in spontaneous fracturing.

■ Decrease in gastrointestinal motility, resulting in constipation.

■ Decrease in the ability to interpret painful stimuli, resulting in risk of injury.

Common psychosocial changes associated with aging include:

■ Prolonged and exaggerated grief, resulting in depression.

■ Physical changes, resulting in disturbed body image.

■ Changes in status, resulting in loss of self-worth.

This list is by no means exhaustive. The nurse should consider many other alterations in his or her assessment of the client. Knowledge of the client's functional capabilities is essential for determining the physiological, psychological, and sociological needs of the elderly individual. Age alone does not preclude the occurrence of all these changes. The aging process progresses at a wide range of variance, and each client must be assessed as a unique individual.

Diagnosis/Outcome Identification

Virtually any nursing diagnosis may be applicable to the aging client, depending on individual needs for assistance. Based on normal changes that occur in the elderly, the following nursing diagnoses may be considered:

Physiologically Related Diagnoses

■ Risk for trauma related to confusion, disorientation, muscular weakness, spontaneous fractures, falls

■ Hypothermia related to loss of adipose tissue under the skin, evidenced by increased sensitivity to cold and body temperature below 98.6°F

■ Decreased cardiac output related to decreased myocardial efficiency secondary to age-related changes, evidenced by decreased tolerance for activity and decline in energy reserve

■ Ineffective breathing pattern related to increase in fibrous tissue and loss of elasticity in lung tissue, evidenced by dyspnea and activity intolerance

■ Risk for aspiration related to diminished cough and laryngeal reflexes

■ Impaired physical mobility related to muscular wasting and weakness, evidenced by need for assistance in ambulation

■ Imbalanced nutrition, less than body requirements, related to inefficient absorption from gastrointestinal tract, difficulty chewing and swallowing, anorexia, difficulty in feeding self, evidenced by wasting syndrome, anemia, weight loss

■ Constipation related to decreased motility; inadequate diet; insufficient activity or exercise, evidenced by decreased bowel sounds; hard, formed stools; or straining at stool

■ Stress urinary incontinence related to degenerative changes in pelvic muscles and structural supports associated with increased age, evidenced by reported or observed dribbling with increased abdominal pressure or urinary frequency

■ Urinary retention related to prostatic enlargement, evidenced by bladder distention, frequent voiding of small amounts, dribbling, or overflow incontinence

■ Disturbed sensory perception related to age-related alterations in sensory transmission, evidenced by decreased visual acuity, hearing loss, diminished sensitivity to taste and smell, or increased touch threshold

■ Insomnia related to age-related decrease in ability to sleep ("sleep decay"), dementia, or medications, evidenced by interrupted sleep, early awakening, or falling asleep during the day

■ Chronic pain related to degenerative changes in joints, evidenced by verbalization of pain or hesitation to use weight-bearing joints

■ Self-care deficit (specify) related to weakness, confusion, or disorientation, evidenced by inability to feed self, maintain hygiene, dress/groom self, or toilet self without assistance

■ Risk for impaired skin integrity related to alterations in nutritional state, circulation, sensation, or mobility

Psychosocially Related Diagnoses

■ Disturbed thought processes related to age-related changes that result in cerebral anoxia, evidenced by short-term memory loss, confusion, or disorientation

■ Complicated grieving related to bereavement overload, evidenced by symptoms of depression

■ Risk for suicide related to depressed mood and feelings of low self-worth

■ Powerlessness related to lifestyle of helplessness and dependency on others, evidenced by depressed mood, apathy, or verbal expressions of having no control or influence over life situation

■ Low self-esteem related to loss of pre-retirement status, evidenced by verbalization of negative feelings about self and life

■ Fear related to nursing home placement, evidenced by symptoms of severe anxiety and

statements such as, "Nursing homes are places to go to die."

■ Disturbed body image related to age-related changes in skin, hair, and fat distribution, evidenced by verbalization of negative feelings about body

■ Ineffective sexuality pattern related to dyspareunia, evidenced by reported dissatisfaction with decrease in frequency of sexual intercourse

■ Sexual dysfunction related to medications (e.g., antihypertensives) evidenced by inability to achieve an erection

■ Social isolation related to total dependence on others, evidenced by expression of inadequacy in or absence of significant purpose in life

■ Risk for trauma (elder abuse) related to caregiver role strain

■ Caregiver role strain related to severity and duration of the care receiver's illness; lack of respite and recreation for the caregiver, evidenced by feelings of stress in relationship with care receiver; feelings of depression and anger; or family conflict around issues of providing care

Outcome Criteria

The following criteria may be used for measurement of outcomes in the care of the elderly client.

The Client:

■ Has not experienced injury.

■ Maintains reality orientation consistent with cognitive level of functioning.

■ Manages own self-care with assistance.

■ Expresses positive feelings about self, past accomplishments, and hope for the future.

■ Compensates adaptively for diminished sensory perception.

Caregivers:

■ Can problem-solve effectively regarding care of the elderly client.

■ Demonstrate adaptive coping strategies for dealing with stress of caregiver role.

■ Openly express feelings.

■ Express desire to join support group of other caregivers.

Planning/Implementation

In Table 35-2, selected nursing diagnoses are presented for the elderly client. Outcome criteria are

Table 35-2 CARE PLAN FOR THE ELDERLY CLIENT

NURSING DIAGNOSIS: RISK FOR TRAUMA

RELATED TO: Confusion, disorientation, muscular weakness, spontaneous fractures, falls

OUTCOME CRITERIA	NURSING INTERVENTIONS	RATIONALE
Short-Term Goals • Client will call for assistance when ambulating or carrying out other activities. • Client will not experience injury. **Long-Term Goal** • Client will not experience injury.	1. The following measures may be instituted: a. Arrange furniture and other items in the room to accommodate client's disabilities. b. Store frequently used items within easy access. c. Keep bed in unelevated position. Pad side rails and headboard if client has history of seizures. Keep bedrails up when client is in bed (if permitted by institutional policy). d. Assign room near nurses' station; observe frequently. e. Assist client with ambulation. f. Keep a dim light on at night. g. If client is a smoker, cigarettes and lighter or matches should be kept at the nurses' station and dispensed only when someone is available to stay with client while he or she is smoking. h. Frequently orient client to place, time, and situation. i. Soft restraints may be required if client is very disoriented and hyperactive.	1. To ensure client safety.

NURSING DIAGNOSIS: DISTURBED THOUGHT PROCESSES

RELATED TO: Age-related changes that result in cerebral anoxia

EVIDENCED BY: Short-term memory loss, confusion, or disorientation

OUTCOME CRITERIA	NURSING INTERVENTIONS	RATIONALE
Short-Term Goal • Client will accept explanations of inaccurate interpretations of the environment within (time to be determined based on client condition) **Long-Term Goal** • Client will interpret the environment accurately and maintain reality orientation to the best of his or her cognitive ability	1. Frequently orient client to reality. Use clocks and calendars with large numbers that are easy to read. Notes and large, bold signs may be useful as reminders. Allow client to have personal belongings. 2. Keep explanations simple. Use face-to-face interaction. Speak slowly and do not shout. 3. Discourage rumination of delusional thinking. Talk about real events and real people. 4. Monitor for medication side effects.	1. To help maintain orientation and aid in memory and recognition. 2. To facilitate comprehension. Shouting may create discomfort, and in some instances, may provoke anger. 3. Rumination promotes disorientation. Reality orientation increases sense of self-worth and personal dignity. 4. Physiological changes in the elderly can alter the body's response to certain medications. Toxic effects may intensify altered thought processes.

Continued

Table 35-2 CARE PLAN FOR THE ELDERLY CLIENT—cont'd

NURSING DIAGNOSIS: SELF-CARE DEFICIT (SPECIFY)
RELATED TO: Weakness, disorientation, confusion, or memory deficits
EVIDENCED BY: Inability to fulfill activities of daily living (ADLs)

OUTCOME CRITERIA	NURSING INTERVENTIONS	RATIONALE

Short-Term Goal
• Client will participate in ADLs with assistance from caregiver.
Long-Term Goals
• Client will accomplish ADLs to the best of his or her ability.
• Unfulfilled needs will be met by caregivers.
	1. Provide a simple, structured environment:
	   a. Identify self-care deficits and provide assistance as required. Promote independent actions as able.
	   b. Allow plenty of time for client to perform tasks.
	   c. Provide guidance and support for independent actions by talking the client through the task one step at a time.
	   d. Provide a structured schedule of activities that do not change from day to day.
	   e. ADLs should follow home routine as closely as possible.
	   f. Allow consistency in assignment of daily caregivers.
		1. To minimize confusion

NURSING DIAGNOSIS: CAREGIVER ROLE STRAIN
RELATED TO: Severity and duration of the care receiver's illness; lack of respite and recreation for the caregiver
EVIDENCED BY: Feelings of stress in relationship with care receiver; feelings of depression and anger; family conflict around issues of providing care

OUTCOME CRITERIA	NURSING INTERVENTIONS	RATIONALE
Short-Term Goal • Caregivers will verbalize understanding of ways to facilitate the caregiver role. **Long-Term Goal** • Caregivers will achieve effective problem-solving skills and develop adaptive coping mechanisms to regain equilibrium.	1. Assess prospective caregivers' ability to anticipate and fulfill client's unmet needs. Provide information to assist caregivers with this responsibility. Ensure that caregivers are aware of available community support systems from which they can seek assistance when required. Examples include adult day-care centers, housekeeping and homemaker services, respite care services, or a local chapter of the Alzheimer's Association. This organization sponsors a nationwide 24-hour hot line to provide information and link families who need assistance with nearby chapters and affiliates. The hotline number is 800-272-0379.	1. Caregivers require relief from the pressures and strain of providing 24-hour care for their loved one. Studies have shown that elder abuse arises out of caregiving situations that place overwhelming stress on the caregivers.
	2. Encourage caregivers to express feelings, particularly anger.	2. Release of these emotions can serve to prevent psychopathology, such as depression or psychophysiological disorders, from occurring.
	3. Encourage participation in support groups composed of members with similar life situations.	3. Hearing others who are experiencing the same problems discuss ways in which they have coped may help caregiver adopt more adaptive strategies. Individuals who are experiencing similar life situations provide empathy and support for each other.

Table 35-2 CARE PLAN FOR THE ELDERLY CLIENT—cont'd

NURSING DIAGNOSIS: LOW SELF-ESTEEM

RELATED TO: Loss of pre-retirement status; early stages of cognitive decline

EVIDENCED BY: Verbalization of negative feelings about self and life

OUTCOME CRITERIA	NURSING INTERVENTIONS	RATIONALE

Short-Term Goal
• Client will verbalize positive aspects of self and past accomplishments.
Long-Term Goal
• Client will participate in group activities in which he or she can experience a feeling of enjoyment and accomplishment (to the best of his or her ability).
	1. Encourage client to express honest feelings in relation to loss of prior status. Acknowledge pain of loss. Support client through process of grieving.
	
	2. If lapses in memory are occurring, devise methods for assisting client with memory deficit. Examples:
	  a. Name sign on door identifying client's room.
	  b. Identifying sign on outside of dining room door.
	  c. Identifying sign on outside of restroom door.
	  d. Large clock, with oversized numbers and hands, appropriately placed.
	  e. Large calendar, indicating one day at a time, with month, day, and year in bold print.
	  f. Printed, structured daily schedule, with one copy for client and one posted on unit wall.
	  g. "News board" on unit wall where current news of national and local interest may be posted.
	
	3. Encourage client's attempts to communicate. If verbalizations are not understandable, express to client what you think he or she intended to say. It may be necessary to reorient client frequently.
	
	4. Encourage reminiscence and discussion of life review (see Box 35-2). Sharing picture albums, if possible, is especially good. Also discuss present-day events.
	
	5. Encourage participation in group activities. May need to accompany client at first, until he or she feels secure that the group members will be accepting, regardless of limitations in verbal communication.
	
	6. Encourage client to be as independent as possible in self-care activities. Provide written schedule of tasks to be performed. Intervene in areas where client requires assistance.
		1. Client may be fixed in anger stage of grieving process, which is turned inward on the self, resulting in diminished self-esteem.
		
		2. These aids may assist client to function more independently, thereby increasing self-esteem.
		
		3. The ability to communicate effectively with others may enhance self-esteem.
		
		4. Reminiscence and life review help client resume progression through the grief process associated with disappointing life events and increase self-esteem as successes are reviewed.
		
		5. Positive feedback from group members will increase self-esteem.
		
		6. The ability to perform independently preserves self-esteem.

Continued

Table 35-2 CARE PLAN FOR THE ELDERLY CLIENT—cont'd

NURSING DIAGNOSIS: DISTURBED SENSORY PERCEPTION
RELATED TO: Age-related alterations in sensory transmission
EVIDENCED BY: Decreased visual acuity, hearing loss, diminished sensitivity to taste and smell, and increased touch threshold

OUTCOME CRITERIA	NURSING INTERVENTIONS*	RATIONALE
Short-Term Goal • Client will not experience injury due to diminished sensory perception. **Long-Term Goal** • Client will attain optimal level of sensory stimulation. • Client will not experience injury due to diminished sensory perception.	1. The following nursing strategies are indicated: 　a. Provide meaningful sensory stimulation to all special senses through conversation, touch, music, or pleasant smells. 　b. Encourage wearing of glasses, hearing aids, prostheses, and other adaptive devices. 　c. Use bright, contrasting colors in the environment. 　d. Provide large-print reading materials, such as books, clocks, calendars, and educational materials. 　e. Maintain room lighting that distinguishes day from night and that is free of shadows and glare. 　f. Teach client to scan the environment to locate objects. 　g. Help client to locate food on plate using "clock" system, and describe food if client is unable to visualize; assist with feeding as needed. 　h. Arrange physical environment to maximize functional vision. 　i. Place personal items and call light within client's field of vision. 　j. Teach client to watch the person who is speaking. 　k. Reinforce wearing of hearing aid; if client does not have an aid, may consider a communication device (e.g., amplifier). 　l. Communicate clearly, distinctly, and slowly, using a low-pitched voice and facing client; avoid overarticulation. 　m. Remove as much unnecessary background noise as possible. 　n. Do not use slang or extraneous words. 　o. As speaker, position self at eye level and no farther than 6 feet away. 　p. Get the client's attention before speaking. 　q. Avoid speaking directly into the client's ear. 　r. If the client does not understand what is being said, rephrase the statement rather than simply repeating it. 　s. Help client select foods from the menu that will ensure discrimination between various tastes and smells.	1. To assist client with diminished sensory perception and because client safety is a nursing priority.

Table 35-2 CARE PLAN FOR THE ELDERLY CLIENT—cont'd

OUTCOME CRITERIA	NURSING INTERVENTIONS	RATIONALE
	t. Ensure that food has been properly cooled so that client with diminished pain threshold is not burned.	
	u. Ensure that bath or shower water is appropriate temperature.	
	v. Use back rubs and massage as therapeutic touch to stimulate sensory receptors.	

The interventions for this nursing diagnosis were adapted from Rogers-Seidl, F. F. (1997). Geriatric nursing care plans (2nd ed.).
St. Louis: Mosby Year Book.

included, along with appropriate nursing interventions and rationale for each.

Reminiscence therapy is especially helpful with elderly clients. This therapeutic intervention is highlighted in Box 35-2.

Evaluation

Reassessment is conducted to determine if the nursing actions have been successful in achieving the objectives of care. Evaluation of the nursing actions for the elderly client may be facilitated by gathering information using the following types of questions:

■ Has the client escaped injury from falls, burns, or other means to which he or she is vulnerable because of age?

■ Can caregivers verbalize means of providing a safe environment for the client?

■ Does the client maintain reality orientation at an optimum for his or her cognitive functioning?

BOX 35-2 Reminiscence Therapy and Life Review with the Elderly

Stanley, Blair, and Beare (2005) stated:

Stimulation of life memories helps older adults to work through their losses and maintain self-esteem. Life review provides older adults with an opportunity to come to grips with guilt and regrets, and to emerge feeling good about themselves. (p. 268)

Studies have indicated that *reminiscence,* or thinking about the past and reflecting on it, may promote better mental health in old age. *Life review* is related to reminiscence, but differs from it in that it is a more guided or directed cognitive process that constructs a history or story in an autobiographical way (Murray, Zentner, & Yakimo, 2009).

Elderly individuals who spend time thinking about the past experience an increase in self-esteem and are less likely to suffer depression. Some psychologists believe that life review may help some people adjust to memories of an unhappy past. Others view reminiscence and life review as ways to bolster feelings of well-being, particularly in older people who can no longer remain active.

Reminiscence therapy can take place on a one-to-one basis or in a group setting. In reminiscence groups, elderly individuals share significant past events with peers. The nurse leader facilitates the discussion of topics that deal with specific life transitions, such as childhood, adolescence, marriage, childbearing, grandparenthood, and retirement. Members share both positive and negative aspects, including personal feelings, about these life-cycle events.

Reminiscence on a one-to-one basis can provide a way for elderly individuals to work through unresolved issues from the past. Painful issues may be too difficult to discuss in the group setting. As the individual reviews his or her life process, the nurse can validate feelings and help the elderly client come to terms with painful issues that may have been long suppressed. This process is necessary if the elderly individual is to maintain (or attain) a sense of positive identity and self-esteem and ultimately achieve the goal of ego integrity as described by Erikson (1963).

A number of creative measures can be used to facilitate life review with the elderly individual. Having the client keep a journal for sharing may be a way to

Continued

BOX 35-2 Reminiscence Therapy and Life Review with the Elderly—cont'd

stimulate discussion (as well as providing a permanent record of past events for significant others). Pets, music, and special foods have a way of provoking memories from the client's past. Photographs of family members and past significant events are an excellent way of guiding the elderly client through his or her autobiographical review.

Care must be taken in the life review to assist clients to work through unresolved issues. Anxiety, guilt,

depression, and despair may result if the individual is unable to work through the problems and accept them. Life review can work in a negative way if the individual comes to believe that his or her life was meaningless. However, it can be a very positive experience for the person who can take pride in past accomplishments and feel satisfied with his or her life, resulting in a sense of serenity and inner peace in the older adult.

■ Can the client distinguish between reality-based and non–reality-based thinking?

■ Can caregivers verbalize ways in which to orient client to reality, as needed?

■ Is the client able to accomplish self-care activities independently to his or her optimum level of functioning?

■ Does the client seek assistance for aspects of self-care that he or she is unable to perform independently?

■ Does the client express positive feelings about himself or herself?

■ Does the client reminisce about accomplishments that have occurred in his or her life?

■ Does the client express some hope for the future?

■ Does the client wear eyeglasses or a hearing aid, if needed, to compensate for sensory deficits?

■ Does the client consistently look at others in the face to facilitate hearing when they are talking to him or her?

■ Does the client use helpful aids, such as signs identifying various rooms, to help maintain orientation?

■ Can the caregivers work through problems and make decisions regarding care of the elderly client?

■ Do the caregivers include the elderly client in the decision-making process, if appropriate?

■ Can the caregivers demonstrate adaptive coping strategies for dealing with the strain of long-term caregiving?

■ Are the caregivers open and honest in expression of feelings?

■ Can the caregivers verbalize community resources to which they can go for assistance with their caregiving responsibilities?

■ Have the caregivers joined a support group?

Summary and Key Points

■ Care of the aging individual presents one of the greatest challenges for nursing.

■ The growing population of individuals ages 65 and older suggests that the challenge will progress well into the 21st century.

■ America is a youth-oriented society. It is not desirable to be old in this culture.

■ In some cultures, the elderly are revered and hold a special place of honor within the society, but in highly industrialized countries such as the United States, status declines with the decrease in productivity and participation in the mainstream of society.

■ Individuals experience many changes as they age. Physical changes occur in virtually every body system.

■ Psychologically, there may be age-related memory deficiencies, particularly for recent events.

■ Intellectual functioning does not decline with age, but length of time required for learning increases.

■ Aging individuals experience many losses, potentially leading to bereavement overload. They are vulnerable to depression and to feelings of low self-worth.

■ The elderly population represents a disproportionately high percentage of individuals who commit suicide.

■ Dementing disorders are the most frequent causes of psychopathology in the elderly. Sleep disorders are very common.

■ The need for sexual expression by the elderly is often misunderstood within our society. Although many physical changes occur at this time of life that alter an individual's sexuality, if he or she has reasonably good health and a willing partner, sexual activity can continue well past the 70s for most people.

■ Retirement has both social and economic implications for elderly individuals. Society often equates an individual's status with occupation, and loss of employment may result in the need for adjustment in the standard of living because retirement income may be reduced by 20 to 40 percent of pre-retirement earnings.

■ Less than 5 percent of the population ages 65 and older live in nursing homes. A profile of the typical elderly nursing home resident is a white woman about 80 years old, widowed, with multiple chronic health conditions. Much stigma is attached to what some still call "rest homes" or "old age homes," and many elderly people still equate them with a place "to go to die."

■ The strain of the caregiver role has become a major dilemma in our society. Elder abuse is sometimes inflicted by caregivers for whom the role has become overwhelming and intolerable. There is an intense need to find assistance for these people, who must provide care for their loved ones on a 24-hour basis. Home health care, respite care, support groups, and financial assistance are needed to ease the burden of this role strain.

■ Caring for elderly individuals requires a special kind of inner strength and compassion. The poem that follows conveys a vital message for nurses.

DavisPlus   Additional info available @ davisplus.fadavis.com

What Do You See, Nurse?

What do you see, nurse, what do you see?
　What are you thinking when you look at me?
A crabbed old woman, not very wise.
　Uncertain of habit, with faraway eyes.
Who dribbles her food and makes no reply
　When you say in a loud voice, "I do wish you'd try."
Who seems not to notice the things that you do
　And forever is losing a stocking or shoe.
Who unresisting or not, lets you do as you will
　With bathing and feeding, the long day to fill.
Is that what you're thinking, is that what you see?
　Then open your eyes, you're not looking at me.
I'll tell you who I am as I sit there so still.
　As I move at your bidding, as I eat at your will.
I'm a small child of ten with a father and a mother,
　Brothers and sisters who love one another.

A young girl at sixteen with wings on her feet
　Dreaming that soon now a lover she'll meet.
A bride soon at twenty—my heart gives a leap
　Remembering the vows that I promised to keep.
At twenty-five, now, I have young of my own
　Who need me to build a secure happy home.
A woman of thirty, my young now grow fast
　Bound to each other with ties that should last.

At forty my young will now soon be gone,
　But my man stays beside me to see I don't mourn.
At fifty once more babies play round my knee.
　Again we know children, my loved one and me.

Dark days are upon me, my husband is dead.
　I look at the future, I shudder with dread.
For my young are all busy rearing young of their own.
　And I think of the years and the love I have known.

I'm an old woman now and nature is cruel.
　Tis her jest to make old age look like a fool.
The body it crumbles, grace and vigor depart.
　There is now just a stone where I once had a heart.
But inside this old carcass a young girl still dwells.
　And now and again my battered heart swells.

I remember the joys, I remember the pain.
　And I'm loving and living life all over again.
I think of the years all too few—gone so fast.
　And accept the stark fact that nothing can last.
So open your eyes, nurse, open and see.
　Not a crabbed old woman—look closer—SEE ME.

Author Unknown

Review Questions
Self-Examination/Learning Exercise

*Select the answer that is **most** appropriate for each of the following questions:*

1. Stanley, age 72, is admitted to the hospital for depression. His son reports that he has periods of confusion and forgetfulness. In her admission assessment, the nurse notices an open sore on Stanley's arm. When she questions him about it he says, "I scraped it on the fence 2 weeks ago. It's smaller than it was." How might the nurse analyze these data?
   a. Stanley was trying to commit suicide.
   b. The delay in healing may indicate that Stanley has developed skin cancer.
   c. A diminished inflammatory response in the elderly increases healing time.
   d. Age-related skin changes and distribution of adipose tissue delay healing in the elderly.

2. What is the most appropriate way to communicate with an elderly person who is deaf in his right ear?
   a. Speak loudly into his left ear.
   b. Speak to him from a position on his left side.
   c. Speak face-to-face in a high-pitched voice.
   d. Speak face-to-face in a low-pitched voice.

3. Why is it important for the nurse to check the temperature of the water before before an elderly individual gets into the shower?
   a. The client may catch cold if the water temperature is too low.
   b. The client may burn himself because of a higher pain threshold.
   c. Elderly clients have difficulty discriminating between hot and cold.
   d. The water must be exactly 98.6°F.

4. Mr. B., age 79, is admitted to the psychiatric unit for depression. He has lost weight and has become socially isolated. His wife died 5 years ago and his son tells the nurse, "He did very well when Mom died. He didn't even cry." Which would be the *priority* nursing diagnosis for Mr. B.?
   a. Complicated grieving.
   b. Imbalanced nutrition: less than body requirements.
   c. Social isolation.
   d. Risk for injury.

5. Mr. B., age 79, is admitted to the psychiatric unit for depression. He has lost weight and has become socially isolated. His wife died 5 years ago and he lives alone. A suicide assessment is conducted. Why is Mr. B. at high risk for suicide?
   a. All depressed people are at high risk for suicide.
   b. Mr. B. is in the age group in which the highest percentage of suicides occur.
   c. Mr. B. is a white man, recently bereaved, living alone.
   d. His son reports that Mr. B. owns a gun.

6. Mr. B., age 79, is admitted to the psychiatric unit for depression. He has lost weight and has become socially isolated. His wife died 5 years ago and his son tells the nurse, "He did very well when Mom died. He didn't even cry." Which would be the *priority* nursing intervention for Mr. B.?
   a. Take blood pressure once each shift.
   b. Ensure that Mr. B. attends group activities.
   c. Encourage Mr. B. to eat all of the food on his food tray.
   d. Encourage Mr. B. to talk about his wife's death.

Continued

7. In group exercise, Mr. B., a 79-year-old man with major depression, becomes tired and short of breath very quickly. This is most likely due to:
   a. Age-related changes in the cardiovascular system.
   b. A sedentary lifestyle.
   c. The effects of pathological depression.
   d. Medication the physician has prescribed for depression.

8. Clara, an 80-year-old woman, says to the nurse, "I'm all alone now. My husband is gone. My best friend is gone. My daughter is busy with her work and family. I might as well just go, too." Which is the best response by the nurse?
   a. "Are you thinking that you want to die, Clara?"
   b. "You have lots to live for, Clara."
   c. "Cheer up, Clara. You have so much to be thankful for."
   d. "Tell me about your family, Clara."

9. An elderly client says to the nurse, "I don't want to go to that crafts class. I'm too old to learn anything." Based on knowledge of the aging process, which of the following is a true statement?
   a. Memory functioning in the elderly most likely reflects loss of long-term memories of remote events.
   b. Intellectual functioning declines with advancing age.
   c. Learning ability remains intact, but time required for learning increases with age.
   d. Cognitive functioning is rarely affected in aging individuals.

10. According to the literature, which of the following is most important for individuals to maintain a healthy, adaptive old age?
    a. To remain socially interactive.
    b. To disengage slowly in preparation of the last stage of life.
    c. To move in with family.
    d. To maintain total independence and accept no help from anyone.

TEST YOUR CRITICAL THINKING SKILLS

Mrs. M., age 76, is seeing her primary physician for her regular 6-month physical examination. Mrs. M.'s husband died 2 years ago, at which time she sold her home in Kansas and came to live in California with her only child, a daughter. The daughter is married and has 3 children (one in college and two teenagers at home). The daughter reports that her mother is becoming increasingly withdrawn, stays in her room, and eats very little. She has lost 13 pounds since her last 6-month visit. The primary physician refers Mrs. M. to a psychiatrist, who hospitalizes her for evaluation. He diagnoses Mrs. M. with Major Depression.

Mrs. M. tells the nurse, "I didn't want to leave my home, but my daughter insisted. I would have been all right. I miss my friends and my church. Back home I drove my car everywhere. But there's too much traffic out here. They sold my car and I have to depend on my daughter or grandkids to take me places. I hate being so dependent! I miss my husband so much. I just sit and think about him and our past life all the time. I don't have any interest in meeting new people. I want to go home!!"

Mrs. M. admits to having some thoughts of dying, although she denies feeling suicidal. She denies having a plan or means for taking her life. "I really don't want to die, but I just can't see much reason for living. My daughter and her family are so busy with their own lives. They don't need me—or even have time for me!" *Answer the following questions about Mrs. M:*

1. What would be the *primary* nursing diagnosis for Mrs. M.?

2. Formulate a short-term goal for Mrs. M.

3. From the assessment data, identify the major problem that may be a long-term focus of care for Mrs. M.

References

Administration on Aging. (2011). *A profile of older Americans: 2010.* Washington, DC: U.S. Department of Health and Human Services.

American Association of Retired Persons. (2010). *Sex, romance, and relationships: AARP survey of midlife and older adults.* Washington, DC: Author.

Beers, M. H., & Jones, T. V. (Eds.). (2004). *The Merck manual of health & aging.* Whitehouse Station, NJ: Merck Research Laboratories.

Blazer, D. (2008). Treatment of seniors. In R. E. Hales, S. C. Yudofsky, & G. O. Gabbard (Eds.), *Textbook of psychiatry* (5th ed., pp. 1449–1469). Washington, DC: American Psychiatric Publishing.

Centers for Disease Control and Prevention. (2010). *Improving and extending quality of life among older Americans: At a glance 2010.* Retrieved October 8, 2010, from http://www.cdc.gov/chronicdisease/resources/publications/AAG/aging.htm

Heiss, G., Wallace, R., Anderson, G. L., Aragak, A., Beresford, S. A. A., Brzyski, R., et al. (2008). Health risks and benefits three years after stopping randomized threatment with estrogen and progestin. *Journal of the American Medical Association, 299,* 1036–1045.

Johnston, C. B., Harper, G. M., & Landefeld, C. S. (2009). Geriatric disorders. In S. J. McPhee & M. A. Papadakis (Eds.), *Current medical diagnosis and treatment* (pp. 56–71). New York: McGraw Hill Medical.

King, B. M. (2009). *Human sexuality today* (6th ed.). Upper Saddle River, NJ: Pearson Prentice Hall.

Masters, W. H., Johnson, V. E., & Kolodny, R. C. (1995). *Human sexuality* (5th ed.). New York: Addison-Wesley Longman.

Murray, R. B., Zentner, J. P., & Yakimo, R. (2009). *Health promotion strategies through the life span* (8th ed.). Upper Saddle River, NJ: Prentice Hall.

National Center for Health Statistics. (2008). *Older Americans 2008: Key indicators of well-being.* Federal Interagency Forum on Aging-Related Statistics. Washington, DC: U.S. Government Printing Office.

National Center for Health Statistics. (2010, December 9). Deaths: Preliminary data for 2008. *National Vital Statistics Reports, 59*(2), 1–72.

National Institute of Mental Health. (2010). *Older adults: Depression and suicide facts.* Retrieved October 8, 2010, from http://www.nimh.nih.gov/health/publications/older-adults-depression-and-suicide-facts-fact-sheet/index.shtml

National Institutes of Health. (2008). *Aging changes in immunity.* Retrieved October 8, 2010, from http://www.nlm.nih.gov/medlineplus/ency/article/004008.htm

O'Connell, H., Chin, A. V., Cunningham, C., & Lawlor, B. A. (2004). Recent developments: Suicide in older people. *British Medical Journal, 329,* 895–899.

Pietraniec-Shannon, M. (2007). Nursing care of older adult patients. In L. S. Williams & P. D. Hopper (Eds.), *Understanding medical-surgical nursing* (3rd ed., pp. 270–288). Philadelphia: F.A. Davis.

Purnell, L. D., & Paulanka, B. J. (2008). *Transcultural health care: A culturally competent approach* (3rd ed.). Philadelphia: F.A. Davis.

Roberts, C. M. (1991). *How did I get here so fast?* New York: Warner Books.

Rogers-Seidl, F. F. (1997). *Geriatric nursing care plans* (2nd ed.). St. Louis: Mosby Year Book.

Sadock, B. J., & Sadock, V. A. (2007). *Synopsis of psychiatry: Behavioral sciences/clinical psychiatry* (10th ed.). Philadelphia: Lippincott Williams & Wilkins.

Srivastava, S., John, O. P., Gosling, S. D., & Potter, J. (2003). Development of personality in early and middle adulthood: Set like plaster or persistent change? *Journal of Personality and Social Psychology, 84,* 1041–1053.

Stanley, M., Blair, K. A., & Beare, P. G. (2005). *Gerontological nursing: Promoting successful aging with older adults* (3rd ed.). Philadelphia: F.A. Davis.

Vaillant, G. E. (2003). *Aging well: Surprising guideposts to a happier life from the landmark Harvard study of adult development.* New York: Little, Brown, & Company.

Classical References

Erikson, E. H. (1963). *Childhood and society* (2nd ed.). New York: WW Norton.

Kübler-Ross, E. (1969). *On death and dying.* New York: Macmillan.

Reichard, S., Livson, F., & Peterson, P. G. (1962). *Aging and personality.* New York: John Wiley & Sons.

@ INTERNET REFERENCES

- Additional sources related to aging may be located at the following websites:
  - http://www.4woman.org/Menopause
  - http://www.aarp.org/
  - http://www.ssa.gov/
  - http://www.nih.gov/nia/
  - http://www.medicare.gov/
  - http://www.seniorlaw.com/
  - http://www.growthhouse.org/cesp.html
  - http://www.agenet.com/
  - http://www.aoa.gov/
  - http://www.nsclc.org/

MOVIE CONNECTIONS

The Hiding Place
On Golden Pond
To Dance With the White Dog

Victims of Abuse or Neglect

CORE CONCEPTS

abuse

battering

incest

neglect

rape

KEY TERMS

acquaintance (date) rape

child sexual abuse

compounded rape reaction

controlled response pattern

cycle of battering

emotional abuse

emotional neglect

expressed response pattern

marital rape

physical neglect

safe house or shelter

sexual exploitation
  of a child

silent rape reaction

statutory rape

OBJECTIVES

After reading this chapter, the student will be able to:

1. Describe epidemiological statistics associated with intimate partner violence, child abuse, and sexual assault.
2. Discuss characteristics of victims and victimizers.
3. Identify predisposing factors to abusive behaviors.
4. Describe physical and psychological effects on the victims of intimate partner violence, child abuse, and sexual assault.
5. Identify nursing diagnoses, goals of care, and appropriate nursing interventions for care of victims of intimate partner violence, child abuse, and sexual assault.
6. Evaluate nursing care of victims of intimate partner violence, child abuse, and sexual assault.
7. Discuss various modalities relevant to treatment of victims of abuse.

HOMEWORK ASSIGNMENT

Please read the chapter and answer the following questions:

1. What neurotransmitters have been implicated in the etiology of aggression and violence?
2. What is the most common reason that women give for staying in an abusive relationship?
3. Describe a compounded rape reaction.
4. What are some adult manifestations of childhood sexual abuse?

CORE CONCEPT

Abuse

The maltreatment of one person by another.

Abuse is on the rise in this society. Books, newspapers, movies, and television inundate their readers and viewers with stories of "man's inhumanity to man" (no gender bias intended).

About 4.8 million intimate partner victimizations occur each year among U.S. women ages 18 and older, and 2.9 million occur among men (Centers for Disease Control and Prevention [CDC], 2009a). More injuries are attributed to intimate partner violence than to all rapes, muggings, and automobile accidents combined.

Rape is vastly underreported in the United States. Because many of these attacks occurring daily go unreported and unrecognized, sexual assault is often considered a silent-violent epidemic. In the United States, 1 in 6 women and 1 in 33 men have reported experiencing an attempted or completed rape at some time in their lives (CDC, 2009b).

An increase in the incidence of child abuse and related fatalities has also been documented. In 2008, an estimated 3.3 million cases of possible child abuse or neglect were reported to child protective services, and about 24 percent of these cases were substantiated (U.S. Department of Health and Human Services [USDHHS], 2010). An estimated 1,740 children died from causes related to abuse or neglect in 2008.

Abuse affects all populations equally. It occurs among all races, religions, economic classes, ages, and educational backgrounds. The phenomenon is cyclical in that many abusers were themselves victims of abuse as children.

Family violence is not a new problem; in fact, it is probably as old as humankind, and has been documented as far back as Biblical times. Child abuse became a mandatory reportable occurrence in the United States in 1968. Responsibility for the protection of elders from abuse rests primarily with the states. In 1987, Congress passed amendments to the Older Americans Act of 1965 that provide for state Area Agencies on Aging to assess the need for elder abuse prevention services. These events have made it possible for individuals who once felt powerless to stop the abuse against them, to come forward and seek advice, support, and protection.

Aside from the individual physical, psychological, and social devastation that violence incurs, there are economic implications as well. The World Health Organization (WHO) reported that, in the United States alone, costs related to interpersonal violence reach 3.3 percent of the gross domestic product (WHO, 2004).

This chapter discusses intimate partner violence, child abuse (including neglect), and sexual assault. Elder abuse is discussed in Chapter 35. Factors that predispose individuals to commit acts of abuse against others, as well as the physical and psychological effects on the victims, are examined.

Nursing of individuals who have experienced abusive behavior from others is presented within the context of the nursing process. Various treatment modalities are described.

Predisposing Factors

What predisposes individuals to be abusive? Although no one really knows for sure, several

theories have been espoused. A brief discussion of ideas associated with biological, psychological, and sociocultural views is presented here.

Biological Theories

Neurophysiological Influences

Various components of the neurological system in both humans and animals have been implicated in both the facilitation and inhibition of aggressive impulses. Areas of the brain that may be involved include the temporal lobe, the limbic system, and the amygdaloid nucleus (Tardiff, 2003).

Biochemical Influences

Studies show that various neurotransmitters—in particular norepinephrine, dopamine, and serotonin—may play a role in the facilitation and inhibition of aggressive impulses (Hollander, Berlin, & Stein, 2008). This theory is consistent with the "fight or flight" arousal described by Selye (1956) in his theory of the response to stress (see Chapter 1). An explanation of these biochemical influences on violent behavior is presented in Figure 36–1.

Genetic Influences

Various genetic components related to aggressive behavior have been investigated. Some studies have linked increased aggressiveness with selective inbreeding in mice, suggesting the possibility of a direct genetic link. Another genetic characteristic that was once thought to have some implication for aggressive behavior was the genetic karyotype XYY. The XYY syndrome has been found to contribute to aggressive behavior in a small percentage of cases (Sadock & Sadock, 2007). The evidence linking this chromosomal aberration to aggressive and deviant behavior has not yet been firmly established.

Disorders of the Brain

Organic brain syndromes associated with various cerebral disorders have been implicated in the predisposition to aggressive and violent behavior (Cummings & Mega, 2003; Sadock & Sadock, 2007; Tardiff, 2003). Brain tumors, particularly in the areas of the limbic system and the temporal lobes; trauma to the brain, resulting in cerebral changes; and diseases, such as encephalitis (or medications that may effect this syndrome) and epilepsy, particularly temporal lobe epilepsy, have all been implicated.

Psychological Theories

Psychodynamic Theory

The psychodynamic theorists imply that unmet needs for satisfaction and security result in an

FIGURE 36–1 Neurobiology of violence.

Neurotransmitters

Neurotransmitters that have been implicated in the etiology of aggression and violence include serotonin (decreases) and norepinephrine and dopamine (increases) (Hollander et al., 2008; Tardiff, 2003).

Associated Areas of the Brain

- Limbic structures: Emotional alterations
- Prefrontal and frontal cortices: Modulation of social judgment
- Amygdala: Anxiety, rage, fear
- Hypothalamus: Stimulates sympathetic nervous system in "fight or flight" response
- Hippocampus: Learning and memory

Medications Used to Modulate Aggression

1. Studies have suggested that selective serotonin reuptake inhibitors (SSRIs) may reduce irritability and aggression consistent with the hypothesis of reduced serotonergic activity in aggression.
2. Mood stabilizers that dampen limbic irritability may be important in reducing the susceptibility to react to provocation or threatening stimuli by overactivation of limbic system structures such as the amygdala (Siever, 2002). Carbamazepine (Tegretol), phenytoin (Dilantin), and divalproex sodium (Depakote) have yielded positive results. Lithium has also been used effectively in violent individuals (Schatzberg, Cole, & DeBattista, 2010).
3. Antiadrenergic agents such as beta blockers (e.g., propranolol) have been shown to reduce aggression in some individuals, presumably by dampening excessive noradrenergic activity (Schatzberg et al., 2010).
4. In their ability to modulate excessive dopaminergic activity, antipsychotics—both typical and atypical—have been helpful in the control of aggression and violence, particularly in individuals with comorbid psychosis

underdeveloped ego and a weak superego. It is thought that, when frustration occurs, aggression and violence supply this individual with a dose of power and prestige that boosts the self-image and validates a significance to his or her life that is lacking. The immature ego cannot prevent dominant id behaviors from occurring, and the weak superego is unable to produce feelings of guilt.

Learning Theory

Children learn to behave by imitating their role models, which are usually their parents. Models are more likely to be imitated when they are perceived as prestigious or influential, or when the behavior is followed by positive reinforcement. Children may have an idealistic perception of their parents during the very early developmental stages but, as they mature, may begin to imitate the behavior patterns of their teachers, friends, and others. Individuals who were abused as children or who witnessed domestic violence as a child are more likely to behave in an abusive manner as adults (Hornor, 2005).

Adults and children alike model many of their behaviors after individuals they observe on television and in movies. Unfortunately, modeling can result in maladaptive as well as adaptive behavior, particularly when children view heroes triumphing over villains by using violence. It is also possible that individuals who have a biological predisposition toward aggressive behavior may be more susceptible to negative role modeling.

Sociocultural Theories

Societal Influences

Although they agree that perhaps some biological and psychological aspects are influential, social scientists believe that aggressive behavior is primarily a product of one's culture and social structure.

American society essentially was founded on a general acceptance of violence as a means of solving problems. The concept of relative deprivation has been shown to have a profound effect on collective violence within a society. Kennedy and associates (1998) have stated:

> Studies have shown that poverty and income are powerful predictors of homicide and violent crime. The effect of the growing gap between the rich and poor is mediated through an undermining of social cohesion, or social capital, and decreased social capital is in turn associated with increased firearm homicide and violent crime. (p. 7)

Indeed, the United States was populated by the violent actions of one group of people over another. Since that time, much has been said and written, and laws have been passed, regarding the civil rights of all people. However, to this day many people would agree that the statement "All men are created equal" is hypocritical in our society.

Societal influences may contribute to violence when individuals realize that their needs and desires are not being met relative to other people (Tardiff, 2003). When poor and oppressed people find that they have limited access through legitimate channels, they are more likely to resort to delinquent behaviors in an effort to obtain desired ends. This lack of opportunity and subsequent delinquency may even contribute to a subculture of violence within a society.

Application of the Nursing Process

Background Assessment Data

Data related to intimate partner violence, child abuse and neglect, and sexual assault are presented in this section. Characteristics of both victim and abuser are addressed. This information may be used as background knowledge in designing plans of care for these clients.

Intimate Partner Violence

> **CORE CONCEPT**
>
> *Battering*
> A pattern of coercive control founded on and supported by physical and/or sexual violence or threat of violence of an intimate partner.

The National Coalition Against Domestic Violence (2010) stated:

> Battering is a pattern of behavior used to establish power and control over another person with whom an intimate relationship is or has been shared through fear and intimidation, often including the threat or use of violence. Battering happens when one person believes they are entitled to control another.

The American Medical Association (2009) defined intimate partner violence as:

> A pattern of coercive behaviors that may include repeated battering and injury, psychological abuse, sexual assault, progressive social isolation, deprivation, and intimidation.

Physical abuse between domestic partners may be known as spouse abuse, domestic or family violence, wife or husband battering, or intimate partner violence (IPV). Data from the U.S. Bureau of Justice Statistics (2009) reflect the following: (1) approximately 83 percent of victims of intimate violence were women, (2) women ages 20 to 24 experienced the highest per capita rates of intimate violence, and (3) intimate partners committed 4 percent of the nonfatal violence against men.

In the same study, approximately 62 percent of women and 64 percent of men reported the victimizations to the police. The most common reason for not reporting was because it was a "private or personal matter."

Profile of the Victim

Battered women represent all age, racial, religious, cultural, educational, and socioeconomic groups. They may be married or single, housewives or business executives. Many women who are battered have low self-esteem, commonly adhere to feminine sex-role stereotypes, and often accept the blame for the batterer's actions. Feelings of guilt, anger, fear, and shame are common. They may be isolated from family and support systems.

Some women who are in violent relationships grew up in abusive homes and may have left those homes, even gotten married, at a very young age in order to escape the abuse. The battered woman views her relationship as male dominant, and as the battering continues, her ability to see the options available to her and to make decisions concerning her life (and possibly those of her children) decreases. The phenomenon of *learned helplessness* may be applied to the woman's progressing inability to act on her own behalf. Learned helplessness occurs when an individual comes to understand that, regardless of his or her behavior, the outcome is unpredictable and usually undesirable.

Profile of the Victimizer

Men who batter usually are characterized as persons with low self-esteem. Pathologically jealous, they present a "dual personality," one to the partner and one to the rest of the world (Meskill & Conner, 2010). They are often under a great deal of stress, but have limited ability to cope with the stress. The typical abuser is very possessive and perceives his spouse as a possession. He becomes threatened when she shows any sign of independence or attempts to share herself and her time with others. Small children are often ignored by the abuser; however, they may also become the targets of abuse as they grow older, particularly if they attempt to protect their mother from abuse. The abuser also may use threats of taking the children away as a tactic of emotional abuse.

The abusing man typically wages a continuous campaign of degradation against his female partner. He insults and humiliates her and everything she does at every opportunity. He strives to keep her isolated from others and totally dependent on him. He demands to know where she is at every moment, and when she tells him he challenges her honesty. He achieves power and control through intimidation.

The Cycle of Battering

In her classic studies of battered women and their relationships, Walker (1979) identified a cycle of predictable behaviors that are repeated over time. The behaviors can be divided into three distinct phases that vary in time and intensity both within the same relationship and among different couples. Figure 36–2 depicts a graphic representation of the **cycle of battering.**

Phase I: The Tension-Building Phase During this phase, the woman senses that the man's tolerance for frustration is declining. He becomes angry with little provocation but, after lashing out at her, may be quick to apologize. The woman may become very nurturing and compliant, anticipating his every whim in an effort to prevent his anger from escalating. She may just try to stay out of his way.

Minor battering incidents may occur during this phase, and in a desperate effort to avoid more serious confrontations, the woman accepts the abuse as legitimately directed toward her. She denies her anger and rationalizes his behavior (e.g., "I need to do better;" "He's under so much stress at work;" "It's the alcohol. If only he didn't drink"). She assumes the guilt for the abuse, even reasoning that perhaps she *did* deserve the abuse, just as her aggressor suggests.

The minor battering incidents continue, and the tension mounts as the woman waits for the impending explosion. The abuser begins to fear that his partner will leave him. His jealousy and possessiveness increase, and he uses threats and brutality to keep her in his captivity. Battering

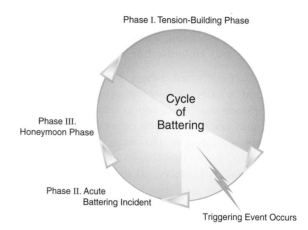

FIGURE 36–2 The cycle of battering.

incidents become more intense, after which the woman becomes less and less psychologically capable of restoring equilibrium. She withdraws from him, which he misinterprets as rejection, further escalating his anger toward her. Phase I may last from a few weeks to many months or even years.

Phase II: The Acute Battering Incident This phase is the most violent and the shortest, usually lasting up to 24 hours. It most often begins with the batterer justifying his behavior to himself. By the end of the incident, however, he cannot understand what has happened, only that in his rage he has lost control over his behavior.

This incident may begin with the batterer wanting to "just teach her a lesson." In some instances, the woman may intentionally provoke the behavior. Having come to a point in phase I in which the tension is unbearable, long-term battered women know that, once the acute phase is behind them, things will be better.

During phase II, women feel their only option is to find a safe place to hide from the batterer. The beating is severe, and many women can describe the violence in great detail, almost as if dissociation from their bodies had occurred. The batterer generally minimizes the severity of the abuse. Help is usually sought only in the event of severe injury or if the woman fears for her life or those of her children.

Phase III: Calm, Loving, Respite ("Honeymoon") Phase In this phase, the batterer becomes extremely loving, kind, and contrite. He promises that the abuse will never recur and begs her forgiveness. He is afraid she will leave him and uses every bit of charm he can muster to ensure this does not happen. He believes he now can control his behavior, and because now he has "taught her a lesson," he believes she will not "act up" again.

He plays on her feelings of guilt, and she desperately wants to believe him. She wants to believe that he *can* change, and that she will no longer have to suffer abuse. During this phase the woman relives her original dream of ideal love and chooses to believe that *this* is what her partner is *really* like.

This loving phase becomes the focus of the woman's perception of the relationship. She bases her reason for remaining in the relationship on this "magical" ideal phase and hopes against hope that the previous phases will not be repeated. This hope is evident even in those women who have lived through a number of horrendous cycles.

Although phase III usually lasts somewhere between the lengths of time associated with phases I and II, it can be so short as to almost pass undetected. In most instances, the cycle soon begins again with renewed tensions and minor battering incidents. In an effort to "steal" a few precious moments of the phase III kind of loving, the battered woman becomes a collaborator in her own abusive lifestyle. Victim and batterer become locked together in an intense, symbiotic relationship.

Why Does She Stay?

Probably the most common response that battered women give for staying is that they fear for their life and/or the lives of their children. As the battering progresses, the man gains power and control through intimidation and instilling fear with threats such as, "I'll kill you and the kids if you try to leave." Challenged by these threats, and compounded by her low self-esteem and sense of powerlessness, the woman sees no way out. In fact, she may try to leave only to return when confronted by her partner and the psychological power he holds over her.

Women have been known to stay in an abusive relationship for many reasons, some of which include the following (Family Violence Law Center, 2003; Meskill & Conner, 2010; National Coalition Against Domestic Violence, 2010):

■ **Fear of retaliation:** Her partner may have told her that if she leaves he will find her and kill her and the children.

■ **For the children:** She may fear losing custody of the children if she leaves.

■ **For financial reasons:** She may have no financial resources, access to the resources, or job skills.

■ **Lack of a support network:** She may be under pressure from family members to stay in the marriage and try to work things out.

■ **Religious reasons:** She may have religious convictions against divorce, believing that she must save the marriage at all costs.

■ **Hopefulness:** She remembers good times and love in the relationship and has hope that her partner will change his behavior and they can have good times again.

Child Abuse

Erik Erikson (1963) stated, "The worst sin is the mutilation of a child's spirit." Children are vulnerable and relatively powerless, and the effects of maltreatment are infinitely deep and long lasting. Child maltreatment typically includes physical or emotional injury, physical or emotional neglect, or sexual acts inflicted upon a child by a caregiver. The Child Abuse Prevention and Treatment Act (CAPTA), as amended and reauthorized in 2003, identifies a minimum set of acts or behaviors that characterize maltreatment (Child Welfare Information Gateway [CWIG], 2008). States may use these as foundations on which to establish state legislation.

Physical Abuse

Physical abuse of a child includes "any nonaccidental physical injury (ranging from minor bruises to severe fractures or death) as a result of punching, beating, kicking, biting, shaking, throwing, stabbing, choking, hitting (with a hand, stick, strap, or other object), burning, or otherwise harming a child, that is inflicted by a parent, caregiver, or other person who has responsibility for the child" (CWIG, 2008). Maltreatment is considered whether or not the caretaker intended to cause harm, or even if the injury resulted from overdiscipline or physical punishment. The most obvious way to detect it is by outward physical signs. However, behavioral indicators also may be evident.

Signs of Physical Abuse Indicators of physical abuse may include any of the following (CWIG, 2007). The child:

- Has unexplained burns, bites, bruises, broken bones, or black eyes.
- Has fading bruises or other marks noticeable after an absence from school.
- Seems frightened of the parents and protests or cries when it is time to go home.
- Shrinks at the approach of adults.
- Reports injury by a parent or another adult caregiver.

Physical abuse may be suspected when the parent or other adult caregiver (CWIG, 2007):

- Offers conflicting, unconvincing, or no explanation for the child's injury.
- Describes the child as "evil," or in some other very negative way.
- Uses harsh physical discipline with the child.
- Has a history of abuse as a child.

IMPLICATIONS OF RESEARCH FOR EVIDENCE-BASED PRACTICE

Sachs, B., Hall, L. A., Lutenbacher, M., & Rayens, M. K. (1999). Potential for abusive parenting by rural mothers with low-birth-weight children. *Image: Journal of Nursing Scholarship, 31,* 21–25.

DESCRIPTION OF THE STUDY: The purpose of this study was to describe factors influencing the potential for abusive parenting by rural mothers of low-birth-weight (LBW) children. The convenience sample in this study included 48 mothers of LBW children, ranging in age from 18 to 39 years, all living in a rural area of the state, and all living with their LBW infant at the time of the study. Average length of the children's hospitalization after birth was 6 weeks, and the average age at time of the study was 9 months. In-home interviews were conducted using structured questionnaires to assess the mothers' everyday stressors, depressive symptoms, functional social support, quality of family relationships, and child abuse potential.

RESULTS OF THE STUDY: According to the questionnaires used for measurement, 54 percent of the mothers indicated a high level of depressive symptoms and 63 percent indicated a high potential for physical child abuse. No significant differences were noted in depressive symptoms and potential for child abuse by birth weight, health status of the child, or time since hospital discharge. Mothers with high child abuse potential reported more everyday stressors and depressive symptoms, less functional social support, and poorer family functioning. Because in this study everyday stressors and the two social support systems (functional social support and quality of family relationships) were examined as predictors of depressive symptoms, it is suggested that everyday stressors exert both a direct and an indirect effect on mothers' potential for child abuse. The strongest predictor of child abuse potential was mothers' depressive symptoms.

IMPLICATIONS FOR NURSING PRACTICE: The researchers concluded that rural mothers of LBW children are at risk for abusive parenting. This study demonstrated the adverse effects of everyday stressors, minimal social resources, and depressive symptoms on mothers' potential for abusive parenting. Nurses should provide attention to the mental health of mothers living in isolated, rural areas. Information should be made available to these mothers regarding community resources that offer social support and child care assistance. Nurses could establish and conduct educational programs to improve parenting skills and promote more positive child health outcomes.

Emotional Abuse

Emotional abuse involves a pattern of behavior on the part of the parent or caregiver that results in serious impairment of the child's social, emotional, or intellectual functioning. Examples of emotional injury include belittling or rejecting the child, ignoring the child, blaming the child for things over which he or she has no control, isolating the child from normal social experiences, and using harsh and inconsistent discipline. Behavioral indicators of emotional injury may include (CWIG, 2007):

- Shows extremes in behavior, such as overly compliant or demanding behavior, extreme passivity, or aggression
- Is either inappropriately adult (e.g., parenting other children) or inappropriately infantile (e.g., frequently rocking or head banging)
- Is delayed in physical or emotional development
- Has attempted suicide
- Reports a lack of attachment to the parent

Emotional abuse may be suspected when the parent or other adult caregiver (CWIG, 2007):

- Constantly blames, belittles, or berates the child.
- Is unconcerned about the child and refuses to consider offers of help for the child's problems.
- Overtly rejects the child.

Physical and Emotional Neglect

> ### CORE CONCEPTS
>
> #### Neglect
> *Physical neglect* of a child includes refusal of or delay in seeking health care, abandonment, expulsion from the home or refusal to allow a runaway to return home, and inadequate supervision.
> *Emotional neglect* refers to a chronic failure by the parent or caregiver to provide the child with the hope, love, and support necessary for the development of a sound, healthy personality.

Indicators of Neglect The possibility of neglect may be considered when the child (CWIG, 2007):

- Is frequently absent from school.
- Begs or steals food or money.
- Lacks needed medical or dental care, immunizations, or glasses.
- Is consistently dirty and has severe body odor.
- Lacks sufficient clothing for the weather.
- Abuses alcohol or other drugs.
- States that there is no one at home to provide care.

The possibility of neglect may be considered when the parent or other adult caregiver (CWIG, 2007):

- Appears to be indifferent to the child.
- Seems apathetic or depressed.
- Behaves irrationally or in a bizarre manner.
- Is abusing alcohol or other drugs.

Sexual Abuse of a Child

Various definitions of **child sexual abuse** are available in the literature. CAPTA defines *sexual abuse* as:

> Employment, use, persuasion, inducement, enticement, or coercion of any child to engage in, or assist any other person to engage in, any sexually explicit conduct or simulation of such conduct for the purpose of producing any visual depiction of such conduct; or the rape, and in cases of caretaker or inter-familial relationships, statutory rape, molestation, prostitution, or other form of sexual exploitation of children, or incest with children. (CWIG, 2008)

Included in the definition is **sexual exploitation of a child,** in which a child is induced or coerced into engaging in sexually explicit conduct for the purpose of promoting any performance, and child sexual abuse, in which a child is being used for the sexual pleasure of an adult (parent or caregiver) or any other person.

> ### CORE CONCEPT
>
> #### Incest
> The occurrence of sexual contacts or interaction between, or sexual exploitation of, close relatives, or between participants who are related to each other by a kinship bond that is regarded as a prohibition to sexual relations (e.g., caregivers, stepparents, stepsiblings) (Sadock & Sadock, 2007).

Indicators of Sexual Abuse Child abuse may be considered a possibility when the child (CWIG, 2007):

- Has difficulty walking or sitting.
- Suddenly refuses to change for gym or to participate in physical activities.
- Reports nightmares or bedwetting.
- Experiences a sudden change in appetite.
- Demonstrates bizarre, sophisticated, or unusual sexual knowledge or behavior.

■ Becomes pregnant or contracts a venereal disease, particularly if under age 14.

■ Runs away.

■ Reports sexual abuse by a parent or another adult caregiver.

Sexual abuse may be considered a possibility when the parent or other adult caregiver (CWIG, 2007):

■ Is unduly protective of the child or severely limits the child's contact with other children, especially of the opposite sex.

■ Is secretive and isolated.

■ Is jealous or controlling with family members.

Characteristics of the Abuser

A number of factors have been associated with adults who abuse or neglect their children. Sadock and Sadock (2007) report that 90 percent of parents who abuse their children were severely physically abused by their own mothers or fathers. Murray, Zentner, and Yakimo (2009) identified the following as additional characteristics that may be associated with abusive parents:

■ Experiencing a stressful life situation (e.g., unemployment; poverty)

■ Having few, if any, support systems; commonly isolated from others

■ Lacking understanding of child development or care needs

■ Lacking adaptive coping strategies; angers easily; has difficulty trusting others

■ Expecting the child to be perfect; may exaggerate any mild difference the child manifests from the "usual"

Flaherty and Stirling (2010) identified a number of factors that place a child at risk for maltreatment. They cited certain characteristics of the child, the parent, and the environment. These characteristics are presented in Table 36-1. When multiple factors coexist, the risk of child abuse increases.

The Incestuous Relationship

A great deal of attention has been given to the study of father-daughter incest. In these cases there is usually an impaired sexual relationship between the parents. Communication between the parents is ineffective, which prevents them from correcting their problems. Typically, the father is domineering, impulsive, and physically abusing; whereas the mother is passive and submissive, and denigrates her role as wife and mother. She is often aware of, or at least strongly suspects, the incestuous behavior between the father and daughter but may believe in or fear her husband's absolute authority over the family. She may deny that her daughter is being harmed and may actually be grateful that her husband's sexual demands are being met by someone other than herself.

TABLE 36-1 Factors and Characteristics That Place a Child at Risk for Maltreatment		
CHILD	**PARENT**	**ENVIRONMENT (COMMUNITY AND SOCIETY)**
Emotional/behavioral difficulties	Low self-esteem	Social isolation
Chronic illness	Poor impulse control	Poverty
Physical disabilities	Substance abuse/alcohol abuse	Unemployment
Developmental disabilities	Young maternal or paternal age	Low educational achievement
Preterm birth	Abused as a child	Single-parent home
Unwanted	Depression or other mental illness	Non–biologically related male living in the home
Unplanned	Poor knowledge of child development or unrealistic expectations of the child Negative perception of normal child behavior	Family or intimate partner violence

From Flaherty, E. G., Stirling, J., & The Committee on Child Abuse and Neglect. (2010). Clinical report—The pediatrician's role in child maltreatment prevention. Pediatrics, 126, 833-841; reprinted with permission.

Onset of the incestuous relationship typically occurs when the daughter is 8 to 10 years of age and commonly begins with genital touching and fondling. In the beginning, the child may accept the sexual advances from her father as signs of affection. As the incestuous behavior continues and progresses, the daughter usually becomes more bewildered, confused, and frightened, never knowing whether her father will be paternal or sexual in his interactions with her.

The relationship may become a love-hate situation on the part of the daughter. She continues to strive for the ideal father-daughter relationship but is fearful and hateful of the sexual demands he places on her. The mother may be alternately caring and competitive as she witnesses her husband's possessiveness and affections directed toward her daughter. Out of fear that his daughter may expose their relationship, the father may attempt to interfere with her normal peer relationships (Sadock & Sadock, 2007).

It has been suggested that some fathers who participate in incestuous relationships may have unconscious homosexual tendencies and have difficulty achieving a stable heterosexual orientation. Conversely, some men have frequent sex with their wives and several of their own children but are unwilling to seek sexual partners outside the nuclear family because of a need to maintain the public facade of a stable and competent patriarch. Although the oldest daughter in a family is most vulnerable to becoming a participant in father-daughter incest, some fathers form sequential relationships with several daughters. If incest has been reported with one daughter, it should be suspected with all of the other daughters (Murray et al., 2009).

The Adult Survivor of Incest

Several common characteristics have been identified in adults who have experienced incest as children. Basic to these characteristics is a fundamental lack of trust resulting from an unsatisfactory parent-child relationship, which causes low self-esteem and a poor sense of identity. Children of incest often feel trapped, for they have been admonished not to talk about the experience and may be afraid, or even fear for their lives, if they are exposed. If they do muster the courage to report the incest, particularly to the mother, they sometimes are not believed. This is confusing to the child, who is then left with a sense of self-doubt and the inability to trust his or her own feelings. The child develops feelings of guilt with the realization over the years that the parents are using him or her in an attempt to solve their own problems.

Childhood sexual abuse is likely to distort the development of a normal association of pleasure with sexual activity (Reeves, 2003). Peer relationships are often delayed, altered, inhibited, or perverted. In some instances, individuals who were sexually abused as children completely retreat from sexual activity and avoid all close interpersonal relationships throughout life. Other adult manifestations of childhood sexual abuse in women include diminished libido, vaginismus, nymphomania, and promiscuity. In male survivors of childhood sexual abuse, impotence, premature ejaculation, exhibitionism, and compulsive sexual conquests may occur. Lerner (2005) suggested that adult survivors of incest are at risk for experiencing symptoms of posttraumatic stress disorder, sexual dysfunction, somatization disorders, compulsive sexual behaviors, depression, anxiety, eating disorders, substance disorders, and intolerance of or constant search for intimacy.

The conflicts associated with pain (either physical or emotional) and sexual pleasure experienced by children who are sexually abused are commonly manifested symbolically in adult relationships. Women who were abused as children commonly enter into relationships with men who abuse them physically, sexually, or emotionally (Bensley, VanEenwyk, & Wynkoop, 2003).

Adult survivors of incest who decide to come forward with their stories usually are estranged from nuclear family members. They are blamed by family members for disclosing the "family secret" and often accused of overreacting to the incest. Frequently the estrangement becomes permanent when family members continue to deny the behavior and the individual is accused of lying. In recent years, a number of celebrities have come forward with stories of their childhood sexual abuse. Some have chosen to make the disclosure only after the death of their parents. Revelation of these past activities can be one way of contributing to the healing process for which incest survivors so desperately strive.

Sexual Assault

CORE CONCEPT

Rape

The expression of power and dominance by means of sexual violence, most commonly by men over women, although men may also be rape victims.

Sexual assault is viewed as any type of sexual act in which an individual is threatened or coerced, or forced to submit against his or her will. Rape, a type of sexual assault, occurs over a broad spectrum of experiences ranging from the surprise attack by a stranger to insistence on sexual intercourse by an acquaintance or spouse. Regardless of the defining source, one common theme always emerges: Rape is an act of aggression, not one of passion.

Acquaintance rape (called **date rape** if the encounter is a social engagement agreed to by the victim) is a term applied to situations in which the rapist is acquainted with the victim. They may be out on a first date, may have been dating for a number of months, or merely may be acquaintances or schoolmates. College campuses are the location for a staggering number of these types of rapes, a great many of which go unreported. An increasing number of colleges and universities are establishing programs for rape prevention and counseling for victims of rape.

Marital rape, which has been recognized only in recent years as a legal category, is the case in which a spouse may be held liable for sexual abuse directed at a marital partner against that person's will. Historically, with societal acceptance of the concept of women as marital property, the legal definition of rape held an exemption within the marriage relationship. In 1993, marital rape became a crime in all 50 states, under at least one section of the sexual offenses code. In 17 states and the District of Columbia, there are no exemptions from rape prosecution granted to husbands. However, in 33 states, there are still some exemptions given to husbands from rape prosecution.

Statutory rape is defined as unlawful intercourse between a person who is over the age of consent and a person who is under the age of consent. The legal age of consent varies from state to state, ranging from age 14 to 18 (King, 2009). An adult who has intercourse with a person who is under the age of consent can be arrested for statutory rape, although the interaction may have occurred between consenting individuals.

Profile of the Victimizer

Older profiles of the individual who rapes were described by Abrahamsen (1960) and Macdonald (1971), who identified the rapist's childhood as "mother-dominated" and the mother as "seductive but rejecting." The behavior of the mother toward the son was described as overbearing, with seductive undertones. Mother and son shared little secrets, and she rescued him when his delinquent acts created problems with others. However, she was quick to withdraw her love and attention when he went against her wishes, a rejection that

was powerful and unyielding. She was domineering and possessive of the son, a dominance that often continued into his adult life. Macdonald (1971) stated:

> The seductive mother arouses overwhelming anxiety in her son with great anger, which may be expressed directly toward her but more often is displaced onto other women. When this seductive behavior is combined with parental encouragement of assaultive behavior, the setting is provided for personality development in the child which may result in sadistic, homicidal sexual attacks on women in adolescence or adult life.

Many rapists report growing up in abusive homes (McCormack, 2002). Even when the parental brutality is discharged by the father, the anger may be directed toward the mother who did not protect her child from physical assault. More recent feminist theories suggest that the rapist displaces this anger on the rape victim because he cannot directly express it toward other men (Sadock & Sadock, 2007). Another feminist view suggests that rape is most common in societies that encourage aggressiveness in males, that have distinct gender roles, and in which men regard women's roles as inferior (King, 2009).

Statistics show that the greatest number of rapists are between the ages of 25 and 44. Of rapists, 51 percent are white, 47 percent are African-American, and the remaining 2 percent come from all other races (Sadock & Sadock, 2007). Many are either married or cohabiting at the time of their offenses. For those with previous criminal activity, the majority of their convictions are for crimes against property rather than against people. Most rapists do not have histories of mental illness.

The Victim

Rape can occur at any age; however, the most recent statistics suggest that the highest-risk age group is 16 to 24 years (U.S. Department of Justice, 2009). Most sexual assault victims are single women, and the attack frequently occurs in or close to the victim's own neighborhood.

Scully (1994), in a study of a prison sample of rapists, found that in "stranger rapes," victims were not chosen for any reason having to do with appearance or behavior, but simply because the individual happened to be in a certain place at a certain time. Scully stated:

> The most striking and consistent factor in all the stranger rapes, whether committed by a lone assailant or a group, is the unfortunate fact that the victim was "just there" in a location unlikely to draw the attention of a

passerby. Almost every one of these men said exactly the same thing, "It could have been any woman," and a few added that because it was dark, they could not even see what their victim looked like very well. (p. 175)

In her study, Scully found that 62 percent of the rapists used a weapon, most frequently a knife. Most suggested that they used the weapon to terrorize and subdue the victim but not to inflict serious injury. The presence of a weapon (real or perceived) appears to be the principal measure of the degree to which a woman resists her attacker.

Rape victims who present themselves for care shortly after the crime has occurred likely may be experiencing an overwhelming sense of violation and helplessness that began with the powerlessness and intimidation experienced during the rape. Burgess (2010) identified two emotional patterns of response that may occur within hours after a rape and with which health-care workers may be confronted in the emergency department or rape crisis center. In the **expressed response pattern,** the victim expresses feelings of fear, anger, and anxiety through such behaviors as crying, sobbing, smiling, restlessness, and tension. In the **controlled response pattern,** the feelings are masked or hidden, and a calm, composed, or subdued affect is seen.

The following manifestations may be evident in the days and weeks after the attack (Burgess, 2010):

- Contusions and abrasions about various parts of the body
- Headaches, fatigue, sleep pattern disturbances
- Stomach pains, nausea and vomiting
- Vaginal discharge and itching, burning upon urination, rectal bleeding and pain
- Rage, humiliation, embarrassment, desire for revenge, and self-blame
- Fear of physical violence and death

The long-term effects of sexual assault depend largely on the individual's ego strength, his or her social support system, and the way he or she was treated as a victim (Burgess, 2010). Various long-term effects include increased restlessness, dreams and nightmares, and phobias (particularly those having to do with sexual interaction). Some women report that it takes years to get over the experience; they describe a sense of vulnerability and a loss of control over their own lives during this period. They feel defiled and unable to wash themselves clean, and some women are unable to remain living alone in their home or apartment.

Some victims develop a **compounded rape reaction,** in which additional symptoms such as depression and suicide, substance abuse, and even psychotic behaviors may be noted (Burgess, 2010). Another variation has been called the **silent rape reaction,** in which the victim tells no one about the assault. Anxiety is suppressed and the emotional burden may become overwhelming. The unresolved sexual trauma may not be revealed until the woman is forced to face another sexual crisis in her life that reactivates the previously unresolved feelings.

Diagnosis/Outcome Identification

Nursing diagnoses are formulated from the data gathered during the assessment phase and with background knowledge regarding predisposing factors to the situation. Some common nursing diagnoses for victims of abuse include:

- Rape-trauma syndrome related to sexual assault evidenced by verbalizations of the attack; bruises and lacerations over areas of body; severe anxiety.
- Powerlessness related to cycle of battering evidenced by verbalizations of abuse; bruises and lacerations over areas of body; fear for her safety and that of her children; verbalizations of no way to get out of the relationship.
- Risk for delayed development related to abusive family situation.

Outcome Criteria

The following criteria may be used to measure outcomes in the care of abuse victims.

The Client Who Has Been Sexually Assaulted:

- Is no longer experiencing panic anxiety.
- Demonstrates a degree of trust in the primary nurse.
- Has received immediate attention to physical injuries.
- Has initiated behaviors consistent with the grief response.

The Client Who Has Been Physically Battered:

- Has received immediate attention to physical injuries.
- Verbalizes assurance of his or her immediate safety.
- Discusses life situation with primary nurse.
- Can verbalize choices from which he or she may receive assistance.

The Child Who Has Been Abused:

■ Has received immediate attention to physical injuries.

■ Demonstrates trust in primary nurse by discussing abuse through the use of play therapy.

■ Is demonstrating a decrease in regressive behaviors.

Planning/Implementation

Table 36-2 provides a plan of care for the client who has been a victim of abuse. Nursing diagnoses are presented, along with outcome criteria, appropriate nursing interventions, and rationales for each.

Concept Care Mapping

The concept map care plan is an innovative approach to planning and organizing nursing care (see Chapter 9). It is a diagrammatic teaching and learning strategy that allows visualization of interrelationships between medical diagnoses, nursing diagnoses, assessment data, and treatments. An example of a concept map care plan for a client who is the victim of abuse is presented in Figure 36–3.

Table 36-2 CARE PLAN FOR VICTIMS OF ABUSE

NURSING DIAGNOSIS: RAPE-TRAUMA SYNDROME
RELATED TO: Sexual assault
EVIDENCED BY: Verbalizations of the attack; bruises and lacerations over areas of body; severe anxiety

OUTCOME CRITERIA	NURSING INTERVENTIONS	RATIONALE
Short-Term Goal • Client's physical wounds will heal without complication. **Long-Term Goal** • Client will begin a healthy grief resolution, initiating the process of physical and psychological healing (time to be individually determined).	1. It is important to communicate the following to the victim of sexual assault: • You are safe here. • I'm sorry that it happened. • I'm glad you survived. • It's not your fault. No one deserves to be treated this way. • You did the best that you could.	1. The woman who has been sexually assaulted fears for her life and must be reassured of her safety. She may also be overwhelmed with self-doubt and self-blame, and these statements instill trust and validate self-worth.
	2. Explain every assessment procedure that will be conducted and why it is being conducted. Ensure that data collection is conducted in a caring, nonjudgmental manner.	2. This may serve to decrease fear/anxiety and increase trust.
	3. Ensure that the client has adequate privacy for all immediate post-crisis interventions. Try to have as few people as possible providing the immediate care or collecting immediate evidence.	3. The post-trauma client is extremely vulnerable. Additional people in the environment increase this feeling of vulnerability and serve to escalate anxiety.
	4. Encourage the client to give an account of the assault. Listen, but do not probe.	4. Nonjudgmental listening provides an avenue for catharsis that the client needs to begin healing. A detailed account may be required for legal follow-up, and a caring nurse, as client advocate, may help to lessen the trauma of evidence collection.
	5. Discuss with the client whom to call for support or assistance. Provide information about referrals for aftercare.	5. Because of severe anxiety and fear, the client may need assistance from others during this immediate post-crisis period. Provide referral information in writing for later reference (e.g., psychotherapist, mental health clinic, community advocacy group).

Table 36-2 CARE PLAN FOR VICTIMS OF ABUSE—cont'd

NURSING DIAGNOSIS: POWERLESSNESS

RELATED TO: Cycle of battering

EVIDENCED BY: Verbalizations of abuse; bruises and lacerations over areas of body; fear for own safety and that of children; verbalizations of no way to get out of the relationship

OUTCOME CRITERIA	NURSING INTERVENTIONS	RATIONALE
Short-Term Goal • Client will recognize and verbalize choices available, thereby perceiving some control over life situation. **Long-Term Goal** • Client will exhibit control over life situation by making decision about what to do regarding living with cycle of abuse.	1. In collaboration with physician, ensure that all physical wounds, fractures, and burns receive immediate attention. Take photographs if the victim will permit. 2. Take the woman to a private area to do the interview. 3. If she has come alone or with her children, assure her of her safety. Encourage her to discuss the battering incident. Ask questions about whether this has happened before, whether the abuser takes drugs, whether she has a safe place to go, and whether she is interested in pressing charges. 4. Ensure that "rescue" efforts are not attempted by the nurse. Offer support, but remember that the final decision must be made by the client. 5. Stress to the victim the importance of safety. She must be made aware of the variety of resources that are available to her. These may include crisis hot lines, community groups for women who have been abused, shelters, counseling services, and information regarding the victim's rights in the civil and criminal justice system. Following a discussion of these available resources, the woman may choose for herself. If her decision is to return to the marriage and home, this choice also must be respected.	1. Client safety is a nursing priority. Photographs may be called in as evidence if charges are filed. 2. If the client is accompanied by the man who did the battering, she is not likely to be truthful about her injuries. 3. Some women will attempt to keep secret how their injuries occurred in an effort to protect the partner or because they are fearful that the partner will kill them if they tell. 4. Making her own decision will give the client a sense of control over her life situation. Imposing judgments and giving advice are nontherapeutic. 5. Knowledge of available choices decreases the victim's sense of powerlessness, but true empowerment comes only when she chooses to use that knowledge for her own benefit.

Continued

Table 36-2 CARE PLAN FOR VICTIMS OF ABUSE—cont'd

NURSING DIAGNOSIS: RISK FOR DELAYED DEVELOPMENT
RELATED TO: Abusive family situation

OUTCOME CRITERIA	NURSING INTERVENTIONS	RATIONALE
Short-Term Goal • Client will develop trusting relationship with nurse and report how evident injuries were sustained. **Long-Term Goal** • Client will demonstrate behaviors consistent with age-appropriate growth and development.	1. Perform complete physical assessment of the child. Take particular note of bruises (in various stages of healing), lacerations, and client complaints of pain in specific areas. Do not overlook or discount the possibility of sexual abuse. Assess for nonverbal signs of abuse: aggressive conduct, excessive fears, extreme hyperactivity, apathy, withdrawal, age-inappropriate behaviors.	1. An accurate and thorough physical assessment is required to provide appropriate care for the client.
	2. Conduct an in-depth interview with the parent or adult who accompanies the child. Consider: If the injury is being reported as an accident, is the explanation reasonable? Is the injury consistent with the explanation? Is the injury consistent with the child's developmental capabilities?	2. Fear of imprisonment or loss of child custody may place the abusive parent on the defensive. Discrepancies may be evident in the description of the incident, and lying to cover up involvement is a common defense that may be detectable in an in-depth interview.
	3. Use games or play therapy to gain child's trust. Use these techniques to assist in describing his or her side of the story.	3. Establishing a trusting relationship with an abused child is extremely difficult. He or she may not even want to be touched. These types of play activities can provide a nonthreatening environment that may enhance the child's attempt to discuss these painful issues.
	4. Determine whether the nature of the injuries warrants reporting to authorities. Specific state statutes must enter into the decision of whether to report suspected child abuse. Individual state statutes regarding what constitutes child abuse and neglect may be found at http://www.childwelfare.gov/systemwide/laws_policies/state/	4. A report is commonly made if there is reason to suspect that a child has been injured as a result of physical, mental, emotional, or sexual abuse. "Reason to suspect" exists when there is evidence of a discrepancy or inconsistency in explaining a child's injury. Most states require that the following individuals report cases of suspected child abuse: all health-care workers, all mental health therapists, teachers, child care providers, firefighters, emergency medical personnel, and law enforcement personnel. Reports are made to the Department of Health and Human Services or a law enforcement agency.

Clinical Vignette: Annette and Charles, both ages 21, have been dating for 2 years. Charles has always been jealous, and gets very angry when Annette even talks to another man. He has hit her several times, hard enough to produce bruises, but never on her face, and she is able to hide the abuse from others. Tonight at a party, Annette danced with another man, and Charles became violent. He punched the man in the face and dragged Annette out to the parking lot. She yelled at him, "This is it! We are through! I don't ever want to see you again!" He started beating her around the face and upper body and yelled, "You can't break up with me! I won't allow it! You belong to me and no one else!" He left her lying in the parking lot. She felt powerless, and in her despondency, opened her purse and swallowed half of a bottle of acetaminophen. When she told her girlfriend, Dana, what had happened, Dana called 911, and Annette was taken to the hospital. She was treated for the overdose, and her wounds were cleaned and dressed. Following physical stability, she was transferred to the psychiatric unit. She tells the nurse, "I can't live like this. He won't let me go! I don't know what to do!" The nurse develops the following concept map care plan for Annette.

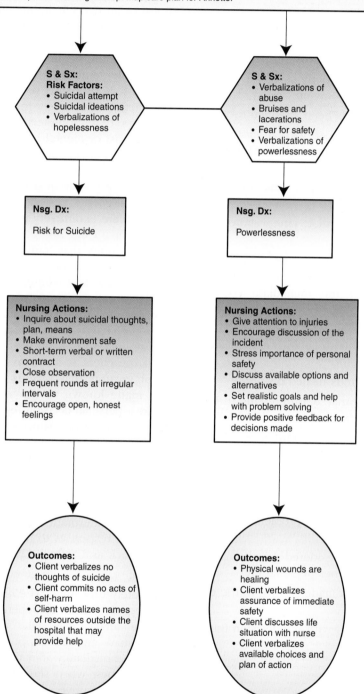

S & Sx:
Risk Factors:
• Suicidal attempt
• Suicidal ideations
• Verbalizations of hopelessness

S & Sx:
• Verbalizations of abuse
• Bruises and lacerations
• Fear for safety
• Verbalizations of powerlessness

Nsg. Dx:
Risk for Suicide

Nsg. Dx:
Powerlessness

Nursing Actions:
• Inquire about suicidal thoughts, plan, means
• Make environment safe
• Short-term verbal or written contract
• Close observation
• Frequent rounds at irregular intervals
• Encourage open, honest feelings

Nursing Actions:
• Give attention to injuries
• Encourage discussion of the incident
• Stress importance of personal safety
• Discuss available options and alternatives
• Set realistic goals and help with problem solving
• Provide positive feedback for decisions made

Outcomes:
• Client verbalizes no thoughts of suicide
• Client commits no acts of self-harm
• Client verbalizes names of resources outside the hospital that may provide help

Outcomes:
• Physical wounds are healing
• Client verbalizes assurance of immediate safety
• Client discusses life situation with nurse
• Client verbalizes available choices and plan of action

FIGURE 36–3   Concept map care plan for a client with physical abuse.

Evaluation

Evaluation of nursing actions to assist victims of abuse must be considered on both a short- and a long-term basis.

Short-term evaluation may be facilitated by gathering information using the following types of questions:

■ Has the individual been reassured of his or her safety?

■ Is this evidenced by a decrease in panic anxiety?

■ Have wounds been properly cared for and provision made for follow-up care?

■ Have emotional needs been attended to?

■ Has trust been established with at least one person to whom the client feels comfortable relating the abusive incident?

■ Have available support systems been identified and notified?

■ Have options for immediate circumstances been presented?

Long-term evaluation may be conducted by health-care workers who have contact with the individual long after the immediate crisis has passed. It may be facilitated by gathering information using the following types of questions:

■ Is the individual able to conduct activities of daily living satisfactorily?

■ Have physical wounds healed properly?

■ Is the client appropriately progressing through the behaviors of grieving?

■ Is the client free of sleep disturbances (nightmares, insomnia); psychosomatic symptoms (headaches, stomach pains, nausea/vomiting); regressive behaviors (enuresis, thumb sucking, phobias); and psychosexual disturbances?

■ Is the individual free from problems with interpersonal relationships?

■ Has the individual considered the alternatives for change in his or her personal life?

■ Has a decision been made relative to the choices available?

■ Is he or she satisfied with the decision that has been made?

Treatment Modalities

Crisis Intervention

The focus of the initial interview and follow-up with the client who has been sexually assaulted is on the rape incident alone. Problems identified but unassociated with the rape are not dealt with at this time. The goal of crisis intervention is to help victims return to their previous lifestyle as quickly as possible.

The client should be involved in the intervention from the beginning. This promotes a sense of competency, control, and decision making. Because an overwhelming sense of powerlessness accompanies the rape experience, active involvement by the victim is both a validation of personal worth and the beginning of the recovery process. Crisis intervention is time limited—usually 6 to 8 weeks. If problems resurface beyond this time, the victim is referred for assistance from other agencies (e.g., long-term psychotherapy from a psychiatrist or mental health clinic).

During the crisis period, attention is given to coping strategies for dealing with the symptoms common to the post-trauma client. Initially the individual undergoes a period of disorganization during which there is difficulty making decisions, extreme or irrational fears, and general mistrust. Observable manifestations may range from stark hysteria, to expression of anger and rage, to silence and withdrawal. Guilt and feelings of responsibility for the rape, as well as numerous physical manifestations, are common. The crisis counselor will attempt to help the victim draw upon previous successful coping strategies to regain control over his or her life.

If the client is a victim of battering, the counselor ensures that various resources and options are made known to the victim so that she may make a personal decision regarding what she wishes to do with her life. Support groups provide a valuable forum for reducing isolation and learning new strategies for coping with the aftermath of physical or sexual abuse. Particularly for the rape victim, the peer support group provides a therapeutic forum for reducing the sense of isolation she may feel in the aftermath of predictable social and interpersonal responses to her experience.

Sadock and Sadock (2007) stated:

Few women emerge from the assault completely unscathed. The manifestations and the degree of damage depend on the violence of the attack itself, the vulnerability of the woman, and the support system available to her immediately after the attack. A rape victim fares best when she receives immediate support and can ventilate her fear and rage to loving family members, sympathetic physicians, and law enforcement officials. Knowing that she has socially acceptable means of recourse, such as the arrest and conviction of the rapist, can help a rape victim. (p. 884)

The Safe House or Shelter

Most major cities in the United States now have **safe houses or shelters** where women can go to be assured of protection for them and their children. These shelters provide a variety of services, and the women receive emotional support from staff and each other. Most shelters provide individual and group counseling; help with bureaucratic institutions such as the police, legal representation, and social services; child care and children's programming; and aid for the woman in making future plans, such as employment counseling and linkages with housing authorities.

The shelters are usually run by a combination of professional and volunteer staff, including nurses, psychologists, lawyers, and others. Women who themselves have been previously abused are often among the volunteer staff members.

Group work is an important part of the service of shelters. Women in residence range from those in the immediate crisis phase to those who have progressed through a variety of phases of the grief process. Those newer members can learn a great deal from the women who have successfully resolved similar problems. Length of stay varies a great deal from individual to individual, depending on a number of factors, such as outside support network, financial situation, and personal resources.

The shelter provides a haven of physical safety for the battered woman and promotes expression of the intense emotions she may be experiencing regarding her situation. A woman often exhibits depression, extreme fear, or even violent expressions of anger and rage. In the shelter, she learns that these feelings are normal and that others have also experienced these same emotions in similar situations. She is allowed to grieve for what has been lost and for what was expected but not achieved. Help is provided in overcoming the tremendous guilt associated with self-blame. This is a difficult step for someone who has accepted responsibility for another's behavior over a long period.

IMPLICATIONS OF RESEARCH FOR EVIDENCE-BASED PRACTICE

Humphreys, J. (2000). Spirituality and distress in sheltered battered women. *Image: Journal of Nursing Scholarship, 32,* 273–278.

DESCRIPTION OF THE STUDY: The purpose of this study was to examine the relationship between spiritual beliefs and psychological distress in sheltered battered women. The convenience sample in this study included 50 women, ages ranging from 19 to 60, who had resided for at least 21 days in one of four battered women's shelters in the San Francisco Bay area. Ethnicity included 20 African Americans, 11 European Americans, 11 Latino Americans, 5 Asian Americans, 1 Native American, and 2 other (mixed or not given). All had been abused by a husband or partner. Psychological distress was measured using the Symptom Checklist-90-Revised (SCL-90-R), a test that is scored and interpreted for nine primary symptom dimensions: somatization, obsessive-compulsiveness, interpersonal sensitivity, depression, anxiety, hostility, phobic anxiety, paranoid ideation, and psychoticism. Spirituality was measured using the Spiritual Perspectives Scale (SPS), a 10-item scale that measures the extent to which one holds certain spiritual views and engages in spiritually related interactions. In the instructions, spirituality is referred to as "an awareness of one's inner self and a sense of connection to a higher being, nature, others, or to some purpose greater than oneself."

RESULTS OF THE STUDY: The women in this study suffered significant psychological distress that was highly correlated with the frequency and severity of battering they had experienced. However, participants who scored higher on the SPS experienced fewer and less intense symptoms in the obsessive-compulsive, interpersonal sensitivity, and hostility dimensions of the SCL-90-R. Eighty percent of the participants indicated a belief in God or a "higher power," and that their spirituality was a significant part of their lives. Some indicated that they strongly relied on their spiritual support for survival in their stressful life situation. Eighty-two percent reported that they thought forgiveness was an important part of their spirituality.

IMPLICATIONS FOR NURSING PRACTICE: The results of this study indicate that spirituality among battered women is a means of reducing psychological stress by a connection with powers beyond oneself. The author cited research studies that concluded that "the role of nurses is not to solve the spiritual problems of clients but to provide an environment where spirituality can be expressed." Suggested nursing interventions include (1) spiritual assessment, (2) identification of resources that have been a source of spiritual

Continued

IMPLICATIONS OF RESEARCH FOR EVIDENCE-BASED PRACTICE—cont'd

support, (3) offering compassionate presence and support, (4) open and honest communication, (5) listening, (6) fostering caring relationships with significant other people in clients' lives, and (7) encouraging prayer and meditation. The author concluded,

"Encouraging battered women to consider personal resources that have been helpful to them in the past, including their spiritual beliefs, may provide benefit to these women who face tremendous demands with limited external resource."

New arrivals at the shelter are given time to experience the relief from the safety and security provided. Making decisions is discouraged during the period of immediate crisis and disorganization. Once the woman's emotions have become more stable, planning for the future begins. Through information from staff and peers, she learns what resources are available to her within the community. Feedback is provided, but the woman makes her own decision about "where she wants to go from here." She is accepted and supported in whatever she chooses to do.

Family Therapy

The focus of therapy with families who use violence is to help them develop democratic ways of solving problems. Studies show that the more a family uses the democratic means of conflict resolution, the less likely they are to engage in physical violence. Families need to learn to deal with problems in ways that can produce mutual benefits for all concerned, rather than engaging in power struggles among family members.

Parents also need to learn more effective methods of disciplining children, aside from physical punishment. Time-out techniques and methods that emphasize the importance of positive reinforcement for acceptable behavior can be very effective. Family members must be committed to consistent use of this behavior modification technique for it to be successful.

Teaching parents about expectations for various developmental levels may alleviate some of the stress that accompanies these changes. Knowing what to expect from individuals at various stages of development may provide needed anticipatory guidance to deal with the crises commonly associated with these stages.

Therapy sessions with all family members together may focus on problems with family communication. Members are encouraged to express honest feelings in a manner that is non-threatening to other family members. Active listening, assertiveness techniques, and respecting the

rights of others are taught and encouraged. Barriers to effective communication are identified and resolved.

Referrals to agencies that promote effective parenting skills (e.g., parent effectiveness training) may be made. Alternative agencies that may relieve the stress of parenting (e.g., "Mom's Day Out" programs, sitter-sharing organizations, and day-care institutions) also may be considered. Support groups for abusive parents may also be helpful, and assistance in locating or initiating such a group may be provided.

Summary and Key Points

- Abuse is the maltreatment of one person by another.

- Intimate partner violence, child abuse, and sexual assault are widespread, and all populations are equally affected.

- Various factors have been theorized as influential in the predisposition to violent behavior. Physiological and biochemical influences within the brain have been suggested, as has the possibility of a direct genetic link.

- Organic brain syndromes associated with various cerebral disorders have been implicated in the predisposition to aggressive and violent behavior.

- Psychoanalytic theorists relate the predisposition to violent behavior to underdeveloped ego and a poor self-concept.

- Learning theorists suggest that children imitate the abusive behavior of their parents. This theory has been substantiated by studies that show that individuals who were abused as children or whose parents disciplined them with physical punishment are more likely to be abusive as adults.

- Societal influences, such as general acceptance of violence as a means of solving problems, also have been implicated.

■ Women who are battered often take blame for their situation. They may have been reared in abusive families and have come to expect this type of behavior.

■ Battered women commonly see no way out of their present situation and may be encouraged by their social support network to remain in the abusive relationship.

■ Child abuse includes physical and emotional abuse, physical and emotional neglect, and sexual abuse of a child.

■ A child may experience many years of abuse without reporting it because of fear of retaliation by the abuser.

■ Some children report incest experiences to their mothers, only to be rebuffed by the mother and told to remain secretive about the abuse.

■ Adult survivors of incest often experience a number of physical and emotional manifestations relating back to the incestuous relationship.

■ Sexual assault is identified as an act of aggression, not passion.

■ Many rapists report growing up in abusive homes, and some theorists relate the predisposition to rape to a "seductive, but rejecting, mother."

■ Rape is a traumatic experience, and many women experience flashbacks, nightmares, rage, physical symptoms, depression, and thoughts of suicide for many years after the occurrence.

■ Treatment modalities for victims of abuse include crisis intervention with the sexual assault victim, safe shelter for battered women, and therapy for families who use violence.

 DavisPlus Additional info available @
davisplus.fadavis.com

Review Questions
Self-Examination/Learning Exercise

*Select the answer that is **most** appropriate for each of the following questions:*

1. Sharon, a woman with multiple cuts and abrasions, arrives at the emergency department (ED) with her three small children. She tells the nurse her husband inflicted these wounds on her. She says, "I didn't want to come. I'm really okay. He only does this when he has too much to drink. I just shouldn't have yelled at him." The best response by the nurse is:
   a. "How often does he drink too much?"
   b. "It is not your fault. You did the right thing by coming here."
   c. "How many times has he done this to you?"
   d. "He is not a good husband. You have to leave him before he kills you."

2. Sharon, a woman with multiple cuts and abrasions, arrives at the ED with her three small children. She tells the nurse her husband inflicted these wounds on her. In the interview, Sharon tells the nurse, "He's been getting more and more violent lately. He's been under a lot of stress at work the last few weeks, so he drinks a lot when he gets home. He always gets mean when he drinks. I was getting scared. So I just finally told him I was going to take the kids and leave. He got furious when I said that and began beating me with his fists." With the nurse's knowledge about the cycle of battering, what does this situation represent?
   a. Phase I; Sharon was desperately trying to stay out of his way and keep everything calm.
   b. Phase I; a minor battering incident for which Sharon assumes all the blame.
   c. Phase II; the acute battering incident that Sharon provoked with her threat to leave.
   d. Phase III; the honeymoon phase where the husband believes that he has "taught her a lesson and she won't act up again."

3. A battered woman presents to the ED with multiple cuts and abrasions. Her right eye is swollen shut. She says that her husband did this to her. The *priority* nursing intervention is:
   a. Tending to the immediate care of her wounds.
   b. Providing her with information about a safe place to stay.
   c. Administering the prn tranquilizer ordered by the physician.
   d. Explaining how she may go about bringing charges against her husband.

4. A woman who has a long history of being battered by her husband is staying at the woman's shelter. She has received emotional support from staff and peers and has been made aware of the alternatives open to her. Nevertheless, she decides to return to her home and marriage. The best response by the nurse to the woman's decision is:
   a. "I just can't believe you have decided to go back to that horrible man."
   b. "I'm just afraid he will kill you or the children when you go back."
   c. "What makes you think things have changed with him?"
   d. "I hope you have made the right decision. Call this number if you need help."

5. Jana, age 5, is sent to the school nurse's office with an upset stomach. She has vomited and soiled her blouse. When the nurse removes her blouse, she notices that Jana has numerous bruises on her arms and torso, in various stages of healing. She also notices some small scars. Jana's abdomen protrudes on her small, thin frame. From the objective physical assessment, the nurse suspects that:
   a. Jana is experiencing physical and sexual abuse.
   b. Jana is experiencing physical abuse and neglect.
   c. Jana is experiencing emotional neglect.
   d. Jana is experiencing sexual and emotional abuse.

6. A school nurse notices bruises and scars on a child's body, but the child refuses to say how she received them. Another way in which the nurse can get information from the child is to:
   a. Have her evaluated by the school psychologist.
   b. Tell her she may select a "treat" from the treat box (e.g., sucker, balloon, junk jewelry) if she answers the nurse's questions.
   c. Explain to her that, if she answers the questions, she may stay in the nurse's office and not have to go back to class.
   d. Use a "family" of dolls to role-play the child's family with her.

7. A school nurse notices bruises and scars on a child's body. The nurse suspects that the child is being physically abused. How should the nurse proceed with this information?
   a. As a health-care worker, report the suspicion to the Department of Health and Human Services.
   b. Check the child again in a week and see if there are any new bruises.
   c. Meet with the child's parents and ask them how the child got the bruises.
   d. Initiate paperwork to have the child placed in foster care.

Review Questions—cont'd
Self-Examination/Learning Exercise

8. Kate is an 18-year-old freshman at the state university. She was extremely flattered when Don, a senior star football player, invited her to a party. On the way home, he parked the car in a secluded area by the lake. He became angry when she refused his sexual advances. He began to beat her and finally raped her. She tried to fight him, but his physical strength overpowered her. He dumped her in the dorm parking lot and left. The dorm supervisor rushed Kate to the emergency department. Kate says to the nurse, "It's all my fault. I shouldn't have allowed him to stop at the lake." The nurse's best response is:
   a. "Yes, you're right. You put yourself in a very vulnerable position when you allowed him to stop at the lake."
   b. "You are not to blame for his behavior. You obviously made some right decisions, because you survived the attack."
   c. "There's no sense looking back now. Just look forward, and make sure you don't put yourself in the same situation again."
   d. "You'll just have to see that he is arrested so he won't do this to anyone else."

9. A young woman who has just undergone a sexual assault is brought into the ED by a friend. The *priority* nursing intervention would be:
   a. Help her to bathe and clean herself up.
   b. Provide physical and emotional support during evidence collection.
   c. Provide her with a written list of community resources for rape victims.
   d. Discuss the importance of a follow-up visit to evaluate for sexually transmitted diseases.

10. A woman who was sexually assaulted 6 months ago by a man with whom she was acquainted has since been attending a support group for rape victims. From this group, she has learned that the most likely reason the man raped her was:
   a. Because he had been drinking, he was not in control of his actions.
   b. He had not had sexual relations with a girl in many months.
   c. He was predisposed to become a rapist by virtue of the poverty conditions under which he was reared.
   d. He was expressing power and dominance by means of sexual aggression and violence.

TEST YOUR CRITICAL THINKING SKILLS

Sandy is a psychiatric RN who works at the safe house for battered women. Lisa has just been admitted with her two small children after she was treated in the emergency department. She had been beaten severely by her husband while he was intoxicated last night. She escaped with her children after he passed out in their bedroom.

In her initial assessment, Sandy learns from Lisa that she has been battered by her husband for 5 years, beginning shortly after their marriage. She explained that she "knew he drank quite a lot before we were married, but thought he would stop after we had kids." Instead, the drinking has increased. Sometimes he doesn't even get home from work until 11 o'clock or midnight, after stopping to drink at the bar with his buddies.

Lately, he has begun to express jealousy and a lack of trust in Lisa, accusing her of numerous infidelities and indiscretions, none of which is true. Lisa says, "If only he wasn't under so much stress on his job, then maybe he wouldn't drink so much. Maybe if I tried harder to make everything perfect for him at home—I don't know. What do you think I should do to keep him from acting this way?"
Answer the following questions related to Lisa:

1. What is an appropriate response to Lisa's question?

2. Identify the priority psychosocial nursing diagnosis for Lisa.

3. What must the nurse ensure that Lisa learns from this experience?

References

American Medical Association. (2009). *Report of the Council on Scientific Affairs: Violence between intimates.* Retrieved October 12, 2010, from http://www.ama-assn.org/ama/no-index/about-ama/13577.shtml

Bensley, L., VanEenwyk, J., & Wynkoop, K. S. (2003). Childhood family violence history and women's risk for intimate partner violence and poor health. *American Journal of Preventive Medicine, 25,* 38–44.

Burgess, A. (2010). Rape violence. *Nursing Spectrum/NurseWeek CE: Course 60025.* Retrieved October 12, 2010, from http://ce.nurse.com/60025/Rape-Violence

Centers for Disease Control and Prevention. (2009a). *Understanding intimate partner violence.* Retrieved October 11, 2010, from http://www.cdc.gov/violenceprevention/pdf/IPV_factsheet-a.pdf

Centers for Disease Control and Prevention. (2009b). *Understanding sexual violence.* Retrieved October 11, 2010, from http://www.cdc.gov/violenceprevention/pdf/SV_factsheet-a.pdf

Child Welfare Information Gateway. (2007). *Recognizing child abuse and neglect: Signs and symptoms.* Retrieved October 12, 2010, from http://www.childwelfare.gov/pubs/factsheets/signs.cfm

Child Welfare Information Gateway. (2008). *What is child abuse and neglect?* Retrieved October 12, 2010, from http://www.childwelfare.gov/pubs/factsheets/whatiscan.cfm

Cummings, J. L., & Mega, M. S. (2003). *Neuropsychiatry and behavioral neuroscience.* New York: Oxford University Press.

Family Violence Law Center. (2003). *Why do women stay in violent relationships?* Retrieved October 12, 2010, from http://www.fvlc.org/pdf_fvlc/English_WhyWomenStay.pdf

Flaherty, E. G., Stirling, J., & The Committee on Child Abuse and Neglect. (2010). Clinical report—The pediatrician's role in child maltreatment prevention. *Periatrics, 126,* 833–841.

Hollander, E., Berlin, H. A., & Stein, D. J. (2008). Impulse-control disorders not elsewhere classified. In R. E. Hales, S. C. Yudofsky, & G. O. Gabbard (Eds.), *Textbook of psychiatry* (5th ed., pp. 777–820). Washington, DC: American Psychiatric Publishing.

Hornor, G. (2005). Domestic violence and children. *Journal of Pediatric Health Care, 19,* 206–212.

Kennedy, B. P., Kawachi, I., Prothrow, S. D., Lochner, K., & Gupta, V. (1998). Social capital, income inequality, and firearm violent crime. *Social Science and Medicine, 47,* 7–17.

King, B. M. (2009). *Human sexuality today* (6th ed.). Upper Saddle River, NJ: Pearson Education.

Lerner, M. (2005). *Adult manifestations of childhood sexual abuse.* New York: The American Academy of Experts in Traumatic Stress.

McCormack, J. (2002, May). Sexual offenders' perceptions of their early interpersonal relationships: An attachment perspective. *Journal of Sex Research, 39,* 85–93.

Meskill, J., & Conner, M. (2010). *Understanding and dealing with domestic violence against women.* Retrieved October 12, 2010, from http://www.oregoncounseling.org/Handouts/DomesticViolenceWomen.htm

Murray, R. B., Zentner, J. P., & Yakimo, R. (2009). *Health promotion strategies through the life span* (8th ed.). Upper Saddle River, NJ: Pearson Education.

National Coalition Against Domestic Violence. (2010). *What is battering?* Retrieved October 12, 2010, from http://www.ncadv.org/learn/TheProblem.php

Reeves, C. R. (2003). *Childhood: It should not hurt.* Huntersville, NC: LTI Publishing.

Sadock, B. J., & Sadock, V. A. (2007). *Synopsis of psychiatry: Behavioral sciences/clinical psychiatry* (10th ed.). Philadelphia: Lippincott Williams & Wilkins.

Schatzberg, A. F., Cole, J. O., & DeBattista, C. (2010). *Manual of clinical psychopharmacology* (7th ed.). Washington, DC: American Psychiatric Publishing.

Scully, D. (1994). *Understanding sexual violence: A study of convicted rapists.* New York: Routledge.

Siever, L. J. (2002, August). Neurobiology of impulsive aggressive personality disordered patients. *Psychiatric Times, 19*(8). Retrieved October 11, 2010, from http://www.psychiatrictimes.com/display/article/10168/47131

Tardiff, K. J. (2003). Violence. In R. E. Hales & S. C. Yudofsky (Eds.), *Textbook of clinical psychiatry* (4th ed., pp. 1485–1509). Washington, DC: American Psychiatric Publishing.

U.S. Bureau of Justice Statistics. (2009). *Intimate partner violence in the U.S.* Retrieved October 12, 2010, from http://bjs.ojp.usdoj.gov/content/intimate/ipv.cfm

U.S. Department of Health and Human Services. (2010). *Child Maltreatment 2008.* Retrieved October 11, 2010, from http://www.acf.hhs.gov/programs/cb/pubs/cm08/cm08.pdf

U.S. Department of Justice. (2009). *National crime victimization survey: Criminal victimization 2008.* Retrieved October 12, 2010, from http://bjs.ojp.usdoj.gov/content/pub/pdf/cv08.pdf

World Health Organization. (2004). The economic dimensions of interpersonal violence. Geneva: Author.

Classical References

Abrahamsen, D. (1960). *The psychology of crime.* New York: John Wiley & Sons.

Erikson, E. H. (1963). *Childhood and society* (2nd ed.). New York: WW Norton.

Macdonald, J. M. (1971). *Rape: Offenders and their victims.* Springfield, IL: Charles C Thomas.

Selye, H. (1956). *The stress of life.* New York: McGraw-Hill.

Walker, L. E. (1979). *The battered woman.* New York: Harper & Row.

@ INTERNET REFERENCES

- Additional information related to child abuse may be located at the following websites:
  - http://www.childwelfare.gov/
  - http://endabuse.org/
  - http://www.child-abuse.com/
  - http://www.nlm.nih.gov/medlineplus/childabuse.html

- Additional information related to sexual assault may be located at the following websites:
  - http://www.vaw.umn.edu/
  - http://www.nlm.nih.gov/medlineplus/sexualassault.html

- Additional information related to intimate partner violence may be located at the following websites:
  - http://www.thehotline.org/
  - http://www.ama-assn.org/ama/no-index/about-ama/13577.shtml
  - http://www.nursingworld.org/MainMenuCategories/ANAMarketplace/ANAPeriodicals/OJIN/TableofContents/Volume72002/No1Jan2002.aspx

MOVIE CONNECTIONS

The Burning Bed (domestic violence) • *Life With Billy* (domestic violence) • *Two Story House* (child abuse) • *The Prince of Tides* (domestic violence) • *Radio Flyer* (child abuse) • *Flowers in the Attic* (child abuse) • *A Case of Rape* (sexual assault) • *The Accused* (sexual assault)

KEY TERMS

case management	diagnosis-related groups (DRGs)	prospective payment
case manager	managed care	shelters
deinstitutionalization	mobile outreach units	storefront clinics

OBJECTIVES

After reading this chapter, the student will be able to:

1. Discuss the changing focus of care in the field of mental health.
2. Define the concepts of care associated with the public health model.
3. Differentiate between the roles of basic level and advanced practice psychiatric/mental health registered nurses.
4. Define the concepts of case management and identify the role of case management in community mental health nursing.
5. Discuss primary prevention of mental illness within the community.
6. Identify populations at risk for mental illness within the community.
7. Discuss nursing intervention in primary prevention of mental illness within the community.
8. Discuss secondary prevention of mental illness within the community.
9. Describe treatment alternatives related to secondary prevention within the community.
10. Discuss tertiary prevention of mental illness within the community as it relates to the seriously mentally ill and homeless mentally ill.
11. Relate historical and epidemiological factors associated with caring for the seriously mentally ill and homeless mentally ill within the community.
12. Identify treatment alternatives for care of the seriously mentally ill and homeless mentally ill within the community.
13. Apply steps of the nursing process to care of the seriously mentally ill and homeless mentally ill within the community.

HOMEWORK ASSIGNMENT

Please read the chapter and answer the following questions:

1. What are *diagnosis-related groups* (DRGs)?
2. Describe and differentiate how interventions at the primary, secondary, and tertiary prevention levels are implemented.
3. Name three common client populations that benefit from psychiatric home health nursing.
4. What is the most common psychiatric diagnosis among mentally ill homeless people?

This chapter explores the concepts of primary and secondary prevention of mental illness within communities. Additional focus is placed on tertiary prevention of mental illness: treatment with community resources of those who suffer from severe and persistent mental illness and homeless persons who are mentally ill. Emphasis is given to the role of the psychiatric nurse in the various treatment alternatives within the community setting.

The Changing Focus of Care

Before 1840, there was no known treatment for individuals who were mentally ill. Because mental illness was perceived as incurable, the only "reasonable" intervention was thought to be removing these ill persons from the community to a place where they would do no harm to themselves or others.

In 1841, Dorothea Dix, a former schoolteacher, began a personal crusade across the land on behalf of institutionalized mentally ill clients. Her efforts resulted in more humane treatment of persons with mental illness and the establishment of a number of hospitals for the mentally ill.

After the movement initiated by Dix, the number of hospitals for persons with mental illness increased, although unfortunately not as rapidly as did the population with mental illness. The demand soon outgrew the supply, and hospitals became overcrowded and understaffed, with conditions that would have sorely distressed Dorothea Dix.

The community mental health movement had its impetus in the 1940s. With establishment of the National Mental Health Act of 1946, the U.S. government awarded grants to the states to develop mental health programs outside of state hospitals. Outpatient clinics and psychiatric units in general hospitals were inaugurated. Then, in 1949, as an outgrowth of the National Mental Health Act, the National Institute of Mental Health (NIMH) was established. The U.S. government has charged this agency with the responsibility for mental health in the United States.

In 1955, the Joint Commission on Mental Health and Illness was established by Congress to identify the nation's mental health needs and to make recommendations for improvement in psychiatric care. In 1961, the Joint Commission published the report, *Action for Mental Health,* in which recommendations were made for treatment of clients with mental illness, training for caregivers, and improvements in education and research on mental illness. With consideration given to these recommendations, Congress passed the Mental Retardation Facilities and Community Mental Health Centers Construction Act (often called the Community Mental Health Centers Act) of 1963. This act called for the construction of comprehensive community health centers, the cost of which would be shared by federal and state governments. The **deinstitutionalization** movement (the closing of state mental hospitals and discharging of individuals with mental illness) had begun.

Unfortunately, many state governments did not have the capability to match the federal funds required for the establishment of these mental health centers. Some communities found it difficult to follow the rigid requirements for services required by the legislation that provided the grant.

In 1980 the Community Mental Health Systems Act, which was to have played a major role in renovation of mental health care, was established. Funding was authorized for community mental health centers, for services to high-risk populations, and for rape research and services. Approval was also granted for the appointment of an associate director for minority concerns at NIMH. However, before this plan could be enacted, the newly inaugurated administration set forth its intention to diminish federal involvement. Budget cuts reduced the number of mandated services, and federal funding for community mental health centers was terminated in 1984.

Meanwhile, costs of care for hospitalized psychiatric clients continued to rise. The problem of the "revolving door" began to intensify. Individuals with severe and persistent mental illness had no place to go when their symptoms exacerbated, except back to the hospital. Individuals without support systems remained in the hospital for extended periods because of lack of appropriate community services. Hospital services were paid for by cost-based, retrospective reimbursement: Medicaid, Medicare, and private health insurance. Retrospective reimbursement encouraged hospital expenditure; the more services provided, the more payment received.

This system of delivery of health care was interrupted in 1983 with the advent of **prospective payment**—the Reagan administration's proposal of cost containment. It was directed at control of Medicare costs by setting forth preestablished amounts that would be reimbursed for specific diagnoses, or **diagnosis-related groups (DRGs).** Since that time, prospective payment has also been integrated by the states (Medicaid) and by some private insurance companies, drastically affecting the amount of reimbursement for health-care services.

Mental health services have been influenced by prospective payment. General hospital services to psychiatric clients have been severely restricted. Clients who present with acute symptoms, such as acute psychosis, suicidal ideations or attempts, or manic exacerbations, constitute the largest segment of the psychiatric hospital census. Clients with less serious illnesses (e.g., moderate depression or adjustment disorders) may be hospitalized, but length of stay has been shortened considerably by the reimbursement guidelines. Clients are being discharged from the hospital with a greater need for aftercare than in the past, when hospital stays were longer.

Deinstitutionalization continues to be the changing focus of mental health care in the United States. Care for the client in the hospital has become cost prohibitive, whereas care for the client in the community is cost effective. The reality of the provision of health-care services today is often more of a political and funding issue than providers would care to admit. Decisions about how to treat are rarely made without consideration of cost and method of payment.

Provision of outpatient mental health services not only is the wave of the future but also has become a necessity today. We must serve the consumer by providing the essential services to assist with health promotion or prevention, to initiate early intervention, and to ensure rehabilitation or prevention of long-term disability.

The Public Health Model

The premise of the model of public health is based largely on the concepts set forth by Gerald Caplan (1964) during the initial community mental health movement. They include primary prevention, secondary prevention, and tertiary prevention. These concepts no longer have relevance only to mental health nursing; rather, they have been widely adapted as guiding principles in many clinical and community settings over a range of medical and nursing specialties.

CORE CONCEPT

Primary prevention
Services aimed at reducing the incidence of mental disorders within the population.

Primary prevention targets both individuals and the environment. Emphasis is twofold:

1. Assisting individuals to increase their ability to cope effectively with stress.
2. Targeting and diminishing harmful forces (stressors) within the environment.

Nursing in primary prevention is focused on the targeting of groups at risk and the provision of educational programs. Examples include:

■ Teaching parenting skills and child development to prospective new parents

■ Teaching physical and psychosocial effects of alcohol/drugs to elementary school students

■ Teaching techniques of stress management to virtually anyone who desires to learn

■ Teaching groups of individuals ways to cope with the changes associated with various maturational stages

■ Teaching concepts of mental health to various groups within the community

■ Providing education and support to unemployed or homeless individuals

■ Providing education and support to other individuals in various transitional periods (e.g., widows and widowers, new retirees, and women entering the workforce in middle life)

These are only a few examples of the types of services nurses provide in primary prevention. Such services can be offered in a variety of settings that are convenient for the public (e.g., churches, schools, colleges, community centers, YMCAs and YWCAs, workplaces of employee organizations, meetings of women's groups, or civic or social organizations such as parent-teacher associations, health fairs, and community shelters).

CORE CONCEPT

Secondary prevention
Interventions aimed at minimizing early symptoms of psychiatric illness and directed toward reducing the prevalence and duration of the illness.

Secondary prevention is accomplished through early identification of problems and prompt initiation of effective treatment. Nursing in secondary prevention focuses on recognition of symptoms and provision of, or referral for, treatment. Examples include:

■ Ongoing assessment of individuals at high risk for illness exacerbation (e.g., during home visits, day care, community health centers, or in any setting where screening of high-risk individuals might occur)

■ Provision of care for individuals in whom illness symptoms have been assessed (e.g., individual or group counseling, medication administration, education and support during period of increased stress [crisis intervention], staffing rape crisis centers, suicide hotlines, homeless shelters, shelters for abused persons, or mobile mental health units)

■ Referral for treatment of individuals in whom illness symptoms have been assessed. Referrals may come from support groups, community mental health centers, emergency services, psychiatrists or psychologists, and day or partial hospitalization. Inpatient therapy on a psychiatric unit of a general hospital or in a private psychiatric hospital may be necessary. Chemotherapy and various adjunct therapies may be initiated as part of the treatment.

Secondary prevention has been addressed extensively in Unit Four of this text. Nursing assessment, diagnosis/outcome identification, planning/implementation, and evaluation were discussed for many of the mental illnesses identified in the *Diagnostic and Statistical Manual of Mental Disorders, Fourth Edition, Text Revision* (DSM-IV-TR) (American Psychiatric Association [APA], 2000). These concepts may be applied in any setting where nursing is practiced.

CORE CONCEPT

Tertiary prevention
Services aimed at reducing the residual defects that are associated with severe and persistent mental illness.

Tertiary prevention is accomplished in two ways:

1. Preventing complications of the illness
2. Promoting rehabilitation that is directed toward achievement of each individual's maximum level of functioning

Historically, individuals with severe and persistent mental illness often experienced long hospitalizations that resulted in loss of social skills and increased dependency. With deinstitutionalization, many of these individuals may never have experienced hospitalization, but they still do not possess adequate skills to live productive lives within the community.

Nursing in tertiary prevention focuses on helping clients learn or relearn socially appropriate behaviors so that they may achieve a satisfying role within the community. Examples include:

■ Consideration of the rehabilitation process at the time of initial diagnosis and treatment planning

■ Teaching the client daily living skills and encouraging independence to his or her maximum ability

■ Referring clients for various aftercare services (e.g., support groups, day treatment programs, partial hospitalization programs, psychosocial rehabilitation programs, group home or other transitional housing)

■ Monitoring effectiveness of aftercare services (e.g., through home health visits or follow-up appointments in community mental health centers)

■ Making referrals for support services when required (e.g., some communities have programs linking individuals with serious mental disorders to volunteers who serve to develop friendships with the individuals and who may assist with household chores, shopping, and other activities of daily living with which the individual is having difficulty, in addition to participating in social activities with the individual)

IMPLICATIONS OF RESEARCH FOR EVIDENCE-BASED PRACTICE

McDevitt, J., Snyder, M., Miller, A., & Wilbur, J. (2006). **Perceptions of barriers and benefits to physical activity among outpatients in psychiatric rehabilitation.** *Journal of Nursing Scholarship,* **38,** 50–55.

DESCRIPTION OF THE STUDY: The purpose of this study was to explore perceived barriers and benefits to physical activity in people with serious and persistent mental illness (SPMI) who were enrolled in

community-based psychiatric rehabilitation. The sample included 34 participants (16 men and 18 women) ages 18 to 50 from two community-based psychiatric rehabilitation centers in a large Midwestern urban area. Ethnic breakdown included 24 African Americans, 7 Whites, and 3 of Hispanic or unknown ethnicity. Four focus groups lasting 50 minutes each were held over a 3-week period, with seven to nine participants in each group. Themes of the focus groups included barriers and benefits of physical activity.

Continued

IMPLICATIONS OF RESEARCH FOR EVIDENCE-BASED PRACTICE—cont'd

RESULTS OF THE STUDY: Barriers to physical activity identified by the study participants included symptoms of the mental illness itself, being medicated, gaining weight, being in a rehabilitation program, and living in urban neighborhoods. They cited symptoms of lethargy and lack of initiative (from either the medication or the illness) and weight gain from the medications as interfering with physical activity. Neighborhood safety concerns and being identified as a person with a mental disorder were also identified. Benefits of physical activity cited included feeling more energetic and less stressed, and improved sleep. Keeping busy and providing distraction from problems were also recognized. Both men and women suggested they would appreciate exercise and activities for same-gender groups.

IMPLICATIONS FOR NURSING PRACTICE: Several recommendations from the participants emerged

from the focus groups. Some of these included the following:

• Need a good leader who encourages, but does not coerce; provides participants with choices
• Groups that provide relevant information that pertains to client health concerns, such as weight gain, and how to address these concerns
• Offer group support, but provide individual options as well.
• Offer a choice of different types of activities, to reduce boredom

The authors of this study stated, "Confronting how attitudes and barriers specific to this population can affect activity and reframing program compliance to include the independent initiation of activity as part of improving health should assist clients of mental health services to become more active" (p. 55).

Nursing care at the tertiary level of prevention can be administered on an individual or group basis and in a variety of settings, such as inpatient hospitalization, day or partial hospitalization, group home or halfway house, shelters, home health care, nursing homes, and community mental health centers.

The Role of the Nurse in Community Mental Health

One emphasis of the National Mental Health Act of 1946 was to increase the supply of mental health professionals. This Act named four major mental health disciplines: psychiatry, clinical psychology, social work, and nursing. To increase the numbers of trained mental health professionals, grants were provided to institutions, and stipends and fellowships were awarded to individuals.

Nurses who work in the field of psychiatry may practice at one of two levels: the psychiatric/mental health registered nurse or the psychiatric/mental health advanced practice registered nurse. These two levels have been differentiated in the *Psychiatric-Mental Health Nursing Scope and Standards of Practice* published by the American Nurses Association (ANA) in 2007.

The Psychiatric/Mental Health Registered Nurse (RN-PMH)

DEFINITION: A registered nurse (RN) who demonstrates competence, including specialized

knowledge, skills, and abilities, obtained through education and experience in caring for persons with mental health issues, mental health problems, and psychiatric disorders (ANA, 2007, p. 16).

EDUCATION: The ANA (2007) stated, "Nurses from a number of educational backgrounds participate and practice in psychiatric nursing settings. Due to the complexity of care in the specialty, the preferred educational preparation is at the baccalaureate level with credentialing by the American Nurses Credentialing Center (ANCC)" (p. 16).

ADDITIONAL CREDENTIALING: In addition to professional licensure by the state, psychiatric/mental health RNs may apply to sit for examinations that certify them as basic-level psychiatric/mental health nurses.

EMPLOYMENT SETTINGS: Inpatient psychiatric hospital unit, day treatment and partial hospitalization programs, community health centers, home health care, long-term care centers.

PROFESSIONAL RESPONSIBILITIES: Health promotion and health maintenance; intake screening, evaluation, and triage; case management; provision of therapeutic and safe environments; promotion of self-care activities; administration of psychobiological treatment regimens and monitoring response and effects; crisis intervention and stabilization; and psychiatric rehabilitation (ANA, 2007, p. 18).

The Psychiatric/Mental Health Advanced Practice Registered Nurse (APRN-PMH)

DEFINITION: A professional nurse who has successfully completed a graduate program of study in a [psychiatric/mental health] nursing specialty that provides specialized knowledge and skills that form the foundation for expanded roles in health care. The ANA (2007) stated, "The APRN-PMH expands the practice of a registered nurse by demonstrating a greater depth and breadth of knowledge, a greater synthesis of data, increased complexity of skills and interventions, and significant role autonomy" (p. 19).

EDUCATION: A master's or doctorate degree in the specialty of psychiatric/mental health nursing, with an advanced practice specialty certification from the ANCC.

ADDITIONAL CREDENTIALING: Master's- or doctorate-prepared nurses may sit for credentialing examinations that certify them as a psychiatric/mental health clinical nurse specialist or nurse practitioner. In addition, some states have special licensure that may be granted to nurses with advanced education that permits them to practice at a more independent level (e.g., Advanced Practice Registered Nurse [APRN] or Advanced Registered Nurse Practitioner [ARNP]) and that makes them eligible for prescriptive authority, inpatient admission privileges, third-party reimbursement, and other specific privileges.

EMPLOYMENT SETTINGS: Inpatient psychiatric hospital units; day treatment and partial hospitalization programs; community mental health centers; private mental health facilities; individual private practice; crisis intervention services; or in the capacity of mental health consultant, supervisor, educator, administrator, or researcher.

PROFESSIONAL RESPONSIBILITIES: In addition to those required at the basic RN level, functions of the APRN-PMH include prescribing psychopharmacological agents, integrative therapy interventions, various forms of psychotherapy, community interventions, case management, consultation and liaison, clinical supervision, expanded advocacy activities, education, and research (ANA, 2007, p. 20).

Case Management

Because of the rising costs of hospitalization and in keeping with the concept of deinstitutionalization, there has become a need for managing the care of clients (particularly those with severe and persistent illnesses) in an outpatient setting. **Case management** was defined and discussed in Chapter 9 of this text. Case management at the secondary level of prevention strives to organize client care so that specific outcomes are achieved within an allotted time frame. Commonly, this time frame is determined by the established protocols for length of stay as defined by the DRGs.

Ideally, case management incorporates concepts of care at the primary, secondary, and tertiary levels of prevention. Various definitions have emerged and should be clarified.

Managed care is a concept designed to control the balance between cost and quality of client care. In a managed-care program, individuals receive health care based on need, as assessed by coordinators of the provider. Managed care exists in many settings, including (but not limited to):

■ Insurance-based programs

■ Employer-based medical provider programs

■ Social service programs

■ The public health sector

Managed care may exist in virtually any setting in which health-care provision is a part of the service; that is, in any setting in which an organization (whether it be private or government based) is responsible for payment of health-care services for a group of people. Examples of managed care are health maintenance organizations (HMOs) and preferred provider organizations (PPOs).

Case management is the method used to achieve managed care. It is the actual coordination of services required to meet the needs of the client. The Case Management Society of America (CMSA) defines case management as "a collaborative process of assessment, planning, facilitation, care coordination, evaluation, and advocacy for options and services to meet an individual's and family's comprehensive health needs through communication and available resources to promote quality cost-effective outcomes" (CMSA, 2010, p. 8). Types of clients who benefit from case management include (but are not limited to):

■ The frail elderly

■ Those who are developmentally disabled

■ Those who are physically handicapped

■ Those who are mentally handicapped

■ Individuals with long-term medically complex problems that require multifaceted, costly care (e.g., high-risk infants, persons with HIV or AIDS, and transplant patients)

■ Individuals who are severely compromised by an acute episode of illness or an acute exacerbation of a severe and persistent illness (e.g., schizophrenia)

The **case manager** is responsible for negotiating with multiple health-care providers to obtain a variety of services for the client. The very nature of nursing that incorporates knowledge about the biological, psychological, and sociocultural aspects related to human functioning makes nurses highly appropriate as case managers. The American Nurse's Credentialing Center (ANCC) now offers accreditation by examination for nursing case management. The applicant must hold a current license as a registered nurse with 2 years of full-time nursing practice experience. In addition, he or she must have functioned as a nursing case manager for a minimum of 2,000 hours of practice within the last 3 years. A number of other professional agencies also now offer programs of accreditation or certification for case management (e.g., Accreditation Commission for Health Care, National Committee for Quality Assurance, American Case Management Association). Some case management programs prefer clinical nurse specialists who have experience working with the specific populations for whom the case management service will be rendered.

Case management is becoming a recommended method of treatment for individuals with a severe and persistent mental illness. This type of care enhances functioning by increasing the individual's ability to solve problems, improving work and socialization skills, promoting leisure-time activities, and endeavoring to diminish dependency on others.

The Community as Client

Primary Prevention

Primary prevention within communities encompasses the twofold emphasis defined earlier in this chapter:

1. Identifying stressful life events that precipitate crises and targeting the relevant populations at high risk.
2. Intervening with these high-risk populations to prevent or minimize harmful consequences.

CORE CONCEPT

Community

A group, population, or cluster of people with at least one common characteristic, such as geographic location, occupation, ethnicity, or health concern (Langley, 2002).

Populations at Risk

One way to view populations at risk is to focus on types of crises that individuals experience in their lives. Two broad categories are maturational crises and situational crises.

Maturational Crises

Maturational crises are crucial experiences that are associated with various stages of growth and development. Erikson (1963) described eight stages of the life cycle during which individuals struggle with developmental "tasks." Crises can occur during any of these stages, although several developmental periods and life-cycle events have been recognized as having increased crisis potential: adolescence, marriage, parenthood, midlife, and retirement.

Adolescence The task for adolescence according to Erikson (1963) is *identity versus role confusion.* This is the time in life when individuals ask questions such as "Who am I?" "Where am I going?" and "What is life all about?"

Adolescence is a transition into young adulthood. It is a very volatile time in most families. Commonly, there is conflict over issues of control. Parents sometimes have difficulty relinquishing even a minimal amount of the control they have had throughout their child's infancy, toddler, and school-age years, at this time when the adolescent is seeking increased independence. It may seem that the adolescent is 25 years old one day and 5 years old the next. An often-quoted definition of an adolescent, by an anonymous author, is: "A toddler with hormones and wheels."

At this time, adolescents are "trying out their wings," although they possess an essential need to know that the parents (or surrogate parents) are available if support is required. Mahler, Pine, and Bergman (1975) have termed this vital concept "emotional refueling," and although they were referring to toddlers when they coined the term, it is highly applicable to adolescents as well. In fact, it is believed that the most frequent immediate precipitant to adolescent suicide is loss, or threat of loss, or abandonment by parents or closest peer relationship.

Adolescents have many issues to deal with and many choices to make. Some of these include issues that relate to self-esteem and body image (in a body that is undergoing rapid changes), peer relationships (with both genders), education and career selection, establishing a set of values and ideals, sexuality and sexual experimentation (including issues of birth control and prevention of sexually transmitted diseases), drug and alcohol abuse, and physical appearance.

Nursing interventions with adolescents at the primary level of prevention focus on providing support and accurate information to ease the difficult transition they are undergoing. Educational offerings can be presented in schools, churches, youth centers, or any location in which groups of teenagers gather. Types of programs may include (but are not limited to):

■ Alateen groups for adolescents with alcoholic parent(s)

■ Other support groups for teenagers who are in need of assistance to cope with stressful situations (e.g., children dealing with divorce of their parents, pregnant teenagers, teenagers coping with abortion, adolescents coping with the death of a parent)

■ Educational programs that inform about and validate bodily changes and emotions about which there may be some concerns

■ Educational programs that inform about nutritional needs specific for this age group

■ Educational programs that inform about sexuality, pregnancy, contraception, and sexually transmitted diseases

■ Educational programs that inform about the use and abuse of alcohol and other drugs

Marriage The "American dream" of the 1950s—especially that of the American woman—was to marry, have two or three children, buy a house in the suburbs, and drive a station wagon. To not be at least betrothed by their mid-20s caused many women to fear becoming an "old maid." Living together without the benefit of marriage was an unacceptable and rarely considered option.

Times have changed considerably since the middle of the 20th century. Today's young women are choosing to pursue careers before entering into marriage, to continue their careers after marriage, or to not marry at all. Many couples are deciding to live together without being married, and, as with most trends, the practice now receives more widespread societal acceptance than it once did.

Why is marriage considered one of the most common maturational crises? Sheehy (1976), in her classic volume about life's passages, wrote:

No two people can possibly coordinate all their developmental crises. The timing of outside opportunities will almost never be the same. But more importantly, each one has an inner life structure with its own idiosyncrasies. Depending on what has gone before, each one will alternate differently between times of feeling full of certainty, hope, and heightened potential and times of feeling vulnerable, unfocused, and scared. (p. 138)

Additional conflicts sometimes also arise when the marriage is influenced by crossovers in religion, ethnicity, social status, or race, although these types of differences have become more individually and societally acceptable than they once were.

Nursing interventions at the primary level of prevention with individuals in this stage of development involve education regarding what to expect at various stages in the marriage. Many high schools now offer courses in marriage and family living in which students role-play through anticipatory marriage and family situations. Nurses could offer these kinds of classes within the community to individuals considering marriage. Too many people enter marriage with the notion that, as sure as the depth of their love, their soon-to-be husband or wife will discontinue his or her "undesirable" traits and change into the perceived ideal spouse. Primary prevention with these individuals involves:

■ Encouraging honest communication

■ Determining what each person expects from the relationship

■ Ascertaining whether or not each individual can accept compromise

This type of intervention can be effective in individual or couple's therapy and in support or educational groups of couples experiencing similar circumstances.

Parenthood Murray, Zentner, and Yakimo (2009) stated:

The coming of the child is a developmental and sometimes situational crisis, a turning point in the couple's life in which old patterns of living must be changed for new ways of living and new values. With the advent of parenthood, a couple is embarking on a journey from which there is no return. To put it simply, parents cannot quit. The child's birth brings finality to many privileges and a permanence of responsibilities. (p. 249)

There is perhaps no developmental stage that creates an upheaval equal to that of the arrival of a child. Even when the child is desperately wanted and pleasurably anticipated, his or her arrival usually results in some degree of chaos within the family system.

Because the family operates as a system, the addition of a new member influences all parts of the system as a whole. If it is a first child, the relationship between the spouses is likely to be affected by the demands of caring for the infant on a 24-hour basis. If there are older children, they may resent the attention showered on the new arrival and show their resentment in a variety of creative ways.

The concept of having a child (particularly the first one) is often romanticized, with little or no consideration given to the realities and responsibilities that accompany this "bundle of joy." Many young parents are shocked to realize that such a tiny human can create so many changes in so many lives. It is unfortunate that, although parenting is one of the most important positions an individual will hold in life, it is one for which he or she is often least prepared.

Nursing intervention at the primary level of prevention with those in the developmental stage of parenthood must begin long before the child is even born. How do we prepare individuals for parenthood? *Anticipatory guidance* is the term used to describe the interventions used to help new parents know what they might expect. Volumes have been written on the subject, but it is also important for expectant parents to have a support person or network with whom they can talk, to express feelings, excitement, and fears. Nurses can provide the following type of information to help ease the transition into parenthood (Mandleco, 2004; Murray, Zentner, & Yakimo, 2009; Spock, 2004):

■ **Prepared childbirth classes:** These classes present what most likely will happen, but with additional information about possible variations from that which is expected.

■ **Information about what to expect after the baby arrives:**
  - *Parent-infant bonding.* Expectant parents should know that it is common for parent-infant bonding not to occur immediately. The strong attachment will occur as parent and infant get to know each other.
  - *Changing husband-wife relationships.* The couple should be encouraged to engage in open honest communication and role-playing of typical situations that are likely to arise after the baby becomes a part of the family.
  - *Clothing and equipment.* Expectant parents need to know what is required to care for a newborn child. Family economics, space available, and lifestyle should be considered.
  - *Feeding.* Advantages and disadvantages of breastfeeding and formula feeding should be presented. The couple should be supported in whatever method is chosen. Anticipatory guidance related to technique should be provided

for one or both methods, as the expectant parents request.
  - *Other expectations.* It is important for expectant parents to receive anticipatory guidance about the infant's sleeping and crying patterns, bathing the infant, care of the circumcision and cord, toys that provide stimulation of the newborn's senses, aspects of providing a safe environment, and when to call the physician.

■ **Stages of Growth and Development.** It is very important for parents to understand what behaviors should be expected at what stage of development. It is also important to know that their child may not necessarily follow the age guidelines associated with these stages. However, a substantial deviation from these guidelines should be reported to their physician.

Midlife What is middle age? A colleague once remarked that, upon turning 50 years of age, she stated, "Now I can say I am officially middle aged . . . until I began thinking about how few individuals I really knew who were 100!"

Midlife crises are not defined by a specific number. Various sources in the literature identify these conflicts as occurring anytime between age 35 and 65.

What is a midlife crisis? This, too, is very individual, but a number of patterns have been identified within three broad categories:

1. An alteration in perception of the self. One's perception of self may occur slowly. One may suddenly become aware of being "old" or "middle aged." Murray and associates (2009) stated:

   Now the person looks in the mirror and sees changes that others may have noticed some time ago. Gray, thinning hair, wrinkles, coarsening features, decreased muscular tone, weight gain, varicosities, and capillary breakage may be the first signs of impending age. (p. 569)

   Other biological changes that occur naturally with the aging process may also affect the crises that occur at this time. In women, a gradual decrease in the production of estrogen initiates the menopause, which results in a variety of physical and emotional symptoms. Some physical symptoms include "hot flashes," vaginal dryness, cessation of menstruation, loss of reproductive ability, night sweats, insomnia, headaches, and minor memory disturbances. Emotional symptoms include anxiety, depression, crying for no reason, and temper outbursts.

Although the menopausal period in men is not as evident as it is in women, most clinicians subscribe to the belief that men undergo a climacteric experience related to the gradual decrease in production of testosterone. Although sperm production diminishes with advancing age, there is usually no complete cessation, as there is of ovum production in women at menopause (Scanlon & Sanders, 2011). Some men experience hot flashes, sweating, chills, dizziness, and heart palpitations (Murray et al., 2009), whereas others may experience severe depression and an overall decline in physical vigor (Sadock & Sadock, 2007). An alteration in sexual functioning is not uncommon (see Chapter 35).

2. **An alteration in perception of others.** A change in relationship with adult children requires a sensitive shift in caring. Wright and Leahey (2009) stated:

The family of origin must relinquish the primary roles of parent and child. They must adapt to the new roles of parent and adult child. This involves renegotiation of emotional and financial commitments. The key emotional process during this stage is for family members to deal with a multitude of exits from and entries into the family system. (p. 101)

These experiences are particularly difficult when parents' values conflict with the relationships and types of lifestyles their children choose. An alteration in perception of one's parents also begins to occur during this time. Having always looked to parents for support and comfort, the middle-aged individual may suddenly find that the roles are beginning to reverse. Aging parents may look to their children for assistance with making decisions regarding their everyday lives and for assistance with chores that they have previously accomplished independently. When parents die, middle-aged individuals must come to terms with their own mortality. The process of recognition and resolution of one's own finitude begins in earnest at this time.

3. **An alteration in perception of time.** Middle age has been defined as the end of youth and the beginning of old age. Individuals often experience a sense that time is running out: "I haven't done all I want to do or accomplished all I intended to accomplish!" Depression and a sense of loss may occur as individuals realize that some of the goals established in their youth may go unmet.

The term "empty nest syndrome" has been used to describe the adjustment period parents experience when the last child leaves home to establish an independent residence. The crisis is often more profound for the mother who has devoted her life to nurturing her family. As the last child leaves, she may perceive her future as uncertain and meaningless.

Some women who have devoted their lives to rearing their children decide to develop personal interests and pursue personal goals once the children are grown. This occurs at a time when many husbands have begun to decrease what may have been a compulsive drive for occupational security during the earlier years of their lives. This disparity in common goals may create conflict between husband and wife. At a time when she is experiencing more value in herself and her own life, he may begin to feel less valued. This may also relate to a decrease in the amount of time and support from the wife to which the husband has become accustomed. This type of role change will require numerous adaptations on the part of both spouses.

Finally, an alteration in one's perception of time may be related to the societal striving for eternal youth. The individual may try to delay the external changes that come with aging by the use of cosmetics, hormone creams, or even surgery. This yearning for youth may take the form of sexual promiscuity or extramarital affairs with much younger individuals, in an effort to prove that one "still has what it takes." Some individuals reach for the trappings of youth with regressive-type behaviors, such as the middle-aged man who buys a motorcycle and joins a motorcycle club, and the 50-year-old woman who wears miniskirts and flirts with her daughter's boyfriends. These individuals may be denying their own past and experience. With a negative view of self, they strongly desire to relive their youth.

Nursing intervention at the primary level of prevention with those in the developmental stage of midlife involves providing accurate information regarding changes that occur during this time of life and support for adapting to these changes effectively. These interventions might include:

■ Nutrition classes to inform individuals in this age group about the essentials of diet and exercise. Educational materials on how to avoid obesity or reduce weight can be included, along with the importance of good nutrition.

■ Assistance with ways to improve health (e.g., quit smoking, cease or reduce alcohol consumption, reduce fat intake).

■ Discussions of the importance of having regular physical examinations, including Pap and breast examinations for women and prostate examinations for men. Monthly breast self-examinations should be taught and yearly mammograms encouraged.

■ Classes on menopause. Provide information about what to expect. Myths that abound regarding this topic should be expelled. Support groups for women (and men) undergoing the menopausal experience should be formed.

■ Support and information related to physical changes occurring in the body during this time of life. Assist with the grief response that some individuals will experience in relation to loss of youth, "empty nest," and sense of identity.

■ Support and information related to care of aging parents. Individuals should be referred to community resources for respite and assistance before strain of the caregiver role threatens to disrupt the family system.

Retirement Retirement, which is often anticipated as an achievement in principle, may be met with a great deal of ambivalence when it actually occurs. Our society places a great deal of importance on productivity and on earning as much money as possible at as young an age as possible. These types of values contribute to the ambivalence associated with retirement. Although leisure has been acknowledged as a legitimate reward for workers, leisure during retirement has never been accorded the same social value. Adjustment to this life-cycle event becomes more difficult in the face of societal values that are in direct conflict with the new lifestyle.

Historically, many women have derived much of their self-esteem from having children, rearing children, and being a "good mother." Likewise, many men have achieved self-esteem through work-related activities—creativity, productivity, and earning money. Termination of these activities can result in a loss of self-worth, and individuals who are unable to adapt satisfactorily may become depressed.

It would appear that retirement is becoming, and will continue to become, more accepted by societal standards. With more and more individuals

retiring earlier and living longer, the growing number of aging persons will spend a significantly longer time in retirement. At present, retirement has become more of an institutionalized expectation, and there appears to be increasing acceptance of it as a social status.

Nursing intervention at the primary level of prevention with the developmental task of retirement involves providing information and support to individuals who have retired or are considering retirement. Support can be on a one-to-one basis to assist these individuals to sort out their feelings regarding retirement. Well-being in retirement is linked to factors such as stable health status and access to health-care services, adequate income, the ability to pursue new goals or activities, extended social network of family and friends, and satisfaction with current living arrangements (Murray et al., 2009).

Support can also be provided in a group environment. Support groups of individuals undergoing the same types of experiences can be extremely helpful. Nurses can form and lead these types of groups to assist retiring individuals through this critical period. These groups can also serve to provide information about available resources that offer assistance to individuals in or nearing retirement, such as information concerning Medicare, Social Security, and Medicaid; information related to organizations that specialize in hiring retirees; and information regarding ways to use newly acquired free time constructively.

Situational Crises

Situational crises are acute responses that occur as a result of an external circumstantial stressor. The number and types of situational stressors are limitless and may be real or exist only in the perception of the individual. Some types of situational crises that put individuals at risk for mental illness include the following.

Poverty A number of studies have identified poverty as a direct correlation to emotional illness. This may have to do with the direct consequences of poverty, such as inadequate and crowded living conditions, nutritional deficiencies, medical neglect, unemployment, or being homeless.

High Rate of Life Change Events Miller and Rahe (1997) found that frequent changes in life patterns due to a large number of significant events occurring in close proximity tend to decrease a person's ability to deal with stress, and physical or emotional illness may be the result. These include life change events such as death of a loved one, divorce, being fired from a job, a change in living conditions, a change in place of employment or residence, physical illness, or a change in body image caused by the loss of a body part or function.

Environmental Conditions Environmental conditions can create situational crises. Tornados, floods, hurricanes, and earthquakes have wreaked devastation on thousands of individuals and families in recent years.

Trauma Individuals who have encountered traumatic experiences must be considered at risk for emotional illness. These include traumatic experiences usually considered outside the range of usual human experience, such as military combat, being a victim of violent personal assault, undergoing torture, being taken hostage or kidnapped, or being the victim of a natural or man-made disaster (APA, 2000).

Nursing intervention at the primary level of prevention with individuals experiencing situational crises is aimed at maintaining the highest possible level of functioning while offering support and assistance with problem solving during the crisis period. Interventions for nursing of clients in crisis include the following:

■ Use a reality-oriented approach. The focus of the problem is on the here and now.

■ Remain with the individual who is experiencing panic anxiety.

■ Establish a rapid working relationship by showing unconditional acceptance, by active listening, and by attending to immediate needs.

■ Discourage lengthy explanations or rationalizations of the situation; promote an atmosphere for verbalization of true feelings.

■ Set firm limits on aggressive, destructive behaviors. At high levels of anxiety, behavior is likely to be impulsive and regressive. Establish at the outset what is acceptable and what is not, and maintain consistency.

■ Clarify the problem that the individual is facing. The nurse does this by describing his or her perception of the problem and comparing it with the individual's perception of the problem.

■ Help the individual determine what he or she believes precipitated the crisis.

■ Acknowledge feelings of anger, guilt, helplessness, and powerlessness, while taking care not to provide positive feedback for these feelings.

■ Guide the individual through a problem-solving process by which he or she may move in the direction of positive life change:
  • Help the individual confront the source of the problem that is creating the crisis response.
  • Encourage the individual to discuss changes he or she would like to make. Jointly determine whether desired changes are realistic.
  • Encourage exploration of feelings about aspects that cannot be changed, and explore alternative ways of coping more adaptively in these situations.
  • Discuss alternative strategies for creating change in situations that can realistically be changed.
  • Weigh benefits and consequences of each alternative.
  • Assist the individual to select alternative coping strategies that will help alleviate future crises.

■ Identify external support systems and new social networks from whom the individual may seek assistance in times of stress.

Nursing at the level of primary prevention focuses largely on education of the consumer to prevent initiation or exacerbation of mental illness. An example of just one type of teaching plan for use in primary prevention situations is presented in Table 37-1.

Secondary Prevention

Populations at Risk

Secondary prevention within communities relates to using early detection and prompt intervention with individuals experiencing mental illness symptoms. The same maturational and situational crises that were presented in the previous section on primary prevention are used to discuss intervention at the secondary level of prevention.

Maturational Crises

Adolescence The need for intervention at the secondary level of prevention in adolescence occurs when disruptive and age-inappropriate behaviors become the norm, and the family can no longer cope adaptively with the situation. All levels of dysfunction are considered—from dysfunctional family coping to the need for hospitalization of the adolescent.

Nursing intervention with the adolescent at the secondary level of prevention may occur in the community setting at community mental health centers, physician's offices, schools, public health departments, and crisis intervention centers. Nurses may work with families to problem-solve and improve coping and communication skills, or they may work on a one-to-one basis with the adolescent in an attempt to modify behavior patterns.

TABLE 37-1 Client Education for Primary Prevention: Drugs of Abuse

CLASS OF DRUGS	EFFECTS	SYMPTOMS OF OVERDOSE	TRADE NAMES	COMMON NAMES	EFFECTS ON THE BODY (CHRONIC OR HIGH-DOSE USE)
CNS Depressants					
Alcohol	Relaxation, loss of inhibitions, lack of concentration, drowsiness, slurred speech, sleep	Nausea, vomiting; shallow respirations; cold, clammy skin; weak, rapid pulse; coma; possible death	Ethyl alcohol, beer, gin, rum, vodka, bourbon, whiskey, liqueurs, wine, brandy, sherry, champagne	Booze, alcohol, liquor, drinks, cocktails, highballs, nightcaps, moonshine, white lightning, firewater	Peripheral nerve damage, skeletal muscle wasting, encephalopathy, psychosis, cardiomyopathy, gastritis, esophagitis, pancreatitis, hepatitis, cirrhosis of the liver, leukopenia, thrombocytopenia, sexual dysfunction
Other (barbiturates and nonbarbiturates)	Same as alcohol	Anxiety, fever, agitation, hallucinations, disorientation, tremors, delirium, convulsions, possible death	Seconal Nembutal Amytal Valium Librium Chloral hydrate Miltown	Red birds Yellow birds Blue birds Blues/yellows Green & whites Mickies Downers	Decreased REM sleep, respiratory depression, hypotension, possible kidney or liver damage, sexual dysfunction
CNS Stimulants					
Amphetamines and related drugs	Hyperactivity, agitation, euphoria, insomnia, loss of appetite	Cardiac arrhythmias, headache, convulsions, hypertension, rapid heart rate, coma, possible death	Dexedrine, Didrex, Tenuate, Prelu-2, Ritalin, Focalin, Provigil	Uppers, pep pills, wakeups, bennies, eye-openers, speed, black beauties, sweet A's	Aggressive, compulsive behavior; paranoia; hallucinations; hypertension
Cocaine	Euphoria, hyperactivity, restlessness, talkativeness, increased pulse, dilated pupils	Hallucinations, convulsions, pulmonary edema, respiratory failure, coma, cardiac arrest, possible death	Cocaine hydrochloride	Coke, flake, snow, dust, happy dust, gold dust, girl, Cecil, C, toot, blow, crack	Pulmonary hemorrhage, myocardial infarction, ventricular fibrillation

Class	Drug	Street names		Psychological effects	Physical effects	Long-term effects
Opioids	Heroin Morphine Codeine Dilaudid Demerol Dolophine Percodan Talwin Opium	Snow, stuff, H, Harry, horse M, morph, Miss Emma Schoolboy Lords Doctors Dollies Perkies Ts Big O, black stuff		Euphoria, lethargy, drowsiness, lack of motivation, constricted pupils	Shallow breathing, slowed pulse, clammy skin, pulmonary edema, respiratory arrest, convulsions, coma, possible death	Respiratory depression, constipation, fecal impaction, hypotension, decreased libido, retarded ejaculation, impotence, orgasm failure
Hallucinogens	LSD PCP Mescaline DMT STP, DOM MDMA Ketamine	Acid, cube, big D Angel dust, hog, peace pill Mesc Businessman's trip Serenity and peace Ecstasy, XTC Special K, Vitamin K, Kit Kat		Visual hallucinations, disorientation, confusion, paranoid delusions, euphoria, anxiety, panic, increased pulse	Agitation, extreme hyperactivity, violence, hallucinations, psychosis, convulsions, possible death	Panic reaction, acute psychosis, flashbacks
Cannabinols	Cannabis Hashish	Marijuana, pot, grass, joint, Mary Jane, MJ Hash, rope, Sweet Lucy		Relaxation, talkativeness, lowered inhibitions, euphoria, mood swings	Fatigue, paranoia, delusions, hallucinations, possible psychosis	Tachycardia, orthostatic hypotension, chronic bronchitis, problems with infertility, amotivational syndrome

Adolescents may be hospitalized for a variety of reasons. The *DSM-IV-TR* (APA, 2000) identifies a number of problems, the severity of which would determine whether the adolescent required inpatient care. Conduct disorders, adjustment disorders, eating disorders, substance-related disorders, depression, and anxiety disorders are the most common diagnoses for which adolescents are hospitalized. Nursing care of adolescents in the hospital setting focuses on problem identification and stabilizing a crisis situation. Once stability has been achieved, clients are commonly discharged to outpatient care. If an adolescent's home situation has been deemed unsatisfactory, the state may take custody and the child is then discharged to a group or foster home. Care plans for intervention with the adolescent at the secondary level of prevention can be found in Chapter 23.

Marriage Problems in a marriage are as far-reaching as the individuals who experience them. Problems that are not uncommon to the disruption of a marriage relationship include substance abuse on the part of one or both partners and disagreements on issues of sex, money, children, gender roles, and infidelity, among others. Murray and associates (2009) stated:

> Marriage to one person and living with the frustrations, conflicts, and boredom that is part of any close and lengthy relationship requires constant work by both parties. (p. 504)

Nursing intervention at the secondary level of prevention with individuals encountering marriage problems may include one or more of the following:

■ Counseling with the couple or with one of the spouses on a one-to-one basis

■ Referral to a couples' support group

■ Identification of the problem and possible solutions; support and guidance as changes are undertaken

■ Referral to a sex therapist

■ Referral to a financial advisor

■ Referral to parent effectiveness training

Murray and associates (2009) stated:

> When marriage fails and bonds are broken, aloneness, anger, mistrust, hostility, guilt, shame, a sense of betrayal, fear, disappointment, loss of identity, anxiety, and depression, alone or in combination, may appear both in the divorcee and the one initiating the divorce. (p. 547)

In Miller and Rahe's (1997) life change questionnaire, only death of a spouse or other family member scored higher than divorce in severity of stress experienced. This is an area in which nurses can intervene to help ease the transition and prevent emotional breakdown. In community health settings, nurses can lead support groups for newly divorced individuals. They can also provide one-to-one counseling for individuals experiencing the emotional chaos engendered by the dissolution of a marriage relationship.

Divorce also has an impact on the children involved. Nurses can intervene with the children of divorce in an effort to prevent dysfunctional behaviors associated with the break-up of a marriage.

Parenthood Intervention at the secondary level of prevention with parents can be required for a number of reasons. A few of these include:

■ Physical, emotional, or sexual abuse of a child

■ Physical or emotional neglect of a child

■ Birth of a child with special needs

■ Diagnosis of a terminal illness in a child

■ Death of a child

Nursing intervention at the secondary level of prevention includes being able to recognize the physical and behavioral signs that indicate possible abuse of a child. The child may be cared for in the emergency department or as an inpatient on the pediatric unit or child psychiatric unit of a general hospital.

Nursing intervention with parents may include teaching effective methods of disciplining children, aside from physical punishment. Methods that emphasize the importance of positive reinforcement for acceptable behavior can be very effective. Family members must be committed to consistent use of this behavior modification technique for it to be successful.

Parents should also be informed about behavioral expectations at the various levels of development. Knowledge of what to expect from children at these various stages may provide needed anticipatory guidance to deal with the crises commonly associated with each stage.

Therapy sessions with all family members together may focus on problems with family communications. Members are encouraged to express honest feelings in a manner that is nonthreatening to other family members. Active listening, assertiveness techniques, and respect for the rights of others are taught and encouraged. Barriers to effective communication are identified and resolved.

Referrals to agencies that promote effective parenting skills may be made (e.g., parent effectiveness training). Alternative agencies that may provide relief from the stress of parenting may also be considered (e.g., "Mom's Day Out" programs, sitter-sharing organizations, and day-care institutions). Support groups for abusive parents may also be helpful, and assistance in locating or initiating such a group may be provided.

The nurse can assist parents who are grieving the loss of a child or the birth of a child with special needs by helping them to express their true feelings associated with the loss. Feelings such as shock, denial, anger, guilt, powerlessness, and hopelessness need to be expressed in order for the parents to progress through the grief response.

Home health-care assistance can be provided for the family of a child with special needs. This can be done by making referrals to other professionals, such as speech, physical, and occupational therapists; medical social workers; psychologists; and nutritionists. If the child with special needs is hospitalized, the home health nurse can provide specific information to hospital staff that may be helpful in providing continuity of care for the client and help in the transition for the family.

Nursing intervention also includes providing assistance in the location of and referral to support groups that deal with loss of a child or birth of a child with special needs. Some nurses may serve as leaders of these types of groups in the community.

Midlife Nursing care at the secondary level of prevention during midlife becomes necessary when the individual is unable to integrate all of the changes that are occurring during this period. An inability to accept the physical and biological changes, the changes in relationships between themselves and their adult children and aging parents, and the loss of the perception of youth may result in depression that the individual may require help to resolve.

Retirement Retirement can also result in depression for individuals who are unable to satisfactorily grieve for the loss of the working aspect of their lives. This is more likely to occur if the individuals have not planned for retirement and if they have derived most of their self-esteem from their employment.

Nursing intervention at the secondary level of prevention with depressed individuals takes place in both inpatient and outpatient settings. Severely depressed clients with suicidal ideations will need close observation in the hospital setting, whereas those with mild to moderate depression may be treated in the community. A plan of care for the client with depression is found in Chapter 27. These concepts apply to the secondary level of prevention and may be used in all nursing care settings.

The physician may elect to use pharmacotherapy with antidepressants. Nurses may intervene by providing information to the client about what to expect from the medication, possible side effects, adverse effects, and how to self-administer the medication.

Situational Crises

Nursing care at the secondary level of prevention with clients undergoing situational crises occurs only if crisis intervention at the primary level failed and the individual is unable to function socially or occupationally. Exacerbation of mental illness symptoms requires intervention at the secondary level of prevention. These disorders were addressed extensively in Unit Four. Nursing assessment, diagnosis and outcome identification, planning and implementation, and evaluation were discussed for many of the mental illnesses identified in the *DSM-IV-TR* (APA, 2000). These skills may be applied in any setting where nursing is practiced.

A case study situation of nursing care at the secondary level of prevention in a community setting is presented in Box 37-1.

Tertiary Prevention

Individuals With Severe and Persistent Mental Illness

Severe and persistent mental illness is characterized by a functional impairment that interferes with vocational capacity, creates serious interpersonal difficulties, or is associated with a suicide plan or attempt (Jans, Stoddard, & Kraus, 2004). These disorders are identified by criteria listed in the *DSM-IV-TR*. Diagnoses include schizophrenia and related disorders, bipolar disorder, autism spectrum disorders, major depressive disorder, panic disorder, obsessive-compulsive disorder, posttraumatic stress disorder, borderline personality disorder, and attention-deficit/hyperactivity disorder (Jans et al., 2004; National Alliance on Mental Illness [NAMI], 2009). Severe and persistent mental disorders affect 5 to 10 million adults and 3 to 5 million children in the United States.

Historical and Epidemiological Aspects

In 1955, more than half a million individuals resided in public mental hospitals. Estimates suggest that this number is fewer than 100,000 today.

BOX 37-1 *Secondary Prevention Case Study: Parenthood*

The identified patient was a petite, doll-like 4-year-old girl named Tanya. She was the older of two children in a Latino American family. The other child was a boy named Joseph, aged 2. The mother was 5 months pregnant with their third child. The family had been referred to the nurse after Tanya was placed in foster care following a report to the Department of Health and Human Services by her nursery school teacher that the child had marks on her body suspicious of child abuse.

The parents, Paulo and Annette, were in their mid-20s. Paulo had lost his job at an aircraft plant 3 months ago and had been unable to find work since. Annette brought in a few dollars from cleaning houses for other people, but the family was struggling to survive.

Paulo and Annette were angry at having to see the nurse. After all, "Parents have the right to discipline their children." The nurse did not focus on the *intent* of the behavior, but instead looked at factors in the family's life that could be viewed as stressors. This family had multiple stressors: poverty, the father's unemployment, the age and spacing of the children, the mother's chronic fatigue from work at home and in other people's homes, and finally, having a child removed from the home against the parents' wishes.

During therapy with this family, the nurse discussed the behaviors associated with various developmental levels. She also discussed possible deviations from these norms and when they should be reported to the physician. The nurse and the family discussed Tanya's behavior, and how it compared with the norms.

The parents also discussed their own childhoods. They were able to relate some of the same types of behaviors that they observed in Tanya. But they both admitted that they came from families whose main method of discipline was physical punishment. Annette had been the oldest child in her large family and had been expected to "keep the younger ones in line." When she had not done so, she was punished with her father's belt. She expressed anger toward her father, although she had never been allowed to express it at the time.

Paulo's father had died when he was a small boy, and Paulo had been expected to be the "man of the family." From the time he was very young, he worked at odd jobs to bring money into the home. Because of this, he had little time for the usual activities of childhood and adolescence. He held much resentment toward the young men who "had everything and never had to work for it."

Paulo and Annette had high expectations for Tanya. In effect, they expected her to behave in a manner well beyond her developmental level. These expectations were based on the reflections of their own childhoods. They were uncomfortable with the spontaneity and playfulness of childhood because they had had little personal experience with these behaviors. When Tanya balked and expressed the verbal assertions common to early childhood, Paulo and Annette interpreted these behaviors as defiance toward them and retaliated with anger in the manner in which they had been parented.

With the parents, the nurse explored feelings and behaviors from their past so that they were able to understand the correlation to their current behaviors. They learned to negotiate ways to deal with Tanya's age-appropriate behaviors. In combined therapy with Tanya, they learned how to relate to her childishness, and even how to enjoy playing with both of their children.

The parents ceased blaming each other for the family's problems. Annette had spent a good deal of her time deprecating Paulo for his lack of support of his family, and Paulo blamed Annette for being "unable to control her daughter." Communication patterns were clarified, and life in the family became more peaceful.

Without a need to "prove himself" to his wife, Paulo's efforts to find employment met with success because he no longer felt the need to turn down jobs that he believed his wife would perceive to be beneath his capabilities. Annette no longer works outside the home, and both she and Paulo participate in the parenting chores. Tanya and her siblings continue to demonstrate age-appropriate developmental progression.

Deinstitutionalization of persons with serious mental illness began in the 1960s as national policy change and with a strong belief in the individual's right to freedom. Other considerations included the deplorable conditions of some of the state asylums, the introduction of neuroleptic medications, and the cost-effectiveness of caring for these individuals in the community setting.

Deinstitutionalization began to occur rapidly and without sufficient planning for the needs of these individuals as they reentered the community. Those who were fortunate enough to have support systems to provide assistance with living arrangements and sheltered employment experiences most often received the outpatient treatment they required. Those without adequate support, however, either managed to survive on a meager existence or were forced to join the ranks of the homeless. Some ended up in nursing homes meant to provide care for individuals with physical disabilities.

Certain segments of our population with severe and persistent mental illness have been left untreated: the elderly, the "working poor," the homeless, and those individuals previously covered by funds that have been cut by various social reforms. These circumstances have promoted in individuals with severe and persistent mental illness a greater number of crisis-oriented emergency department visits and hospital admissions, and repeated confrontations with law enforcement officials.

In 2002, President George W. Bush established the New Freedom Commission on Mental Health. This commission was charged with the task of conducting a comprehensive study of the United States mental health service delivery system. They were to identify unmet needs and barriers to services and recommend steps for improvement in services and support for individuals with serious mental illness. In July 2003, the commission presented its final report to the President (President's New Freedom Commission on Mental Health, 2003). The Commission identified the following five barriers:

1. **Fragmentation and gaps in care exist for children.** About 7 to 9 percent of all children (ages 9 to 17) have a serious emotional disturbance (SED). The Commission found that services for children are even more fragmented than those for adults, with more uncoordinated funding and differing eligibility requirements. Only a fraction of children with SED appear to have access to school-based or school-linked mental health services. Children with SED who are identified for special education services have higher levels of absenteeism, higher drop-out rates, and lower levels of academic achievement than students with other disabilities.

2. **Fragmentation and gaps in care exist for adults with serious mental illness.** The commission expressed concern that so many adults with serious mental illness are homeless, dependent on alcohol or drugs, and unemployed, and go without treatment. According to the World Health Organization (WHO), neuropsychiatric conditions account for 13 percent of the total Disability Adjusted Life Years (DALYs) lost due to all disease and injuries in the world, and are expected to increase by 15 percent by the year 2020 (WHO, 2004). The Commission identified public attitudes and the stigma associated with mental illness as major barriers to treatment. Stigma is often internalized by individuals with mental illness, leading to hopelessness, lower self-esteem, and isolation. Stigma deprives these individuals of the support they need to recover.

3. **High unemployment and disability exist for people with serious mental illness.** Undetected, untreated, and poorly treated mental disorders interrupt careers, leading many individuals into lives of disability, poverty, and long-term dependence. The commission found a 90 percent unemployment rate among adults with serious mental illness—the worst level of employment of any group of people with disabilities. Some surveys have shown that many individuals with serious mental illness *want* to work, and could, with modest assistance. However, the largest "program" of assistance the United States has for people with mental illness is disability payments. Sadly, societal stigma is also reflected in employment discrimination against people with mental illness.

4. **Older adults with mental illnesses are not receiving care.** The commission reported that about 5 to 10 percent of older adults have major depression, yet most are not properly recognized and treated. The report stated:

Older people are reluctant to get care from specialists. They feel more comfortable going to their primary care physician. Still, they are often more sensitive to the stigma of mental illness, and do not readily bring up their sadness and despair. If they acknowledge problems, they are more likely than young people to describe physical symptoms. Primary care doctors may see their suffering as "natural" aging, or treat their reported physical distress instead of the underlying mental disorder. What is often missed is the deep impact of depression on older people's capacity to function in ways that are seemingly effortless for others.

5. **Mental health and suicide prevention are not yet national priorities.** The fact that the United States has failed to prioritize mental health puts many lives at stake. Families struggle to maintain equilibrium while communities strain (and often fail) to provide needed assistance for adults and children who suffer from mental illness. Over 30,000 lives are lost annually to suicide. About 90 percent of those who take their life have a mental disorder. Many individuals who commit suicide have not had the care in the months before their death that would help them to affirm life. Both the

American Psychiatric Association and the National Mental Health Association have called on the U.S. Congress to pass parity legislation. Lack of equal access to insurance coverage is conspicuous evidence of the low priority placed on mental health treatment.

The Commission outlined the following goals and recommendations for mental health reform:

Goal 1. Americans will understand that mental health is essential to overall health.

Commission recommendations:

■ Advance and implement a national campaign to reduce the stigma of seeking care and a national strategy for suicide prevention.

■ Address mental health with the same urgency as physical health.

Goal 2. Mental health care will be consumer and family driven.

Commission recommendations:

■ Develop an individualized plan of care for every adult with a serious mental illness and child with a serious emotional disturbance.

■ Involve consumers and families fully in orienting the mental health system toward recovery.

■ Align relevant federal programs to improve access and accountability for mental health services.

■ Create a comprehensive state mental health plan.

■ Protect and enhance the rights of people with mental illness.

Goal 3. Disparities in mental health services will be eliminated.

Commission recommendations:

■ Improve access to quality care that is culturally competent.

■ Improve access to quality care in rural and geographically remote areas.

Goal 4. Early mental health screening, assessment, and referral to services will be common practice.

Commission recommendations:

■ Promote the mental health of young children.

■ Improve and expand school mental health programs.

■ Screen for co-occurring mental and substance use disorders and link with integrated treatment strategies.

■ Screen for mental disorders in primary health care, across the life span, and connect to treatment and supports.

Goal 5. Excellent mental health care will be delivered and research will be accelerated.

Commission recommendations:

■ Accelerate research to promote recovery and resilience, and ultimately to cure and prevent mental illnesses.

■ Advance evidence-based practices using dissemination and demonstration projects, and create a public-private partnership to guide their implementation.

■ Improve and expand the workforce providing evidence-based mental health services and supports.

■ Develop the knowledge base in four understudied areas: mental health disparities, long-term effects of medications, trauma, and acute care.

Goal 6. Technology will be used to access mental health care and information.

Commission recommendations:

■ Use health technology and telehealth to improve access and coordination of mental health care, especially for Americans in remote areas or in underserved populations.

■ Develop and implement integrated electronic health record and personal health information systems.

Since the release of this report, a number of organizations have released plans for implementing some of these recommendations. Von Esenwein and associates (2005) conducted a follow-up survey of organizations represented at the 19th annual Rosalynn Carter Symposium on Mental Health Policy (which was held in 2003 just following release of the report). In this survey, nearly half of the respondents reported that at least one change had been made in their organization in response to the commission's report. Von Esenwein and associates (2005) reported:

Factors most consistently identified as contributing to successful implementation of the recommendations of the New Freedom Commission were willingness to change within the organization, partnerships with community agencies, and availability of public funding. The most common barriers cited were financial constraints, other competing priorities within the organization, and lack of local political support. (p. 606)

If the proposals outlined in the report became reality, it would surely mean improvement in the care of individuals with severe and persistent mental illness. Many nurse leaders see this period of health-care reform as an opportunity for nurses to expand their roles and assume key positions in education, prevention, assessment, and referral. Nurses are, and will continue to be, in key positions to assist individuals with severe and persistent mental illness to remain as independent as possible, to manage their illness within the community setting, and to strive to minimize the number of hospitalizations required.

Treatment Alternatives

Community Mental Health Centers The goal of community mental health centers in caring for individuals with severe and persistent mental illness is to improve coping ability and prevent exacerbation of acute symptoms. A major obstacle in meeting this goal has been the lack of advocacy or sponsorship for clients who require services from a variety of sources. This has placed responsibility for health care on an individual with mental illness who is often barely able to cope with everyday life. Case management has become a recommended method of treatment for individuals with severe and persistent mental illness. Ling (2010) stated:

> Nurses may be uniquely qualified to be case managers because of their holistic and broad-based background, understanding of health care, and role in patient education and referrals. Case management is an area of practice that offers nurses an opportunity to build on their clinical knowledge, communication, and nursing process skills to function in an expanded patient care role.

Ling (2010) identified six essential activities and nursing role functions that blend with the steps of the nursing process to form a framework for nursing case management. The essential activities include:

■ **Assessment.** During the assessment process, the nurse gathers pertinent information about a client's situation and ability to function. Information may be obtained through physical examination, client interview, medical records, and reports from significant others. Ling stated, "The case manager's goal is to obtain accurate information about the patient's status and identify factors that may significantly affect the patient's recovery and care."

■ **Planning.** A service care plan is devised with client participation. The plan should include mutually agreed-on goals, specific actions directed toward goal achievement, and selection of essential resources and services through collaboration among health-care professionals, the client, and the family or significant others.

■ **Implementation.** In this phase, the client receives the needed services from the appropriate providers. In some instances the nursing case manager is also a provider of care, whereas in others, he or she is only the coordinator of care.

■ **Coordination.** The case manager organizes, secures, integrates, and modifies the resources necessary to accomplish the case management goals (CMSA, 2010). This coordination effort involves the client, the physician, any other pertinent health-care providers, and family members or significant others concerned with the client's care. The case manager ensures that all tests and treatments are conducted according to schedule, and maintains close communication with all health-care providers to ensure that client care is proceeding according to the plan.

■ **Monitoring.** The case manager monitors the effectiveness of the care plan by gathering pertinent information from various sources at regular intervals to determine the client's response and progress (CMSA, 2010). If problems are identified, immediate adjustments are made.

■ **Evaluation.** The case manager evaluates the client's responses to interventions and progress toward preestablished goals. Regular contact is maintained with client, family or significant others, and direct service providers. Ongoing coordination of care continues until outcomes have been achieved. If the expected outcomes are not achieved, the case manager reevaluates the plan to determine the reason, and takes steps to intervene and modify the existing plan.

A case study of nursing case management within a community mental health center is presented in Box 37-2.

Program of Assertive Community Treatment (PACT) The National Alliance on Mental Illness (NAMI) defines PACT as a service-delivery model that provides comprehensive, locally based treatment to people with serious and persistent mental illnesses (NAMI, 2010). PACT is a type of case management program that provides highly individualized services directly to consumers. It is a team approach, and includes members from psychiatry,

BOX 37-2 **Nursing Case Management in the Community Mental Health Center: A Case Study**

Michael, 73 years old with a history of multiple psychiatric admissions, has lived in various adult foster homes and boarding houses for the past 10 years. He was originally diagnosed as having Schizophrenia, but he was recently rediagnosed as having Bipolar Disorder, Mania. His symptoms are well controlled with lithium 300 mg three times a day, which is prescribed by the outpatient psychiatrist.

The nurse practitioner/case manager in the outpatient clinic coordinates Michael's care, advocates for his needs, and counsels him regarding his health problems. She orders routine blood tests to assess his lithium levels. When Michael experienced visual disturbances, she referred him for an emergency eye evaluation. He was found to have a retinal detachment and was sent to a local Department of Veterans Affairs (VA) hospital for emergency surgery. After his eye surgery, the nurse practitioner arranged transportation to his follow-up visits with the eye doctor and instructed him about his eye care and instillation of his eyedrops. Michael did not like putting drops in his eye and tended to neglect doing it. Because he also had glaucoma and required ongoing treatment with pilocarpine and timolol maleate eyedrops twice daily, he needed a great deal of education and reassurance to continue using the eyedrops.

In addition to routine quarterly visits for ongoing case management, the nurse practitioner also performs his annual health assessment, consisting of history, review of systems, mental status examination, and physical assessment. During Michael's last physical examination, the nurse practitioner detected a thyroid mass and referred him for a complete evaluation, including thyroid function tests, a thyroid scan, and evaluation by a surgeon and an endocrinologist. She discussed his thyroid problem with the surgeon and the endocrinologist, and they determined that Michael would best benefit from thyroid replacement (i.e., levothyroxine sodium 0.1 mg daily).

Because Michael eats all of his meals in restaurants, the nurse was concerned about his diet. A brief diet review revealed that his diet was low in vitamin C. He was then instructed in which foods and juices he should include in his daily menu. The nurse practitioner discussed ways that Michael could get the best nutrition for the least cost.

Michael currently is living in a boarding house and is totally responsible for taking his own medication, attending to his activities of daily living, and managing his own money. He has very limited income and depends on donations for many of his clothing needs.

Despite his age, he is quite active and alert. He attends many VA-sponsored social activities and does daily volunteer work at the VA, such as pushing wheelchairs, running errands, and escorting other veterans to clinic appointments. His nurse case manager arranged for him to receive free lunches as a reward for some of his volunteer activities.

Nursing case management has helped this elderly gentleman with severe and persistent psychiatric illness and many years of hospitalization to live independently within the community setting.

From Pittman, D. C. (1989). Nursing case management: Holistic care for the deinstitutionalized chronically mentally ill. Journal of Psychosocial Nursing, 27(11), 23–27, with permission.

social work, nursing, substance abuse, and vocational rehabilitation. The PACT team provides these services 24 hours a day, 7 days a week, 365 days a year.

NAMI (2010) identified the primary goals of PACT as follows:

■ To lessen or eliminate the debilitating symptoms of mental illness each individual client experiences

■ To minimize or prevent recurrent acute episodes of the illness

■ To meet basic needs and enhance quality of life

■ To improve functioning in adult social and employment roles

■ To enhance an individual's ability to live independently in his or her own community

■ To lessen the family's burden of providing care

The PACT team provides treatment, rehabilitation, and support services to individuals with severe and persistent mental illness who are unable on their own to receive treatment from a traditional model of case management. The team is usually able to provide most services with minimal referrals to other mental health programs or providers. Services are provided within community settings, such as a person's home, local restaurants, parks, nearby stores, and any other place that the individual requires assistance with living skills.

Studies have shown that PACT clients spend significantly less time in hospitals and more time in independent living situations, have less time unemployed, earn more income from competitive employment, experience more positive social relationships, express greater satisfaction with life, and are less symptomatic (NAMI, 2010). Only about half of the states currently have PACT programs established or under pilot testing. NAMI (2010) stated:

> Despite the documented treatment success of PACT, only a fraction of those with the greatest needs have access to this uniquely effective program. In the United States, adults with severe and persistent mental illnesses constitute one-half to 1 percent of the adult population. It is estimated that 10 to 20 percent of this group could be helped by the PACT model if it were available.

Day/Evening Treatment (Partial Hospitalization Programs) Day or evening treatment programs (also called partial hospitalization) are designed to prevent institutionalization or to ease the transition from inpatient hospitalization to community living. Various types of treatment are offered. Many include therapeutic community (milieu) activities; individual, group, and family therapies; psychoeducation; alcohol and drug education; crisis intervention; therapeutic recreational activities; and occupational therapy. Many programs offer medication administration and monitoring as part of their care. Some programs have established medication clinics for individuals on long-term psychopharmacological therapy. These clinics may include educational classes and support groups for individuals with similar conditions and treatments.

Partial hospitalization programs generally offer a comprehensive treatment plan formulated by an interdisciplinary team of psychiatrists, psychologists, nurses, occupational and recreational therapists, and social workers. Nurses take a leading role in the administration of partial hospitalization programs. They lead groups, provide crisis intervention, conduct individual counseling, act as role models, and make necessary referrals for specialized treatment. Use of the nursing process provides continual evaluation of the program, and modifications can be made as necessary.

Partial hospitalization programs have proven to be an effective method of preventing hospitalization for many individuals with severe and persistent mental illness. They are a way of transitioning these individuals from the acute care setting back into the mainstream of the community. For some individuals who have been deinstitutionalized, they provide structure, support, opportunities for socialization, and an improvement in their overall quality of life.

Community Residential Facilities Community residential facilities for persons with severe and persistent mental illness are known by many names: group homes, halfway houses, foster homes, boarding homes, sheltered care facilities, transitional housing, independent living programs, social rehabilitation residences, and others. These facilities differ by the purpose for which they exist and the activities that they offer.

Some of these facilities provide food, shelter, housekeeping, and minimal supervision and assistance with activities of daily living. Others may also include a variety of therapies and serve as a transition between hospital and independent living. In addition to the basics, services might include individual and group counseling, medical care, job training or employment assistance, and leisure-time activities.

A wide variety of personnel staff these facilities. Some facilities have live-in professionals who are available at all times, some have professional staff who are on call for intervention during crisis situations, and some are staffed by volunteers and individuals with little knowledge or background for understanding and treating persons with severe and persistent mental illness.

The concept of transitional housing for individuals with serious mental illness is sound and has proved in many instances to be a successful means of therapeutic support and intervention for maintaining them within the community. However, without guidance and planning, transition to the community can be futile. These individuals may be ridiculed and rejected by the community. They may be targets of unscrupulous individuals who take advantage of their inability to care for themselves satisfactorily. These behaviors may increase maladaptive responses to the demands of community living and exacerbate the mental illness. A period of structured reorientation to the community in a living situation that is supervised and monitored by professionals is more likely to result in a successful transition for the individual with severe and persistent mental illness.

Psychiatric Home Health Care For the individual with serious mental illness who no longer lives in a structured, supervised setting, home health care may be the element that helps to keep him or her living independently. To receive home health care, individuals must validate their homebound status for the prospective payer (Medicare, Medicaid, most insurance companies, and Department of Veterans Affairs [VA] benefits). An acute psychiatric diagnosis is not enough to qualify for the service.

The client must show that he or she is unable to leave the home without considerable difficulty or the assistance of another person. The plan of treatment and subsequent charting must explain why the client's psychiatric disorder keeps him or her at home and justify the need for home services.

Homebound clients most often have diagnoses of depression, dementia, anxiety disorders, bipolar affective disorder, and schizophrenia. Many elderly clients are homebound because of medical conditions that impair mobility and necessitate home care.

Nurses who provide psychiatric home care must have an in-depth knowledge of psychopathology, psychopharmacology, and how medical and physical problems can be influenced by psychiatric impairments. These nurses must be highly adept at performing biopsychosocial assessments. They must be sensitive to changes in behavior that signal that the client is decompensating psychiatrically or medically so that early intervention may be implemented.

Another important job of the psychiatric home health nurse is monitoring compliance with the regimen of psychotropic medications. Some clients who are receiving injectible medications remain on home health care only until they can be placed on oral medications. Those clients receiving oral medications require close monitoring for compliance and assistance with the uncomfortable side effects of some of these drugs. Medication noncompliance is responsible for approximately two thirds of psychiatric hospital readmissions. Home health nurses can assist clients with this problem by helping them to see the relationship between control of their psychiatric symptoms and compliance with their medication regimen.

Client populations that benefit from psychiatric home health nursing include:

■ **Elderly clients.** These individuals may not have a psychiatric diagnosis, but they may be experiencing emotional difficulties that have arisen from medical, sociocultural, or developmental factors. Depressed mood and social isolation are common.

■ **Persons with severe and persistent mental illness.** These individuals have a history of psychiatric illness and hospitalization. They require long-term medications and continual supportive care. Common diagnoses include recurrent major depression, schizophrenia, and bipolar disorder.

■ **Individuals in acute crisis situations.** These individuals are in need of crisis intervention and/or short-term psychotherapy.

The American Nurses Association (ANA) (2008) defined home health nursing as,

. . . nursing practice applied to patients of all ages in the patient's residences, which may include private homes, assisted living, or personal care facilities. Patients and their families and other caregivers are the focus of home health nursing practice. The goal of care is to maintain or improve the quality of life for patients and their families and other caregivers, or to support patients in their transition to end of life. (p. 3)

Medicare requires that psychiatric home nursing care be provided by "psychiatrically trained nurses," which they define as, "nurses who have special training and/or experience beyond the standard curriculum required for a registered nurse" (Centers for Medicare & Medicaid Services [CMS], 2005).

The guidelines that cover psychiatric nursing services are not well defined by CMS. This has presented some reimbursement problems for psychiatric nurses in the past. The CMS statement regarding psychiatric nursing services is presented in Box 37-3.

Preparation for psychiatric home health nursing, in addition to the registered nurse licensure, should include several years of psychiatric inpatient

---

BOX 37-3 CMS Guidelines for Psychiatric Home Nursing Care

PSYCHIATRIC EVALUATION, THERAPY, AND TEACHING

The evaluation, psychotherapy, and teaching needed by a patient suffering from a diagnosed psychiatric disorder that requires active treatment by a psychiatrically trained nurse and the costs of the psychiatric nurse's services may be covered as a skilled nursing service. Psychiatrically trained nurses are nurses who have special training and/or experience beyond the standard curriculum required for a registered nurse. The services of the psychiatric nurse are to be provided under a plan of care established and reviewed by a physician.

From Centers for Medicare & Medicaid Services. (2005). Medicare Benefit Policy Manual. Baltimore, MD: Author.

treatment experience. It is also recommended that the nurse have medical-surgical nursing experience, because of common client physical comorbidity and the holistic nursing perspective. Additional training and experience in psychotherapy is viewed as an asset. However, psychotherapy is not the primary focus of psychiatric home nursing care. In fact, most reimbursement sources do not pay for exclusively insight-oriented therapy. Crisis intervention, client education, and hands-on care are common interventions in psychiatric home nursing care.

The psychiatric home health nurse provides comprehensive nursing care, incorporating interventions for physical and psychosocial problems into the treatment plan. The interventions are based on the client's mental and physical health status, cultural influences, and available resources.

The nurse is accountable to the client at all times during the therapeutic relationship. Nursing interventions are carried out with appropriate knowledge and skill, and referrals are made when the need is outside the scope of nursing practice. Continued collaboration with other members of the health-care team (e.g., psychiatrist, social worker, psychologist, occupational therapist, and/or physical therapist) is essential for maintaining continuity of care.

A case study of psychiatric home health care and the nursing process is presented in Box 37-4. A plan of care for Mrs. C. (the client in the case study) is presented in Table 37-2. Nursing diagnoses are presented, along with outcome criteria, appropriate nursing interventions, and rationale for each.

BOX 37-4 Psychiatric Home Health Care and the Nursing Process: A Case Study

ASSESSMENT

Mrs. C., age 76, has been living alone in her small apartment for 6 months since the death of her husband, to whom she had been married for 51 years. Mrs. C. had been an elementary school teacher for 40 years, retiring at age 65 with an adequate pension. She and her husband had no children. A niece looks in on Mrs. C. regularly. It was she who contacted Mrs. C.'s physician when she observed that Mrs. C. was not eating properly, was losing weight, and seemed to be isolating herself more and more. She had not left her apartment in weeks. Her physician referred her to psychiatric home health care.

On her initial visit, Carol, the psychiatric home health nurse, conducted a preliminary assessment revealing the following information about Mrs. C.:

1. Blood pressure 90/60 mm Hg.
2. Height 5'5"; weight 102 lb.
3. Poor skin turgor; dehydration.
4. Subjective report of occasional dizziness.
5. Subjective report of loss of 20 pounds since the death of her husband.
6. Oriented to time, place, person, and situation.
7. Memory (remote and recent) intact.
8. Flat affect.
9. Mood is dysphoric and tearful at times, but client is cooperative.
10. Denies thoughts to harm self, but states, "I feel so alone; so useless."
11. Subjective report of difficulty sleeping.
12. Subjective report of constipation.

DIAGNOSIS/OUTCOME IDENTIFICATION

The following nursing diagnoses were formulated for Mrs. C.:

1. Complicated grieving related to death of husband evidenced by symptoms of depression such as withdrawal, anorexia, weight loss, difficulty sleeping, dysphoric/tearful mood.
2. Risk for injury related to dizziness and weakness from lack of activity, low blood pressure, and poor nutritional status.
3. Social isolation related to depressed mood and feelings of worthlessness evidenced by staying home alone, refusing to leave her apartment.

Outcome Criteria

The following criteria were selected as measurement of outcomes in the care of Mrs. C.:

1. Experiences no physical harm/injury.
2. Is able to discuss feelings about husband's death with nurse.
3. Sets realistic goals for self.

Continued

BOX 37-4 Psychiatric Home Health Care and the Nursing Process: A Case Study—cont'd

4. Is able to participate in problem solving regarding her future.
5. Eats a well-balanced diet with snacks to restore nutritional status and gain weight.
6. Drinks adequate fluid daily.
7. Sleeps at least 6 hours per night and verbalizes feeling well rested.
8. Shows interest in personal appearance and hygiene, and is able to accomplish self-care independently.
9. Seeks to renew contact with previous friends and acquaintances.
10. Verbalizes interest in participating in social activities.

PLANNING/IMPLEMENTATION

A plan of care for Mrs. C. is presented in Table 37-2.

EVALUATION

Mrs. C. started the second week taking trazodone (Desyrel) 150 mg at bedtime. Her sleep was enhanced and within 2 weeks she showed a noticeable improvement in mood. She began to discuss how angry she felt about being all alone in the world. She admitted that she had felt anger toward her husband but experienced guilt and tried to suppress that anger. As she was assured that these feelings were normal, they became easier for her to express.

The nurse arranged for a local teenager to do some weekly grocery shopping for Mrs. C. and contacted the local Meals on Wheels program, which delivered her noon meal to her every day. Mrs. C. began to eat more and slowly to gain a few pounds. She still has an occasional problem with constipation but verbalizes improvement with the addition of vegetables, fruit, and a daily stool softener prescribed by her physician.

Mrs. C. used her walker until she felt she was able to ambulate without assistance. She reports that she no longer experiences dizziness, and her blood pressure has stabilized at around 100/70 mm Hg.

Mrs. C. has joined a senior citizens group and attends activities weekly. She has renewed previous friendships and formed new acquaintances. She sees her physician monthly for medication management and visits a local adult day health center for regular blood pressure and weight checks. Her niece still visits regularly, but her favorite relationship is the one she has formed with her constant canine companion, Molly, whom Mrs. C. rescued from the local animal shelter and who continually demonstrates her unconditional love and gratitude.

Table 37-2 CARE PLAN FOR PSYCHIATRIC HOME HEALTH CARE OF DEPRESSED ELDERLY (MRS. C.)

NURSING DIAGNOSIS: COMPLICATED GRIEVING

RELATED TO: Death of husband

EVIDENCED BY: Symptoms of depression such as withdrawal, anorexia, weight loss, difficulty sleeping, and dysphoric/tearful mood

OUTCOME CRITERIA	NURSING INTERVENTIONS	RATIONALE
Short-Term Goal • Mrs. C. will discuss any angry feelings she has about the loss of her husband. **Long-Term Goal** • Mrs. C. will demonstrate adaptive grieving behaviors and evidence of progression toward resolution.	1. Assess Mrs. C.'s position in the grief process. 2. Develop a trusting relationship by showing empathy and caring. Be honest and keep all promises. Show genuine positive regard. 3. Explore feelings of anger and help Mrs. C. direct them toward the source. Help her understand it is appropriate and acceptable to have feelings of anger and guilt about her husband's death.	1. Accurate baseline data are required to plan accurate care for Mrs. C. 2. These interventions provide the basis for a therapeutic relationship. 3. Knowledge of acceptability of the feelings associated with normal grieving may help to relieve some of the guilt that these responses generate.

Table 37-2 CARE PLAN FOR PSYCHIATRIC HOME HEALTH CARE OF DEPRESSED ELDERLY (MRS. C.)—cont'd

OUTCOME CRITERIA	NURSING INTERVENTIONS	RATIONALE
	4. Encourage Mrs. C. to review honestly the relationship she had with her husband. With support and sensitivity, point out reality of the situation in areas where misrepresentations may be expressed.	4. Mrs. C. must give up an idealized perception of her husband. Only when she is able to see both positive and negative aspects about the relationship will the grieving process be complete.
	5. Determine if Mrs. C. has spiritual needs that are going unfulfilled. If so, contact spiritual leader for intervention with Mrs. C.	5. Recovery may be blocked if spiritual distress is present and care is not provided.
	6. Refer Mrs. C. to physician for medication evaluation.	6. Antidepressant therapy may help Mrs. C. to function while confronting the dynamics of her depression.

NURSING DIAGNOSIS: RISK FOR INJURY

RELATED TO: Dizziness and weakness from lack of activity, low blood pressure, and poor nutritional status

OUTCOME CRITERIA	NURSING INTERVENTIONS	RATIONALE
Short-Term Goals • Mrs. C. will use walker when ambulating. • Mrs. C. will not experience physical harm or injury. Long-Term Goal • Mrs. C. will not experience physical harm or injury.	1. Assess vital signs at every visit. Report to physician should they fall below baseline.	1. Client safety is a nursing priority.
	2. Encourage Mrs. C. to use walker until strength has returned.	2. The walker will help prevent Mrs. C. from falling.
	3. Visit Mrs. C. during mealtimes and sit with her while she eats. Encourage her niece to do the same. Ensure that easy-to-prepare, nutritious foods for meals and snacks are available in the house and that they are items that Mrs. C. likes.	3. She is more likely to eat what is convenient and what she enjoys.
	4. Contact local meal delivery service (e.g., Meals on Wheels) to deliver some of Mrs. C.'s meals.	4. This would ensure that she receives at least one complete and nutritious meal each day.
	5. Weigh Mrs. C. each week.	5. Weight gain is a measurable, objective means of assessing whether Mrs. C. is eating.
	6. Ensure that diet contains sufficient fluid and fiber.	6. Adequate dietary fluid and fiber will help to alleviate constipation. She may also benefit from a daily stool softener.

Continued

Table 37-2 CARE PLAN FOR PSYCHIATRIC HOME HEALTH CARE OF DEPRESSED ELDERLY (MRS. C.)—cont'd

NURSING DIAGNOSIS: SOCIAL ISOLATION
RELATED TO: Depressed mood and feelings of worthlessness
EVIDENCED BY: Staying home alone, refusing to leave apartment

OUTCOME CRITERIA	NURSING INTERVENTIONS	RATIONALE
Short-Term Goal • Mrs. C. will discuss with nurse feelings about past social relationships and those she may like to renew. **Long-Term Goal** • Mrs. C. will renew contact with friends and participate in social activities.	1. As nutritional status is improving and strength is gained, encourage Mrs. C. to become more active. Take walks with her; help her perform simple tasks around her house. 2. Assess lifelong patterns of relationships. 3. Help her identify present relationships that are satisfying and activities that she considers interesting. 4. Consider the feasibility of a pet. 5. Suggest possible alternatives that Mrs. C. may consider as she seeks to participate in social activities. These may include foster grandparent programs, senior citizens centers, church activities, craft groups, and volunteer activities. Help her to locate individuals with whom she may attend some of these activities.	1. Increased activity enhances both physical and mental status. 2. Basic personality characteristics will not change. Mrs. C. will very likely keep the same style of relationship development that she had in the past. 3. She is the person who truly knows what she likes, and these personal preferences will facilitate success in reversing social isolation. 4. There are many documented studies of the benefits to elderly individuals of companion pets. 5. She is more likely to attend and participate if she does not have to do so alone.

Care for the Caregivers Another aspect of psychiatric home health care is to provide support and assistance to primary caregivers. When family is the provider of care on a 7-day-a-week, 24-hour-a-day schedule for a loved one with a severe and persistent mental disorder, it can be very exhausting and very frustrating. A care plan for primary caregivers is presented in Table 37-3.

The Homeless Population

Historical and Epidemiological Aspects

In 1992, Dr. Richard Lamb, a recognized expert in the field of severe and persistent mental illness, wrote:

Alec Guinness, in his memorable role as a British Army colonel in *Bridge on the River Kwai*, exclaims at the end of the film when he finally realizes he has been working to help the enemy, "What have I done?" As a vocal advocate and spokesman for deinstitutionalization and community treatment of severely mentally ill patients for well over two decades, I often find myself asking that same question.

The number of homeless in the United States has been estimated at somewhere between 250,000 and 4 million. It is difficult to determine the true scope of the problem because even the statisticians who collect the data have difficulty defining homeless persons. They have sometimes been identified as, "those people who sleep in shelters or public spaces." This approach results in underestimates because available shelter services are insufficient to meet the numbers of homeless people (U.S. Conference of Mayors [USCM], 2008).

Table 37-3 CARE PLAN FOR PRIMARY CAREGIVERS OF CLIENT WITH SEVERE AND PERSISTENT MENTAL ILLNESS

NURSING DIAGNOSIS: CAREGIVER ROLE STRAIN

RELATED TO: Severity and duration of the care receiver's illness and lack of respite and recreation for the caregivers

EVIDENCED BY: Feelings of stress in relationship with care receiver, feelings of depression and anger, family conflict around issues of providing care

OUTCOME CRITERIA	NURSING INTERVENTIONS	RATIONALE
Short-Term Goal • Caregivers will verbalize understanding of ways to facilitate the caregiver role. **Long-Term Goal** • Caregivers will demonstrate effective problem-solving skills and develop adaptive coping mechanisms to regain equilibrium.	1. Assess prospective caregivers' abilities to anticipate and fulfill client's unmet needs. Provide information to assist caregivers with this responsibility. Ensure that caregivers encourage client to be as independent as possible.	1. Caregivers may be unaware of what the client can realistically accomplish. They may be unaware of the nature of the illness.
	2. Ensure that caregivers are aware of available community support systems from which they may seek assistance when required. Examples include respite care services, day treatment centers, and adult day-care centers.	2. Caregivers require relief from the pressures and strain of providing 24-hour care for their loved one. Studies have shown that abuse arises out of caregiving situations that place overwhelming stress on the caregivers.
	3. Encourage caregivers to express feelings, particularly anger.	3. Release of these emotions can serve to prevent psychopathology, such as depression or psychophysiological disorders, from occurring.
	4. Encourage participation in support groups comprising members with similar life situations. Provide information about support groups that may be helpful: a. National Alliance on Mental Illness (NAMI) (800) 950-NAMI b. American Association on Intellectual and Developmental Disabilities (AAIDD) (800) 424-3688 c. Alzheimer's Association (800) 272-3900	4. Hearing others who are experiencing the same problems discuss ways in which they have coped may help caregivers adopt more adaptive strategies. Individuals who are experiencing similar life situations provide empathy and support for each other.

According to the Stewart B. McKinney Act, a person is considered homeless who:

lacks a fixed, regular, and adequate nighttime residence; and...has a primary night-time residency that is: (A) a supervised publicly or privately operated shelter designed to provide temporary living accommodations, (B) an institution that provides a temporary residence for individuals intended to be institutionalized, or (C) a public or private place not designed for, or ordinarily used as, a regular sleeping accommodation for human beings. (National Coalition for the Homeless [NCH], 2009d)

Two methods of counting the homeless are commonly used (NCH, 2009c). The *point-in-time* method attempts to count all the people who are literally homeless on a given day or during a given week. The second method (called *period prevalence counts*) examines the number of people who are homeless over a given period of time. This second method may result in a more accurate count because the extended time period would allow for including the people who are homeless one day (or week) but find employment and affordable housing later, removing them from the homeless count. At the same time during this extended period, others would lose housing and become homeless.

Who Are the Homeless?

The homeless are increasingly a heterogeneous group. The NCH (2009d) provided the following demographics.

Age Studies have produced a variety of statistics related to age of the homeless: 39 percent are younger than 18 years of age; individuals between the ages of 25 and 34 make up 25 percent; and 6 percent are ages 55 to 64.

Gender More men than women are homeless. The NCH (2009d) reported that 76 percent of the homeless population are single individuals. Within this largest segment of homeless individuals, 67.5 percent are men and 32.5 percent are female.

Families Families with children are among the fastest growing segments of the homeless population. They make up 23 percent of the homeless population, but research indicates that this number is higher in rural areas, where families, single mothers, and children account for the largest group of homeless people.

Ethnicity The homeless population is estimated to be 45 percent African American, 37 percent Caucasian, 13 percent Hispanic, 3 percent Native American, and 2 percent Asian (USCM, 2007). The ethnic makeup of homeless populations varies according to geographic location.

Mental Illness and Homelessness

The USCM (2008) survey revealed that approximately 26 percent of the homeless population suffers from some form of mental illness. Who are these individuals, and why are they homeless? Some blame the deinstitutionalization movement. Persons with mental illness who were released from state and county mental hospitals and who did not have families with whom they could reside sought residence in board-and-care homes of varying quality. Halfway houses and supportive group living arrangements were helpful but scarce. Many of those with families returned to their homes, but because families received little if any instruction or support, the consequences of their mentally ill loved one returning to live at home were often turbulent, resulting in the individual frequently leaving home.

Types of Mental Illness Among the Homeless A number of studies have been conducted, primarily in large, urban areas, that have addressed the most common types of mental illness identified among homeless individuals. Schizophrenia is frequently described as the most common diagnosis. Other prevalent disorders include bipolar disorder, substance abuse and dependence, depression, personality disorders, and organic mental disorders. Many exhibit psychotic symptoms, many are former residents of long-term care institutions for the mentally ill, and many have such a strong desire for independence that they isolate themselves in an effort to avoid being identified as a part of the mental health system. Many of them are clearly a danger to themselves or others, yet they often do not even see themselves as ill.

Contributing Factors to Homelessness Among the Mentally Ill

Deinstitutionalization As previously stated, deinstitutionalization is frequently implicated as a contributing factor to homelessness among the mentally ill. Deinstitutionalization began out of expressed concern by mental health professionals and others who described the "deplorable conditions" under which mentally ill individuals were housed.

The advent of psychotropic medications and the community mental health movement began a growing philosophical view that mentally ill individuals receive better and more humanitarian treatment in the community than in state hospitals far removed from their homes. It was believed that commitment and institutionalization in many ways deprived these individuals of their civil rights. Not the least of the motivating factors for deinstitutionalization was the financial burden these clients placed on state governments.

In fact, deinstitutionalization has not failed completely. About 50 percent of the mentally ill population—those who have insight into their illness and need for medication—have done reasonably well. It is individuals from the other 50 percent, those who lack such insight and who frequently stop taking their medication, that often end up on the streets.

However, because the vast increases in homelessness did not occur until the 1980s, the release of severely mentally ill people from institutions cannot be solely to blame. A number of other factors have been implicated.

Poverty Cuts in various government entitlement programs have depleted the allotments available for individuals with severe and persistent mental illness living in the community. The job market is prohibitive for individuals whose behavior is incomprehensible or even frightening to many. The stigma and discrimination associated with mental illness may be diminishing slowly, but it is highly visible to those who suffer from its effects.

A Scarcity of Affordable Housing The National Coalition for the Homeless (NCH, 2009e) stated:

> A lack of affordable housing and the limited scale of housing assistance programs have contributed to the current housing crisis and to homelessness. The lack of affordable housing has [led] to high rent burdens (rents which absorb a high proportion of income), overcrowding, and substandard housing. These phenomena, in turn, have not only forced many people to become homeless; they have put a large and growing number of people at risk of becoming homeless. Recently, foreclosures have increased the number of people who experience homelessness. [An NCH] report found that there was a 32% jump in the number of foreclosures between April 2008 and April 2009.

In addition, the number of single-room-occupancy (SRO) hotels has diminished drastically. These SRO hotels provided a means of relatively inexpensive housing, and although some people believe that these facilities nurtured isolation, they provided adequate shelter from the elements for their occupants. So many individuals currently frequent the shelters of our cities that there is concern that the shelters are becoming mini-institutions for individuals with serious mental illness.

Other Factors Several other factors that may contribute to homelessness have been identified (NCH, 2009e). They include the following:

- **Lack of affordable health care.** For families barely able to scrape together enough money to pay for day-to-day living, a catastrophic illness can create the level of poverty that starts the downward spiral to homelessness.

- **Domestic Violence.** The NCH (2009e) reported that domestic violence is a primary cause of homelessness, with approximately 63 percent of homeless women having experienced domestic violence in their adult lives. Battered women are often forced to choose between an abusive relationship and homelessness.

- **Addiction Disorders.** For individuals with alcohol or drug addictions, in the absence of appropriate treatment, the chances increase for being forced into life on the street. The

following have been cited as obstacles to addiction treatment for homeless persons: lack of health insurance, lack of documentation, waiting lists, scheduling difficulties, daily contact requirements, lack of transportation, ineffective treatment methods, lack of supportive services, and cultural insensitivity.

Community Resources for the Homeless

Interfering Factors Among the many issues that complicate service planning for the homeless mentally ill is this population's penchant for mobility. Frequent relocation confounds service delivery and interferes with providers' efforts to ensure appropriate care. Some individuals with serious mental illness may be affected by homelessness only temporarily or intermittently. These individuals are sometimes called the "episodically homeless." Others move around within neighborhoods or cities as needs change and based on whether or not they can obtain needed services. A large number of the homeless mentally ill population exhibits continuous unbounded movement over wide geographical areas.

Not all of the homeless mentally ill population are mobile. Some studies have indicated that a large percentage remains in the same location over a number of years. Health-care workers must identify movement patterns of homeless people in their area to at least try to bring the best care possible to this unique population. This may indeed mean delivering services to those individuals who do not seek out services on their own.

Health Issues Life as a homeless person can have severe consequences in terms of health. Exposure to the elements, poor diet, sleep deprivation, risk of violence, injuries, and little or no health care lead to a precarious state of health and exacerbate any preexisting illnesses. One of the major afflictions is alcoholism. It has been estimated that about 40 percent of homeless individuals abuse alcohol. Compared to other homeless individuals, those who abuse alcohol are at greater risk for neurological impairment, heart disease and hypertension, chronic lung disease, gastrointestinal (GI) disorders, hepatic dysfunction, and trauma.

Thermoregulation is a health problem for all homeless individuals because of their exposure to all kinds of weather. It is a compounded problem for the homeless alcoholic who spends much time in an altered level of consciousness.

It is difficult to determine whether mental illness is a cause or an effect of homelessness. Some behaviors that may seem deviant to some people may in actuality be adaptations to life on the street.

It has been suggested that some homeless individuals may even seek hospitalization in psychiatric institutions in an attempt to get off the streets for a while.

Tuberculosis is a serious problem among individuals who are homeless (Haddad, Wilson, Ijak, Marks, & Moore, 2005). Crowded shelters provide ideal conditions for spread of respiratory infections among their inhabitants. The risk of acquiring tuberculosis is also increased by the prevalence of alcoholism, drug addiction, HIV infection, and poor nutrition among homeless individuals.

Dietary deficiencies are a continuing problem for homeless individuals. Not only is the homeless person commonly in a poor nutritional state, but also the condition itself exacerbates a number of other health problems. Homeless people suffer from higher mortality rates and a greater number of serious disorders than their counterparts in the general population.

Sexually transmitted diseases, such as gonorrhea and syphilis, are a serious problem for the homeless. One of the most serious sexually transmitted diseases prevalent among homeless individuals is HIV infection. Street life is precarious for individuals whose systems are immunosuppressed by HIV. Rummaged food scraps are often spoiled, and exposure to the elements is a continuous threat. Individuals with HIV infection who stay in shelters often are exposed to the infectious diseases of others, which can be life threatening in their vulnerable condition.

IMPLICATIONS OF RESEARCH FOR EVIDENCE-BASED PRACTICE

Rew, L., Fouladi, R. T., & Yockey, R. D. (2002). Sexual health practices of homeless youth. *Journal of Nursing Scholarship, 34,* **139–145.**

DESCRIPTION OF THE STUDY: The purpose of this study was to describe the sexual health practices of homeless adolescents, examine relationships among variables in a conceptual model of sexual health practices, and determine direct and indirect effects of population characteristics, cognitive-perceptual factors, and behavioral factors on sexual health practices among homeless adolescents. A survey was administered to a convenience sample of 414 homeless young men (244) and women (170) ages 16 to 20 years, the majority of whom were Anglo American. Likert scale questionnaires were administered seeking information regarding sexually transmitted diseases (STDs), knowledge about AIDS, self-efficacy to use condoms, future time perspective, intentions to use condoms, social support, sexual health practices, assertive communication, and background information.

RESULTS OF THE STUDY: Thirty-five percent of the sample reported homosexual or bisexual orientation, and sexual orientation was reported as a reason for leaving home. Over half reported a history of sexual abuse, and nearly 1 in 4 had been treated for gonorrhea. Seven percent had been treated for HIV, 8 percent for chlamydia, and 3.6 percent for syphilis, and 32 percent had received one or more immunizations to prevent hepatitis B. Future time perspective scores were low, a finding that was not surprising knowing the daily challenges of living on the street. Perceived social support scores were also low, again being an expected finding due to lack of socially supportive environments of homes, parents, and schools. The mean safe-sex behavior score was higher than those in a study of university males. The authors speculated that this may indicate that participants were exposed to safe-sex messages more frequently at the street outreach center than were the university males. Those participants who had higher scores in perceived social support and assertive communication also had higher scores in self-efficacy to use condoms.

IMPLICATIONS FOR NURSING PRACTICE: The authors suggested that the correlation of self-efficacy to use condoms with social support and assertive communication may indicate that an intervention directed at the enhancement of assertive communication skills and social support might result in increased self-efficacy, which could in turn increase safe-sex behaviors. The authors stated:

> The relationship of intention to use condoms with future time perspective, social connectedness, and self-efficacy to use condoms, but also with sexual health responsibility indicates yet another domain in which to intervene with homeless adolescents. Interventions that focus on enhancing sexual health responsibility (e.g., seeking health care services if one suspects an STD or refusing to engage in sexual intercourse with someone known to have HIV) could have positive effects on these youth.

This study provides information that can be used by nurses who work with the homeless population, in an effort to change risky behavior and promote positive health-care habits under frequently unfavorable conditions.

HIV disease is increasing among the homeless population. The NCH (2009a) reported that an estimated 3.4 percent of the homeless population are HIV-positive, compared to 0.4 percent within the general population. It is estimated that up to 50 percent of persons living with HIV infection are expected to need housing assistance of some kind during their lifetimes.

Homeless children have special health needs. The NCH (2009b) reported that children without a home have higher rates of asthma, ear infections, stomach problems, and speech problems than their counterparts who are not homeless. They also experience more mental health problems, such as anxiety, depression, and withdrawal. They are twice as likely to experience hunger and four times as likely to have delayed development.

Types of Resources Available

Homeless Shelters The system of **shelters** for the homeless in the United States varies widely, from converted warehouses that provide cots or floor space on which to sleep overnight to significant operations that provide a multitude of social and health care services. They are run by volunteers and paid professionals and are sponsored by churches, community governments, and a variety of social agencies.

It is impossible, then, to describe a "typical" shelter. One profile may be described as the provision of lodging, food, and clothing to individuals who are in need of these services. Some shelters also provide medical and psychiatric evaluations, first aid and other health-care services, and referral for case management services by nurses or social workers.

Individuals who seek services from the shelter are generally assigned a bed or cot, issued a set of clean linen, provided a place to shower, shown laundry facilities, and offered a meal in the shelter kitchen or dining hall. Most shelters attempt to separate dormitory areas for men and women, with various consequences for those who violate the rules.

Shelters cover expenses through private and corporate donations, church sponsorships, and government grants. From the outset, shelters were conceptualized as "temporary" accommodations for individuals who needed a place to spend the night. Realistically, they have become permanent lodging for homeless individuals with little hope for improving their situation. Some individuals use shelters for their mailing address.

Shelters provide a safe and supportive environment for homeless individuals who have no other place to go. Some homeless people who inhabit shelters use the resources offered to improve their lot in life, whereas others become hopelessly dependent on the shelter's provisions. To a few, the availability of a shelter may even mean the difference between life and death.

Health-Care Centers and Storefront Clinics Some communities have established "street clinics" to serve the homeless population. Many of these clinics are operated by nurse practitioners who work in consultation with physicians in the area. In recent years, some of these clinics have provided clinical sites for nursing students in their community health rotation. Some have been staffed by faculties of nursing schools that have established group practices in the community setting.

A wide variety of services are offered at these clinics, including administering medications, assessing vital signs, screening for tuberculosis and other communicable diseases, giving immunizations and flu shots, changing dressings, and administering first aid. Physical and psychosocial assessments, health education, and supportive counseling are also frequent interventions.

Nursing in **storefront clinics** for the homeless provides many special challenges, not the least of which is poor working conditions. These clinics often operate under severe budgetary constraints with inadequate staffing, supplies, and equipment, in rundown facilities located in high-crime neighborhoods. Frustration is often high among nurses who work in these clinics, as they are seldom able to see measurable progress in their homeless clients. Maintenance of health management is virtually impossible for many individuals who have no resources outside the health-care setting. When return appointments for preventive care are made, the lack of follow-through is high.

Mobile Outreach Units Outreach programs literally reach out to the homeless in their own environment in an effort to provide health care. Volunteers and paid professionals form teams to drive or walk around and seek out homeless individuals who are in need of assistance. They offer coffee, sandwiches, and blankets in an effort to show concern and establish trust. If assistance can be provided at the site, it is done so. If not, every effort is made to ensure that the individual is linked with a source that can provide the necessary services.

Mobile outreach units provide assistance to homeless individuals who are in need of physical or psychological care. The emphasis of outreach programs is to accommodate the homeless who refuse to seek treatment elsewhere. Most target the mentally ill segment of the population. When trust has been established, and the individual agrees to come to the team's office, medical and psychiatric treatment is initiated. Involuntary hospitalization is initiated when an individual is deemed harmful to self or others, or otherwise meets the criteria for being considered "gravely disabled."

The Homeless Client and the Nursing Process

A case study demonstrating the nursing process with a homeless client is presented in Box 37-5.

BOX 37-5 Case Study: Nursing Process With a Homeless Client

ASSESSMENT

Joe, age 65, is brought to the Community Health Clinic by two of his peers, who report: "He just had a fit. He needs a drink bad!" Joe is dirty and unkempt, has visible tremors of the upper extremities, and is weak enough to require assistance when ambulating. He is cooperative as the nurse completes the intake assessment. He is coherent, although thought processes are slow. He is disoriented to time and place. He appears somewhat frightened as he scans the unfamiliar surroundings. He is unable to tell the nurse when he had his last drink. He reports no physical injury, and none is observable.

Joe carries a small bag with a few personal items inside, including a Department of Veterans Affairs (VA) benefit card, identifying him as a veteran of the Vietnam War. The nurse finds a cot for Joe to lie down, ensures that his vital signs are stable, and telephones the number on the VA card. The clinic nurse discovers that Joe is well known to the admissions personnel at the VA. He has a 35-year history of schizophrenia, with numerous hospitalizations. At the time of his last discharge, he was taking fluphenazine (Prolixin) 10 mg twice a day. He told the clinic nurse that he took the medication for a few months after he got out of the hospital but then did not have the prescription refilled. He could not remember when he had last taken fluphenazine.

Joe also has a long history of alcohol-related disorders and has participated in the VA substance rehabilitation program three times. He has no home address and receives his VA disability benefit checks at a shelter address. He reports that he has no family. The nurse makes arrangements for VA personnel to drive Joe from the clinic to the VA hospital, where he is admitted for detoxification. She sets up a case management file for Joe and arranges with the hospital to have Joe return to the clinic after discharge.

DIAGNOSIS/OUTCOME IDENTIFICATION

The following nursing diagnosis was formulated for Joe:

Ineffective health maintenance related to ineffective coping skills evidenced by abuse of alcohol, lack of follow-through with neuroleptic medication, and lack of personal hygiene.

Ongoing criteria were selected as outcomes for Joe. They include:

- Follows the rules of the group home and maintains his residency status.
- Attends weekly sessions of group therapy at the VA day treatment program.
- Attends weekly sessions of Alcoholics Anonymous and maintains sobriety.
- Reports regularly to the health clinic for injections of fluphenazine.
- Volunteers at the VA hospital 3 days a week.
- Secures and retains permanent employment.

PLANNING/IMPLEMENTATION

During Joe's hospitalization, the clinic nurse remained in contact with his case. Joe received complete physical and dental examinations and treatment during his hospital stay. The clinic nurse attended the treatment team meeting for Joe as his outpatient case manager. It was decided at the meeting to try giving Joe injections of fluphenazine decanoate because of his history of noncompliance with his daily oral medications. The clinic nurse would administer the injection every 4 weeks.

At Joe's follow-up clinic visit, the nurse explains to Joe that she has found a group home where he may live with others who have personal circumstances similar to his. At the group home, meals will be provided and the group home manager will ensure that Joe's basic needs are fulfilled. A criterion for remaining at the residence is for Joe to remain alcohol free. Joe is agreeable to these living arrangements.

With Joe's concurrence, the clinic nurse also performs the following interventions:

- Goes shopping with Joe to purchase some new clothing, allowing Joe to make decisions as independently as possible.
- Helps Joe move into the group home and introduces him to the manager and residents.
- Helps Joe change his address from the shelter to the group home so that he may continue to receive his VA benefits.
- Enrolls Joe in the weekly group therapy sessions of the day treatment facility connected with the VA hospital.
- Helps Joe locate the nearest Alcoholics Anonymous group and identifies a sponsor who will ensure that Joe gets to the meetings.

BOX 37-5 Case Study: Nursing Process With a Homeless Client—cont'd

- Sets up a clinic appointment for Joe to return in 4 weeks for his fluphenazine injection; telephones Joe 1 day in advance to remind him of his appointment.
- Instructs Joe to return to or call the clinic if any of the following symptoms occur: sore throat, fever, nausea and vomiting, severe headache, difficulty urinating, tremors, skin rash, or yellow skin or eyes.
- Assists Joe in securing transportation to and from appointments.
- Encourages Joe to set realistic goals for his life and offers recognition for follow-through.
- When Joe is ready, discusses employment alternatives with him; suggests the possibility of starting with a volunteer job (perhaps as a VA hospital volunteer).

EVALUATION
Evaluation of the nursing process with the homeless mentally ill must be highly individualized. Statistics show that chances for relapse with this population are high. Therefore, it is extremely important that outcome criteria be realistic so as not to set the client up for failure.

Summary and Key Points

■ The trend in psychiatric care is shifting from that of inpatient hospitalization to a focus of outpatient care within the community. This trend is largely due to the need for greater cost-effectiveness in the provision of medical care to the masses.

■ The community mental health movement began in the 1960s with the closing of state hospitals and the deinstitutionalization of many individuals with severe and persistent mental illness.

■ Mental health care within the community targets primary prevention (reducing the incidence of mental disorders within the population), secondary prevention (reducing the prevalence of psychiatric illness by shortening the course of the illness), and tertiary prevention (reducing the residual defects that are associated with severe and persistent mental illness).

■ Primary prevention focuses on identification of populations at risk for mental illness, increasing their ability to cope with stress, and targeting and diminishing harmful forces within the environment.

■ The focus of secondary prevention is accomplished through early identification of problems and prompt initiation of effective treatment.

■ Tertiary prevention focuses on preventing complications of the illness and promoting rehabilitation that is directed toward achievement of the individual's maximum level of functioning.

■ Registered nurses serve as providers of psychiatric/mental health care in the community setting.

■ Nurses provide outpatient care for individuals with severe and persistent mental illness in community mental health centers, in day and evening treatment programs, in partial hospitalization programs, in community residential facilities, and with psychiatric home health care.

■ Homeless persons with mental illness provide a special challenge for the community mental health nurse. Care is provided within homeless shelters, at health-care centers or storefront clinics, and through mobile outreach programs.

 DavisPlus

Additional info available @
davisplus.fadavis.com

Review Questions
Self-Examination/Learning Exercise

*Select the answer that is **most** appropriate for each of the following questions:*

1. Which of the following represents a nursing intervention at the primary level of prevention?
   a. Teaching a class in parent effectiveness training.
   b. Leading a group of adolescents in drug rehabilitation.
   c. Referring a married couple for sex therapy.
   d. Leading a support group for battered women.

2. Which of the following represents a nursing intervention at the secondary level of prevention?
   a. Teaching a class about menopause to middle-aged women.
   b. Providing support in the emergency room to a rape victim.
   c. Leading a support group for women in transition.
   d. Making monthly visits to the home of a client with schizophrenia to ensure medication compliance.

3. Which of the following represents a nursing intervention at the tertiary level of prevention?
   a. Serving as case manager for a mentally ill homeless client.
   b. Leading a support group for newly retired men.
   c. Teaching prepared childbirth classes.
   d. Caring for a depressed widow in the hospital.

4. John, a homeless person, has just come to live in the shelter. The shelter nurse is assigned to his care. Which of the following is a *priority* intervention on the part of the nurse?
   a. Referring John to a social worker.
   b. Developing a plan of care for John.
   c. Conducting a behavioral and needs assessment on John.
   d. Helping John apply for Social Security benefits.

5. John, a homeless person, has a history of paranoid schizophrenia and noncompliance with medications. Which of the following medications might be the best choice of neuroleptic for John?
   a. Haldol.
   b. Navane.
   c. Lithium carbonate.
   d. Prolixin decanoate.

6. Ann is a psychiatric home health nurse. She has just received an order to begin regular visits to Mrs. W., a 78-year-old widow who lives alone. Mrs. W.'s primary care physician has diagnosed her as depressed. Which of the following criteria would qualify Mrs. W. for home health visits?
   a. Mrs. W. never learned to drive and has to depend on others for her transportation.
   b. Mrs. W. is physically too weak to travel without risk of injury.
   c. Mrs. W. refuses to seek assistance as suggested by her physician, "because I don't have a psychiatric problem."
   d. Mrs. W. says she would prefer to have home visits than go to the physician's office.

Review Questions—cont'd
Self-Examination/Learning Exercise

7. Ann is a psychiatric home health nurse. She has just received an order to begin regular visits to Mrs. W., a 78-year-old widow who lives alone. Mrs. W.'s primary care physician has diagnosed her as depressed. Based on a needs assessment, which of the following problems would Ann address during her first visit?
   a. Complicated grieving.
   b. Social isolation.
   c. Risk for injury.
   d. Sleep pattern disturbance.

8. Mrs. W. (a 78-year-old depressed widow) says to her home health nurse, "What's the use? I don't have anything to live for anymore." Which is the best response on the part of the nurse?
   a. "Of course you do, Mrs. W. Why would you say such a thing?"
   b. "You seem so sad. I'm going to do my best to cheer you up."
   c. "Let's talk about why you are feeling this way."
   d. "Have you been thinking about harming yourself in any way?"

9. The physician orders trazodone (Desyrel) for Mrs. W. (a 78-year-old widow with depression), 150 mg to take at bedtime. Which of the following statements about this medication would be appropriate for the home health nurse to make in teaching Mrs. W. about trazadone?
   a. "You may feel dizzy when you stand up, so go slowly when you get up from sitting or lying down."
   b. "You must be sure and not eat any chocolate while you are taking this medicine."
   c. "We will need to draw a sample of blood to send to the lab every month while you are on this medication."
   d. "If you don't feel better right away with this medicine, the doctor can order a different kind for you."

10. Three predominant client populations have been identified as benefiting most from psychiatric home health care. Which of the following is *not* included among this group?
    a. Elderly individuals.
    b. Individuals living in poverty.
    c. Individuals with severe and persistent mental illness.
    d. Individuals in acute crisis situations.

References

American Nurses Association. (2007). *Psychiatric-mental health nursing: Scope and standards of practice.* Silver Spring, MD: Author.

American Nurses Association. (2008). *Home health nursing: Scope and standards of practice.* Silver Spring, MD: Author.

American Psychiatric Association. (2000). *Diagnostic and statistical manual of mental disorders* (4th ed.). *Text revision.* Washington, DC: American Psychiatric Publishing.

Case Management Society of America. (2010). *Standards of practice for case management.* Little Rock, AR: Author.

Centers for Medicare & Medicaid Services. (2005). *Medicare Benefit Policy Manual.* Baltimore, MD: Author.

Haddad, M. G., Wilson, T. W., Ijaz, K., Marks, S. M., & Moore, M. (2005). Tuberculosis and homelessness in the United States, 1994–2003. *Journal of the American Medical Association, 293,* 2762–2766.

Jans, L., Stoddard, S., & Kraus, L. (2004). *Chartbook on mental health and disability in the United States.* An InfoUse Report. Washington, DC: U.S. Department of Education, National Institute on Disability and Rehabilitation Research.

Lamb, H. R. (1992). Perspectives on effective advocacy for homeless mentally ill persons. *Hospital and Community Psychiatry, 43,* 1209–1212.

Langley, C. (2002). Community-based nursing practice: An overview in the United States. In J. M. Sorrell & G. M. Redmond (Eds.), *Community-based nursing practice: Learning through students' stories* (pp. 3–19). Philadelphia: F.A. Davis.

Ling, C. (2010). *Case management basics.* Nursing Spectrum/NurseWeek Continuing Education Course #60102. Retrieved

October 23, 2010, from http://ce.nurse.com/ 60102/
Case-Management-Basics/

Mandleco, B. L. (2004). *Growth & development handbook: Newborn through adolescent.* New York: Delmar Learning.

Miller, M. A., & Rahe, R. H. (1997). Life changes scaling for the 1990s. *Journal of Psychosomatic Research, 43,* 279–292.

Murray, R. B., Zentner, J. P., & Yakimo, R. (2009). *Health promotion strategies through the life span* (8th ed.). Upper Saddle River, NJ: Prentice Hall.

National Alliance on Mental Illness. (2009). *NAMI Public Policy Platform* (8th ed.). Arlington, VA: Author.

National Alliance on Mental Illness. (2010). *PACT: Program of assertive community treatment.* Retrieved October 23, 2010 from http://www.nami.org/

National Coalition for the Homeless. (2009a). *HIV/AIDS and homelessness.* Retrieved October 24, 2010, from http://www.nationalhomeless.org/

National Coalition for the Homeless. (2009b). *Homeless families with children.* Retrieved October 24, 2010, from http://www.nationalhomeless.org/

National Coalition for the Homeless. (2009c). *How many people experience homelessness?* Retrieved October 24, 2010, from http://www.nationalhomeless.org/

National Coalition for the Homeless. (2009d). *Who is homeless?* Retrieved October 24, 2010, from http://www.national-homeless.org/

National Coalition for the Homeless. (2009e). *Why are people homeless?* Retrieved October 24, 2010, from http://www.nationalhomeless.org/

Pittman, D. C. (1989). Nursing case management: Holistic care for the deinstitutionalized chronically mentally ill. *Journal of Psychosocial Nursing, 27*(11), 23–27.

President's New Freedom Commission on Mental Health. (2003). *Achieving the promise: Transforming mental health care in America.* Retrieved October 24, 2010, from http://www.mentalhealthcommission.gov/

Sadock, B. J., & Sadock, V. A. (2007). *Synopsis of psychiatry: Behavioral sciences/clinical psychiatry* (10th ed.). Philadelphia: Lippincott Williams & Wilkins.

Scanlon, V. C., & Sanders, T. (2011). *Essentials of anatomy and physiology* (6th ed.). Philadelphia: F.A. Davis.

Spock, B. (2004). *Baby and child care* (8th ed.). New York: Simon & Schuster.

U.S. Conference of Mayors. (2007). *A status report on hunger and homelessness in America's cities: 2007.* Washington, DC: Author.

U.S. Conference of Mayors. (2008). *A status report on hunger and homelessness in America's cities: 2008.* Washington, DC: Author.

Von Esenwein, S. A., Bornemann, T., Ellingson, L., Palpant, R., Randolph, L., & Druss, B. G. (2005). A survey of mental health leaders one year after the President's New Freedom Commission Report. *Psychiatric Services, 56,* 605–607.

World Health Organization. (2004). *Prevention of mental disorders: Effective interventions and policy options.* Retrieved October 23, 2010, from http://www.who.int/mental_health/evidence/en/prevention_of_mental_disorders_sr.pdf

Wright, L. M., & Leahey, M. (2009). *Nurses and families: A guide to family assessment and intervention* (5th ed.). Philadelphia: F.A. Davis.

Classical References

Caplan, G. (1964). *Principles of preventive psychiatry.* New York: Basic Books.

Erikson, E. (1963). *Childhood and society* (2nd ed.). New York: WW Norton.

Mahler, M., Pine, F., & Bergman, A. (1975). *The psychological birth of the human infant.* New York: Basic Books.

Sheehy, G. (1976). *Passages: Predictable crises of adult life.* New York: Bantam Books.

Forensic Nursing CHAPTER

38

CORE CONCEPT
forensic

KEY TERMS

colposcope

forensic nursing

sexual assault nurse examiner (SANE)

OBJECTIVES
After reading this chapter, the student will be able to:

1. Define the terms *forensic* and *forensic nursing.*
2. Discuss historical perspectives of forensic nursing.
3. Identify areas of nursing within which forensic nurses may practice.
4. Describe forensic nursing specialties.
5. Apply the nursing process within the role of clinical forensic nursing in trauma care.
6. Apply the nursing process within the role of forensic psychiatric nursing in correctional facilities.

HOMEWORK ASSIGNMENT
Please read the chapter and answer the following questions:

1. When deaths occur in the emergency department, it is critical to determine if the death was natural or unnatural. What is the difference?
2. What is a colposcope?
3. Name four reasons that are identified as rationales for imprisonment for criminal behavior.
4. In what ways is HIV infection commonly spread in prisons?

The many roles of nurses continue to increase with the ever-expanding health service delivery system. **Forensic nursing** is an example of a nursing role that is rapidly increasing in its scope of practice. Nurses practicing in this unique specialty may apply their skills to the care of both victims and perpetrators of crime and in a variety of settings, including primary care facilities, hospitals, and correctional institutions. This chapter focuses on defining forensic nursing within varied aspects of the role. A discussion of historical perspectives is included, and care of the client is presented within the context of the nursing process.

What Is Forensic Nursing?

CORE CONCEPT

Forensic
Pertaining to the law; legal.

The International Association of Forensic Nurses (IAFN) and the American Nurses Association (ANA) defined *forensic nursing* as "the practice of nursing globally when health and legal systems intersect" (ANA & IAFN, 2009, p. 3).

Bellfield and Catalano (2009) offered the following:

> Forensic nursing is an emerging field that forms an alliance between nursing, law enforcement, and the forensic sciences. The term *forensic* means anything belonging to, or pertaining to, the law. Forensic nurses provide a continuum of care to victims and their families beginning in the emergency room or crime scene and leading to participation in the criminal investigation and the courts of law. (p. 446)

Hancock (2010) suggested that:

> Forensic nursing is the application of clinical and scientific knowledge to questions of law, and the civil or criminal investigation for survivors of traumatic injury and/or patient treatment involving court-related issues.

Because this area of nursing is a continuing pioneering effort, roles, definitions, and educational programs are still being formulated.

Historical Perspectives

Forensic nursing has its roots in Alberta, Canada, around 1975, where nurses served as investigators for medical examiners in the field of death investigation. They were valued for their biomedical education, their sensitivity in dealing with family members, and their ability to substitute in the role of the medical examiner when required. These are qualities that were often found to be lacking in medically untrained criminal investigative personnel.

The discipline has made great advances since that time. The role of forensic nursing has expanded from concerns solely with death investigation to include the living—the survivors of violent crime—as well as the perpetrators of criminal acts. In 1992, seventy-four nurses, primarily sexual assault nurse examiners, met to form the International Association of Forensic Nurses. By 1997, this organization had grown to more than 1,000 members. It currently boasts a membership of more than 3,000 nurses from 20 countries (Lynch, 2011).

Violence has reached epidemic proportions in the United States and has been identified as a major public health problem. It is with this in mind that the health care system and the legal system have joined in an attempt to respond to the increasing needs of crime victims. Stokowski (2008b) stated, "The zone where healthcare needs intersect with the law is expanding, and forensic nurses have stepped in to become leaders in the healthcare response to violence."

The Context of Forensic Nursing Practice

The IAFN (2010) has identified a variety of assignments within which the forensic nurse may practice. Some of these include the following:

■ **Interpersonal Violence**
  - Domestic violence
  - Sexual assault
  - Child abuse and neglect
  - Elder mistreatment
  - Human trafficking

■ **Death Investigation**
  - Examination of the body
  - Scene investigation

■ **Mass Disasters**

■ **Forensic Mental Health**

■ **Correctional Nursing**

■ **Legal Nurse Consulting**

■ **Public Health and Safety**
  - Environmental hazards
  - Drug and alcohol abuse
  - Epidemiological issues

■ **Emergency/Trauma Services**
  - Automobile and pedestrian accidents
  - Work-related injuries
  - Suicide attempts

IMPLICATIONS OF RESEARCH FOR EVIDENCE-BASED PRACTICE

Shelton, D. (2009). Leadership, education, achievement, and development: A nursing intervention for prevention of youthful offending behavior. *Journal of the American Psychiatric Nurses Association, 14,* 429–441.

DESCRIPTION OF THE STUDY: The purpose of this study was to examine a theoretically designed community-based program aimed at reducing the risk of first-time involvement by minority youth with the juvenile justice system. One hundred forty-six youths

IMPLICATIONS OF RESEARCH FOR EVIDENCE-BASED PRACTICE—cont'd

(90 male and 56 female) between the ages of 10 and 14 participated in the 3-year study. All were African American and were attending middle school. Members of both the intervention group ($n = 77$) and the control group ($n = 69$) were from an impoverished rural community, were having behavioral difficulties in school or at home, and were identified as "at-risk for delinquency." The study intervention, LEAD (leadership, education, achievement, and development), is a psychoeducational program that uses creative arts and instructional activities designed to assist the youth with self-awareness in relation to family and community. The authors stated, "The project uses empowering techniques and education strategies to emphasize development of self-esteem and consideration of less risky behaviors" (p. 433). The treatment participants met in groups for 14 weeks each semester and in a community-led group during the summer. Comparisons were made with an after-school program control group. Pre- and post-tests were administered to measure self-esteem, resilience, behavioral control, and protective factors (self-efficacy and self-control).

RESULTS OF THE STUDY: In all four areas of study, the LEAD program participants showed larger increases in post-test scores compared to pretest scores. Although the control group also indicated higher post-test scores, the increases were smaller compared to the treatment group. In evaluating the program, participants were asked if they would recommend the program to a friend, if the program was helpful in learning

to control their behavior, and, if they had a chance, whether they would ever participate in a program like this again. Participants in the LEAD program responded more positively on all evaluation items than did the after-school control youth. The communities that partnered with the study program responded that the researchers "had indeed tapped into the youth population that had been targeted for services: kids who were at risk of getting into trouble for any number of reasons, and most of all, because they were 'Black, poor, and not being served by other youth programs'" (p. 438).

IMPLICATIONS FOR NURSING PRACTICE: Becoming involved in programs such as the one described in this study is well within the scope of nursing practice. Programs that target at-risk youths have long-range, positive outcomes for participants by attempting to prevent offending behaviors that can have life-changing consequences for young people. The authors concluded:

> Community development is hard work. The number of man-hours and the level of patience required will be tolerated only by those who are believers in prevention. It does work. Compared to the expected thousands of dollars spent to incarcerate one child per year, LEAD is a great alternative. What it does take is time, the thing young people need the most from us but that seems to be so very hard to give. (p. 440)

Forensic Nursing Specialties*

Clinical Forensic Nursing

Clinical forensic nursing is the management of crime victims from trauma to trial. Nurses working in clinical forensics collect evidence through assessment of living victims, survivors of traumatic injury, or those whose death is pronounced in the clinical environment. Clinical forensic nursing involves making judgments related to patient treatment associated with court-related issues. The clinical forensic nurse assesses victims of child and elder abuse and domestic violence. Forensic nurses are asked to differentiate between conditions that simulate accidental injury and those that are purposely inflicted. An essential skill required by

the forensic nurse is the ability to assess patterned injury by differentiating marks such as defense wounds, grab marks, and fingernail marks. Clinical forensic nurses focus on observation of the communication and interaction patterns of suspected abuse victims and perpetrators. Many nurses come to forensic nursing from acute care settings of emergency department nursing, critical care nursing, and perioperative nursing.

In the coroner's office, death notification entails stabilization of the family situation and grief support, skills that are basic to nursing practice. Expert skills in physical assessment, clinical history taking and interviewing, and use of technology have helped advance this nursing role.

Because of their awareness of the effects of violence in society and their ability to assess situations in which potential for violence exists, clinical forensic nurses are often called upon for consultation. By identifying risk factors and cues for violence in health-care and workplace settings, these

---

*This section adapted from Hufft and Peternelj-Taylor (2003) and Bellfield and Catalano (2009), with permission.

nurses can assist in the development of strategies, policies, and protocols to manage risk and reduce violence and injury. They also assist in the debriefing or resolution of violent events in a workplace or community.

The Sexual Assault Nurse Examiner (SANE)

The **sexual assault nurse examiner (SANE)** is a clinical forensic registered nurse who has received specialized training to provide care to the sexual assault victim. His or her responsibilities include interviewing the victim, completing the physical examination, collecting specimens for forensic evidence, and documenting the findings. SANEs also provide emotional support for victims and family members. When the case goes to court, the SANE testifies as an expert legal witness about how evidence was collected and the physical and psychological condition of the client. The SANE may offer an opinion as to whether a crime occurred.

Forensic Psychiatric Nursing

Forensic psychiatric nurses integrate psychiatric/mental health nursing philosophy and practice with knowledge of the criminal justice system and assessment of the sociocultural influences on the individual client, the family, and the community, to provide comprehensive psychiatric and mental health nursing. Forensic psychiatric nurses work with mentally ill offenders and with victims of crime. They help victims cope with their emotional wounds and assist in the assessment and care of perpetrators. They focus on identification and change of behaviors that link criminal offenses or reactions to them. These nurses assist perpetrators and victims of crime in dealing with the courts and other aspects of the criminal justice system, minimizing further victimization and promoting functional abilities.

Functional applications of forensic psychiatric nursing include assessment of inmates for physical fitness, criminal responsibility, disposition, and early release. Forensic psychiatric nurses also provide mental health treatment for convicted offenders and those who are not found criminally responsible. In the criminal justice system, forensic psychiatric nurses deal with destructive, aggressive, and socially unacceptable behavior. These nurses provide interventions that encourage individuals to exercise self-control, foster individual change in behavior, and, in the process, protect other members of society and property.

There has been an increase in the involvement of forensic psychiatric nurses (especially those prepared for advanced practice) in the assessment and treatment of forensic psychiatric patients. These practitioners are involved in the development and refining of clinical roles in forensic psychiatric nursing and are in a position to promote intervention strategies that increase the likelihood of rehabilitation and reintegration of the forensic client into society.

Forensic Correctional Nursing

Forensic correctional nurses work in secure settings, providing treatment, rehabilitation, and health promotion to clients who have been charged with or convicted of crimes. Settings include jails, state and federal prisons, and halfway houses. Correctional facilities reflect the demographics of the general population, with an increasingly aging incarcerated population who have age-related health-care problems. Forensic correctional nurses provide health care for inmates in correctional facilities such as juvenile centers, jails, and prisons. They manage acute and chronic illness, develop health-care plans, dispense medications, and perform health screenings and health education. Forensic correctional nurses conduct psychiatric assessments and respond to emergency situations. The role of the forensic correctional nurse offers a high level of autonomy compared with other nursing roles.

Legal Nurse Consultant

The legal nurse consultant is a licensed registered nurse who critically evaluates and analyzes health-care issues in medically related lawsuits. Because the legal system is involved, nurses acting as consultants are considered to be practicing forensics. Nurses uniquely combine their medical expertise with legal knowledge to assess compliance with accepted standards of health-care practice.

Legal nurse consultants work in collaboration with attorneys and other legal and health-care professionals. They may have independent practices, work in the hospital setting in risk management, or be employed by law firms or health insurance companies.

Forensic Nurse Death Investigator

A death investigator is a professional with experiential and scientific knowledge who can accurately determine the cause of death. The forensic nurse death investigator is a registered nurse with specialized education who is functioning in the death investigator's role. Forensic nurse death investigators respond to scenes of deaths or accidents and work in collaboration with law enforcement. At the scene, they examine the body, pronounce death, and take tissue and blood samples. They take pictures of the body and evidence at the scene. Nurse death investigators must be able to recognize and integrate other evidence collected during the investigation, such as patterns of injury, types of wounds, and estimated time of death. They are responsible for record-keeping and arranging for the transport of the body to the morgue or to the coroner's office to undergo autopsy for further examination. Nurse death investigators work with the forensic pathologist to collect additional evidence in the laboratory during autopsy.

Nurses in General Practice

In addition to nurses in specialty practice, nurses in general practice find forensic nursing knowledge of growing importance. Forensic applications in the acute care setting emphasize the use of forensic knowledge and awareness of criminal justice implications for assessment, documentation of care, and reporting of information to police or other law enforcement agencies. Nurses who work in emergency departments and in critical care units are often in positions to preserve evidence of what might be a criminal offense. Victims of automobile accidents or apparent accidental overdoses are not always what they appear to be. Knowledge of what to look for and how to collect evidence, in addition to knowing whom to call and when, can be valuable in finding out what really happened in such cases. Clients often come into acute care settings with what are first thought to be injuries that are the result of an accident. However, preservation of evidence such as stomach contents, clothing residue, or marks on the skin surface can provide a very different picture—one of injury caused by a self-inflicted wound or violence perpetrated by another.

This chapter focuses on two specialties in forensic nursing: the clinical forensic nurse specialist in trauma care settings and the psychiatric forensic nurse in correctional facilities. The ANA and IAFN (2009) Standards of Practice and Standards of Professional Performance for forensic nursing are presented in Box 38-1.

BOX 38-1 Standards of Practice and Standards of Professional Performance for Forensic Nursing

STANDARDS OF PRACTICE

Standard 1. Assessment
  The forensic nurse collects comprehensive data pertinent to the patient's health or the situation.

Standard 2. Diagnosis
  The forensic nurse analyzes the assessment data to determine the diagnoses or issues.

Standard 3. Outcome Identification
  The forensic nurse identifies expected outcomes for a plan individualized to the patient or the situation.

Standard 4. Planning
  The forensic nurse develops a plan that prescribes strategies and alternatives to attain expected outcomes.

Standard 5. Implementation
  The forensic nurse implements the identified plan.

  Standard 5A. Coordination of Care
  The forensic nurse coordinates care delivery.

  Standard 5B. Health Teaching and Health Promotion
  The forensic nurse employs strategies to promote health and a safe environment.

  Standard 5C. Consultation
  The Forensic Advanced Practice Registered Nurse and the nursing role specialist provide consultation to influence the identified plan, enhance the abilities of others, and effect change.

  Standard 5D. Prescriptive Authority and Treatment
  The Forensic Advanced Practice Registered Nurse uses prescriptive authority, procedures, referrals, treatments, and therapies in accordance with state and federal laws and regulations.

Standard 6. Evaluation
  The forensic nurse evaluates progress towards attainment of outcomes.

STANDARDS OF PROFESSIONAL PERFORMANCE

Standard 7. Quality of Care
  The forensic nurse systematically evaluates the quality and effectiveness of forensic nursing practice.

Continued

BOX 38-1 Standards of Practice and Standards of Professional Performance for Forensic Nursing—cont'd

Standard 8. Education

The forensic nurse attains knowledge and competency that reflect current nursing practice.

Standard 9. Professional Practice Evaluation

The forensic nurse evaluates one's own nursing practice in relation to professional practice standards and guidelines, relevant statutes, rules, and regulations.

Standard 10. Collegiality

The forensic nurse interacts with and contributes to the professional development of peers and colleagues.

Standard 11. Collaboration

The forensic nurse collaborates with patient, family, and others in the conduct of nursing practice.

Standard 12. Ethics

The forensic nurse integrates ethical provisions into all areas of practice.

Standard 13. Research

The forensic nurse integrates research findings into practice.

Standard 14. Resource Utilization

The forensic nurse considers factors related to safety, effectiveness, cost, and impact on practice in the planning and delivery of nursing services.

Standard 15. Leadership

The forensic nurse provides leadership in the professional practice setting and the profession.

From American Nurses Association and International Association of Forensic Nurses. (2009). *Forensic nursing: Scope and standards of practice.* Silver Spring, MD: American Nurses Association, with permission.

Application of the Nursing Process in Clinical Forensic Nursing in Trauma Care

Assessment

Forensic nurse examiners (FNEs) are included as valuable members of trauma units in many emergency departments. Dougherty (2011) stated,

> In addition to performing sexual assault examinations, these nursing specialists provide other services such as formal assessments for abuse and neglect, forensic photography, wound identification, evidence collection, and expert testimony. (p. 155)

All traumatic injuries in which liability is suspected are considered within the scope of forensic nursing. Reports to legal agencies are required to ensure follow-up investigation; however, the protection of clients' rights remains a nursing priority.

McPeck (2002) reported on the performance of forensic nurses in the aftermath of the September 11, 2001, attack on New York City and Washington, DC. He stated:

> [Forensic nurses] worked as mortuary assistants to collect and process biological and evidentiary remains of the victims. The forensic nurses provided clinical care and support

for about 2,000 police officers, firefighters, and emergency workers who were at Ground Zero at any one time. Forensic nurses are trained to intervene in crises and offer that kind of mental support. (p. 25)

With the rise of violence in our society, the role of the clinical forensic nurse in the care of trauma clients in the emergency department is expanding. The forensic clinical nurse specialist may be the ideal liaison between legal and medical agencies.

Lynch (2011) identified several areas of assessment in which the clinical forensic nurse specialist may become involved. Some of these include the preservation of evidence, investigation of wound characteristics, and deaths in the emergency department.

Preservation of Evidence

Intentional traumas in the emergency department may be crime related or self-inflicted. Crime-related evidence is essential and must be safeguarded in a manner consistent with the investigation. Brown (2010a) identified common types of evidence as clothing, bullets, gunshot powder on the skin, bloodstains, hairs, fibers, grass, and any other type of debris that is found on the individual, such as fragments of glass, paint, and wood. Often this type of evidence is destroyed in the clinical setting when health-care personnel are unaware of its potential value in an investigation. It is important that this type of evidence be saved and documented in all medical or accident instances that have legal implications.

Investigation of Wound Characteristics

When clients present to the emergency department with wounds from undiagnosed trauma, it is important for the clinical forensic nurse specialist to make a detailed documentation of the injuries. Failure to do so may interfere with the administration of justice should legal implications later arise. The following categories of medicolegal injuries are identified (Besant-Matthews, 2011; Brown, 2010a):

■ Sharp force injuries: includes stab wounds and other wounds resulting from penetration with a sharp object.

■ Blunt force injuries: includes cuts and bruises resulting from the impact of a blunt object against the body.

■ Dicing injuries: multiple, minute cuts and abrasions caused by contact with shattered glass (e.g., often occur in motor vehicle accidents)

■ Patterned injuries: specific injuries that reflect the pattern of the weapon used to inflict the injury.

■ Bite mark injuries: a type of patterned injury inflicted by human or animal.

■ Defense wounds: injuries that reflect the victim's attempt to defend himself or herself from attack.

■ Hesitation wounds: usually superficial, sharp force wounds; often found perpendicular to the lower part of the body and may reflect self-inflicted wounds.

■ Fast-force injuries: usually gunshot wounds; may reflect various patterns of injury.

Nurses managing the client's care in the emergency department must be able to make assessments about the type of wound, the weapon involved, and an estimate of the length of time between the injury and presentation for treatment.

Deaths in the Emergency Department

When deaths occur in the emergency department as a result of abuse or accident, evidence must be retained, the death must be reported to legal authorities, and an investigation is conducted. It is therefore essential that the nurse carefully document the appearance, condition, and behavior of the victim upon arrival at the hospital. The information gathered from the client and family (or others accompanying the client) may serve to facilitate the postmortem investigation and may be used during criminal justice proceedings.

The critical factor is to be able to determine if the cause of death is natural or unnatural. *Natural* deaths occur because of disease pathology of the internal organs or the degenerative aging process (Lynch & Koehler, 2011). In the emergency department, most deaths are sudden and unexpected. Those that are considered natural most commonly involve the cardiovascular, respiratory, and central nervous systems. Deaths that are considered *unnatural* include those from trauma, from self-inflicted acts, or from injuries inflicted by another. Legal authorities must be notified of all deaths related to unnatural circumstances.

Nursing Diagnosis

Clinical forensic nurse specialists in the trauma care setting analyze the information gathered during assessment of the client to formulate nursing diagnoses. Common nursing diagnoses relevant to forensic clients in the emergency department include:

■ Impaired tissue integrity

■ Risk for post-trauma syndrome

■ Fear

■ Anxiety

■ Risk for self-mutilation

■ Risk for suicide

■ Risk for complicated grieving

Planning/Implementatation
Preservation of Evidence

When a trauma victim is admitted to the emergency department, the most obvious priority intervention is medical stabilization. This priority must be balanced against the need to protect rapidly deteriorating physical evidence that can determine if a crime has occurred.

Wounds must be examined to speculate about the type of weapon used and to estimate age of the wound. Clothing must be checked for blood, semen, gunshot residue, or trace materials such as hair, fibers, and other debris. Clothing that is removed from a victim should not be shaken, so any evidence that may be adhering to it is not lost. Each separate item of clothing should be carefully placed in a paper bag, sealed, dated, timed, and signed. Plastic bags should never be used because of the tendency for condensation to occur. This promotes the growth of mold and the decay of biological tissue, which results in contamination of the evidence (Brown, 2010a; Saferstein, 2011).

When the trauma is sexual assault, a SANE may be called to the emergency department. SANEs usually work on-call, and because most sexual assault victims are women, female nurses are employed as SANEs. Male victims of sexual assault also most often prefer to work with a female SANE, because the perpetrators are usually men and because of the subsequent mistrust of men following the attack.

Ledray (2001) suggested the following essential components of a forensic examination of the sexual assault survivor in the emergency department.

Treatment and Documentation of Injuries

Emergency department (ED) staff typically performs the initial assessments when a sexual assault victim arrives. Obtaining vital signs and treatment of serious injuries often occur before the arrival of the SANE. Unless the injuries are life threatening, the forensic examination should occur before medical treatment is administered so as not to destroy physical evidence that is needed to establish that a sexual crime has occurred.

It is often expected that a sexual assault survivor must exhibit cuts and bruises in the genital or nongenital area. It has been estimated that there are no visible physical injuries in 40 to 60 percent of sexual assaults (American Medical Association [AMA], 1999). Absence of physical trauma does not necessarily mean that no force was used and that consent was given. This, however, is the case often used by defense attorneys in court. The AMA (1999) suggested the use of a traumagram—a diagram of a nude figure on which the locations of visible injuries are made. A written description of the color, size, and location of each wound, abrasion, and laceration is then documented. With the client's permission, photographs of the wounds should be taken for accurate documentation.

The nurse may use a **colposcope** to examine for tears and abrasions inside the vaginal area. A colposcope is an instrument that contains a magnifying lens and a light source, and to which a 35-mm camera can be attached.

Some states have legally mandated procedures, and some acute care settings also have established protocols, for gathering evidence in cases of sexual assault. In some instances, "rape kits" are available for collecting specimens and laboratory samples in a competent manner that is consistent with legal requirements and that will not interfere with the victim's option to pursue criminal charges. In addition to the vaginal examination, oral and rectal examinations may be conducted. Fingernail scrapings and body, head, and pubic hair samples should also be collected. Client hair samples are important to be able to differentiate them from those of the assailant. As previously stated, all evidence should be sealed in paper, *not* plastic, bags to prevent the possible growth of mildew from accumulation of moisture inside the plastic container, and subsequent contamination of the evidence.

Some states may require a urine specimen to test for pregnancy or screen for drugs. It is best, if possible, to wait until the initial internal examination is complete before collecting the urine sample. However, the AMA (1999) stated, "Patients needing to urinate before the internal examination should be allowed to do so, with a notation being made in the medical record."

Maintaining the Proper Chain of Custody

Stokowski (2008a) stated, "*Chain of custody* is a legal process referring to the paper trail that assures the integrity and security of the evidence." Unless the proper chain of custody has been maintained, the evidence cannot be used successfully in a court of law to convict an assailant. To preserve and maintain the chain of custody, each item of evidence is sealed and labeled with the client's name, a description and source of the item, name of the person who sealed the evidence, and date and time it was sealed. Stokowski (2008a) stated,

> Collected evidence must remain on the person of the nurse, in plain view, or in a secure location to maintain the chain of custody. Evidence should never be left unattended or handled by patients, parents, support persons, or caseworkers. Sealed and correctly labeled evidence kits or bags may be stored in a secure location until they are transferred to law enforcement officials. The best place to store evidence is in a locked drop box and locked refrigerator, located in a limited access room that requires a key entry.

Treatment and Evaluation of Sexually Transmitted Diseases

The AMA (1999) recommended that counseling about, and prophylaxis for, sexually transmitted diseases (STDs) be given to sexual assault victims. Conducted within 72 hours of the attack, several tests and interventions are available. Prophylactic antibiotics may be given to prevent chlamydia, gonorrhea, trichomoniasis, and bacterial vaginosis according to guidelines from the Centers for Disease Control and Prevention (CDC, 2002). They also recommend post-exposure prophylaxis using hepatitis B immunoglobulin. Information also should be provided describing symptoms of STDs for which there are no preventive measures. Because incubation periods vary, the importance of follow-up testing must be emphasized.

There is no proven prophylactic intervention for human HIV infection, and this is a serious concern for sexual assault victims. Even though the CDC (2002) reported that the risk for acquiring HIV infection through sexual assault is low in most cases, some states mandate testing for HIV as part of the sexual assault protocol. The AMA (1999) stated, "Baseline testing can diagnose or rule out preexisting HIV infection, but repeated testing after 6 months and again in 1 year is recommended, particularly when the assailant is known to be HIV positive or the serostatus is unknown" (p. 15).

Pregnancy Risk Evaluation and Prevention

It is important that sexual assault victims receive information related to risks and interventions for prevention of conception as a result of the assault. Evaluation of pregnancy risk is based on the client's ability to relay accurate information about the occurrence of her last menses so that an estimate can be made of time of ovulation. A combined regimen of ethinyl estradiol and levonorgestrel (Ovral) has been available for a number of years. Two tablets are taken at the time of treatment and two tablets are taken 12 hours later. An antiemetic, such as trimethobenzamide (Tigan), may be given to prevent nausea and vomiting, the most common side effects of the medication. A progestin-only contraceptive (Plan B One-Step; Next Choice) is available over-the-counter to individuals 18 years of age and by prescription to those less than age 18. These single-medication treatments appear to be somewhat more effective than the combined-medication treatment, and consequently have become the emergency contraceptive of choice. Some studies have shown the risk of pregnancy is reduced by 88 percent with the single-medication treatment and by 75 percent with the combined-medication contraceptive (Office of Population Research, 2010). The effectiveness of both methods decreases as the time between the assault and administration of the first dose increases.

Crisis Intervention and Arrangements for Follow-Up Counseling

In the hours immediately following the sexual assault, the rape victim experiences an overwhelming sense of violation and helplessness that began with the powerlessness and intimidation experienced during the rape. Burgess (2010) has identified two emotional response patterns that may occur within hours after a rape and that health-care workers may encounter in the emergency department or rape crisis center. In the *expressed response pattern,* the victim expresses feelings of fear, anger, and anxiety through such behaviors as crying, sobbing, smiling, restlessness, and tension. In the *controlled response pattern,* the feelings are masked or hidden, and a calm, composed, or subdued affect is seen. Brown (2010b) suggested that helping the victim to regain a sense of control—that is, helping her to make decisions about what she wants to do—can be an effective method of enhancing recovery. Brown (2010b) stated:

> Lack of control during a rape or sexual assault creates special needs in victims. These women need to feel in control [of everything that happens in the ED]. Any hint of lack of control can trigger an uncooperative, difficult, or anxious response, and they may be lost to follow-up. Providing as much control as possible for these women in clinical situations within safety guidelines may greatly increase their comfort level.

This is also an important time to ensure that the victim understands that she is not to blame for what has happened. She may be blaming herself and feeling guilty for certain behaviors, such as drinking or walking alone late at night, that may have placed her in a vulnerable position. It is important to communicate the following to the victim of sexual assault:

■ You are safe here.

■ I'm sorry that it happened.

■ I'm glad you survived.

■ It's not your fault. No one deserves to be treated this way.

■ You did the best that you could.

Before she leaves the emergency department, the individual should be advised about the importance of returning for follow-up counseling. She should be given the names of individuals to call for support. Often a survivor will not follow up with aftercare because she is too ashamed or is fearful of having to relive the nightmare of the attack by sharing the information in group or individual counseling. For this reason, it may be important for the nurse to get permission from the individual to allow a counselor to call her to make a follow-up appointment.

Deaths in the Emergency Department

The emergency department becomes the scene of legal investigation when death occurs in the trauma care setting. Evidence is preserved and the body is protected until the investigation has been completed. Lynch (2011) stated,

> The medical examiner and the crime laboratory rely on the attending staff to provide an accurate and detailed description of wounds, to collect and preserve admission or postmortem blood and body fluids, and to recognize and recover trace evidence. The forensic nurse examiner on duty will be responsible for gathering essential documents, contacting appropriate authorities and agencies, ensuring notification of death, and intervening with the decedent's family. (p. 203)

Anatomical Gifts

When a sudden and unexpected death occurs in the trauma care setting, the clinical forensic nurse may become involved in organ/tissue donation. Some states now require that a request for organ/tissue donation be made of the family when a death occurs under certain circumstances. This is a very painful period for family members, and nurses may feel it is an inappropriate time to present the information associated with an anatomical request. However, most nurses employed in trauma care recognize that organ/tissue recovery for transplantation is a requisite component of their work. Shafer (2011) stated,

> The forensic nurse examiner (FNE) can serve as a bridge between families of the bereaved and the medical examiner. Time spent with grieving families, helping them to cope with the events surrounding the death of their loved one, is certainly a role in which the FNE, as a nurse, would excel. Organ and tissue donation are often the only comfort that a family gains in an otherwise tragic situation. The FNE works closely with the organ recovery coordinator by coordinating information in donation situations, and she or he works jointly with other healthcare professionals by assisting families in moving forward through their loss. (p. 596)

Evaluation

Evaluation of the clinical forensic nursing process in the trauma care setting involves ongoing measurement of the diagnostic criteria aimed at resolution of identified real or potential problems.

The following types of questions may provide assistance in the evaluation process:

■ Have the physical and psychological needs of the survivors who present themselves to the emergency department been met?

■ Has the evidence in potential criminal investigations been handled such that it can be used in a credible manner?

■ Has the sexual assault survivor received information related to choices pertaining to STDs, pregnancy, and follow-up counseling?

■ In the instance of sudden and unexpected death in the emergency department, have the needs of the grieving family been met?

■ Has the importance of anatomical donations been communicated?

The role of the clinical forensic nurse in trauma care continues to expand. With the widespread prevalence of societal violence, clinical forensic nurses potentially may intervene in the examination of victims of all types of abuse situations. The clinical forensic nurse specialist must also strive to be proactive, beginning with educating emergency department staff in the philosophy and interventions of clinical forensic nursing practice. Within the community, proactive responsibilities may include providing information about environmental hazards and issues that may affect public health and safety. Effectiveness of these changes provides measurement for ongoing evaluation.

Application of the Nursing Process in Forensic Psychiatric Nursing in Correctional Facilities

Assessment

Notwithstanding the positive intentions of deinstitutionalization, some negative consequences may have ensued. Raphael and Stoll (2010) stated:

> The deinstitutionalization of the mentally ill juxtaposed against the increase in incarceration rates and the current high incidence of severe mental illness behind bars begs the question of whether the mentally ill have been trans-institutionalized from mental hospitals to prisons and jails. To the extent that the untreated mentally ill are more likely to commit crime, and that deinstitutionalization was not offset by sufficient expansion of outpatient mental health services, the closing of U.S. mental hospitals may have contributed to the drastic increase in U.S. incarceration rates

over the past several decades, with prisons and jails becoming de facto mental institutions. (p. 2)

It was believed that deinstitutionalization increased the freedom of mentally ill individuals in accordance with the principle of "least restrictive alternative." Because of inadequate community-based services, however, many of these individuals drifted into poverty and homelessness, increasing their vulnerability to criminalization. Because the bizarre behavior of mentally ill individuals living on the street is sometimes offensive to community standards, law enforcement officials have the authority to protect the welfare of the public and the safety of the individual by initiating emergency hospitalization. Legal criteria for commitment are so stringent in most cases, however, that arrest becomes an easier way of getting the mentally ill person off the street if a criminal statute has been violated. According to the Bureau of Justice Statistics, more than half of all prison and jail inmates have some form of mental health problem (James & Glaze, 2006). Some of these individuals are incarcerated as a result of the increasingly popular "guilty but mentally ill" verdict. With this verdict, the individual is deemed mentally ill, yet is held criminally responsible for his or her actions. He or she is incarcerated and receives special treatment, if needed, but no different from that available for and needed by any prisoner.

The U.S. Department of Justice has reported that U.S. prisons and jails held more than 2 million inmates in 2009 (West, 2010). The report stated that 34 percent of those incarcerated were white, 39 percent were African American, 21 percent were Hispanic, and 6 percent were American Indians, Alaska Natives, Asians, Pacific Islanders, or of two or more races. Men accounted for 87 percent of the total.

Care of the mentally-ill offender population is a highly specialized area of nursing practice. The rationale of imprisonment for criminal behavior has been identified as:

■ Retribution to society

■ Deterrence of future crimes

■ Rehabilitation and repentance

■ Protection of society

If an institution bases its orientation on retribution and deterrence of criminal activity, the prison will reflect a punishment-oriented atmosphere. If rehabilitation and repentance are accepted as a basis for change, mental health programs that encourage reflection and insight may be a part of the correctional setting. Because at times these basic objectives may seem incompatible with each other, nurses who work in correctional facilities may struggle with a cognitive dissonance founded in their basic nursing value system.

IMPLICATIONS OF RESEARCH FOR EVIDENCE-BASED PRACTICE

Yurkovich, E., & Smyer, T. (2000, June). Health maintenance behaviors of individuals with severe and persistent mental illness in a state prison. _Journal of Psychosocial Nursing and Mental Health Services, 38_(6), 20–31.

DESCRIPTION OF THE STUDY: The purpose of this study was to define health and health-seeking behaviors of incarcerated individuals experiencing severe and persistent mental illness (SPMI) in a state prison. The researchers conducted a comparative analysis of these findings to two studies that explored the same questions with individuals experiencing SPMI and attending two different community treatment centers. The researchers also examined strategies used by inmates with SPMI to prevent loss of control and maintain health in the prison environment. Information was gathered by in-depth interview using a semi-structured interview guide, participant observation,

and review of inmates' charts. Nineteen prisoners with SPMI participated. Age range was 21 to 56 and educational level ranged from 4 to 18 years. Fifteen prisoners had committed crimes against persons and 4 had committed crimes against property. Criminal activity was related to substance abuse in 15 of the cases. All interviews were conducted in a room set aside for the researchers in the prison infirmary.

RESULTS OF THE STUDY: Individuals in the community are able to define their environment through use of health-care providers and the trusted informal system of peers, friends, and relatives. Individuals with SPMI in the corrections facility do not have this connection. Negative response from other inmates to the behavior of inmates with SPMI reduces their ability to seek an appropriate level of assistance and maintain a healthy status. Some comparisons from the study are as follows:

Continued

IMPLICATIONS OF RESEARCH FOR EVIDENCE-BASED PRACTICE—cont'd

VARIABLE	COMMUNITY-BASED INDIVIDUALS	INMATES WITH SPMI
Relationships	Maintains a balance within family	Maintains relationships based on purpose (e.g., to provide protection or prevent abuse)
Feelings	Controls negative feelings and prevents destructive outcome when feeling angry (e.g., leave hostile environment)	Control of negative feelings by self-imposed solitude, lockdown, or withdrawal from socialization areas
Attitude	Builds self-esteem through purpose or goal completion	Lack of opportunity for building self-esteem
Functional Behaviors	Performs ADLs and participates in treatment center activities	Lacks opportunities to perform and participate

The prisoners demonstrated a need for education about their illnesses and medications. They demonstrated little insight into how stress and poor physical health affected their mental illness.

IMPLICATIONS FOR NURSING PRACTICE: The authors stated, "This study communicates a message from prisoners with SPMI that tells health care providers how they struggle to maintain a healthy status within a toxic environment and what they need to support this process. Nurses within a correctional setting have a responsibility to assist individuals with SPMI to interpret their environment, define role behaviors, and determine how to maintain wellness within the prison system."

Assessing Mental Health Needs of the Incarcerated

Is the provision of mental health care within the custodial environment possible? Or are clinical care concerns incompatible with security issues? What special knowledge and skills must a psychiatric nurse possess to be successful in caring for the mentally ill offender?

Psychiatric diagnoses commonly identified in incarcerated individuals include schizophrenia, bipolar disorder, major depression, substance use disorders, and personality disorders, and many have dual diagnoses. Common psychiatric behaviors include hallucinations, suspiciousness, thought disorders, anger/agitation, and impulsivity. Denial of problems is a common behavior among this population. Use of substances and medication noncompliance are common obstacles to rehabilitation. Substance abuse has been shown to have a strong correlation with recidivism among the prison population. Many individuals report that they were under the influence of illegal substances at the time of their criminal actions. Detoxification frequently occurs in jails and prisons, and some deaths have occurred from the withdrawal syndrome because of inadequate treatment during this process.

Although many people use the terms *prison* and *jail* interchangeably, there is a fundamental difference between the two. Local jails are usually administered by city or county officials and house defendants awaiting a trial, sentencing, or transfer to a prison. They commonly confine defendants convicted of misdemeanor, and for periods of less than a year. In contrast, prisons, which are run by state or federal administrations, are correctional facilities that house individuals convicted of major crimes or felonies and who are serving sentences that are usually in excess of a year. A large portion of offenders who are mentally ill, particularly the acutely psychotic, never reach the prison system. Frequent arrests for minor offenses may lead to numerous jail incarcerations, a sense of loss of control, and a continual state of crisis. The National Center on Institutions and Alternatives (2009) reported that the suicide rate in county jails is several times greater than that of the general population, while the suicide rate in prisons remains slightly higher than in the community.

Special Concerns

Overcrowding and Violence

Numerous studies have shown that crowding affects the level of violence in prisons. The prison system is not capable of handling the burden of large numbers of prisoners for which it has become responsible, and many of the infractions by prisoners are violent in nature. The growing number of prisoners is thought to be related to the increasing war on drugs, longer mandatory sentencing, and the "three strikes and you're out" laws. As this population continues to grow, the solution seems to be to continue to construct larger and larger complexes to house the growing numbers of inmates. The unfortunate truth lies in the fact that violent behavior often proves to be resourceful for the individuals who use it in prison.

Inmate violence directed toward prison staff is also a common occurrence. Light (1991) reported the most frequently cited motives as: inmate resistance to officer's commands, protest of unjust treatment, resistance to searches and attempt to remove contraband, and staff intervention in fights between inmates. Actual or implied verbal threats and swearing are the common everyday language of most offender clients. Nurses who work in correctional facilities must be able to adjust to the commonality of physical and verbal aggression if they are to prevail in this chosen area of specialization.

Sexual Assault

On September 4, 2003, President George W. Bush signed into law the Prison Rape Elimination Act of 2003. This legislation requires the Bureau of Justice Statistics (BJS) to develop new national data collections on the incidence and prevalence of sexual violence within correctional facilities (Beck, Harrison, & Adams, 2007). Currently, it is estimated that at least 13 percent of inmates in the United States have been sexually assaulted in prison, with many of them suffering repeated assaults (Cornell University Law School, 2010). The majority of these assaults go unreported because the consequences of "ratting" on fellow prisoners are often far more serious than the rape itself.

Rape in prison is viewed as an act of dominance and power, rather than one that is sexually motivated, and the majority of both victims and victimizers are heterosexuals. The typical victim is a young person convicted of a nonviolent crime. They are most likely to be first-time offenders who are small, weak, shy, and inexperienced with prison life. In some instances, sexual assault is used as a means of punishment and social control when the victim is believed to have violated certain unwritten prison codes. Gang rape is not uncommon, and severe physical injury is often the result if the victim attempts to defend himself.

HIV Infection in the Prison Population

The AIDS rate is more than three times higher in state and federal prisons than in the general U.S. population (CDC), 2009). In addition to sexual conduct, other means of HIV transmission among inmates include fights that result in lacerations, bites, or bleeding. Body piercing and tattooing are popular in prison, and clean instruments for these activities are not available. Intravenous drug use results in sharing of unsterilized injection equipment.

HIV has placed an enormous financial burden on a prison system that was already financially distressed. Some terminally ill prisoners with advanced HIV disease are being granted early compassionate release to family or hospice care and with access to community health services (Kantor, 2006).

The most recent approach to prevention of HIV transmission has shifted from segregation to education. Education of the prison population about HIV is difficult because as many as 50 percent of American prisoners are functionally illiterate, and many do not speak English (Kantor, 2006). Educational programs to meet the communication needs of this special population would be required.

Female Offenders

Women comprise approximately 10 percent of the total population in prisons and jails (West, 2010). As a minority group, they appear to be discriminated against within the prison system. Their facilities are usually more isolated, making it more difficult for family visits. In some instances, separate institutions do not exist, making it necessary to house male and female offenders in co-correctional facilities. Men are given a greater number of opportunities regarding education and vocational training services. McClellan (2002) stated:

> My first study of women prisoners uncovered striking disparity: women prisoners were cited more often for disciplinary infractions than were men. Rules scrupulously enforced in women's institutions were routinely ignored in men's. Although their infractions were less serious in nature, women were punished more severely than men. Operating under the same set of court-mandated formal rules, prisons display two gender-differentiated systems of surveillance and control. (p. 36)

Many women are single mothers who are unable to make adequate provision for their children while they serve their time in prison and who often lose custody of their children to the state. Prison health care is mostly inadequate, and the unique health needs of women often go unmet. Many of these women had very little before they were incarcerated, and have come to expect that little is what they deserve. Many report long histories of sexual and emotional abuse throughout their lives. Depression and acting-out behaviors are common in women's prisons.

Nursing Diagnosis

Forensic psychiatric nurse specialists in correctional facilities analyze the information gathered during assessment of the client to formulate nursing diagnoses. Common nursing diagnoses relevant to forensic clients in correctional facilities include:

- Defensive coping
- Complicated grieving
- Anxiety/fear
- Disturbed thought processes
- Powerlessness
- Low self-esteem
- Risk for self-mutilation
- Risk for self-directed or other-directed violence
- Ineffective coping
- Risk for infection
- Rape-trauma syndrome

Planning/Implementation

Psychiatric nurses who work in correctional facilities must be armed with extraordinary psychosocial skills and the knowledge to apply them in the most appropriate manner.

Development of a Therapeutic Relationship

Incarcerated individuals have difficulty trusting anyone associated with authority, including nurses. For most of these individuals, this likely relates back to very early stages of development and lack of nurturing.

Aside from the added difficulty of dealing with this special population, development of a therapeutic relationship in the correctional facility encompasses the same phases of interaction as it does with other clients. Chapter 7 of this text discusses the dynamics of this process at length.

Preinteraction Phase

During this phase, the nurse must examine his or her feelings, fears, and anxieties about working with prisoners, and in particular violent offenders—perhaps murderers, rapists, or pedophiles. This is the phase in which the nurse must determine whether he or she is able to separate the *person* from the *behavior* and provide the unconditional positive regard that Rogers (1951) believed identified each individual as a worthwhile and unique human being.

Orientation (Introductory) Phase

This is the phase in which the nurse works to establish trust with the client. This is a lengthy and intense process with the prisoner population. The characteristics that have been identified as significant to the development of a therapeutic nurse-client relationship—rapport, trust, and genuineness—are commonly met with suspicion on the part of the offender. Empathy may be used as a tool for manipulating the nurse. It is therefore imperative that limits be established and enforced by all of the nursing staff. Testing of limits is commonplace, so consequences for violation must be consistently administered. Splitting treatment team members against each other is a common ploy among inmates.

Touch and self-disclosure, two elements used in the establishment of trust with clients, are most commonly unacceptable with the prisoner population. A handshake may be appropriate, but any other form of touch between nurse and inmate of the opposite gender is usually restricted in most settings. Self-disclosure is commonly used to convey empathy and to promote trust by helping the client view the nurse as an ordinary human being. With the prisoner population, however, the client may seek personal information about the nurse in an effort to maintain control of the relationship. Nurses must maintain awareness of the situation and ensure that personal boundaries are not being violated.

Communication within the correctional facility may prove to be a challenge for the nurse. Slang terminology is commonplace and changes rapidly. Some of these terms are presented in Box 38-2.

Working Phase

Nursing skills are implemented during the working phase of the relationship, and promoting behavioral change is the primary goal. This is extremely difficult with offenders who commonly deny problems and resist change. Transference and counter-transference issues (see Chapter 7) are more common in working with this population than with other psychiatric clients. Issues are discussed in the treatment team meetings, and ongoing modifications are made as required. Following are some of

BOX 38-2 Glossary of Prison Slang

Ad-Seg. Administrative segregation. A prisoner placed on ad-seg is being investigated and will go into isolation (the "hole") until the investigation is complete.

Beef. Criminal charges. As, "I caught a burglary beef this time around." Also used to mean a problem. "I have a beef with that guy."

Big Yard. The main recreation yard.

Bit. Prison sentence, usually relatively short. "I got a three-year bit." (opposite of *jolt*)

Bitch, bitched (v). To be sentenced as a "habitual offender."

Blocks. Cellhouses.

Books. Administratively controlled account ledger that lists each prisoner's account balance.

Bone Yard. The visiting trailers, used for overnight visits of wives and/or families.

Bum Beef. A false accusation. Also, a wrongful conviction.

Catch a Ride. To ask a friend with drugs to get you high. "Hey man, can I catch a ride?"

The Chain. The bus transports that bring prisoners to prison. One is shackled and chained when transported. As, "I've been riding the chain," or "I just got in on the chain," or "Is there anyone we know on the chain?"

Check-In. Someone who has submitted to pressure, intimidation, debts, etc., and no longer feels secure in the prison population and "checks in" to a protective custody (PC) unit.

Chi-Mo. Child molester; also "chester," "baby-raper," "short-eyes" (as "he has short-eyes," meaning he goes after young children). The worst of the *rapo* class in the eyes of *convicts*.

Convict. Guys who count in prison; loyal to the code; aren't stool pigeons; their word is good. (opposite of *inmate*)

C.U.S. Custody unit supervisor/cellhouse supervisor.

De-Seg. Disciplinary segregation. When a person is on de-seg, he is in isolation (the "hole") for an infraction.

Ding. A disrespectful term for a mentally ill prisoner.

Dry Snitching. To inform on someone indirectly by talking loudly or performing suspicious actions when officers are in the area.

Dummy Up; Get on the Dummy. To shut up, to pipe down, to be quiet, especially about one's knowledge of a crime.

E.P.R.D. Earliest possible release date.

Fish. A new arrival, a first-timer, a bumpkin, not wise to prison life.

Gate Money. Money the state gives a prisoner upon his release.

Gate Time. At most prisons they yell "gate time," meaning prisoners can get in or out of their cells. See *lock-up*.

Hacks/Hogs/Pigs/Snouts/Screws/Cops/Bulls. The guards; called "Corrections Officers" by themselves and *inmates.*

Heat Wave. Being under constant suspicion, thereby bringing attention to those around you.

Hit It. Go away, leave, get lost

Hold Your Mud. Do not tell, even under pressure of punishment.

The Hole. An isolation ("segregation") cell, used as punishment for offenses.

House. Cell.

Hustle. A professional criminal's avocation. Also refers to any scheme to obtain money or drugs while in prison.

I.K. Inmate kitchen.

I.M.U. Intensive Management Unit. Administration's name for "segregation" or "the hole."

Inmate. Derogatory term for prisoners. Used by guards, administrators, other inmates, or new arrivals who don't know the language yet. (Opposite of *convict*)

Jacket. Prison file containing all information on a prisoner. "He's a child molester; it's in his jacket." Also reputation. Prisoners can put false jackets on other prisoners to discredit them.

Jolt. A long sentence. ("I got a life jolt.") (Opposite of *bit*)

Jumping-Out. Turning to crime. "I've been jumping out since I was a kid."

Keister. To hide something in the anal cavity.

Lag. A *convict*, as in, "He's an old lag, been at it all his life."

Lifer or "All Day." Anyone doing a life sentence. A life *jolt.*

Continued

BOX 38-2 Glossary of Prison Slang—cont'd

Lock-Down. When prisoners are confined to their cells.

Lock-Up. Free movement period for prisoners. (See also *gate time*)

Lop. Same as *inmate*.

Mule. A person who smuggles drugs into the institution.

On the Leg. A prisoner who is always chatting with and befriending guards.

Paper. A small quantity of drugs packaged for selling.

P.C. Protective custody. Also as in "He's a PC case," meaning weak or untrustworthy.

Point/Outfit. Syringe.

Pruno. Homemade wine.

Punk. Derogatory term meaning homosexual or weak individual.

Rapo. Anyone with a sex crime—generally looked down on by *convicts.*

Rat/Snitch/Stool Pigeon. n., informant. v., to inform.

Stand Point. Watch for "the man" (guard).

Tag/Write-Up. Infraction of institution rules.

The Bag/Sack. Dope.

Tom or George. Meaning "no good" (Tom) or "okay" (George). Used in conversation to indicate if someone or something is okay or not.

Turned Out. To be forced into homosexual acts, or to turn someone out to do things for you; to use someone for your own needs.

White Money. Currency within the institution.

Yard-In/Yard-Out. Closing of the recreation yard (yard-in). Recreation yard opens (yard-out).

---

the interventions associated with psychiatric forensic nursing in correctional institutions.

Counseling and Supportive Psychotherapy Nurses may work with inmates who are experiencing feelings of powerlessness and grief. Women who have left children behind may fear the permanent loss of custody or of never seeing them again. Helping these individuals work through a period of mourning is an important nursing intervention.

Nurses may also counsel victims of sexual assault. Victims of sexual assault in prison often experience the symptoms associated with rape-trauma syndrome. Feelings of helplessness and vulnerability, coupled with shame, humiliation, and embarrassment, are characteristic. Internalized rage can become paralytic. Perception of gender identity may even be compromised.

These individuals often become withdrawn and isolated and are at high risk for suicide. The nurse can recognize these symptoms and intervene as required. All unusual behavior should be shared with the treatment team. Interventions for treating specific behaviors (such as depression and suicide, psychotic

behaviors, and antisocial behaviors) are located in Units 3 and 4 of this text.

Crisis Intervention Behaviors such as aggression, self-mutilation, suicide attempts, acute psychotic episodes, and post-trauma responses require that the nurse be proficient in crisis intervention. Feelings of helplessness and loss of control are pervasive in the prison population. The chaotic, overburdened prison system lacks the resources to provide the kind of services needed to prevent the continual state of crisis these conditions engender. Suicide risk is higher in jails and prisons than it is in the community. Noncompliance with prison rules, feelings of hopelessness, psychopathology, substance abuse, and overcrowded conditions all contribute to the potential for violence. Threatening behaviors must be reported immediately to all members of the treatment team. A strong foundation in crisis intervention theory and techniques is mandatory for nurses who work in correctional institutions.

Education Opportunities for teaching abound in the correctional facility. As was mentioned previously, however, because of the level of education of many incarcerated individuals, and because many of them speak little English, the teaching plan must be highly individualized. Many have no desire or motivation to learn and resist cooperating with these efforts. Important educational endeavors with these clients include:

- **Health Teaching.** Most criminals are not in good physical condition when they reach prison. They have lived rough lives of smoking, poor diets, substance abuse, and minimal health care. This is an opportunity for nurses to provide information about ways to achieve optimum wellness.

- **HIV/AIDS Education.** Kantor (2006) stated:

   All persons entering prison must be informed in clear, simple terms, *and in their own language,* about how to avoid transmission of HIV and other communicable diseases. Educational programs can reduce fears about HIV and its transmission among staff members and inmates. Individual counseling, peer counseling, support groups, and special programs for women, designed by and for prisoners, have been successful in a number of institutions and seem to be the best educational tools.

   Some correctional institutions now provide condoms to inmates, but this remains a point of controversy between legal and public health officials.

- **Stress Management.** Nurses can present information and demonstration of stress management techniques. They can help individuals practice reduction of anxiety without resorting to medications or substances.

- **Substance Abuse.** The Federal Bureau of Prisons (2010) has established a comprehensive substance abuse treatment strategy in an effort to change inmates' criminal and drug-using behaviors. This strategy begins with drug abuse education and ends with a strong community transition component. The individuals receive information about alcohol and drugs and the physical, social, and psychological impact of abusing these substances. Since its inception, this program has proved highly successful in decreasing recidivism and relapse rates among its participants.

   Nurses can participate in substance abuse treatment programs by providing client education (e.g., the effects of substances on the body; the consequences of sharing needles). They can also form support groups for individuals who abuse substances if one does not exist in the institution. A large percentage of the prison population has a history of substance abuse, and many correlate the commission of their crimes with substance use. This is an important area of need for nursing intervention in the correctional system.

Termination Phase

Ideally, the termination phase of the nurse-client relationship ensures therapeutic closure. This is not always possible in the correctional environment. Prisoners are transferred from one institution to another, and from one part of an institution to another, for a variety of reasons, not the least of which are safety and security of self or others. When possible, it is important for nurses to initiate termination with clients so that at least some semblance of closure can be achieved and a review of goal attainment can be accomplished. Community facilities for mentally ill ex-offenders are few, and recidivism is rampant. Johnson (2010) stated:

   The majority of mentally ill offenders need the basic elements of case management. Psychiatric nurses in correctional settings often act as case managers, beginning prerelease planning upon the initial contact with inmates. Continuation of any treatment and medication from jail and transition to the community-based treatment in a swift manner is critical to success. Unfortunately resources in this area are often lacking. Many inmates may not have predetermined release dates, thereby leading to releases at all hours of the day and night. Prerelease planning and coordination with community-based programs are necessary to promote continuity of care and prevent recidivism. Nurses are vital members of the interdisciplinary team and play significant roles in the assessment, planning, implementation, and evaluation of the case management plan to best meet the needs of patients.

Evaluation

Evaluation of the psychiatric forensic nursing process in the correctional environment involves ongoing measurement of the diagnostic criteria aimed at resolution of identified real or potential problems. The following types of questions may provide assistance in the evaluation process:

- Has a degree of trust been established in the nurse-client relationship?

- Has violence by the offender to self or others been prevented?

- If victimization has occurred, has appropriate care and support been provided to the survivor?

■ Have limits been set on inappropriate behaviors, and has consistency of consequences for violation of the limits been administered by all staff?

■ Have educational programs been established to provide information about health and wellness, HIV/AIDS, stress management, and substance abuse?

Evaluation is an ongoing process and must be assumed by the entire treatment team. Modification of the treatment plan as required is part of the ongoing evaluation process, and positive change within the system is the ultimate outcome. Nurses who work in correctional facilities are "pioneers" within the nursing profession. To share the knowledge gleaned from this specialty area is an important part of the nursing process.

Summary and Key Points

■ Forensic nursing, which is a growing area within the profession, is composed of a variety of areas of expertise.

■ Forensic nurses take care of both victims and perpetrators of crime in a variety of settings, including primary care facilities, hospitals, and correctional institutions.

■ The International Association of Forensic Nurses, founded in 1992, now has more than 3,000 members.

■ Forensic nursing specialties include clinical forensic nursing, the sexual assault nurse examiner, forensic psychiatric nursing, forensic correctional nursing, legal nurse consultant, and forensic nurse death investigator.

■ Nurses in general practice also find forensic nursing knowledge of importance in their practices, particularly in emergency departments and intensive care units.

■ Forensic nurses in trauma care are involved with preservation of evidence, investigation of wound characteristics, and management of responsibilities associated with deaths that occur in the emergency department, including assisting with requests for anatomical gifts.

■ Forensic psychiatric nursing in correctional facilities involves care of the mentally ill offender population, as well as the emotional needs of all incarcerated individuals.

■ Interventions for the forensic psychiatric nurse include establishment of a therapeutic relationship; providing counseling and supportive psychotherapy; intervening in crises; and providing education concerning health and wellness issues, HIV/AIDS, stress management, and substance abuse.

■ The number of educational offerings pertaining to forensic nursing is growing. Some content is taught in traditional nursing courses, and some colleges and universities are establishing forensic nursing courses as electives.

■ Forensic nursing is fertile ground for nursing research, and the complex nature of the specialty lends itself well to those nurses who seek a challenge within the profession.

 Additional info available @ davisplus.fadavis.com

TEST YOUR CRITICAL THINKING SKILLS

Kim is a 27-year-old woman who recently moved from a small town in Texas to work in the city of Dallas as a reporter for one of the major newspapers. She is 5'6" tall and weighs 115 lb. To keep in shape she likes to jog, which she did regularly in her hometown. She doesn't know anyone in Dallas and has been lonely for her family since arriving. But she has moved into a small apartment in a quiet neighborhood and hopes to meet young people soon though her work and church.

On the first Saturday morning after she moved into her new apartment, Kim decided to get up early and go jogging. It was still dark out, but Kim was not afraid. She had been jogging alone in the dark many times in her hometown. She donned her jogging clothes and headed down the quiet street toward a nearby park. As she entered the park, an individual came out from behind a dense clump of bushes, put a knife to her throat, and ordered her to the ground. She was raped and beaten unconscious. She remained in that condition until sunrise, when she was found by another jogger who called emergency services, and Kim was taken to the nearest emergency department. Upon regaining consciousness, Kim was hysterical, but a sexual assault nurse examiner (SANE) was called to the scene, and Kim was assigned to a quiet area of the hospital, where the post-rape examination was initiated.

Answer the following questions related to Kim:

1. What are the initial nursing interventions for Kim?

2. What treatments must the nurse ensure that Kim is aware are available for her?

3. What nursing diagnosis would the nurse expect to focus on with Kim in follow-up care?

Review Questions
Self-Examination/Learning Exercise

*Select the answer that is **most** appropriate for each of the following questions:*

1. Deaths that occur in the emergency department (ED) will be identified as *natural* or *unnatural*. Which of the following would be considered a natural death?
   a. A young man who died in a motorcycle accident.
   b. A young woman who was a victim of domestic violence.
   c. A middle-aged man who died of myocardial infarction.
   d. An elderly female victim who fell down a flight of stairs.

2. A young woman has been transported to the ED by emergency services. She has been physically beaten and sexually assaulted. Which of the following is the *priority* nursing intervention for this client?
   a. Take photographs of the injuries.
   b. Ensure stability of her physical injuries.
   c. Check her clothing for evidence of blood or semen.
   d. Notify her nearest relative.

3. Psychiatric behaviors observed to be common among mentally ill offenders include which of the following? (Select all that apply.)
   a. Denial of problems.
   b. Thought disorders.
   c. Self-mutilative behaviors.
   d. Dissociative behaviors.
   e. Anger and impulsivity.

4. When a victim of physical and sexual assault is admitted to the ED, his or her clothing is an important aspect of potential criminal evidence. Which of the following are correct procedures in the preservation of clothing as evidence? (Select all that apply.)
   a. Remove the clothing from the victim.
   b. Shake the clothing to remove anything that is adhering to it.
   c. Place each separate piece of clothing into a plastic bag.
   d. Seal each bag.
   e. Date, time, and sign each bag.

5. Which of the following is a true statement about the populations in U.S. prisons and jails?
   a. Females constitute about half of the total inmate population.
   b. HIV disease is more prevalent in the general population than in the inmate population.
   c. There is a disparity in U.S. prisons in the treatment of male and female prisoners.
   d. About a third of the U.S. prison and jail population has some form of mental health problem.

6. The forensic psychiatric nurse is working with a client who fatally injured a person while driving in an intoxicated condition. He says to the nurse, "It had nothing to do with my drinking. I've been drinking since I was 12 years old! I can handle my liquor just fine!" In preparing a care plan for this client, the nurse selects which of the following nursing diagnoses to address this problem?
   a. Defensive coping.
   b. Ineffective coping.
   c. Disturbed thought processes.
   d. Ineffective denial.

Continued

Review Questions—cont'd
Self-Examination/Learning Exercise

7. In attempting to establish a trusting relationship with an individual incarcerated in a correctional facility, the nurse must recognize which of the following to be a true statement?
   a. The offender population responds readily to genuineness on the part of the nurse.
   b. Touch is an important element of the nurse-client relationship with individuals in a correctional facility.
   c. In establishing a therapeutic relationship with an offender-client, the nurse may use self-disclosure to promote trust and convey empathy to the client.
   d. Empathy is essential to development of a trusting relationship, but may be used as manipulation by the prisoner population.

8. A woman is admitted to the ED with multiple physical injuries, and reports that she was mugged on the street by two men who beat her up and stole her purse. She has multiple bruises and abrasions on her arms, and notable cuts on the palms of her hands. The nurse recognizes the wounds on the woman's hands as most probably which of the following types?
   a. Blunt force injuries from impact of a blunt object.
   b. Defense wounds from her attempt to defend herself.
   c. Dicing injuries caused by contact with shattered glass.
   d. Fast-force injuries, probably caused by gunshot wounds.

9. Which of the following types of care may be given to a female sexual assault victim in the emergency department? (Select all that apply.)
   a. Prophylactic treatment for gonorrhea.
   b. Prophylactic treatment for HIV infection.
   c. Emergency prevention for conception as a result of the assault.
   d. Crisis intervention in the hours immediately following the assault.
   e. Arrangements for follow-up counseling.

10. Because follow-up counseling is crucial to the healing process for a sexual assault victim, and because these individuals often fail to follow up after they leave the ED, which of the following is the most effective way to ensure that the client receives the appropriate aftercare?
   a. Tell her that she needs to call the counselor's office and make an appointment as soon as possible.
   b. Make an appointment for her and give her the date and time written on an appointment card.
   c. Obtain permission from the client to have a follow-up counselor call her.
   d. Contact significant others to tell them that they need to ensure that the client sees a follow-up counselor.

References

American Medical Association. (1999). *Strategies for the treatment and prevention of sexual assault*. Chicago, IL: Science and Public Health Advocacy Programs.

American Nurses Association and International Association of Forensic Nurses. (2009). *Forensic nursing: Scope and standards of practice*. Silver Spring, MD: American Nurses Association.

Beck, A. J., Harrison, P. M., & Adams, D. B. (2007). *Sexual violence reported by correctional authorities, 2006*. Bureau of Justice Statistics Special Report, August 2007. Washington, DC: Bureau of Justice Statistics.

Bellfield, B., & Catalano, J. T. (2009). Developments in current nursing practice. In J. T. Catalano (Ed.), *Nursing now! Today's issues, tomorrow's trends* (5th ed., pp. 446–464). Philadelphia: F.A. Davis.

Besant-Matthews, P. E. (2011). Blunt, sharp, and firearm injuries. In V. A. Lynch (Ed.), *Forensic nursing science* (2nd ed., pp. 290–313). St. Louis: Mosby.

Brown, K. (2010a). Evidence collection and preservation in a healthcare setting. *Nursing Spectrum/Nurseweek CE: Course CE296-60*. Retrieved October 26, 2010, from http://ce.nurse.com/CE296-60/Evidence-Collection-and-Preservation-in-a-Healthcare-Setting/

Brown, K. (2010b). Sexual assault and rape: The nursing role. *Nursing spectrum/ Nurseweek CE: Course CE253-60*. Retrieved October 27, 2010, from http://ce.nurse.com/CE253-60/Sexual-Assault-and-Rape-The-Nursing-Role/

Burgess, A. (2010). Rape violence. *Nursing Spectrum/NurseWeek CE: Course 60025*. Retrieved October 27, 2010, from http://ce.nurse.com/60025/Rape-Violence

Centers for Disease Control and Prevention. (2002). Sexually transmitted diseases treatment guidelines 2002. *MMWR Recommendations and Reports, 51*(RR-6), 1–84.

Centers for Disease Control and Prevention. (2009). *HIV testing implementation guidance for correctional settings*. Retrieved October 29, 2010, from http://www.cdc.gov/hiv/topics/testing/resources/guidelines/correctional-settings/pdf/Correctional_Settings_Guidelines.pdf

Cornell University Law School. (2010). *U.S. Code, Title 42, Section 15601*. Cornell University Law School Legal Information Institute. Retrieved October 28, 2010, from http://www.law.cornell.edu/uscode/html/uscode42/usc_sec_42_00015601----000-.html

Dougherty, C. M. (2011). Evidence collection in the emergency department. In V. A. Lynch (Ed.), *Forensic nursing science* (2nd ed., pp. 155–167). St. Louis: Mosby.

Federal Bureau of Prisons. (2010). *Substance abuse treatment*. Retrieved October 30, 2010, from http://www.bop.gov/inmate_programs/substance.jsp

Hancock, P. (2010). Forensic nursing. *UFCW 141 Nurses*. Retrieved October 25, 2010, from http://www.ufcw141nurses.org/forensic%20ns.htm

Hufft, A., & Peternelj-Taylor, C. (2003). Forensic nursing: A specialty for the twenty-first century. In J. T. Catalano (Ed.). *Nursing now! Today's issues, tomorrow's trends* (3rd ed.). Philadelphia: F.A. Davis.

International Association of Forensic Nurses. (2010). *Areas of forensic nursing practice*. Retrieved October 25, 2010, from http://iafn.org/displaycommon.cfm?an=1&subarticlenbr=529

James, D. J., & Glaze, L. E. (2006). *Mental health problems of prison and jail inmates*. Bureau of Justice Statistics Special Report, September 2006. Washington, DC: Bureau of Justice Statistics.

Johnson, J. D. (2010). Psychiatric nursing in the correctional setting. *Nursing Spectrum/Nurseweek CE: Course CE522*. Retrieved October 30, 2010, from http://www.ce.nurse.com/CE522/Psychiatric-Nursing-in-the-Correctional-Setting/

Kantor, E. (2006). HIV transmission and prevention in prisons. *HIV InSite Knowledge Base*. Retrieved October 31, 2010, from http://hivinsite.ucsf.edu/InSite?page=kb-07&doc=kb-07-04-13

Ledray, L. E. (2001). Evidence collection and care of the sexual assault survivor: The SANE-SART response. *Violence Against Women*. Retrieved October 26, 2010, from http://www.mincava.umn.edu/documents/commissioned/2forensicevidence/2forensicevidence.html

Light, S. (1991). Assaults on prison officers: Interactional themes. *Justice Quarterly, 8*, 243–261.

Lynch, V. A. (2011). Global expansion and future perspective. In V. A. Lynch (Ed.), *Forensic nursing science* (2nd ed., pp. 617–629). St. Louis: Mosby

Lynch, V. A., & Koehler, S. A. (2011). Forensic investigation of death. In V. A. Lynch (Ed.), *Forensic nursing science* (2nd ed., pp. 179–194). St. Louis: Mosby.

McClellan, D. S. (2002). Coming to the aid of women in U.S. prisons. *Monthly Review, 54*(2), 33–44.

McPeck, P. (2002, January 21). Down to a science. *NurseWeek*, pp. 24–25.

National Center on Institutions and Alternatives. (2009). *Jail suicide prevention*. Retrieved October 28, 2010, from http://www.ncianet.org/suicideprevention/index.asp

Office of Population Research. (2010). *Emergency contraception*. Office of Population Research, Princeton University. Retrieved October 28, 2010, from http://ec.princeton.edu/emergency-contraception.html

Raphael, S., & Stoll, M. A. (2010). *Assessing the contribution of the deinstitutionalization of the mentally ill to growth in the U.S. incarceration rate*. Berkeley: The University of California, Goldman School of Public Policy (Berkley) and School of Public Affairs (Los Angeles).

Saferstein, R. (2011). Principles of forensic evidence collection and preservation. In V. A. Lynch (Ed.), *Forensic nursing science* (2nd ed., pp. 54–60). St. Louis: Mosby.

Shafer, T. J. (2011). Organ donation and tissue transplantation. In V. A. Lynch (Ed.). *Forensic nursing science* (2nd ed., pp. 581–597). St. Louis: Mosby.

Stokowski, L.A. (2008a). Forensic nursing: Part 1. Evidence collection for nurses. *MedscapeNursing, 2008*. Retrieved October 26, 2010, from http://cme.medscape.com/viewprogram/8908

Stokowski, L. A. (2008b). Forensic nursing: Part 2. Inside forensic nursing. *MedscapeNursing, 2008*. Retrieved October 25, 2010, from http://www.medscape.com/viewarticle/571555

West, H. C. (2010). *Prison inmates at midyear 2009*. Bureau of Justice Statistics. Retrieved October 27, 2010, from http://bjs.ojp.usdoj.gov/content/pub/pdf/pim09st.pdf

Classical Reference

Rogers, C. R. (1951). *Client centered therapy*. Boston: Houghton Mifflin.

@ INTERNET REFERENCES

- Additional sources related to forensic nursing may be located at the following websites:
  - http://www.forensiceducation.com/
  - http://www.iafn.org/
  - http://www.amrn.com/
  - http://nursing.advanceweb.com/common/Editorial/Editorial.aspx?CC=40302
  - http://www.forensicnursemag.com/

The Bereaved Individual

39

CORE CONCEPTS

grief

loss

CHAPTER OUTLINE

Objectives

Homework Assignment

Theoretical Perspectives on Loss and
   Bereavement

Length of the Grief Response

Anticipatory Grief

Maladaptive Responses to Loss

Application of the Nursing Process

Additional Assistance

Summary and Key Points

Review Questions

KEY TERMS

advance directive

anticipatory grieving

bereavement overload

delayed grief

hospice

luto

mourning

shiva

velorio

OBJECTIVES

After reading this chapter, the student will be able to:

1. Describe various types of loss that trigger the grief response in individuals.
2. Discuss theoretical perspectives of grieving as proposed by Elisabeth Kübler-Ross, John Bowlby, George Engel, and J. William Worden.
3. Differentiate between normal and maladaptive responses to loss.
4. Discuss grieving behaviors common to individuals at various stages across the life span.
5. Describe customs associated with grief in individuals of various cultures.
6. Formulate nursing diagnoses and goals of care for individuals experiencing the grief response.
7. Describe appropriate nursing interventions for individuals experiencing the grief response.
8. Identify relevant criteria for evaluating nursing care of individuals experiencing the grief response.
9. Describe the concept of hospice care for people who are dying and their families.
10. Discuss the use of advance directives for individuals to provide directions about their future medical care.

HOMEWORK ASSIGNMENT

Please read the chapter and answer the following questions:

1. What type of maladaptive response to loss occurs when an individual becomes fixed in the anger stage of grief? What clinical disorder is associated with this occurrence?
2. Describe the phenomenon of bereavement overload.
3. With what types of behaviors is grief manifested in school-age children?
4. According to Engel, when is the grief response thought to be resolved?

CORE CONCEPT

Loss

The experience of separation from something of personal importance.

Loss is anything that is perceived as such by the individual. The separation from loved ones or the giving up of treasured possessions, for whatever reason; the experience of failure, either real or perceived; or life events that create change in a familiar pattern of existence—all can be experienced as loss, and all can trigger behaviors associated with the grieving process. Loss and bereavement are universal events encountered by all beings that experience emotions. Following are examples of some notable forms of loss:

■ A significant other (person or pet), through death, divorce, or separation for any reason.

■ Illness or debilitating conditions. Examples include (but are not limited to) diabetes, stroke, cancer, rheumatoid arthritis, multiple sclerosis, Alzheimer's disease, hearing or vision loss, and spinal cord or head injuries. Some of these conditions not only incur a loss of physical and/or emotional wellness, but may also result in the loss of personal independence.

■ Developmental/maturational changes or situations, such as menopause, andropause, infertility, "empty nest," aging, impotence, or hysterectomy.

■ A decrease in self-esteem due to inability to meet self-expectations or the expectations of others (even if these expectations are only perceived by the individual as unfulfilled). This includes a loss of potential hopes and dreams.

■ Personal possessions that symbolize familiarity and security in a person's life. Separation from these familiar and personally valued external objects represents a loss of material extensions of the self.

CORE CONCEPT

Grief

Deep mental and emotional anguish that is a response to the subjective experience of loss of something significant.

Some texts differentiate the terms **mourning** and grief by describing mourning as the psychological process (or stages) through which the individual passes on the way to successful adaptation to the loss of a valued object. Grief may be viewed as the subjective states that accompany mourning, or the emotional work involved in the mourning process. For purposes of this text, grief work and the process of mourning are collectively referred to as the *grief response*.

This chapter examines human responses to the experience of loss. Care of bereaved individuals is presented in the context of the nursing process.

Theoretical Perspectives on Loss and Bereavement

Stages of Grief

Behavior patterns associated with the grief response include many individual variations. However, sufficient similarities have been observed to warrant characterization of grief as a syndrome that has a predictable course with an expected resolution. Early theorists, including Kübler-Ross (1969), Bowlby (1961), and Engel (1964), described behavioral stages through which individuals advance in their progression toward resolution. A number of variables influence one's progression through the grief process. Some individuals may reach acceptance, only to revert back to an earlier stage; some may never complete the sequence; and some may never progress beyond the initial stage.

A more contemporary grief specialist, J. William Worden (2009), offered a set of tasks that must be processed in order to complete the grief response. He suggested that it is possible for a person to accomplish some of these tasks and not others, resulting in an incomplete bereavement, and thus impairing further growth and development. A comparison of the similarities among these four models is presented in Table 39-1.

Elisabeth Kübler-Ross

These well-known stages of the grief process were identified by Kübler-Ross in her extensive work with dying patients. Behaviors associated with each of these stages can be observed in individuals experiencing the loss of any concept of personal value.

■ **Stage I: Denial.** In this stage the individual has difficulty believing that the loss has occurred. He or she may say, "No, it can't be true!" or "It's just not possible." This stage may protect the individual against the psychological pain of reality.

■ **Stage II: Anger.** This is the stage when reality sets in. Feelings associated with this stage

TABLE 39-1 Stages and Tasks of the Normal Grief Response: A Comparison of Models by Elisabeth Kübler-Ross, John Bowlby, George Engel, and William Worden

STAGES/TASKS				POSSIBLE TIME DIMENSION	BEHAVIORS
Kübler-Ross	Bowlby	Engel	Worden		
I. Denial	I. Numbness/ protest	I. Shock/disbelief	I. Accepting the reality of the loss	Occurs immediately on experiencing the loss. Usually lasts no more than a few weeks.	Individual has difficulty believing that the loss has occurred.
II. Anger	II. Disequilibrium	II. Developing awareness		In most cases begins within hours of the loss. Peaks within a few weeks.	Anger is directed toward self or others. Ambivalence and guilt may be felt toward the lost entity.
III. Bargaining					The individual fervently seeks alternatives to improve current situation.
		III. Restitution			Attends to various rituals associated with the culture in which the loss has occurred.
IV. Depression	III. Disorganization and despair	IV. Resolution of the loss	II. Processing the pain of grief	Very individual. Commonly 6 to 12 months. Longer for some.	The actual work of grieving. Preoccupation with the lost entity. Feelings of helplessness and loneliness occur in response to realization of the loss. Feelings associated with the loss are confronted.
			III. Adjusting to a world without the lost entity	Ongoing.	How the environment changes depends on the roles the lost entity played in the life of the bereaved person. Adaptations will have to be made as the changes are presented in daily life. New coping skills will have to be developed.
V. Acceptance	IV. Reorganization	V. Recovery	IV. Finding an enduring connection with the lost entity in the midst of embarking on a new life.		Resolution is complete. The bereaved person experiences a reinvestment in new relationships and new goals. The lost entity is not purged or replaced, but relocated in the life of the bereaved. At this stage, terminally ill persons express a readiness to die.

include sadness, guilt, shame, helplessness, and hopelessness. Self-blame or blaming of others may lead to feelings of anger toward the self and others. The anxiety level may be elevated, and the individual may experience confusion and a decreased ability to function independently. He or she may be preoccupied with an idealized image of what has been lost. Numerous somatic complaints are common.

■ **Stage III: Bargaining.** At this stage in the grief response, the individual attempts to strike a bargain with God for a second chance, or for more time. The person acknowledges the loss, or impending loss, but holds out hope for additional alternatives, as evidenced by statements such as, "If only I could. . ." or "If only I had. . . ."

■ **Stage IV: Depression.** In this stage, the individual mourns for that which has been or will be lost. This is a very painful stage, during which the individual must confront feelings associated with having lost someone or something of value (called *reactive* depression). An example might be the individual who is mourning a change in body image. Feelings associated with an impending loss (called *preparatory* depression) are also confronted. Examples include permanent lifestyle changes related to the altered body image or even an impending loss of life itself. Regression, withdrawal, and social isolation may be observed behaviors with this stage. Therapeutic intervention should be available, but not imposed, and with guidelines for implementation based on client readiness.

■ **Stage V: Acceptance.** At this time, the individual has worked through the behaviors associated with the other stages and accepts or is resigned to the loss. Anxiety decreases, and methods for coping with the loss have been established. The client is less preoccupied with what has been lost and increasingly interested in other aspects of the environment. If this is an impending death of self, the individual is ready to die. The person may become very quiet and withdrawn, seemingly devoid of feelings. These behaviors are an attempt to facilitate the passage by slowly disengaging from the environment.

John Bowlby

John Bowlby hypothesized four stages in the grief process. He implies that these behaviors can be observed in all individuals who have experienced the loss of something or someone of value, even in babies as young as 6 months of age.

■ **Stage I: Numbness or Protest.** This stage is characterized by a feeling of shock and disbelief that the loss has occurred. Reality of the loss is not acknowledged.

■ **Stage II: Disequilibrium.** During this stage, the individual has a profound urge to recover what has been lost. Behaviors associated with this stage include a preoccupation with the loss, intense weeping and expressions of anger toward the self and others, and feelings of ambivalence and guilt associated with the loss.

■ **Stage III: Disorganization and Despair.** Feelings of despair occur in response to realization that the loss has occurred. Activities of daily living become increasingly disorganized, and behavior is characterized by restlessness and aimlessness. Efforts to regain productive patterns of behavior are ineffective and the individual experiences fear, helplessness, and hopelessness. Somatic complaints are common. Perceptions of visualizing or being in the presence of that which has been lost may occur. Social isolation is common, and the individual may feel a great deal of loneliness.

■ **Stage IV: Reorganization.** The individual accepts or becomes resigned to the loss. New goals and patterns of organization are established. The individual begins a reinvestment in new relationships and indicates a readiness to move forward within the environment. Grief subsides and recedes into valued remembrances.

George Engel

■ **Stage I: Shock and Disbelief.** The initial reaction to a loss is a stunned, numb feeling and refusal by the individual to acknowledge the reality of the loss. Engel states that this stage is an attempt by the individual to protect the self "against the effects of the overwhelming stress by raising the threshold against its recognition or against the painful feelings evoked thereby."

■ **Stage II: Developing Awareness.** This stage begins within minutes to hours of the loss. Behaviors associated with this stage include excessive crying and regression to a state of helplessness and a childlike manner. Awareness of the loss creates feelings of emptiness, frustration, anguish, and despair. Anger may be directed toward the self or toward others in the environment who are held accountable for the loss.

■ **Stage III: Restitution.** In this stage, the various rituals associated with loss within a culture are performed. Examples include funerals, wakes, special attire, a gathering of friends and family, and religious practices customary to the spiritual beliefs of the bereaved. Participation in these rituals is thought to assist the individual to accept the reality of the loss and to facilitate the recovery process.

■ **Stage IV: Resolution of the Loss.** This stage is characterized by a preoccupation with the loss. The concept of the loss is idealized, and the individual may even imitate admired qualities of the lost entity. Preoccupation with the loss gradually decreases over a year or more, and the individual eventually begins to reinvest feelings in others.

■ **Stage V: Recovery.** Obsession with the loss has ended, and the individual is able to go on with his or her life.

J. William Worden

Worden views the bereaved person as active and self-determining rather than a passive participant in the grief process. He proposes that bereavement includes a set of tasks that must be reconciled in order to complete the grief process. Worden's four tasks of mourning are as follows:

■ **Task I. Accepting the Reality of the Loss.** When something of value is lost, it is common for individuals to refuse to believe that the loss has occurred. Behaviors include misidentifying individuals in the environment for their lost loved one, retaining possessions of the lost loved one as though he or she has not died, and removing all reminders of the lost loved one so as not to have to face the reality of the loss. Worden (2009) stated,

Coming to an acceptance of the reality of the loss takes time since it involves not only an intellectual acceptance but also an emotional one. The bereaved person may be intellectually aware of the finality of the loss long before the emotions allow full acceptance of the information as true. (p. 42)

Belief and denial are intermittent while grappling with this task. It is thought that traditional rituals such as the funeral help some individuals move toward acceptance of the loss.

■ **Task II. Processing the Pain of Grief.** Pain associated with a loss includes both physical pain and emotional pain. This pain must be acknowledged and worked through. To avoid or suppress it serves only to delay or prolong the grieving process. People do this by refusing to allow themselves to think painful thoughts, by idealizing or avoiding reminders of the lost entity, and by using alcohol or drugs. The intensity of the pain and the man-

ner in which it is experienced are different for all individuals. However, the commonality is that it *must* be experienced. Failure to do so generally results in some form of depression that commonly requires therapy, which then focuses on working through the pain of grief that the individual failed to work through at the time of the loss. In this very difficult Task II, individuals must "allow themselves to process the pain—to feel it and to know that one day it will pass" (Worden, 2009, p. 45).

■ **Task III. Adjusting to a World Without the Lost Entity.** It usually takes a number of months for a bereaved person to realize what his or her world will be like without the lost entity. In the case of a lost loved one, how the environment changes will depend on the types of roles that person fulfilled in life. In the case of a changed lifestyle, the individual will be required to make adaptations to his or her environment in terms of the changes as they are presented in daily life. In addition, those individuals who had defined their identity through the lost entity will require an adjustment to their own sense of self. Worden (2009) stated,

The coping strategy of redefining the loss in such a way that it can redound to the benefit of the survivor is often part of the successful completion of Task III. (p. 47)

If the bereaved person experiences failures in his or her attempt to adjust in an environment without the lost entity, feelings of low self-esteem may result. Regressed behaviors and feelings of helplessness and inadequacy are not uncommon. Worden (2009) stated,

[Another] area of adjustment is to one's sense of the world. Loss through death can challenge one's fundamental life values and philosophical beliefs—beliefs that are influenced by our families, peers, education, and religion as well as life experiences. The bereaved person searches for meaning in the loss and its attendant life changes in order to make sense of it and to regain some control of his or her life. (pp. 48–49)

To be successful in Task III, bereaved individuals must develop new skills to cope and adapt to their new environment without the lost entity. Successful achievement of this task determines the outcome of the mourning process—that of continued growth or a state of arrested development.

■ **Task IV. Finding an Enduring Connection With the Lost Entity in the Midst of Embarking on a New Life.** This task allows for the bereaved person to identify a special place for the lost entity. Individuals need not purge from their history or find a replacement for that which has been lost. Instead, there is a kind of continued presence of the lost entity that only becomes *relocated* in the life of the bereaved. Successful completion of Task IV involves letting go of past attachments and forming new ones. However, there is also the recognition that, although the relationship between the bereaved and what has been lost is changed, it is nonetheless still a relationship. Worden (2009) suggested that one never loses memories of a significant relationship. He stated,

For many people, Task IV is the most difficult one to accomplish. They get stuck at this point in their grieving and later realize that their life in some way stopped at the point the loss occurred. (p. 52)

Worden (2009) related the story of a teenaged girl who had a difficult time adjusting to the death of her father. After 2 years, when she began to finally fulfill some of the tasks associated with successful grieving, she wrote these words that express rather clearly what bereaved people in Task IV are struggling with: "There are other people to be loved, and it doesn't mean that I love Dad any less" (p. 52).

Length of the Grief Process

Stages of grief allow bereaved persons an orderly approach to the resolution of mourning. Each stage presents tasks that must be overcome through a painful experiential process. Engel (1964) has stated that successful resolution of the grief response is thought to have occurred when a bereaved individual is able "to remember comfortably and realistically both the pleasures and disappointments of [that which is lost]." The length of the grief process depends on the individual and can last for a number of years without being maladaptive. The acute phase of normal grieving usually lasts about 6 to 8 weeks—longer in older adults—but complete resolution of the grief response may take much longer. Sadock and Sadock (2007) stated,

Ample evidence suggests that the bereavement process does not end within a prescribed interval; certain aspects persist indefinitely for many otherwise high-functioning, normal individuals. Common manifestations of protracted grief

occur intermittently. Most grief does not fully resolve or permanently disappear; rather grief becomes circumscribed and submerged only to reemerge in response to certain triggers. (p. 64)

A number of factors influence the eventual outcome of the grief response. The grief response can be more difficult if:

■ The bereaved person was strongly dependent on or perceived the lost entity as an important means of physical and/or emotional support.

■ The relationship with the lost entity was highly ambivalent. A love-hate relationship may instill feelings of guilt that can interfere with the grief work.

■ The individual has experienced a number of recent losses. Grief tends to be cumulative, and if previous losses have not been resolved, each succeeding grief response becomes more difficult.

■ The loss is that of a young person. Grief over loss of a child is often more intense than it is over the loss of an elderly person.

■ The state of the person's physical or psychological health is unstable at the time of the loss.

■ The bereaved person perceives (whether real or imagined) some responsibility for the loss.

The grief response may be facilitated if:

■ The individual has the support of significant others to assist him or her through the mourning process.

■ The individual has the opportunity to prepare for the loss. Grief work is more intense when the loss is sudden and unexpected. The experience of *anticipatory grieving* is thought to facilitate the grief response that occurs at the time of the actual loss.

Worden (2009) stated,

There is a sense in which mourning can be finished, when people regain an interest in life, feel more hopeful, experience gratification again, and adapt to new roles. There is also a sense in which mourning is never finished. [People must understand] that mourning is a long-term process and that the culmination will not be a pre-grief state. (p. 77)

Anticipatory Grief

Anticipatory grieving is the experiencing of the feelings and emotions associated with the normal grief response before the loss actually occurs. One dissimilar aspect relates to the fact that conventional grief tends to diminish in intensity with the passage of time. Anticipatory grief can become more intense as the expected loss becomes imminent.

Although anticipatory grief is thought to facilitate the actual mourning process following the loss, there may be some problems. In the case of a dying person, difficulties can arise when the family members complete the process of anticipatory grief, and detachment from the dying person occurs prematurely. The person who is dying experiences feelings of loneliness and isolation as the psychological pain of imminent death is faced without family support. Another example of difficulty associated with premature completion of the grief response is one that can occur on the return of persons long absent and presumed dead (e.g., soldiers missing in action or prisoners of war). In this instance, resumption of the previous relationship may be difficult for the bereaved person.

Anticipatory grieving may serve as a defense for some individuals to ease the burden of loss when it actually occurs. It may prove to be less functional for others who, because of interpersonal, psychological, or sociocultural variables, are unable in advance of the actual loss to express the intense feelings that accompany the grief response.

IMPLICATIONS OF RESEARCH FOR EVIDENCED-BASED PRACTICE

Bratcher, J. R. (2010). How do critical care nurses define a "good death" in the intensive care unit? *Critical Care Nursing Quarterly, 33*(1), 87–99.

DESCRIPTION OF THE STUDY: The purpose of this study was to explore and describe the characteristics of a good death as defined by critical care nurses working in the intensive care unit (ICU). The number of deaths in the ICU is likely to increase as the population ages and the use of life-prolonging technologies expands. Research has indicated a growing awareness of inadequacies with end-of-life (EOL) care in the ICU. The author stated, "Findings from the Committee on Care at the End of Life demonstrated that people suffer needlessly at the EOL; physicians and nurses lack basic training necessary to provide EOL care; economic, cultural, and organizational structures in the US healthcare system encumbers the delivery of good EOL care; and knowledge to guide care for patients at the EOL is deficient" (p. 87).

RESULTS OF THE STUDY: The study group consisted of 15 registered nurses (5 males; 10 females) working in the medical-surgical ICU at a Department of Veterans Affairs hospital in a midsized urban city. Ages ranged from 36 to 59, and years in nursing ranged from 3 to 26. Eight participants had associate degrees and 7 had baccalaureate degrees. Personal interviews were conducted by the author and lasted up to 60 minutes. Interviews were taped and transcribed verbatim. Each interview started with the question, "How do you define a good death in the ICU?" Nurses were encouraged to recall personal situations with specific patients who they believed had experienced a good death. A great deal of diversity was revealed in the participants' descriptions of a good death. Following are various themes that emerged. The number in parentheses indicates the number of nurses who identified each theme in their interview.

- Patient does not die alone (11) (includes allowing patient's pet)
- Patient does not suffer (10) (includes those who suggested patient's death is quick)
- Acceptance of death by patient and/or loved ones (8)
- Patient dies with dignity (3) (implying with solemnity, peace, and respect)
- Religious/spiritual/cultural needs are met (3)
- Patient's and/or family's wishes are honored (3)
- Patient was not successfully resuscitated, but staff tried their best (2)
- Music is allowed (1)
- Environment is quiet (1)
- Staff does not panic (1)
- Family does not panic (1) or scream or cry out loud in distress (1)

IMPLICATIONS FOR NURSING PRACTICE: The results of this study offer information applicable to EOL care in the critical care setting. The author suggested that there is a need to recognize that palliative care in the ICU can coexist with curative care. The author concluded, "Critical care nurses have an opportunity to provide excellent EOL care for their patients, but they must first understand what constitutes a good death; obtaining this information will help facilitate compassionate EOL care, which will ultimately improve the nursing care of dying patients and their families in the ICU" (p. 97).

Maladaptive Responses to Loss

When, then, is the grieving response considered to be maladaptive? Three types of pathological grief reactions have been described. These include delayed or inhibited grief, an exaggerated or distorted grief response, and chronic or prolonged grief.

Delayed or Inhibited Grief

Delayed or inhibited grief refers to the absence of evidence of grief when it ordinarily would be expected. Many times, cultural influences, such as the expectation to keep a "stiff upper lip," cause the delayed response.

Delayed or inhibited grief is potentially pathological because the person is simply not dealing with the reality of the loss. He or she remains fixed in the denial stage of the grief process, sometimes for many years. When this occurs, the grief response may be triggered, sometimes many years later, when the individual experiences a subsequent loss. Sometimes the grief process is triggered spontaneously or in response to a seemingly insignificant event. Overreaction to another person's loss may be one manifestation of **delayed grief.**

The recognition of delayed grief is critical because, depending on the profoundness of the loss, the failure of the mourning process may prevent assimilation of the loss and thereby delay a return to satisfying living. Delayed grieving most commonly occurs because of ambivalent feelings toward the lost entity, outside pressure to resume normal function, or perceived lack of internal and external resources to cope with a profound loss.

Distorted (Exaggerated) Grief Response

In the distorted grief reaction, all of the symptoms associated with normal grieving are exaggerated. Feelings of sadness, helplessness, hopelessness, powerlessness, anger, and guilt, as well as numerous somatic complaints, render the individual dysfunctional in terms of management of daily living. Murray, Zentner, and Yakimo (2009) described an exaggerated grief reaction in the following way:

> An intensification of grief to the point that the person is overwhelmed, demonstrates prolonged maladaptive behavior, manifests excessive symptoms and extensive interruptions in healing, and does not progress to integration of the loss, finding meaning in the loss, and resolution of the mourning process. (p. 706)

When the exaggerated grief reaction occurs, the individual remains fixed in the anger stage of the grief response. This anger may be directed toward others in the environment to whom the individual may be attributing the loss. However, many times the anger is turned inward on the self. When this occurs, depression is the result. Depressive mood disorder is a type of exaggerated grief reaction.

Chronic or Prolonged Grieving

Some authors have discussed a chronic or prolonged grief response as a type of maladaptive grief response. Care must be taken in making this determination because, as was stated previously, length of the grief response depends on the individual. An adaptive response may take years for some people. A prolonged process may be considered maladaptive when certain behaviors are exhibited. Prolonged grief may be a problem when behaviors such as maintaining personal possessions aimed at keeping a lost loved one alive (as though he or she will eventually reenter the life of the bereaved) or disabling behaviors that prevent the bereaved from adaptively performing activities of daily living are in evidence. Another example is of a widow who refused to participate in family gatherings following the death of her husband. For many years until her own death, she took a sandwich to the cemetery on holidays, sat on the tombstone, and ate her "holiday meal" with her husband. Other bereaved individuals have been known to set a place at the table for the deceased loved one long after the completed mourning process would have been expected.

Normal Versus Maladaptive Grieving

Several authors have identified one crucial difference between normal and maladaptive grieving: the loss of self-esteem. Marked feelings of worthlessness are indicative of depression rather than uncomplicated bereavement. Corr, Nabe, and Corr (2008) stated, "Normal grief reactions do not include the loss of self-esteem commonly found in most clinical depression" (p. 215). Cheong, Herkov, and Goodman (2010) affirmed,

> Although both conditions may have depressed mood, loss of appetite, sleep disturbance, and decreased energy, people with depression usually experience a sense of worthlessness, guilt and/or low self-esteem that is not common in normal grief reactions.

It is thought that this major difference between normal grieving and a maladaptive grieving response (the feeling of worthlessness or low self-esteem) ultimately precipitates depression. A summary of differences between normal grieving and clinical depression is presented in Table 39-2.

TABLE 39-2 Normal Grief Reactions versus Symptoms of Clinical Depression

NORMAL GRIEF	CLINICAL DEPRESSION
Self-esteem intact	Self-esteem is disturbed
May openly express anger	Usually does not directly express anger
Experiences a mixture of "good and bad days"	Persistent state of dysphoria
Able to experience moments of pleasure	Anhedonia is prevalent
Accepts comfort and support from others	Does not respond to social interaction and support from others
Maintains feeling of hope	Feelings of hopelessness prevail
May express guilt feelings over some aspect of the loss	Has generalized feelings of guilt
Relates feelings of depression to specific loss experienced	Does not relate feelings to a particular experience
May experience transient physical symptoms	Expresses chronic physical complaints

Sources: Cheong, Herkov, and Goodman (2010); Corr, Nabe, and Corr (2008); and Sadock and Sadock (2007).

Application of the Nursing Process

Background Assessment Data: Concepts of Death—Developmental Issues

All individuals have their own unique concept of death, which is influenced by past experiences with death as well as age and level of emotional development. This section addresses the various perceptions of death according to developmental age.

Children

Birth to Age 2

Infants are unable to recognize and understand death, but they can experience the feelings of loss and separation. Infants who are separated from their mother may become quiet, lose weight, and sleep less. Children at this age will likely sense changes in the atmosphere of the home where a death has occurred. They often react to the emotions of adults by becoming more irritable and crying more.

Ages 3 to 5

Preschoolers and kindergartners have some understanding about death but often have difficulty distinguishing between fantasy and reality. They believe death is reversible, and their thoughts about death may include magical thinking. For example, they may believe that their thoughts or behaviors caused a person to become sick or to die.

Children of this age are capable of understanding at least some of what they see and hear from adult conversations or media reports. They become

frightened if they feel a threat to themselves or their loved ones. They are concerned with safety issues and require a great deal of personal reassurance that they will be protected. Regressive behaviors, such as loss of bladder or bowel control, thumb sucking, and temper tantrums, are common. Changes in eating and sleeping patterns may also occur.

Ages 6 to 9

Children at this age are beginning to understand the finality of death. They are able to understand a more detailed explanation of why or how a person died, although the concept of death is often associated with old age or with accidents. They may believe that death is contagious and avoid association with individuals who have experienced a loss by death. Death is often personified, in the form of a "bogey man" or a monster—someone who takes people away or someone whom they can avoid if they try hard enough. It is difficult for them to perceive their own death. Normal grief reactions at this age include regressive and aggressive behaviors, withdrawal, school phobias, somatic symptoms, and clinging behaviors.

Ages 10 to 12

Preadolescent children are able to understand that death is final and eventually affects everyone, including themselves. They are interested in the physical aspects of dying and the final disposition of the body. They may ask questions about how the death will affect them personally. Feelings of anger, guilt, and depression are common. Peer relationships and school performance may be disrupted. There may be a preoccupation with the loss and a withdrawal into the self. They will require reassurance of their own safety and self-worth.

Adolescents

Adolescents are usually able to view death on an adult level. They understand death to be universal and inevitable; however, they have difficulty tolerating the intense feelings associated with the death of a loved one. They may or may not cry. They may withdraw into themselves or attempt to go about usual activities in an effort to avoid dealing with the pain of the loss. Some teens exhibit acting-out behaviors, such as aggression and defiance. It is often easier for adolescents to discuss their feelings with peers than with their parents or other adults. Some adolescents may show regressive behaviors, whereas others react by trying to take care of their loved ones who are also grieving. In general, individuals of this age group have an attitude of immortality. Although they understand that their own death is inevitable, the concept is so far-reaching as to be imperceptible.

Adults

The adult's concept of death is influenced by experiential, cultural, and religious backgrounds (Murray et al., 2009). Behaviors associated with grieving in the adult were discussed in the section on "Theoretical Perspectives on Loss and Bereavement."

Elderly Adults

Bateman (1999) stated,

> For the older adult, the later years have been described by philosophers and poets as the 'season of loss.' Loss of one's occupational role upon retirement, loss of control and competence, loss in some life experiences, loss of material possessions, and loss of dreams, loved ones, and friends must be understood and accepted if the older adult is to adapt effectively. (p. 144)

By the time individuals reach their 60s and 70s, they have experienced numerous losses, and mourning has become a lifelong process. Those who are most successful at adapting earlier in life will similarly cope better with the losses and grief inherent in aging. Unfortunately, with the aging process comes a convergence of losses, the timing of which makes it impossible for the aging individual to complete the grief process in response to one loss before another occurs. Because grief is cumulative, this can result in **bereavement overload,** the person is less able to adapt and reintegrate, and mental and physical health is jeopardized (Halstead, 2005). Bereavement overload has been

implicated as a predisposing factor in the development of depressive disorder in the elderly person.

Background Assessment Data: Concepts of Death—Cultural Issues

As previously stated, bereavement practices are greatly influenced by cultural and religious backgrounds. It is important for health-care professionals to have an understanding of these individual differences in order to provide culturally sensitive care to their clients. Clinicians must be able to identify and appreciate what is culturally expected or required, because failure to carry out expected rituals may hinder the grief process and result in unresolved grief for some bereaved individuals. Box 39-1 provides a set of guidelines for assessing culturally specific death rituals. Following is a discussion of selected culturally specific death rituals.

African Americans

Customs of bereaved African Americans are similar to those of the dominant American culture of the same religion and social class, with a blending of cultural practices from the African heritage. Most African American Christians are affiliated with the Baptist and Methodist denominations (Campinha-Bacote, 2008). Campinha-Bacote (2008) stated,

> One response to hearing about a death of a family member or close member in the African American culture is "falling-out," which is manifested by sudden collapse and paralysis and the inability to see or speak. However, the individual's hearing and understanding remain intact. Health care practitioners must understand the African American culture to recognize this condition as a cultural response to

---

BOX 39-1 Guidelines for Assessing Culturally Specific Death Rituals

DEATH RITUALS AND EXPECTATIONS

1. Identify culturally specific death rituals and expectations.
2. Explain death rituals and mourning practices.
3. What are specific burial practices, such as cremation?

RESPONSES TO DEATH AND GRIEF

4. Identify cultural responses to death and grief.
5. Explore the meaning of death, dying, and the afterlife.

From Purnell, L. D. (2008). The Purnell model for cultural competence. In L. D. Purnell & B. J. Paulanka (Eds.), Transcultural health care: A culturally competent approach (3rd ed., pp. 19–55). Philadelphia: F.A. Davis.

the death of a family member or other severe emotional shock and not as a medical condition requiring emergency intervention. (p. 68)

Funeral services may differ from the traditional European American service with ceremonies and rituals modified by the musical rhythms and patterns of speech and worship that are unique to African Americans. Feelings are expressed openly and publicly at the funeral, and eulogies are extremely important. Services usually conclude with a viewing of the body and burial at a cemetery. Burial rather than cremation is usually chosen (Asante, 2010).

Many African Americans attempt to maintain a strong connection with their loved ones who have died. This connection may take the form of communication with the deceased's spirit through mediums who are believed to possess this special capability.

Asian Americans

Chinese Americans

Death and bereavement in the Chinese tradition are centered on ancestor worship. Chinese people have an intuitive fear of death and avoid references to it. Wang and Purnell (2008) stated,

> Many Chinese are hesitant to purchase life insurance because of their fear that it is inviting death. The color white is associated with death and is considered bad luck. Black is also a bad luck color. (p. 138)

In the traditional Chinese culture, people often do not express their emotions openly. Mourners are recognized by black armbands and white strips of cloth tied around their heads (Wang & Purnell, 2008). The dead are honored by placing food, money for the person's spirit, or articles made of paper around the coffin.

Japanese Americans

The dominant religion among the Japanese is Buddhism. On death of a loved one, the body is prepared by close family members. This is followed by a 2-day period of visitation by family and friends, during which there is prayer, burning of incense, and presentation of gifts. Funeral ceremonies are held at the Buddhist temple, and cremation is common. The mourning period is 49 days, the end of which is marked by a family prayer service and the serving of special rice dishes. It is believed that, at this time, the departed has joined those already in the hereafter. Perpetual prayers may be donated through a gift to the temple (Turale & Ito, 2008).

Vietnamese Americans

Buddhism is the predominant religion among the Vietnamese. Attitudes toward death are influenced by the Buddhist emphasis on cyclic continuity and reincarnation. Many Vietnamese people believe that birth and death are predestined.

Most Vietnamese people prefer to die at home, and most do not approve of autopsy. Cremation is common. The final moments before the funeral procession are a time of prayer for the immediate family. Individuals in mourning wear white clothing for 14 days. During the following year, men wear black armbands and women wear white headbands (Purnell, 2008). The 1-year anniversary of an individual's death is commemorated. Clergy should only be called at the request of the client or family, and is usually associated with last rites, especially by Vietnamese people who practice Catholicism. For this reason, hospital visitation by clergy may be very upsetting to clients. Receiving flowers also may be distressing, as flowers usually are reserved for the rites of the dead (Stauffer, 2008).

Filipino Americans

Following a death in the Filipino community, a wake is held with family and friends. This wake usually takes place in the home of the deceased and lasts up to a week before the funeral. A large proportion of Filipinos are Catholic. Pacquiao (2008) stated,

> Among Catholics, 9 days of novenas are held in the home or in the church. These special prayers ask God's blessing for the deceased. Depending upon the economic resources of the family, food and refreshments are served after each prayer day. Sometimes the last day of the novena takes on the atmosphere of a *fiesta* or a celebration. Filipino families in the United States follow variations of this ritual according to their social and economic circumstances. (p. 189)

Most follow the traditional custom of wearing dark clothing—black armbands for men and black dresses for women—for 1 year after the death, at which time ritualistic mourning officially ends. Emotional outbursts of uncontrolled crying are common expressions of grief. Fainting as a bereavement practice is not uncommon (Pacquiao, 2008). Burial of the body is most common, but cremation is acceptable.

Jewish Americans

Traditional Judaism believes in an afterlife, where the soul continues to flourish, although today, many dispute this interpretation (Purnell & Selekman,

2008). However, most Jewish people show little concern about life after death and focus is concentrated more on how one conducts one's present life. Taking one's own life is forbidden, and ultraconservative Jewish people may deny the person who commits suicide full burial honors; however, the more liberal view is to emphasize the needs of the survivors.

A dying person is never left alone. At death, the face is covered with a cloth, and the body is treated with respect. Autopsy is only allowed if it is required by law, the deceased person has requested it, or it may save the life of another (Purnell & Selekman, 2008).

For the funeral, the body is wrapped in a shroud and placed in a wooden, unadorned casket. No wake and no viewing are part of a Jewish funeral. Cremation is prohibited. Purnell and Selekman (2008) stated,

> After the funeral, mourners are welcomed to the home of the closest relative. Water to wash one's hands before entering is outside the front door, symbolic of cleansing the impurities associated with contact with the dead. The water is not passed from person to person, just as it is hoped that the tragedy is not passed. At the home, a meal is served to all the guests. This "meal of condolence" or "meal of consolation" is traditionally provided by the neighbors and friends. (p. 288)

The 7-day period beginning with the burial is called **shiva.** During this time, mourners do not work, and no activity is permitted that diverts attention from thinking about the deceased. Mourning lasts 30 days for a relative and 1 year for a parent, at which time a tombstone is erected and a graveside service is held (Purnell & Selekman, 2008).

Mexican Americans

Most Mexican Americans view death as a natural part of life. The predominant religion is Catholic, and many of the death rituals are a reflection of these religious beliefs. A vigil by family members is kept over the sick or dying person. Following the death, large numbers of family and friends gather for a **velorio,** a festive watch over the body of the deceased person (Zoucha & Zamarripa, 2008). Evening group prayers (*novenario*) are held for 9 days following the burial (Salazar, 2009).

Mourning is called **luto** and is symbolized by wearing black, black and white, or dark clothing and by subdued behavior. Often the bereaved refrain from attending movies or social events and from listening to radio or watching television. For middle-aged or elderly Mexican Americans, the period of bereavement may last for 2 years or more. These mourning behaviors do not indicate a sign of respect for the dead; instead, they demonstrate evidence that the individual is grieving for a loved one. Burial is more common than cremation, and often the body is buried within 24 hours of death, which is required by law in Mexico (Zoucha & Zamarripa, 2008).

Native Americans

More than 500 Native-American tribes are now recognized by the U.S. government. Although many of the tribal traditions have been modified throughout the years, some of the traditional Native American values have been preserved.

The Navajo of the Southwest, the largest Native American tribe in the United States, do not bury the body of a deceased person for 4 days after death. Beliefs require that a cleansing ceremony take place before burial to prevent the spirit of the dead person from trying to assume control of someone else's spirit (Purnell, 2009). The dead are buried with their shoes on the wrong feet and rings on their index fingers. The Navajo generally do not express their grief openly and are reluctant to touch the body of a dead person. Purnell (2009) stated,

> One death taboo involves talking with clients concerning a fatal disease or illness. Effective discussions require that the issue be presented in the third person, as if the illness or disorder occurred with someone else. [The health care provider must] never suggest that the client is dying. To do so would imply that the provider wishes the client dead. If the client does die, it would imply that the provider may have evil powers. (p. 314)

Nursing Diagnosis/Outcome Identification

From analysis of the assessment data, appropriate nursing diagnoses are formulated for the client and family experiencing grief and loss. From these identified diagnoses, accurate planning of nursing care is executed. Possible nursing diagnoses for grieving persons include:

■ Risk for complicated grieving related to loss of a valued entity/concept; loss of a loved one

■ Risk for spiritual distress related to complicated grief process

The following criteria may be used for measurement of outcomes in the care of the grieving client:

The client:

■ Acknowledges awareness of the loss.

■ Is able to express feelings about the loss.

■ Verbalizes stages of the grief process and behaviors associated with each.

■ Expresses personal satisfaction and support from spiritual practices.

Planning/Implementation

Table 39-3 provides a plan of care for the grieving person. Selected nursing diagnoses are presented, along with outcome criteria, appropriate nursing interventions, and rationales for each.

Evaluation

In the final step of the nursing process, a reassessment is conducted to determine if the nursing actions have been successful in achieving the objectives of care. Evaluation of the nursing actions for the grieving client may be facilitated by gathering information using the following types of questions:

■ Has the client discussed the recent loss with staff and family members?

■ Is the client able to verbalize feelings and behaviors associated with each stage of the grieving process and recognize his or her own position in the process?

■ Has obsession with and idealization of the lost entity subsided?

■ Is anger toward the loss expressed appropriately?

■ Is the client able to participate in usual religious practices and feel satisfaction and support from them?

■ Is the client seeking out interaction with others in an appropriate manner?

■ Is the client able to verbalize positive aspects about his or her life, past relationships, and prospects for the future?

Table 39-3 CARE PLAN FOR THE GRIEVING PERSON

NURSING DIAGNOSIS: RISK FOR COMPLICATED GRIEVING

RELATED TO: Loss of a valued entity/concept; loss of a loved one

EVIDENCED BY: Feelings of sadness, anger, guilt, self-reproach, anxiety, loneliness, fatigue, helplessness, shock, yearning, and numbness

OUTCOME CRITERIA	NURSING INTERVENTIONS	RATIONALE
Short-Term Goals • Client will acknowledge awareness of the loss. • Client will express feelings about the loss. • Client will verbalize own position in the grief process. **Long-Term Goal** • Client will progress through the grief process in a healthful manner toward resolution.	1. Assess the client's stage in the grief process. 2. Develop trust. Show empathy, concern, and unconditional positive regard. 3. Help the client actualize the loss by talking about it: "When did it happen?" "How did it happen?" and so forth. 4. Help the client identify and express feelings. Some of the more problematic feelings include: a. **Anger.** The anger may be directed at the deceased or at God, displaced onto others, or retroflected inward on the self. Encourage the client to examine this anger and validate the appropriateness of this feeling.	1. Accurate baseline data are required to provide appropriate assistance. 2. Developing trust provides the basis for a therapeutic relationship. 3. Reviewing the events of the loss can help the client come to full awareness of the loss. 4. Until the client can recognize and accept personal feelings regarding the loss, grief work cannot progress. a. Many people will not admit to angry feelings, believing it is inappropriate and unjustified. Expression of this emotion is necessary to prevent fixation in this stage of grief.

Table 39-3 CARE PLAN FOR THE GRIEVING PERSON—cont'd

OUTCOME CRITERIA	NURSING INTERVENTIONS	RATIONALE
	b. **Guilt.** The client may feel that he or she did not do enough to prevent the loss. Help the client by reviewing the circumstances of the loss and the reality that it could not be prevented.	b. Feelings of guilt prolong resolution of the grief process.
	c. **Anxiety and helplessness.** Help the client to recognize the way that life was managed before the loss. Help the client to put the feelings of helplessness into perspective by pointing out ways that he or she managed situations effectively without help from others. Role-play life events and assist with decision-making situations.	c. The client may have fears that he or she may not be able to carry on alone.
	5. Interpret normal behaviors associated with grieving and provide the client with adequate time to grieve.	5. Understanding of the grief process will help prevent feelings of guilt generated by these responses. Individuals need adequate time to adjust to the loss and all its ramifications. This involves getting past birthdays and anniversaries of which the deceased was a part.
	6. Provide continuing support. If this is not possible by the nurse, then offer referrals to support groups. Support groups of individuals going through the same experiences can be very helpful for the grieving individual.	6. The availability of emotional support systems facilitates the grief process.
	7. Identify pathological defenses that the client may be using (e.g., drug/alcohol use, somatic complaints, social isolation). Assist the client in understanding why these are not healthy defenses and how they delay the process of grieving.	7. The bereavement process is impaired by behaviors that mask the pain of the loss.
	8. Encourage the client to make an honest review of the relationship with the lost entity. Journal keeping is a facilitative tool with this intervention.	8. Only when the client is able to see both positive and negative aspects related to the loss will the grieving process be complete.

Continued

Table 39-3 CARE PLAN FOR THE GRIEVING PERSON—cont'd

NURSING DIAGNOSIS: RISK FOR SPIRITUAL DISTRESS
RELATED TO: Complicated grief process
EVIDENCED BY: Anger toward God, questioning meaning of own existence, inability to participate in usual religious practices

OUTCOME CRITERIA	NURSING INTERVENTIONS	RATIONALE
Short-Term Goal • Client will identify meaning and purpose in life, moving forward with hope for the future. **Long-Term Goal** • Client will express achievement of support and personal satisfaction from spiritual practices.	1. Be accepting and nonjudgmental when the client expresses anger and bitterness toward God. Stay with the client. 2. Encourage the client to ventilate feelings related to meaning of own existence in the face of current loss. 3. Encourage the client as part of grief work to reach out to previously used religious practices for support. Encourage the client to discuss these practices and how they provided support in the past. 4. Assure the client that he or she is not alone when feeling inadequate in the search for life's answers. 5. Contact spiritual leader of client's choice, if he or she requests.	1. The nurse's presence and nonjudgmental attitude increase the client's feelings of self-worth and promote trust in the relationship. 2. The client may believe he or she cannot go on living without the lost entity. Catharsis can provide relief and put life back into realistic perspective. 3. The client may find comfort in religious rituals with which he or she is familiar. 4. Validation of the client's feelings and assurance that they are shared by others offer reassurance and an affirmation of acceptability. 5. These individuals serve to provide relief from spiritual distress and often can do so when other support persons cannot.

Additional Assistance

Hospice

Hospice is a program that provides palliative and supportive care to meet the special needs of people who are dying and their families. Hospice care provides physical, psychological, spiritual, and social care for the person for whom aggressive treatment is no longer appropriate. Various models of hospice exist, including freestanding institutions that provide both inpatient and home care, those affiliated with hospitals and nursing homes in which hospice services are provided within the institutional setting, and hospice organizations that provide home care only. Historically, the hospice movement in the United States has evolved mainly as a system of home-based care.

Hospice helps clients achieve physical and emotional comfort so that they can concentrate on living life as fully as possible. Clients are urged to stay active for as long as they are able—to take part in activities they enjoy, and to focus on the quality of life.

The National Hospice and Palliative Care Organization (NHPCO) (2000) has published standards of care based on principles that are directed at the hospice program concept. These principles of care are presented in Box 39-2.

Hospice follows an interdisciplinary team approach to provide care for the terminally ill individual within the healthcare institution or in the familiar surroundings of the home environment. The interdisciplinary team consists of nurses, attendants (homemakers, home health aides), physicians, social workers, volunteers, and other health-care workers from other disciplines as required for individual clients.

The hospice approach is based on seven components: the interdisciplinary team, pain and symptom management, emotional support to client and family, pastoral and spiritual care, bereavement counseling, 24-hour on-call nurse/counselor, and

BOX 39-2 Principles of Care—National Hospice and Palliative Care Organization

ACCESS, RIGHTS AND ETHICS

Access: The hospice offers palliative care to terminally ill patients and their families regardless of age, gender, nationality, race, creed, sexual orientation, disability, diagnoses, availability of primary caregiver or ability to pay.

Rights: The hospice respects and honors the rights of each patient and family it serves.

Ethics: The hospice assumes responsibility for ethical decision-making and behavior related to the provision of hospice care.

BEREAVEMENT CARE AND SERVICES

Addressing issues related to loss, grief and bereavement begins at the time of admission to the hospice with the initial assessment and continues throughout the course of care. Bereavement services are provided to help patients, families and caregivers cope with the multitude of losses that occur during the illness and eventual death of the patient. Bereavement services are offered based on a number of factors including the individual assessment, intensity of grief, coping ability of the survivors and their needs, as perceived by each patient, family and caregiver.

CLINICAL CARE AND SERVICES

The desired outcomes of hospice intervention are safe and comfortable dying, self-determined life closure and effective grieving, all as determined by the patient and family/caregivers. The interdisciplinary team identifies, assists and respects the desires of the patient and family/caregivers in the facilitation of these outcomes through treatment, prevention and promotion of strategies based on continuous assessment.

COORDINATION AND CONTINUITY OF CARE

The hospice provides coordinated and uninterrupted service and assures continuity of care across settings from admission through discharge and subsequent bereavement care.

HUMAN RESOURCES

Hospice organizational leaders ensure that the number and qualifications of staff and volunteers are appropriate to the scope of care and services provided by the hospice program.

INTERDISCIPLINARY TEAM

The hospice interdisciplinary team, in collaboration with the patient, family and caregiver, develops and maintains a patient, family and caregiver-directed, individualized, safe and coordinated plan of palliative care.

LEADERSHIP AND GOVERNANCE

Hospice has an organizational leadership structure that permits and facilitates action and decision-making by those individuals closest to any issue or process.

MANAGEMENT OF INFORMATION

The hospice identifies and collects information needed to operate in an efficient manner. Such information is handled in a manner that respects the patient's, family's and hospice's confidentiality.

PERFORMANCE IMPROVEMENT AND OUTCOMES MEASUREMENT

The hospice defines a systematic, planned approach to improving performance. This approach is authorized and supported by the governing body and leaders.

SAFETY AND INFECTION CONTROL

The hospice provides for the safety of all staff and promotes the development and maintenance of a safe environment for patients and families served.

Adapted from National Hospice and Palliative Care Organization. (2000). Standards of Practice for Hospice Programs. Alexandria, VA: Author. Item No. 711077, available from NHPCO 1-800-646-6460.

staff support. These are the ideal, and not all hospice programs may include all of these services.

Interdisciplinary Team

Nurses

A registered nurse usually acts as case manager for care of hospice clients. The nurse assesses the client's and family's needs, establishes the goals of care, supervises and assists caregivers, evaluates care, serves as client advocate, and provides educational information as needed to client, family, and caregivers. He or she also provides physical care when needed, including IV therapy.

Attendants

These individuals are usually the members of the team who spend the most time with the client. They assist with personal care and all activities of daily living. Without these daily attendants, many individuals would be unable to spend their remaining days in their home. Attendants may be noncertified and provide basic housekeeping services; they may be certified nursing assistants who assist with personal care; or they may be licensed vocational or practical nurses who provide more specialized care, such as dressing changes or tube feedings.

Physicians

The client's primary physician and the hospice medical consultant have input into the care of the hospice client. Orders may continue to come from the primary physician, whereas pain and symptom management may come from the hospice consultant. Ideally, these physicians attend weekly client care conferences and provide in-service education for hospice staff as well as others in the medical community.

Social Workers

The social worker assists the client and family members with psychosocial issues, including those associated with the client's condition, financial issues, legal needs, and bereavement concerns. The social worker provides information on community resources from which client and family may receive support and assistance. Some of the functions of the nurse and social worker may overlap at times.

Trained Volunteers

Volunteers are vital to the hospice concept. They provide services that may otherwise be financially impossible. They are specially selected and extensively trained, and they provide services such as transportation, companionship, respite care, recreational activities, and light housekeeping, and in general are sensitive to the needs of families in stressful situations.

Rehabilitation Therapists

Physical therapists may assist hospice clients in an effort to minimize physical disability. They may assist with strengthening exercises and provide assistance with special equipment needs. Occupational therapists may help the debilitated client learn to accomplish activities of daily living as independently as possible. Other consultants, such as speech therapists, may be called upon for the client with special needs.

Dietitian

A nutritional consultant may be helpful to the hospice client who is experiencing nausea and vomiting, diarrhea, anorexia, and weight loss. A nutritionist can ensure that the client is receiving the proper balance of calories and nutrients.

Counseling Services

The hospice client may require the services of a psychiatrist or psychologist if there is a history of mental illness, or if dementia or depression has become a problem. Other types of counseling services are available to provide assistance in dealing with the special needs of each client.

Pain and Symptom Management

Improved quality of life at all times is a primary goal of hospice care. Thus, a major intervention for all caregivers is to ensure that the client is as comfortable as possible, whether experiencing pain or other types of symptoms common in the terminal stages of an illness.

Emotional Support

Members of the hospice team encourage clients and families to discuss the eventual outcome of the disease process. Some individuals find discussing issues associated with death and dying uncomfortable, and if so, their decision is respected. However, honest discussion of these issues provides a sense of relief for some people, and they are more realistically prepared for the future. It may even draw some clients and families closer together during this stressful time.

Pastoral and Spiritual Care

Hospice philosophy supports the individual's right to seek guidance or comfort in the spiritual practices most suited to that person. The hospice team members help the client obtain the spiritual support and guidance for which he or she expresses a preference.

Bereavement Counseling

Hospice provides a service to surviving family members or significant others after the death of their loved one. This is usually provided by a bereavement counselor, but when one is not available, volunteers with special training in bereavement care may be of service. A grief support group may be helpful for the bereaved and provide a safe place for them to discuss their own fears and concerns about the death of a loved one.

Twenty-Four-Hour On-Call

The standards of care set forth by the NHPCO state that care shall be available 24 hours a day, 7 days a week. A nurse or counselor is usually available by phone or for home visits around the clock. The knowledge that emotional or physical support is available at any time, should it be required, provides considerable support and comfort to significant others or family caregivers.

Staff Support

Team members (all who work closely and frequently with the client) often experience emotions similar to those of the client or their family and/or significant others. They may experience anger, frustration, or fears of death and dying—all of which must be addressed through staff support groups, team conferences, time off, and adequate and effective supervision. Burnout is a common problem among hospice staff. Stress can be reduced, trust enhanced, and team functioning more effective if lines of communication are kept open among all members (medical director through volunteer), if information is readily accessible through staff conferences and in-service education, and if staff know they are appreciated and feel good about what they are doing.

Advance Directives

The term **advance directive** refers to either a living will or a durable power of attorney for health care (also called a health-care proxy). Either document allows an individual to provide directions about his or her future medical care.

IMPLICATIONS OF RESEARCH FOR EVIDENCED-BASED PRACTICE

Douglas, R., & Brown, H. N. (2002). Patients' attitudes toward advance directives. *Journal of Nursing Scholarship, 34(1)*, 61–65.

DESCRIPTION OF THE STUDY: This study was conducted to investigate hospitalized patients' attitudes toward advance directives. It explored patients' reasons for completing or not completing advance directive forms, and examined demographic differences between patients who did and did not complete advance directive forms. Subjects consisted of a convenience sample of 30 hospitalized patients. Criteria required that the patients (1) speak English, (2) be at least 18 years of age, (3) be oriented to time and place, and (4) have been approached by an RN regarding advance directives, as documented in the patient chart. Data were collected over a 3-week period in the oncology and medical telemetry units of a teaching hospital in central North Carolina. Interviews were conducted using an adapted advance directive attitude survey (ADAS) in which subjects were asked five general questions regarding perceptions of personal health, whether they had ever received information on advance directives, whether they had ever completed an advance directive, and whether they had ever had a discussion with either their primary physician or family members about end-of-life care. Demographic data were also obtained. The tool was based on a 4-point Likert scale from 1 (strongly disagree) to 4 (strongly agree). Higher scores indicated more favorable attitudes toward advance directives.

RESULTS OF THE STUDY: Subjects ranged in age from 24 to 85 years, with a mean age of 57 years. Nineteen were Caucasian, 10 were African American, and 1 was Hispanic. Ten had completed grade school or junior high, 13 completed high school, 4 completed college, and 3 had master's degrees or beyond. Twelve subjects had been diagnosed with cancer; 5 with respiratory disorders; 4 with sickle cell disease; 3 with cardiac disorders; 2 with vascular disorders; and 1 each with gastrointestinal, musculoskeletal, neurological, and dermatological disorders. Twenty-three subjects had received information on advance directives and 7 said they had received no information. Thirteen of the subjects had completed advance directives and 17 had not.

Participants with the highest mean scores were African American, female, ages 35 to 49 years, with a high school education. No subject in the 20 to 30 age group had completed an advanced directive, whereas 62 percent of subjects over age 65 had done so. The two people with the lowest scores both disagreed with the statement that an advance directive would make sure that their family knew what treatment they desired and they would receive the treatment they desired. The 13 participants who had completed advance directives cited the following reasons for doing so: (1) desire not to be placed on life support, (2) desire to name someone to make decisions in event of incapacitation, (3) desire to make decisions easier for spouse or family, (4) failing health, and (5) advancing age. The 17 who had not completed advance directives cited the following reasons: (1) keep putting it off, (2) not necessary at this point in my life, (3) uncomfortable making decisions about life support, (4) never heard of advance directives before, (5) form was too long, (6) trust husband to make those decisions, and (7) advance directives are unnecessary.

IMPLICATIONS FOR NURSING PRACTICE: The authors suggested that nurses need to explain what advance directives are when asking patients if they have an advance directive. They stated, "[Nurses] can explore alternative ways to educate patients about advance directives (e.g., videotape), and follow up with patients who have requested information to see if they have additional questions or need assistance completing an advance directive." They also suggest that nurses need to inform physicians when patients have advance directives. As patient advocates, nurses have the responsibility for making sure that patients understand the purpose of advance directives and what is involved in completing an advance directive, and for ensuring that patients' end-of-life care is executed according to their wishes.

A living will is a written document made by a competent individual that provides instructions that should be used when that individual is no longer able to express his or her wishes for health-care treatment. The durable power of attorney for health care is a written form that gives another person legal power to make decisions regarding health care when an individual is no longer capable of making such decisions. Some states have adopted forms that combine the intent of the durable power of attorney for health care (i.e., to have a proxy) and the intent of the living will (i.e., to state choices for end-of-life medical treatment).

Doctors usually follow clearly stated directives. It is important that the physician be informed that an advance directive exists and what the specific wishes of the client are. In most states, health-care professionals are legally bound to honor the client's wishes (Norlander, 2008). In 1991, the U.S. Congress passed the *Patient Self-Determination Act.* This legislation requires that all health-care facilities that receive Medicare or Medicaid funds must advise clients of their rights to refuse treatment, must make advance directives available to clients on admission, and must keep records of whether a client has an advance directive or a designated health-care proxy (Sadock & Sadock, 2007).

Catalano (2009) pointed out that, unless a natural death act has been enacted into law by a state, the living will has no mechanism of legal enforcement. These laws have been called "pull the plug" statutes and have various names in different states, such as "Removal of Life Support Systems Act" (Connecticut), "Natural Death Act" (Washington), "Declaration of Death Act" (New Jersey), and "Medical Treatment Decision Act" (Arizona) (Mantel, 2010). Catalano (2009) stated,

> In some states, a living will is considered only advisory and the physician has the right to comply with the living will or treat the client as the physician deems most appropriate. There is no protection for nurses or other health care practitioners against criminal or civil liability in the execution of living wills in states without a natural death act. (p. 161)

Norlander (2008, p. 20) suggested the following reasons why advance directives sometimes are not honored:

■ The advance directive is not available at the time treatment decisions need to be made. This is especially true in emergency situations.

■ The advance directive is not clear. Statements such as "no heroic measures" can be interpreted in many different ways.

■ The health-care proxy is unsure of the client's wishes.

Advance directives allow the client to be in control of decisions at the end of life. It is also a way to spare family and loved ones the burden of making choices without knowing what is most important to the person who is dying.

Summary and Key Points

■ Loss is the experience of separation from something of personal importance.

■ Loss is anything that is perceived as such by the individual.

■ Loss of any concept of value to an individual can trigger the grief response.

■ Elisabeth Kübler-Ross identified five stages that individuals pass through on their way to resolution of a loss. These are denial, anger, bargaining, depression, and acceptance.

■ John Bowlby described similar stages that he identified in the following manner: stage I, numbness or protest; stage II, disequilibrium; stage III, disorganization and despair; and stage IV, reorganization.

■ George Engel's stages include shock and disbelief, developing awareness, restitution, resolution of the loss, and recovery.

■ J. William Worden, a more contemporary clinician, has proposed that bereaved individuals must accomplish a set of tasks in order to complete the grief process. These four tasks are accepting the reality of the loss, processing the pain of grief, adjusting to a world without the lost entity, and finding an enduring connection with the lost entity in the midst of embarking on a new life.

■ The length of the grief process is highly individual, and it can last for a number of years without being maladaptive.

■ The acute stage of the grief process usually lasts a couple of months, but resolution usually lasts much longer.

■ Kübler-Ross suggested that a calendar year of experiencing significant events and anniversaries without the lost entity may be required.

■ Anticipatory grieving is the experiencing of the feelings and emotions associated with the normal grief process in response to anticipation of the loss.

■ Anticipatory grieving is thought to facilitate the grief process when the actual loss occurs.

■ Three types of pathological grief reactions have been described. These are as follows:

- Delayed or inhibited grief, in which there is absence of evidence of grief when it ordinarily would be expected.
- Distorted or exaggerated grief response, in which the individual remains fixed in the anger stage of the grief process and all of the symptoms associated with normal grieving are exaggerated.
- Chronic or prolonged grieving, in which the individual is unable to let go of grieving behaviors after a extended period of time and in which behaviors are evident that indicate the bereaved individual is not accepting that the loss has occurred.

■ Several authors have identified one crucial difference between normal and maladaptive grieving: the loss of self-esteem.

■ Feelings of worthlessness are indicative of depression rather than uncomplicated bereavement.

■ Very young children do not understand death, but often react to the emotions of adults by becoming more irritable and crying more. They often believe death is reversible.

■ School-age children understand the finality of death. Grief behaviors may reflect regression or aggression, school phobias, or sometimes a withdrawal into the self.

■ Adolescents are usually able to view death on an adult level. Grieving behaviors may include withdrawal or acting out. Although they understand that their own death is inevitable, the concept is so far-reaching as to be imperceptible.

■ By the time a person reaches the 60s or 70s, he or she has experienced numerous losses. Because grief is cumulative, this can result in bereavement overload. Depression is a common response.

■ Nurses must be aware of the death rituals and grief behaviors common to various cultures. Some of these rituals associated with African Americans, Asian Americans, Filipino Americans, Jewish Americans, Mexican Americans, and Native Americans were presented in this chapter.

■ Hospice is a program that provides palliative and supportive care to meet the special needs of people who are dying and their families.

■ The term *advance directive* refers to either a living will or a durable power of attorney for health care. Advance directives allow clients to be in control of decisions at the end of life and spare family and loved ones the burden of making choices without knowing what is most important to the person who is dying.

 DavisPlus — Additional info available @ davisplus.fadavis.com

Review Questions
Self-Examination/Learning Exercise

*Select the answer that is **most** appropriate for each of the following questions:*

1. Which of the following is most likely to initiate a grief response in an individual?
   a. Death of the pet dog.
   b. Being told by her doctor that she has begun menopause.
   c. Failing an examination.
   d. A only.
   e. All of the above.

2. Nancy, who is dying of cancer, says to the nurse, "I just want to see my new grandbaby. If only God will let me live until she is born. Then I'll be ready to go." This is an example of which of Kübler-Ross's stages of grief?
   a. Denial.
   b. Anger.
   c. Bargaining.
   d. Acceptance.

Continued

Review Questions—cont'd
Self-Examination/Learning Exercise

3. Gloria, a recent widow, states, "I'm going to have to learn to pay all the bills. Hank always did that. I don't know if I can handle all of that." This is an example of which of the tasks described by Worden?
   a. Task I. Accepting the reality of the loss.
   b. Task II. Processing the pain of grief.
   c. Task III. Adjusting to a world without the lost entity.
   d. Task IV. Finding an enduring connection with the lost entity in the midst of embarking on a new life.

4. Engel identifies which of the following as successful resolution of the grief process?
   a. When the bereaved person can talk about the loss without crying.
   b. When the bereaved person no longer talks about the lost entity.
   c. When the bereaved person puts all remembrances of the loss out of sight.
   d. When the bereaved person can discuss both positive and negative aspects about the lost entity.

5. Which of the following is thought to facilitate the grief process?
   a. The ability to grieve in anticipation of the loss.
   b. The ability to grieve alone without interference from others.
   c. Having recently grieved for another loss.
   d. Taking personal responsibility for the loss.

6. When Frank's wife of 34 years dies, he is very stoic, handles all the funeral arrangements, doesn't cry or appear sad, and comforts all of the other family members in their grief.
   Two years later, when Frank's best friend dies, Frank has sleep disturbances, difficulty concentrating, loss of weight, and difficulty performing on his job. This is an example of which of the following maladaptive responses to loss?
   a. Delayed grieving.
   b. Distorted grieving.
   c. Prolonged grieving.
   d. Exaggerated grieving.

7. A major difference between normal and maladaptive grieving has been identified by which of the following?
   a. There are no feelings of depression in normal grieving.
   b. There is no loss of self-esteem in normal grieving.
   c. Normal grieving lasts no longer than 1 year.
   d. In normal grief the person does not show anger toward the loss.

8. Which grief reaction can the nurse anticipate in a 10-year-old child?
   a. Statements that the deceased person will soon return.
   b. Regressive behaviors, such as loss of bladder control.
   c. A preoccupation with the loss.
   d. Thinking that they may have done something to cause the death.

9. Which of the following is a correct statement when attempting to distinguish normal grief from clinical depression?
   a. In clinical depression, anhedonia is prevalent.
   b. In normal grieving, the person has generalized feelings of guilt.
   c. The person who is clinically depressed relates feelings of depression to a specific loss.
   d. In normal grieving, there is a persistent state of dysphoria.

Review Questions—cont'd
Self-Examination/Learning Exercise

10. Which of the following is *not* true regarding grieving by an adolescent?
    a. Adolescents may not show their true feelings about the death.
    b. Adolescents tend to have an immortal attitude.
    c. Adolescents do not perceive death as inevitable.
    d. Adolescents may exhibit acting out behaviors as part of their grief.

References

Asante, M. K. (2010). *Contours of the African American culture.* Retrieved November 1, 2010, from http://africawithin.com/asante/contours.htm

Bateman, A. L. (1999). Understanding the process of grieving and loss: A critical social thinking perspective. *Journal of the American Psychiatric Nurses Association, 5*(5), 139–147.

Campinha-Bacote, J. (2008). People of African American heritage. In L. D. Purnell & B. J. Paulanka (Eds.), *Transcultural health care* (3rd ed., pp. 56–74). Philadelphia: F.A. Davis.

Catalano, J. T. (2009). *Nursing Now! Today's issues, tomorrow's trends* (5th ed.). Philadelphia: F.A. Davis.

Cheong, J., Herkov, M., & Goodman, W. (2010). Frequently asked questions about depression. *PsychCentral.* Retrieved November 1, 2010, from http://psychcentral.com/library/depression_faq.htm

Corr, C. A., Nabe, C. M., & Corr, D. M. (2008). *Death and dying: Life & living* (6th ed.). Florence, KY: Cengage Learning.

Halstead, H. L. (2005). Spirituality in older adults. In M. Stanley, K. A. Blair, & P. G. Beare (Eds.), *Gerontological nursing: A health promotion/protection approach* (3rd ed., pp. 313–318). Philadelphia: F.A. Davis.

Mantel, D. L. (2010). Laws on death and dying. *Advance for long-term care management.* Retrieved November 2, 2010, from http://long-term-care.advanceweb.com/Article/Laws-On-Death-Dying-2.aspx

Murray, R. B., Zentner, J. P., & Yakimo, R. (2009). *Health promotion strategies through the life span* (8th ed.). Upper Saddle River, NJ: Prentice Hall.

National Hospice and Palliative Care Organization. (2000). *Standards of Practice for hospice programs.* Alexandria, VA: Author.

Norlander, L. (2008). *To comfort always: A nurse's guide to end-of-life care.* Indianapolis, IN: Sigma Theta Tau International.

Pacquiao, D. F. (2008). People of Filipino heritage. In L. D. Purnell & B. J. Paulanka (Eds.), *Transcultural health care: A culturally competent approach* (3rd ed., pp. 175–195) Philadelphia: F.A. Davis.

Purnell, L. D. (2008). People of Vietnamese heritage. In L. D. Purnell & B. J. Paulanka (Eds.), *Transcultural health care: A culturally competent approach* (3rd ed., pp. 401–402). Philadelphia: F.A. Davis.

Purnell, L. D. (2009). People of Navajo Indian heritage. *Guide to culturally competent health care* (2nd ed., pp. 397–398). Philadelphia: F.A. Davis.

Purnell, L. D. (2008). The Purnell model for cultural competence. In L. D. Purnell & B. J. Paulanka (Eds.), *Transcultural health care: A culturally competent approach* (3rd ed., pp. 19–55). Philadelphia: F.A. Davis.

Purnell, L. D., & Selekman, J. (2008). People of Jewish heritage. In L. D. Purnell & B. J. Paulanka (Eds.),

Transcultural health care: A culturally competent approach (3rd ed., pp. 278–292). Philadelphia: F.A. Davis.

Sadock, B. J., & Sadock, V. A. (2007). *Synopsis of psychiatry: Behavioral sciences/clinical psychiatry* (10th ed.). Philadelphia: Lippincott Williams & Wilkins.

Salazar, M. L. (2009). *Life in death: Mexican American grave decorating and funerary rituals.* Unpublished thesis, Department of Anthropology, Texas State University, San Marcos, TX.

Stauffer, R.Y. (2008). Vietnamese Americans. In J. N. Giger & R. E. Davidhizar (Eds.), *Transcultural nursing: Assessment and intervention* (5th ed., pp. 494–536). St. Louis: Mosby.

Turale, S., & Ito, M. (2008). People of Japanese heritage. In L. D. Purnell & B. J. Paulanka (Eds.), *Transcultural health care: A culturally competent approach* (3rd ed., pp. 260–277). Philadelphia: F.A. Davis.

Wang, Y., & Purnell, L. D. (2008). People of Chinese heritage. In L. D. Purnell & B. J. Paulanka (Eds.), *Transcultural health care* (3rd ed., pp. 129–144). Philadelphia: F.A. Davis.

Worden, J. W. (2009). *Grief counseling and grief therapy: A handbook for the mental health practitioner* (4th ed.). New York: Springer.

Zoucha, R., & Zamarripa, C. A. (2008). People of Mexican heritage. In L. D. Purnell & B. J. Paulanka (Eds.), *Transcultural health care: A culturally competent approach* (3rd ed., pp. 309–324). Philadelphia: F.A. Davis.

Classical References

Bowlby, J. (1961). Processes of mourning. *International Journal of Psychoanalysis, 42,* 22.

Engel, G. (1964). Grief and grieving. *American Journal of Nursing, 64,* 93.

Kübler-Ross, E. (1969). *On death and dying.* New York: Macmillan.

@ INTERNET REFERENCES

- Additional information about bereavement may be located at the following websites:
  - http://www.journeyofhearts.org/
  - http://www.nhpco.org/
  - http://www.hospicefoundation.org/
  - http://www.bereavement.org/
  - http://www.caringinfo.org/
  - http://www.aahpm.org/
  - http://www.hpna.org/

Appendix A

Answers to Chapter Review Questions

CHAPTER 1. The Concept of Stress Adaptation
1. b   **2.** d   **3.** a   **4.** b   **5.** c   **6.** c, d, b, a

CHAPTER 2. Mental Health/Mental Illness: Historical and Theoretical Concepts
1. c   **2.** d   **3.** b   **4.** a   **5.** b   **6.** d   **7.** c
8. a, b, c, d   **9.** c   **10.** b

CHAPTER 3. Theoretical Models of Personality Development
1. b   **2.** c   **3.** d   **4.** b   **5.** b   **6.** b   **7.** a
8. c   **9.** a   **10.** b

CHAPTER 4. Concepts of Psychobiology
1. d   **2.** d   **3.** a   **4.** b   **5.** c   **6.** a   **7.** d
8. c   **9.** b   **10.** a   **11.** d   **12.** a   **13.** c

CHAPTER 5. Ethical and Legal Issues in Psychiatric/Mental Health Nursing
1. b   **2.** a   **3.** c   **4.** b   **5.** c   **6.** d   **7.** a, b, d
8. b, d   **9.** a, b   **10.** c

CHAPTER 6. Cultural and Spiritual Concepts Relevant to Psychiatric/Mental Health Nursing
1. c   **2.** d   **3.** a   **4.** d   **5.** b   **6.** c   **7.** c
8. b   **9.** b   **10.** a   **11.** a   **12.** d

CHAPTER 7. Relationship Development
1. c   **2.** a   **3.** a, b, c   **4.** b, e   **5.** b   **6.** d
7. c   **8.** b   **9.** d   **10.** a, c, d

CHAPTER 8. Therapeutic Communication
1. b   **2.** a   **3.** d   **4.** c   **5.** a   **6.** b   **7.** d
8. a   **9.** a, b, d   **10.** b

CHAPTER 9. The Nursing Process in Psychiatric/Mental Health Nursing
1. b   **2.** a   **3.** d   **4.** a   **5.** c   **6.** b
7. a, b, c, d   **8.** d   **9.** c   **10.** a, c, d

CHAPTER 10. Therapeutic Groups
1. b   **2.** d   **3.** a   **4.** c   **5.** c   **6.** d   **7.** c
8. b   **9.** d   **10.** a

CHAPTER 11. Intervention With Families
1. b   **2.** c   **3.** a   **4.** b   **5.** d   **6.** c   **7.** b
8. c   **9.** d   **10.** a

CHAPTER 12. Milieu Therapy—The Therapeutic Community
1. a, b, c   **2.** b   **3.** c   **4.** b   **5.** a   **6.** d   **7.** c
8. b   **9.** a, b, d, e   **10.** a, b, c

CHAPTER 13. Crisis Intervention
1. c   **2.** d   **3.** a   **4.** b   **5.** c   **6.** a   **7.** d
8. b   **9.** b   **10.** d   **11.** c   **12.** c   **13.** e

CHAPTER 14. Relaxation Therapy
1. a, b, e   **2.** a, b, d   **3.** a   **4.** c   **5.** d

CHAPTER 15. Assertiveness Training
1. c   **2.** a   **3.** b   **4.** a   **5.** a   **6.** c   **7.** d
8. a   **9.** c   **10.** b

CHAPTER 16. Promoting Self-Esteem
1. b   **2.** a   **3.** d   **4.** c   **5.** a   **6.** c   **7.** b
8. d   **9.** b   **10.** a

CHAPTER 17. Anger/Aggression Management
1. b, c   **2.** c   **3.** a   **4.** a, b, d   **5.** c
6. a, b, c   **7.** c   **8.** b   **9.** b, c, d, e   **10.** a, b, c

CHAPTER 18. The Suicidal Client
1. b   **2.** a   **3.** c   **4.** a   **5.** d   **6.** c   **7.** c
8. b   **9.** a, b, c   **10.** b

CHAPTER 19. Behavior Therapy
1. a   **2.** a   **3.** b   **4.** c   **5.** a   **6.** b   **7.** d
8. f, b, d, a, e, c

CHAPTER 20. Cognitive Therapy
1. c   **2.** a   **3.** d   **4.** b   **5.** c   **6.** a   **7.** d
8. a   **9.** b   **10.** c

CHAPTER 21. Electroconvulsive Therapy
1. c   **2.** b   **3.** a   **4.** c   **5.** d   **6.** a   **7.** c
8. d   **9.** b   **10.** c

CHAPTER 22. Complementary Therapies
1. a, c, e, f   **2.** a, b, d   **3.** c, d   **4.** a, d, e
5. c   **6.** d   **7.** a   **8.** b   **9.** a, b, c   **10.** c

CHAPTER 23. **Disorders Usually First Diagnosed in Infancy, Childhood, or Adolescence**
1. b   **2.** c   **3.** a   **4.** b   **5.** b   **6.** b, c, d   **7.** c
8. d   **9.** a   **10.** b

CHAPTER 24. **Delirium, Dementia, and Amnestic Disorders**
1. c, e   **2.** d   **3.** b   **4.** a, b, e   **5.** b
6. a, c, e   **7.** d   **8.** c   **9.** a   **10.** b   **11.** c, e

CHAPTER 25. **Substance-Related Disorders**
1. a   **2.** c   **3.** b   **4.** b   **5.** a   **6.** c   **7.** a
8. b   **9.** d   **10.** a

CHAPTER 26. **Schizophrenia and Other Psychotic Disorders**
1. b   **2.** b   **3.** c   **4.** d   **5.** d   **6.** a   **7.** c
8. b   **9.** c   **10.** d

CHAPTER 27. **Mood Disorders—Depression**
1. c   **2.** b   **3.** a   **4.** d   **5.** b, c   **6.** a, b, c, e
7. a   **8.** c   **9.** b   **10.** d

CHAPTER 28. **Mood Disorders—Bipolar Disorder**
1. b   **2.** c   **3.** a   **4.** a, c, d   **5.** b   **6.** d   **7.** b
8. c   **9.** a = 3, b = 1, c = 4, d = 2   **10.** c

CHAPTER 29. **Anxiety Disorders**
1. d   **2.** c   **3.** d   **4.** a   **5.** b   **6.** c   **7.** b
8. c   **9.** a   **10.** d

CHAPTER 30. **Somatoform and Dissociative Disorders**
1. a   **2.** b   **3.** d   **4.** b   **5.** c   **6.** d   **7.** b
8. a   **9.** b   **10.** d

CHAPTER 31. **Issues Related to Human Sexuality and Gender Identity**
1. b   **2.** c   **3.** a, b, c, d   **4.** a   **5.** b   **6.** d
7. b   **8.** d   **9.** c   **10.** a, b, d, e

CHAPTER 32. **Eating Disorders**
1. c   **2.** a   **3.** b   **4.** b   **5.** c   **6.** b   **7.** c
8. b   **9.** c   **10.** a

CHAPTER 33. **Adjustment and Impulse Control Disorders**
1. b   **2.** b   **3.** c   **4.** a   **5.** d   **6.** c   **7.** a
8. d   **9.** b   **10.** c   **11.** a, b, c   **12.** d

CHAPTER 34. **Personality Disorders**
1. d   **2.** a   **3.** b   **4.** d   **5.** a   **6.** b   **7.** c
8. c   **9.** d   **10.** b

CHAPTER 35. **The Aging Individual**
1. c   **2.** d   **3.** b   **4.** a   **5.** c   **6.** d   **7.** a
8. a   **9.** c   **10.** a

CHAPTER 36. **Victims of Abuse or Neglect**
1. b   **2.** c   **3.** a   **4.** d   **5.** b   **6.** d   **7.** a
8. b   **9.** b   **10.** d

CHAPTER 37. **Community Mental Health Nursing**
1. a   **2.** b   **3.** a   **4.** c   **5.** d   **6.** b   **7.** c
8. d   **9.** a   **10.** b

CHAPTER 38. **Forensic Nursing**
1. c   **2.** b   **3.** a, b, e   **4.** a, d, e   **5.** c   **6.** d
7. d   **8.** b   **9.** a, c, d, e   **10.** c

CHAPTER 39. **The Bereaved Individual**
1. e   **2.** c   **3.** c   **4.** d   **5.** a   **6.** a   **7.** b
8. c   **9.** a   **10.** c

Chapters on the Website:

Psychopharmacology
1. a   **2.** c   **3.** d   **4.** b   **5.** c   **6.** b   **7.** a
8. b   **9.** d   **10.** b

Client Education
1. a   **2.** c   **3.** d   **4.** c   **5.** a   **6.** b   **7.** c
8. d   **9.** a   **10.** b

Psychological Factors Affecting Medical Conditions
1. a, d   **2.** c   **3.** d   **4.** b   **5.** c   **6.** a   **7.** b
8. d   **9.** b   **10.** d

Appendix B

Mental Status Assessment

Gathering the correct information about the client's mental status is essential to the development of an appropriate plan of care. The mental status examination is a description of all the areas of the client's mental functioning. The following are the components that are considered critical in the assessment of a client's mental status. Examples of interview questions and criteria for assessment are included.

Identifying Data

1. Name
2. Gender
3. Age
   a. How old are you?
   b. When were you born?
4. Race/culture
   a. What country did you (your ancestors) come from?
5. Occupational/financial status
   a. How do you make your living?
   b. How do you obtain money for your needs?
6. Educational level
   a. What was the highest grade level you completed in school?
7. Significant other
   a. Are you married?
   b. Do you have a significant relationship with another person?
8. Living arrangements
   a. Do you live alone?
   b. With whom do you share your home?
9. Religious preference
   a. Do you have a religious preference?
10. Allergies
    a. Are you allergic to anything?
    b. Foods? Medications?
11. Special diet considerations
    a. Do you have any special diet requirements?
    b. Diabetic? Low sodium?
12. Chief complaint
    a. For what reason did you come for help today?
    b. What seems to be the problem?
13. Medical diagnosis

General Description

Appearance

1. Grooming and dress
   a. Note unusual modes of dress.
   b. Evidence of soiled clothing?
   c. Use of makeup?
   d. Neat; unkempt?
2. Hygiene
   a. Note evidence of body or breath odor.
   b. Condition of skin, fingernails?
3. Posture
   a. Note if standing upright, rigid, slumped over.
4. Height and weight
   a. Perform accurate measurements.
5. Level of eye contact
   a. Intermittent?
   b. Occasional and fleeting?
   c. Sustained and intense?
   d. No eye contact?
6. Hair color and texture
   a. Is hair clean and healthy looking?
   b. Greasy, matted, tangled?
7. Evidence of scars, tattoos, or other distinguishing skin marks
   a. Note any evidence of swelling or bruises.
   b. Birth marks?
   c. Rashes?
8. Evaluation of client's appearance compared with chronological age.

Motor Activity

1. Tremors
   a. Do hands or legs tremble?
      - Continuously?
      - At specific times?
2. Tics or other stereotypical movements
   a. Any evidence of facial tics?
   b. Jerking or spastic movements?
3. Mannerisms and gestures
   a. Specific facial or body movements during conversation?
   b. Nail biting?
   c. Covering face with hands?
   d. Grimacing?
4. Hyperactivity
   a. Gets up and down out of chair.
   b. Paces.
   c. Unable to sit still.
5. Restlessness or agitation
   a. Lots of fidgeting.
   b. Clenching hands.
6. Aggressiveness
   a. Overtly angry and hostile.
   b. Threatening.
   c. Uses sarcasm.
7. Rigidity
   a. Sits or stands in a rigid position.
   b. Arms and legs appear stiff and unyielding.
8. Gait patterns
   a. Any evidence of limping?
   b. Limitation of range of motion?
   c. Ataxia?
   d. Shuffling?
9. Echopraxia
   a. Evidence of mimicking the actions of others?
10. Psychomotor retardation
    a. Movements are very slow.
    b. Thinking and speech are very slow.
    c. Posture is slumped.
11. Freedom of movement (range of motion)
    a. Note any limitation in ability to move.

Speech Patterns

1. Slowness or rapidity of speech
   a. Note whether speech seems very rapid or slower than normal.
2. Pressure of speech
   a. Note whether speech seems frenzied.
   b. Unable to be interrupted?
3. Intonation
   a. Are words spoken with appropriate emphasis?
   b. Are words spoken in monotone, without emphasis?
4. Volume
   a. Is speech very loud? Soft?
   b. Is speech low-pitched? High-pitched?
5. Stuttering or other speech impairments
   a. Hoarseness?
   b. Slurred speech?
6. Aphasia
   a. Difficulty forming words
   b. Use of incorrect words
   c. Difficulty thinking of specific words
   d. Making up words (neologisms)

General Attitude

1. Cooperative/uncooperative
   a. Answers questions willingly.
   b. Refuses to answer questions.
2. Friendly/hostile/defensive
   a. Is sociable and responsive.
   b. Is sarcastic and irritable.
3. Uninterested/apathetic
   a. Refuses to participate in interview process.
4. Attentive/interested
   a. Actively participates in interview process.
5. Guarded/suspicious
   a. Continuously scans the environment.
   b. Questions motives of interviewer.
   c. Refuses to answer questions.

Emotions

Mood

1. Depressed; despairing
   a. An overwhelming feeling of sadness
   b. Loss of interest in regular activities
2. Irritable
   a. Easily annoyed and provoked to anger.
3. Anxious
   a. Demonstrates or verbalizes feeling of apprehension.

4. Elated

   a. Expresses feelings of joy and intense pleasure.

   b. Is intensely optimistic.

5. Euphoric

   a. Demonstrates a heightened sense of elation.

   b. Expresses feelings of grandeur ("Everything is wonderful!").

6. Fearful

   a. Demonstrates or verbalizes feeling of apprehension associated with real or perceived danger.

7. Guilty

   a. Expresses a feeling of discomfort associated with real or perceived wrongdoing.

   b. May be associated with feelings of sadness and despair

8. Labile

   a. Exhibits mood swings that range from euphoria to depression or anxiety.

Affect

1. Congruence with mood

   a. Outward emotional expression is consistent with mood (e.g., if depressed, emotional expression is sadness, eyes downcast, may be crying).

2. Constricted or blunted

   a. Minimal outward emotional expression is observed.

3. Flat

   a. There is an absence of outward emotional expression.

4. Appropriate

   a. The outward emotional expression is what would be expected in a certain situation (e.g., crying upon hearing of a death).

5. Inappropriate

   a. The outward emotional expression is incompatible with the situation (e.g., laughing upon hearing of a death).

Thought Processes

Form of Thought

1. Flight of ideas

   a. Verbalizations are continuous and rapid, and flow from one to another.

2. Associative looseness

   a. Verbalizations shift from one unrelated topic to another.

3. Circumstantiality

   a. Verbalizations are lengthy and tedious, and because of numerous details, are delayed reaching the intended point.

4. Tangentiality

   a. Verbalizations are lengthy and tedious, and never reach an intended point.

5. Neologisms

   a. The individual is making up nonsensical-sounding words, which only have meaning to him or her.

6. Concrete thinking

   a. Thinking is literal; elemental.

   b. Absence of ability to think abstractly.

   c. Unable to translate simple proverbs.

7. Clang associations

   a. Speaks in puns or rhymes; uses words that sound alike but have different meanings.

8. Word salad

   a. Uses a mixture of words that have no meaning together; sounds incoherent.

9. Perseveration

   a. Persistently repeats the last word of a sentence spoken to the person (e.g., Nurse: "George, it's time to go to lunch." George: "lunch, lunch, lunch, lunch").

10. Echolalia

   a. Persistently repeats what another person says.

11. Mutism

   a. Does not speak (either cannot or will not).

12. Poverty of speech

   a. Speaks very little; may respond in monosyllables.

13. Ability to concentrate and disturbance of attention

   a. Does the person hold attention to the topic at hand?

   b. Is the person easily distractible?

   c. Is there selective attention (e.g., blocks out topics that create anxiety)?

Content of Thought

1. Delusions (Does the person have unrealistic ideas or beliefs?)

   a. Persecutory: A belief that someone is out to get him or her is some way (e.g., "The FBI will be here at any time to take me away.").

b. Grandiose: An idea that he or she is all-powerful or of great importance (e.g., "I am the king...and this is my kingdom! I can do anything!").

c. Reference: An idea that whatever is happening in the environment is about him or her (e.g., "Just watch the movie on TV tonight. It is about my life.").

d. Control or influence: A belief that his or her behavior and thoughts are being controlled by external forces (e.g., "I get my orders from Channel 27. I do only what the forces dictate.").

e. Somatic: A belief that he or she has a dysfunctional body part (e.g., "My heart is at a standstill. It is no longer beating.").

f. Nihilistic: A belief that he or she, or a part of the body, or even the world does not exist or has been destroyed (e.g., "I am no longer alive.").

2. Suicidal or homicidal ideas

a. Is the individual expressing ideas of harming self or others?

3. Obsessions

a. Is the person verbalizing about a persistent thought or feeling that he or she is unable to eliminate from the consciousness?

4. Paranoia/suspiciousness

a. Continuously scans the environment.

b. Questions motives of interviewer.

c. Refuses to answer questions.

5. Magical thinking

a. Is the person speaking in a way that indicates his or her words or actions have power? (e.g., "If you step on a crack, you break your mother's back!")

6. Religiosity

a. Is the individual demonstrating obsession with religious ideas and behavior?

7. Phobias

a. Is there evidence of irrational fears (of a specific object, or a social situation)?

8. Poverty of content

a. Is little information conveyed by the client because of vagueness or stereotypical statements or clichés?

Perceptual Disturbances

1. Hallucinations (Is the person experiencing unrealistic sensory perceptions?)

a. Auditory (Is the individual hearing voices or other sounds that do not exist?)

b. Visual (Is the individual seeing images that do not exist?)

c. Tactile (Does the individual feel unrealistic sensations on the skin?)

d. Olfactory (Does the individual smell odors that do not exist?)

e. Gustatory (Does the individual have a false perception of an unpleasant taste?)

2. Illusions

a. Does the individual misperceive or misinterpret real stimuli within the environment? (Sees something and thinks it is something else?)

3. Depersonalization (altered perception of the self)

a. The individual verbalizes feeling "outside the body;" visualizing him- or herself from afar.

4. Derealization (altered perception of the environment)

a. The individual verbalizes that the environment feels "strange or unreal." A feeling that the surroundings have changed.

Sensorium and Cognitive Ability

1. Level of alertness/consciousness

a. Is the individual clear-minded and attentive to the environment?

b. Or is there disturbance in perception and awareness of the surroundings?

2. Orientation: Is the person oriented to the following?

a. Time

b. Place

c. Person

d. Circumstances

3. Memory

a. Recent (Is the individual able to remember occurrences of the past few days?)

b. Remote (Is the individual able to remember occurrences of the distant past?)

c. Confabulation (Does the individual fill in memory gaps with experiences that have no basis in fact?

4. Capacity for abstract thought

a. Can the individual interpret proverbs correctly?

   • "What does 'no use crying over spilled milk' mean?"

Impulse Control

1. Ability to control impulses. (Does psychosocial history reveal problems with any of the following?)

a. Aggression

b. Hostility

c. Fear

d. Guilt

e. Affection

f. Sexual feelings

Judgment and Insight

1. Ability to solve problems and make decisions

    a. What are your plans for the future?

    b. What do you plan to do to reach your goals?

2. Knowledge about self

    a. Awareness of limitations

    b. Awareness of consequences of actions

    c. Awareness of illness

      • "Do you think you have a problem?"

      • "Do you think you need treatment?"

3. Adaptive/maladaptive use of coping strategies and ego defense mechanisms (e.g., rationalizing maladaptive behaviors, projection of blame, displacement of anger)

Appendix C

DSM-IV-TR Classification: Axes I and II Categories and Codes*

Disorders Usually First Diagnosed in Infancy, Childhood, or Adolescence

Mental Retardation

Note: These are coded on Axis II.

317	Mild Mental Retardation
318.0	Moderate Retardation
318.1	Severe Retardation
318.2	Profound Mental Retardation
319	Mental Retardation, Severity Unspecified

Learning Disorders

315.00	Reading Disorder
315.1	Mathematics Disorder
315.2	Disorder of Written Expression
315.9	Learning Disorder Not Otherwise Specified (NOS)

Motor Skills Disorder

315.4	Developmental Coordination Disorder

Communication Disorders

315.31	Expressive Language Disorder
315.32	Mixed Receptive-Expressive Language Disorder
315.39	Phonological Disorder
307.0	Stuttering
307.9	Communication Disorder NOS

Pervasive Developmental Disorders

299.00	Autistic Disorder
299.80	Rett's Disorder
299.10	Childhood Disintegrative Disorder
299.80	Asperger's Disorder
299.80	Pervasive Developmental Disorder NOS

*Reprinted with permission from the *Diagnostic and Statistical Manual of Mental Disorders, Fourth Edition, Text Revision*. Copyright 2000, American Psychiatric Association.

Attention-Deficit and Disruptive Behavior Disorders

314.xx	Attention-Deficit/Hyperactivity Disorder
314.01	Combined Type
314.00	Predominantly Inattentive Type
314.01	Predominantly Hyperactive-Impulsive Type
314.9	Attention-Deficit/Hyperactivity Disorder NOS
312.xx	Conduct Disorder
.81	Childhood-Onset Type
.82	Adolescent-Onset Type
.89	Unspecified Onset
313.81	Oppositional Defiant Disorder
312.9	Disruptive Behavior Disorder NOS

Feeding and Eating Disorders of Infancy or Early Childhood

307.52	Pica
307.53	Rumination Disorder
307.59	Feeding Disorder of Infancy or Early Childhood

Tic Disorders

307.23	Tourette's Disorder
307.22	Chronic Motor or Vocal Tic Disorder
307.21	Transient Tic Disorder
307.20	Tic Disorder NOS

Elimination Disorders

—	Encopresis
787.6	With Constipation and Overflow Incontinence
307.7	Without Constipation and Overflow Incontinence
307.6	Enuresis (Not due to a General Medical Condition)

Other Disorders of Infancy, Childhood, or Adolescence

309.21	Separation Anxiety Disorder
313.23	Selective Mutism

313.89 Reactive Attachment Disorder of Infancy or Early Childhood

307.3 Stereotypic Movement Disorder

313.9 Disorder of Infancy, Childhood, or Adolescence NOS

Delirium, Dementia, and Amnestic and Other Cognitive Disorders

Delirium

293.0 Delirium due to... *(indicate the General Medical Condition)*

— Substance Intoxication Delirium *(refer to Substance-Related Disorders for substance-specific codes)*

— Substance Withdrawal Delirium *(refer to Substance-Related Disorders for substance-specific codes)*

— Delirium due to Multiple Etiologies *(code each of the specific etiologies)*

780.09 Delirium NOS

Dementia

294.xx Dementia of the Alzheimer's Type, With Early Onset

   .10 Without Behavioral Disturbance

   .11 With Behavioral Disturbance

294.xx Dementia of the Alzheimer's Type, With Late Onset

   .10 Without Behavioral Disturbance

   .11 With Behavioral Disturbance

290.xx Vascular Dementia

   .40 Uncomplicated

   .41 With Delirium

   .42 With Delusions

   .43 With Depressed Mood

294.1x Dementia due to HIV Disease

294.1x Dementia due to Head Trauma

294.1x Dementia due to Parkinson's Disease

294.1x Dementia due to Huntington's Disease

294.1x Dementia due to Pick's Disease

294.1x Dementia due to Creutzfeldt-Jakob Disease

294.1x Dementia due to *(indicate the General Medical Condition not listed above)*

— Substance-Induced Persisting Dementia *(refer to Substance-Related Disorders for substance-specific codes)*

— Dementia due to Multiple Etiologies *(code each of the specific etiologies)*

294.8 Dementia NOS

Amnestic Disorders

294.0 Amnestic Disorder due to *(indicate the General Medical Condition)*

— Substance-Induced Persisting Amnestic Disorder *(refer to Substance-Related Disorders for substance-specific codes)*

294.8 Amnestic Disorder NOS

Other Cognitive Disorders

294.9 Cognitive Disorder NOS

Mental Disorders due to a General Medical Condition Not Elsewhere Classified

293.89 Catatonic Disorder due to *(indicate the General Medical Condition)*

310.1 Personality Change due to *(indicate the General Medical Condition)*

293.9 Mental Disorder NOS due to *(indicate the General Medical Condition)*

Substance-Related Disorders

Alcohol-Related Disorders
Alcohol Use Disorders

303.90 Alcohol Dependence

305.00 Alcohol Abuse

Alcohol-Induced Disorders

303.00 Alcohol Intoxication

291.81 Alcohol Withdrawal

291.0 Alcohol Intoxication Delirium

291.0 Alcohol Withdrawal Delirium

291.2 Alcohol-Induced Persisting Dementia

291.1 Alcohol-Induced Persisting Amnestic Disorder

291.x Alcohol-Induced Psychotic Disorder

   .5 With Delusions

   .3 With Hallucinations

291.89 Alcohol-Induced Mood Disorder

291.89 Alcohol-Induced Anxiety Disorder

291.89 Alcohol-Induced Sexual Dysfunction

291.89 Alcohol-Induced Sleep Disorder

291.9 Alcohol-Related Disorder NOS

Amphetamine (or Amphetamine-Like)-Related Disorders
Amphetamine Use Disorders

304.40 Amphetamine Dependence

305.70 Amphetamine Abuse

Amphetamine-Induced Disorders

292.89 Amphetamine Intoxication

292.0 Amphetamine Withdrawal

292.81 Amphetamine Intoxication Delirium

292.xx Amphetamine-Induced Psychotic
Disorder

   .11 With Delusions

   .12 With Hallucinations

292.84 Amphetamine-Induced Mood Disorder

292.89 Amphetamine-Induced Anxiety Disorder

292.89 Amphetamine-Induced Sexual
Dysfunction

292.89 Amphetamine-Induced Sleep Disorder

292.9 Amphetamine-Related Disorder NOS

Caffeine-Related Disorders

Caffeine-Induced Disorders

305.90 Caffeine Intoxication

292.89 Caffeine-Induced Anxiety Disorder

292.89 Caffeine-Induced Sleep Disorder

292.9 Caffeine-Related Disorder NOS

Cannabis-Related Disorders

Cannabis Use Disorders

304.30 Cannabis Dependence

305.20 Cannabis Abuse

Cannabis-Induced Disorders

292.89 Cannabis Intoxication

292.81 Cannabis Intoxication Delirium

292.xx Cannabis-Induced Psychotic Disorder

   .11 With Delusions

   .12 With Hallucinations

292.89 Cannabis-Induced Anxiety Disorder

292.9 Cannabis-Related Disorder NOS

Cocaine-Related Disorders

Cocaine Use Disorders

304.20 Cocaine Dependence

305.60 Cocaine Abuse

Cocaine-Induced Disorders

292.89 Cocaine Intoxication

292.0 Cocaine Withdrawal

292.81 Cocaine Intoxication Delirium

292.xx Cocaine-Induced Psychotic Disorder

   .11 With Delusions

   .12 With Hallucinations

292.84 Cocaine-Induced Mood Disorder

292.89 Cocaine-Induced Anxiety Disorder

292.89 Cocaine-Induced Sexual Dysfunction

292.89 Cocaine-Induced Sleep Disorder

292.9 Cocaine-Related Disorder NOS

Hallucinogen-Related Disorders

Hallucinogen Use Disorders

304.50 Hallucinogen Dependence

305.30 Hallucinogen Abuse

Hallucinogen-Induced Disorders

292.89 Hallucinogen Intoxication

292.89 Hallucinogen Persisting Perception
Disorder (Flashbacks)

292.81 Hallucinogen Intoxication Delirium

292.xx Hallucinogen-Induced Psychotic Disorder

   .11 With Delusions

   .12 With Hallucinations

292.84 Hallucinogen-Induced Mood Disorder

292.89 Hallucinogen-Induced Anxiety Disorder

292.9 Hallucinogen-Related Disorder NOS

Inhalant-Related Disorders

Inhalant Use Disorders

304.60 Inhalant Dependence

305.90 Inhalant Abuse

Inhalant-Induced Disorders

292.89 Inhalant Intoxication

292.81 Inhalant Intoxication Delirium

292.82 Inhalant-Induced Persisting Dementia

292.xx Inhalant-Induced Psychotic Disorder

   .11 With Delusions

   .12 With Hallucinations

292.84 Inhalant-Induced Mood Disorder

292.89 Inhalant-Induced Anxiety Disorder

292.9 Inhalant-Related Disorder NOS

Nicotine-Related Disorders

Nicotine Use Disorders

305.1 Nicotine Dependence

Nicotine-Induced Disorders

292.0 Nicotine Withdrawal

292.9 Nicotine-Related Disorder NOS

Opioid-Related Disorders

Opioid Use Disorders

304.00 Opioid Dependence

305.50 Opioid Abuse

Opioid-Induced Disorders

292.89 Opioid Intoxication

292.0 Opioid Withdrawal

292.81 Opioid Intoxication Delirium

292.xx Opioid-Induced Psychotic Disorder

   .11 With Delusions

   .12   With Hallucinations

292.84   Opioid-Induced Mood Disorder

292.89   Opioid-Induced Sexual Dysfunction

292.89   Opioid-Induced Sleep Disorder

292.9   Opioid-Related Disorder NOS

Phencyclidine (or Phencyclidine-Like)-Related Disorders

Phencyclidine Use Disorders

304.60   Phencyclidine Dependence

305.90   Phencyclidine Abuse

Phencyclidine-Induced Disorders

292.89   Phencyclidine Intoxication

292.81   Phencyclidine Intoxication Delirium

292.xx   Phencyclidine-Induced Psychotic Disorder

   .11   With Delusions

   .12   With Hallucinations

292.84   Phencyclidine-Induced Mood Disorder

292.89   Phencyclidine-Induced Anxiety Disorder

292.9   Phencyclidine-Related Disorder NOS

Sedative-, Hypnotic-, or Anxiolytic-Related Disorders

Sedative, Hypnotic, or Anxiolytic Use Disorders

304.10   Sedative, Hypnotic, or Anxiolytic Dependence

305.40   Sedative, Hypnotic, or Anxiolytic Abuse

Sedative-, Hypnotic-, or Anxiolytic-Induced Disorders

292.89   Sedative, Hypnotic, or Anxiolytic Intoxication

292.0   Sedative, Hypnotic, or Anxiolytic Withdrawal

292.81   Sedative, Hypnotic, or Anxiolytic Intoxication Delirium

292.81   Sedative, Hypnotic, or Anxiolytic Withdrawal Delirium

292.82   Sedative-, Hypnotic-, or Anxiolytic-Induced Persisting Dementia

292.83   Sedative-, Hypnotic-, or Anxiolytic-Induced Persisting Amnestic Disorder

292.xx   Sedative-, Hypnotic-, or Anxiolytic-Induced Psychotic Disorder

   .11   With Delusions

   .12   With Hallucinations

292.84   Sedative-, Hypnotic-, or Anxiolytic-Induced Mood Disorder

292.89   Sedative-, Hypnotic-, or Anxiolytic-Induced Anxiety Disorder

292.89   Sedative-, Hypnotic-, or Anxiolytic-Induced Sexual Dysfunction

292.89   Sedative-, Hypnotic-, or Anxiolytic-Induced Sleep Disorder

292.9   Sedative-, Hypnotic-, or Anxiolytic-Related Disorder NOS

Polysubstance-Related Disorder

304.80   Polysubstance Dependence

Other (or Unknown) Substance-Related Disorders

Other (or Unknown) Substance Use Disorders

304.90   Other (or Unknown) Substance Dependence

305.90   Other (or Unknown) Substance Abuse

Other (or Unknown) Substance-Induced Disorders

292.89   Other (or Unknown) Substance Intoxication

292.0   Other (or Unknown) Substance Withdrawal

292.81   Other (or Unknown) Substance-Induced Delirium

292.82   Other (or Unknown) Substance-Induced Persisting Dementia

292.83   Other (or Unknown) Substance-Induced Persisting Amnestic Disorder

292.xx   Other (or Unknown) Substance-Induced Psychotic Disorder

   .11   With Delusions

   .12   With Hallucinations

292.84   Other (or Unknown) Substance-Induced Mood Disorder

292.89   Other (or Unknown) Substance-Induced Anxiety Disorder

292.89   Other (or Unknown) Substance-Induced Sexual Dysfunction

292.89   Other (or Unknown) Substance-Induced Sleep Disorder

292.9   Other (or Unknown) Substance-Related Disorder NOS

Schizophrenia and Other Psychotic Disorders

295.xx   Schizophrenia

   .30   Paranoid type

   .10   Disorganized type

   .20   Catatonic type

   .90   Undifferentiated type

   .60   Residual type

295.40   Schizophreniform Disorder

295.70   Schizoaffective Disorder

297.1   Delusional Disorder

298.8   Brief Psychotic Disorder

297.3   Shared Psychotic Disorder

293.xx Psychotic Disorder due to *(indicate the General Medical Condition)*

  .81 With Delusions

  .82 With Hallucinations

  — Substance-Induced Psychotic Disorder *(refer to Substance-Related Disorders for substance-specific codes)*

298.9   Psychotic Disorder NOS

Mood Disorders

(Code current state of Major Depressive Disorder or Bipolar I Disorder in fifth digit: 0 = unspecified; 1 = mild; 2 = moderate; 3 = severe, without psychotic features; 4 = severe, with psychotic features; 5 = in partial remission; 6 = in full remission.)

Depressive Disorders

296.xx Major Depressive Disorder

  .2x Single episode

  .3x Recurrent

300.4   Dysthymic Disorder

311   Depressive Disorder NOS

Bipolar Disorders

296.xx Bipolar I Disorder

  .0x Single Manic Episode

  .40 Most Recent Episode Hypomanic

  .4x Most Recent Episode Manic

  .6x Most Recent Episode Mixed

  .5x Most Recent Episode Depressed

  .7   Most Recent Episode Unspecified

296.89 Bipolar II Disorder *(specify current or most recent episode: Hypomanic or Depressed)*

301.13 Cyclothymic Disorder

296.80 Bipolar Disorder NOS

293.83 Mood Disorder due to *(indicate the General Medical Condition)*

  — Substance-Induced Mood Disorder *(refer to Substance-Related Disorders for substance-specific codes)*

296.90 Mood Disorder NOS

Anxiety Disorders

300.01 Panic Disorder Without Agoraphobia

300.21 Panic Disorder With Agoraphobia

300.22 Agoraphobia Without History of Panic Disorder

300.29 Specific Phobia

300.23 Social Phobia

300.3   Obsessive-Compulsive Disorder

309.81 Posttraumatic Stress Disorder

308.3   Acute Stress Disorder

300.02 Generalized Anxiety Disorder

293.89 Anxiety Disorder due to *(indicate the General Medical Condition)*

  — Substance-Induced Anxiety Disorder *(refer to Substance-Related Disorders for substance-specific codes)*

300.00 Anxiety Disorder NOS

Somatoform Disorders

300.81 Somatization Disorder

300.82 Undifferentiated Somatoform Disorder

300.11 Conversion Disorder

307.xx Pain Disorder

  .80 Associated With Psychological Factors

  .89 Associated With Both Psychological Factors and a General Medical Condition

300.7   Hypochondriasis

300.7   Body Dysmorphic Disorder

300.82 Somatoform Disorder NOS

Factitious Disorders

300.xx Factitious Disorder

  .16 With Predominantly Psychological Signs and Symptoms

  .19 With Predominantly Physical Signs and Symptoms

  .19 With Combined Psychological and Physical Signs and Symptoms

300.19 Factitious Disorder NOS

Dissociative Disorders

300.12 Dissociative Amnesia

300.13 Dissociative Fugue

300.14 Dissociative Identity Disorder

300.6   Depersonalization Disorder

300.15 Dissociative Disorder NOS

Sexual and Gender Identity Disorders

Sexual Dysfunctions

Sexual Desire Disorders

302.71 Hypoactive Sexual Desire Disorder

302.79 Sexual Aversion Disorder

Sexual Arousal Disorders

302.72 Female Sexual Arousal Disorder

302.72 Male Erectile Disorder

Orgasmic Disorders

302.73 Female Orgasmic Disorder

302.74 Male Orgasmic Disorder

302.75 Premature Ejaculation

Sexual Pain Disorders

302.76 Dyspareunia (Not due to a General Medical Condition)

306.51 Vaginismus (Not due to a General Medical Condition)

Sexual Dysfunction due to a General Medical Condition

625.8 Female Hypoactive Sexual Desire Disorder due to *(indicate the General Medical Condition)*

608.89 Male Hypoactive Sexual Desire Disorder due to *(indicate the General Medical Condition)*

607.84 Male Erectile Disorder due to *(indicate the General Medical Condition)*

625.0 Female Dyspareunia due to *(indicate the General Medical Condition)*

608.89 Male Dyspareunia due to *(indicate the General Medical Condition)*

625.8 Other Female Sexual Dysfunction due to *(indicate the General Medical Condition)*

608.89 Other Male Sexual Dysfunction due to *(indicate the General Medical Condition)*

— Substance-Induced Sexual Dysfunction *(refer to Substance-Related Disorders for substance-specific codes)*

302.70 Sexual Dysfunction NOS

Paraphilias

302.4 Exhibitionism

302.81 Fetishism

302.89 Frotteurism

302.2 Pedophilia

302.83 Sexual Masochism

302.84 Sexual Sadism

302.3 Transvestic Fetishism

302.82 Voyeurism

302.9 Paraphilia NOS

Gender Identity Disorders

302.xx Gender Identity Disorder

  .6 In Children

  .85 In Adolescents or Adults

302.6 Gender Identity Disorder NOS

302.9 Sexual Disorder NOS

Eating Disorders

307.1 Anorexia Nervosa

307.51 Bulimia Nervosa

307.50 Eating Disorder NOS

Sleep Disorders

Primary Sleep Disorders
Dyssomnias

307.42 Primary Insomnia

307.44 Primary Hypersomnia

347 Narcolepsy

780.59 Breathing-Related Sleep Disorder

307.45 Circadian Rhythm Sleep Disorder

307.47 Dyssomnia NOS

Parasomnias

307.47 Nightmare Disorder

307.46 Sleep Terror Disorder

307.46 Sleepwalking Disorder

307.47 Parasomnia NOS

Sleep Disorders Related to Another Mental Disorder

307.42 Insomnia Related to *(indicate the Axis I or Axis II Disorder)*

307.44 Hypersomnia Related to *(indicate the Axis I or Axis II Disorder)*

Other Sleep Disorders

780.xx Sleep Disorder due to *(indicate the General Medical Condition)*

  .52 Insomnia type

  .54 Hypersomnia type

  .59 Parasomnia type

  .59 Mixed type

— Substance-Induced Sleep Disorder *(refer to Substance-Related Disorders for substance-specific codes)*

Impulse Control Disorders Not Elsewhere Classified

312.34 Intermittent Explosive Disorder

312.32 Kleptomania

312.33 Pyromania

312.31 Pathological Gambling

312.39 Trichotillomania

312.30 Impulse Control Disorder NOS

Adjustment Disorders

309.xx Adjustment Disorder

  .0 With Depressed Mood

.24 With Anxiety

.28 With Mixed Anxiety and Depressed Mood

.3 With Disturbance of Conduct

.4 With Mixed Disturbance of Emotions and Conduct

.9 Unspecified

Personality Disorders

Note: These are coded on Axis II.

301.0 Paranoid Personality Disorder

301.20 Schizoid Personality Disorder

301.22 Schizotypal Personality Disorder

301.7 Antisocial Personality Disorder

301.83 Borderline Personality Disorder

301.50 Histrionic Personality Disorder

301.81 Narcissistic Personality Disorder

301.82 Avoidant Personality Disorder

301.6 Dependent Personality Disorder

301.4 Obsessive-Compulsive Personality Disorder

301.9 Personality Disorder NOS

Other Conditions That May Be a Focus of Clinical Attention

Psychological Factors Affecting Medical Condition

316 *Choose name based on nature of factors:*

Mental Disorder Affecting Medical Condition

Psychological Symptoms Affecting Medical Condition

Personality Traits or Coping Style Affecting Medical Condition

Maladaptive Health Behaviors Affecting Medical Condition

Stress-Related Physiological Response Affecting Medical Condition

Other or Unspecified Psychological Factors Affecting Medical Condition

Medication-Induced Movement Disorders

332.1 Neuroleptic-Induced Parkinsonism

333.92 Neuroleptic Malignant Syndrome

333.7 Neuroleptic-Induced Acute Dystonia

333.99 Neuroleptic-Induced Acute Akathisia

333.82 Neuroleptic-Induced Tardive Dyskinesia

333.1 Medication-Induced Postural Tremor

333.90 Medication-Induced Movement Disorder NOS

Other Medication-Induced Disorder

995.2 Adverse Effects of Medication NOS

Relational Problems

V61.9 Relational Problem Related to a Mental Disorder or General Medical Condition

V61.20 Parent-Child Relational Problem

V61.10 Partner Relational Problem

V61.8 Sibling Relational Problem

V62.81 Relational Problem NOS

Problems Related to Abuse or Neglect

V61.21 Physical Abuse of Child

V61.21 Sexual Abuse of Child

V61.21 Neglect of Child

— Physical Abuse of Adult

V61.12 (if by partner)

V62.83 (if by person other than partner)

— Sexual Abuse of Adult

V61.12 (if by partner)

V62.83 (if by person other than partner)

Additional Conditions That May Be a Focus of Clinical Attention

V15.81 Noncompliance With Treatment

V65.2 Malingering

V71.01 Adult Antisocial Behavior

V71.02 Childhood or Adolescent Antisocial Behavior

V62.89 Borderline Intellectual Functioning (coded on Axis II)

780.9 Age-Related Cognitive Decline

V62.82 Bereavement

V62.3 Academic Problem

V62.2 Occupational Problem

313.82 Identity Problem

V62.89 Religious or Spiritual Problem

V62.4 Acculturation Problem

V62.89 Phase of Life Problem

Additional Codes

300.9 Unspecified Mental Disorder (nonpsychotic)

V71.09 No Diagnosis or Condition on Axis I

799.9 Diagnosis or Condition Deferred on Axis I

V71.09 No Diagnosis on Axis II

799.9 Diagnosis Deferred on Axis II

Appendix D

NANDA Nursing Diagnoses: Taxonomy II

Domains, Classes, and Diagnoses

Domain 1: Health Promotion

Class 1: Health Awareness

Class 2: Health Management
  Approved Diagnoses:
  Ineffective self health management
  Ineffective family therapeutic regimen management
  Ineffective health maintenance
  Impaired home maintenance
  Readiness for enhanced self health management
  Readiness for enhanced nutrition
  Readiness for enhanced immunization status
  Self neglect

Domain 2: Nutrition

Class 1: Ingestion
  Approved Diagnoses:
  Ineffective infant feeding pattern
  Impaired swallowing
  Imbalanced nutrition: Less than body requirements
  Imbalanced nutrition: More than body requirements
  Risk for imbalanced nutrition: More than body requirements

Class 2: Digestion

Class 3: Absorption

Class 4: Metabolism
  Approved Diagnoses:
  Risk for impaired liver function
  Risk for unstable blood glucose level
  Neonatal jaundice

Class 5: Hydration
  Approved Diagnoses:
  Deficient fluid volume
  Risk for deficient fluid volume
  Excess fluid volume
  Readiness for enhanced fluid balance
  Risk for electrolyte imbalance
  Risk for imbalanced fluid volume

Domain 3: Elimination and Exchange

Class 1: Urinary Function
  Approved Diagnoses:
  Impaired urinary elimination
  Urinary retention
  Functional urinary incontinence
  Stress urinary incontinence
  Urge urinary incontinence
  Reflex urinary incontinence
  Risk for urge urinary incontinence
  Readiness for enhanced urinary elimination
  Overflow urinary incontinence

Class 2: Gastrointestinal Function
  Approved Diagnoses:
  Bowel incontinence
  Diarrhea
  Constipation
  Risk for constipation
  Perceived constipation
  Dysfunctional gastrointestinal motility
  Risk for dysfunctional gastrointestinal motility

Class 3: Integumentary Function

Class 4: Respiratory Function
  Approved Diagnoses:
  Impaired gas exchange
  Ineffective airway clearance
  Impaired spontaneous ventilation

Domain 4: Activity/Rest

Class 1: Sleep/Rest
  Approved Diagnoses:
  Sleep deprivation
  Readiness for enhanced sleep
  Insomnia
  Disturbed sleep pattern

Class 2: Activity/Exercise
Approved Diagnoses:

Risk for disuse syndrome

Impaired physical mobility

Impaired bed mobility

Impaired wheelchair mobility

Impaired transfer ability

Impaired walking

Deficient diversional activity

Delayed surgical recovery

Sedentary lifestyle

Class 3: Energy Balance
Approved Diagnoses:

Energy field disturbance

Fatigue

Class 4: Cardiovascular/Pulmonary Responses
Approved Diagnoses:

Decreased cardiac output

Impaired spontaneous ventilation

Ineffective breathing pattern

Activity intolerance

Risk for activity intolerance

Dysfunctional ventilatory weaning response

Risk for decreased cardiac tissue perfusion

Risk for ineffective cerebral tissue perfusion

Risk for ineffective gastrointestinal perfusion

Risk for tissue perfusion

Ineffective peripheral tissue perfusion

Risk for shock

Risk for bleeding

Class 5: Self-Care
Approved Diagnoses:

Dressing self-care deficit

Bathing self-care deficit

Feeding self-care deficit

Toileting self-care deficit

Readiness for enhanced self-care

Domain 5: Perception/Cognition

Class 1: Attention
Approved Diagnoses:

Unilateral neglect

Class 2: Orientation
Approved Diagnoses:

Impaired environmental interpretation syndrome

Wandering

Class 3: Sensation/Perception
Approved Diagnoses:

Disturbed sensory perception (specify: visual, auditory, kinesthetic, gustatory, tactile)

Class 4: Cognition
Approved Diagnoses:

Deficient knowledge

Readiness for enhanced knowledge

Acute confusion

Chronic confusion

Impaired memory

Disturbed thought processes

Readiness for enhanced decision making

Risk for acute confusion

Ineffective activity planning

Class 5: Communication
Approved Diagnoses:

Impaired verbal communication

Readiness for enhanced communication

Domain 6: Self-Perception

Class 1: Self-Concept
Approved Diagnoses:

Disturbed personal identity

Powerlessness

Risk for powerlessness

Hopelessness

Risk for loneliness

Readiness for enhanced self-concept

Readiness for enhanced power

Risk for compromised human dignity

Readiness for enhanced hope

Class 2: Self-Esteem
Approved Diagnoses:

Chronic low self-esteem

Situational low self-esteem

Risk for situational low self-esteem

Class 3: Body Image
Approved Diagnoses:

Disturbed body image

Domain 7: Role Relationships

Class 1: Caregiving Roles
Approved Diagnoses:

Caregiver role strain

Risk for caregiver role strain

Impaired parenting

Risk for impaired parenting

Readiness for enhanced parenting

Class 2: Family Relationships
Approved Diagnoses:

Interrupted family processes

Readiness for enhanced family processes

Dysfunctional family processes

Risk for impaired attachment

Class 3: Role Performance
Approved Diagnoses:

Effective breastfeeding

Ineffective breastfeeding

Interrupted breastfeeding

Ineffective role performance

Parental role conflict

Impaired social interaction

Readiness for enhanced relationship

Domain 8: Sexuality

Class 1: Sexual Identity
Class 2: Sexual Function
Approved Diagnoses:

Sexual dysfunction

Ineffective sexuality pattern

Class 3: Reproduction
Approved Diagnoses:

Readiness for enhanced childbearing process

Risk for disturbed maternal/fetal dyad

Domain 9: Coping/Stress Tolerance

Class 1: Post-Trauma Responses
Approved Diagnoses:

Relocation stress syndrome

Risk for relocation stress syndrome

Rape-trauma syndrome

Post-trauma syndrome

Risk for post-trauma syndrome

Class 2: Coping Responses
Approved Diagnoses:

Fear

Anxiety

Death anxiety

Chronic sorrow

Ineffective denial

Ineffective coping

Disabled family coping

Compromised family coping

Defensive coping

Ineffective community coping

Readiness for enhanced coping (individual)

Readiness for enhanced family coping

Readiness for enhanced community coping

Risk for complicated grieving

Stress overload

Risk-prone health behavior

Grieving

Complicated grieving

Impaired individual resilience

Risk for compromised resilience

Readiness for enhanced resilience

Class 3: Neurobehavioral Stress
Approved Diagnoses:

Autonomic dysreflexia

Risk for autonomic dysreflexia

Disorganized infant behavior

Risk for disorganized infant behavior

Readiness for enhanced organized infant behavior

Decreased intracranial adaptive capacity

Domain 10: Life Principles

Class 1: Values
Approved Diagnoses:

Readiness for enhanced hope

Class 2: Beliefs
Approved Diagnoses:

Readiness for enhanced spiritual well-being

Readiness for enhanced hope

Class 3: Value/Belief/Action Congruence
Approved Diagnoses:

Spiritual distress

Risk for spiritual distress

Decisional conflict (specify)

Noncompliance (specify)

Risk for impaired religiosity

Impaired religiosity

Readiness for enhanced religiosity

Moral distress

Readiness for enhanced decision making

Domain 11: Safety/Protection

Class 1: Infection
Approved Diagnoses:

Risk for infection

Readiness for enhanced immunization status

Class 2: Physical Injury
Approved Diagnoses:

Impaired oral mucous membrane

Risk for injury

Risk for perioperative positioning injury

Risk for falls

Risk for trauma

Impaired skin integrity

Risk for impaired skin integrity

Impaired tissue integrity

Impaired dentition

Risk for suffocation

Risk for aspiration

Ineffective airway clearance

Risk for peripheral neurovascular dysfunction

Ineffective protection

Risk for sudden infant death syndrome

Risk for vascular trauma

Class 3: Violence
Approved Diagnoses:

Risk for self-mutilation

Self-mutilation

Risk for other-directed violence

Risk for self-directed violence

Risk for suicide

Class 4: Environmental Hazards
Approved Diagnoses:

Risk for poisoning

Risk for contamination

Contamination

Class 5: Defensive Processes
Approved Diagnoses:

Latex allergy response

Risk for latex allergy response

Readiness for enhanced immunization status

Class 6: Thermoregulation
Approved Diagnoses:

Risk for imbalanced body temperature

Ineffective thermoregulation

Hypothermia

Hyperthermia

Domain 12: Comfort

Class 1: Physical Comfort
Approved Diagnoses:

Acute pain

Chronic pain

Nausea

Readiness for enhanced comfort

Impaired comfort

Class 2: Environmental Comfort
Approved Diagnoses:

Readiness for enhanced comfort

Impaired comfort

Class 3: Social Comfort
Approved Diagnoses:

Social isolation

Impaired comfort

Domain 13: Growth/Development

Class 1: Growth
Approved Diagnoses:

Delayed growth and development

Risk for disproportionate growth

Adult failure to thrive

Class 2: Development
Approved Diagnoses:

Delayed growth and development

Risk for delayed development

From NANDA International. (2009). *NANDA Nursing Diagnoses: Definitions & Classification 2009–2011*. Hoboken, NJ: Wiley-Blackwell, with permission.

Appendix E

Assigning Nursing Diagnoses to Client Behaviors

Following is a list of client behaviors and the NANDA nursing diagnoses that correspond to the behaviors and that may be used in planning care for the client exhibiting the specific behavioral symptoms.

BEHAVIORS	NANDA NURSING DIAGNOSES
Aggression; hostility	Risk for injury; Risk for other-directed violence
Anorexia or refusal to eat	Imbalanced nutrition: Less than body requirements
Anxious behavior	Anxiety (Specify level)
Confusion; memory loss	Confusion, acute/chronic; Disturbed thought processes; Impaired memory
Delusions	Disturbed thought processes
Denial of problems	Ineffective denial
Depressed mood or anger turned inward	Complicated grieving
Detoxification; withdrawal from substances	Risk for injury
Difficulty accepting new diagnosis or recent change in health status	Risk-prone health behavior
Difficulty making important life decision	Decisional conflict (specify)
Difficulty sleeping	Insomnia; Disturbed sleep pattern
Difficulty with interpersonal relationships	Impaired social interaction
Disruption in capability to perform usual responsibilities	Ineffective role performance
Dissociative behaviors (depersonalization; derealization)	Disturbed sensory perception (kinesthetic)
Expresses anger at God	Spiritual distress
Expresses feelings of disgust about body or body part	Disturbed body image
Expresses lack of control over personal situation	Powerlessness
Fails to follow prescribed therapy	Ineffective self health management; Noncompliance
Flashbacks, nightmares, obsession with traumatic experience	Post-trauma syndrome
Hallucinations	Disturbed sensory perception (auditory; visual)
Highly critical of self or others	Low self-esteem (chronic; situational)
HIV positive; altered immunity	Ineffective protection

BEHAVIORS	NANDA NURSING DIAGNOSES
Inability to meet basic needs	Self-care deficit (feeding; bathing; dressing; toileting)
Loose associations or flight of ideas	Impaired verbal communication
Loss of a valued entity, recently experienced	Risk for complicated grieving
Manic hyperactivity	Risk for injury
Manipulative behavior	Ineffective coping
Multiple personalities; gender identity disturbance	Disturbed personal identity
Orgasm, problems with; lack of sexual desire; erectile dysfunction	Sexual dysfunction
Overeating, compulsive	Risk for imbalanced nutrition: More than body requirements
Phobias	Fear
Physical symptoms as coping behavior	Ineffective coping
Potential or anticipated loss of significant entity	Grieving
Projection of blame; rationalization of failures; denial of personal responsibility	Defensive coping
Ritualistic behaviors	Anxiety (severe); ineffective coping
Seductive remarks; inappropriate sexual behaviors	Impaired social interaction
Self-inflicted injuries (non–life-threatening)	Self-mutilation; Risk for self-mutilation
Sexual behaviors (difficulty, limitations, or changes in; reported dissatisfaction)	Ineffective sexuality pattern
Stress from caring for chronically ill person	Caregiver role strain
Stress from locating to new environment	Relocation stress syndrome
Substance use as a coping behavior	Ineffective coping
Substance use (denies use is a problem)	Ineffective denial
Suicidal gestures/threats; suicidal ideation	Risk for suicide; Risk for self-directed violence
Suspiciousness	Disturbed thought processes; ineffective coping
Vomiting, excessive, self-induced	Risk for deficient fluid volume
Withdrawn behavior	Social isolation

Appendix F

Controlled Drug Categories and Pregnancy Categories

DEA Controlled Substances Schedules

Classes or schedules are determined by the Drug Enforcement Agency (DEA), an arm of the U.S. Department of Justice, and are based on the potential for abuse and dependence liability (physical and psychological) of the medication. Some states may have stricter prescription regulations. Physicians, dentists, podiatrists, and veterinarians may prescribe controlled substances. Nurse practitioners and physician's assistants may prescribe controlled substances with certain limitations.

Schedule I (C-I)

Potential for abuse is so high as to be unacceptable. May be used for research with appropriate limitations. Examples are LSD and heroin.

Schedule II (C-II)

High potential for abuse and extreme liability for physical and psychological dependence (amphetamines, opioid analgesics, dronabinol, certain barbiturates). Outpatient prescriptions must be in writing. In emergencies, telephone orders may be acceptable if a written prescription is provided within 72 hours. No refills are allowed.

Schedule III (C-III)

Intermediate potential for abuse (less than C-II) and intermediate liability for physical and psychological dependence (certain nonbarbiturate sedatives, certain nonamphetamine CNS stimulants, and limited dosages of certain opioid analgesics). Outpatient prescriptions can be refilled 5 times within 6 months from date of issue if authorized by prescriber. Telephone orders are acceptable.

Schedule IV (C-IV)

Less abuse potential than Schedule III with minimal liability for physical or psychological dependence (certain sedative-hypnotics, certain antianxiety agents, some barbiturates, benzodiazepines, chloral hydrate, and pentazocine). Outpatient prescriptions can be refilled 6 times within 6 months from date of issue if authorized by prescriber. Telephone orders are acceptable.

Schedule V (C-V)

Minimal abuse potential. Number of outpatient refills determined by prescriber. Some products (cough suppressants with small amounts of codeine, antidiarrheals containing paragoric) may be available without prescription to patients at least 18 years of age.

FDA Pregnancy Categories

Category A Adequate, well-controlled studies in pregnant women have not shown an increased risk of fetal abnormalities.

Category B Animal studies have revealed no evidence of harm to the fetus, however, there are no adequate and well-controlled studies in pregnant women.
OR
Animal studies have shown an adverse effect, but adequate and well-controlled studies in pregnant women have failed to demonstrate a risk to the fetus.

Category C Animal studies have shown an adverse effect and there are no adequate and well-controlled studies in pregnant women.
OR
No animal studies have been conducted and there are no adequate and well-controlled studies in pregnant women.

Category D   Studies, adequate well-controlled or observational, in pregnant women have demonstrated a risk to the fetus. However, the benefits of therapy may outweigh the potential risk.

Category X   Studies, adequate well-controlled or observational, in animals or pregnant women have demonstrated positive evidence of fetal abnormalities. The use of the product is contraindicated in women who are or may become pregnant.

From Deglin, J. H., & Vallerand, A. H. (2009). Davis's Drug Guide for Nurses (11th ed.). Philadelphia: F.A. Davis, with permission.

Appendix G

Sample Client Teaching Guides

Benzodiazepines

Patient Medication Instruction Sheet

Patient Name_____ **Drug Prescribed**_____
Directions for Use_____

Examples and Uses of This Medicine:

Benzodiazepines are used to treat moderate to severe anxiety: alprazolam [Xanax], chlordiazepoxide [Librium], clonazepam [Klonopin], clorazepate [Tranxene], diazepam [Valium], lorazepam [Ativan], and oxazepam. Some are used to treat insomnia (sleeplessness): flurazepam [Dalmane], temazepam [Restoril], estazolam, quazepam [Doral], and triazolam [Halcion]. Some are used for muscle spasms and to treat seizure disorders.

Before Using This Medicine, Be Sure to Tell Your Doctor if You:

- Are allergic to any medicine
- Have glaucoma
- Are pregnant, plan to be, or are breastfeeding
- Are taking any other medications

Side Effects of This Medicine:

REPORT THE FOLLOWING SIDE EFFECTS TO YOUR DOCTOR IMMEDIATELY

- Mental confusion or depression
- Hallucinations (seeing, hearing, or feeling things not there)
- Skin rash or itching
- Sore throat and fever
- Unusual excitement, nervousness, irritability, or trouble sleeping

SIDE EFFECTS THAT MAY OCCUR BUT NOT REQUIRE A DOCTOR'S ATTENTION UNLESS THEY PERSIST LONGER THAN A FEW DAYS:

- Blurred vision, or other changes in vision
- Clumsiness, dizziness, lightheadedness, or slurred speech
- Constipation, diarrhea, nausea, vomiting, or stomach pain
- Difficulty in urination
- Drowsiness, headache, or unusual tiredness or weakness

Other Instructions While Taking This Medication:

- Take this medicine only as your doctor has directed. Do not take more of it or do not take it more often than prescribed. If large doses are taken for a prolonged period of time, it may become habit-forming.
- If you are taking this medicine several times a day and you forget a dose, if it is within an hour or so of the missed dose, go ahead and take it. Otherwise, wait and take the next dose at regular time. Do not double up on a dose if you forget one. Just keep taking the prescribed dosage.
- Do not stop taking the drug abruptly. To do so might produce serious withdrawal symptoms, such as depression, insomnia, anxiety, abdominal and muscle cramps, tremors, vomiting, sweating, convulsions, and delirium. Discuss with the doctor before stopping this medication.
- Do not consume other CNS depressants (including alcohol) while taking this medication.
- Do not take nonprescription medication without approval from physician.
- Rise slowly from the sitting or lying position to prevent a sudden drop in blood pressure.

Buspirone (BuSpar)

Patient Medication Instruction Sheet

Patient Name_____
Directions for Use_____

Uses of This Medicine:

BuSpar is used in the treatment of anxiety disorders. It is also sometimes used to treat the symptoms of premenstrual syndrome.

- Are allergic to any medicine
- Are pregnant, plan to be, or are breastfeeding
- Are taking any other medications

Side Effects of This Medicine:

REPORT THE FOLLOWING SIDE EFFECTS TO
YOUR DOCTOR IMMEDIATELY:

- Mental confusion or depression
- Hallucinations (seeing, hearing, or feeling things not there)
- Skin rash or itching
- Unusual excitement, nervousness, irritability, or trouble sleeping
- Persistent headache
- Involuntary movements of the head or neck muscles

SIDE EFFECTS THAT MAY OCCUR BUT NOT
REQUIRE A DOCTOR'S ATTENTION UNLESS THEY
PERSIST LONGER THAN A FEW DAYS:

- Dizziness; lightheadedness
- Drowsiness
- Nausea
- Fatigue
- Headache that subsides

Other Instructions While Taking This Medication:

- Take this medicine only as your doctor has directed. Do not take more of it or do not take it more often than prescribed.
- If you are taking this medicine several times a day and you forget a dose, if it is within an hour or so of the missed dose, go ahead and take it. Otherwise, wait and take the next dose at regular time. Do not double up on a dose if you forget one. Just keep taking the prescribed dosage.
- Do not consume CNS depressants (including alcohol) while taking this medication.
- Do not take nonprescription medication without approval from physician.
- Rise slowly from the sitting or lying position to prevent a sudden drop in blood pressure.

Tricyclic Antidepressants

Patient Medication Instruction Sheet

Patient Name_____ Drug Prescribed_____
Directions for Use_____

Examples and Uses of This Medicine:

Tricyclic antidepressants are used to treat symptoms of depression: amitriptyline, amoxapine, desipramine [Norpramin], doxepin [Sinequan], imipramine [Tofranil], nortriptyline [Aventyl], protriptyline [Vivactil], and trimipramine [Surmontil]. Doxepin is used to treat depression with anxiety. Clomipramine [Anafranil] is used to treat obsessive-compulsive disorder. Imipramine is also used to treat enuresis (bedwetting) in children.

Before Using This Medicine, Be Sure
to Tell Your Doctor if You:

- Are allergic to any medicine
- Have glaucoma
- Have a history of heart problems or high blood pressure
- Are pregnant, plan to be, or are breastfeeding
- Are taking any other medications
- Have a history of seizures

Side Effects of This Medicine:

REPORT THE FOLLOWING SIDE EFFECTS TO
YOUR DOCTOR IMMEDIATELY:

- Seizures
- Difficulty urinating
- Irregular heartbeat or chest pain
- Hallucinations
- Skin rash
- Sore throat and fever
- Unusual amount of restlessness and excitement
- Confusion; disorientation

SIDE EFFECTS THAT MAY OCCUR BUT MAY NOT
REQUIRE A DOCTOR'S ATTENTION:

- Drowsiness
- Dry mouth
- Nausea
- Sensitivity to the sun (may burn easily)
- Headache
- Constipation

Other Instructions While Taking This Medication:

- Continue to take the medication even though you still have symptoms. It may take as long as 4 weeks before you start feeling better.
- Use caution when driving or operating dangerous machinery. Drowsiness and dizziness can occur. If these side effects don't go away or get worse, report them to the doctor.

- Do not stop taking the drug abruptly. To do so might produce withdrawal symptoms, such as nausea, vertigo, insomnia, headache, malaise, and nightmares. Tell the doctor when you want to stop taking it.
- Use sunblock lotion and wear protective clothing when spending time outdoors.
- Rise slowly from a sitting or lying position to prevent a sudden drop in blood pressure.
- Take frequent sips of water, chew sugarless gum, or suck on hard candy if dry mouth is a problem.
- You may take this medication with food if nausea is a problem.
- Do not drink alcohol while taking this medication.
- Do not consume other medications (including over-the-counter medications) without the physician's approval while taking this medication. Many medications contain substances that, in combination with tricyclic antidepressants, could be dangerous.

Selective Serotonin Reuptake Inhibitors (SSRIs)

Patient Medication Instruction Sheet

Patient Name_____ Drug Prescribed_____
Directions for Use_____

Examples and Uses of This Medicine:

SSRIs are used to treat symptoms of depression: citalopram [Celexa], escitalopram [Lexapro], fluoxetine [Prozac], paroxetine [Paxil], vilazodone [Viibryd], and sertraline [Zoloft]. Some are used to treat obsessive-compulsive disorder: fluvoxamine [Luvox], fluoxetine, [Prozac], paroxetine [Paxil], and sertraline [Zoloft]. Also bulimia nervosa: fluoxetine [Prozac]; panic disorder and premenstrual dysphoric disorder: fluoxetine [Prozac; Serafem], sertraline [Zoloft] and paroxetine [Paxil]; posttraumatic stress disorder: paroxetine [Paxil] and sertraline [Zoloft]; generalized anxiety disorder: escitalopram [Lexapro] and paroxetine [Paxil]; and social anxiety disorder: paroxetine [Paxil], sertraline [Zoloft], and fluvoxamine [Luvox].

Before Using This Medicine, Be Sure to Tell Your Doctor if You:

- Are allergic to any medicine
- Are pregnant, plan to be, or are breastfeeding
- Are taking any other medications
- Have diabetes

Side Effects of This Medicine:

REPORT THE FOLLOWING SIDE EFFECTS TO YOUR DOCTOR IMMEDIATELY:
- Skin rash
- Fever
- Unusual excitement, nervousness, irritability, or trouble sleeping
- Loss of appetite and weight loss
- Seizures
- Difficulty breathing
- Increased sensitivity to sunburn

SIDE EFFECTS THAT MAY OCCUR BUT MAY NOT REQUIRE A DOCTOR'S ATTENTION:
- Drowsiness
- Dizziness
- Nausea
- Headache
- Impotence or loss of sexual desire (this should be reported to physician if it is troubling to the patient)

Other Instructions While Taking This Medication:

- Continue to take the medication even though you still have symptoms. It may take as long as 4 weeks before you start feeling better.
- Use caution when driving or operating dangerous machinery. Drowsiness and dizziness can occur. If these side effects don't go away or get worse, report them to the doctor.
- Use sunblock lotion and wear protective clothing when spending time outdoors.
- Rise slowly from a sitting or lying position to prevent a sudden drop in blood pressure.
- Take frequent sips of water, chew sugarless gum, or suck on hard candy if dry mouth is a problem.
- You may take this medication with food if nausea is a problem.
- Avoid drinking alcohol while taking this medication.
- Do not consume other medications (including over-the-counter medications) without the physician's approval while taking this medication. Many medications contain substances that, in combination with SSRI antidepressants, could be dangerous.

Monoamine Oxidase Inhibitors (MAOIs)

Patient Medication Instruction Sheet

Patient Name_____ **Drug Prescribed** _____
Directions for Use_____

Examples and Uses of This Medicine:

MAOIs are used to treat the symptoms of depression: isocarboxazid [Marplan], phenelzine [Nardil], tranylcypromine [Parnate], and selegiline transdermal system [Emsam].

Before Using This Medicine, Be Sure to Tell Your Doctor if You:

- Are allergic to any medicine
- Have a history of liver or kidney disease
- Have been diagnosed with pheochromocytoma
- Have a history of severe or frequent headaches
- Are pregnant, plan to be, or are breastfeeding
- Have a history of hypertension
- Have a history of heart disease
- Are taking (or have taken in the last 2 weeks) *any* other medication

Side Effects of This Medicine:

REPORT THE FOLLOWING SIDE EFFECTS TO YOUR DOCTOR IMMEDIATELY:

- Severe, pounding headache
- Rapid or pounding heartbeat
- Stiff or sore neck
- Chest pain
- Nausea and vomiting
- Seizures

THE FOLLOWING SIDE EFFECTS SHOULD ALSO BE REPORTED TO THE DOCTOR:

- Dark urine
- Yellowing of eyes or skin
- Hallucinations
- Fainting
- Hyperexcitability
- Confusion
- Fever
- Skin rash
- Disorientation

SIDE EFFECTS THAT MAY OCCUR BUT MAY NOT REQUIRE A DOCTOR'S ATTENTION:

- Constipation
- Diarrhea (unless severe and persistent)
- Dizziness
- Dry mouth
- Fatigue
- Drowsiness
- Nausea
- Decreased sexual ability

Other Instructions While Taking This Medication:

- Continue to take the medication even though you still have symptoms. It may take as long as 4 weeks before you start feeling better.
- Use caution when driving or operating dangerous machinery. Drowsiness and dizziness can occur.
- Do not stop taking the drug abruptly. To do so might produce withdrawal symptoms, such as nausea, vertigo, insomnia, headache, malaise, and nightmares. Tell the doctor when you want to stop taking it.
- Rise slowly from a sitting or lying position to prevent a sudden drop in blood pressure.
- Take frequent sips of water, chew sugarless gum, or suck on hard candy if dry mouth is a problem.
- You may take this medication with food if nausea is a problem. Do not drink alcohol.
- Do not consume other medications (including over-the-counter medications) without the physician's approval while taking this medication. Many medications contain substances that, in combination with MAOI antidepressants, could be dangerous.
- Do not consume the following foods or medications while taking MAOIs (or for 2 weeks after you stop taking them): aged cheese, raisins, red wine (especially Chianti), beer, chocolate, colas, coffee, tea, sour cream, beef/chicken livers, game meat, canned figs, soy sauce, meat tenderizer (MSG), pickled herring, smoked/processed meats (lunchmeats, sausage, pepperoni), yogurt, yeast products, broad beans, sauerkraut, cold remedies, diet pills, or nasal decongestants. To do so could cause a life-threatening condition.
- Be sure to tell any doctor or dentist that you see that you are taking this medication.
- Follow package directions carefully when applying the selegiline transdermal patch.

Heterocyclic Antidepressants

Patient Medication Instruction Sheet

Patient Name_____ Drug Prescribed_____
Directions for Use_____

Examples and Uses of This Medicine:

Heterocyclic antidepressanats are used to treat symptoms of depression: maprotiline, mirtazapine [Remeron], trazodone [Desyrel], bupropion [Wellbutrin], and nefazodone. Maprotiline is also used to treat anxiety associated with depression. Trazodone is also used to treat insomnia and panic disorder. Bupropion has been shown to be effective in the treatment of attention-deficit/hyperactivity disorder and as a smoking deterrent (Zyban).

Before Using This Medicine, Be Sure to Tell Your Doctor if You:

- Are allergic to any medicine
- Have an eating disorder
- Have a history of heart problems
- Are pregnant, plan to be, or are breastfeeding
- Are taking any other medications
- Have a history of seizures or high blood pressure

Side Effects of This Medicine:

REPORT THE FOLLOWING SIDE EFFECTS TO YOUR DOCTOR IMMEDIATELY:

- Seizures
- Fever, chills
- Sore throat
- Prolonged erection (trazodone)
- Unusual amount of restlessness and excitement
- Irregular heartbeat or chest pain
- Hallucinations
- Skin rash
- Jaundice, anorexia, GI complaints, malaise (signs of liver dysfunction [nefazodone])

SIDE EFFECTS THAT MAY OCCUR BUT NOT REQUIRE A DOCTOR'S ATTENTION UNLESS THEY PERSIST LONGER THAN A FEW DAYS:

- Drowsiness
- Dizziness
- Dry mouth
- Constipation
- Headache
- Nausea

Other Instructions While Taking This Medication:

- Continue to take the medication even though you still have symptoms. It may take as long as 4 weeks before you start feeling better.
- Use caution when driving or operating dangerous machinery. Drowsiness and dizziness can occur. If these side effects don't go away or get worse, report them to the doctor.
- Do not stop taking the drug abruptly. To do so might produce withdrawal symptoms, such as nausea, vertigo, insomnia, headache, malaise, and nightmares. Tell the doctor when you want to stop taking it.
- Rise slowly from a sitting or lying position to prevent a sudden drop in blood pressure.
- Take frequent sips of water, chew sugarless gum, or suck on hard candy if dry mouth is a problem.
- You may take this medication with food if nausea is a problem.
- Do not drink alcohol while taking this medication.
- Do not consume other medications (including over-the-counter medications) without the physician's approval while taking this medication. Many medications contain substances that, in combination with heterocyclic antidepressants, could be dangerous.

Serotonin-Norepinephrine Reuptake Inhibitors (SNRIs)

Patient Medication Instruction Sheet

Patient Name_____ Drug Prescribed_____
Directions for Use_____

Examples and Uses of This Medicine:

SNRIs are used to treat symptoms of depression: venlafaxine [Effexor], duloxetine [Cymbalta], and desvenlafaxine [Pristiq]. Venlafaxine is also used to treat generalized anxiety disorder, social anxiety disorder, and panic disorder. It has also been effective in treatment of hot flashes, premenstrual dysphoric disorder, and posttraumatic stress disorder. Duloxetine is also used to treat diabetic peripheral neuropathic pain, fibromyalgia, and generalized anxiety disorder.

Before Using This Medicine, Be Sure to Tell Your Doctor if You:

- Are allergic to any medicine
- Have glaucoma

- Have a history of seizures
- Are pregnant, plan to be, or are breastfeeding
- Are taking any other medications
- Have a history of heart disease

Side Effects of This Medicine:

REPORT THE FOLLOWING SIDE EFFECTS TO YOUR DOCTOR IMMEDIATELY:

- Skin rash
- Seizures
- Unusual amount of restlessness or excitement
- Irregular heartbeat or chest pain

SIDE EFFECTS THAT MAY OCCUR BUT NOT REQUIRE A DOCTOR'S ATTENTION UNLESS THEY PERSIST LONGER THAN A FEW DAYS:

- Dizziness
- Headache
- Constipation
- Dry mouth
- Drowsiness
- Insomnia
- Sexual dysfunction (should be reported to the physician if it is troubling to the patient)
- Nausea

Other Instructions While Taking This Medication:

- Continue to take the medication even though you still have symptoms. It may take as long as 4 weeks before you start feeling better.
- Use caution when driving or operating dangerous machinery. Drowsiness and dizziness can occur. If these side effects don't go away or get worse, report them to the doctor.
- Do not stop taking the drug abruptly. To do so might produce withdrawal symptoms, such as nausea, vertigo, insomnia, headache, malaise, and nightmares. Tell the doctor when you want to stop taking it.
- Rise slowly from a sitting or lying position to prevent a sudden drop in blood pressure.
- Take frequent sips of water, chew sugarless gum, or suck on hard candy if dry mouth is a problem.
- You may take this medication with food if nausea is a problem.
- Do not drink alcohol while taking this medication.
- Do not consume other medications (including over-the-counter medications) without the physician's approval while taking this medication.

Many medications contain substances that, in combination with SNRI antidepressants, could be dangerous.

Lithium

Patient Medication Instruction Sheet

Patient Name_____

Directions for Use_____

Uses of This Medicine:

Lithium is used for treatment of manic episodes associated with bipolar disorder. Taking lithium regularly also prevents manic episodes or causes fewer, less serious manic episodes in a person with bipolar disorder.

Before Using This Medicine, Be Sure to Tell Your Doctor if You:

- Are allergic to any medicine
- Have heart, kidney, or thyroid disease
- Are pregnant, plan to be, or are breastfeeding
- Are taking any other medication, particularly diuretics, haloperidol, NSAIDs, fluoxetine, or carbamazepine

Side Effects of This Medicine:

REPORT THE FOLLOWING SIDE EFFECTS TO YOUR DOCTOR IMMEDIATELY:

- Lack of coordination
- Persistent nausea and vomiting
- Slurred speech
- Blurred vision
- Ringing in the ears
- Jerking of arms and legs
- Severe diarrhea
- Confusion

SIDE EFFECTS THAT MAY OCCUR BUT MAY NOT REQUIRE A DOCTOR'S ATTENTION UNLESS THEY PERSIST:

- Mild hand tremors
- GI upset; nausea
- Diarrhea
- Dizziness
- Dry mouth

Other Instructions While Taking This Medication:

- Take this medicine exactly as it is prescribed. Do not take more of it or more often than it is prescribed. Sometimes it takes several weeks of taking this medication before you begin to feel better. At some point, your doctor may make an adjustment in the dosage.

■ Do not drive or operate dangerous machinery until your response to the medication is adjusted. Drowsiness or dizziness can occur.

■ Do not stop taking the medication even if you are feeling fine and don't think you need it. Symptoms of mania can occur.

■ Take this medication with food or milk to lessen stomach upset, unless otherwise directed by your doctor.

■ Use a normal amount of salt in your food. Drink 8 to 10 glasses of water each day. Avoid drinks that contain caffeine (that have a diuretic effect). Have blood tests taken to check lithium level every month, or as advised by physician.

■ Avoid consuming alcoholic beverages and nonprescription medications without approval from physician.

■ Use extra care in hot weather and during activities that cause you to sweat heavily, such as hot baths, saunas, or exercising. The loss of too much water and salt from your body can lead to serious side effects from this medicine.

■ Be sure to get enough salt and water in the diet during times of sickness that can deplete the body of water, such as high fever, nausea and vomiting, and diarrhea.

■ Carry card at all times identifying the name of medications being taken.

Antipsychotics (Conventional)

Patient Medication Instruction Sheet

Patient Name_____ **Drug Prescribed**_____
Directions for Use_____

Examples:

■ Chlorpromazine

■ Perphenazine

■ Thioridazine

■ Thiothixene (Navane)

■ Fluphenazine

■ Prochlorperazine

■ Trifluoperazine

■ Loxapine

■ Haloperidol (Haldol)

■ Pimozide (Orap)

Uses of This Medicine:

These medications are used in the management of schizophrenia and other psychotic disorders. Chlorpromazine is also used in bipolar mania. Selected agents are used to treat nausea and vomiting: chlorpromazine, perphenazine, haloperidol [Haldol], and prochlorperazine; pediatric behavior problems: chlorpromazine and haloperidol [Haldol]; intractable hiccoughs: chlorpromazine and haloperidol [Haldol]; and Tourette's disorder: haloperidol [Haldol] and pimozide [Orap].

Before Using This Medicine, Be Sure to Tell Your Doctor if You:

■ Are allergic to any medicine

■ Have history of seizures

■ Have liver or heart disease

■ Have any blood disorders

■ Are pregnant, plan to be, or are breastfeeding

■ Are taking any other medications (either prescription or over-the-counter)

■ Have any other medical problem

Side Effects of This Medicine:

REPORT THE FOLLOWING SIDE EFFECTS TO YOUR DOCTOR IMMEDIATELY:

■ Difficulty urinating

■ Shuffling walk

■ Yellow eyes and skin

■ Wormlike movements of the tongue

■ Fainting

■ Skin rash

■ Sore throat

■ Seizures

■ Fever

■ Muscle spasms or stiffness

■ Excitement or restlessness

■ Jerky movements of head, face, or neck

■ Unusual bleeding; easy bruising

■ Unusually fast heartbeat

SIDE EFFECTS THAT MAY OCCUR BUT MAY NOT REQUIRE A DOCTOR'S ATTENTION:

■ Dry mouth

■ Nausea

■ Weight gain

■ Blurred vision

■ Decreased sweating

■ Dizziness

■ Constipation

- Increased sensitivity to sunburn
- Drowsiness

Other Instructions While Taking This Medication:

- Use caution when driving or operating dangerous machinery. Drowsiness and dizziness can occur.
- Do not stop taking the drug abruptly after long-term use. To do so might produce withdrawal symptoms, such as nausea, vomiting, gastritis, headache, tachycardia, insomnia, and tremulousness.
- Use sunblock lotion and wear protective clothing when spending time outdoors. Skin is more susceptible to sunburn, which can occur in as little as 30 minutes.
- Rise slowly from a sitting or lying position to prevent a sudden drop in blood pressure.
- Take frequent sips of water, chew sugarless gum, or suck on hard candy, if experiencing a problem with dry mouth.
- Dress warmly in cold weather and avoid extended exposure to very high or low temperatures. Body temperature is harder to maintain with this medication.
- Do not drink alcohol while on antipsychotic therapy. These drugs potentiate each other's effects.
- Do not consume other medications (including over-the-counter products) without physician's approval. Many medications contain substances that interact with antipsychotics in a way that may be harmful.
- Continue to take medication, even if feeling well and as though it is not needed. Symptoms may return if medication is discontinued.
- Some of these medications may turn the urine pink to red or reddish brown. This is harmless.

Antipsychotics (Atypical)

Patient Medication Instruction Sheet

Patient Name_____ **Drug Prescribed**_____
Directions for Use_____

Examples:

- Risperidone (Risperdal)
- Clozapine (Clozaril)
- Olanzapine (Zyprexa)
- Quetiapine (Seroquel)
- Ziprasidone (Geodon)

- Aripiprazole (Abilify)
- Paliperidone (Invega)
- Iloperidone (Fanapt)
- Asenapine (Saphris)
- Lurasidone (Latuda)

Uses of This Medicine:

These medications are used in the management of schizophrenia and other psychotic disorders. Selected agents are used to treat bipolar mania: ziprasidone [Geodon], olanzapine [Zyprexa], quetiapine [Seroquel], risperidone [Risperdal], asenapine [Saphris], and aripiprazole [Abilify]. Aripiprazole (Abilify) is also used as adjunctive therapy in resistant depression.

Before Using This Medicine, Be Sure to Tell Your Doctor if You:

- Are allergic to any medicine
- Have history of seizures
- Have liver or heart disease
- Have any blood disorders
- Are pregnant, plan to be, or are breastfeeding
- Are taking any other medications (either prescription or over-the-counter)
- Have any other medical problem

Side Effects of This Medicine:

REPORT THE FOLLOWING SIDE EFFECTS TO YOUR DOCTOR IMMEDIATELY:

- Difficulty urinating
- Shuffling walk
- Yellow eyes and skin
- Wormlike movements of the tongue
- Fainting
- Skin rash
- Sore throat
- Seizures
- Fever
- Muscle spasms or stiffness
- Excitement or restlessness
- Jerky movements of head, face, or neck
- Unusual bleeding; easy bruising
- Unusually fast heartbeat

SIDE EFFECTS THAT MAY OCCUR BUT MAY NOT REQUIRE A DOCTOR'S ATTENTION:

- Dry mouth
- Nausea
- Weight gain

- Blurred vision
- Decreased sweating
- Dizziness
- Constipation
- Increased sensitivity to sunburn
- Drowsiness

Other Instructions While Taking This Medication:

- Use caution when driving or operating dangerous machinery. Drowsiness and dizziness can occur.

- Do not stop taking the drug abruptly after long-term use. To do so might produce withdrawal symptoms, such as nausea, vomiting, gastritis, headache, tachycardia, insomnia, and tremulousness.

- Use sunblock lotion and wear protective clothing when spending time outdoors. Skin is more susceptible to sunburn, which can occur in as little as 30 minutes.

- Rise slowly from a sitting or lying position to prevent a sudden drop in blood pressure.

- Take frequent sips of water, chew sugarless gum, or suck on hard candy, if you have dry mouth.

- Dress warmly in cold weather and avoid extended exposure to very high or low temperatures. Body temperature is harder to maintain with this medication.

- Do not drink alcohol while on antipsychotic therapy. These drugs potentiate each other's effects.

- Do not consume other medications (including over-the-counter products) without physician's approval. Many medications contain substances that interact with antipsychotics in a way that may be harmful.

- Continue to take medication, even if feeling well and as though it is not needed. Symptoms may return if medication is discontinued.

- Report weekly (if receiving clozapine therapy) to have blood levels drawn and to obtain a weekly supply of the drug.

Agents for Attention-Deficit/ Hyperactivity Disorder (ADHD)

Patient Medication Instruction Sheet

Patient Name_____ **Drug Prescribed**_____
Directions for Use_____

Examples and Uses of This Medicine:

These central nervous system (CNS) stimulants are used in the treatment of attention-deficit/ hyperactivity disorder (ADHD) in children and adults: dextroamphetamine sulfate [Dexedrine], methamphetamine [Desoxyn], lisdexamphetamine [Vyvanse], dextroamphetamine/amphetamine mixture [Adderall], dexmethylphenidate [Focalin], methylphenidate [Ritalin and others]. Atomoxetine [Strattera], the antidepressant bupropion [Wellbutrin], and the alpha-adrenergic agonists clonidine [Catapres] and guanfacine [Intuniv] are also used to treat ADHD.

Before Using This Medicine, Be Sure to Tell Your Doctor if You:

- Are allergic to any medicine
- Have glaucoma
- Have a history of tics or Tourette's disorder
- Have a history of heart disease
- Have a history of hyperthyroidism
- Have any other medical problem
- Are pregnant, plan to be, or are breastfeeding
- Are taking any other medications
- Have arteriosclerosis
- Have high blood pressure
- Have taken an MAOI within 14 days

Side Effects of This Medicine:

REPORT THE FOLLOWING SIDE EFFECTS TO YOUR DOCTOR IMMEDIATELY:

- Insomnia
- Rapid, pounding heartbeat
- Restlessness or agitation
- Slurred speech/confusion
- Severe, persistent headache
- Skin rash
- Fainting
- Sudden vision changes
- Shortness of breath
- Seizures
- Chest/arm pain
- Yellow skin/eyes

SIDE EFFECTS THAT MAY OCCUR BUT MAY NOT REQUIRE A DOCTOR'S ATTENTION:

- Dry mouth
- Dizziness
- Constipation
- Anorexia

- Nausea
- Headache

Other Instructions While Taking This Medication:

- Use caution in driving or operating dangerous machinery. Dizziness can occur.

- Do not stop taking the drug abruptly. To do so can cause fatigue and mental depression. Abrupt withdrawal from alpha-adrenergic agonists can result in nervousness and anxiety, and increase in blood pressure. Tell the physician if you wish to discontinue this medication.

- Take CNS stimulants, bupropion, or atomoxetine no later than 6 hours before bedtime to prevent insomnia.

- Do not take other medications (including over-the-counter drugs) without physician's approval. Many medications contain substances that, in combination with CNS stimulants, can be harmful.

- Diabetic clients should monitor blood sugar two or three times a day or as instructed by the physician. Be aware of need for possible alteration in insulin requirements because of changes in food intake, weight, and activity.

- Do not double up on the medication if doses are missed. Ensure that bupropion doses are taken at least 4 to 6 hours apart.

- Avoid consumption of large amounts of caffeinated products (coffee, tea, colas, chocolate). They may increase restlessness and stimulation.

Mood Stabilizing Agents (Anticonvulsants)

Patient Medication Instruction Sheet

Patient Name_____ Drug Prescribed_____
Directions for Use_____

Examples and Uses of This Medicine:

These medications are used in the treatment of seizure disorders and bipolar disorder: carbamazepine [Tegretol], clonazepam [Klonopin], valproic acid [Depakote], lamotrigine [Lamictal], gabapentin [Neurontin], topiramate [Topamax], and oxcarbazepine [Trileptal]. Selected agents are used for migraine prophylaxis: valproic acid, gabapentin, topiramate; and in panic disorder: clonazepam.

Before Using This Medicine, Be Sure to Tell Your Doctor if You:

- Are allergic to any medicine
- Have glaucoma

- Have a history of kidney disease
- Have a history of heart disease
- Have a history of liver disease
- Are pregnant, plan to be, or are breastfeeding
- Are taking any other medications
- Have taken an MAOI within 14 days
- Have high blood pressure
- Have any other medical problem

Side Effects of This Medicine:

REPORT THE FOLLOWING SIDE EFFECTS TO YOUR DOCTOR IMMEDIATELY:

- Easy bruising
- Unusual bleeding
- Pale stools or dark urine
- Diminished vision or eye pain (with topiramate)
- Suspected pregnancy
- Skin rash
- Yellow skin or eyes
- Sore throat or fever
- Abdominal pain
- Severe nausea and vomiting

SIDE EFFECTS THAT MAY OCCUR BUT MAY NOT REQUIRE A DOCTOR'S ATTENTION:

- Drowsiness
- Dizziness
- Constipation
- Headache
- Nausea
- Blurred vision
- Impaired concentration
- Increased sensitivity to the sun

Other Instructions While Taking This Medication:

- Use caution in driving or operating dangerous machinery. Dizziness can occur.

- Do not stop taking the drug abruptly. To do so may cause serious adverse reactions. Tell the physician if you wish to discontinue this medicine.

- Use sunblock lotion and protective clothing to protect from sunburn.

- Women taking oral contraceptives may need to choose another form of birth control, as their effectiveness is compromised with carbamazepine or topiramate.

- Do not take alcohol or other CNS depressants while you are taking this medication.

- Do not take other medications (including over-the-counter drugs) without physician's approval.

- Take medication as prescribed by physician. Do not take larger dose or more frequently than prescribed.

- Carry identification describing medication regimen.

Depression

What Is Depression?

It is normal to feel "blue" sometimes. In fact, feelings of sadness or disappointment are quite common, particularly in response to a loss, a failure, or even a change. Depression is different than just feeling "blue" or unhappy. The severity of the feelings, how long they last, and the presence of other symptoms are some of the factors that separate normal sadness from depression. Depression is more common in women that it is in men, and the probability increases with age.

What Are the Symptoms of Depression? (From the National Institute of Mental Health)

- Persistent sad, anxious or "empty" feeling

- Loss of interest or pleasure in ordinary activities, including sex

- Decreased energy, fatigue, feeling "slowed down"

- Sleep problems (insomnia, oversleeping, early-morning waking)

- Eating problems (loss of appetite or weight, weight gain)

- Difficulty concentrating, remembering, or making decisions

- Recurring aches and pains that don't respond to treatment

- Irritability

- Excessive crying

- Feelings of hopelessness or pessimism

- Feelings of guilt, worthlessness, or helplessness

- Thoughts of death or suicide; a suicide attempt

What Causes Depression?

The causes of depression are not fully known. It is most likely caused by a combination of factors.

- **Genetic.** A lot of research has been done to determine if depression is hereditary. Although no direct mode of hereditary transmission has been discovered, it has been found that depression does run in families. You are more likely to get depressed if a close biological relative has or has had the illness.

- **Biological.** Depression is thought to be caused by a chemical imbalance in the brain. Neurotransmitters called serotonin, norepinephrine, and dopamine have been found to be deficient in people with depressive symptoms.

- **Hormonal.** In women, the female hormones estrogen and progesterone most likely play a role in depression. These hormones contribute to premenstrual depression, postpartum depression, and depression associated with menopause.

- **Medication side effects.** Some medications, such as steroids, hormones, cancer chemotherapy, and antiparkinsonian agents, cause depression as a side effect.

- **Nutritional deficiencies.** Deficiencies in vitamins B_1, B_6, B_{12}, and C, and niacin, iron, folic acid, zinc, calcium, and potassium may produce symptoms of depression.

How Is Depression Diagnosed?

A mental health specialist, such as a psychiatrist, social worker, or psychologist, is the best source for a diagnosis of depression. A pencil-and-paper screening test may be administered, but generally depression is diagnosed based on symptoms and other criteria.

What Is the Treatment for Depression?

Patients with depression have a number of treatment options, including psychotherapy and antidepressant medication. It has been found that either of these options may be effective; however, a combination of the two has been shown to be more effective than either treatment alone. For those who fail to improve with medications and/or psychotherapy, other techniques, such as electroconvulsive therapy (ECT), have proven to be safe and effective for treating depressive symptoms.

Other Contacts:

International Foundation for Research and Education on Depression (iFred), P.O. Box 17598, Baltimore, MD 21297; http://www.ifred.org/

Depression and Bipolar Support Alliance (DBSA), 730 N. Franklin St., Suite 501, Chicago, IL 60654, 1-800-826-3632; http://www.ndmda.org/

National Alliance on Mental Illness, 3803 North Fairfax Dr., Suite 100, Arlington, VA 22203, 1-800-950-6264; http://www.nami.org/

Bipolar Disorder

What Is Bipolar Disorder?

Bipolar disorder is sometimes called manic-depressive illness. It is indicated by moods that swing between two opposite extremes:

- Periods of mania (when the mood is elevated and the person is very excited or irritable)
- Periods of depression (when the person is sad and withdrawn)

What Are the Symptoms of Bipolar Disorder?

The symptoms of bipolar disorder, depression, are similar to those experienced by a person who gets depressed (but does not have bipolar disorder). They are sadness, fatigue, sleep problems, weight changes, inability to concentrate, loss of interest or pleasure in life, and thoughts or attempts of suicide.

Symptoms of bipolar disorder, mania, include being very excited, irritable, distracted, and unable to sleep. Individuals with bipolar mania have thoughts that race through their head, and sometimes they believe things that are not true. They talk excessively and move about constantly. They may be angry and suspicious, and can become violent. Some manic people spend a lot of money and abuse substances. Some manic patients may have thoughts of suicide. Some people have mixed symptoms in which they experience symptoms of depression part of the day and symptoms of mania part of the day.

Bipolar disorder affects men and women equally. It can occur in childhood, adolescence, adulthood, or late in life.

What Causes Bipolar Disorder?

- **Genetic.** Bipolar disorder has a strong hereditary factor. It occurs more often within families, and individuals who have close biological relatives with the illness are more likely to get the disorder themselves.
- **Biological.** Bipolar disorder is thought to be caused by a chemical imbalance in the brain. Neurotransmitters called dopamine and norepinephrine have been found to be elevated in people with manic symptoms.
- **Medication side effects.** Certain medications, such as steroids, amphetamines, antidepressants, and high doses of anticonvulsants and narcotics have the potential for initiating a manic episode.

How Is Bipolar Disorder Diagnosed?

Bipolar disorder is often difficult to diagnose, and an individual with symptoms should be seen by a mental health professional. A careful history, taken with the help of family if possible, of any and all episodes of depression, mania, or both, must be completed. Patients often deny problems with mania. Other illnesses, such as attention-deficit/hyperactivity disorder, schizophrenia, substance abuse, thyroid disorders, adrenal disorders, and certain neurological disorders, which can all cause mood swings, must be ruled out.

What Is the Treatment for Bipolar Disorder?

The goals of treating bipolar disorder are to:
- Treat the episodes of mania and depression when they occur.
- Decrease the number of episodes that occur.
- Help the patient function as effectively as possible between episodes.

Treatment is with mood-stabilizing drugs, such as lithium, valproic acid, carbamazepine, clonazepam, gabapentin, topiramate, oxcarbazepine, or lamotrigine. Antipsychotic medications, such as risperidone, olanzapine, aripiprazole, chlorpromazine, ziprasidone, asenapine, or quetiapine, are sometimes given. Psychotherapy has been shown to be helpful in patients with bipolar disorder to assist in the management of everyday stressors and to help prevent relapse.

Other Contacts:

Depression and Bipolar Support Alliance (DBSA), 730 Franklin St., Suite 501, Chicago, IL 60654, 1-800-826-3632; http://www.ndmda.org/

National Alliance on Mental Illness, 3803 North Fairfax Dr., Suite 100, Arlington, VA 22203, 1-800-950-6264; http://www.nami.org/

Posttraumatic Stress Disorder (PTSD)

What Is PTSD?

PTSD is an anxiety disorder, the symptoms of which occur following exposure to an extreme traumatic stressor. The stressor that triggers these symptoms is outside the norm of human experience, and includes events such as military combat, violent personal assault, being kidnapped or taken hostage, terrorist attack, being tortured, being a prisoner of war, natural or man-made disasters, severe automobile accidents, or being diagnosed with a life-threatening illness (*DSM-IV-TR,* 2000).

What Are the Symptoms of PTSD?

■ Recurrent and distressing thoughts about the event

■ Nightmares about the event and sleeping problems

■ Flashbacks and reliving the event

■ Inability to remember parts of the event

■ Avoids people or activities that remind of the event

■ Guilt for surviving when others died

■ Difficulty concentrating

■ Irritability or outbursts of anger

■ Exaggerated startle response

■ Decreased interest or participation in activities

■ Emotional withdrawal

What Causes PTSD?

No one really knows why some people develop PTSD while others do not. Some theories include:

■ Conditioned learning (People learn throughout their lives to respond to stress in certain ways.)

■ Ineffective coping strategies (Some people naturally have stronger ability to cope than others.)

■ Extreme severity and long duration of the stressor (It is thought that the more severe the stressor is and the longer it lasts, the more likely the person is to develop PTSD.)

■ Absence of support systems (Whether a person has significant others in his or her life to offer support in time of extreme stress affects the outcome of the response.)

■ Presence of preexisting psychopathology (Some individuals who already have an emotional problem may be more likely to develop PTSD in response to an extreme stressor.)

■ People with a family history of anxiety disorders, who have a history of childhood abuse or neglect, or who experienced early separation from parents seem more highly predisposed to develop PTSD.

How Is PTSD Diagnosed?

A physical examination to rule out physical illness is conducted. The patient must tell the physician about any anxiety disorders or depression within the family, and mention any other contributing factors, such as a history of having experienced a traumatic event. PTSD is best diagnosed by a mental health professional.

What Is the Treatment for PTSD?

Group therapy and family therapy are effective treatments for PTSD in association with prescribed medications. Cognitive-behavioral therapy and eye movement desensitization and reprocessing are also recommended. The following medications have been useful in individuals with PTSD:

■ Sertraline (Zoloft) and paroxetine (Paxil) have been approved by the FDA for treatment of PTSD. Other SSRIs (fluoxetine [Prozac], citalopram [Celexa], escitalopram [Lexapro], and fluvoxamine [Luvox]) have also been used.

■ Other antidepressants have also been effective: bupropion (Wellbutrin), mirtazapine (Remeron), nefazodone, and venlafaxine (Effexor).

■ Tricyclic and MAOI antidepressants have been successful with some individuals.

■ Benzodiazepines may relieve anxiety, but are not recommended because they are addictive.

■ The antihypertensives propranolol (Inderal) and clonidine (Catapres), as well as lithium and carbamazepine (Tegretol), have been successful in alleviating nightmares, intrusive recollections, insomnia, startle responses, and angry outbursts associated with PTSD.

Other Contacts:

International Society for Traumatic Stress Studies, 60 Revere Dr., Suite 500, Northbrook, IL 60062, 847-480-9028; http://www.istss.org/

National Alliance on Mental Illness, 3803 North Fairfax Dr., Suite 100, Arlington, VA 22203, 1-800-950-6264; http://www.nami.org/

Obsessive-Compulsive Disorder (OCD)

What Is OCD?

OCD is an anxiety disorder in which a person has recurring thoughts or images (called **obsessions**) and/or repetitive, ritualistic-type behaviors that the individual is unable to keep from doing (called **compulsions**). An individual with OCD may try to suppress these thoughts or behaviors, but is unable to do so. The individual knows that the thoughts or behaviors are irrational, but feels powerless to stop.

What Are the Symptoms of OCD?

The most common obsessions include:

- Repeated thoughts about contamination (e.g., may lead to fear of shaking hands or touching objects)
- Repeated doubts (e.g., repeatedly wondering if they locked the door or turned off an appliance)
- A need to have things in a certain order (e.g., feels intense anxiety when things are out of place)
- Thoughts of aggression (e.g., to hurt a loved one)
- Sexual imagery (e.g., recurring pornographic image)

The most common compulsions include:

- Washing and cleaning (e.g., excessive hand washing or housecleaning)
- Counting (e.g., counting the number of times that something is done)
- Checking (e.g., checking something that one has done, over and over)
- Requesting or demanding assurances from others
- Repeating actions (e.g., going in and out of a door, or up and down from a chair)
- Ordering (e.g., arranging and rearranging clothes or other items)

The obsessions and compulsions seem to be worse in the face of emotional stress.

What Causes OCD?

The exact causes of OCD are unclear. There appear to be certain contributing factors to the disorder. These include:

- **Biochemical.** OCD may be caused by a disturbance in the chemistry of the brain involving the neurotransmitter serotonin.
- **Genetics.** OCD seems to run in families. Researchers are still looking for specific genetic factors that may contribute to an inherited risk.
- **Learning theory.** Some clinicians believe that OCD may be the result of certain patterns of learned behavior in one's early family development.

How Is OCD Diagnosed?

OCD has differing degrees of severity. Some people are able to hide their illness or learn to live with it. In other instances, individuals may not be able to do anything but carry out their rituals, thereby causing a great deal of interference in their lives. Most individuals wait until the illness is severe enough that it is interfering with their social or occupational functioning before they seek treatment. A diagnosis should be made by a mental health professional.

What Is the Treatment for OCD?

Antidepressants have been used with success in the treatment of OCD. Clomipramine (Anafranil) was first to be approved by the FDA for this purpose. Because of their effectiveness and low side-effect profile, the SSRIs have become the first line of treatment for OCD. Other antidepressants that have also shown to be effective include venlafaxine (Effexor) and mirtazapine (Remeron).

In addition to medication, psychosocial techniques, such as cognitive-behavioral therapy, individual psychotherapy, and relaxation training, have been helpful for some individuals with OCD.

Other Contacts:

The International OCD Foundation, PO Box 961029, Boston, MA 02196, 617-973-5801; http://www.ocfoundation.org/

National Alliance on Mental Illness, 3803 North Fairfax Dr., Suite 100, Arlington, VA 22203, 1-800-950-6264; http://www.nami.org/

Panic Disorder

What Is Panic Disorder?

Panic disorder is characterized by periodic attacks of anxiety, feelings of terror, and intense physical discomfort. They usually last about 15 to 30 minutes. The individual feels nervous and fearful between attacks. The attacks can occur spontaneously or in response to a particular situation. They may occur daily, then remit for months, or they may occur weekly for months at a time.

What Are the Symptoms of Panic Disorder?

- Fast, pounding heartbeat
- Shortness of breath
- Nausea
- Fear of going insane
- Chills or hot flashes
- Sweating
- A choking feeling
- Dizziness
- Fear of dying
- Trembling or shaking

- Chest pain
- Feelings of unreality
- Numbness

What Causes Panic Disorder?

The exact cause of panic disorder is unclear. There appear to be certain contributing factors to the disorder:

- **Biochemical.** Panic disorder may be caused by a disturbance in the chemistry of the brain involving the neurotransmitter norepinephrine.
- **Genetics.** Panic disorder seems to run in families. Many people with panic disorder have close relatives with the disorder.
- **Psychodynamics.** This theory suggests that panic disorder may be caused by the inability to solve the early childhood conflict of dependence vs. independence.

How Is Panic Disorder Diagnosed?

A physical examination to rule out physical illness is conducted. The patient should report any anxiety disorders or depression in other family members and other contributing factors, such as excessive caffeine use, recent life changes, or stressful events. Panic disorder is best diagnosed by a mental health professional.

What Is the Treatment for Panic Disorder?

A combination of psychosocial therapy and medication is the treatment of choice for panic disorder. Medications include: benzodiazepines (alprazolam [Xanax], lorazepam [Ativan], and clonazepam [Klonopin]). Care must be used in taking these medications, because they are addictive. Antidepressants such as the SSRIs are particularly effective and are often first-line treatment for panic disorder. The tricyclics clomipramine [Anafranil] and imipramine [Tofranil] have also been successful in treating this disorder. Individual psychotherapy, cognitive-behavioral therapy, and relaxation training are helpful.

Other Contacts:

Anxiety Disorders Association of America, 8730 Georgia Ave., Silver Spring, MD 20910, 240-485-1001; http://www.adaa.org/

National Anxiety Foundation, 3135 Custer Dr., Lexington, KY 40517, 606-272-7166 or 1-800-755-1576; http://lexington-on-line.com/naf.html

National Alliance on Mental Illness, 3803 North Fairfax Dr., Suite 100, Arlington, VA 22203, 1-800-950-6264; http://www.nami.org/

Eating Disorders

What Are Eating Disorders?

The categories of eating disorders include anorexia nervosa, bulimia nervosa, and binge eating. These disorders deal with food obsessions, distorted body images, and obsessional thinness. In reality, they have little to do with food and more to do with psychological and emotional factors. Ninety percent of eating disorders are in women.

What Are the Symptoms of Eating Disorders?

In **anorexia nervosa,** individuals have an intense fear of gaining weight. They see themselves as fat, even though they may only weigh 85 percent or less of expected weight. They may eat very little, and they sometimes self-induce vomiting after eating. They exercise excessively. Women generally stop having periods. Blood pressure and temperature are low and the heartbeat is slow. In **bulimia nervosa,** the individual eats huge amounts of food and follows with self-induced vomiting (purging). They often abuse laxatives and diuretics. Their weight is usually within normal range. In **binge eating disorder,** the individual eats huge amounts of food, but does not purge. Weight gain can progress to obesity.

What Causes Eating Disorders?

- **Genetics.** Eating disorders appear to run in families. There is thought to be a hereditary link.
- **Biological.** Eating disorders may be associated with a disturbance in the chemistry of the brain involving the neurotransmitters serotonin and norepinephrine.
- **Family dynamics.** Some clinicians believe that eating behaviors become maladaptive when there are issues of power and control within the family. Perfectionism is expected by the parents in order for the child to earn their love and affection. Distorted eating patterns may be viewed by the adolescent as a way to gain and remain in control.

How Are Eating Disorders Diagnosed?

Denial (on the part of both the parent and the child) is common in eating disorders. The disorder may progress to a serious condition before treatment is sought. In anorexia nervosa, the individual may be emaciated, not having periods, and may have a distorted self-image. In bulimia, the diagnosis is made if there are at least two bulimic episodes per week for 3 months. Lab work is completed: blood count, electrolytes, protein levels, ECG, and chest x-ray. A bone-density test may be administered.

What is the Treatment for Eating Disorders?

Hospitalization for nutritional stabilization is common for anorexia and sometimes for bulimia. For the anorexic person, behavior modification with weight gain is the goal. Cognitive-behavioral therapy, interpersonal psychotherapy, and family therapy are used, along with medication. Medications for eating disorders include antidepressants (the SSRIs) for anorexia, bulimia, and binge eating; appetite stimulants for anorexia; and anorexiants for obesity.

Other Contacts:

National Association of Anorexia Nervosa and Associated Disorders, P.O. Box 640, Naperville, IL 60566, 630-577-1330; http://www.anad.org/

National Eating Disorders Association, 603 Stewart Street, Suite 803, Seattle, WA 98101, 206-382-3587; http://www.nationaleatingdisorders.org/

Schizophrenia

What Is Schizophrenia?

Schizophrenia is a severe, chronic, and often disabling brain disease. It causes severe mental disturbances that disrupt normal thought, speech, and behavior. It can affect anyone at any age, but most cases develop between adolescence and age 30. Schizophrenia impairs a person's ability to think clearly, make decisions, and relate to others.

What Are the Symptoms of Schizophrenia?

■ Delusions (false ideas)

■ Hallucinations (hearing, seeing, or feeling things that are not there)

■ Confused thinking

■ Speech that does not make sense

■ Lack of feeling or emotional expression

■ Lack of pleasure or interest in life

■ Lack of ability to complete activities

■ Suspiciousness

■ Difficulty socializing with others

What Causes Schizophrenia?

The cause of schizophrenia is unknown. Several theories exist:

■ **Genetics.** Genetics appears to play a role, as schizophrenia seems to run in families.

■ **Biochemical.** An excess of the neurotransmitter dopamine is thought to play a role in the cause of the disorder. Abnormalities in other neurotransmitters have also been suggested.

■ **Brain abnormalities.** Structural and cellular changes in the brain have been noted in people with schizophrenia.

■ **Other.** Scientists are currently investigating maternal prenatal viral infections and mild brain damage to the child from complications during birth as contributing to the development of schizophrenia.

How Is Schizophrenia Diagnosed?

To be diagnosed with schizophrenia, a person must have psychotic, "loss-of-reality" symptoms for at least 6 months and show increasing difficulty in normal functioning. The doctor will rule out other problems that cause psychotic symptoms, such as drugs, mania, major depression, autistic disorder, or personality disorders. Diagnosis should be made by a mental health professional.

What Is the Treatment for Schizophrenia?

Hospitalization may be necessary to treat severe delusions or hallucinations or inability for self-care. A combination of psychosocial therapy and medication has been effective in treating schizophrenia. Individual psychotherapy, behavior therapy, social skills training, and family therapy are appropriate, along with antipsychotic medication. Conventional antipsychotics include chlorpromazine, fluphenazine, haloperidol [Haldol], thiothixene [Navane], prochlorperazine, trifluoperazine, perphenazine, thioridazine, loxapine, and pimozide [Orap]. Newer atypical antipsychotics have fewer side effects and include risperidone [Risperdal], clozapine [Clozaril], olanzapine [Zyprexa], quetiapine [Seroquel], ziprasidone [Geodon], paliperidone [Invega], iloperidone [Fanapt], asenapine [Saphris], lurasidone [Latuda], and aripiprazole [Abilify]. Medications must be taken daily for maintenance of symptoms. Certain ones may be taken by injection at 1- to 4-week intervals.

Other Contacts:

National Alliance on Mental Illness, 3803 North Fairfax Dr., Suite 100, Arlington, VA 22203, 1-800-950-6264; http://www.nami.org/

World Fellowship for Schizophrenia and Allied Disorders, 19 MacPherson Ave., Toronto, Ontario M5R 1W7, Canada; http://www.world-schizophrenia.org/

Alzheimer's Disease

What Is Alzheimer's Disease?

Alzheimer's disease is a type of dementia characterized by a loss of intellectual abilities involving impairment of memory, judgment, abstract thinking, and coordination of movement and changes in personality. An estimated 4 million people in the United States have Alzheimer's disease.

What Are the Symptoms of Alzheimer's Disease?

Early Stages

- Forgetfulness (loses things; forgets names)
- Confusion with performing simple tasks
- Confusion about month or season
- Difficulty making decisions
- Increasing loss of interest in activities
- Depression; anger
- Difficulty completing sentences or finding the right words
- Reduced and/or irrelevant conversation
- Visibly impaired movement or coordination, including slowing of movements, halting gait, and reduced sense of balance

Later Stages

- Unable to dress, groom, and toilet self
- Forgets names of close relatives
- Withdrawal; apathy
- Disorientation to surroundings
- Urinary and fecal incontinence
- Wandering
- Loss of language skills

What Causes Alzheimer's Disease?

- **Genetics.** Hereditary factors appear to play a role in the development of Alzheimer's disease.
- **Biological.** Imbalance in the neurotransmitter acetylcholine. Levels of serotonin and norepinephrine may also be affected.
- **Brain changes.** Twisted nerve cell fibers, called neurofibrillary tangles, and a high concentration of plaques of a protein known as beta amyloid are found in the brains of people with Alzheimer's disease.
- **Head injury.** Injury to the head can accelerate the development of Alzheimer's disease in people who are susceptible to it.
- **Down syndrome.** People with Down syndrome are especially susceptible to Alzheimer's disease.

How Is Alzheimer's Disease Diagnosed?

Family members report difficulties with memory, language, behavior, reasoning, and orientation. The physician then conducts a history and physical examination. Diagnostic laboratory tests are performed. CT scans or MRI may be used to rule out tumors or stroke. The neurologist will perform a mental status examination and possibly other cognitive and functional ability tests.

What Is the Treatment for Alzheimer's Disease?

Treatment for Alzheimer's disease involves assistance with hygiene, dressing, grooming, toileting, and food preparation. Safety is an important issue, particularly as the individual begins to have difficulty with balance and coordination, and if he or she tends to wander. Individuals with Alzheimer's disease require help with all activities of daily living, and as the disease progresses, usually require institutionalization. Some medications have been approved for treating the symptoms of Alzheimer's disease. These include: memantine (Namenda), tacrine (Cognex), donepezil (Aricept), rivastigmine (Exelon), and galantamine (Reminyl). These medications have been shown to slow the progression of cognitive, functional, and behavioral symptoms in some individuals with Alzheimer's disease.

Other Contacts:

Alzheimer's Association, 225 N. Michigan Ave, Fl. 17, Chicago, IL 60601, 1-800-272-3900; http://www.alz.org/

Alzheimer's Disease Education and Referral Center, PO Box 8250, Silver Spring, MD 20907, 1-800-438-4380; http://www.nia.nih.gov/alzheimers/

Alcoholism

What Is Alcoholism?

Alcoholism is a disease in which an individual is dependent upon alcohol. About 9 million persons in the United States have this disease. It is a lifelong illness, and is incurable, and the only effective management is total abstinence from alcohol.

What Are the Symptoms of Alcoholism?

Alcoholism may begin with social drinking or drinking to relieve stress and tension. As the individual continues to drink, tolerance develops, and the amount required to achieve the desired effect increases steadily. This progresses to blackouts—periods of drinking time that the individual is unable to remember. The disease has now progressed to the point that the individual requires alcohol to prevent withdrawal symptoms, yet denial of problems is common. Binges occur leading to physical illness and/or loss of consciousness. Abstaining from alcohol at this point can lead to tremors, hallucinations, convulsions, and severe agitation. Chronic alcoholism leads to many serious physical problems involving the heart, brain, and gastrointestinal system.

What Causes Alcoholism?

- **Genetic.** Alcoholism is thought to have a strong hereditary component.
- **Biological.** There may be a connection between alcoholism and certain neurotransmitters that form addictive substances in the brain when they combine with the products of alcohol metabolism.
- **Social learning.** Drinking alcohol may be learned early in the family of origin, thereby leading to a problem with drinking.
- **Cultural.** The incidence of alcohol abuse and dependence is higher in some cultures than others.

How Is Alcoholism Diagnosed?

Alcoholism is diagnosed when the use of alcohol interferes with any aspect of the individual's life. The individual continues to drink even though he or she understands the negative consequences. When dependence occurs, the individual develops a tolerance and requires more and more of the substance. A syndrome of withdrawal symptoms occurs when the individual stops drinking or drastically cuts down on the amount consumed.

What Is the Treatment for Alcoholism?

- **Rehabilitation Programs.** Help the individual get dry and, through therapy, to work toward achieving and maintaining sobriety.
- **Alcoholics Anonymous.** Self-help support groups made up of alcoholics who work to help each other achieve and maintain sobriety.

- **Medications.** Disulfiram (Antabuse) is a deterrent therapy. Individuals who drink alcohol while taking this drug become very ill. Naltrexone (ReVia), nalmefene (Revex), and acamprosate (Campral) have been used with some success in the treatment of alcoholism.

Other Contacts:

Alcoholics Anonymous, P.O. Box 459, New York, NY 10163, 212-870-3400; http://www.aa.org/

National Institutes of Health, National Institute on Alcohol Abuse and Alcoholism, 5635 Fishers Lane, MSC 9304, Bethesda, MD 20892, 301-443-3860; http://www.niaaa.nih.gov/

Attention-Deficit/Hyperactivity Disorder (ADHD)

What Is ADHD?

ADHD is a behavior disorder that is characterized by hyperactivity, impulsiveness, inattention, or a combination of these behaviors that are more frequent and severe than would be expected for the age. It is usually not diagnosed before age 4, and is more common in boys than it is in girls. ADHD can also be a disorder in adults.

What Are the Symptoms of ADHD?

There are three subtypes of the disorder:

1. **ADHD, Inattentive type:** has difficulty paying attention; does not listen when spoken to; is easily distracted; does not follow through on instructions; has difficulty organizing tasks and activities.
2. **ADHD, Hyperactive-Impulsive type:** has trouble sitting still; gets up out of seat at times when expected to remain seated; cannot play quietly; talks excessively; blurts out answers before questions are completed; has difficulty waiting turn; often interrupts or intrudes on others.
3. **ADHD, Combined type:** displays a combination of behaviors associated with the above two types.

What Causes ADHD?

- **Genetics.** Hereditary factors appear to play a role in the development of ADHD.
- **Biochemical.** Abnormal levels of dopamine, norepinephrine, and serotonin have been implicated as a cause of ADHD.
- **Perinatal factors.** Perinatal factors implicated: problem pregnancies and difficult deliveries;

maternal smoking and use of alcohol or other drugs during pregnancy; exposure during pregnancy to environmental toxins.

- **Environmental factors.** Exposure to environmental lead may be an influential factor.
- **Early family life.** A chaotic family environment, maternal mental disorder, paternal criminality, and family history of alcoholism, sociopathic behaviors, or hyperactivity may be contributing factors to ADHD.

How Is ADHD Diagnosed?

ADHD is difficult to diagnose. A mother's description of her child's behavior can be the most accurate and reliable guide for diagnosing ADHD. A detailed history of the child's behavior will be matched against a standardized checklist used to define the disorder. The physician will inquire about problem behaviors at home and school, sibling relationships, recent life changes, family history of ADHD, eating and sleeping patterns, and speech and language development. A medical history will be taken of the child, and also of the mother's pregnancy and delivery. A physical examination will be conducted. Screening tests may be used to test neurological, intellectual, and emotional development.

What Is the Treatment for ADHD?

Behavior modification and family therapy, in combination with medication, is used to treat ADHD. Medications include: CNS stimulants, including methylphenidate [Ritalin]; dexmethylphenidate [Focalin]; dextroamphetamine [Dexadrine]; methamphetamine [Desoxyn]; lisdexamfetamine [Vyvanse], and dextroamphetamine/amphetamine mixture [Adderall]. Other medications used for ADHD include atomoxetine [Strattera], the antidepressant bupropion [Wellbutrin], and the alpha-adrenergic agonists clonidine [Catapres] and guanfacine [Intuniv].

Other Contacts:

National Institute of Mental Health, 6001 Executive Blvd, Rm 8184, MSC 9663, Bethesda, MD 20892, 866-615-6464; http://www.nimh.nih.gov/health/topics/attention-deficit-hyperactivity-disorder-adhd/index.shtml

National Attention Deficit Disorder Association, 15000 Commerce Pkwy, Suite C, Mount Laurel, NJ 08054, 856-439-9099; http://www.add.org/

Glossary

A

abandonment. A unilateral severance of the professional relationship between a health-care provider and a client without reasonable notice at a time when there is still a need for continuing health care.

abreaction. "Remembering with feeling"; bringing into conscious awareness painful events that have been repressed, and re-experiencing the emotions that were associated with the events.

abuse. To use wrongfully or in a harmful way. Improper treatment or conduct that may result in injury.

acquired immunodeficiency syndrome (AIDS). A condition in which the immune system becomes deficient in its efforts to prevent opportunistic infections, malignancies, and neurological disease. It is caused by the human immunodeficiency virus (HIV), which is passed from one individual to another through body fluids.

acupoints. In Chinese medicine, acupoints represent areas along the body that link pathways of healing energy.

acupressure. A technique in which the fingers, thumbs, palms, or elbows are used to apply pressure to certain points along the body. This pressure is thought to dissolve any obstructions in the flow of healing energy and to restore the body to a healthier functioning.

acupuncture. A technique in which hair-thin, sterile, disposable, stainless-steel needles are inserted into points along the body to dissolve obstructions in the flow of healing energy and restore the body to a healthier functioning.

adaptation. Restoration of the body to homeostasis following a physiological and/or psychological response to stress.

adjustment. The process of modifying one's behavior in changed circumstances or an altered environment in order to fulfill psychological, physiological, and social needs.

adjustment disorder. A maladaptive reaction to an identifiable psychosocial stressor that occurs within 3 months after onset of the stressor. The individual shows impairment in social and occupational functioning, or exhibits symptoms that are in excess of a normal and expectable reaction to the stressor.

advance directive. A legal document that a competent individual may sign to convey to wishes regarding future health-care decisions intended for a time when the individual is no longer capable of informed consent. It may include one or both of the following: (1) a living will, in which the individual identifies the type of care that he or she does or does not wish to have performed, and (2) a durable power of attorney for health care, in which the individual names another person who is given the right to make health-care decisions for the individual who is incapable of doing so.

advocacy. The act of pleading for, supporting, or representing a cause or individual. Advocacy in nursing applies to any act in which the nurse is serving in the best interests of the patient, from simple procedures such as hand washing to protect the patient from infection to complex ethically and morally charged issues in which certain clients are unable to advocate for themselves. Nurses also advocate for their patients indirectly by serving in organizations that support and serve to improve health care for all individuals, and by participating in policy-making legislation that affects health care of the public.

affect. The behavioral expression of emotion; may be appropriate (congruent with the situation); inappropriate (incongruent with the situation); constricted or blunted (diminished range and intensity); or flat (absence of emotional expression).

affective domain. A category of learning that includes attitudes, feelings, and values.

aggression. Harsh physical or verbal actions intended (either consciously or unconsciously) to harm or injure another.

aggressiveness. Behavior that defends an individual's own basic rights by violating the basic rights of others (as contrasted with **assertiveness**).

agoraphobia. The fear of being in places or situations from which escape might be difficult (or embarrassing) or in which help might not be available in the event of a panic attack.

agranulocytosis. Extremely low levels of white blood cells. Symptoms include sore throat, fever, and malaise. This may be a side effect of long-term therapy with some antipsychotic medications.

AIDS. See **acquired immunodeficiency syndrome (AIDS).**

akathisia. Restlessness; an urgent need for movement. A type of extrapyramidal side effect associated with some antipsychotic medications.

akinesia. Muscular weakness; or a loss or partial loss of muscle movement; a type of extrapyramidal side effect associated with some antipsychotic medications.

Alcoholics Anonymous (AA). A major self-help organization for the treatment of alcoholism. It is based on a 12-step program to help members attain and maintain sobriety. Once individuals have achieved sobriety, they in turn are expected to help other alcoholic persons.

allopathic medicine. Traditional medicine. The type traditionally, and currently, practiced in the United States and taught in U.S. medical schools.

alternative medicine. Practices that differ from usual traditional (allopathic) medicine.

altruism. One curative factor of group therapy (identified by Yalom) in which individuals gain self-esteem through mutual sharing and concern. Providing assistance and support to others creates a positive self-image and promotes self-growth.

altruistic suicide. Suicide based on behavior of a group into which an individual is excessively integrated.

amenorrhea. Cessation of the menses; may be a side effect of some antipsychotic medications.

amnesia. An inability to recall important personal information that is too extensive to be explained by ordinary forgetfulness.

amnesia, continuous. The inability to recall events occurring after a specific time up to and including the present.

amnesia, generalized. The inability to recall anything that has happened during the individual's entire lifetime.

amnesia, localized. The inability to recall all incidents associated with a traumatic event for a specific time period following the event (usually a few hours to a few days).

amnesia, selective. The inability to recall only certain incidents associated with a traumatic event for a specific time period following the event.

amnesia, systematized. The inability to remember events that relate to a specific category of information, such as one's family, a particular person, or an event.

amphetamine. A racemic sympathomimetic amine that acts as a central nervous system stimulant. It (and its derivatives, such as methamphetamine and dextroamphetamine) is a commonly abused substance, but has therapeutic use in the treatment of narcolepsy and attention-deficit/hyperactivity disorder.

andropause. A term used to identify the male climacteric. Also called *male menopause*. A syndrome of symptoms related to the decline of testosterone levels in men. Some symptoms include depression, weight gain, insomnia, hot flashes, decreased libido, mood swings, decreased strength, and erectile dysfunction.

anger. An emotional response to one's perception of a situation. Anger has both positive and negative functions.

anger management. The use of various techniques and strategies to control responses to anger-provoking situations. The goal of anger management is to reduce both the emotional feelings and the physiological arousal that anger engenders.

anhedonia. The inability to experience or even imagine any pleasant emotion.

anomic suicide. Suicide that occurs in response to changes that occur in an individual's life that disrupt cohesiveness from a group and cause that person to feel he or she is without support from the formerly cohesive group.

anorexia. Loss of appetite.

anorexiants. Drugs that suppress appetite.

anorgasmia. Inability to achieve orgasm.

anosmia. Inability to smell.

anticipatory grief. A subjective state of emotional, physical, and social responses to an anticipated loss of a valued entity. The grief response is repeated once the loss actually occurs, but it may not be as intense as it might have been if anticipatory grieving has not occurred.

antisocial personality disorder. A pattern of socially irresponsible, exploitative, and guiltless behavior, evident in the tendency to fail to conform to the law, develop stable relationships, or sustain consistent employment; exploitation and manipulation of others for personal gain is common.

anxiety. Vague diffuse apprehension that is associated with feelings of uncertainty and helplessness.

aphasia. Inability to communicate through speech, writing, or signs, caused by dysfunction of brain centers.

aphonia. Inability to speak.

apraxia. Inability to carry out motor activities despite intact motor function.

arbitrary inference. A type of thinking error in which the individual automatically comes to a conclusion about an incident without the facts to support it, or even sometimes despite contradictory evidence to support it.

ascites. Excessive accumulation of serous fluid in the abdominal cavity, occurring in response to portal hypertension caused by cirrhosis of the liver.

assault. An act that results in a person's genuine fear and apprehension that he or she will be touched without consent. Nurses may be guilty of assault for threatening to place an individual in restraints against his or her will.

assertive behavior. Behavior that enables individuals to act in their own best interests, to stand up for themselves without undue anxiety, to express their honest feelings comfortably, or to exercise their own rights without denying those of others.

assessment. A systematic, dynamic process by which the registered nurse, through interaction with the patient, family, groups, communities, populations, and health-care providers, collects and analyzes data. Assessment may include the following dimensions: physical, psychological, sociocultural, spiritual, cognitive, functional abilities, developmental, economic, and lifestyle (ANA, 2010).

associative looseness. Sometimes called loose associations, a thinking process characterized by speech in which ideas shift from one unrelated subject to another. The individual is unaware that the topics are unconnected.

ataxia. Muscular incoordination.

attachment theory. The hypothesis that individuals who maintain close relationships with others into old age are more likely to remain independent and less likely to be institutionalized than those who do not.

attitude. A frame of reference around which an individual organizes knowledge about his or her world. It includes an emotional element and can have a positive or negative connotation.

autism. A focus inward on a fantasy world, while distorting or excluding the external environment; common in schizophrenia.

autism spectrum disorders. A group of disorders that are characterized by impairment in several areas of development, including social interaction skills and interpersonal communication. Included in this category are autistic disorder, Rett's disorder, childhood disintegrative disorder, pervasive developmental disorder not otherwise specified, and Asperger's disorder (APA, 2000).

autistic disorder. The withdrawal of an infant or child into the self and into a fantasy world of his or her own creation. There is marked impairment in interpersonal functioning and communication and in imaginative play. Activities and interests are restricted and may be considered somewhat bizarre.

autocratic. A leadership style in which the leader makes all decisions for the group. Productivity is very high with this type of leadership, but morale is often low because of the lack of member input and creativity.

autoimmunity. A condition in which the body produces a disordered immunological response against itself. In this situation, the body fails to differentiate between what is normal and what is a foreign substance. When this occurs, the body produces antibodies against normal parts of the body to such an extent as to cause tissue injury.

automatic thoughts. Thoughts that occur rapidly in response to a situation, and without rational analysis. They are often negative and based on erroneous logic.

autonomy. Independence; self-governance. An ethical principle that emphasizes the status of persons as autonomous moral agents whose right to determine their destinies should always be respected.

aversive stimulus. A stimulus that follows a behavioral response and decreases the probability that the behavior will recur; also called *punishment.*

axon. The cellular process of a neuron that carries impulses away from the cell body.

B

battering. A pattern of repeated physical assault, usually of a woman by her spouse or intimate partner. Men are also battered, although this occurs much less frequently.

battery. The unconsented touching of another person. Nurses may be charged with battery should they participate in the treatment of a client without his or her consent and outside of an emergency situation.

behavior modification. A treatment modality aimed at changing undesirable behaviors, using a system of reinforcement to bring about the modifications desired.

behavior therapy. A form of psychotherapy, the goal of which is to modify maladaptive behavior patterns by reinforcing more adaptive behaviors.

behavioral objectives. Statements that indicate to an individual what is expected of him or her. Behavioral objectives are a way of measuring learning outcomes, and are based on the affective, cognitive, and psychomotor domains of learning.

belief. A belief is an idea that one holds to be true. It can be rational, irrational, taken on faith, or a stereotypical idea.

beneficence. An ethical principle that refers to one's duty to benefit or promote the good of others.

bereavement overload. An accumulation of grief that occurs when an individual experiences many losses over a short period of time and is unable to resolve one before another is experienced. This phenomenon is common among the elderly.

binge and purge. A syndrome associated with eating disorders, especially bulimia, in which an individual consumes thousands of calories of food at one sitting (binging), and then purges through the use of laxatives or self-induced vomiting.

bioethics. The term used with ethical principles that refer to concepts within the scope of medicine, nursing, and allied health.

biofeedback. The use of instrumentation to become aware of processes in the body that usually go unnoticed and to bring them under voluntary control (e.g., the blood pressure or pulse); used as a method of stress reduction.

bipolar disorder. Characterized by mood swings from profound depression to extreme euphoria (mania), with intervening periods of normalcy. Psychotic symptoms may or may not be present.

body image. One's perception of his or her own body. It may also be how one believes others perceive his or her body. (See also **physical self.**)

borderline personality disorder. A disorder characterized by a pattern of intense and chaotic relationships, with affective instability, fluctuating and extreme attitudes regarding other people, impulsivity, direct and indirect self-destructive behavior, and lack of a clear or certain sense of identity, life plan, or values.

boundaries. The level of participation and interaction between individuals and between subsystems. Boundaries denote physical and psychological space individuals identify as their own. They are sometimes referred to as limits. Boundaries are appropriate when they permit appropriate contact with others while preventing excessive interference. Boundaries may be clearly defined (healthy) or rigid or diffuse (unhealthy).

bulimia. Excessive, insatiable appetite.

C

cachexia. A state of ill health, malnutrition, and wasting; extreme emaciation.

cannabis. The dried flowering tops of the hemp plant. It produces euphoric effects when ingested or smoked and is commonly used in the form of marijuana or hashish.

carcinogen. Any substance or agent that produces or increases the risk of developing cancer in humans or lower animals.

case management. A health-care delivery process, the goals of which are to provide quality health care, decrease fragmentation, enhance the client's quality of life, and contain costs. A case manager coordinates the client's care from admission to discharge and sometimes following discharge. Critical pathways of care are the tools used for the provision of care in a case management system.

case manager. The individual responsible for negotiating with multiple health-care providers to obtain a variety of services for a client.

catastrophic thinking. Always thinking that the worst will occur without considering the possibility of more likely, positive outcomes.

catatonia. A type of schizophrenia that is typified by stupor or excitement. Stupor is characterized by extreme psychomotor retardation, mutism, negativism, and posturing; excitement by psychomotor agitation, in which the movements are frenzied and purposeless.

catharsis. One curative factor of group therapy (identified by Yalom), in which members in a group can express both positive and negative feelings in a nonthreatening atmosphere.

cell body. The part of the neuron that contains the nucleus and is essential for the continued life of the neuron.

Centers for Medicare and Medicaid Services (CMS). The division of the U.S. Department of Health and Human Services responsible for Medicare funding.

child sexual abuse. Any sexual act, ranging from indecent exposure or improper touching to penetration (sexual intercourse), that is carried out with a child.

chiropractic medicine. A system of alternative medicine based on the premise that the relationship between structure and function in the human body is a significant health factor and that such relationships between the spinal column and the nervous system are important because the normal transmission and expression of nerve energy are essential to the restoration and maintenance of health.

Christian ethics. The ethical philosophy that states one should treat others as moral equals, and recognize the equality of other persons by permitting them to act as we do when they occupy a position similar to ours; sometimes referred to as "the ethic of the golden rule."

circadian rhythm. A 24-hour biological rhythm controlled by a "pacemaker" in the brain that sends messages to other systems in the body. Circadian rhythm influences various regulatory functions, including the sleep-wake cycle, body temperature regulation, patterns of activity such as eating and drinking, and hormonal and neurotransmitter secretion.

circumstantiality. In speaking, the delay of an individual to reach the point of a communication, owing to unnecessary and tedious details.

civil law. Law that protects the private and property rights of individuals and businesses.

clang association. A pattern of speech in which the choice of words is governed by sounds. Clang associations often take the form of rhyming.

classical conditioning. A type of learning that occurs when an unconditioned stimulus (UCS) that produces an unconditioned response (UCR) is paired with a conditioned stimulus (CS), until the CS alone produces the same response, which is then called a conditioned response (CR). Pavlov's example: food (i.e., UCS) causes salivation (i.e., UCR); ringing bell (i.e., CS) with food (i.e., UCS) causes salivation (i.e., UCR), ringing bell alone (i.e., CS) causes salivation (i.e., CR).

codependency. An exaggerated dependent pattern of learned behaviors, beliefs, and feelings that make life painful. It is a dependence on people and things outside the self, along with neglect of the self to the point of having little self-identity.

cognition. Mental operations that relate to logic, awareness, intellect, memory, language, and reasoning powers.

cognitive. Relating to the mental processes of thinking and reasoning.

cognitive development. A series of stages described by Piaget through which individuals progress, demonstrating at each successive stage a higher level of logical organization than at each previous stage.

cognitive domain. A category of learning that involves knowledge and thought processes within the individual's intellectual ability. The individual must be able to synthesize information at an intellectual level before the actual behaviors are performed.

cognitive maturity. The capability to perform all mental operations needed for adulthood.

cognitive therapy. A type of therapy in which the individual is taught to control thought distortions that are considered to be a factor in the development and maintenance of emotional disorders.

colposcope. An instrument that contains a magnifying lens and to which a 35-mm camera can be attached. A colposcope is used to examine for tears and abrasions inside the vaginal area of a sexual assault victim.

common law. Laws that are derived from decisions made in previous cases.

communication. An interactive process of transmitting information between two or more entities.

community. A group of people living close to and depending to some extent on each other.

compensation. An ego defense mechanism identified by the covering up of a real or perceived weakness by emphasizing a trait one considers more desirable.

complementary medicine. Practices that differ from usual traditional (allopathic) medicine, but may in fact supplement it in a positive way.

compounded rape reaction. Symptoms that are in addition to the typical rape response of physical complaints, rage, humiliation, fear, and sleep disturbances. They include depression and suicide, substance abuse, and even psychotic behaviors.

compulsions. Unwanted repetitive behavior patterns or mental acts (e.g., praying, counting, repeating words silently) that are intended to reduce anxiety, not to provide pleasure or gratification (APA, 2000). They may be performed in response to an obsession or in a stereotyped fashion.

concept mapping. A diagrammatic teaching and learning strategy that allows students and faculty to visualize interrelationships between medical diagnoses, nursing diagnoses, assessment data, and treatments. A diagram of client problems and interventions.

concrete thinking. Thought processes that are focused on specifics rather than on generalities and immediate issues rather than eventual outcomes. Individuals who are experiencing concrete thinking are unable to comprehend abstract terminology.

conditioned response. In classical conditioning, a response that is a *learned* response (not reflexive) following repeated exposure to a target stimulus.

conditioned stimulus. In classical conditioning, an unrelated stimulus that is presented to a subject with a target stimulus, and that, with repeated exposure, comes to elicit the same response as the original target stimulus.

confabulation. Creating imaginary events to fill in memory gaps.

confidentiality. The right of an individual to the assurance that his or her case will not be discussed outside the boundaries of the health-care team.

contextual stimuli. Conditions present in the environment that support a focal stimulus and influence a threat to self-esteem.

contingency contracting. A written contract between individuals used to modify behavior. Benefits and consequences for fulfilling the terms of the contract are delineated.

controlled response pattern. The response to rape in which feelings are masked or hidden, and a calm, composed, or subdued affect is seen.

counselor. One who listens as the client reviews feelings related to difficulties he or she is experiencing in any aspect of life; one of the nursing roles identified by H. Peplau.

countertransference. In psychoanalytic theory, countertransference refers to the counselor's behavioral and emotional responses to the client. These responses may be related to unresolved feelings toward significant others from the counselor's past, or they may be generated in response to the client's behavior toward the counselor.

covert sensitization. An aversion technique used to modify behavior that relies on the individual's imagination to produce unpleasant symptoms. When the individual is about to succumb to undesirable behavior, he or she visualizes something that is offensive or even nauseating in an effort to block the behavior.

criminal law. Law that provides protection from conduct deemed injurious to the public welfare. It provides for punishment of those found to have engaged in such conduct.

crisis. Psychological disequilibrium in a person who confronts a hazardous circumstance that constitutes an important problem that, for the time, he or she can neither escape nor solve with usual problem-solving resources.

crisis intervention. An emergency type of assistance in which the intervener becomes a part of the individual's life situation. The focus is to provide guidance and support to help mobilize the resources needed to resolve the crisis and restore or generate an improvement in previous level of functioning. Usually lasts no longer than 6 to 8 weeks.

critical pathways of care. An abbreviated plan of care that provides outcome-based guidelines for goal achievement within a designated length of time.

culture. A particular society's entire way of living, encompassing shared patterns of belief, feeling, and knowledge that guide people's conduct and are passed down from generation to generation.

curandera. A female folk healer in the Latino culture.

curandero. A male folk healer in the Latino culture.

cycle of battering. Three phases of predictable behaviors that are repeated over time in a relationship between a batterer and a victim: tension-building phase; the acute battering incident; and the calm, loving, respite (honeymoon) phase.

cyclothymic disorder. A chronic mood disturbance involving numerous episodes of hypomania and depressed mood, of insufficient severity or duration to meet the criteria for bipolar disorder.

D

date rape. A situation in which the rapist is known to the victim. This may occur during dating or with acquaintances or schoolmates.(Also called *acquaintance rape.*)

decatastrophizing. In cognitive therapy, with this technique the therapist assists the client to examine the validity of a negative automatic thought. Even if some validity exists, the client is then encouraged to review ways to cope adaptively, moving beyond the current crisis situation.

defamation of character. An individual may be liable for defamation of character by sharing with others information about a person that is detrimental to that person's reputation.

deinstitutionalization. The removal of mentally ill individuals from institutions and the subsequent plan to provide care for these individuals in the community setting.

delayed grief. The absence of evidence of grief when it ordinarily would be expected.

delirious mania. A grave form of mania characterized by severe clouding of consciousness and representing an intensification of the symptoms associated with mania. The symptoms of delirious mania have become relatively rare since the availability of antipsychotic medications.

delirium. A state of mental confusion and excitement characterized by disorientation to time and place, often with hallucinations, incoherent speech, and a continual state of aimless physical activity.

delusions. False personal beliefs, not consistent with a person's intelligence or cultural background. The individual continues to have the belief in spite of obvious proof that it is false and/or irrational.

dementia. Global impairment of cognitive functioning that is progressive and interferes with social and occupational abilities.

dendrites. The cellular processes of a neuron that carry impulses toward the cell body.

denial. Refusal to acknowledge the existence of a real situation and/or the feelings associated with it.

density. The number of people in a given environmental space, influencing interpersonal interaction.

dependence. A compulsive or chronic requirement. The need is so strong as to generate distress (either physical or psychological) if left unfulfilled.

depersonalization. An alteration in the perception or experience of the self so that the feeling of one's own reality is temporarily lost.

depression. An alteration in mood that is expressed by feelings of sadness, despair, and pessimism. There is a loss of interest in usual activities, and somatic symptoms may be evident. Changes in appetite and sleep patterns are common.

derealization. An alteration in the perception or experience of the external world so that it seems strange or unreal.

detoxification. The process of withdrawal from a substance on which one has become dependent.

diagnosis-related groups (DRGs). A system used to determine prospective payment rates for reimbursement of hospital care based on the client's diagnosis.

Diagnostic and Statistical Manual of Mental Disorders, Fourth Edition, Text Revision (DSM-IV-TR). Standard nomenclature of emotional illness published by the American Psychiatric Association (APA) and used by all health-care practitioners. It classifies mental illness and presents guidelines and diagnostic criteria for various mental disorders.

dichotomous thinking. In this type of thinking, situations are viewed in all-or-nothing, black-or-white, good-or-bad terms.

directed association. A technique used to help clients bring into consciousness events that have been repressed. Specific thoughts are guided and directed by the psychoanalyst.

disaster. A natural or man-made occurrence that overwhelms the resources of an individual or community, and increases the need for emergency evacuation and medical services.

discriminative stimulus. A stimulus that precedes a behavioral response and predicts that a particular reinforcement will occur. Individuals learn to discriminate between various stimuli that will produce the responses they desire.

disengagement. In family theory, disengagement refers to extreme separateness among family members. It is promoted by rigid boundaries or lack of communication among family members.

disengagement theory. The hypothesis that there is a process of mutual withdrawal of aging persons and society from each other that is correlated with successful aging. This theory has been challenged by many investigators.

displacement. Feelings are transferred from one target to another that is considered less threatening or neutral.

disruptive behavior disorders. A disturbance of conduct severe enough to produce significant impairment in social, occupational, or academic functioning because of symptoms that range from oppositional defiant to moderate and severe conduct disturbances (Shahrokh & Hales, 2003).

dissociation. The splitting off of clusters of mental contents from conscious awareness, a mechanism central to hysterical conversion and dissociative disorder (Shahrokh & Hales, 2003).

distraction. In cognitive therapy, when dysfunctional cognitions have been recognized, activities are identified that can be used to distract the client and divert him or her from the intrusive thoughts or depressive ruminations that are contributing to the client's maladaptive responses.

disulfiram. A drug that is administered to individuals who abuse alcohol as a deterrent to drinking. Ingestion of alcohol while disulfiram is in the body results in a syndrome of symptoms that can produce a great deal of discomfort, and can even result in death if the blood alcohol level is high.

domains of learning. Categories in which individuals learn or gain knowledge and demonstrate behavior. There are three domains of learning: affective, cognitive, and psychomotor.

double-bind communication. An emotionally distressing situation in which an individual receives conflicting messages in the communication process, whereby one message is negated by another. This creates a condition in which a successful response to one message results in a failed response to the other.

dual diagnosis. A client has a dual diagnosis when it is determined that he or she has a coexisting substance disorder and mental illness. Treatment is designed to target both problems.

dyspareunia. Pain during sexual intercourse.

dysthymic disorder. A depressive neurosis. The symptoms are similar to, if somewhat milder than, those ascribed to major depression. There is no loss of contact with reality.

dystonia. Involuntary muscular movements (spasms) of the face, arms, legs, and neck; may occur as an extrapyramidal side effect of some antipsychotic medications.

E

echolalia. The parrot-like repetition, by an individual with loose ego boundaries, of the words spoken by another.

echopraxia. An individual with loose ego boundaries attempting to identify with another person by imitating movements that the other person makes.

ego. One of the three elements of the personality identified by Freud as the rational self or "reality principle." The ego seeks to maintain harmony between the external world, the id, and the superego.

ego defense mechanisms. Strategies employed by the ego for protection in the face of threat to biological or psychological integrity. (See individual defense mechanisms.)

egoistic suicide. The response of an individual who feels separate and apart from the mainstream of society.

electroconvulsive therapy (ECT). A type of somatic treatment in which electrical current is applied to the brain through electrodes placed on the temples. A grand mal seizure produces the desired effect. This is used with severely depressed patients refractory to antidepressant medications.

emaciated. The state of being excessively thin or physically wasted.

emotional abuse. A pattern of behavior on the part of the parent or caregiver that results in serious impairment of the child's social, emotional, or intellectual functioning.

emotional neglect. A chronic failure by the parent or caregiver to provide the child with the hope, love, and support necessary for the development of a sound, healthy personality.

empathy. The ability to see beyond outward behavior, and sense accurately another's inner experiencing. With empathy, one can accurately perceive and understand the meaning and relevance in the thoughts and feelings of another.

enmeshment. Exaggerated connectedness among family members. It occurs in response to diffuse boundaries in which there is overinvestment, overinvolvement, and lack of differentiation between individuals or subsystems.

esophageal varices. Veins in the esophagus become distended because of excessive pressure from defective blood flow through a cirrhotic liver.

essential hypertension. Persistent elevation of blood pressure for which there is no apparent cause or associated underlying disease.

ethical dilemma. A situation that arises when, on the basis of moral considerations, an appeal can be made for taking each of two opposing courses of action.

ethical egoism. An ethical theory espousing that what is "right" and "good" is what is best for the individual making the decision.

ethics. A branch of philosophy dealing with values related to human conduct, to the rightness and wrongness of certain actions, and to the goodness and badness of the motives and ends of such actions.

ethnicity. The concept of people identifying with each other because of a shared heritage.

evaluation. The process of determining the progress toward attainment of expected outcomes, including the effectiveness of care (ANA, 2010).

exhibitionism. A paraphilic disorder characterized by a recurrent urge to expose one's genitals to a stranger.

expressed response pattern. Pattern of behavior in which the victim of rape expresses feelings of fear, anger, and anxiety through such behavior as crying, sobbing, smiling, restlessness, and tenseness (in contrast to the rape victim who withholds feelings in the **controlled response pattern**).

extinction. In behavior therapy, the gradual decrease in frequency or disappearance of a response when the positive reinforcement is withheld.

extrapyramidal symptoms (EPS). A variety of responses that originate outside the pyramidal tracts and in the basal ganglion of the brain. Symptoms may include tremors, chorea, dystonia, akinesia, akathisia, and others. May occur as a side effect of some antipsychotic medications.

F

false imprisonment. The deliberate and unauthorized confinement of a person within fixed limits by the use of threat or force. A nurse may be charged with false imprisonment by placing a patient in restraints against his or her will in a nonemergency situation.

family. Two or more individuals who depend on one another for emotional, physical, and economic support. The members of the family are self-defined. (Kaakinen, Hanson, & Denham, 2010).

family structure. A family system in which the structure is founded on a set of invisible principles that influence the interaction among family members. These principles are established over time and become the "laws" that govern the conduct of various family members.

family system. A system in which the parts of the whole may be the marital dyad, parent-child dyad, or sibling groups. Each of these subsystems is further divided into subsystems of individuals.

family therapy. A type of therapy in which the focus is on relationships within the family. The family is viewed as a system in which the members are interdependent, and a change in one creates change in all.

fetishism. A paraphilic disorder characterized by recurrent sexual urges and sexually arousing fantasies involving the use of nonliving objects.

"fight-or-flight" syndrome. A syndrome of physical symptoms that result from an individual's real or perceived notion that harm or danger is imminent.

flexible boundary. A personal boundary is flexible when, because of unusual circumstances, individuals can alter limits that they have set for themselves. Flexible boundaries are healthy boundaries.

flooding. Sometimes called *implosion therapy,* this technique is used to desensitize individuals to phobic stimuli. The individual is "flooded" with a continuous presentation (usually through mental imagery) of the phobic stimulus until it no longer elicits anxiety.

focal stimulus. A situation of immediate concern that results in a threat to self-esteem.

Focus Charting®. A type of documentation that follows a data, action, and response (DAR) format. The main perspective is a client "focus," which can be a nursing diagnosis, a client's concern, a change in status, or a significant event in the client's therapy. The focus cannot be a medical diagnosis.

folk medicine. A system of health care within various cultures that is provided by a local practitioner, not professionally trained, but who uses techniques specific to that culture in the art of healing.

forensic. Pertaining to the law; legal.

forensic nursing. The application of forensic science combined with the biopsychological education of the registered nurse in the scientific investigation, evidence collection and preservation, analysis, prevention, and treatment of trauma- and/or death-related medical-legal issues.

free association. A technique used to help individuals bring to consciousness material that has been repressed. The individual is encouraged to verbalize whatever comes into his or her mind, drifting naturally from one thought to another.

frotteurism. A paraphilic disorder characterized by the recurrent preoccupation with intense sexual urges or fantasies involving touching or rubbing against a nonconsenting person.

fugue. A sudden unexpected travel away from home or customary work locale with the assumption of a new identity and an inability to recall one's previous identity; usually occurring in response to severe psychosocial stress.

G

gains. The reinforcements an individual receives for somaticizing.

Gamblers Anonymous (GA). An organization of inspirational group therapy, modeled after Alcoholics Anonymous (AA), for individuals who desire to, but cannot, stop gambling.

gender. The condition of being either male or female.

gender identity disorder. A sense of discomfort associated with an incongruence between biologically assigned gender and subjectively experienced gender.

general adaptation syndrome. The general biological reaction of the body to a stressful situation, as described by Hans Selye. It occurs in three stages: the alarm reaction stage, the stage of resistance, and the stage of exhaustion.

generalized anxiety disorder. A disorder characterized by chronic (at least 6 months), unrealistic, and excessive anxiety and worry.

genetics. Study of the biological transmission of certain characteristics (physical and/or behavioral) from parent to offspring.

genogram. A graphic representation of a family system. It may cover several generations. Emphasis is on family roles and emotional relatedness among members. Genograms facilitate recognition of areas requiring change.

genotype. The total set of genes present in an individual at the time of conception, and coded in the DNA.

genuineness. The ability to be open, honest, and "real" in interactions with others; the awareness of what one is experiencing internally and the ability to project the quality of this inner experiencing in a relationship.

geriatrics. The branch of clinical medicine specializing in the care of the elderly and concerned with the problems of aging.

gerontology. The study of normal aging.

geropsychiatry. The branch of clinical medicine specializing in psychopathology of the elderly.

gonorrhea. A sexually transmitted disease caused by the bacterium *Neisseria gonorrhoeae* and resulting in inflammation of the genital mucosa. Treatment is through the use of antibiotics, particularly penicillin. Serious complications occur if the disease is left untreated.

"granny-bashing." Media-generated term for abuse of the elderly.

"granny-dumping." Media-generated term for abandoning elderly individuals at emergency departments, nursing homes, or other facilities—literally leaving them in the hands of others when the strain of caregiving becomes intolerable.

grief. A subjective state of emotional, physical, and social responses to the real or perceived loss of a valued entity. Change and failure can also be perceived as losses. The grief response consists of a set of relatively predictable behaviors that describe the subjective state that accompanies mourning.

grief, exaggerated. A reaction in which all of the symptoms associated with normal grieving are exaggerated out of proportion. Pathological depression is a type of exaggerated grief.

grief, inhibited. The absence of evidence of grief when it ordinarily would be expected.

group. A collection of individuals whose association is founded on shared commonalities of interest, values, norms, or purpose. Membership in a group is generally by chance (born into the group), by choice (voluntary affiliation), or by circumstance (the result of life-cycle events over which an individual may or may not have control).

group therapy. A therapy group, founded in a specific theoretical framework, led by a person with an advanced degree in psychology, social work, nursing, or medicine. The goal is to encourage improvement in interpersonal functioning.

gynecomastia. Enlargement of the breasts in men; may be a side effect of some antipsychotic medications.

H

hallucinations. False sensory perceptions not associated with real external stimuli. Hallucinations may involve any of the five senses.

hepatic encephalopathy. A brain disorder resulting from the inability of the cirrhotic liver to convert ammonia to urea for excretion. The continued rise in serum ammonia results in progressively impaired mental functioning, apathy, euphoria or depression, sleep disturbances, increasing confusion, and progression to coma and eventual death.

histrionic personality disorder. Conscious or unconscious overly dramatic behavior for the purpose of drawing attention to oneself.

HIV-associated dementia (HAD). A neuropathological syndrome, possibly caused by chronic HIV encephalitis and myelitis and manifested by cognitive, behavioral, and motor symptoms that become more severe with progression of the disease.

home care. A wide range of health and social services that are delivered at home to recovering, disabled, chronically or terminally ill persons in need of medical, nursing, social, or therapeutic treatment and/or assistance with essential activities of daily living.

homocysteine. An amino acid produced by the catabolism of methionine. Elevated levels may be linked to increased risk of cardiovascular disease.

homosexuality. A sexual preference for persons of the same gender.

hospice. A program that provides palliative and supportive care to meet the special needs arising out of the physical, psychosocial, spiritual, social, and economic stresses that are experienced during the final stages of illness and during bereavement.

humors. The four body fluids described by Hippocrates: blood, black bile, yellow bile, and phlegm. Hippocrates associated insanity and mental illness with these four fluids.

hyperactivity. Excessive psychomotor activity that may be purposeful or aimless, accompanied by physical movements and verbal utterances that are usually more rapid than normal. Inattention and distractibility are common with hyperactive behavior.

hypersomnia. Excessive sleepiness or seeking excessive amounts of sleep.

hypertensive crisis. A potentially life-threatening syndrome that results when an individual taking monoamine oxidase (MAO) inhibitors eats a product high in tyramine. Symptoms include severe occipital headache, palpitations, nausea and vomiting, nuchal rigidity, fever, sweating, marked increase in blood pressure, chest pain, and coma. Foods with tyramine include aged cheeses or other aged, overripe, and fermented foods; broad beans; pickled herring; beef or chicken liver; preserved meats; beer and wine; yeast products; chocolate; caffeinated drinks; canned figs; sour cream; yogurt; soy sauce; and some over-the-counter cold medications and diet pills.

hypnosis. A treatment for disorders brought on by repressed anxiety. The individual is directed into a state of subconsciousness and assisted, through suggestions, to recall certain events that he or she cannot recall while conscious.

hypochondriasis. The unrealistic preoccupation with fear of having a serious illness.

hypomania. A mild form of mania. Symptoms are excessive hyperactivity, but not severe enough to cause marked impairment in social or occupational functioning or to require hospitalization.

hysteria. A polysymptomatic disorder characterized by recurrent, multiple somatic complaints often described dramatically.

I

id. One of the three components of the personality identified by Freud as the "pleasure principle." The id is the locus of instinctual drives; is present at birth; and compels the infant to satisfy needs and seek immediate gratification.

identification. An attempt to increase self-worth by acquiring certain attributes and characteristics of an individual one admires.

illusion. A misperception of a real external stimulus.

implosion therapy. See **flooding.**

impulsive. The urge or inclination to act without consideration of the possible consequences of one's behavior.

incest. Sexual exploitation of a child under 18 years of age by a relative or nonrelative who holds a position of trust in the family.

informed consent. Permission granted to a physician by a client to perform a therapeutic procedure, prior to which information about the procedure has been presented to the client with adequate time given for consideration about the pros and cons.

insomnia. Difficulty initiating or maintaining sleep.

insulin coma therapy. The induction of a hypoglycemic coma aimed at alleviating psychotic symptoms; a dangerous procedure, questionably effective, no longer used in psychiatry.

integration. The process used with individuals with dissociative identity disorder in an effort to bring all the personalities together into one; usually achieved through hypnosis.

intellectualization. An attempt to avoid expressing actual emotions associated with a stressful situation by using the intellectual processes of logic, reasoning, and analysis.

interdisciplinary care. A concept of providing care for a client in which members of various disciplines work together with common goals and shared responsibilities for meeting those goals.

intimate distance. The closest distance that individuals will allow between themselves and others. In the United States, this distance is 0 to 18 inches.

intoxication. A physical and mental state of exhilaration and emotional frenzy or lethargy and stupor.

introjection. The beliefs and values of another individual are internalized and symbolically become a part of the self, to the extent that the feeling of separateness or distinctness is lost.

isolation. The separation of a thought or a memory from the feeling tone or emotions associated with it (sometimes called *emotional isolation*).

J

justice. An ethical principle reflecting that all individuals should be treated equally and fairly.

K

Kantianism. The ethical principle espousing that decisions should be made and actions taken out of a sense of duty.

kleptomania. A recurrent failure to resist impulses to steal objects not needed for personal use or monetary value.

Korsakoff's psychosis. A syndrome of confusion, loss of recent memory, and confabulation in alcoholics, caused by a deficiency of thiamine. It often occurs together with Wernicke's encephalopathy and may be termed *Wernicke-Korsakoff syndrome*.

L

la belle indifference. A symptom of conversion disorder in which there is a relative lack of concern that is out of keeping with the severity of the impairment.

laissez-faire. A leadership type in which the leader lets group members do as they please. There is no direction from the leader. Member productivity and morale may be low, owing to frustration from lack of direction.

lesbian. A female homosexual.

libel. An action with which an individual may be charged for sharing with another individual, in writing, information that is detrimental to someone's reputation.

libido. Freud's term for the psychic energy used to fulfill basic physiological needs or instinctual drives such as hunger, thirst, and sexuality.

limbic system. The part of the brain that is sometimes called the "emotional brain." It is associated with feelings of fear and anxiety; anger and aggression; love, joy, and hope; and with sexuality and social behavior.

long-term memory. Memory for remote events, or those that occurred many years ago. The type of memory that is preserved in the elderly individual.

loss. The experience of separation from something of personal importance.

luto. In the Mexican-American culture, the period of mourning following the death of a loved one, which is symbolized by wearing black, black and white, or dark clothing and by subdued behavior.

M

magical thinking. A primitive form of thinking in which an individual believes that thinking about a possible occurrence can make it happen.

magnification. A type of thinking in which the negative significance of an event is exaggerated.

maladaptation. A failure of the body to return to homeostasis following a physiological and/or psychological response to stress, disrupting the individual's integrity.

malpractice. The failure of one rendering professional services to exercise that degree of skill and learning commonly applied under all the circumstances in the community by the average prudent reputable member of the profession, with the result of injury, loss, or damage to the recipient of those services or to those entitled to rely upon them.

managed care. A concept purposefully designed to control the balance between cost and quality of care. Examples of managed care are health maintenance organizations (HMOs) and preferred provider organizations (PPOs). The amount and type of health care that the individual receives is determined by the organization providing the managed care.

mania. A type of bipolar disorder in which the predominant mood is elevated, expansive, or irritable. Motor activity is frenzied and excessive. Psychotic features may or may not be present.

marital rape. Sexual violence directed at a marital partner against that person's will.

marital schism. A state of severe chronic disequilibrium and discord within the marital dyad, with recurrent threats of separation.

marital skew. A marital relationship in which there is lack of equal partnership. One partner dominates the relationship and the other partner.

masochism. Sexual stimulation derived from being humiliated, beaten, bound, or otherwise made to suffer.

Medicaid. A system established by the federal government to provide medical care benefits for indigent Americans. The Medicaid program is jointly funded by state and federal governments, and coverage varies significantly from state to state.

Medicare. A system established by the federal government to provide medical care benefits for elderly Americans.

meditation. A method of relaxation in which an individual sits in a quiet place and focuses total concentration on an object, word, or thought.

melancholia. A severe form of major depressive episode. Symptoms are exaggerated, and interest or pleasure in virtually all activities is lost.

menopause. The period marking the permanent cessation of menstrual activity; usually occurs at approximately 48 to 51 years of age.

mental health. The successful adaptation to stressors from the internal or external environment, evidenced by thoughts, feelings, and behaviors that are age-appropriate and congruent with local and cultural norms.

mental illness. Maladaptive responses to stressors from the internal or external environment, evidenced by thoughts, feelings, and behaviors that are incongruent with the local and cultural norms, and interfere with the individual's social, occupational, and/or physical functioning.

mental imagery. A method of stress reduction that employs the imagination. The individual focuses imagination on a scenario that is particularly relaxing to him or her (e.g., a scene on a quiet seashore, a mountain atmosphere, or floating through the air on a fluffy white cloud).

meridians. In Chinese medicine, pathways along the body in which the healing energy (*qi*) flows, and which are links between acupoints.

migraine personality. Personality characteristics that have been attributed to the migraine-prone person. The characteristics include perfectionistic, overly conscientious, somewhat inflexible, neat and tidy, compulsive, hard worker, intelligent, exacting, and places a very high premium on success, setting high (sometimes unrealistic) expectations on self and others.

milieu. French for "middle;" the English translation connotes "surroundings, or environment."

milieu therapy. Also called therapeutic community, or therapeutic environment, this type of therapy consists of a scientific structuring of the environment in order to effect behavioral changes and to improve the individual's psychological health and functioning.

minimization. A type of thinking in which the positive significance of an event is minimized or undervalued.

mobile outreach units. Programs in which volunteers and paid professionals drive or walk around and seek out homeless individuals who need assistance with physical or psychological care.

modeling. Learning new behaviors by imitating the behaviors of others.

mood. An individual's sustained emotional tone, which significantly influences behavior, personality, and perception.

moral behavior. Conduct that results from serious critical thinking about how individuals ought to treat others; reflects respect for human life, freedom, justice, or confidentiality.

moral-ethical self. That aspect of the personal identity that functions as observer, standard setter, dreamer, comparer, and most of all evaluator of who the individual says he or she is. This component of the personal identity makes judgments that influence an individual's self-evaluation.

mourning. The psychological process (or stages) through which the individual passes on the way to successful adaptation to the loss of a valued entity.

multidisciplinary care. A concept of providing care for a client in which individual disciplines provide specific services for the client without formal arrangement for interaction between the disciplines.

N

narcissism. Self-love or self-admiration.

narcissistic personality disorder. A disorder characterized by an exaggerated sense of self-worth. These individuals lack empathy and are hypersensitive to the evaluation of others.

narcolepsy. A disorder in which the characteristic manifestation is sleep attacks. The individual cannot prevent falling asleep, even in the middle of a sentence or performing a task.

natural law theory. The ethical theory that has as its moral precept to "do good and avoid evil" at all costs. Natural law ethics are grounded in a concern for the human good, that is based on people's ability to live according to the dictates of reason.

negative reinforcement. Increasing the probability that a behavior will recur by removal of an undesirable reinforcing stimulus.

negativism. Strong resistance to suggestions or directions; exhibiting behaviors contrary to what is expected.

Neglect of a child. *Physical neglect* of a child includes refusal of or delay in seeking health care, abandonment, expulsion from the home or refusal to allow a runaway to return home, and inadequate supervision. *Emotional neglect* refers to a chronic failure by the parent or caregiver to provide the child with the hope, love, and support necessary for the development of a sound, healthy personality.

negligence. The failure to do something that a reasonable person, guided by those considerations that ordinarily regulate human affairs, would do, or doing something that a prudent and reasonable person would not do.

neologism. New words that an individual invents that are meaningless to others, but have symbolic meaning to the psychotic person.

neuroendocrinology. The study of hormones functioning within the neurological system.

neuroleptic. Antipsychotic medication used to prevent or control psychotic symptoms.

neuroleptic malignant syndrome (NMS). A rare but potentially fatal complication of treatment with neuroleptic drugs. Symptoms include severe muscle rigidity, high fever, tachycardia, fluctuations in blood pressure, diaphoresis, and rapid deterioration of mental status to stupor and coma.

neuron. A nerve cell; consists of a cell body, an axon, and dendrites.

neurosis. An unconscious conflict that produces anxiety and other symptoms and leads to maladaptive use of defense mechanisms.

neurotic disorder. A psychiatric disturbance, characterized by excessive anxiety and/or depression, disrupted bodily functions, unsatisfying interpersonal relationships, and behaviors that interfere with routine functioning. There is no loss of contact with reality.

neurotransmitter. A chemical that is stored in the axon terminals of the presynaptic neuron. An electrical impulse through the neuron stimulates the release of the neurotransmitter into the synaptic cleft, which in turn determines whether or not another electrical impulse is generated.

nonassertive. Individuals who are nonassertive (sometimes called passive) seek to please others at the expense of denying their own basic human rights.

nonmaleficence. The ethical principle that espouses abstaining from negative acts toward another, including acting carefully to avoid harm.

nursing diagnosis. A clinical judgment about individual, family, or community responses to actual and potential health problems/life processes. Nursing diagnoses provide the basis for selection of nursing interventions to achieve outcomes for which the nurse is accountable.

Nursing Interventions Classification (NIC). A comprehensive, research-based, standardized classification of interventions that nurses perform.

Nursing Outcomes Classification (NOC). A comprehensive, standardized classification of patient/client outcomes developed to evaluate the effects of nursing interventions (Moorhead et al., 2008).

nursing process. A dynamic, systematic process by which nurses assess, diagnose, identify outcomes, plan, implement, and evaluate nursing care. It has been called "nursing's scientific methodology." Nursing process gives order and consistency to nursing intervention.

O

obesity. The state of having a body mass index of 30 or above.

object constancy. The phase in the separation/individuation process when the child learns to relate to objects in an effective, constant manner. A sense of separateness is established, and the child is able to internalize a sustained image of the loved object or person when out of sight.

obsessions. Unwanted, intrusive, persistent ideas, thoughts, impulses, or images that cause marked anxiety or distress. The most common ones include repeated thoughts about contamination, repeated doubts, a need to have things in a particular order, aggressive or horrific impulses, and sexual imagery (APA, 2000).

obsessive-compulsive disorder. Recurrent thoughts or ideas (obsessions) that an individual is unable to put out of his or her mind, and actions that an individual is unable to refrain from performing (compulsions). The obsessions and compulsions are severe enough to interfere with social and occupational functioning.

oculogyric crisis. An attack of involuntary deviation and fixation of the eyeballs, usually in the upward position. It may last for several minutes or hours and may occur as an extrapyramidal side effect of some antipsychotic medications.

operant conditioning. The learning of a particular action or type of behavior that is followed by a reinforcement.

opioids. A group of compounds that includes opium, opium derivatives, and synthetic substitutes.

orgasm. A peaking of sexual pleasure, with release of sexual tension and rhythmic contraction of the perineal muscles and pelvic reproductive organs.

osteoporosis. A reduction in the mass of bone per unit of volume that interferes with the mechanical support function of bone. This process occurs because of demineralization of the bones, and is escalated in women about the time of menopause.

outcomes. End results that are measurable, desirable, and observable, and translate into observable behaviors (ANA, 2010).

overgeneralization. Also called "absolutistic thinking." With overgeneralization, sweeping conclusions are made based on one incident—an "all or nothing" type of thinking.

overt sensitization. A type of aversion therapy that produces unpleasant consequences for undesirable behavior. An example is the use of disulfiram therapy with alcoholics, which induces an undesirable physical response if the individual has consumed any alcohol.

P

palilalia. Repeating one's own sounds or words (a type of vocal tic associated with Tourette's disorder).

panic. A sudden overwhelming feeling of terror or impending doom. This most severe form of emotional anxiety is usually accompanied by behavioral, cognitive, and physiological signs and symptoms considered to be outside the expected range of normalcy.

panic disorder. A disorder characterized by recurrent panic attacks, the onset of which are unpredictable, and manifested by intense apprehension, fear, or terror, often associated with feelings of impending doom, and accompanied by intense physical discomfort.

paradoxical intervention. In family therapy, "prescribing the symptom." The therapist requests that the family continue to engage in the behavior that they are trying to change. Tension is relieved, and the family is able to view more clearly the possible solutions to their problem.

paralanguage. The gestural component of the spoken word. It consists of pitch, tone, and loudness of spoken messages, the rate of speaking, expressively placed pauses, and emphasis assigned to certain words.

paranoia. A term that implies extreme suspiciousness. Paranoid schizophrenia is characterized by persecutory delusions and hallucinations of a threatening nature.

paraphilia. Repetitive behavior or fantasy that involves nonhuman objects, real or simulated suffering or humiliation, or nonconsenting partners.

parasomnia. Unusual or undesirable behaviors that occur during sleep (e.g., nightmares, sleep terrors, and sleepwalking).

passive-aggressive behavior. Behavior that defends an individual's own basic rights by expressing resistance to social and occupational demands. Sometimes called *indirect aggression,* this behavior takes the form of sly, devious, and undermining actions that express the opposite of what the person is really feeling.

pathological gambling. A failure to resist impulses to gamble, and gambling behavior that compromises, disrupts, or damages personal, family, or vocational pursuits.

pedophilia. Recurrent urges and sexually arousing fantasies involving sexual activity with a prepubescent child.

peer assistance programs. A program established by the American Nurses Association to assist impaired nurses. The individuals who administer these efforts are nurse members of the state associations, as well as nurses who are in recovery themselves.

perseveration. Persistent repetition of the same word or idea in response to different questions.

personal distance. The distance between individuals who are having interactions of a personal nature, such as a close conversation. In the U.S. culture, personal distance is approximately 18 to 40 inches.

personal identity. An individual's self-perception that defines his or her functions as observer, standard setter, and self-evaluator. It strives to maintain a stable self-image and relates to what the individual strives to become.

personal self. See **personal identity.**

personality. Deeply ingrained patterns of behavior, which include the way one relates to, perceives, and thinks about the environment and oneself.

personalization. Taking complete responsibility for situations without considering that other circumstances may have contributed to the outcome.

pharmacoconvulsive therapy. The chemical induction of a convulsion, used in the past for the reduction of psychotic symptoms; a type of therapy no longer used in psychiatry.

phencyclidine. An anesthetic used in veterinary medicine; used illegally as a hallucinogen, referred to as PCP or angel dust.

phenotype. Characteristics of physical manifestations that identify a particular genotype. Examples of phenotypes include eye color, height, blood type, language, and hairstyle. Phenotypes may be genetic or acquired.

phobia. An irrational fear.

physical neglect of a child. The failure on the part of the parent or caregiver to provide for a child's basic needs, such as food, clothing, shelter, medical-dental care, and supervision.

physical self. A personal appraisal by an individual of his or her physical being; includes physical attributes, functioning, sexuality, wellness-illness state, and appearance.

PIE charting. More specifically called "APIE," this method of documentation has an assessment, problem, intervention, and evaluation (APIE) format and is a problem-oriented system used to document nursing process.

positive reinforcement. A reinforcement stimulus that increases the probability that the behavior will recur.

postpartum depression. Depression that occurs during the postpartum period. It may be related to hormonal changes, tryptophan metabolism, or alterations in membrane transport during the early postpartum period. Other predisposing factors may also be influential.

posttraumatic stress disorder (PTSD). A syndrome of symptoms that develop following a psychologically distressing event that is outside the range of usual human experience (e.g., rape, war). The individual is unable to put the experience out of his or her mind, and has nightmares, flashbacks, and panic attacks.

posturing. The voluntary assumption of inappropriate or bizarre postures.

preassaultive tension state. Behaviors predictive of potential violence. They include excessive motor activity, tense posture, defiant affect, clenched teeth and fists, and other arguing, demanding, and threatening behaviors.

precipitating event. A stimulus arising from the internal or external environment that is perceived by an individual as taxing or exceeding his or her resources and endangering his or her well-being.

predisposing factors. A variety of elements that influence how an individual perceives and responds to a stressful event. Types of predisposing factors include genetic influences, past experiences, and existing conditions.

Premack principle. This principle states that a frequently occurring response (R1) can serve as a positive reinforcement for a response (R2) that occurs less frequently. For example, a girl may talk to friends on the phone (R2) only if she does her homework (R1).

premature ejaculation. Ejaculation that occurs with minimal sexual stimulation or before, upon, or shortly after penetration and before the person wishes it.

premenstrual dysphoric disorder. A disorder that is characterized by depressed mood, anxiety, mood swings, and decreased interest in activities during the week prior to menses and subsiding shortly after the onset of menstruation.

presenile. Pertaining to premature old age as judged by mental or physical condition. In presenile-onset dementia, initial symptoms appear at age 65 or younger.

priapism. Prolonged painful penile erection, may occur as an adverse effect of some antidepressant medications, particularly trazodone.

primary dementia. Dementia, such as Alzheimer's disease, in which the dementia itself is the major sign of some organic brain disease not directly related to any other organic illness.

primary gain. The receipt of positive reinforcement for somaticizing by being able to avoid difficult situations because of physical complaint.

primary prevention. Reduction of the incidence of mental disorders within the population by helping individuals to cope more effectively with stress and by trying to diminish stressors within the environment.

privileged communication. A doctrine common to most states that grants certain privileges under which health-care professionals may refuse to reveal information about and communications with clients.

problem-oriented recording (POR). A system of documentation that follows a subjective data, objective data, assessment, plan, implementation, and evaluation (SOAPIE) format. It is based on a list of identified patient problems to which each entry is directed.

prodromal syndrome. A syndrome of symptoms that often precede the onset of aggressive or violent behavior. These symptoms include anxiety and tension, verbal abuse and profanity, and increasing hyperactivity.

progressive relaxation. A method of deep muscle relaxation in which each muscle group is alternately tensed and relaxed in a systematic order, with the person concentrating on the contrast of sensations experienced from tensing and relaxing.

projection. Attributing to another person feelings or impulses unacceptable to oneself.

prospective payment. The program of cost containment within the health-care profession directed at setting forth preestablished amounts that would be reimbursed for specific diagnoses.

pseudocyesis. A condition in which an individual has nearly all the signs and symptoms of pregnancy but is not pregnant; a conversion reaction.

pseudodementia. Symptoms of depression that mimic those of dementia.

pseudohostility. A family interaction pattern characterized by a state of chronic conflict and alienation among family members. This relationship pattern allows family members to deny underlying fears of tenderness and intimacy.

pseudomutuality. A family interaction pattern characterized by a facade of mutual regard with the purpose of denying underlying fears of separation and hostility.

pseudoparkinsonism. A side effect of some antipsychotic medications. Symptoms mimic those of Parkinson's disease, such as tremor, shuffling gait, drooling, and rigidity.

psychiatric home care. Care provided by psychiatric nurses in the client's home. Psychiatric home care nurses must have physical and psychosocial nursing skills to meet the demands of the client population they serve.

psychobiology. The study of the biological foundations of cognitive, emotional, and behavioral processes.

psychodrama. A specialized type of group therapy that employs a dramatic approach in which patients become "actors" in life situation scenarios. The goal is to resolve interpersonal conflicts in a less-threatening atmosphere than the real-life situation would present.

psychodynamic nursing. Being able to understand one's own behavior, to help others identify felt difficulties, and to apply principles of human relations to the problems that arise at all levels of experience.

psychoimmunology. The study of the implications of the immune system in psychiatry.

psychomotor domain. A category of learning in which the behaviors are processed and demonstrated. The information has been intellectually processed, and the individual is displaying motor behaviors.

psychomotor retardation. Extreme slowdown of physical movements. Posture slumps; speech is slowed; digestion becomes sluggish. Common in severe depression.

psychophysiological. Referring to psychological factors contributing to the initiation or exacerbation of a physical condition. Either a demonstrable organic pathology or a known pathophysiological process is involved.

psychosis. A mental state in which there is a severe loss of contact with reality. Symptoms may include delusions, hallucinations, disorganized speech patterns, and bizarre or catatonic behaviors.

psychosomatic. See **psychophysiological.**

psychotic disorder. A serious psychiatric disorder in which there is a gross disorganization of the personality, a marked disturbance in reality testing, and the impairment of interpersonal functioning and relationship to the external world.

psychotropic medication. Medication that affects psychic function, behavior, or experience.

public distance. Appropriate interactional distance for speaking in public or yelling to someone some distance away. U.S. culture defines this distance as 12 feet or more.

purging. The act of attempting to rid the body of calories by self-induced vomiting or excessive use of laxatives or diuretics.

pyromania. An inability to resist the impulse to set fires.

Q

qi. In Chinese medicine, the healing energy that flows through pathways in the body called *meridians*. (Also called "chi").

R

rape. The expression of power and dominance by means of sexual violence, most commonly by men over women, although men may also be rape victims. Rape is considered an act of aggression, not of passion.

rapport. The development between two people in a relationship of special feelings based on mutual acceptance, warmth, friendliness, common interest, a sense of trust, and a nonjudgmental attitude.

rationalization. Attempting to make excuses or formulate logical reasons to justify unacceptable feelings or behaviors.

reaction formation. Preventing unacceptable or undesirable thoughts or behaviors from being expressed by exaggerating opposite thoughts or types of behaviors.

receptor sites. Molecules that are situated on the cell membrane of the postsynaptic neuron that will accept only molecules with a complementary shape. These complementary molecules are specific to certain neurotransmitters that determine whether an electrical impulse will be excited or inhibited.

reciprocal inhibition. Also called counterconditioning, this technique serves to decrease or eliminate a behavior by introducing a more adaptive behavior, but one that is incompatible with the unacceptable behavior (e.g., introducing relaxation techniques to an anxious person; relaxation and anxiety are incompatible behaviors).

reframing. Changing the conceptual or emotional setting or viewpoint in relation to which a situation is experienced and placing it in another frame that fits the "facts" of the same concrete situation equally well or even better, and thereby changing its entire meaning. The behavior may not actually change, but the consequences of the behavior may change because of a change in the meaning attached to the behavior.

regression. A retreat to an earlier level of development and the comfort measures associated with that level of functioning.

relaxation. A decrease in tension or intensity, resulting in refreshment of body and mind. A state of refreshing tranquility.

religion. A set of beliefs, values, rites, and rituals adopted by a group of people. The practices are usually grounded in the teachings of a spiritual leader.

religiosity. Excessive demonstration of or obsession with religious ideas and behavior; common in schizophrenia.

reminiscence therapy. A process of life review by elderly individuals that promotes self-esteem and provides assistance in working through unresolved conflicts from the past.

repression. The involuntary blocking of unpleasant feelings and experiences from one's awareness.

residual stimuli. Certain beliefs, attitudes, experiences, or traits that may contribute to an individual's low self-esteem.

retarded ejaculation. Delayed or absent ejaculation, even though the man has a firm erection and has had more than adequate stimulation.

retrograde ejaculation. Ejaculation of the seminal fluid backward into the bladder; may occur as a side effect of antipsychotic medications.

right. That which an individual is entitled (by ethical, legal, or moral standards) to have, or to do, or to receive from others within the limits of the law.

rigid boundaries. A person with rigid boundaries is "closed" and difficult to bond with. Such a person has a narrow perspective on life, sees things one way, and cannot discuss matters that lie outside his or her perspective.

ritualistic behavior. Purposeless activities that an individual performs repeatedly in an effort to decrease anxiety (e.g., hand washing); common in obsessive-compulsive disorder.

S

sadism. Recurrent urges and sexually arousing fantasies involving acts (real, not simulated) in which the psychological or physical suffering (including humiliation) of the victim is sexually exciting.

safe house or shelter. An establishment set up by many cities to provide protection for battered women and their children.

scapegoating. Occurs when hostility exists in a marriage dyad and an innocent third person (usually a child) becomes the target of blame for the problem.

schemas (also called *core beliefs*). Cognitive structures that consist of the individual's fundamental beliefs and assumptions, which develop early in life from personal experiences and identification with significant others. These concepts are reinforced by further learning experiences and in turn, influence the formation of other beliefs, values, and attitudes.

schizoid personality disorder. A profound defect in the ability to form personal relationships or to respond to others in any meaningful, emotional way.

schizotypal personality disorder. A disorder characterized by odd and eccentric behavior, not decompensating to the level of schizophrenia.

secondary dementia. Dementia that is caused by or related to another disease or condition, such as HIV disease or a cerebral trauma.

secondary gain. The receipt of positive reinforcement for somaticizing through added attention, sympathy, and nurturing.

secondary prevention. Health care that is directed at reduction of the prevalence of psychiatric illness by shortening the course (duration) of the illness. This is accomplished through early identification of problems and prompt initiation of treatment.

selective abstraction (sometimes referred to as "mental filter"). A type of thinking in which a conclusion is drawn based on only a selected portion of the evidence.

self-concept. The composite of beliefs and feelings that one holds about oneself at a given time, formed from perceptions of others' reactions. The self-concept consists of the physical self, or body image; the personal self, or identity; and the self-esteem.

self-consistency. The component of the personal identity that strives to maintain a stable self-image.

self-esteem. The degree of regard or respect that individuals have for themselves. It is a measure of worth that they place on their abilities and judgments.

self-expectancy. The component of the personal identity that is the individual's perception of what he or she wants to be, to do, or to become.

self-ideal. See **self-expectancy**.

senile. Pertaining to old age and the mental or physical weakness with which it is sometimes associated. In senile-onset dementia, the first symptoms appear after age 65.

sensate focus. A therapeutic technique used to treat individuals and couples with sexual dysfunction. The technique involves touching and being touched by another and focusing attention on the physical sensations encountered thereby. Clients gradually move through various levels of sensate focus that progress from nongenital touching to touching that includes the breasts and genitals; touching done in a simultaneous, mutual format rather than by one person at a time; and touching that extends to and allows eventually for the possibility of intercourse.

seroconversion. The development of evidence of antibody response to a disease or vaccine. The time at which antibodies may be detected in the blood.

sexual assault nurse examiner (SANE). A clinical forensic registered nurse who has received specialized training to provide care to the sexual assault victim.

sexual exploitation of a child. The inducement or coercion of a child into engaging in sexually explicit conduct for the purpose of promoting any performance (e.g., child pornography).

sexuality. The constitution and life of an individual relative to characteristics regarding intimacy. It reflects the totality of the person and does not relate exclusively to the sex organs or sexual behavior.

shaman. The Native American "medicine man" or folk healer.

shaping. In learning, one shapes the behavior of another by giving reinforcements for increasingly closer approximations to the desired behavior.

shelters. A variety of places designed to help the homeless, ranging from converted warehouses that provide cots or floor space on which to sleep overnight to significant operations that provide a multitude of social and health-care services.

"ship of fools." The term given during the Middle Ages to sailing boats filled with severely mentally ill people who were sent out to sea with little guidance and in search of their lost rationality.

shiva. In the Jewish-American culture, following the death of a loved one, *shiva* is the 7-day period beginning with the burial. During this time, mourners do not work, and no activity is permitted that diverts attention from thinking about the deceased.

short-term memory. The ability to remember events that occurred very recently. This ability deteriorates with age.

silent rape reaction. The response of a rape victim in which he or she tells no one about the assault.

slander. An action with which an individual may be charged for orally sharing information that is detrimental to a person's reputation.

social distance. The distance considered acceptable in interactions with strangers or acquaintances, such as at a cocktail party or in a public building. U.S. culture defines this distance as 4 to 12 feet.

social phobia. The fear of being humiliated in social situations.

social skills training. Educational opportunities through role-play for the person with schizophrenia to learn appropriate social interaction skills and functional skills that are relevant to daily living.

Socratic questioning (also called *guided discovery*). When the therapist questions the client with Socratic questioning, the client is asked to describe feelings associated with specific situations. Questions are stated in a way that may stimulate in the client a recognition of possible dysfunctional thinking and produce a dissonance about the validity of the thoughts.

somatization. A method of coping with psychosocial stress by developing physical symptoms.

specific phobia. A persistent fear of a specific object or situation, other than the fear of being unable to escape from a situation (agoraphobia) or the fear of being humiliated in social situations (social phobia).

spirituality. The human quality that gives meaning and sense of purpose to an individual's existence. Spirituality exists within each individual regardless of belief system and serves as a force for interconnectedness between the self and others, the environment, and a higher power.

splitting. A primitive ego defense mechanism in which the person is unable to integrate and accept both positive and negative feelings. In the view of these individuals, people—including themselves—and life situations are either all good or all bad. This trait is common in borderline personality disorder.

statutory law. A law that has been enacted by legislative bodies, such as a county or city council, state legislature, or the U.S. Congress.

statutory rape. Unlawful intercourse between a person who is over the age of consent and a person who is under the age of consent. Legal age of consent varies from state to state. An individual can be arrested for statutory rape even when the interaction has occurred between consenting individuals.

stereotyping. The process of classifying all individuals from the same culture or ethnic group as identical.

stimulus. In classical conditioning, that which elicits a response.

stimulus generalization. The process by which a conditioned response is elicited from all stimuli *similar* to the one from which the response was learned.

store-front clinics. Establishments that have been converted into clinics that serve the homeless population.

stress. A state of disequilibrium that occurs when there is a disharmony between demands occurring within an individual's internal or external environment and his or her ability to cope with those demands.

stress management. Various methods used by individuals to reduce tension and other maladaptive responses to stress in their lives; includes relaxation exercises, physical exercise, music, mental imagery, or any other technique that is successful for a person.

stressor. A demand from within an individual's internal or external environment that elicits a physiological and/or psychological response.

sublimation. The rechanneling of personally and/or socially unacceptable drives or impulses into activities that are more tolerable and constructive.

subluxation. The term used in chiropractic medicine to describe vertebrae in the spinal column that have become displaced, possibly pressing on nerves and interfering with normal nerve transmission.

substance abuse. Use of psychoactive drugs that poses significant hazards to health and interferes with social, occupational, psychological, or physical functioning.

substance dependence. Physical dependence is identified by the inability to stop using a substance despite attempts to do so; a continual use of the substance despite adverse consequences; a developing tolerance; and the development of withdrawal symptoms upon cessation or decreased intake. Psychological dependence is said to exist when a substance is perceived by the user to be necessary to maintain an optimal state of personal well-being, interpersonal relations, or skill performance.

substitution therapy. The use of various medications to decrease the intensity of symptoms in an individual who is withdrawing from, or experiencing the effects of excessive use of, substances.

subsystems. The smaller units of which a system is composed. In family systems theory, the subsystems are composed of husband-wife, parent-child(ren), or sibling-sibling.

sundowning. A phenomenon in dementia in which the symptoms seem to worsen in the late afternoon and evening.

superego. One of the three elements of the personality identified by Freud that represents the conscience and the culturally determined restrictions that are placed on an individual.

suppression. The voluntary blocking from one's awareness of unpleasant feelings and experiences.

surrogate. One who serves as a substitute figure for another.

symbiotic relationship. A type of "psychic fusion" that occurs between two people; it is unhealthy in that severe anxiety is generated in either or both if separation is indicated. A symbiotic relationship is normal between infant and mother.

sympathy. The actual sharing of another's thoughts and behaviors. Differs from **empathy,** in that with empathy one experiences an objective understanding of what another is feeling, rather than actually sharing those feelings.

synapse. The junction between two neurons. The small space between the axon terminals of one neuron and the cell body or dendrites of another is called the synaptic cleft.

syphilis. A sexually transmitted disorder caused by the spirochete *Treponema pallidum* and resulting in a chancre on the skin or mucous membranes of the sexual organs. If left untreated, it may become systemic. End-stage disease can have profound effects, such as blindness or insanity.

systematic desensitization. A treatment for phobias in which the individual is taught to relax and then asked to imagine various components of the phobic stimulus on a graded hierarchy, moving from that which produces the least fear to that which produces the most.

T

tangentiality. The inability to get to the point of a story. The speaker introduces many unrelated topics, until the original topic of discussion is lost.

tardive dyskinesia. Syndrome of symptoms characterized by bizarre facial and tongue movements, a stiff neck, and difficulty swallowing. It may occur as an adverse effect of long-term therapy with some antipsychotic medications.

technical expert. Peplau's term for one who understands various professional devices and possesses the clinical skills necessary to perform the interventions that are in the best interest of the client.

temperament. A set of inborn personality characteristics that influence an individual's manner of reacting to the environment, and ultimately influences his or her developmental progression.

territoriality. The innate tendency of individuals to "own" space. Individuals lay claim to areas around them as their own. This phenomenon can have an influence on interpersonal communication.

tertiary gain. The receipt of positive reinforcement for somaticizing by causing the focus of the family to switch to the individual and away from conflict that may be occurring within the family.

tertiary prevention. Health care that is directed toward reduction of the residual effects associated with severe or chronic physical or mental illness.

therapeutic communication. Caregiver verbal and nonverbal techniques that focus on the care receiver's needs and advance the promotion of healing and change. Therapeutic communication encourages exploration of feelings and fosters understanding of behavioral motivation. It is nonjudgmental, discourages defensiveness, and promotes trust.

therapeutic community. Also called *milieu therapy,* this approach strives to manipulate the environment so that all aspects of the client's hospital experience are considered therapeutic.

therapeutic group. Differs from group therapy in that there is a lesser degree of theoretical foundation. Focus is on group relations, interactions between group members, and the consideration of a selected issue. Leaders of therapeutic groups do not require the degree of educational preparation required of group therapy leaders.

therapeutic relationship. An interaction between two people (usually a caregiver and a care receiver) in which input from both participants contributes to a climate of healing, growth promotion, and/or illness prevention.

thought-stopping technique. A self-taught technique that an individual uses each time he or she wishes to eliminate intrusive or negative, unwanted thoughts from awareness.

time out. An aversive stimulus or punishment during which the individual is removed from the environment where the unacceptable behavior is being exhibited.

token economy. In behavior modification, a type of contracting in which the reinforcers for desired behaviors are presented in the form of tokens, which may then be exchanged for designated privileges.

tolerance. The need for increasingly larger or more frequent doses of a substance in order to obtain the desired effects originally produced by a lower dose.

tort. The violation of a civil law in which an individual has been wronged. In a tort action, one party asserts that wrongful conduct on the part of the other has caused harm, and compensation for harm suffered is sought.

transference. Transference occurs when a client unconsciously displaces (or "transfers") to the nurse or therapist feelings formed toward a person from his or her past.

transgenderism. A disorder of gender identity or gender dysphoria (unhappiness or dissatisfaction with one's gender) of the most extreme variety. The individual, despite having the anatomical characteristics of a given gender, has the self-perception of being of the opposite gender, and may seek to have gender changed through surgical intervention.

transvestic fetishism. Recurrent urges and sexually arousing fantasies involving dressing in the clothes of the opposite gender.

triangles. A three-person emotional configuration that is considered the basic building block of the family system. When anxiety becomes too great between two family members, a third person is brought in to form a triangle. Triangles are dysfunctional in that they offer relief from anxiety through diversion rather than through resolution of the issue.

trichotillomania. The recurrent failure to resist impulses to pull out one's own hair.

type A personality. The personality characteristics attributed to individuals prone to coronary heart disease, including excessive competitive drive, chronic sense of time urgency, easy anger, aggressiveness, excessive ambition, and inability to enjoy leisure time.

type B personality. The personality characteristics attributed to individuals who are not prone to coronary heart disease; includes characteristics such as ability to perform even under pressure but without the competitive drive and constant sense of time urgency experienced by the type A personality. Type Bs can enjoy their leisure time without feeling guilty, and they are much less impulsive than type A individuals; that is, they think things through before making decisions.

type C personality. The personality characteristics attributed to the cancer-prone individual. Includes characteristics such as suppression of anger, calm, passive, puts the needs of others before his or her own, but holds resentment toward others for perceived "wrongs."

type D personality. Personality characteristics attributed to individuals who are at increased risk of cardiovascular morbidity and mortality. The characteristics include a combination of negative emotions and social inhibition.

tyramine. An amino acid found in aged cheeses or other aged, overripe, and fermented foods; broad beans; pickled herring; beef or chicken liver; preserved meats; beer and wine; yeast products; chocolate; caffeinated drinks; canned figs; sour cream; yogurt; soy sauce; and some over-the-counter cold medications and diet pills. If foods high in tyramine content are consumed while an individual is taking MAO inhibitors, a potentially life-threatening syndrome called hypertensive crisis can result.

U

unconditional positive regard. Carl Rogers' term for the respect and dignity of an individual regardless of his or her unacceptable behavior.

unconditioned response. In classical conditioning, a reflexive response to a specific target stimulus.

unconditioned stimulus. In classical conditioning, a specific stimulus that elicits an unconditioned, reflexive response.

undoing. A mechanism used to symbolically negate or cancel out a previous action or experience that one finds intolerable.

universality. One curative factor of groups (identified by Yalom) in which individuals realize that they are not alone in a problem and in the thoughts and feelings they are experiencing. Anxiety is relieved by the support and understanding of others in the group who share similar experiences.

utilitarianism. The ethical theory that espouses "the greatest happiness for the greatest number." Under this theory, action would be taken based on the end results that will produce the most good (happiness) for the most people.

V

vaginismus. Involuntary constriction of the outer one third of the vagina that prevents penile insertion and intercourse.

values. Personal beliefs about the truth, beauty, or worth of a thought, object, or behavior, that influence an individual's actions.

values clarification. A process of self-discovery by which people identify their personal values and their value rankings. This process increases awareness about why individuals behave in certain ways.

velorio. In the Mexican-American culture, following the death of a loved one, the *velorio* is a festive watch by family and friends over the body of the deceased person before burial.

veracity. An ethical principle that refers to one's duty to always be truthful.

voyeurism. Recurrent urges and sexually arousing fantasies involving the act of observing unsuspecting people, usually strangers, who are either naked, in the process of disrobing, or engaging in sexual activity.

W

waxy flexibility. A condition by which the individual with schizophrenia passively yields all movable parts of the body to any efforts made at placing them in certain positions.

Wernicke's encephalopathy. A brain disorder caused by thiamine deficiency and characterized by visual disturbances, ataxia, somnolence, stupor, and, without thiamine replacement, death.

withdrawal. The physiological and mental readjustment that accompanies the discontinuation of an addictive substance.

word salad. A group of words that are put together in a random fashion without any logical connection.

Y

yin and yang. The fundamental concept of Asian health practices. Yin and yang are opposite forces of energy such as negative/positive, dark/light, cold/hot, hard/soft, and feminine/masculine. Food, medicines, and herbs are classified according to their yin and yang properties and are used to restore a balance, thereby restoring health.

yoga. A system of beliefs and practices, the ultimate goal of which is to unite the human soul with the universal spirit. In Western countries, yoga uses body postures, along with meditation and breathing exercises, to achieve a balanced, disciplined workout that releases muscle tension, tones the internal organs, and energizes the mind, body, and spirit, so that natural healing can occur.

References

American Nurses' Association. (ANA). (2010). *Nursing: Scope and standards of Ppractice* (2nd ed.). Silver Spring, MD: Author.

American Psychiatric Association. (2000). *Diagnostic and statistical manual of mental disorders* (4th ed.). *Text revision*. Washington, DC: American Psychiatric Publishing.

Kaakinen, J. R., Hanson, S. M. H., & Denham, S. A. (2010). Family health care nursing: An introduction. In J. R. Kaakinen, V. Gedaly-Duff, D. P. Coehlo, & S. M. H. Hanson (Eds.), *Family health care nursing* (4th ed., pp. 3–33). Philadelphia: F.A. Davis.

Moorhead, S., Johnson, M., Maas, M., & Swanson, E. (2008). *Nursing Ooutcomes Cclassification (NOC)* (4th ed.). St. Louis, MO: Mosby Elsevier.

Shahrokh, N. C., & Hales, R. E. (2003). *American psychiatric glossary* (8th ed.). Washington, DC: American Psychiatric Publishing.

Index

Page numbers followed by f denote figures; those followed by t denote tables.

A

AA (Alcoholics Anonymous), 191, 490, 498, 500–501, 506, 912, 1002
Abandonment, 1001
  fear of, 241–242, 798
  "granny-dumping," 839, 1008
  and object loss theory of depression, 564
Abilify. *See* Aripiprazole
Abnormal Involuntary Movement Scale (AIMS), 546–547
Abreaction, 693, 1001
Absolutistic thinking, 335
Abuse, 856–877. *See also* Aggression; Anger; Violence
  biological theories of, 857
  care plan for victim of, 868t–870t
    concept map, 868, 871f
  of child, 861–865, 875 (*See also* Child abuse)
  definition of, 856, 874, 1001
  economic implications of, 857
  of elderly persons, 839–841, 844 (*See also* Elder abuse)
  emotional, 839–841, 863, 1007
  epidemiology of, 857
  of intimate partner, 856, 859–861, 860f, 874
  learning theory of, 840, 858–859, 874
  nursing process in, 859–872
  predisposing factors for, 857–859, 874
  psychodynamic theory of, 857–858, 874
  self-esteem and, 287
  sexual assault, 865–867
  of substances, 456 (*See also* Substance-related disorders)
  treatment for victims of, 872–874, 875
    crisis intervention, 872
    family therapy, 874
    safe house or shelter, 873–874
    support groups, 872
Acamprosate, 503
Acceptance, in grief response, 24, 940t, 941
Acculturation, 105
Acetaldehyde, 460
Acetylcholine, 60f, 62t, 63
  in aggressive behavior, 297
  in Alzheimer's disease, 63, 73t, 425, 426f, 446
  changes with aging, 831
  in depression, 561, 563, 600
  in elderly persons, 447

  in mania, 600
  psychotropic drug effects on, 79t
  in schizophrenia, 516, 517f
  in sleep, 71
  in Tourette's disorder, 407
Acetylcholinesterase, 63
Acquired immunodeficiency syndrome (AIDS), 727, 731t, 1001. *See also* Human immunodeficiency virus (HIV) disease
ACT (Assertive Community Treatment), 537–538, 899–901
ACTH (adrenocorticotropic hormone), 67, 67t, 68, 830
Active avoidance, 644
Active listening, 156, 158, 161
Activity intolerance, risk for, 348t
Activity scheduling, 338
Activity theory of aging, 828–829
Acupoints, 362, 1001
Acupressure, 362, 371, 1001
Acupuncture, 357, 362, 371, 1001
Adaptation. *See also* Transactional model of stress/adaptation
  anxiety and, 17
  definition of, 5, 1001
  diseases of, 4, 9
  general adaptation syndrome, 3–4, 9, 1008
  genetic factors and, 7
  to retirement, 837–838
  to stress, 2, 7–8, 9
    mental health and, 16
    psychological, 17–26
  to tasks of aging, 828, 832
Adaptive coping strategies, 8–9, 10
Adderall; Adderall XR. *See* Dextroamphetamine/amphetamine mixture
Addison's disease, 68, 563
Adenohypophysis, 57, 65
  hormones released by, 57, 67–69, 67t
  target organs of, 66f, 67t
ADH (antidiuretic hormone), 55, 65, 66t, 830
ADHD. *See* Attention-deficit/hyperactivity disorder (ADHD)
Adipex-P. *See* Phentermine
Adjustment, 1001
Adjustment disorder, 762–768, 779–780, 1001
  with anxiety, 764
  biological theory of, 764
  classification of, 763–764
  client/family education in, 777

  concept map care plan for, 768, 769f
  with depressed mood, 764
  diagnostic criteria for, 764
  with disturbance of conduct, 764
  epidemiology of, 763, 780
  historical aspects of, 763
  with mixed disturbance of emotions and conduct, 764
  nursing process in, 763–768
  psychosocial theories of, 764–765
  symptoms of, 763
  transactional model of stress/adaptation in, 765, 766f
  treatment of, 777–778, 780
    behavior therapy, 778
    crisis intervention, 778
    family therapy, 778
    individual psychotherapy, 778
    pharmacological, 778
    self-help groups, 778
  unspecified, 764
Adolescents
  anorexia nervosa in, 739, 740
  anxiety disorders in
    generalized anxiety disorder, 636
    obsessive-compulsive disorder, 642
    social phobia, 638
  bipolar disorder in, 600–603
  body dysmorphic disorder in, 671
  bulimia nervosa in, 739
  concepts of death, 947, 957
  conduct disorder in, 397–402, 401t–402t
  conversion disorder in, 671
  depression in, 567
  development of self-esteem in, 283
  developmental tasks of, 39–40, 39t, 283, 886
  dissociative disorders in, 671
  educational programs for, 887
  family predictors of antisocial behavior in, 808
  family with, 202t, 203
  gender identity disorder in, 722–723, 724
  group therapy for, 415–416
  human papillomavirus vaccines for, 701
  informed consent for treatment of, 95
  inhalant abuse by, 473
  intermittent explosive disorder in, 770, 778
  kleptomania in, 771
  nursing intervention for prevention of offending behavior in, 918–919

G

O